Perinatal *and* Pediatric Respiratory Care

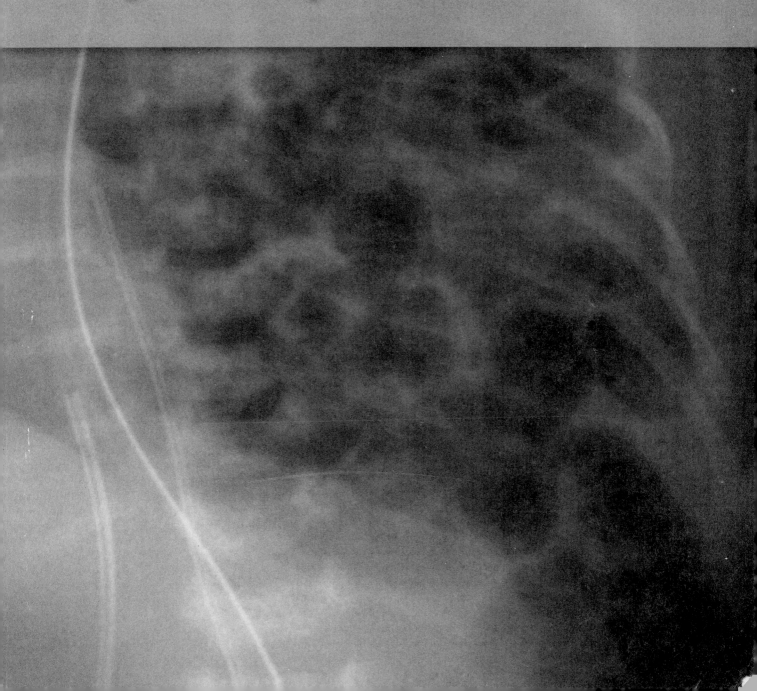

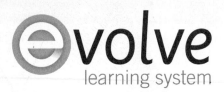
learning system

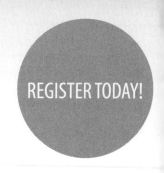
REGISTER TODAY!

To access your Student Resources, visit the web address below:

http://evolve.elsevier.com/Walsh/perinatal/

Evolve Student Resources for *Perinatal and Pediatric Respiratory Care*, 3/e, offer the following features

Evolve Free Resources

- Answers to Assessment Questions and Clinical Scenarios
- NBRC Neonatal/Pediatric Specialty (NPS) Exam Correlation Guide
- Additional Ventilator Content
- Credits
- Weblinks

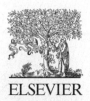
ELSEVIER

THIRD EDITION

Perinatal *and* Pediatric Respiratory Care

Brian K. Walsh, MBA, BS, RRT-NPS, RPFT, FAARC
Director of Respiratory Care
Children's Medical Center
Dallas, Texas

Michael P. Czervinske, RRT-NPS
Director of Clinical Education
Department of Respiratory Care Education
School of Allied Health
University of Kansas Medical Center
Kansas City, Kansas

Robert M. DiBlasi, RRT-NPS
Clinical Research Coordinator
Seattle Children's Hospital Research Institute
Department of Developmental Therapeutics
Department of Respiratory Therapy
Children's Hospital and Regional Medical Center
Seattle, Washington

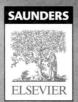

SAUNDERS

ELSEVIER

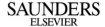

SAUNDERS
ELSEVIER

11830 Westline Industrial Drive
St. Louis, Missouri 63146

PERINATAL AND PEDIATRIC RESPIRATORY CARE, ISBN 978-1-4160-2448-4
THIRD EDITION

Library of Congress Cataloging-in-Publication Data
Perinatal and pediatric respiratory care / [edited by] Brian K. Walsh, Michael P. Czervinske,
  Robert M. DiBlasi. – 3rd ed.
    p. ; cm.
  Includes bibliographical references and index.
  ISBN 978-1-4160-2448-4 (pbk. : alk. paper) 1. Pediatric respiratory diseases. 2. Perinatology. I. Walsh,
Brian K. II. Czervinske, Michael P. III. DiBlasi, Robert M.
  [DNLM: 1. Respiratory Tract Diseases. 2. Child. 3. Infant. 4. Respiratory Therapy. WS 280 P445 2010]
RJ431.P47 2010
  618.92'2–dc22   2009014211

ISBN: 978-1-4160-2448-4

Publisher: Jeanne Olson
Managing Editor: Billie Sharp
Senior Developmental Editor: Mindy Hutchinson
Publishing Services Manager: Catherine Jackson
Senior Project Manager: Karen M. Rehwinkel
Designer: Jessica Williams

**Working together to grow
libraries in developing countries**

www.elsevier.com | www.bookaid.org | www.sabre.org

ELSEVIER   BOOK AID International   Sabre Foundation

Printed in the United States of America

Last digit is the print number: 9 8 7 6 5 4 3

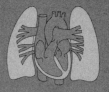

To my wife Stephanie, whose silent love speaks volumes through me;
to my children Trey and Keagan, for the laughter and pure joy you bring to my life.
Finally, to my God, who has blessed me beyond belief.

BKW

To my family, close and far.
Also, to all of our pets, and to the memory of George and Joey.

MPC

To my loving wife Cori and my beautiful daughter Sophia,
you truly are my only sunshine;
and to my mentors,
Sally Whitten, Gary Hamelin, Walter Chop,
Peter Richardson, John Salyer, and Dr. Tom Hansen
your words will always echo in my ears;
and in memory of my mother who said to me:
"Son, you often take the back roads, but you always seem to get there."

RMD

Robert G. Aucoin, PharmD
Children's Center
Our Lady of the Lakes Regional Medical Center
Baton Rouge, Louisiana

Sherry L. Barnhart, AS, RRT
Respiratory Care Services
Arkansas Children's Hospital
Little Rock, Arkansas

Craig Patrick Black, PhD, RRT-NPS
Associate Professor, Respiratory Care Program
College of Health Science and Human Service
The University of Toledo;
Staff Therapist
St. Vincent Mercy Medical Center
Toledo, Ohio

Kathleen D. Bongiovanni, MS
Research Technician
Center for Developmental Therapeutics
Seattle Children's Hospital Research Institute
Seattle, Washington

Teodor D. Butiu, MD, FAAP
Pediatric Critical Care
Northern Maine Medical Center
Fort Kent, Maine

Ira Cheifetz, MD, FCCM, FAARC
Associate Professor of Pediatrics
Division Chief, Pediatric Critical Care Medicine
Duke Children's Hospital
Durham, North Carolina

David N. Crotwell, RRT
Respiratory Care Service
Children's Hospital and Regional Medical Center
Seattle, Washington

Kristina H. Deeter, MD, FAAP
Fellow, Pediatric Critical Care Medicine
Seattle Children's Hospital
University of Washington
Seattle, Washington

Okan Elidemir, MD
Pediatric Pulmonologist
Texas Children's Hospital
Houston, Texas

Katherine Fedor, RRT-NPS, CPFT
Cleveland Clinic Foundation
Cleveland, Ohio

James B. Fink, PhD, RRT, FAARC
Adjunct Professor, Respiratory Care Program
Georgia State University
Atlanta, Georgia, California

Julie Lynn Fitzgerald, MD
Critical Care Medicine
Department of Pediatrics
University of Chicago Hospitals
Chicago, Illinois

Michael A. Gentile, RRT, FAARC, FCCM
Associate in Research
Division of Pulmonary and Critical Care Medicine
Duke University Medical Center
Durham, North Carolina

Cynthia L. Gibson, MD
Medical Director, Pediatric Hospitalist,
Pediatric Critical Care Physician
Department of Pediatrics
INOVA Fairfax Hospital for Children
Falls Church, Virginia

Jay S. Greenspan, MD
Associate Professor, Pediatrics
Thomas Jefferson University Hospital
Philadelphia, Pennsylvania

Douglas R. Hansell, BS, RRT
Director of Pulmonary Services
Vanderbilt Children's Hospital
Nashville, Tennessee

Mary E. Hartman, MD, MPH
Associate in Pediatric Critical Care Medicine
Children's Hospital at Duke
Duke University Medical Center
Durham, North Carolina

J. David Ingram, MD
Assistant Professor, Pediatric Radiology
University of Colorado Health Science Center
Department of Radiology
The Children's Hospital
Denver, Colorado

Cynthia Jacobus, BS, RRT
Clinical Specialist
Department of Respiratory Care
Texas Children's Hospital
Houston, Texas

Ian N. Jacobs, MD
Director, The Center for Pediatric Airway Disorders
Children's Hospital of Philadelphia
Associate Professor, Otorhinolaryngology: Head
and Neck Surgery
University of Pennsylvania School of Medicine
Philadelphia, Pennsylvania

Patrice Johnson, BS, RRT
Director, Respiratory Care
Children's Mercy Hospital
Kansas City, Missouri

Maridee Jones, RRT, FAARC, ARNT
Wesley Medical Center
Preoperative Assessment Clinic
Wichita, Kansas

Karl Kalavantavanich, MD
Attending Physician
Department of Pediatrics
Ramathibodi Hospital
Mahidol University
Bangkok, Thailand

Thomas J. Kallstrom, BS, RRT, AE-C, FAARC
Chief Operating Officer
American Association for Respiratory Care
Irving, Texas

Pradip Kamat, MD
Pediatric Critical Care
Childrens Healthcare Atlanta
Atlanta, Georgia

David Kaufman, MD
Department of Pediatrics
University of Virginia Health System
Charlottesville, Virginia

Scott Keckler, MD
Resident in General Surgery
University of Kansas Medical Center
Kansas City, Kansas

Antoun Y. Khabbaz, MD
Department of OB/GYN
University of Illinois
Champaign, Illinois

Scott M. Kirley, RRT
Pulmonary Division
Department of Pediatrics, College of Medicine
University of South Florida
Tampa, Florida

Tracy Koogler, MD
Associate Professor, Pediatrics
University of Chicago Hospitals
Chicago, Illinois

George B. Mallory, Jr., MD
Director, Lung Transplant Program
Associate Professor of Pediatrics
Baylor College of Medicine
Texas Children's Hospital
Houston, Texas

Paul Mathews, PhD, RRT, FCCM, FCCP, FAARC
Associate Professor Respiratory Care
University of Kansas Medical Center
School of Allied Health
Kansas City, Kansas

Eugene D. McGahren, MD
Pediatric Surgery and Pediatrics
University of Virginia Health Systems
Charlottesville, Virginia

John K. McGuire, MD
Pediatric Critical Care Medicine
Seattle Children's Hospital
University of Washington School of Medicine
Seattle, Washington

Keith S. Meredith, MD, MS
Neonatology Medical Director
Phoenix Perinatal Associates/Obstetrix Medical Group
Phoenix, Arizona

Peter H. Michelson, MD, MS
Associate Professor of Pediatrics
Duke University Medical Center
Durham, North Carolina

Thomas L. Miller, PhD
Nemours Research Lung Center
Alfred I. duPont Hospital for Children
Wilmington, Delaware

Ronald P. Mlcak, PhD, RRT, FAARC
Associate Professor, Respiratory Care
School of Allied Health Science
University of Texas Medical Branch
Director, Respiratory Care
Shriners Hospital for Children
Galveston, Texas

Charles L. Paxson, Jr., MD, FAAP
Director, Newborn Education
Neonatology Division, Department of Pediatrics
University of Kansas Medical Center
Kansas City, Kansas

Mary M. Pettignano, RRT, MMSc
Winter Park, Florida

Robert Pettignano, MD, FAAP, FccM
Pediatrics Intensivist
Nemours Children's Clinic Orlando
Division of Pediatric Critical Care
Arnold Palmer Hospital for Children and Women
Orlando, Florida

J. Gerald Quirk, MD, PhD
Professor and Chairman
University Associates in Obstetrics
and Gynecology, Inc
Department of Obstetrics and Gynecology
East Setauket, New York

Peter Richardson, PhD
Research Associate Professor
Pulmonology Division
Department of Pediatrics
University of Washington
Center for Developmental Therapeutics
Seattle Children's Hospital Research Institute
Seattle, Washington

Bradley M. Rodgers, MD
University of Virginia Children's Hospital
Department of Pediatric Surgery
Charlottesville, Virginia

Mark Rogers, BS, RCP, RRT
Clinical Applications Manager
Advanced Product Development
VIASYS Healthcare
Yorba Linda, California

Bruce K. Rubin, MEngr, MD, FRCP(C), FCCP
Professor and Vice-Chair Basic Research
Department of Pediatrics
Professor of Medicine,
Physiology, and Pharmacology
Wake Forest University School of Medicine
Winston-Salem, North Carolina

John Salyer, RRT
Respiratory Care Service
Children's Hospital and Regional Medical Center
Seattle, Washington

Thomas H. Schaffer, PhD
Director, Nemours Research Lung Center
Alfred I. duPont Hospital for Children
Wilmington, Delaware

Marc G. Schecter, MD
Assistant Professor, Pediatrics
Section of Pulmonology
Baylor College of Medicine
Houston, Texas

Dennis E. Schellhaese, MD
Associate Professor
Pediatric Pulmonology
Arkansas Children's Hospital
Little Rock, Arkansas

Bruce M. Schnapf, DO
Chief, Pediatric Pulmonary
Department of Pediatrics
College of Medicine
University of South Florida
Tampa, Florida

Kurt P. Schropp, MD
Chief, Pediatric Surgery
University of Kansas Medical Center
Kansas City, Kansas

Craig M. Schramm, MD
Associate Professor Pediatrics
University of Connecticut Health Center
Pediatric Pulmonary
Connecticut Children's Medical Center
Hartford, Connecticut

Garry Sitler, RRT
Director
Intensive Care Transport Team
Texas Children's Hospital
Houston, Texas

Anthony D. Slonim, MD, DrPH
Children's National Medical Center
Washington, District of Columbia

Kim Stevenson, RRT
Clinical Specialist, PICU
Children's Mercy Hospital
Kansas City, Missouri

Paul C. Stillwell, MD
Executive Vice President, Medical Affairs
Pulmonology
Phoenix Children's Hospital
Phoenix, Arizona

W. Gerald Teague, MD
Medical Director, Respiratory Care Services
Children's Healthcare of Atlanta at Egleston
Atlanta, Georgia

Jennifer L. Turi, MD
Associate in Pediatrics
Pediatric Critical Care Medicine
Duke Children's Hospital
Durham, North Carolina

Nico Vehse, MD
Pediatric Pulmonary Fellow
Division of Allergy and Pulmonology
University of Virginia Children's Hospital
Charlottesville, Virginia

Pearl Yu, MD
Director, Pediatric Sleep Disorders Program
Division of Pediatric Respiratory Medicine
University of Virginia Children's Hospital
Charlottesville, Virginia

Santina A. Zanelli, MD
Division of Neonatology
Department of Pediatrics
University of Virginia Health System
Charlottesville, Virginia

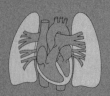

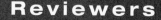

Reviewers

Terrell Ashe, RRT, RCP
Clinical Manager
Respiratory Care Services
Athens Regional Medical Center
Athens, Georgia

Kathy Boyle, MEd, MS, RRT-NPS
Coordinator, Respiratory Care Program
Southeast Arkansas College
Pine Bluff, Arkansas

Tabitha Carney, PharmD
Clinical Pharmacist
Pediatrics and Neonatology
Emory Healthcare
Atlanta, Georgia

Margaret-Ann Carno, PhD, MBA, RNC, CCRN
Assistant Clinical Professor
Nursing and Pediatrics
University of Rochester School of Nursing
Rochester, New York

Heidi V. Connolly, MD
Assistant Professor, Pediatrics
Pediatric Critical Care and Sleep Medicine
Fellowship Training Program Director
Pediatric Critical Care Associate Director
University of Rochester
Rochester, New York

Tim Douds, BS, RRT, NPS
Respiratory Care Manager
Gwinnet Women's Pavilion
Gwinnett Hospital
Lawrenceville, Georgia

Dana Evans, BHS, RRT-NPS, AE-C
School of Health Professions
University of Missouri-Columbia
Columbia, Missouri

Robert Joyner, Jr., PhD, RRT
Salisbury University
Salisbury, Maryland

Steven C. Mason, RRT, NPS
Respiratory Care Practitioner
Department of Respiratory Care Services
Massachusetts General Hospital
Boston, Massachusetts

Timothy Op'tHolt, EdD, RRT, AEC, FAARC
University of South Alabama
Mobile, Alabama

Clement L. Ren, MD
Associate Professor of Pediatrics
Division of Pediatric Pulmonology
University of Rochester
Rochester, New York

Ruben D. Restrepo, MD, RRT
University of Texas Health Science Center
San Antonio, Texas

Robert Sinkin, MD, MPH, FAAP, FATS
Professor of Pediatrics
Division Chief, Neonatology
University of Virginia Children's Hospital
Charlottesville, Virginia

Preface

Since the first edition published in 1995, *Perinatal and Pediatric Respiratory Care* has been a foundational neonatal and pediatric respiratory care textbook. We are proud to continue that tradition with the third edition.

The fundamental role of the pediatric respiratory therapist (RT) continues to be redefined on a daily basis. Dr. Dean Hess, editor-in-chief of the journal *Respiratory Care,* has described today's respiratory therapist as "a technologist, a clinician, and a physiologist." RTs specializing in the care of children are an integral part of an autonomous healthcare team. These individuals can be described as highly technical and have become more involved in critical roles as experts in critical and acute care, ECMO, air and ground transport, discharge coordination, home-care, education, and research. All roles that encompass the respiratory care of children require an individual who remains current with the changing face of this profession. The proliferation of new surgical interventions, discoveries in applied translational and clinical research, devices and mechanical ventilator technologies, and strategies that are currently being implemented into practice require dynamic, self-driven clinicians who are dedicated to remaining current with all of these aspects. Increases in premature and multiple births, as well as paradigm shifts in strategies focused at reducing hospital costs and healthcare spending, have led to the growth and development of many neonatal special care or intensive care units across the nation. RTs working outside of free-standing children's and university hospitals, many of whom have typically cared for adults, are now frequently called to support newborns at high-risk deliveries or to manage pediatric patients in respiratory distress. With these expanding roles, practitioners are faced with more technically challenging decisions in which critical thinking skills, coupled with better understanding of disease-specific management strategies and technologically advanced equipment, could impact patient outcomes.

We believe that *Perinatal and Pediatric Respiratory Care,* third edition, will provide you the tools and knowledge to improve the respiratory care of neonates, infants, and children regardless of your education, experience, or the environment in which you work.

AUDIENCE

Although principally designed as a textbook for the respiratory care student and practitioners new to the field, this book is also intended to be detailed enough to serve as a current desk-top reference for the experienced practitioner engaged in mastering the practice of respiratory care in infants and children, regardless of professional discipline. This textbook may also serve as a study guide for the National Board for Respiratory Care's (NBRC) specialty examination concerning the respiratory care of neonatal and pediatric patients. For convenience, the Evolve Resources for this edition include a correlation guide for the NBRC's Neonatal/Pediatric Respiratory Care Specialty Examination.

New to this Edition

The publisher and editors of this textbook have taken a more focused approach at satisfying some of the essential features that are needed to help guide educators and students at the collegiate level. This third edition introduces the following:

- Two new editors, researchers in pediatric respiratory care, who bring additional experience from the east and west coasts of the United States. The addition of these new editors, combined with 22 new contributors, adds new perspective and knowledge to this project.
- Revisions to all of the chapters reflect the latest updates in scientific literature.
- A new chapter entitled **Pediatric Thoracic Trauma** has improved the well-rounded character of the book.
- Measurable learning objectives have been added to the beginning of each chapter. The objectives are designed to succinctly guide the student to key areas of importance and mastery of chapter content.
- Each chapter now concludes with a series of multiple-choice assessment questions. Answers can be found on the Evolve website.

LEARNING AIDS

Evolve Resources—http://evolve.elsevier.com/Walsh/perinatal/

Evolve is an interactive learning environment designed to work in coordination with this text. Instructors may use Evolve to provide an internet-based course component that reinforces and expands the concepts presented in class. Evolve may be used to publish the class syllabus, outlines, and lecture notes; set up "virtual office hours" and e-mail communication; share important dates and information through the online class calendar; and encourage student participation through chat rooms and discussion boards. Evolve allows instructors to post exams and manage their grade books online.

For the Instructor

For the instructor, Evolve offers valuable resources to help them prepare their courses including:

- A test bank of approximately 800 questions in ExamView
- An image collection of the figures from the book available in jpeg and PowerPoint formats
- PowerPoint presentations for each chapter

For Students

For students, Evolve offers valuable resources to help them succeed in their courses including:

- Answers to Assessment Questions and Clinical Scenarios
- Correlation guides for the NBRC's Neonatal/Pediatric Respiratory Care Specialty Examination
- Additional content on ventilators commonly used for neonatal and pediatric care
- Weblinks to topics of interest to respiratory therapy students and practitioners

For more information, visit http://evolve.elsevier.com/Walsh/perinatal/ or contact an Elsevier sales representative.

ACKNOWLEDGMENTS

We would like to thank all of the contributors to this edition of *Perinatal and Pediatric Respiratory Care*. It is their work that laid yet again the foundation for this edition. We thank them for their patience and the professional quality of each chapter's content. We would also like to thank William Wojchiechowski for his work writing the test bank and Linda Cochran for the PowerPoint presentations.

We would also like to include a special and warm appreciation to Sherry L. Barnhart, one of the editors in the first and second edition of this book who could no longer participate in the editor role. She deserves our gratitude, especially since it was Sherry's work that kindled the original concept of this textbook. Sherry, we thank you for your dedication and continued support by contributing chapters and professional interest.

Additionally we want to thank the developmental publishing staff, especially Senior Developmental Editor Mindy Hutchinson, who tirelessly attempted to keep us in line and on target for publication. We continued to be awed by your wonderful attitude and never-ending supply of positive instruction, in spite of many delays and changes along this journey. We also thank Karen Rehwinkel, Senior Project Manager, for her calm patience and attention to detail.

Last, but by no means least, we especially thank our spouses for their love, support, and encouragement to persevere through this project. We are blessed beyond words.

Brian K. Walsh
Michael P. Czervinske
Robert M. DiBlasi

Contents

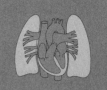

Chapter **1**

Fetal Lung Development

BRUCE M. SCHNAPF • SCOTT M. KIRLEY

OUTLINE

Stages of Lung Development
    Embryonal Stage
    Pseudoglandular Stage
    Canalicular Stage
    Saccular Stage
    Alveolar Stage

Postnatal Lung Growth
Factors Affecting Prenatal and Postnatal Lung Growth
Abnormal Lung Development
Pulmonary Hypoplasia
Alveolar Cell Development and Surfactant Production
Fetal Lung Liquid

LEARNING OBJECTIVES

After reading this chapter the reader will be able to:

- List the five stages of fetal development and the gestational age at which they occur
- Explain why knowing the key steps of each stage of fetal development is important
- Identify the gestational age during which extrauterine viability occurs, and explain why it cannot occur earlier

- Identify several conditions that lead to abnormal development and lung injury
- Discuss the role of the type II pneumocyte in surfactant production
- Discuss the various functions of surfactant
- Explain how fetal lung liquid differs from amniotic fluid and outline how it is cleared during and after labor

At birth, the lungs must immediately supply oxygen to the infant. Fetal lung development is such that, at this crucial moment, the lungs have reached only that degree of morphologic, physiologic, and biochemical maturity necessary for basic functioning. In other words, lung development is not complete at birth: the newborn lung undergoes further differentiation and growth.[1,2] Functionally, fetal lung development is not complete until the alveoli possess an adequate surface area for gas exchange. The pulmonary vascular system must also have sufficient capacity to transport an adequate amount of blood through the lungs for carbon dioxide and oxygen exchange. The alveoli need to be structurally and functionally stable, and elastic and resilient enough to undergo the stretching associated with tidal breathing and crying.

Much has been learned about the normal development of the human lung. In the 1960s, Reid formulated the laws of development of the human lung:

- The bronchial tree develops by week 16 of intrauterine life.
- After birth the alveoli develop in increasing numbers until the age of 8 years, and increase in size until growth of the chest wall is finished.
- Preacinar arteries and veins develop after the airway has been established; intra-acinar vessels develop after the alveoli are generated.[3]

Although these facts are known, renewed interest in the mechanics of fetal lung development has been kindled by the desire to understand and prevent chronic lung injury in premature infants. This interest is centered on the biochemical and genetic mechanisms of cellular repair in the immature lung that permit recovery of injured lungs in premature infants. Another topic of focus concerns the complex process of geometric growth and alveolar development.[4-6]

As stated earlier, birth does not signal the end of lung development. A remarkably complex process of growth occurs after birth, accommodating differing proportions of airway size, alveolar size, and surface area. The term infant, with approximately 50 million alveoli, has the potential to add another 250 million alveoli and increase its total alveolar surface area from approximately 3 to 70 m^2 at maturity. More than 40 different cell types, with many different functions, are found in the lung. Adding to this complexity are growth factors, which are responsible for normal cell and structural development and affect various aspects of prenatal and postnatal lung function, growth, and structure.

STAGES OF LUNG DEVELOPMENT

In humans, there are five well-recognized stages of lung development: embryonal, pseudoglandular, canalicular, saccular, and alveolar (Table 1-1).[7-9]

Embryonal Stage

The first stage is the embryonal period, which covers primitive development and is generally regarded as encompassing the first 2 months of gestation. The lung begins to emerge as a bud from the pharynx 26 days after conception (Figure 1-1). This lung bud elongates and forms two bronchial buds and the trachea, which then separate from the esophagus through the development of the tracheoesophageal septum. Further subdivisions occur in an irregular, dichotomous way until the end of the embryonal stage. By this time, the major airways have developed. Various growth factors and fibroblasts mediate morphogenesis of the tubular epi-

TABLE 1-1

Classification of Stages of Human Intrauterine Lung Growth

Stage	Time of Occurrence	Significance
Embryonal	Day 26 to day 52	Development of trachea and major bronchi
Pseudoglandular	Day 52 to week 16	Development of remaining conducting airways
Canalicular	Week 17 to week 26	Development of vascular bed and framework of respiratory acini
Saccular	Week 26 to week 36	Increased complexity of saccules
Alveolar	Week 36 to term	Development of alveoli

thelium, which results in airway branching: 10 on the right and nine on the left.[1] The left and right pulmonary arteries form plexuses even before the heart descends into the thorax. Left and right pulmonary veins start to develop at about week 5 as a single evagination in the sinoatrial portion of the heart.

During this phase, the respiratory epithelium develops from the foregut bud, an endodermal layer construct (the endoderm is the innermost layer of the three primary germ layers: endoderm, mesoderm, and ectoderm), and interacts with the bronchial mesoderm (the middle primary germ layer). The mesenchyme, a network of embryonic connective tissue in the mesoderm, will eventually give rise to the pulmonary interstitium, smooth muscle, blood vessels, and cartilage.[10] The mesenchyme determines the nature of airway branching by a complex interaction of epithelial cells with the bronchial mesoderm.[11] The surrounding mesenchyme is composed of cells that have not differentiated into cartilage or other fully developed connective tissue cells. The mesenchyme and epithelium are separated from each other by a basal lamina that contains type I collagen at the sites of branching.

The diaphragm also develops during the embryonal stage of lung development. Complete development of the diaphragm occurs by approximately week 7 of gestation.

Pseudoglandular Stage

The next stage is the pseudoglandular phase, named after the distinct glandular appearance of the developing lung. This stage extends to week 16 of gestation, during which time the conducting airways continue to develop. In this stage, there is extensive subdivision of the conducting airway system. The branching pattern

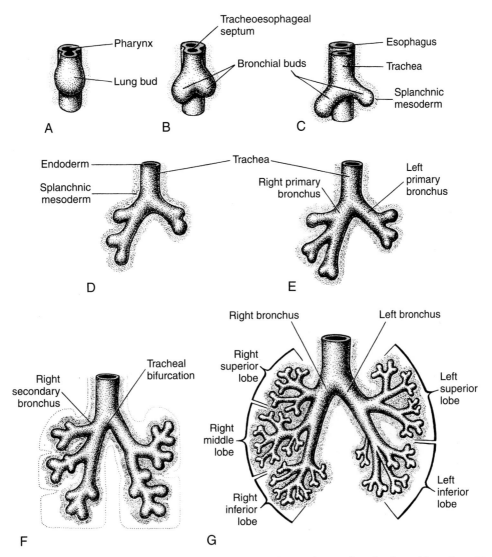

FIGURE 1-1 Embryonal stage of lung development: the trachea and major bronchi at **A** to **C,** 4 weeks; **D** and **E,** 5 weeks; **F,** 6 weeks; **G,** 8 weeks.

that occurs in both lungs determines the pattern in the adult lung.[12] The subsequent growth of these airways is in size only. The most peripheral structures are the terminal bronchioles, which likely differentiate into the respiratory bronchioles and alveolar ducts.[13] Once the pattern is laid, the subsequent growth of these airways is in size only. The gas-exchanging part of the lung, consisting of the pulmonary acini, or terminal respiratory units, may also be laid down completely during the pseudoglandular phase. Various growth factors and chemical mediators also begin to transdifferentiate the primordial tracheal epithelium into respiratory type II epithelial cells required for alveolar development.[1]

During the pseudoglandular phase, cilia appear on the surface of the epithelium of the trachea and the mainstem bronchi at 10 weeks of gestation and are pres-ent on the epithelial cells of the peripheral airways by 13 weeks of gestation. Goblet cells appear in the bronchial epithelium at 13 to 14 weeks of gestation, and submucosal glands arise as solid buds from basal layers of the surface epithelium at 15 to 16 weeks of gestation. Smooth muscle cells derived from the primitive mesenchyme surrounding the airways can be seen at the end of week 7 of gestation and by week 12 form the posterior wall of the large bronchi. The development of cartilage has been documented at 24 weeks of gestation and may be present earlier. Cartilage may be present in about 10 to 14 airway generations at 24 weeks of gestation. The cartilage is immature at this stage. Lymphatics appear first in the hilar region of the lung during week 8 of gestation and in the lung itself by week 10. This phase has been termed *pseudoglandular* because random histologic sections show the appearance of multiple, apparently round structures resembling glands. They are separated from each other by mesenchyme and its derivatives. The cells lining the spaces are columnar and contain glycogen. By the end of this stage, airways, arteries, and veins have developed in the pattern corresponding to that found in the adult.

Maturation of the immune system begins before birth. By 14 weeks of gestation, T lymphocytes can be found in the respiratory system. Fetal immune responses to allergens develop early and can be detected in cord blood. The potential routes of exposure are via the placenta (transplacental) or the fetal gut (by the swallowing of amniotic fluid). However, the relative importance of the two is not fully understood.[3]

Canalicular Stage

The canalicular phase follows the pseudoglandular stage and lasts from approximately 17 weeks to about 26 weeks of gestation. This stage is so named because of the appearance of vascular channels, or capillaries, which begin to grow by forming a capillary network around the air passages.[14] Some of the capillaries extend into the epithelium. The capillaries develop at 20 weeks of gestation and by 22 weeks have increased in number. Satisfactory gas exchange cannot occur until the capillaries have sufficient surface area and are close enough to the airspaces for efficient gas transfer. This development, along with the appearance of surfactant, is therefore critical to the extrauterine survival of the immature fetus. The survival of the fetus becomes possible during the canalicular stage, at 22 to 24 weeks of gestation.

Pulmonary acinar units are also formed during the canalicular period (Figure 1-2). Each acinus consists of a respiratory bronchiole (which contains no cartilage in its wall), alveolar ducts, and alveolar sacs. It follows that primitive lobules will have formed by the beginning of the canalicular period. Each lobule will contain three to five terminal bronchioles; approximately 25,000 terminal bronchioles will be found in the adult lung. If the primitive acinar units are all formed by the end of the canalicular period, this would imply that the full complement of 25,000 terminal bronchioles should be present by 28 weeks of gestation.

Thinning of the extracellular matrix, or mesenchyme, continues through the canalicular period. By 20 to 22 weeks of gestation, type I and type II epithelial cells can be differentiated in the human fetal lung. The type II cells retain the cytoplasmic shape of their precursors. Lamellar bodies, crucial to surfactant formation, and glycogen begin to appear in the type II cell cytoplasm. The type I cells begin their flattening process and elongate. The conducting airways have now developed smooth muscle.

By the end of the canalicular period, the developing air–blood barrier is thin enough to support gas exchange. Blood vessels grow alongside conducting airways, which are also undergoing muscularization, to a peripheral position that is more distant than in the adult.[15] The bronchial artery system may be as critical for lung development as the pulmonary arteries, although the role of the bronchial arteries in lung differentiation and growth is not clear.[16] It has been suggested that the most peripheral parts of the developing lung are

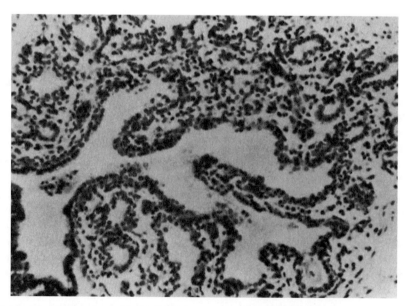

FIGURE 1-2 Canalicular stage of lung development at 22 weeks of gestation. A terminal bronchiole (*bottom left*) leads into a prospective acinus. Note that branches are sparse.

supplied only by the pulmonary arterial vasculature.[15] The epithelial cells at this point are capable of producing fetal lung liquid.

Saccular Stage

The saccular period was formerly thought to be the last stage of lung development before birth. However, because alveoli are now known to form before birth, the termination of the saccular period is now arbitrarily set at 35 to 36 weeks of gestation. At the beginning of this phase, at about 26 weeks of gestation, the terminal structures are referred to as *saccules* and are relatively smooth-walled, cylindrical structures. They then become subdivided by ridges known as *secondary crests* (Figure 1-3). As the crests protrude into the saccules, part of the capillary net is drawn in with them, forming a double capillary layer.[17,18] Further septation between the crests results in smaller spaces, which have been termed *subsaccules*. Exactly when these subsaccular structures become alveoli is a matter of judgment (Figure 1-4). Some have advocated that any structure bordered on three sides should be termed an *alveolus*. Alveoli can be seen as early as 32 weeks of gestation and are present at 36 weeks of gestation in all fetuses (Figure 1-5). During the saccular phase, there is a marked increase in the potential gas-exchanging surface area.

Alveolar Stage

Clearly distinction between the saccular and alveolar stages is difficult and arbitrary. Hislop, Wigglesworth, and Desai[19] claim that alveoli are present at 29 weeks of gestation; Langston and coworkers[7] believe that 36 weeks of gestation is the earliest point at which subsaccules and alveoli can be distinguished. Alveolar maturation and proliferation are primarily a postnatal event, extending beyond birth with rapid growth up to 18 months postgestation.[1] Alveologenesis is characterized by a complex interaction of epithelial, fibroblast, and vascular growth factors with extracellular matrix components.

At birth, the number of alveoli is highly variable, ranging from 20 to 150 million. The accepted mean number of alveoli, as described in the literature, is also variable, given as 50 million by Langston and colleagues[7] and 150 million by Hislop, Wigglesworth, and Desai.[19] It has been estimated that only 15% to 20% of the adult number of alveoli are present at birth, and thus alveologenesis is largely a postnatal event. Hislop, Wigglesworth, and Desai[19] believe that almost half the total number of alveoli are present at birth. The important point is that alveolarization is rapidly progressing during the period of development from late fetal to early neonatal life and may be complete by a year or so after birth.

POSTNATAL LUNG GROWTH

Normal lung growth is a continuous process that begins early in gestation and extends through infancy and childhood. Major structural development occurs in late gestation and continues over the first years of postnatal life.[20,21] As stated earlier, estimates of alveolar number at birth vary widely, and the average of 50 million is generally accepted. These alveoli provide a total gas-exchanging surface of approximately 3 to 4 m². More than 80%

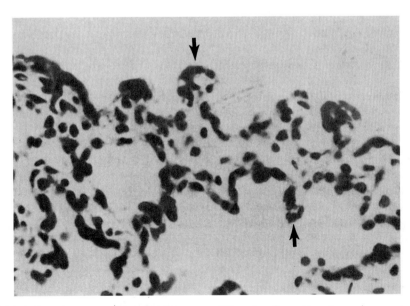

FIGURE 1-3 Saccular stage of lung development at 29 weeks of gestation. Secondary crests *(arrows)* begin to divide saccules into smaller compartments.

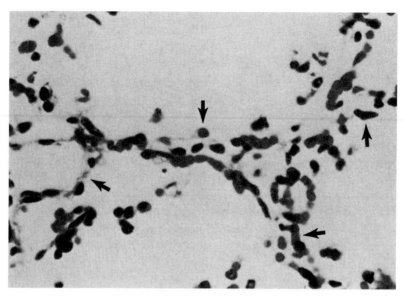

FIGURE 1-4 Alveolar stage of lung development at 36 weeks of gestation. Note the double capillary network *(solid arrows, center and right)* and the single capillary layer *(arrow at left).*

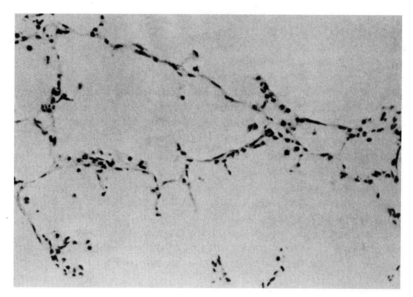

FIGURE 1-5 Alveolar stage of lung development at 36 weeks of gestation: thin-walled alveoli are present.

of the eventual total number of alveoli—about 300 million—will form after birth. Lung volume will increase 23-fold, alveolar number will increase 6-fold, alveolar surface area will increase 21-fold, and lung weight will increase 20-fold. Lung volume increases disproportionally to alveolar number.

As the human infant doubles in body weight by 6 months and triples by 1 year, oxygen uptake will increase proportionally; this is matched by an increase in alveolar growth. The area of the air–tissue interface increases in a linear relationship to body surface area.[22] Alveolar

volume and alveolar surface area increase in proportion to each other. However, alveolar number and alveolar diameter do not change proportionally. Most of the postnatal formation of alveoli in the infant occurs over the first 1.5 years of life.[23,24] Thereafter, the lung continues to grow in proportion to body growth.

Boyden and Tompsett[25] have described a mechanism of alveolar formation. They observed an extension of the gas-exchange region with transformation of the respiratory bronchioles into alveolar ducts and of terminal bronchioles into respiratory bronchioles.

Lateral pouches from these transformed respiratory bronchioles formed new alveoli. It was proposed that new alveolar formation occurs in this manner into later childhood and that this is the likely mechanism for new alveolar formation throughout life. At 2 years of age, the number of alveoli varies substantially among individuals. After 2 years of age, boys have more alveoli than do girls. After the end of alveolar multiplication, the alveoli continue to increase in size until thoracic growth is completed.[21]

FACTORS AFFECTING PRENATAL AND POSTNATAL LUNG GROWTH

Several factors are responsible for stimulating both normal and compensatory lung growth. It is generally accepted that pneumonectomy (removal of one entire lung) causes the remaining lung to grow, both in size and weight, and compensate for the missing lung.[25,26] Both alveolar multiplication and lengthening of alveolar septa probably occur. After pneumonectomy, disproportionate growth of alveoli and airways takes place, although some compensation through increased length and conducting airway volume has been reported.[27] There is no evidence that new conducting airways can form once branching is completed by the beginning of the canalicular period, at about week 17 of gestation.

Several studies have examined the effects of an altered metabolic rate on the growing lung. This occurs in hypoxia, starvation, and hyperoxia. The effects of hypoxia on the growing lung have been studied in 3- to 4-week-old rat pups, and in fetal rats by exposing the mother to 10% oxygen.[28,29] Fetal exposure to hypoxia resulted in a decrease in body weight and smaller lungs that remained appropriate for body weight.

Prenatal and postnatal nutritional deprivation can affect various aspects of lung function, growth, and structure. Kerr and associates[30] starved growing rats to produce emphysematous changes in their lungs and postulated that connective tissue, specifically collagen, was altered in the alveolar septa. Enlargement of airspaces is found with starvation and affects alveolar duct size as well as alveoli without apparent alveolar septal destruction.[31] Changes in connective tissue elements, pulmonary surfactant, ultrastructural features, and elastic recoil occur in adult rats after a few weeks of caloric restriction.[32,33] The structural alterations are not reversible after a short period of refeeding, whereas surfactant-associated functional changes are.

High concentrations of oxygen are toxic to pulmonary tissue. This damage is a causative factor in the development of bronchopulmonary dysplasia and associated abnormal lung repair after oxygen treatment of infants with hyaline membrane disease. The premature infant's antioxidant defense mechanisms are inadequate to prevent lung injury secondary to exposure to high concentrations of oxygen. In addition, young rats exposed to 40% oxygen have suppressed lung growth.[29,34,35] Also, DNA synthesis is suppressed by an increase in oxygen tension, and lung repair is adversely affected by high levels of oxygen.[36]

Pregnant rats exposed to cigarette smoke have been studied. These animals produced growth-retarded fetuses with a reduced lung-to-body weight ratio, decreased DNA content, and structural abnormalities.[37] The affected fetuses demonstrated reduced lung volume, a decrease in the number of saccules, an increase in saccular size, and a decrease in surface area. These changes are thought to result in part from a decrease in lung elastic tissue.

Other clinical factors have been cited as causing diminished lung growth. These conditions can be divided into four categories:
- Chest wall compression as occurs in diaphragmatic hernia, that is, an abnormal opening in the prenatal diaphragm that allows some of the abdominal organs to move into the chest and exert pressure on the developing lungs; chest wall abnormalities; and probably hydrops fetalis, that is, abnormal fluid accumulation in the fetus, often hydrothorax and ascites.
- Oligohydramnios, that is, reduced amniotic fluid for an extended period, with or without renal anomalies, is associated with lung hypoplasia.[38-40] The mechanisms by which amniotic fluid volume influences lung growth remain unclear. Possible explanations include mechanical restriction of the chest wall, interference with fetal breathing, or failure to produce fetal lung liquid. These clinical and experimental observations possibly point to a common denominator, lung stretch, as being a major growth stimulant.
- Diminished respiration has been shown to have a severe effect on lung growth. This effect could be mediated through a lack of stretch of the developing lung parenchyma.[41]
- A variety of hormonal or metabolic abnormalities may alter lung growth and structure. Leprechaunism, associated with abnormal carbohydrate metabolism, results in dysmorphic lungs with a decreased number of terminal bronchioles, dilated alveolar ducts and saccules, and enlarged airspaces.[42] Experimental diabetes produced by streptozotocin administration to 3-week-old rats resulted in diminished airspace size, increased alveolar number, and a marked effect on pulmonary connective tissue metabolism.[43,44]

An example of altered lung development is seen in children with Down syndrome. Although fetal lung growth is normal, postnatal lung growth is characterized by larger and fewer alveoli than normal.[45]

ABNORMAL LUNG DEVELOPMENT

Structural development of the lung may be altered by a number of conditions affecting the lungs in utero or by postnatal events.[46,47] Complex relationships exist among humoral, hormonal, and physical forces acting on the developing lung, altering its growth in ways that are poorly understood. Growth retardation of the fetal lung may affect size and weight but not maturation of airways and alveoli, whereas malnutrition may slow functional rather than structural maturation.[46]

Timing or dating of adverse events influencing fetal lung development is important in considering the approach to treatment and prognosis. Abnormalities occurring in the embryonic period are often associated with renal agenesis or dysplastic kidneys; branching of the lungs may also be affected. Abnormalities occurring later in development, such as diaphragmatic hernia, may affect the lungs during the pseudoglandular period, or before 16 weeks of gestation, and thereby decrease airway branching. If abnormalities occur during the second trimester of pregnancy, completion of pulmonary vascularization and acinar development may not proceed, and hypoplasia in the gas-exchanging area may result. Abnormal influences occurring during the last trimester of pregnancy, such as premature birth and hyaline membrane disease, may alter subsequent alveolar growth and differentiation, ultimately leading to a decrease in alveolar number.

PULMONARY HYPOPLASIA

Pulmonary hypoplasia, or failure of the lungs to develop in utero, is a relatively common abnormality of lung development, with a number of clinical associations and anatomic correlates. Hypoplasia may be considered to be present when there are too few cells, too few alveoli, or too few airways. The incidence of pulmonary hypoplasia diagnosed at autopsy is between 10% and 25% of all cases.[47-50]

The best-studied condition associated with hypoplasia is diaphragmatic hernia. The incidence of diaphragmatic hernia is about 1 in 4000 births. The range of abnormalities reported is wide and is probably related to variations in the severity and timing of the onset of lung compression.[51] Compression of the lung before 16 weeks of gestation causes incomplete branching of the conducting airways, terminal airways, or both. Early and severe compression results in severe hypoplasia, reducing the weight of the affected lung to less than half that of the contralateral lung. The affected lung demonstrates fewer, smaller alveoli, a decreased gas-exchanging surface area, and a proportionate decrease in pulmonary vasculature.

Other forms of lung compression may result in hypoplasia. Causes include osteogenesis imperfecta, hypophosphatasia,[52] and thoracic dystrophies. In addition to chest wall anomalies, pleural effusion, ascites, intrathoracic tumors, and extralobar sequestration may cause lung compression.

Pulmonary hypoplasia occurs in oligohydramnios as a result of leakage of amniotic fluid. It was first described by Potter in association with renal agenesis.[38] Experimental evidence supports the conclusion that the amount of lung liquid present in the fetus is a major determinant of lung growth, because chronic tracheal drainage produces pulmonary hypoplasia, and tracheal ligation produces lungs with increased tissue mass.[53] It has been shown that experimental oligohydramnios causes pulmonary hypoplasia, which can be more or less severe depending on its timing.[48,54]

Several experimental studies suggest that lung growth alteration may be caused by various hormonal imbalances.[55-59] Changes caused by endocrine effects may cause lung compression or diminished lung liquid and respiration. Glucocorticoid administration has been shown to accelerate lung maturation but may also affect lung growth. Type II epithelial cell maturation is induced both functionally and anatomically by this drug. Depending on the dose, glucocorticoids may reduce the rate of DNA synthesis and thus produce hypoplasia. Thyroidectomy in fetal sheep produces pulmonary hypoplasia and diminished type II cell differentiation. Maternal growth hormone apparently plays little role in fetal growth, but the effect of maternal administration of growth hormone on fetal lung growth has not been studied. Maternal experimental diabetes results in diminished tissue maturity in the fetus.[60]

ALVEOLAR CELL DEVELOPMENT AND SURFACTANT PRODUCTION

As the primordial epithelium evolves, the epithelial lining undergoes cellular division and differentiation into the highly specialized type I and type II pneumocytes. Type I pneumocytes are flat (squamous) cells serving as a thin, gas-permeable membrane for the diffusion of gases and as a barrier against water and solute leakage.[61] They account for more than 97% of the alveolar surface area, primarily as a result of their size, shape, and large cellular surface.[62]

Despite its smaller surface area, the cuboidal-appearing type II pneumocyte is the principal structure involved in surfactant production, storage, secretion, and reuse. Surfactant storage occurs in the lamellar bodies inside type II pneumocytes. An additional function of the type II pneumocyte, discovered by pulse-labeling with [³H]thymidine, is to differentiate into type I pneumocytes.[63]

Type II pneumocytes contain the precursors required for surfactant synthesis and osmiophilic lamellar bodies that function as the storage apparatus for the synthesized surfactant.[9,62] Through a continuous process of exocytosis, the lamellar bodies release their contents of tubular myelin into the alveolar hypophase (the thin liquid lining of the internal surface of the alveoli). The liberated tubular myelin unravels and disperses to form a monolayer at the air–liquid interface.[63]

The primary role of mammalian surfactant is to lower the surface tension within the alveolus, specifically at the air–liquid interface. This allows the delicate structure of the alveolus to expand when filled with air. Without surfactant, the alveolus remains collapsed because of the high surface tension of the moist alveolar surface. Surfactant is composed predominantly of an intricate blend of phospholipids, neutral lipids, and proteins. See Chapter 16 (Surfactant Replacement) for more information about surfactant composition.

Various chemical and mechanical stimulatory mechanisms leading to increased surfactant precursor production have been identified and include, but are not limited to, β-adrenergic agonists, prostaglandins, epidermal growth factor, and mechanical ventilation. Late gestational analysis of phosphatidylglycerol was shown to be a sensitive indicator of lung maturity and is associated with a previous rise in phosphatidylcholine.[64]

FETAL LUNG LIQUID

Fetal lungs are secretory organs that make breathing-like movements but serve no respiratory function before birth. They secrete about 250 to 300 ml of liquid per day. Thus the fetal airways are not collapsed but filled with fluid from the canalicular period until delivery and the initiation of ventilation. This liquid flows from the terminal respiratory units through the conducting airways and into the oropharynx, where it is either swallowed or expelled into the amniotic sac. The presence of fetal lung fluid is essential for normal lung development. This luminal fluid is high in chloride and low in bicarbonate, with a negligible concentration of protein.[65,66] Active transport of chloride ions across the fetal pulmonary epithelium generates an electric potential difference and causes liquid to flow from the lung microcirculation through the interstitium and into the airspaces.[67] The pulmonary circulation, rather than the bronchial circulation, is the major source of this liquid. The balance between production and drainage of this liquid has an important effect on lung development. During fetal breathing, there is a small but steady movement of fluid outward from the trachea. The net movement of fluid away from the lungs has been measured at about 15 ml/hour and was about five times higher during periods of fetal breathing than during apnea.[68] Prolonged outflow obstruction expands the lungs and leads to a decrease in type II cells.[69] In contrast, unimpeded removal of lung liquid decreases lung size, increases apparent tissue density, and stimulates proliferation of type II cells.[53]

The clearance of fetal lung fluid is essential for normal neonatal respiratory adaptation. However, several studies have shown that both the rate of liquid formation and the volume within the lumen of the fetal lung normally decrease before birth.[70-72] It is unknown what causes the reduction in fetal lung secretions before birth. Hormonal changes, which occur in the fetus just before and during labor, may have an important role in triggering this process. The influence of catecholamines on fetal lung liquid volume has been investigated. It has been shown that injecting β-adrenergic agonists into pregnant rabbits reduces the amount of water in the lungs of their pups.[73] Epinephrine has been shown to inhibit secretion of fetal lung liquid.[74] Other hormones, such as arginine vasopressin and prostaglandin E_2, which are secreted around the time of birth, may reduce production of lung luminal liquid.[75,76]

Removal of lung liquid continues after birth. When breathing begins, air inflation shifts residual liquid from the lumen into distensible perivascular spaces around large pulmonary blood vessels and bronchi. Accumulation of liquid in these connective tissue spaces, which are distant from the sites of respiratory gas exchange, allows time for small blood vessels and lymphatics to remove the displaced liquid with little or no impairment of neonatal lung function at this critical juncture.[77,78] The clearance of the fluid from the interstitial spaces occurs over many hours.

ASSESSMENT QUESTIONS

See Evolve Resources for answers.

1. Which of the following are stages of human lung development?
   - I. Embryonal
   - II. Canalicular
   - III. Blastocystic
   - IV. Chorionic
   - V. Saccular
   - A. I, II, and III
   - B. I, II, and V
   - C. I, II, and IV
   - D. I, III, and IV
   - E. I, IV, and V

Continued

2. The initial lung bud emerges from which of the following?
   A. Esophagus
   B. Trachea
   C. Umbilical cord
   D. Pharynx
   E. Mesoderm layer
3. The bronchial tree is formed at which gestational age?
   A. Embryonal
   B. Canalicular
   C. Pseudoglandular
   D. Saccular
   E. Alveolar
4. The alveolar epithelial lining undergoes cell division into type I and type II pneumocytes. Which of the following correctly describe the pneumocytes?
   I. Type I pneumocytes account for more than 97% of the alveolar surface area.
   II. Type II pneumocytes form a gas-permeable membrane for diffusion of gases.
   III. Surfactant production occurs in the lamellar bodies of type II pneumocytes, which release surfactant by exocytosis.
   IV. Type I pneumocytes are responsible for surfactant production and storage.
   V. Type I pneumocytes are squamous in shape and optimized for gas exchange; type II pneumocytes are cube-shaped and may differentiate into type I cells.
   A. I, II, IV, and V
   B. I, III, and V
   C. I, IV, and V
   D. II, IV, and V
   E. III and IV
5. What are the minimal developmental features required for an immature human fetus to survive outside the uterus?
   I. 32 weeks of gestation
   II. Sufficient alveolar and vascular surface area for gas exchange
   III. Sufficient endoplasmic reticulum production
   IV. 22 to 24 weeks of gestation
   V. Completion of the canalicular stage of lung development
   A. I, II, III, and IV
   B. I and V
   C. II, III, and V
   D. II, IV, and V
   E. III, IV, and V
6. Which of the following best describe(s) fetal lung liquid?
   A. It lowers surface tension within the alveoli.
   B. It maintains the structure of the airway lumen and developing alveoli, preventing complete collapse.
   C. With fetal breathing movement it continuously flows out of the lungs and is swallowed or excreted into the amniotic fluid.
   D. A and B
   E. B and C

7. Estimates of the exact number of alveoli at birth vary widely, but investigators agree that
   A. The surface area of gas exchange increases inversely with age.
   B. Normal structural development is complete before the first breath.
   C. Normal lung growth is a continuous process that extends into adulthood.
   D. Gas exchange surface area grows proportionally with an increase in oxygen consumption and body surface area.
   E. Extension of gas exchange occurs with transformation of alveolar ducts and terminal bronchioles into respiratory bronchioles.
8. Which is the lung development stage formerly thought to be the last stage before birth, and characterized by relatively smooth-walled, cylindrical structures subdivided by ridges known as secondary crests?
   A. Alveolar stage
   B. Saccular stage
   C. Terminal stage
   D. Trophoblast stage
   E. Canalicular stage
9. Pulmonary hypoplasia is a relatively common abnormality of lung development with a number of clinical associations including:
   A. Lung tissue compression
   B. Oligohydramnios
   C. Maternal diabetes
   D. All of the above
   E. A and C only
10. Reid's laws of human lung development state that
   I. The bronchial tree develops by week 16 of intrauterine life.
   II. Preacinar vasculature develops after the airway has been established, and intra-acinar vasculature develops after the alveoli are generated.
   III. Alveolar development is complete when there is sufficient gas exchange surface area to support extrauterine life.
   IV. The esophageal lung bud arises from the embryonic mesoderm to form the tracheal bronchial tree.
   V. Alveoli increase in number until 8 years of age and grow in size until chest wall growth is complete.
   A. I and IV
   B. I, II, and V
   C. I, III, IV, and V
   D. II, and III
   E. II, III, and V

References

1. Burri PH: Structural aspects of prenatal and postnatal development and growth of the lung. In: McDonald JA, editor: *Lung growth and development*, New York, Marcel Dekker, 1997, pp 1-35.

2. Boyden EA: Development and growth of the airways. In Hodson WA, editor: *Development of the lung*, New York, Marcel Dekker, 1977, pp 3-35.

3. Reid L: The embryology of the lung. In DeReuek AV, Porter R, editors: *Development of the lung*, Boston, Little, Brown, 1967, pp 109-130.

4. Sheffield M, Mabry S, Thibeault DW et al: Pulmonary nitric oxide synthases and nitrotyrosine: findings during lung development and in chronic lung disease of prematurity, *Pediatrics* 2006;118:1056.

5. Kreiger PA, Ruchelli ED, Mahboubi S et al: Fetal pulmonary malformations: defining histopathology, *Am J Surg Pathol* 2006;30:643.

6. Bourbon J, Boucherat O, Chailley-Heu B et al: Control mechanisms of lung alveolar development and their disorders in bronchopulmonary dysplasia, *Pediatr Res* 2005;57:38R.

7. Langston C, Kida K, Reed M et al: Human lung growth in late gestation and in the neonate, *Am Rev Respir Dis* 1984;129:607.

8. Liggins GC: Growth of the fetal lung, *J Dev Physiol* 1984;97:237.

9. Xu J, Tian J, Grumelli SM, Haley KJ et al: Stage-specific effects of cAMP signaling during distal lung epithelial development, *J Biol Chem* 2006;281:38894.

10. Loosli CG, Potter EL: Pre- and postnatal development of the respiratory portion on the human lung, *Am Rev Respir Dis* 1959;80:5.

11. Spooner BS, Wessells MK: Mammalian lung development: interactions in primordium formation and bronchial morphogenesis, *J Exp Zool* 1970;175:445.

12. Hislop AA, Reid L: Growth and development of the respiratory system: anatomical development. In Davies JA, Dobbing J, editors: *Scientific foundation of paediatrics*, London, Heinemann Medical Books, 1974, pp 214-254.

13. Hoh K, Hoh H: A study of cartilage development in pulmonary hypoplasia, *Pediatr Pulmonol* 1988;8:65.

14. Thurlbeck WM: Prematurity and the developing lung, *Clin Perinatol* 1992;19:497.

15. Hislop A, Reid L: Formation of the pulmonary vasculature. In Hodson WA, editor: *Development of the lung*, New York, Marcel Dekker, 1979, pp 37-86.

16. Boyden EA: The time lag in the development of bronchial arteries, *Anat Rec* 1970;166:611.

17. Cooney TP, Thurlbeck WM: The radial alveolar count method of Emery and Methal—a reappraisal. II. Intra-uterine and early post-natal lung growth, *Thorax* 1982;37:580.

18. Bruce MC, Honaker CE, Cross RJ: Lung fibroblasts undergo apoptosis following alveolarization, *Am J Respir Cell Mol Biol* 1999;20:228.

19. Hislop A, Wigglesworth JS, Desai R: Alveolar development in the human fetus and infant, *Early Hum Dev* 1986;13:1.

20. Reid L: The lung: its growth and remodelling in health and disease, *Am J Roentgenol* 1977;129:777.

21. Thurlbeck WM: The state of the art: postnatal growth and development of the lung, *Am Rev Respir Dis* 1975;111:803.

22. Dunnill MS: Postnatal growth of the lung, *Thorax* 1962;17:329.

23. Zeltner TB, Burri PH: The postnatal development and growth of the human lung. II. Morphology, *Respir Physiol* 1987;67:269.

24. Zeltner TB, Burri PH: The postnatal development and growth of the human lung. I. Morphometry, *Respir Physiol* 1987;67:247.

25. Boyden EA, Tompsett DH: The changing patterns in the developing lungs of infants, *Acta Anat (Basel)* 1965;61:164.

26. Cagle PT, Thurlbeck WM: Postpneumonectomy and compensatory lung growth, *Am Rev Respir Dis* 1988;138:1314.

27. Boatman ES: A morphometric and morphological study of the lungs of rabbits after unilateral pneumonectomy, *Thorax* 1977;32:406.

28. Bartlett D, Remmers JE: Effects of high altitude exposure on the lungs of young rats, *Respir Physiol* 1971;13:116.

29. Burri PH, Weibel ER: Morphometric estimation of pulmonary diffusion capacity. II. Effect of Po_2 on the growing lung: adaptation of the growing rat to hypoxia and hyperoxia, *Respir Physiol* 1971;11:247.

30. Kerr JS, Riley DJ, Lanza-Jacoby S et al: Nutritional emphysema in the rat: influence of protein depletion and impaired lung growth, *Am Rev Respir Dis* 1985;131:644.

31. Harkema JR, Mauderly JL, Gregory RE et al: A comparison of starvation and elastase models of emphysema in the rat, *Am Rev Respir Dis* 1984;129:584.

32. Sahebjami H, Vassallo CL: Effects of starvation and refeeding on lung mechanics and morphometry, *Am Rev Respir Dis* 1979;119:443.

33. Sahebjami H, Vassallo CL, Wirman JA: Lung mechanics and ultrastructure in prolonged starvation, *Am Rev Respir Dis* 1978;117:77.

34. Bartlett D: Postnatal growth of the mammalian lung: influence of low and high oxygen tensions, *Respir Physiol* 1970;9:58.

35. Butcher JR, Roberts RJ: The development of the newborn rat lung in hyperoxia: a dose–response study of lung growth, maturation, and changes in antioxidant enzyme activities, *Pediatr Res* 1981;15:999.

36. Witschi HR, Haschek WM, Klein-Szanto AJ et al: Potentiation of diffuse lung damage by oxygen: determining of variables, *Am Rev Respir Dis* 1981;123:98.

37. Collins MH, Moessinger AC, Kleinerman J et al: Fetal lung hypoplasia associated with maternal smoking: a morphometric analysis, *Pediatr Res* 1985;19:408.

38. Potter EL: Bilateral renal agenesis, *J Pediatr* 1946;29:68.

39. King JC, Mitzner W, Butterfield AB et al: Effect of induced oligohydramnios on fetal lung development, *Am J Obstet Gynecol* 1986;154:823.

40. Perlman M, Williams J, Hirsch M: Neonatal pulmonary hypoplasia after prolonged leakage of amniotic fluid, *Arch Dis Child* 1976;51:349.

41. Nagai A, Thurlbeck WM, Deboeck C et al: The effects of maternal CO_2 breathing in lung development of fetuses in the rabbit: morphologic and morphometric studies, *Am Rev Respir Dis* 1988;135:130.

42. Thurlbeck WM, Cooney TP: Dysmorphic lungs in a case of leprechaunism: case report and review of literature, *Pediatr Pulmonol* 1988;5:100.
43. Ofulue AF, Kida K, Thurlbeck WM: Experimental diabetes and the lung. I. Changes in growth, morphometry, and biochemistry, *Am Rev Respir Dis* 1988;137:162.
44. Ofulue AF, Thurlbeck WM: Experimental diabetes and the lung. II. In vivo connective tissue metabolism, *Am Rev Respir Dis* 1988;138:284.
45. Cooney TP, Wentworth PJ, Thurlbeck WM: Diminished radial count is found only postnatally in Down's syndrome, *Pediatr Pulmonol* 1988;5:204.
46. Lipsett J, Tamblyn M, Madigan K et al: Restricted fetal growth and lung development: a morphometric analysis of pulmonary structure, *Pediatr Pulmonol* 2006;41:1138.
47. Reale FR, Easterly JR: Pulmonary hypoplasia: a morphometric study of the lungs of infants with diaphragmatic hernia, anencephaly, and renal malformations, *Pediatrics* 1973;52:91.
48. Moessinger AC, Abbey-Mensah M, Driscoll JM et al: Pulmonary hypoplasia, a disorder on the rise? [abstract], *Pediatr Res* 1983;17:327A.
49. Moessinger AC, Collins MH, Blanc WA et al: Oligohydramnios-induced lung hypoplasia: the influence of timing and duration, *Pediatr Res* 1986;20:951.
50. Page DV, Stocker JT: Anomalies associated with pulmonary hypoplasia, *Am Rev Respir Dis* 1982;125:216.
51. George DK, Cooney TP, Chiu BK et al: Hypoplasia and immaturity of the terminal lung unit (acinus) in congenital diaphragmatic hernia, *Am Rev Respir Dis* 1987;136:947.
52. Silver MM, Vilos GA: Pulmonary hypoplasia in neonatal hypophosphatasia, *Pediatr Pathol* 1988;84:83.
53. Alcorn D, Adamson TM, Lambert TF et al: Morphological effects of chronic tracheal ligation and drainage in fetal lamb lung, *J Anat* 1977;123:649.
54. Blatchford KG, Thurlbeck WM: Lung growth and maturation in experimental oligohydramnios in the rat, *Pediatr Pulmonol* 1987;3:328.
55. Crone RK, Davies P, Liggins GC et al: The effects of hypophysectomy, thyroidectomy, and postoperative infusion of cortisol or adrenocorticotrophin on the structure of the ovine fetal lung, *J Dev Physiol* 1983;5:281.
56. Erenberg A, Rhodes ML, Weinstein MM et al: The effect of fetal thyroidectomy on ovine fetal lung maturation, *Pediatr Res* 1979;13:230.
57. Liggins GC, Kitterman JA, Campos GA et al: Pulmonary maturation in the hypophysectomized ovine fetus: differential responses to adrenocorticotrophin and cortisol, *J Dev Physiol* 1981;3:1.
58. Morishige WK, John NS: Influence of glucocorticoids on postnatal lung development in the rat: possible modulation by thyroid hormone, *Endocrinology* 1982;111:1587.
59. Pinkerton KE, Kendall JZ, Randall GC et al: Hypophysectomy and porcine fetal lung development, *Am J Respir Cell Mol Biol* 1989;1:319.
60. Sosenko IRS, Frantz ID III, Roberts RJ et al: Morphologic disturbance of lung maturation in fetuses of alloxan diabetic rats, *Am Rev Respir Dis* 1980;122:687.
61. Schneeberger EE: Alveolar type I cells. In Crystal RG, West JB, editors: *The lung: scientific foundations*, New York, Raven Press, 1991, pp 1677-1685.
62. Notter RH, Shapiro DL: Lung surfactants for replacement therapy: biochemical, biophysical, and clinical aspects, *Clin Perinatol* 1987;433.
63. Adamson YR, Bowden DH: The type II cell as a progenitor of alveolar epithelial regeneration, *Lab Invest* 1974;30:35.
64. Kresch MJ, Gross I: The biochemistry of fetal lung development, *Clin Perinatol* 1987;14:481.
65. Mescher EJ, Platzker AC, Ballard PL et al: Ontogeny of tracheal fluid, pulmonary surfactant, and plasma corticoids in the fetal lamb, *J Appl Physiol* 1975;39:1017.
66. Adams FH, Fujiwara T, Rowshan G: The nature and origin of the fluid in the fetal lamb lung, *J Pediatr* 1963;63:881.
67. Olver RE, Strang LB: Ion fluxes across the pulmonary epithelium and the secretion of lung liquid in the foetal lamb, *J Physiol* 1974;241:327.
68. Harding R, Sigger JN, Wickham PJ et al: The regulation of flow of pulmonary fluid in fetal sheep, *Respir Physiol* 1984;57:47.
69. Carmal JA, Friedman F, Adams FH: Fetal tracheal ligation and lung development, *Am J Dis Child* 1965;109:452.
70. Kitterman JA, Ballard PL, Clements JA et al: Tracheal fluid in fetal lambs: spontaneous decrease prior to birth, *J Appl Physiol* 1979;47:985.
71. Dickson KA, Maloney JE, Berger PJ: Decline in lung liquid volume before labor in fetal lambs, *J Appl Physiol* 1986;61:2266.
72. Brown MJ, Olver RE, Ramsden CA et al: Effects of adrenaline and of spontaneous labour on the secretion and absorption of lung liquid in the foetal lamb, *J Physiol* 1983;344:137.
73. Enhorning G, Chamberlain D, Contreras C et al: Isoxsuprine-induced release of pulmonary surfactant in the rabbit fetus, *Am J Obstet Gynecol* 1977;129:197.
74. Lawson EE, Brown ER, Torday JS et al: The effect of epinephrine on tracheal fluid flow and surfactant efflux in fetal sheep, *Am Rev Respir Dis* 1978;118:1023.
75. Bland RD et al: Vasopressin decreases lung water in fetal lambs [abstract], *Pediatr Res* 1985;19:399A.
76. Kitterman JA: Fetal lung development, *J Dev Physiol* 1984;6:67.
77. Bland RD, Hansen TN, Haberkern CM et al: Lung fluid balance in lambs before and after birth, *J Appl Physiol* 1982;53:992.
78. Bland RD, McMillan DD, Bressack MA et al: Clearance of liquid from lungs of newborn rabbits, *J Appl Physiol* 1980;49:171.

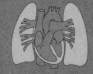

Chapter 2

Fetal Gas Exchange and Circulation

MICHAEL P. CZERVINSKE

OUTLINE

Maternal–Fetal Gas Exchange
Cardiovascular Development
    Early Development
    Chamber Development
    Maturation

Fetal Circulation and Fetal Shunts
Transition to Extrauterine Life

LEARNING OBJECTIVES

After reading this chapter the reader will be able to:
- Discuss the identifiable stages of heart development and explain the development of the heart chambers
- Identify the origin of congenital heart anomalies named after the developmental structures that occur during heart development
- Name the three fetal shunts and discuss their role during fetal circulation

- Explain the direction of blood flow and relative vascular pressures in the placenta, umbilical vein, three fetal shunts, right heart chambers, left heart chambers, pulmonary artery, lungs, aorta, and umbilical arteries
- Describe the cardiac and pulmonary sequences of events that occur when transitioning from fetal to extrauterine life, including the changes in fetal shunts

The rapidly growing embryo and fetus must develop a network to circulate nutrients and provide gas exchange. The fetus depends on the mother's circulation for gas exchange; however, the maternal and fetal vascular networks are separate systems, and no blood is shared between the two. The growing embryo quickly develops a myocardial pump and vascular system to provide fetal circulation.

MATERNAL–FETAL GAS EXCHANGE

As the fertilized egg, or *zygote*, travels to the uterus, it undergoes various degrees of cell division, but has no nutrient source as in a bird egg. So the developing cells, at this point termed the *blastocyst*, must implant into the uterine lining for nourishment. The outer surrounding layer of the blastocyst is the *trophoblast*, which combines with tissues from the endometrium to form the *chorionic membrane* around the blastocyst.[1] Inside the blastocyst, a group of cells arrange on one side in the shape of a figure eight. The central portion is the *embryonic disk*, which forms the three embryonic germ layers: the *ectoderm* and the *endoderm*, followed by the *mesoderm*.[2] Box 2-1 lists the tissue systems that arise from the three germ layers.

The outer or top loop of the figure eight envelops the embryonic structure and forms the *amniotic sac*, while the inner or bottom loop forms the *yolk sac*. The yolk sac soon degenerates and incorporates into the embryo, giving way for the amniotic sac to grow. Suspended in the cavity of the blastocyst, the amniotic sac then

Box 2-1	Origin of the Various Tissue Systems From the Three Embryonic Germ Layers*

ECTODERM
- Central nervous system: brain and spinal cord
- Peripheral nervous system: cranial nerves and spinal nerves
- Sensory epithelia of the eyes, inner ears, and nose
- Glandular tissues: posterior pituitary gland, adrenal medulla
- Skin: epidermal layer
- Specializations of the skin: sweat and sebaceous glands, hair follicles, nails, mammary glands
- Teeth: enamel

MESODERM
- Cardiovascular system: heart and blood vessels
- Lymphatic system vessels
- All connective tissue: general connective tissue, and cartilage, bone, bone marrow, and blood cells
- All muscle tissue: skeletal, cardiac, and smooth
- Skin: dermis and hypodermis
- Kidneys and ureters, spleen
- Reproductive tissues (not including the germ cells)
- The three major body cavities: pericardium, left and right pleura, and peritoneum
- Serous linings of organs within the body cavities
- Teeth: dentine, cementum, and pulp

ENDODERM
- Digestive system: stomach, small and large intestines, and epithelial lining of the entire digestive system except parts of the mouth and pharynx, and anus (which are supplied by the ectoderm)
- Respiratory system: pharynx, lungs, and epithelial lining of the trachea and lungs
- Urinary system: bladder, and lining of the urethra
- Liver and pancreas, and epithelial lining of all glands that open into the digestive system
- Tonsils, thymus, thyroid, parathyroid
- Epithelial lining of auditory tube and tympanic cavity

* Adapted from Moore KL, Persaud TVN, editors: *The developing human: clinically oriented embryology*, ed 6, Philadelphia: WB Saunders; 1998. pp 63-82.

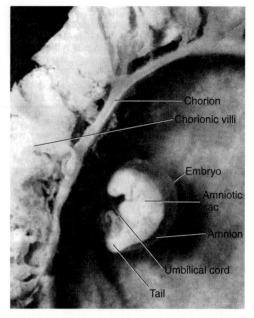

FIGURE 2-1 Implanted human embryo, approximately day 28, showing the relationship of the chorion, amnion, and chorionic villi. The umbilical cord and tail are difficult to differentiate in this view.

surrounds the entire embryo. The embryo attaches to the outer layer through the *umbilical stalk,* and later the *umbilical cord.* The umbilical cord connects to the finger-like projections in the outer lining of the *chorion,* or *chorionic villi* (Figure 2-1). Within the chorionic villi a capillary network forms and connects to the umbilical stalk. The villi intertwine into the blood-filled lacunar cavities of the endometrium of the maternal uterus.[1] Oxygen, carbon dioxide, and nutrients diffuse through the vast capillary surface area of this indirect connection between mother and fetus. As fetal development continues, the region of this interface becomes limited to the discus-shaped *placenta,* because the amniotic sac completely fills the chorionic cavity. The umbilical cord connects the placenta to the fetus with one large vein and two smaller arteries. As the cord grows, the vessels tend to spiral.[3] Wharton's jelly, a gelatinous substance inside the umbilical cord, helps protect the vessels and prevents the cord from kinking.

CARDIOVASCULAR DEVELOPMENT

During the third gestational week, the heart is the first organ formed during fetal development. By 8 weeks of gestation, the normal fetal heart is fully functional, complete with all chambers, valves, and major vessels. In addition, the fetal heart must adapt to accommodate the circulatory configuration required while in the fluid-filled uterine environment. As the embryonic heart changes are described, note which of them may result in the cardiac anomalies discussed in Chapter 30 (Congenital Cardiac Defects). Table 2-1 lists the timing of the key cardiac developments.

Early Development

During early embryonic development, small cellular pools, referred to as *angiogenic clusters* or *blood islands,* supply nutrition to the growing embryo. These clusters coalesce to form two heart tubes lined with specialized

TABLE 2-1

Timetable of Significant Events During Fetal Heart Development

Time of Gestation	Event
Early Development	
Week 3	
Day 16	Angiogenic clusters (blood islands) appear
Day 18	Heart tubes form
Day 21	Heart tubes fuse
Chamber Development	
Week 4	
Day 22	Fusion of heart tubes complete
	Heart begins to beat
	Bidirectional blood flow begins
Day 23	Folding, looping, ballooning begin
Day 25	Atrial septation begins with growth of septum primum
Day 28	Ventricular septation starts
	Endocardial cushions form
	Unidirectional blood flow begins
Week 5	
Day 32	Septum secundum starts
Week 6	
Day 37	Foramen ovale complete
Maturation	
Week 7	
Day 46	Ventricle formation complete
Day 49	Four chambers complete
	Valve formation matures
Week 8	
Day 52	Aorta/pulmonary artery complete separation
Day 56	Valve formation complete

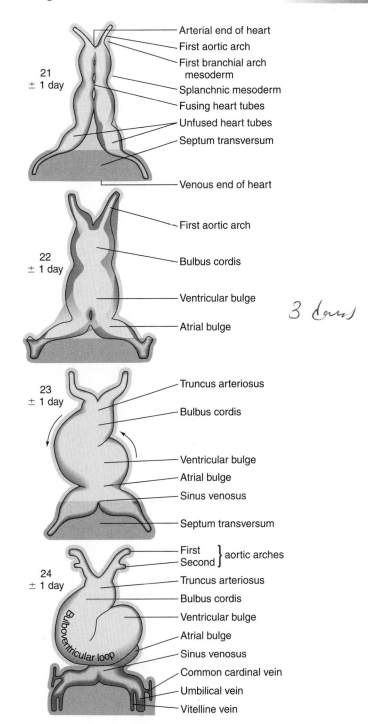

FIGURE 2-2 Formation of the primordial heart chambers after fusion of the heart tubes at a gestational age of 3 weeks.

myocardial tissue.[4] On approximately day 18, the heart tubes fold into what will become the thoracic cavity. At this point, they become close enough to fuse, and grow into a complete single-chamber tubular structure by day 21. The cardiovascular system forms primarily from the mesoderm layer, but myocardial tissue has a diverse origin related to the recruitment of myocytes from surrounding tissue types during embryogenesis.[5] By day 22 cardiac contractions are detectable and bidirectional tidal blood flow begins.[3]

Chamber Development

Dramatic changes begin to occur during the fourth week of gestation. The heart tubes continue to merge into three recognizable structures: the *bulbus cordis,* the *ventricular bulge,* and the *atrial bulge,* which empty into the *sinus venosus,* which receives oxygenated, nutrient-rich blood from the placenta (Figure 2-2). These structures continue to bend, fold, and dilate by incorporating components from surrounding tissue structures as the *truncus arteriosus* (which connects the heart to the future arterial system) becomes recognizable.[6] Note that initially the atrial bulge is inferior to the ventricular bulge. Between days 23 and 28 a process referred to as *dextral looping* occurs, whereby the ventricular bulge balloons into a C-shaped loop that pushes the atrial bulge in a superior direction (see Figure 2-2). Subsequently, the embryonic heart appears as a twisted S shape, and the ventricular structure merges with the bulbus cordis to form a one-ventricle structure known as the *bulboventric-ular loop,* which continues to dilate.[7]

Simultaneous with the external changes, the *septum primum* begins the separation of the primitive atrium, followed shortly by growth of the *endocardial cushions,* which will separate the atria from the ventricles. During this time, the left atrium incorporates the primordial pulmonary veins as four pulmonary veins empty into the primordial left atrium. The right horn of the sinus venosus grows in dominance and merges into the future right atrium from the inferior and superior vena cava. By the end of the fourth week, the dilating ventricular spaces fold into each other and force the ventricular septal bud upward at the base of the bulboventricular loop (see Figure 2-3).[8] By this time, blood flow matures into a unidirectional path as the myocardium continues to

strengthen by recruiting myocytes from the surrounding mesenchymal tissue.[5, 9]

During weeks 5 and 6 the internal and external structures continue to mature rapidly. Between the atria, the *septum secundum* begins to appear. By week 6, the septum secundum and a flap from the septum primum form the *foramen ovale,* one of the fetal shunts discussed later in this chapter (Figures 2-4 and 2-5). The atrioventricular canal continues to mature, and the endocardial cushions separate the ventricular spaces from the atrium. The muscular portion of the ventricular septum continues to grow into the ventricular space as the two ventricles dilate. Ridges also appear opposite each other in the bulbus cordis and truncus. They grow toward each other and fuse into a spiraling *aorticopulmonary septum,* which ultimately separates into the aorta and pulmonary arteries.[9] A fetal heart rate of about 95 beats per minute becomes discernible during this period and increases by approximately 4 beats per day until heart development is complete.[10]

Maturation

Continuing maturation of the internal and external structures characterizes weeks 7 and 8. The ventricles finish forcing the ventricular septum up from its base. A small intraventricular foramen remains, and blood flows between the two ventricles until the endocardial cushions

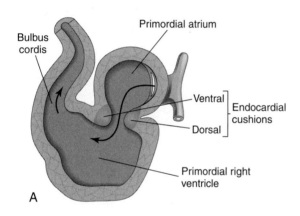

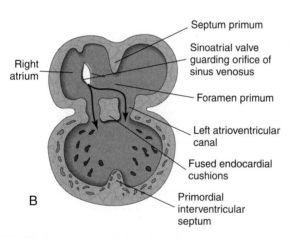

FIGURE 2-3 **A,** Sagittal view of the developing heart during week 4, showing the position of the atrium, bulbus cordis, ventricles, and endocardial cushions merging from the ventral and dorsal sides. **B,** Traditional view of the developing heart during weeks 4 to 5, showing budding interventricular septum, fused endocardial cushions. septum primum, and the left and right atria. The ventricular septum continues to fold and grow upward between the ventricles.

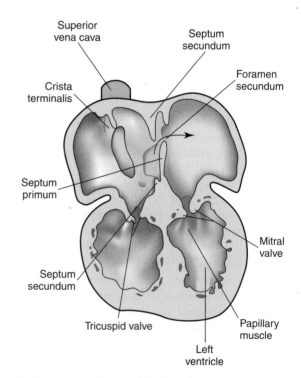

FIGURE 2-4 Frontal view of the fetal heart between weeks 5 and 6, showing the development of the four chambers nearing completion. The *arrow* shows the one-way path through the foramen ovale.

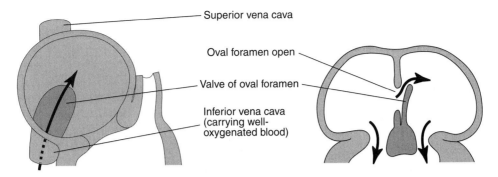

Superior vena cava

Oval foramen open

Valve of oval foramen

Inferior vena cava
(carrying well-
oxygenated blood)

FIGURE 2-5 Frontal view *(right)* and side view *(left)* schematics of the foramen ovale. The septum primum forms the flap, and the septum secundum remains open to form the foramen ovale. The *arrows* show the one-way path through the foramen ovale.

fuse with the ventricular septum (see Figure 2-4). At the end of the seventh week, tissue from remnants of the bulbus cordis and tissue from the endocardial cushions grow into the ventricular foramen, closing it as they merge with the muscular ventricular septum. The tricuspid and mitral valves form from specialized tissue surrounding the two atrioventricular openings. The aorticopulmonary septum divides the bulbus cordis and truncus into an aortic and pulmonary trunk. As these outflow tracts continue to mature, the semilunar valves form at the base of each structure.[6] Early in the eighth week the outflow tracts and valves are completely developed. At this stage, development of the cardiac structures is complete, and blood flows through the fetal circulation pathway. The heart continues to develop, increasing proportionately more in length than width, paralleling embryonic growth.[11,12]

FETAL CIRCULATION AND FETAL SHUNTS

Fetal circulation differs from circulation after the infant is born. Figure 2-6 illustrates fetal circulation and the three fetal shunts that must close after birth. The mother's lungs and liver perform most of the functions required by the same organs in the fetus. The fetal circulation pathway allows for shunting of blood flow around the fetal liver and lungs. Shunting most of the blood volume through the fetal heart allows pumping the required large quantities of fetal blood to the placenta, which is the interface between the maternal and fetal organ systems.[12]

Oxygenated blood travels from the placenta to the fetus through the umbilical vein. The *ductus venosus,* the first fetal shunt, appears continuous with the umbilical vein, shunting approximately 30% to 50% of the oxygen-rich blood around the fetal liver. The amount of shunting through the ductus venosus appears to decrease with gestational age.[13] The shunted oxygen-rich blood empties into the inferior vena cava and mixes with venous blood as it flows to the right atrium. Even though some

admixture takes place, this volume of blood contains the highest oxygen saturations available to the fetus.

In the right atrium most of the blood flow from the inferior vena cava crosses through the foramen ovale into the left atrium. The foramen ovale, the second fetal shunt, is formed during septation of the atria as described previously. The septum primum acts as a one-way valve over the ostium secundum (see Figure 2-5). The remainder of the blood in the right atrium mixes with desaturated blood from the superior vena cava and empties into the right ventricle. Blood flow in the right ventricle contains slightly higher oxygen content than blood from the superior vena cava, which is pumped into the pulmonary artery to the developing lungs.

The pulmonary vascular resistance (PVR) in utero remains high. Likely mechanisms include physical compression of the vessels resulting from relatively low lung volumes and low oxygen concentrations, because the lungs are devoid of air. Both of these mechanisms help induce chemical mediators, which maintain a high resistive tone in the pulmonary vascular bed.[14] Approximately 13% to 25% of the fetal blood flow reaches the lungs, slightly more than previously calculated.[12,15]

Blood from the pulmonary veins empties into the left atrium and then flows into the left ventricle, out the aortic valve, and into the ascending aorta, where it supplies blood with the highest oxygen content to the head, right arm, and coronary circulation. The high PVR causes most of the pulmonary artery blood flow from the right ventricle to bypass the lungs, flowing through the *ductus arteriosus,* the third fetal shunt, into the aorta. Because large quantities of blood are required to flow to the placenta, this permits the right ventricle and left ventricle to pump almost in parallel. The path of fetal circulation and percentage of oxygen saturation in various locations is illustrated in Figure 2-6.[16]

The deoxygenated blood from the upper torso returns to the right atrium via the superior vena cava. Finally, blood in the descending and abdominal aorta flows

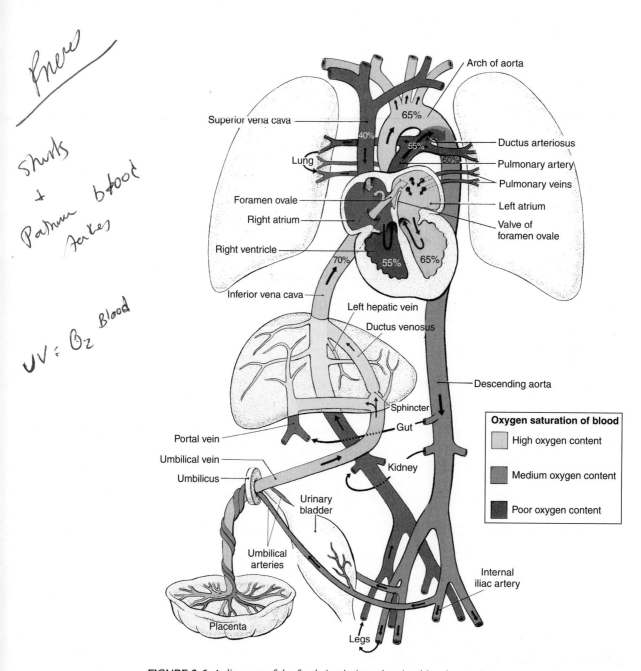

FIGURE 2-6 A diagram of the fetal circulation, showing blood containing oxygen and nourishment moving from the placenta to the fetal heart and through the three fetal shunts: the ductus venosus, the foramen ovale, and the ductus arteriosus.

through the two umbilical arteries and back to the placenta for oxygenation. Initially 17% to 20% of the fetal cardiac output flows through the umbilical arteries, but as the fetus matures this rises to 33%.[17] The placenta contains as much as half of the fetal blood volume. Because of the large vascular surface area of the placenta, impedance is extremely low and normal blood flow remains stable.[12]

TRANSITION TO EXTRAUTERINE LIFE

Clamping the umbilical vessels removes the low-pressure system of the placenta from fetal circulation. During the first breath, several factors drastically improve pulmonary blood flow and reduce the PVR.[18] Inflating the lungs initiates gas exchange, which increases and directly dilates pulmonary arterioles. Rising arterial oxygen pressure (Pao_2) also stimulates the release of endogenous pulmonary vasodilating factors.[19] Stretching of the pulmonary units also physically stretches open vascular units as well as stimulates the release of other vasodilating compounds. Besides vasodilation, lung inflation results in the inhibition of vasoconstricting agents produced by the lung to facilitate fetal circulation.[18]

Once the PVR decreases and the cord is clamped, pressures in the right side of the heart decrease and pressures in the left side increase. Because the foramen ovale flap allows blood to flow only from right to left, it closes when the pressures in the left atrium become greater than those in the right atrium. Closing the foramen ovale further facilitates the increase of blood flow to the lungs during the transitional period, and is necessary to maintain normal extrauterine circulation.

Because the pressure in the aorta also increases and becomes greater than the pressure in the pulmonary artery, the amount of shunting through the ductus arteriosus decreases. The functional closure of the ductus arteriosus usually occurs rapidly as the result of sudden increases in oxygenation and changes in prostaglandin levels.[20] Normally, constriction starts to occur at birth, and 20% of the ductus closes within 24 hours, with 80% closed in 48 hours, and 100% by 96 hours after birth.[21] Anatomic closure of the ductus begins in the last trimester as endothelial tissue begins to proliferate into the lumen of the ductus, forming bulges known as *intimal mounds*. Initially assisted by vasoconstriction, the ductal lumen closes completely as gestational and postgestational age advances.[22] By 2 to 4 weeks of age, the anatomic closure is complete and blood flow normalizes to the adult pattern of circulation.[21]

ASSESSMENT QUESTIONS

See Evolve Resources for answers.

1. Which of the following are true statements concerning the development of the circulatory system?
    - I. Heart development is completed by about 32 weeks of gestation.
    - II. Heart development, other than growth, is complete when valve formation is complete.
    - III. Angiogenic clusters form the primitive vascular network in the earliest stages of the embryo.
    - IV. The right myocardial fibers begin contracting before the left side to provide blood flow to the lungs.

ASSESSMENT QUESTIONS—cont'd

   - V. At about 3 weeks, two heart tubes fuse into what will become the basic structure of the four-chamber heart.
   - A. I, III, and V
   - B. II and III
   - C. II, III, and IV
   - D. II, IV, and V
   - E. III and IV

2. Which of the following are recognizable structures during development of the heart after the heart tubes fuse?
    - I. Sinus venosus
    - II. Bulbus cordis
    - III. Ductus arteriosus
    - IV. Ventricular bulge
    - V. Truncus arteriosus
   - A. I and III
   - B. I, II, IV, and V
   - C. II, III, and V
   - D. II, III, IV, and V
   - E. III, IV, and V

3. How does oxygenated blood leave the placenta and travel to the fetus?
   - A. Through the aortic artery
   - B. Through the umbilical vein
   - C. Through the umbilical artery
   - D. Through the spiral artery
   - E. Through the ductus arteriosus

4. How is most of the fetal blood entering the main pulmonary artery shunted to the aorta?
   - A. Through the foramen ovale
   - B. Through the ductus venosus
   - C. Through the ductus arteriosus
   - D. Through the superior vena cava
   - E. Through the iliac arteries

5. How is most of the fetal blood entering via the umbilical vein shunted to the inferior vena cava?
   - A. Through the foramen ovale
   - B. Through the ductus venosus
   - C. Through the ductus arteriosus
   - D. Through the superior vena cava
   - E. Through the iliac arteries

6. Circulatory changes required in the transitional stage at birth correspond with which of the following?
    - I. A decrease in pulmonary vascular resistance
    - II. A decrease in systemic vascular resistance
    - III. A decrease in pulmonary artery pressure
    - IV. An increase in left ventricular pressure
    - V. An increase in pulmonary blood
   - A. I and IV
   - B. I, II, IV, and V
   - C. I, III, IV, and V
   - D. II, III, and V
   - E. III, IV, and V

Continued

ASSESSMENT QUESTIONS—cont'd

7. How is most of the fetal blood entering via the right atrium shunted to the left atrium?
- **A.** Through the foramen ovale
- **B.** Through the ductus venosus
- **C.** Through the ductus arteriosus
- **D.** Through the superior vena cava
- **E.** Through the aorto-iliac shunt

8. When discussing fetal circulation which of the following is/are true?
- **A.** Fetal shunts help to shunt the best oxygenated blood to the head.
- **B.** Pressure gradients related to blood flow are the opposite of those in an adult.
- **C.** Fetal shunts help to bypass the lungs.
- **D.** The placenta has low vascular resistance.
- **E.** All of the above

9. What *one* set of actions causes the systemic circulation to transition from a low-resistance system to a high-resistance system?
- **A.** Clamping the umbilical cord and creating a short period of hypoxia
- **B.** Getting a higher concentration of oxygen into the lungs with the first breath
- **C.** Clamping the umbilical cord, thus preventing blood flow to the placenta
- **D.** Pulmonary hypertension from a change in blood flow direction
- **E.** Expulsion of the placenta at birth

10. Anatomic narrowing of the ductus arteriosus begins in the last trimester by which process?
- **A.** The formation of bulges known as intimal mounds
- **B.** The release of tolazoline compounds
- **C.** Ductal termination
- **D.** The formation of the aortic valve
- **E.** Activating thrombokinins

References

1. Kingdom JC, Kaufmann P: Oxygen and placental vascular development, *Adv Exp Med Biol* 1999;474:259.
2. Moore KL, Persaud TVN, editors: *The developing human: clinically oriented embryology*, ed 6, Philadelphia: WB Saunders; 1998, pp 63–82.
3. England MA, editor: *Color atlas of life before birth: normal fetal development*, ed 2, Chicago: Year-Book Medical; 1996, pp 40–41.
4. Gourdie RG, Kubalak S, Mikawa T: Conducting the embryonic heart: orchestrating development of specialized cardiac tissues, *Trends Cardiovasc Med* 1999;9:8.
5. Eisenberg LM, Markwald RR: Cellular recruitment and the development of the myocardium, *Dev Biol* 2004;274:225.
6. Moorman A, Webb S, Brown NA et al: Development of the heart. 1. Formation of the cardiac chambers and arterial trunks, *Heart* 2003;89:806.
7. Bartman T, Hove J: Mechanics and function in heart morphogenesis, *Dev Dyn* 2005;233:373.
8. England MA, editor: *Color atlas of life before birth: normal fetal development*, ed 2, Chicago, Year-Book Medical Publishers, 1996, p 102.
9. Moore KL, Persaud TVN, editors: *The developing human: clinically oriented embryology*, ed 6, Philadelphia: WB Saunders; 1998, pp 349–403.
10. Tezuka N Sato S, Kanasugi H et al: Embryonic heart rates: development in early first trimester and clinical evaluation, *Gynecol Obstet Invest* 1991;32:210.
11. Marecki B: The formation of heart-proportion in fetal ontogenesis, *Z Morphol Anthropol* 1992;79:197.
12. Kiserud T, Acharya G: The fetal circulation, *Prenat Diagn* 2004;24:1049.
13. Kiserud T: Fetal venous circulation: an update on hemodynamics, *J Perinat Med* 2000;28:90.
14. Heymann MA: Control of the pulmonary circulation in the fetus and during the transitional period to air breathing, *Eur J Obstet Gynecol Reprod Biol* 1999;84:127.
15. Lakshminrusimha S, Steinhorn RH: Pulmonary vascular biology during neonatal transition, *Clin Perinatol* 1999;26:333.
16. Rudolph AM: *Congenital diseases of the heart*, Chicago: Year Book Medical; 1974.
17. Goldkrand JW, Morre DH, Lenz SU et al: Volumetric flow in the umbilical artery: normative data, *J Matern Fetal Med* 2000;9:224.
18. Rudolph AM: The development of concepts of the ontogeny of the pulmonary circulation. In Weir EK, Archer SL, Reeves JT, editors: *The fetal and neonatal pulmonary circulations*, Armonk, NY: Futura Publishing; 2000.
19. Hageman JR, Caplan MS: An introduction to the structure and function of inflammatory mediators for clinicians, *Clin Perinatol* 1995;22:251.
20. Hammerman C: Patent ductus arteriosus: clinical relevance of prostaglandins and prostaglandin inhibitors in PDA pathophysiology and treatment, *Clin Perinatol* 1995;22:457.
21. Lim MK Hanretty K, Houston AB et al: Intermittent ductal patency in healthy newborn infants: demonstration by colour Doppler flow mapping, *Arch Dis Child* 1992;67:1217.
22. Mirro R, Gray P: Aortic and pulmonary blood velocities during the first 3 days of life, *Am J Perinatol* 1986;3:333.

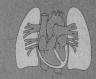

Chapter 3

Antenatal Assessment and High-risk Delivery

ANTOUN Y. KHABBAZ • J. GERALD QUIRK

OUTLINE

Maternal History and Risk Factors
    Preterm Birth
    Cervical Insufficiency
    Toxic Habits in Pregnancy
    Hypertension and Diabetes Mellitus
    Infectious Diseases
    Fetal Membranes, Umbilical Cord, and Placenta
    Disorders of Amniotic Fluid Volume
    Mode of Delivery

Antenatal Assessment
    Ultrasound
    Amniocentesis
    Nonstress Test and Contraction Stress Test
    Fetal Biophysical Profile
Intrapartum Monitoring
High-risk Conditions
    Preterm Labor
    Postterm Pregnancy

LEARNING OBJECTIVES

After reading this chapter the reader will be able to:
- Identify various high-risk conditions and their adverse effects on pregnancy
- Describe current methods used for antenatal and intrapartum assessment of fetal well-being
- Explain preterm labor and postterm pregnancy evaluation and management
- Recommend techniques for taking care of the newborn during the neonatal period

The transition from intrauterine life to the outside world is critical. It involves major physiologic changes and requires medical attention for an optimal outcome. Cooperation and communication among all members of the health care team are essential to identify potential problems and to intervene in a timely manner. Maternal history, antenatal assessment (as dictated by maternal–fetal risk factors), and intrapartum monitoring are all-important in identifying the fetus or newborn at risk of decompensation during the perinatal period. This chapter outlines the essentials of antenatal assessment and touches briefly on the management of some high-risk conditions: preterm delivery and postterm pregnancy.

MATERNAL HISTORY AND RISK FACTORS

At the initial prenatal visit, the obstetrician obtains a comprehensive maternal history and performs a physical examination. Risk factors are identified and included in an initial problem list that serves as a quick summary for future reference. Subsequent periodic visits serve the purpose of identifying new obstetric risks that will necessitate special interventions. The following sections discuss commonly encountered maternal–fetal risk factors with their impact on obstetric care and perinatal outcome.

Preterm Birth

Other than major congenital anomalies, *preterm birth* (birth before 37 weeks of gestation) is the greatest cause of neonatal morbidity and mortality. Preterm birth can be the consequence of preterm labor, preterm premature rupture of the fetal membranes, or obstetric intervention mandated by fetal jeopardy or maternal clinical status. Interestingly enough, prior preterm delivery is one of the most important risk factors for subsequent preterm labor. With one prior preterm birth, a woman carries a 15% risk of subsequent preterm delivery; this risk increases to 32% with a history of two previous preterm births.[1] Risk factors, diagnosis, and treatment of preterm labor are discussed in the section Preterm Labor, later in this chapter.

Cervical Insufficiency

Patients with risk factors for cervical insufficiency are recommended for evaluation by ultrasound examination of the cervix starting at 16 weeks of gestation. Intervention in the form of *cervical cerclage,* that is, placing a suture around the cervical canal, should be offered in case of evidence of cervical shortening or funneling of the cervix before fetal viability. An elective cerclage (usually performed at 14 weeks of gestation, after confirmation of absence of gross congenital anomalies in the fetus by ultrasound) should be considered for patients with a history of three or more unexplained mid-trimester pregnancy losses or preterm deliveries.[2]

Toxic Habits in Pregnancy

Maternal habits should be assessed early in the course of gestation. Smoking, alcohol use, and illicit drug use in pregnancy can cause well-described adverse effects on the fetus. The American College of Obstetricians and Gynecologists (Washington, DC) estimates that the prevalence of substance abuse in pregnant women is about 10%.[3]

Alcohol

Alcohol is a potent *teratogen,* an agent or factor that causes malformation of the fetus. Fetal alcohol syndrome, first described in 1973 by Jones and colleagues[4] and associated with maternal use of alcohol during pregnancy, is characterized by mental retardation and prenatal and postnatal growth restriction, as well as by brain, cardiac, spinal, and craniofacial anomalies. It is usually

seen among children of women who consume four to six drinks daily throughout pregnancy.[5] However, no safe range for drinking alcohol during pregnancy has been established.

Smoking

Smoking during pregnancy can cause several adverse effects. Carbon monoxide and nicotine, the main ingredients responsible, mediate their effects by decreasing the availability of oxygen to the fetus and placenta. A strong association occurs between cigarette smoking and lower birth weight.[6] The mean birth weight of infants of women who smoke during pregnancy is about 200 g less than that of infants of nonsmokers. Smoking is also associated with a higher incidence of premature preterm rupture of membranes,[7] placental abruption (i.e., separation of the placenta before birth of the newborn) and placenta previa (i.e., blockage of the cervix),[8] and risk of infant death from sudden infant death syndrome.[9]

Cocaine

Cocaine has a potent sympathomimetic action and hence is a potent constrictor of blood vessels. It can cause numerous maternal medical complications that include myocardial infarction, stroke, seizures, bowel ischemia, and death. Cocaine is also associated with adverse pregnancy sequelae: placental abruption, preterm delivery, and growth restriction.[10] It is also thought to cause congenital malformations of the limbs, heart, brain, and genitourinary tract. Finally, infants born to women who abuse opiates or amphetamines during pregnancy tend to have significant withdrawal symptoms after birth and to be small for gestational age.

The obstetrician–gynecologist can have an impact on prevention of substance abuse in pregnancy by identifying patients at risk, educating patients about the effects of drugs, and referring patients already abusing drugs.

Hypertension and Diabetes Mellitus

The obstetrician frequently encounters patients with hypertension and diabetes mellitus presenting for prenatal care.

Hypertension

Hypertensive disease complicates 12% to 22% of pregnancies in the United States and is second only to embolism as a cause of maternal mortality.[11] Perinatal morbidity and mortality are increased secondary to intrauterine growth restriction, placental abruption, and preterm delivery. Preeclampsia is traditionally described as a triad of hypertension, proteinuria (protein in the urine), and generalized edema. It is commonly cited that preeclampsia

complicates approximately 5% to 8% of pregnancies. Predisposing factors include the following:
- Nulliparity (never having given birth to a child)
- Advanced maternal age
- Chronic hypertension
- Chronic renal disease
- Diabetes mellitus
- Twin gestation
- Molar pregnancy
- Hydrops fetalis (total body edema [anasarca] with pleural and pericardial effusion)

Preeclampsia remains a poorly understood disease despite extensive research. Immunologic mechanisms, genetic predisposition, dietary deficiencies, vasoactive substances, and endothelial dysfunction have all been implicated in the pathophysiology of preeclampsia.[12] Severe preeclampsia is diagnosed in the presence of:
- Systolic blood pressure higher than 160 mm Hg
- Diastolic blood pressure higher than 110 mm Hg
- Proteinuria: more than 5 g per 24-hour urine collection
- Pulmonary edema
- Intrauterine growth restriction
- Oliguria: urine output less than 500 ml^3 in 24 hours
- Thrombocytopenia: platelet count less than 100,000/ml
- Headache
- Epigastric or right upper quadrant abdominal pain
- Hepatocellular dysfunction
- Grand mal seizure: definition of eclampsia

Treatment of preeclampsia is by delivery of the fetus. Magnesium sulfate is used to prevent seizures, and antihypertensive agents such as hydralazine and labetalol are usually used to control severe hypertension. The recurrence rate of preeclampsia is about 25%.[13] Calcium, magnesium, and zinc supplementation and use of low-dose aspirin have been studied for prevention of pregnancy-induced hypertension, with conflicting results thus far.

Diabetes

Diabetes in pregnancy is classified broadly as pregestational or gestational.

Pregestational Diabetes. Women with pregestational diabetes are at increased risk for adverse maternal and fetal outcomes. Adverse maternal outcomes include increased risk of developing diabetic ketoacidosis, proliferative retinopathy, and preeclampsia/eclampsia. Close maternal metabolic surveillance focused on attaining normal blood glucose levels throughout pregnancy has significantly decreased the risk of these outcomes.

Adverse fetal outcomes include unexplained fetal death in the third trimester of pregnancy and major fetal structural malformations. Close maternal metabolic surveillance coupled with close fetal biophysical evaluation has significantly decreased the risk of fetal death as well as the necessity of delivering a fetus prematurely because of abnormal test results. The rate of fetal structural malformations in infants born to pregestational diabetic women can be as high as 10% to 15% compared with a rate of 1% to 2% for infants of otherwise normal women. The most frequently encountered defects include malformations of the cardiovascular system including both the heart and great vessels and the central nervous system including the brain and spinal cord. No amount of maternal metabolic surveillance or fetal biophysical assessment after the period of fetal organogenesis will decrease this risk. Therefore it is recommended strongly that women with diabetes mellitus receive counseling and treatment with the goal of achieving optimal glycemic control before they become pregnant.

Gestational Diabetes Mellitus. Gestational diabetes mellitus (GDM) is abnormal glucose tolerance that occurs or is first recognized during pregnancy. The frequency of this disorder varies according to the ethnic background of the woman but is said to complicate about 3% of pregnancies in the United States. Poor blood sugar control in these women is associated with an increased risk of macrosomia (birth weight greater than 4000 g), traumatic vaginal delivery, and preterm delivery, and with a small increased risk for fetal death in selected women. After delivery, the infants are at increased risk for metabolic disturbances in the neonatal period; these include hypoglycemia, hypocalcemia, hyperkalemia, hyperbilirubinemia, and idiopathic respiratory distress syndrome. In the long term, women with GDM are at risk of developing type 2, or adult-onset, diabetes; nearly 50% will be diagnosed with type 2 diabetes within 10 years.

Among pregnant women, selective screening based on risk factors identifies only half. Thus, at the present time, it is recommended that all pregnant women be screened for gestational diabetes with the 1-hour glucose challenge test administered between 24 and 28 weeks of gestation. For those with an abnormal screening result, the diagnosis of GDM is made when there are two abnormal values on a 3-hour, 100-g oral glucose tolerance test.

Maternal glycemic control and fetal biophysical status are monitored in a manner similar to protocols for managing the pregnancy complicated by pregestational diabetes. With good maternal glycemic control, pregnancies complicated by GDM can proceed to full term with a normal delivery; cesarean delivery is reserved for traditional obstetric indications. Insulin has traditionally been the drug of choice for achieving glycemic control in patients with gestational diabetes. Glyburide has been studied for the treatment of gestational diabetes with promising results.[14]

Infectious Diseases

A number of infectious agents can affect pregnancy outcome. Among the most important in the United States are group B *Streptococcus* (GBS), herpes simplex virus (HSV), human immunodeficiency virus (HIV), and hepatitis B virus (HBV).

Group B *Streptococcus*

As many as 10% to 40% of pregnant women are colonized with GBS. Their infants are at risk for death or severe morbidity if they are born prematurely or after prolonged rupture of the fetal membranes.

In the past, two approaches were adopted for the prevention of early-onset GBS disease: culture-based and risk-based approaches. More recently, and based on a large retrospective cohort study, the American College of Obstetricians and Gynecologists has recommended the culture-based approach because of its superiority in prevention of GBS disease.[15]

Vaginal/rectal cultures are usually obtained at 35 to 37 weeks of gestation. Patients with positive cultures should be treated with antibiotics from the time of membrane rupture or from the onset of labor. Penicillin is the drug of choice, with ampicillin being a good alternative. In the case of allergy to penicillin, sensitivity to clindamycin and erythromycin should be performed. Vancomycin is indicated in the case of resistance to clindamycin and erythromycin or in case of absent sensitivity studies. Patients who present in labor or with rupture of membranes with unknown GBS status should be given antibiotic prophylaxis in case of intrapartum fever, prolonged membrane rupture (more than 18 h), or preterm delivery (less than 37 wk of gestation). Note finally that antibiotic prophylaxis for GBS disease should be given to all patients with GBS bacteriuria during the current pregnancy or with a previous infant with invasive GBS disease.[15]

Herpes Simplex Virus

Women who have primary or recurrent HSV outbreaks during pregnancy are at risk for infecting their baby if the outbreak occurs at the time of membrane rupture or the onset of labor. In this circumstance, the virus can ascend to infect the fetus; therefore cesarean delivery is undertaken as soon as possible after membrane rupture or after the onset of labor.

Hepatitis B Virus and Human Immunodeficiency Virus

At this time, all pregnant women should be screened for HIV and HBV infection. Both viruses can cause disease in the fetus.

HIV. In the general obstetric population in the United States, the frequency of HIV infection is about 1 per 1000.

The prevalence is as high as 1% to 1.5% in inner-city populations.[16] Approximately 30% of the exposed fetuses will also acquire the infection.[17] Zidovudine (an antiretroviral drug) used during pregnancy, during labor, and as chemoprophylaxis for 6 weeks in exposed newborns is associated with a decrease in perinatal HIV transmission to 8.3%.[18] When care includes both zidovudine therapy and a scheduled cesarean delivery, the risk is approximately 2%.[19] Nursing should be discouraged in HIV-positive women because the virus is secreted in breast milk.

HBV. Infants of women infected with HBV become infected at delivery. When these infants are treated with anti–hepatitis B immunoglobulin and are begun on vaccination within the first 12 hours of life, 95% of neonatal infections are prevented. Cesarean delivery of these newborns has no advantage.[20] Cytomegalovirus, rubella, *Toxoplasma, Listeria,* mycobacteria, and *Treponema pallidum* (syphilis) can all affect the mother, fetus, and fetoplacental unit significantly. Early diagnosis and treatment of the pregnancy complicated by infection with *Listeria, Toxoplasma,* or syphilis can result in normal pregnancy outcomes.

Fetal Membranes, Umbilical Cord, and Placenta

In utero, the fetus is contained in the sterile fluid-filled amniotic sac. If the membranes that compose the external lining of the amniotic sac rupture before term (before 37 weeks of gestation) or before the onset of normal labor at term, the fetal environment is no longer sterile, increasing the risk of fetal infection. At the same time, the volume of fluid in the sac decreases. This may cause compression of the umbilical cord, resulting in compromised blood flow between the placenta and fetus. The causes of premature rupture of the fetal membranes are generally not known but are responsible for nearly 50% of preterm births in the United States. Preterm rupture of the fetal membranes can be seen as being responsible for all of the problems faced by most prematurely born infants.

Abnormalities of the umbilical cord and placenta can have profound effects on fetal development and pregnancy outcome. The umbilical cord has a mean length of 55 cm and contains three vessels: two arteries and one vein. The two arteries arising from the end of the fetal aorta bring relatively deoxygenated blood from the fetus to the placenta, while the single umbilical vein returns oxygenated blood from the placenta to the fetus. In 3% of pregnancies, the umbilical cord contains a single umbilical artery. A single umbilical artery cord is associated with fetal structural and chromosomal anomalies as well as fetal growth restriction.[21]

The length of the umbilical cord has long been recognized to be of clinical significance. A short cord predisposes to placental abruption and uterine inversion.

A long cord is associated with cord prolapse (delivery of the cord before the infant, with compromise of blood flow from compression), cord knots, and nuchal cords (cord wrapped around the infant's neck). Marginal cord insertion (on the edge of the placenta) is of little clinical importance. Velamentous insertion of the cord (in which the umbilical vessels cross the fetal membranes unsupported by placenta or cord structure) may be associated with risk of rupture of a fetal vessel at the time of rupture of membranes, resulting in fetal exsanguination.

Placental abruption can cause fetal distress and death in addition to serious vaginal bleeding and coagulopathy. It is usually associated with[22]
- Hypertensive disease in pregnancy
- Advanced maternal age
- Multiparity *more than one baby previous births.*
- Preterm premature rupture of membranes
- Trauma
- Cigarette smoking
- Cocaine abuse
- Uterine leiomyoma (benign tumor of the uterus) behind the placental implantation site

Placenta previa occurs when the placenta covers the cervical os. Cesarean delivery is usually required. Placenta previa is associated with
- Advanced maternal age
- Multiparity
- Prior cesarean delivery
- Multiple gestation

Disorders of Amniotic Fluid Volume

Early in pregnancy, amniotic fluid is derived from the fetal membranes that compose the amniotic sac. Later, the majority of amniotic fluid is the product of fetal urination, with little contribution from the fetal skin. Fetal swallowing is an important mechanism for absorption of amniotic fluid. The fetal lungs help circulate the amniotic fluid. The amniotic fluid index is calculated by measuring the length of the largest vertical pocket of fluid in each of the four equal uterine quadrants at the time of ultrasound examination. It is the most commonly used method for quantification of amniotic fluid.

Oligohydramnios, too little amniotic fluid or an amniotic fluid index below 5 cm, is usually associated with congenital anomalies (especially renal agenesis or urinary tract obstruction), fetal growth restriction or demise, postterm pregnancy (pregnancy continuing beyond 42 weeks from the first day of the pregnant woman's last menstrual period [more than 294 d]), ruptured membranes, uteroplacental insufficiency, and use of prostaglandin synthase inhibitors. When oligohydramnios occurs early in gestation, it can cause lung hypoplasia and limb deformities. When renal agenesis occurs in association with oligohydramnios, it is always fatal and is called *Potter's syndrome*. Later in gestation, oligohydramnios is usually associated with adverse perinatal outcomes secondary to compression of the umbilical cord. In labor, there is an increase in variable decelerations (due to cord compression) and an increase in cesarean delivery rates.[23]

Polyhydramnios, too much amniotic fluid, or an amniotic fluid index higher than 24 cm, is frequently associated with fetal malformations that might affect swallowing of amniotic fluid (e.g., anencephaly, esophageal atresia, and tracheoesophageal fistula). It is also associated with hydrops fetalis, twin gestation (with twin–twin transfusion syndrome), and maternal diabetes. Polyhydramnios overdistends the uterus and can lead to premature rupture of membranes or preterm labor as well as risk for cord prolapse.

Mode of Delivery

Most deliveries occur spontaneously by the vaginal route. Typically, infants born vaginally are delivered head first (vertex presentation). However, there are times when assisted vaginal delivery (with forceps or vacuum) or abdominal delivery (cesarean) is needed. Breech presentation (legs or buttocks first) occurs in 3% to 4% of all births.

Breech Presentation

The breech position creates a situation in which there is greater potential for complications at the time of delivery. Predisposing factors for breech presentation include multiparity, previous breech delivery, uterine anomalies, fetal anomalies, multiple gestation, and polyhydramnios. The Term Breech Trial Collaborative Group conducted a multicenter randomized controlled trial of planned cesarean versus planned vaginal delivery for breech presentation at term. It concluded that planned cesarean delivery is preferred because of less risk for perinatal mortality or serious morbidity and no increase in serious maternal complications.[24] Two small randomized controlled trials published earlier have not found planned cesarean delivery of substantial benefit to the fetus.[25,26] At present, the American College of Obstetricians and Gynecologists recommends that patients with persistent breech presentation at term in a singleton gestation should have a planned cesarean delivery. This recommendation does not apply to patients who present with breech presentation in labor and with imminent delivery.[27] Transverse lie, in which the fetus is oriented transversely inside the uterus, is another malpresentation that requires cesarean delivery.

Assisted Vaginal Delivery

Obstetric forceps is an instrument used to cradle and guide the fetal head while applying traction to expedite delivery. The vacuum extractor is a suction device that holds the head tightly and allows traction to be applied. Indications for forceps or vacuum use include maternal cardiac, pulmonary, or neurologic disease (contraindicating the pushing process); maternal exhaustion in labor; and nonreassuring fetal status.

Cesarean Delivery

Cesarean delivery is the operative delivery of the fetus through the abdominal wall. It accounted for 26% of all births in the United States in 2003.[28]

Major indications for cesarean delivery include the following:
- Previous cesarean delivery
- Failure to progress in labor
- Malpresentation (breech or transverse)
- Placenta previa
- Non reassuring fetal status

Although cesarean delivery might be the least traumatic method of delivery of the fetus, it is associated with the following:
- An increased risk of significant blood loss
- Anesthesia complications
- Intraoperative bladder or bowel injuries
- Postoperative wound infection
- Endomyometritis
- Thromboembolic events

The syndrome of transient tachypnea of the newborn (wet lung or type II respiratory distress syndrome [see Chapter 27, Neonatal Pulmonary Disorders]), which includes the clinical features of cyanosis, grunting, and tachypnea during the first hours of life, is more commonly seen in infants delivered by cesarean. The preferred explanation for the clinical features is delayed absorption of fetal lung fluid.[29]

ANTENATAL ASSESSMENT

To ascertain the pregnancy at risk for an adverse outcome, one must begin with a thorough history and physical examination. Technological advances have made it possible to make many assessments of fetal condition. Both invasive and noninvasive methods of evaluating fetal structure and function are used with regularity. It is possible to view fetal anatomy, measure fetal biochemical and genetic status, assess fetal biophysical status, evaluate uteroplacental function, and determine the ability of the fetus and placenta to function during the normal stresses of labor. Depending on the characteristics of any given pregnancy, most perinatal centers are capable of performing detailed antepartum assessment.[30]

Ultrasound

One of the most widely used methods of noninvasive assessment is ultrasonography (Figure 3-1). Using

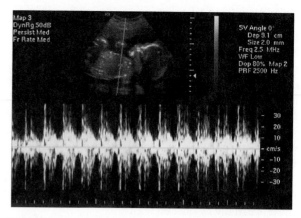

FIGURE 3-1 Ultrasound picture of a fetus at 23 weeks of gestation *(top),* with a Doppler study of the fetal heart *(bottom).* Dop, Doppler; Fr, frame; Freq, frequency; PRF, pulse-repetition frequency; SV, sample volume; WF, wall filter. (Courtesy Frank Fox, RDMS.)

ultrahigh-frequency sound waves to obtain real-time images, and with transabdominal or transvaginal transducers, the clinician can diagnose multifetal pregnancy and evaluate fetal anatomy, growth, and position. One can also localize the placenta within the uterus, measure amniotic fluid volume, estimate fetal growth over time, and assess fetal biophysical status. In addition, Doppler flow studies measure blood flow to fetal organs. This measurement permits early identification of fetuses at risk, enabling opportune delivery or transport to sophisticated perinatal centers. Ultrasonography is also invaluable for guiding the physician while performing amniocentesis, umbilical blood sampling, and other invasive procedures.

Three-dimensional ultrasound imaging has been introduced to the obstetrics field. It offers better visualization of fetal organs (especially the face, heart, and spine) than the conventional two-dimensional ultrasound imaging. Outcome studies are underway, accompanied by an increase in the use of three-dimensional ultrasound imaging among obstetricians and maternal fetal specialists.[31]

Amniocentesis

The most commonly performed invasive procedure to assess fetal condition is amniocentesis. In this procedure, under sterile conditions, a needle is inserted through the skin and uterine wall to obtain a sample of fluid from the amniotic sac. Depending on the reason for performing the procedure, the concentration of many substances in the fluid can be measured. For example, as the fetal lung matures, pulmonary surfactant is secreted from the fetal lung into the amniotic fluid, where its concentration can be measured. Women with Rh isoimmunization (i.e., Rh-negative women producing antibody to the Rh factor on the red blood cells of their Rh-positive fetus) are at risk for delivering babies with severe anemia secondary to hemolysis. The degree of hemolysis is correlated with the concentration of bilirubin (a by-product of hemoglobin degradation) urinated by the fetus into the amniotic fluid. If the concentration of bilirubin in the amniotic fluid is markedly elevated, interventions to assist the fetus (preterm delivery or intrauterine fetal transfusion) can be undertaken. Fetal cells isolated from amniotic fluid can be used to assess for fetal chromosomal abnormalities (e.g., trisomy 21), fetal enzyme deficiencies (e.g., Tay-Sachs), and certain discrete genetic mutations (e.g., sickle cell disease).

Nonstress Test and Contraction Stress Test

Fetal well-being is highly dependent on placental function. Assessment of placental function is commonly done by monitoring the fetal heart rate (FHR) response when the fetus moves spontaneously (nonstress test [NST]) or in reaction to induced uterine contractions (contraction stress test [CST]). For both tests, the FHR is monitored continuously. In the normally oxygenated fetus (as with a child or adult), cardiac output rises to support physical activity. This rise in cardiac output can be mediated by an increase in either heart rate or stroke volume. In the fetus, cardiac output rises by increasing the heart rate.

A reactive NST (Figure 3-2) requires at least two accelerations in fetal heart rate, each of at least 15 beats per minute and lasting at least 15 seconds, associated with maternal perception of fetal movement over a period of 20 minutes. A reactive NST is highly correlated with normal uteroplacental function. If no change in maternal clinical status transpires, this result predicts normal fetal survival when this test is performed within 1 week of delivery.[32]

The CST is conducted by continuously monitoring the FHR while uterine contractions are stimulated by intravenous infusion into the mother of a dilute solution of oxytocin. In a normal pregnancy, fetal Po_2 (partial pressure of oxygen) decreases with each uterine contraction, and then rapidly returns to normal. A fetal Po_2 drop below 12 mm Hg, resulting in slowing of the FHR, indicates uteroplacental insufficiency. This slowing of the FHR in response to uterine contractions is called a *late deceleration*. A *negative CST* is one in which no late decelerations of the FHR develop with a frequency of three contractions, each lasting 40 to 60 seconds, per 10 minutes. A *positive CST* is diagnosed when late decelerations follow at least 50% of contractions. A *suspicious CST* is one in which late decelerations are inconsistent (follow less than 50% of contractions). Assuming no change in maternal clinical status, a negative CST predicts fetal survival if performed within 1 week of delivery. An abnormal CST must prompt further evaluation or delivery.

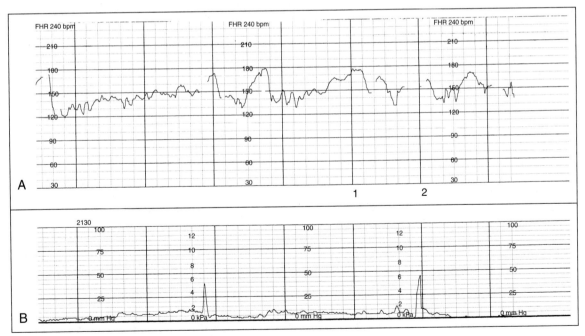

FIGURE 3-2 A nonstress test recording, produced with a cardiotocograph. **A,** The fetal heart rate (FHR) is recorded with an ultrasound probe as changes in beats per minute (bpm) over time. **B,** Uterine contractions (UC) are recorded with a pressure transducer as changes in pressure (mm Hg) over time. In this case the nonstress test is *reactive*, indicating normal uteroplacental function.

Fetal Biophysical Profile

The so-called fetal biophysical profile (BPP) (Table 3-1) assesses placental function and fetal well-being.[33] The BPP has been likened to the Apgar score (a quick method to assess the health of a newborn baby, based on the scoring of five factors [see Chapter 4]). In producing a BPP, five determinants of fetal status are assessed and given a score of 0 to 2. Four are assessed by ultrasonography. They include fetal breathing, fetal tone, fetal gross body movement, and amniotic fluid volume. The fifth determinant is the NST. A BPP score of 8 to 10 is considered normal and reassuring; a score of 6 is equivocal and is generally repeated within 24 hours; BPP scores of 0 to 4 are clearly abnormal and are associated with poor perinatal outcomes and require careful evaluation and usually immediate delivery.[34]

INTRAPARTUM MONITORING

Evidence suggests that the use of continuous FHR monitoring during labor in uncomplicated pregnancies has little to no impact on neonatal outcome.[35] Despite this finding, its use has become routine in the United States. Its utility in high-risk patients is valuable. The response of the FHR to uterine contractions does provide information concerning the status of the fetus during labor. FHR responses to uterine contractions and their likely etiologies are described in Figures 3-3, 3-4, and 3-5.

On many obstetric services, when persistent severe variable or late decelerations of the FHR are diagnosed, fetal scalp blood is obtained via transvaginal fetal scalp puncture, and blood gas measurements can be obtained. Scalp blood pH greater than 7.25 is considered reassuring; values of 7.15 or less signal high risk of fetal acidemia. Many clinicians believe that scalp blood gas assessment in the face of an abnormal FHR pattern more precisely defines the fetus at risk and can thus prevent unnecessary forceps and cesarean deliveries.

An alternative to scalp blood gas assessment is fetal scalp stimulation. Using the underlying rationale of the NST, transvaginal stimulation of the fetal scalp to induce fetal movement results in acceleration of the fetal heart rate and reassures the clinician that the fetus is not hypoxemic or acidemic.[35] Table 3-2 lists normal values for fetal scalp blood and umbilical cord blood gases.

Fetal oxygenation as determined by fetal pulse oximetry has been studied for intrapartum fetal assessment. A randomized controlled trial of intrapartum fetal pulse oximetry revealed a decrease in the number of cesarean deliveries performed for nonreassuring fetal heart tracing. The fetal pulse oximetry did not change the overall cesarean delivery rate.[36] More randomized controlled trials comparing fetal pulse oximetry with conventional fetal surveillance techniques are underway.

HIGH-RISK CONDITIONS

Preterm Labor

Preterm labor is defined as labor before 37 weeks of gestation. It complicates about 8% of pregnancies and is associated with significant neonatal morbidity, including sepsis, respiratory distress syndrome, intraventricular hemorrhage, retinopathy of prematurity, bronchopulmonary dysplasia, necrotizing enterocolitis, visual and hearing problems, and cerebral palsy. The smaller the infant is, the more the risks increase.

TABLE 3-1

Biophysical Profile Scoring

Biophysical Variable	Normal (Score = 2)	Abnormal (Score = 0)
Fetal breathing movements	At least one episode of FBM, lasting at least 30 sec, in 30 min	No FBM or no episode lasting >30 sec in 30 min
Gross body movements	At least three discrete body/limb movements (episodes of active continuous movement, considered as a single movement) in 30 min	Two or fewer episodes of body/limb movements in 30 min
Fetal tone	At least one episode of active extension with return to flexion of fetal limb or trunk; opening and closing of hand considered normal tone	Either slow extension with return to partial flexion movement of limb in full extension, or absent fetal movement
Reactive FHR	At least two episodes of FHR acceleration of >15 bpm and lasting at least 15 sec associated with fetal movement in 20 min	Fewer than two episodes of acceleration of FHR or acceleration of <15 bpm in 40 min
Qualitative AFV	At least one pocket of AF that measures at least 1 cm in two perpendicular planes	Either no AF pockets or a pocket <1 cm in two perpendicular planes

AF, Amniotic fluid; AFV, amniotic fluid volume; bpm, beats per minute; FBM, fetal breathing movements; FHR, fetal heart rate.
Modified from Manning FA et al: Fetal biophysical profile score and the nonstress test: a comparative trial, Obstet Gynecol 1984;64:326.

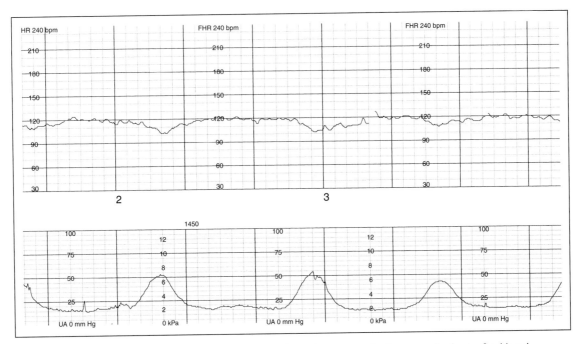

FIGURE 3-3 Early decelerations (coinciding with uterine contraction) are usually due to fetal head compression and pose little threat to the fetus.

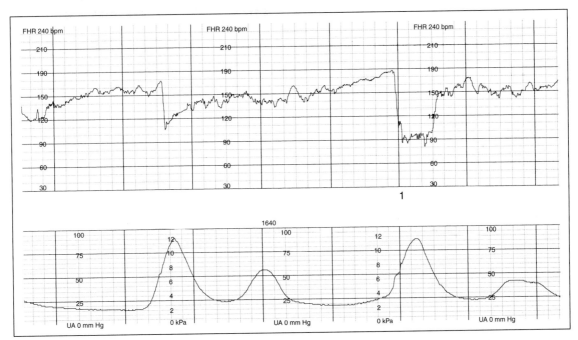

FIGURE 3-4 Variable decelerations are the most common. They are due to cord compression and have different configurations. Repetitive severe variable decelerations are associated with increased risk of fetal hypoxia.

Risk factors for preterm delivery include the following:
- Previous preterm delivery
- Premature rupture of membranes
- Genital infections: *Chlamydia, Gardnerella vaginalis*
- Nongenital infections: pyelonephritis, pneumonia
- Chorioamnionitis: infection of fetal membranes and amniotic fluid
- Conditions that overdistend the uterus: multiple gestations, increased amount of amniotic fluid
- Placental conditions: placental abruption or placenta previa

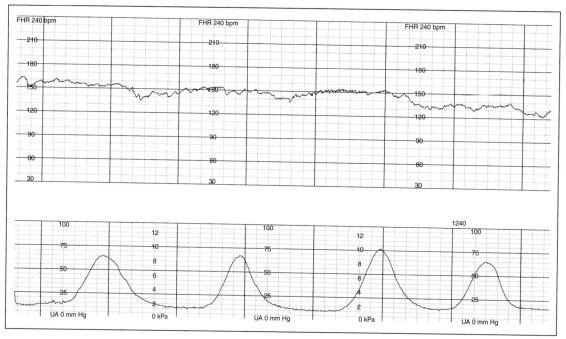

FIGURE 3-5 Late decelerations are due to uteroplacental insufficiency. They usually begin at the peak of the contraction and are associated with fetal distress.

TABLE 3-2

Normal Values for Fetal Scalp Blood and Umbilical Cord Blood Gases

	FETAL SCALP DURING LABOR		UMBILICAL CORD AT BIRTH		ARTERIAL SAMPLE AFTER BIRTH		
	First-stage Labor	Second-stage Labor	Umbilical Artery	Umbilical Vein	5-10 Min	30 Min	60 Min
pH	7.33	7.29	7.24	7.32	7.21	7.30	7.33
P_{CO_2} (mm Hg)	44	46	49	38	46	38	36
P_{O_2} (mm Hg)	22	16	16	27	50	54	63
Bicarbonate (mEq/L)	20	17	19	20	17	18	19

P_{CO_2}, Carbon dioxide pressure; P_{O_2}, oxygen pressure.
Data from Beard RW, Nathanielsz PW: *Fetal physiology and medicine,* New York: Marcel Dekker; 1984 and from Koch G, Wendel H: Adjustment of arterial blood gases and acid–base balance in the normal newborn infant during the first week of life, *Biol Neonate* 1968;12:136.

• Abnormalities of the uterine cavity: uterine septum or fibroids
• Fetal anomalies
• Cervical insufficiency

Signs of preterm labor include back pain, menstrual-like pains, pelvic heaviness, vaginal discharge, and vaginal bleeding. Diagnosis of labor is based on having six contractions in a 1-hour period associated with cervical changes: cervical dilation (opening wider) and cervical effacement (thinning out). Several approaches to prevention of preterm labor have been studied. These include serial cervical examinations, home uterine activity monitoring, prophylactic use of oral *tocolytics* (drugs used to stop labor), and bed rest. None has been shown to be clearly effective.

Fetal fibronectin (a glycoprotein produced in the chorion) seems to be expressed in cervical and vaginal secretions in cases of preterm labor. It has been studied as a marker of preterm labor in symptomatic patients. The absence of fetal fibronectin is a strong predictor that preterm delivery is unlikely to happen within 1 to 2 weeks, with a negative predictive value exceeding 95% in some studies.[37] Its use may be beneficial in providing reassurance to asymptomatic women who have high-risk factors for preterm delivery.[38]

Once preterm labor is diagnosed, prompt measures should be taken to try to stop labor and prevent an early delivery. Intravenous hydration is commonly the first approach used. It does not seem to be of clinical significance in a well-hydrated patient.[39] Excessive hydration should be avoided, because it might potentiate the risk of pulmonary edema that is usually associated with tocolytic use. Some of the tocolytics used are as follows:

Most commonly used:
- Magnesium sulfate
- β-Mimetic agents
- Indomethacin (a prostaglandin inhibitor)

Less commonly used:
- Nifedipine (calcium channel blocker)
- Nitroglycerin (nitric oxide donor drug)
- Atosiban (oxytocin antagonist)
- Combination therapy

Magnesium sulfate is usually given as an initial intravenous bolus of 4 to 6 g followed by intravenous infusion at 2 to 4 g/hour. Its main mechanism of action seems to be by decreasing free intracellular calcium ion concentration, resulting in decreased electrical potential of the cell. Magnesium sulfate is contraindicated in patients with hypocalcemia, renal failure, and myasthenia gravis. Potential toxic effects include pulmonary edema, respiratory depression, cardiac arrest, muscular paralysis, and profound hypotension.[40] Loss of deep tendon reflexes usually precedes the above-mentioned complications. It is frequently checked to monitor patients receiving magnesium sulfate therapy. Magnesium blood level can also be assessed. Toxic effects are rarely seen with levels less than 8 mg/dl.

β-Mimetic drugs (terbutaline and ritodrine) can also cause uterine relaxation and are commonly used tocolytic agents. They decrease the electrical potential of the cell by increasing calcium binding to the intracellular sarcoplasmic reticulum, an effect mediated by cyclic adenosine monophosphate. They are contraindicated in patients with poorly controlled diabetes, thyrotoxicosis, and maternal cardiac disease. Potential side effects include hyperglycemia, hypokalemia, hypotension, pulmonary edema, dysrhythmias, and myocardial ischemia. β-Mimetic drugs are administered intravenously. The rate of infusion is slowly titrated upward until a clinical response is obtained. Maternal pulse rate correlates with the blood concentration of the drug, and is typically used to assess the adequacy of the dosage. A pulse rate higher than 120 beats per minute should be avoided.

Indomethacin (a prostaglandin inhibitor) reduces the synthesis of prostaglandins by inhibiting cyclooxygenase. It is contraindicated in patients with asthma, gastrointestinal bleeding, renal failure, coronary artery disease, and oligohydramnios. Its major potential complications include renal failure, gastrointestinal bleeding, and hepatitis (with chronic use). It can cause oligohydramnios, and when used after 32 weeks of gestation it may induce closure of the ductus arteriosus in the fetus, leading to heart failure and hydrops. Indomethacin is used orally or via the rectal route. Ultrasound is used to periodically assess the amniotic fluid volume when indomethacin is used.

Tocolytics are widely used for the treatment of preterm labor. Studies have failed to show much success beyond delaying delivery for 48 hours.[41,42] Adjunctive therapy with corticosteroids for induction of fetal lung maturity is beneficial and justifies the use of tocolytics.

All women between 24 and 34 weeks of gestation with preterm labor and intact membranes are candidates for antenatal corticosteroid therapy.[43] Patients with preterm labor and ruptured membranes benefit from corticosteroid therapy between 24 and 32 weeks of gestation. Betamethasone and dexamethasone are most commonly used for antenatal corticosteroid therapy. Maximal benefit occurs 48 hours after initiation of therapy and lasts for 7 days. Corticosteroids reduce respiratory distress syndrome and neonatal morbidity by 50%.[44] This effect is due to induction of proteins that regulate the production of surfactant by type II cells in the fetal lungs. Corticosteroids also decrease the incidence of intracranial hemorrhage, probably by promoting maturation of the germinal matrix in the fetal brain. Repeat corticosteroid courses should not be used routinely because of the possible risk of adverse neurodevelopmental outcome.[43]

Prevention of preterm delivery in patients with previous preterm deliveries is currently being studied. A study using weekly intramuscular injection of 17α-hydroxyprogesterone caproate showed promising results in decreasing the rate of recurrent preterm birth.[45] Other progesterone formulations and other routes of administration are being studied. Preliminary results are promising. Long term safety studies are underway.

Postterm Pregnancy

Postterm pregnancy complicates from 3% to 12% of pregnancies. The most frequent reason for a diagnosis of postdate gestation is inaccurate dating due to either irregular ovulation or inaccurate recall of last menstrual period. Inaccurate dating is frequently encountered in patients who become pregnant after discontinuation of birth control pills. These patients tend to experience a delay in ovulation of 2 or more weeks. Less common causes of postterm pregnancy are fetal anencephaly, placental sulfatase deficiency, and abdominal pregnancy. Most postterm pregnancies are of unknown cause; deficiency of prostaglandin production or refractoriness of the cervix to endogenous prostaglandins could be the cause.[46]

Postterm pregnancy may be associated with maternal and neonatal problems. A woman may suffer from anxiety of being past her due date and still undelivered. She is at higher risk of obstetric trauma (i.e., vaginal and cervical laceration) from delivery of a large infant. Physically, she is at increased risk of long-term sequelae of incontinence and pelvic relaxation. The infant may suffer from oligohydramnios, macrosomia, meconium aspiration (inhalation of fecal discharge into the fetal lungs), and placental insufficiency. After reaching a maximum of about 1 liter at 37 weeks of gestation, amniotic fluid volume decreases gradually. The decrease in amniotic fluid may result in cord compression, fetal hypoxia, and a higher incidence of cesarean delivery for FHR abnormalities. Intrapartum amnioinfusion, the installation of fluid into the amniotic cavity, significantly improves neonatal outcome and lessens the rate of cesarean section in the presence of oligohydramnios.[47]

Fetal macrosomia, that is, a birth weight greater than 4000 g, increases the risk of cesarean delivery for dystocia (abnormal or difficult childbirth) and increases the risk of birth trauma during vaginal delivery due to shoulder dystocia (when the anterior shoulder of the infant cannot pass below the mother's hip bone, or requires significant manipulation to pass the pubic symphysis), resulting in brachial plexus palsy.

Meconium aspiration is another significant problem. Meconium passage in utero is common after 42 weeks of gestation. It is frequently associated with fetal hypoxia. Meconium becomes more concentrated in the amniotic fluid when associated with oligohydramnios. Aspiration of meconium may lead to obstruction of the respiratory passages and interference with surfactant function (see Chapter 4).[46] However, the infant should only be intubated after delivery and meconium should be aspirated from below the vocal cord for a better outcome if the infant is limp and cynotic. A recent meta-analysis of prospective clinical trials of intrapartum amnioinfusion for meconium-stained fluid revealed significant improvement in neonatal outcome and a lower cesarean delivery rate.[48]

Placental insufficiency is another hazard to the fetus. When the placenta "ages," it fails to provide the fetus with substantial nutritional requirements. This may result in fetal intrauterine growth restriction. In labor, poor beat-to-beat variability, late decelerations, and bradycardia may be signs of fetal compromise due to placental insufficiency.

To decrease fetal risk of adverse outcome, two strategies are widely used: antenatal surveillance and induction of labor. There is a lack of evidence that antenatal testing improves neonatal outcome. However, it became standard practice because of its universal acceptance. Because of the lack of evidence, it is not clear when to start antenatal surveillance. There are wide variations of practice regarding what method of testing to use (NST, CST, or BPP) and how often to perform testing. Furthermore, it is unclear whether labor induction results in a better outcome when compared with antenatal surveillance. The American College of Obstetricians and Gynecologists recommends labor induction for pregnancies at 41 weeks or more when the cervix is favorable. When the cervix is unfavorable, cervical ripening followed by labor induction and fetal antenatal surveillance are acceptable options.[49]

Labor induction can be achieved with various medications when the cervix is favorable for induction. Intravenous infusion of oxytocin is most commonly used. Oxytocin is started at a rate of 1 or 2 milliunits/minute and increased periodically until an adequate pattern of uterine contractions is achieved. Possible side effects include water retention with long use of high doses (usually more than 20 milliunits/min). This can result in hyponatremia with seizures and coma. Oxytocin also causes hypotension when administered rapidly as an intravenous bolus. Uterine rupture and amniotic fluid embolism have been cited with oxytocin use.

When the cervix is unfavorable for induction, its texture, dilation, and effacement can be improved by several modalities. Mechanical methods include placement of a Foley catheter balloon or osmotic dilator (Laminaria tents) into the cervical canal. Laminaria tents are thought to act by absorbing water from the cervix, rendering it softer and more dilated. Their use for cervical ripening was associated with increased maternal and neonatal infection rate.[50] Pharmacologic agents have also been used for cervical ripening. Prostaglandin E_2 cervical gel (Prepidil) and vaginal insert (Cervidil) are widely used. They act by causing dissolution of collagen fibers in the cervix. The most common side effects include maternal fever, nausea, vomiting, and diarrhea. Misoprostol (Cytotec) is a prostaglandin E_1 analog that is approved by the Food and Drug Administration for the prevention of ulcers that occur during long-term treatment with nonsteroidal antiinflammatory drugs. Because of its uterotonic effect, it has been increasingly used for cervical ripening and labor induction. Its popularity stems from its effectiveness, low cost, and stability at room temperature.[51] Safety concerns have been raised in view of reports of uterine rupture occurring after misoprostol induction in patients with previous uterine scars,[52] or multiparous patients.[53]

ASSESSMENT QUESTIONS

See Evolve Resources for answers.

1. All of the following are criteria for diagnosis of severe preeclampsia *except:*
   A. Headache
   B. Diastolic blood pressure higher than 110 mm Hg
   C. Generalized edema
   D. Intrauterine growth restriction

ASSESSMENT QUESTIONS—cont'd

2. Cesarean delivery is indicated for which of the following maternal infections:
   A. Group B *Streptococcus*
   B. Hepatitis B
   C. Hepatitis C
   D. Ano-genital herpes simplex virus
3. Polyhydramnios is associated with all of the following *except:*
   A. Gestational diabetes
   B. Anencephaly
   C. Twin–twin transfusion syndrome
   D. Use of prostaglandin synthase inhibitors
4. Late decelerations are usually caused by:
   A. Uteroplacental insufficiency
   B. Fetal anemia
   C. Umbilical cord compression
   D. Fetal head compression
5. The earliest sign of magnesium sulfate toxicity is:
   A. Hypotension and tachycardia
   B. Loss of deep tendon reflexes
   C. Respiratory depression
   D. Acute renal failure
6. When used for labor induction, misoprostol is contraindicated for patients with:
   A. Postterm pregnancy
   B. Preeclampsia
   C. Previous cesarean section
   D. Nulliparous pregnancy
7. All of the following are true about the use for induction of fetal lung maturity *except:*
   A. Corticosteroids are contraindicated for patients with premature rupture of membranes.
   B. Betamethasone and dexamethasone are the most commonly used corticosteroids.
   C. Corticosteroid use is associated with a decreased risk of fetal intracranial hemorrhage.
   D. Corticosteroid therapy reduces risk of respiratory distress syndrome by 50%.

References

1. Carr-Hill RA, Hall MH: The repetition of spontaneous preterm labor, *Br J Obstet Gynaecol* 1985;92:921.
2. American College of Obstetricians and Gynecologists: Cervical insufficiency. ACOG Practice Bulletin 48. Washington DC: American College of Obstetricians and Gynecologists; 2003.
3. American College of Obstetricians and Gynecologists: Substance abuse in pregnancy. ACOG Technical Bulletin 195. Washington DC: American College of Obstetricians and Gynecologists; 1994.
4. Jones KL et al: Patterns of malformation in offspring of chronic alcoholic mothers, *Lancet* 1973;1:1267.
5. Committee on Substance Abuse and Committee on Children with Disabilities: Fetal alcohol syndrome and fetal alcohol effects, *Pediatrics* 1993;91:1004.
6. Hammoud AO et al: Smoking in pregnancy revisited: findings from a large population-based study, *Am J Obstet Gynecol* 2005;192:1856.
7. Harfer JH et al: Risk factors for preterm premature rupture of membranes: a multicenter case control study, *Am J Obstet Gynecol* 1990;163:130.
8. Naeye RL: Abruptio placentae and placenta previa: frequency, perinatal mortality, and cigarette smoking, *Obstet Gynecol* 1980;55:701.
9. Taylor JA, Sanderson M: A reexamination of the risk factors for sudden infant death syndrome, *J Pediatr* 1995;126:887.
10. Shiono PH et al: The impact of cocaine and marijuana use on low birth weight and preterm birth: a multicenter study, *Am J Obstet Gynecol* 1995;172:19.
11. American College of Obstetricians and Gynecologists: Diagnosis and management of preeclampsia and eclampsia. Practice Bulletin 33. Washington DC: American College of Obstetricians and Gynecologists; 2002.
12. Cunningham FG, Leveno KJ, Bloom SL, Hauth JC, Gilstrap LC, Wenstrom KD, editors: *Williams obstetrics,* ed 22, New York: The McGraw–Hill Companies; 2005, pp 768-770.
13. Sibai BM, El-Nazer A, Gonzalez-Ruiz AR: Severe preeclampsia–eclampsia in young primigravida women: subsequent pregnancy outcome and remote prognosis, *Am J Obstet Gynecol* 1986;155:1011.
14. Langer O et al: Insulin and glyburide therapy: dosage, severity level of gestational diabetes, and pregnancy outcome, *Am J Obstet Gynecol* 2005;192:134.
15. American College of Obstetricians and Gynecologists: Prevention of early-onset group B streptococcal disease in newborns. Committee Opinion 279. Washington DC: American College of Obstetricians and Gynecologists; 2002.
16. Guinan ME, Hardy A: Epidemiology of AIDS in women in the United States, *JAMA* 1987;257:2039.
17. MacGregor SN: Human immunodeficiency virus infection in pregnancy, *Clin Perinatol* 1997;18:33.
18. Connor EM et al: Pediatric AIDS Clinical Trials Group Protocol 076 Study Group: Reduction of maternal-infant transmission of HIV-1 with zidovudine treatment, *N Engl J Med* 1994;331:1173.
19. European Mode of Delivery Collaboration: Elective caesarean section versus vaginal delivery in prevention of vertical HIV transmission: a randomized clinical trial, *Lancet* 1999;353:1035.
20. Duff P: Maternal and perinatal infection. In Gabbe SG, Niebyl JR, Simpson JL, editors: *Obstetrics: normal and problem pregnancies,* ed 4, New York: Churchill Livingstone; 1996. p 1316.
21. Rinehart BK et al: Single umbilical artery is associated with an increased incidence of structural and chromosomal anomalies and growth restriction, *Am J Perinatol* 2000;17:229.
22. Cunningham FG, Leveno KJ, Bloom SL, Hauth JC, Gilstrap LC, Wenstrom KD editors: *Williams obstetrics,* ed 22, New York: The McGraw-Hill Companies; 2005, pp 813-814.
23. Baron C, Morgan MA, Garite TJ: The impact of amniotic fluid volume assessed intrapartum on perinatal outcome, *Am J Obstet Gynecol* 1995;173:167.
24. Hannah ME et al: Planned caesarean section versus planned vaginal birth for breech presentation at term: a randomized multicentre trial, *Lancet* 2000;356:1375.

25. Collea JV, Chein C, Quilligan EJ: The randomized management of term frank breech presentation: a study of 208 cases, *Am J Obstet Gynecol* 1990;137:235.

26. Gimovsky ML et al: Randomized management of the non-frank breech presentation at term: a preliminary report, *Am J Obstet Gynecol* 1983;146:34.

27. American College of Obstetricians and Gynecologists: Mode of term singleton breech delivery. Committee Opinion 265. Washington DC: American College of Obstetricians and Gynecologists; 2001.

28. Martin JA et al: Births: final data for 2003, *Natl Vital Stat Rep* 2005;54:1.

29. Rosenberg AA: The neonate. In Gabbe SG, Niebyl JR, Simpson JL, editors: *Obstetrics: normal and problem pregnancies*, ed 3, New York: Churchill Livingstone; 1997, pp 663-664.

30. Blocking A: Observations of biophysical activities in the normal fetus, *Clin Perinatol* 1989;16:583.

31. Timor-Tritsch IE, Platt LD: Three-dimensional ultrasound experiences in obstetrics, *Curr Opin Obstet Gynecol* 2002;14:569.

32. Druzin ML: Antepartum fetal heart rate monitoring: state of the art, *Clin Perinatol* 1989;16:627.

33. Manning FA et al: Fetal biophysical profile score and the nonstress test: a comparative trial, *Obstet Gynecol* 1984;64:326.

34. Vintzileos AM, Campbell WA: Fetal biophysical scoring: current status, *Clin Perinatol* 1989;16:661.

35. American College of Obstetricians and Gynecologists: Intrapartum fetal heart rate monitoring postop. Practice Bulletin 62. Washington DC: American College of Obstetricians and Gynecologists; 2005.

36. Kuhnert M, Schmidt S: Intrapartum management of non reassuring fetal heart rate patterns: a randomized controlled trial of fetal pulse oximetry, *Am J Obstet Gynecol* 2004;191:1989.

37. Lockwood CJ et al: Fetal fibronectin in cervical and vaginal secretions as a predictor of preterm delivery, *N Engl J Med* 1991;325:669.

38. Andersen HF: Use of fetal fibronectin in women at risk for preterm delivery, *Clin Obstet Gynecol* 2000;43:746.

39. Pircon RA et al: Controlled trial of hydration and bed rest versus bed rest alone in the evaluation of preterm uterine contractions, *Am J Obstet Gynecol* 1989;161:775.

40. American College of Obstetricians and Gynecologists: Management of preterm labor. Practice Bulletin 4. Washington DC: American College of Obstetricians and Gynecologists; 2003.

41. King JF et al: Betamimetics in preterm labor: an overview of the randomized controlled trials, *Br J Obstet Gynaecol* 1988;95:211.

42. Cox SM, Sherman ML, Leveno KJ: Randomized investigation of magnesium sulfate for prevention of preterm birth, *Am J Obstet Gynecol* 1990;163:767.

43. American College of Obstetricians and Gynecologists: Antenatal corticosteroid therapy for fetal maturation. Committee Opinion 402. Washington DC: American College of Obstetricians and Gynecologists; 2008.

44. NIH Consensus Development Panel on the Effect of Corticosteroids for Fetal Maturation on Perinatal Outcomes: Effect of corticosteroids for fetal maturation on perinatal outcomes, *JAMA* 1995;273:413.

45. Meis PJ et al: Prevention of recurrent preterm delivery by 17α-hydroxyprogesterone caproate, *N Engl J Med* 2003;348:2379.

46. Spellacy WN: Postdate pregnancy. In Scott JR, Di Saia PJ, Hammond CB, Spellacy WN, editors: *Danforth's obstetrics and gynecology*, ed 8, Philadelphia: Lippincott Williams & Wilkins; 1999, pp 287-292.

47. Pitt C et al: Prophylactic amnioinfusion for intrapartum oligohydramnios: a meta-analysis of randomized controlled trials, *Obstet Gynecol* 2000;95:861.

48. Pierce J, Gaudier FL, Sanchez-Ramos L: Intrapartum amnioinfusion for meconium-stained fluid: meta-analysis of prospective clinical trials, *Obstet Gynecol* 2000;95:1051.

49. American College of Obstetricians and Gynecologists: Management of postterm pregnancy. Practice Bulletin 55. Washington DC: American College of Obstetricians and Gynecologists; 2004.

50. Krammer J et al: Pre-induction cervical ripening: a randomized comparison of two methods, *Obstet Gynecol* 1995;85:614.

51. Wing DA et al: Misoprostol: an effective agent for cervical ripening and labor induction, *Am J Obstet Gynecol* 1995;172:4844.

52. Wing DA, Lovett K, Paul RH: Disruption of prior uterine incision following misoprostol for labor induction in women with previous cesarean delivery, *Obstet Gynecol* 1998;91:828.

53. Khabbaz AY et al: Rupture of an unscarred uterus with misoprostol induction: case report and review of the literature, *J Matern Fetal Med* 2001;10:141.

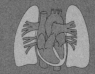

Chapter 4

Neonatal Assessment and Resuscitation

CRAIG PATRICK BLACK

OUTLINE

Preparation
Stabilizing the Neonate
    Drying and Warming
    Clearing the Airway
    Providing Stimulation
Assessing the Neonate
    Respiration
    Heart Rate
    Skin Color

    Apgar Score
    Apgar Score in the Very Low Birth Weight Infant
Resuscitating the Neonate
    Oxygen Administration
    Ventilation
    Chest Compressions
    Medications
    Postresuscitation Care
    Ethical Considerations

LEARNING OBJECTIVES

After reading this chapter the reader will be able to:

- List steps for initial assessment of the newborn to determine the need for neonatal resuscitation and name the criteria indicating infants not requiring delivery room resuscitation
- List steps to be taken in the first 30 seconds for an infant who requires resuscitation
- Describe care to be given to infants born with meconium staining
- Describe the Apgar scoring system and how and when it is performed on the newborn
- Describe how resuscitation for the very low birth weight infant differs from that for the term infant
- List three means for delivery of positive-pressure ventilation to the newborn and the advantages and disadvantages of each

- Demonstrate proper technique for delivery of positive-pressure ventilation
- List the circumstances under which a newborn will require intubation
- Describe the proper delivery room treatment of an infant with suspected diaphragmatic hernia
- List circumstances under which external chest compressions will be required for a newborn and demonstrate the two techniques for delivery of external chest compressions
- List medications, their purpose, and appropriate doses and routes of administration for their delivery to the newborn during resuscitation
- Describe circumstances under which resuscitation efforts should not be undertaken or should be stopped once they are undertaken

[handwritten: no firm to breathe]

he first few moments of an infant's life are the most critical. At this time the newborn must make the transition from intrauterine to extrauterine life. Most infants enter extrauterine life with crying and vigorous activity. However, of the approximately 4 million babies born in the United States each year, 7.3% are low birth weight, or 1500 to 2500 g, and 1.3% are very low birth weight, or less than 1500 g.[1] Adverse maternal and fetal conditions contribute to the need to initiate resuscitative efforts in approximately 6% to 10% of all deliveries.[2]

The key to successful neonatal resuscitation lies in rapid and skillful assessment of the newborn's condition followed by interventions appropriate to that condition. Infants who meet the following four criteria generally will not require resuscitation and can be quickly dried, placed on the mother's abdomen, and covered with dry, warm linen to maintain temperature[3]:

- Infants born at full-term gestation
- Amniotic fluid clear with no evidence of infection
- Crying or normal breathing
- Good muscle tone

For those infants requiring resuscitation current methods are directed toward[3]

- Providing warmth and stimulation
- Providing oxygen and removing carbon dioxide by positive-pressure ventilation
- Maintaining circulation by external cardiac massage
- Using volume expanders to combat shock
- Infrequently, using cardiotonic medications

Proper care of the newborn can be divided into four phases: preparation, stabilization, assessment, and resuscitation.

PREPARATION

Neonatal resuscitation guidelines require skilled personnel to function as a team in an appropriately equipped delivery room. Successful delivery room resuscitation depends on the rapid availability of skilled personnel trained in neonatal assessment and resuscitation and in advanced preparation, including the availability of equipment to

- Maintain warmth
- Provide and maintain an airway
- Obtain vascular access
- Provide resuscitative drugs

Ideally, a detailed history of perinatal problems associated with an infant who may require resuscitation (Box 4-1) should be available. If this information cannot be obtained, the neonatal resuscitation team will be better prepared if they at least know

- If the mother is in premature labor
- The approximate gestational age of the infant
- The number of babies expected
- If meconium is present in the amniotic fluid

Box 4-1 — Perinatal Factors Associated With Increased Risk of Neonatal Depression

ANTEPARTUM (FETOMATERNAL)
- Maternal diabetes
- Postterm status (born at greater than 42 weeks of gestation)
- Maternal infection (especially group B *Streptococcus*, or herpes)
- Hemorrhage
- Substance abuse
- No prenatal care
- Age greater than 35 years
- Multifetal gestation
- Diminished fetal activity
- Maternal anemia or Rh isoimmunization*
- Oligohydramnios or polyhydramnios*
- Small fetus for maternal dates
- Previous fetal or neonatal death
- Immature pulmonary maturity studies
- Chronic or pregnancy-induced hypertension
- Preterm labor or premature rupture of membranes
- Other maternal illness (e.g., cardiovascular, thyroid, neurologic)
- Drug therapy (e.g., magnesium, adrenergic blockers, lithium)
- Congenital abnormalities

[handwritten: Mg for mom]

INTRAPARTUM
- Maternal or fetal infection
- Prolapsed cord
- Prolonged labor
- Maternal sedation
- Operative or device-assisted delivery
- Meconium-stained delivery
- Prolonged rupture of membranes
- Breech or other abnormal presentation
- Indices of fetal distress (e.g., abnormal heart rate)

See Chapter 3, Antenatal Assessment and High-risk Delivery.

STABILIZING THE NEONATE

Stabilizing the newborn starts with proper positioning, followed by drying and warming. Immediately after delivery place the infant on a preheated radiant warmer, and position the infant with the neck slightly flexed (Figure 4-1). Placing a small roll under the shoulders often attains the correct position.

Drying and Warming

Preventing heat loss is critical when caring for a newborn, because cold stress increases oxygen consumption and impedes effective resuscitation. If possible, deliver the infant in a warm, draft-free area.[4] Heat loss can be greatly reduced by rapidly drying the infant's

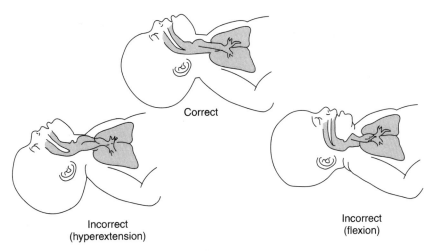

Correct

Incorrect
(hyperextension)

Incorrect
(flexion)

FIGURE 4-1 Correct and incorrect head positions for resuscitation.

skin, immediately removing wet linens, and wrapping the infant in prewarmed blankets.[5] If the infant is less than 1500 g, wrapping the newborn in a topical polyethylene film reduces evaporative heat loss but permits radiant heat transfer.[6] Wrapping a very low birth weight infant in polyethylene at delivery reduces the risk of a decrease in postnatal temperature and may reduce mortality.[7] Hyperthermia should also be avoided because increased body temperature causes increased oxygen consumption.[8]

Clearing the Airway

Once positioned, suction the infant to clear secretions. Positioning the infant and clearing secretions open the infant's airway. Suspect airway obstruction if the newborn's respiratory efforts are not effective. Immediately reposition the head and clear the airway of the obstruction. Use either a bulb syringe or a suction catheter, and limit each pass to 3 to 5 seconds at a time, clearing the mouth first and then the nose. Remember to monitor heart rate for possible bradycardia during suctioning.[9] Aggressive pharyngeal or stomach suctioning may cause laryngeal spasm and vagal stimulation with bradycardia and may delay the onset of spontaneous breathing.[5,9] To avert injury and atelectasis, as well as interference with the infant's ability to establish adequate ventilation, avoid excessive suctioning of clear fluid from the nasopharynx.[2] In the absence of meconium or blood, limit mechanical suctioning with a catheter to a depth of 5 cm from the lips for 5 seconds. Negative pressure of the suction apparatus should not exceed 90 to 100 mm Hg.[5]

Attempts to suction meconium from the pharynx or trachea before birth, during birth, or postpartum increase the likelihood of severe aspiration pneumonia.[3] Some obstetricians orally and nasally suction meconium-stained infants after delivery of the head, but before delivery of the shoulders. However, a large, multicenter,

randomized trial showed no benefit from this practice.[10] Therefore, current recommendations for infants with meconium are that

- No intrapartum suctioning should occur
- Infants who are vigorous at birth (strong respiratory effort, heart rate > 100 beats/min, good muscle tone) should not receive tracheal suctioning
- Infants who are not vigorous (no or poor respiratory effort, heart rate < 100 beats/min, poor muscle tone) may receive direct laryngotracheal suctioning[3]

For direct laryngotracheal suctioning, intubate the infant and apply suction directly to the endotracheal tube with the help of a meconium aspirator (Figure 4-2). Constantly apply suction while removing the tube from the airway. Repeat the intubation and suctioning procedure until meconium is no longer visible in the airway or until resuscitation is required.

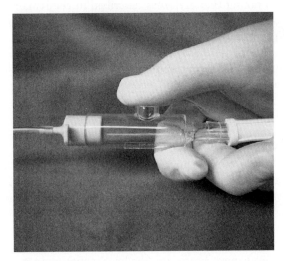

FIGURE 4-2 Meconium aspirator, with an endotracheal tube attached to one end and a suction source attached at the other end.

If positive-pressure ventilation is required, reintubate with a clean endotracheal tube after meconium has been removed with repeated suctioning attempts. Perform subsequent suctioning by passing a suction catheter through the endotracheal tube. If the newborn heart rate is less than 100 and ventilatory effort is poor or nonexistant, positive-pressure ventilation should be performed, even if some meconium remains in the airway. Do not suction the stomach until vital signs are stable and the infant has been fully resuscitated.

Providing Stimulation

If the newborn does not respond to the extrauterine environment with a strong cry, good respiratory effort, and the movement of all extremities, the infant requires stimulation. Flicking the bottoms of the feet, gently rubbing the back, and drying with a towel are all acceptable methods of stimulation. Slapping, shaking, spanking, and holding the newborn upside down are contraindicated and potentially dangerous to the infant.[11]

Basic or advanced life support should be initiated if the newborn does not establish effective, spontaneous respirations after brief stimulation. Tactile stimulation should stimulate spontaneous breathing in an infant who is in primary apnea. If the infant has already had more than one apneic episode prior to or during labor and delivery, in all likelihood it will not resume spontaneous respirations without positive-pressure ventilation.[8]

ASSESSING THE NEONATE

Immediately after birth, the initial assessment process includes evaluating the newborn's respirations, heart rate, and skin color, deciding what action to take, and then taking that action as described in the remaining sections of this chapter. Perform a quick visual inspection to detect external structural anomalies, lesions, or trauma. Initial positioning, clearing of the airway, and initiation of drying and stimulation should be completed within the first 30 seconds, followed immediately by assessment of respiratory effort, heart rate, and color (Figure 4-3).

Respiration

An appropriate respiratory response within the first 30 seconds is either spontaneous crying or strong, quiet ventilation with adequate rate and depth. Shallow, slow, or absent respirations necessitate immediate initiation of positive-pressure ventilation (see Figure 4-3). Recall, however, that the presence of respirations does not guarantee adequate heart rate. Shallow respirations may primarily ventilate anatomic dead space and thus provide inadequate alveolar ventilation. Initiate positive-pressure ventilation if the infant is apneic or gasping or if ventilatory effort is ineffective. If the respiratory response is appropriate, heart rate is evaluated next.

Heart Rate

Determine heart rate by (1) feeling the pulse by lightly grasping the base of the umbilical cord, (2) listening to the apical beat with a stethoscope, or (3) feeling the brachial or femoral pulse. Heart rate is a critical determinant of the resuscitation sequence and should be more than 100 beats/minute. If the heart rate is less than 100 beats/minute, positive-pressure ventilation should be started immediately. Frequently, effective positive-pressure ventilation alone will result in heart rate accelerating to more than 100 beats/minute. If the heart rate is 60 beats/minute or less and adequate ventilation is being provided, chest compressions should be initiated immediately.

Skin Color

Color is not as sensitive an indicator of the infant's condition as is heart rate. Many infants demonstrate acrocyanosis (blue extremities only) shortly after birth. This condition is common in the first few minutes of life because of sluggish peripheral circulation; oxygen therapy is unnecessary. On occasion, despite adequate ventilation and a heart rate greater than 100 beats/minute, an infant may continue to be cyanotic. If central cyanosis is present in an infant with spontaneous respirations and a heart rate greater than 100 beats/minute, free-flow oxygen should be given until the cause of the cyanosis is determined.

Apgar Score

Introduced in 1952 by Virginia Apgar, the Apgar score (Table 4-1) is an evaluation of newborns based on five factors: heart rate, respiratory effort, muscle tone, reflex irritability, and skin color.[12] Historically, proponents of the Apgar score have encouraged evaluation of newborns immediately after birth. It has also been used as a predictive index of neonatal mortality and neurologic or developmental outcome and continues to be used as the best-established index of immediate postnatal health.[13,14] The Apgar score obtained 1 minute after delivery provides an immediate evaluation of the infant and guides the appropriate clinical intervention at that time. However, do not postpone immediate therapeutic interventions or resuscitation to assign an Apgar score at 1 minute. In infants significantly compromised at birth, begin appropriate resuscitative efforts immediately, because any delay in proper medical treatment may prove disastrous.

Scoring again at 5 minutes of age gives information about the infant's ability to recover from the stress of

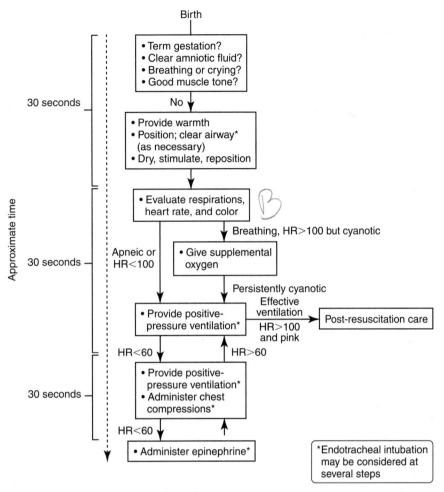

FIGURE 4-3 Algorithm for resuscitation of the newborn. HR, Heart rate (beats/min).

TABLE 4-1			
Apgar Scoring			
		APGAR SCORE	
Parameter	**0**	**1**	**2**
Heart rate	None	<100 beats/min	>100 beats/min
Respiratory rate	None	Weak, irregular	Strong cry
Skin color	Pale blue	Body pink, extremities blue	Completely pink
Reflex irritability (response to stimulation)	No response	Grimace	Cry, cough, or sneeze
Muscle tone	Limp tone	Some flexion	Well flexed

birth and adapt to extrauterine life. When the 5-minute Apgar score is less than 7, additional scores are usually obtained at 5-minute intervals until the score is greater than 7. Survival of the infant is unlikely if the score remains 0 after 10 minutes of resuscitation.[15]

Apgar Score in the Very Low Birth Weight Infant

Three of the assessment criteria used in the Apgar score—muscle tone, respiratory effort, and reflex irritability—reflect the neonate's level of developmental maturity as well as its cardiopulmonary status. Muscle tone is typically flaccid in the infant with less than 28 weeks of gestation. Respiratory effort and regulation of respiration also decrease with declining gestational age. Primitive reflexes that are present in the full-term infant, such as sucking and rooting, are variably present or absent as gestational age declines.[16]

The most important of the signs is heart rate, which indicates life or death. Failure of the heart rate to respond to resuscitation is an ominous prognostic sign.[13] Heart rate appears to be least affected by developmental maturity but may still be inadequate because of developmental difficulties in establishing cardiorespiratory function at birth.

In the immediate newborn period, skin color has the weakest correlation with the other four components of the Apgar score. Also, color does not reliably correlate with umbilical arterial pH, carbon dioxide pressure, and base excess.[16] Although the Apgar score may be limited in predicting morbidity and short-term mortality in preterm infants, it remains the best tool for identifying infants needing cardiopulmonary resuscitation.[13]

RESUSCITATING THE NEONATE

Once the need for resuscitation is determined, begin immediately. Ensure that the infant is dry and warm and that the airway is open. Resuscitation consists of administering oxygen, assisting ventilation, and initiating cardiopulmonary resuscitation and cardiotonic drugs as indicated.

Oxygen Administration

If central cyanosis is present, as assessed by examining the lips and mucous membranes, but ventilation is adequate with a heart rate greater than 100 beats/minute, administer 100% free-flow oxygen through a mask toward the infant's mouth and nose. If a mask is not available, use a funnel, or cup the hands around the oxygen tubing. Holding the oxygen one-half inch from the nose at a flow of 6 to 8 L/minute provides approximately 60% to 80% oxygen.[2] Gradually withdraw the oxygen as the infant's color improves.

Research has raised questions concerning the routine use of 100% oxygen versus room air for neonatal resuscitation. Different studies have yielded conflicting results supporting the use of 100% oxygen versus some air in both human[3,17-19] and animal studies.[20] Oxygen can be a toxic drug and has the potential to cause lung injury. Therefore, oxygen should be used judiciously in newborns, avoiding prolonged and unnecessarily high concentrations.[21,22]

While in the delivery room, continuous positive airway pressure (CPAP) may provide benefit to an infant with mild to moderate respiratory distress. Theory suggests this intervention may keep lungs open, avoiding the potentially harmful collapse and reexpansion of terminal air spaces (see Chapter 18, Newborn Continuous Positive Airway Pressure). CPAP also has a well-documented effect on apnea.[23] In some studies, early CPAP in the delivery room reduced the number of premature infants requiring mechanical ventilation.[23-25] To initiate CPAP in the delivery room, use a mask–bag setup with attached manometer to monitor applied pressure; however, place the infant on a nasal apparatus designed for CPAP administration as soon as practical.

Ventilation

Indications for assisted ventilation include apnea or gasping after stimulation, or a heart rate less than 100 beats/minute. The recommended ventilation rate is from 40 to 60 breaths/minute.[3] In the delivery room, ventilation is usually accomplished with a manual resuscitation bag and mask, although T-piece resuscitators are being used with increasing frequency.

Appropriate-sized face masks for preterm, term, and large newborns must be available in the delivery room and at the bedside. A properly sized mask fits the contours of the face and has little dead space (less than 5 ml). The mask should be large enough to form a seal around the mouth and nose but should not cover the eyes or overlap the chin. For best results, the mask should be clear and should have a cushioned rim.[2,5]

Proper technique is essential when performing mask ventilation (Figure 4-4). Place the fingers on the anterior margin of the mandible, and lift the face into the mask. Placing the fingers onto the soft tissue under the mandible will collapse the floor of the mouth and obstruct the airway by pushing the tongue against the roof of the mouth (Figure 4-5).[26] Even if the neonate is intubated, an appropriate-sized face mask must always be readily available, especially during transport.

Three types of apparatus can effectively deliver positive-pressure breaths in the neonate: a self-inflating resuscitation bag, a flow-inflating (anesthesia) bag, and a T-piece resuscitator. Advantages and disadvantages of each are summarized in Table 4-2. Appropriate initial inflation pressures range between 20 and 40 cm H_2O for unresponsive term infants and between 20 and 25 cm H_2O for preterm infants. Once adequate chest rise is noted inflation pressures should be decreased to the minimum required to keep chest rise satisfactory. Breaths should be delivered at a rate of 40 to 60 breaths/minute. No published evidence suggests an optimal inspiratory time.[3]

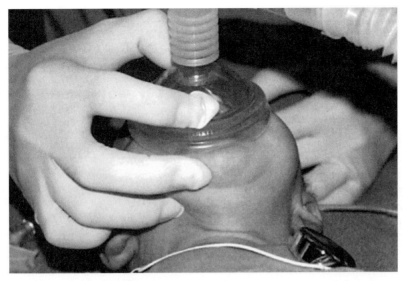

FIGURE 4-4 Correct technique for holding a mask to the face of a newborn. Note that fingers do not touch the neck or soft tissue under the chin.

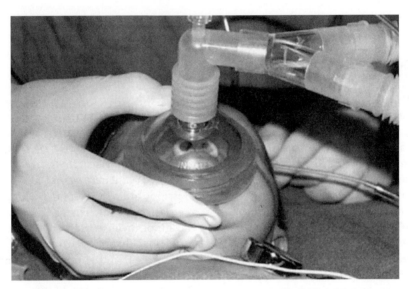

FIGURE 4-5 Incorrect technique for holding a mask to the face of a newborn. Note that the fingers are touching the neck and soft tissue under the chin, causing airway obstruction.

The self-inflating bag refills without supplementary gas flow through an intake valve. Thus, it must be hooked to an O_2 source and have an attached oxygen reservoir to deliver high concentrations of oxygen. Also, take note that many self-inflating bags do not effectively deliver free-flow oxygen through the mask.[27] The appropriate-sized bag for a neonate has a volume of 450 to 750 ml. Some bags are equipped with a pressure-limited pop-off valve, usually preset at 30 to 35 cm H_2O. Because pressures higher than the preset pop-off may be required for initial breaths a pop-off bypass device may be needed. Also, addition of a positive end-expiratory pressure (PEEP) valve is required to deliver CPAP through self-inflating bags. Finally, connect an in-line manometer to monitor pressure delivered with each breath.

The flow-inflating (anesthesia) bag inflates only with pressure and flow from a compressed gas source of air, oxygen, or both. Successful use of this type of resuscitation bag requires appropriate gas flow (8 to 10 L/min), correct adjustment of the flow control valve, and careful attention to a tight seal at the face mask. To control all these factors, more training is required than with a self-inflating bag.[28] Adjust the flow and the flow control valve to allow

TABLE 4-2

Advantages and Disadvantages of Three Devices for Delivering Positive-pressure Ventilation to Neonates

Device	Advantages	Disadvantages
Self-inflating resuscitation bag	Refills after squeeze even with no compressed gas source	Inflates even without a good face seal
	Pressure-release valve makes overinflation less likely	Requires an O_2 reservoir to provide high O_2 concentration
		Does not deliver free-flow O_2 through the mask
		Delivers PEEP/CPAP only with the addition of a PEEP valve
Flow-inflating resuscitation bag	Delivers exact O_2 concentration from source	Requires a tight seal between the mask and the infant's face
	Easy to determine whether there is a good seal with the face mask	Requires a compressed gas source
	Delivers free-flow O_2	Does not always have a pressure-release valve
T-piece resuscitator	Consistent breath-to-breath pressures delivered	Requires a compressed gas source
	Reliable control of PIP and PEEP	Lung compliance cannot be "felt"
	Reliable delivery of 100% O_2	Requires pressures to be set before use
	Operator does not become fatigued	Changing pressures during resuscitation is awkward

CPAP, Continuous positive airway pressure; PEEP, positive end-expiratory pressure; PIP, peak inspiratory pressure.
From Kattwinkel J et al: Textbook of neonatal resuscitation, ed 5, Dallas, Tex: American Academy of Pediatrics/American Heart Association; 2006.

neither overdistention nor bag deflation with subsequent breaths. Using anesthesia bags requires constant monitoring of baseline and peak ventilation pressures through an adapter attached to a pressure manometer.

The anesthesia bag offers the advantage of being able to provide more precise control of oxygen concentration, a greater range of peak inspiratory pressures, and the ability to deliver free-flow oxygen and/or CPAP through the mask. Neither style of resuscitation bag offers an advantage in terms of consistent ventilation.[29]

At least two different mechanical resuscitators (T-piece resuscitator) are available commercially. These devices require an external gas source and have the advantage of delivering predictable, consistent peak inspiratory pressure, positive end-expiratory pressure, and inspiratory time and may be helpful in avoiding inadvertent overdistention of the lungs. At the present time no evidence exists to suggest the superiority of any one of these methods.[30] Furthermore, evidence also suggests that in the hands of a well-trained clinician, effective ventilation can be achieved with any of the three devices described above.[3]

Positive-pressure ventilation should result in bilateral expansion of the lungs with chest wall motion and auscultation of bilateral breath sounds, a heart rate greater than 100 beats/minute, and progressive improvement in the infant's color. Failure to move the chest with positive-pressure ventilation may indicate a poorly positioned or leaking mask, an obstructed airway, inadequate inspiratory pressure, the presence of a pneumothorax), or some other respiratory compromise. Avoid overdistention and hyperventilation to minimize the risk of lung and brain injury.[2] Once the heart rate reaches 100 beats/minute, observe the infant for signs of adequate spontaneous respiration and clinical stability at least once every 30 seconds until the infant's condition stabilizes and positive-pressure ventilation can be discontinued.

Endotracheal intubation is indicated when (1) bag-mask ventilation is ineffective; (2) tracheal suctioning is required, especially of thick meconium in a neonate with depressed or ineffective ventilatory effort; (3) chest compressions are required; (4) prolonged positive-pressure ventilation is anticipated; or (5) endotracheal administration of medications is required.[3] When suspecting a congenital diaphragmatic hernia, *immediately* perform endotracheal intubation to minimize overdistention of the stomach resulting from bag–mask ventilation if the infant is clearly unable to sustain adequate ventilation on its own with only the addition of supplemental oxygen. In addition, a nasogastric tube to decompress the bowel and allow the lungs to inflate *should always be placed in these infants.*[4]

Intubation is an elective procedure and should be performed under the preceding conditions only after preoxygenation and initial stabilization of the infant have been performed with bag–mask ventilation. Appropriate size of endotracheal tube, correct tube placement, verification, secure fastening, and monitoring are all essential in the successful resuscitation of the neonate (see Chapter 15, Airway Management, for details). Head position does affect the endotracheal tube position. Maintain a midline head position to avoid accidental extubation or mainstem intubation.

Chest Compressions

Cardiopulmonary resuscitation in the delivery room requiring chest compressions and medications is an infrequent occurrence. In one large study, chest compressions and medications were given to 39 (0.12%) of 30,839 infants delivered.[31]

Providing adequate ventilation is the primary factor in the effective resuscitation of a neonate. Most neonates will respond once ventilation is established. After 30 seconds of effective positive-pressure ventilation with 100% O_2, if the heart rate remains less than 60 beats/minute, begin chest compressions. Chest compressions and positive-pressure ventilation must be coordinated with 1 breath for every 3 chest compressions, delivered at a rate of 30 breaths and 90 chest compressions per minute.[3]

The two accepted techniques for delivering chest compressions are the thumb method and the two-finger technique. The thumb method consists of holding the torso of the infant, with both hands encircling with the thumbs on the sternum, and the fingers under the infant. The fingers support the back, and the thumbs are used to compress the sternum. The advantage of the thumb method is better coronary perfusion pressure.[2] The disadvantage is interference with access to the infant's torso for other procedures.[3]

In the second method, the two-finger technique, the index and middle fingers are used to compress the chest. The other hand supports the back if a firm surface is not available.

With both techniques the compressions should be applied on the lower third of the sternum. Compress to approximately one third of the anteroposterior diameter of the chest to generate a palpable pulse.[5] Resuscitation should be a coordinated effort, with compressions and ventilation delivered at a 3:1 ratio, approximately 90 compressions to 30 ventilations.[3] Heart rate should be reassessed every 30 seconds and compressions discontinued when the heart rate exceeds 60 beats/minute.

Medications

Medications and the dosages recommended for neonatal resuscitation have been extrapolated mainly from adult and animal research.[31] Neonatal anatomy and physiology differ from animal and adult physiology, with the potential for unrecognized effects and hazards. More research is necessary on the effects of emergency medications in the neonate.

Epinephrine

Epinephrine is an endogenous catecholamine with both α-adrenergic- and β-adrenergic–stimulating properties; in cardiac arrest, α-adrenergic–mediated vasoconstriction may be the more important action. This vasoconstriction elevates the perfusion pressure during chest compression, enhancing delivery of oxygen to the heart and brain. In addition, epinephrine enhances the contractile state of the heart, stimulates spontaneous contractions, and increases the heart rate. Epinephrine is indicated in asystole or with a spontaneous heart rate of 60 beats/minute or less, after at least 30 seconds of ventilation with 100% oxygen and chest compressions.

An epinephrine dose of 0.01 to 0.03 mg/kg body weight (0.1 to 0.3 ml/kg of a 1:10,000 solution) may be repeated every 3 to 5 minutes if required. Some children and adults who do not respond to standard doses of epinephrine may respond to doses as high as 0.2 mg/kg. However, the routine use of this dose in neonates is not recommended. Neonates most often have hemodynamically significant bradycardia, and scientific dose-response data are lacking for the use of epinephrine in neonates or in neonatal animal models for this rhythm. Further, this dose has been associated with prolonged periods of hypertension after administration. Because the newborn, especially the premature infant, has a vascular germinal matrix (an area of the brain at high risk for the development of hemorrhage after hypertension), the risk of intracranial hemorrhage may be increased.[2,5,21,31]

Epinephrine is given either intravenously or through an endotracheal tube, although the intravenous route is strongly preferred.[3] Although giving epinephrine by the endotracheal route is expeditious and the drug is absorbed systemically, low plasma concentrations result. Data from animal models and a single adult human study suggest that if the typical intravenous dose of epinephrine is administered by the endotracheal route, the resulting serum concentration will be approximately 10% of that achieved by the intravenous route.[21,31] Thus, doses as high as 0.1 mg/kg may be considered for endotracheal tube administration before obtaining intravenous access.[3] Use a concentration of 1:10,000 (0.1 mg/ml) epinephrine and administer every 3 to 5 minutes during the treatment of pulseless arrest.

Volume Expanders

Volume expanders may be necessary to resuscitate a newborn with hypovolemia, which should be suspected in any neonate who fails to respond to resuscitation. Intravascular volume expansion may present a risk for intracranial hemorrhage in an asphyxiated neonate, particularly if the newborn is significantly preterm. However, volume expanders are indicated when acute blood loss is suspected or the neonate responds poorly to resuscitation or appears to be in shock.[3,8]

Blood volume expansion may be accomplished with 10 ml/kg of normal saline, lactated Ringer's solution, or O-negative blood cross-matched with the mother's blood (when severe hemorrhage or fetal anemia is present).[8] The volume expander may be given as a rapid infusion over 5 to 10 minutes through an umbilical vein catheter.

Naloxone

Naloxone hydrochloride, administered to reverse narcotic-induced respiratory depression, is a narcotic antagonist that does not possess direct respiratory depressant activity. Naloxone is indicated in the neonate for reversal of respiratory depression induced by narcotics given to the mother within 4 hours of delivery; however, administration should occur only after the heart rate and color are satisfactory and is not recommended for the delivery room.[3] Because the duration of action of narcotics may exceed that of naloxone, continued monitoring is essential. Also, naloxone may induce a withdrawal reaction in a newborn with a narcotic-dependent mother and should be avoided in this situation.[32]

The initial dose of naloxone, 0.1 mg/kg for infants of every gestational age, may be repeated every 2 to 3 minutes as needed.[3,5] Recurrent doses may be necessary to prevent recurrent apnea in the neonate. Naloxone should be given intravenously; endotracheal administration is not recommended.[8]

Sodium Bicarbonate

Administration of sodium bicarbonate as a part of neonatal resuscitation is controversial. Its use is recommended cautiously by some[8,21] whereas it is not mentioned at all in the most recent neonatal resuscitation guidelines prepared and issued by the American Heart Association and the American Academy of Pediatrics.[3] It may be indicated when a newborn with prolonged respiratory arrest does not respond to other therapy.[3,31] A dose of 1 to 2 mEq/kg of a 0.5-mEq/ml solution may be given by slow intravenous push after adequate ventilation and perfusion have been established. Higher concentrations have been associated with higher risks of hypernatremia and intracranial hemorrhage.[2,3,5,21,31] Regardless, it should be given only after adequate ventilation has first corrected any respiratory acidosis. Furthermore, volume expanders to reverse metabolic acidosis may be more effective and less likely to cause hyperosmolarity than sodium bicarbonate.[21]

Postresuscitation Care

Optimal care of the neonate after resuscitation requires frequent reassessment and careful monitoring, including appropriateness of therapy and determination of arterial pH and blood gas levels. Physiologic stability should be maintained by (1) treatment of hypotension with volume expanders or pressors, (2) appropriate fluid therapy, and (3) treatment of seizures. During the first hours after resuscitation, the patient must be monitored closely for hypoglycemia and hypocalcemia. Also, radiographic documentation of the appropriate placement of intravascular lines and the endotracheal tube should be obtained.[6,22]

Ethical Considerations

The issue of whether to initiate resuscitation arises with the birth of extremely premature infants or those with congenital birth defects. With advances in technology and improved medications, however, very low birth weight infants who previously would have died now can survive. Survival with normal neurodevelopmental outcome has been documented in infants weighing less than 1 pound (454 g).[21,33,34]

Initiating resuscitative efforts does not preclude withdrawing life support later. In fact, later withdrawal of support allows more time to gain better clinical information and to counsel a family on expected outcomes. Extremely premature infants or those with anencephaly may have no chance of survival, however, and they may be the exception to this recommendation, although clinicians may wish to give consideration to the possibility of organ donation in the latter situation. However, if a decision is made to initiate resuscitation, it should be initiated promptly and aggressively; there is no advantage to delayed, graduated, or partial support if the infant survives. Worse outcomes may result because of this approach.[5]

Research shows that infants with no heart beat or respiratory effort after 10 minutes of resuscitative effort have high rates of mortality, or if they survive high rates of severe neurological damage and developmental delay.[35] "After 10 minutes of continuous and adequate resuscitative efforts, discontinuation of resuscitation may be justified if there are no signs of life."[3]

ASSESSMENT QUESTIONS

See Evolve Resources for answers.

1. Infants *not* requiring delivery room resuscitation will show all of the following characteristics *except:*
   A. Born at full-term gestation
   B. Heart rate of 80 to 100 beats/minute
   C. Crying or normal breathing
   D. Amniotic fluid clear with no indication of infection

Continued

2. Which of the following actions is the initial step in stabilizing an infant?
   A. Proper positioning under a radiant warmer
   B. Suctioning of mouth and nose with a bulb syringe
   C. Determining the heart rate
   D. Determining the Apgar score

3. What is the proper procedure to implement for an infant known to have experienced meconium aspiration before birth?
   A. The obstetrician should suction the mouth, nose, and pharynx after delivery of the head, but before delivery of the shoulders.
   B. Intubate immediately and aspirate the trachea, using a meconium aspirator regardless of whether the infant is vigorous.
   C. Treat the infant exactly as if meconium was not present.
   D. Intubate and suction only if the infant is not vigorous; otherwise, follow the normal resuscitation procedures .

4. The ideal heart rate for a term newborn is _____ per minute.
   A. 60 to 80 beats
   B. 80 to 100 beats
   C. 100 to 120 beats
   D. 120 to 140 beats

5. Appropriate stimulation of a newborn includes all of the following *except*:
   A. Flicking the bottoms of the feet
   B. Gently shaking the shoulders
   C. Drying with a warm towel
   D. Gently rubbing the back

6. The Apgar score includes all of the following criteria *except*:
   A. Color
   B. Evaluation of the Moro reflex
   C. Heart rate
   D. Reflex irritability

7. The best indicator of an infant's overall cardiopulmonary status immediately after birth is
   A. Heart rate
   B. Apgar score
   C. Color
   D. Respiratory effort

8. Chest compressions should be initiated on a newborn when
   A. Heart rate is less than 100 beats/minute
   B. Heart rate is less than 80 beats/minute
   C. Heart rate is less than 60 beats/minute
   D. Only when heart rate is completely absent

9. When delivering positive-pressure ventilation, the recommended breath rate is
   A. 20-40 breaths/minute
   B. 40-60 breaths/minute
   C. 60-80 breaths/minute
   D. At least 100 breaths/minute

10. The self-inflating bag is ideal for neonatal resuscitation because it
    A. Always provides 100% O_2 when hooked to an O_2 source
    B. Can easily and dependably be used to deliver free-flow or "blow-by" O_2 as well as positive-pressure ventilation through the mask
    C. Does not require a PEEP valve to deliver CPAP by mask
    D. Requires the least experience and training for the individual using it

11. The one procedure that should always be carried out immediately after the birth of an infant known or suspected to have a diaphragmatic hernia is
    A. Intubation and suctioning of the trachea as the first step in resuscitation
    B. Prompt use of bag–mask ventilation to ensure adequate gas exchange
    C. Placement of a nasogastric tube hooked to suction
    D. Procurement of an X-ray of the chest and abdomen

12. The single most effective step in the resuscitation of a newborn is to
    A. Administer epinephrine down the endotracheal tube
    B. Administer external chest compressions at a rate of 100/minute
    C. Vigorously dry and stimulate immediately after birth
    D. Establish and maintain adequate ventilation

13. The preferred way to administer epinephrine during neonatal resuscitation is by
    A. The intravenous route
    B. Down the endotracheal tube
    C. Intramuscular injection
    D. Subcutaneous injection

14. According to guidelines described in the chapter, "After ___ minutes of continuous and adequate resuscitative efforts, discontinuation of resuscitation may be justified if there are no signs of life."
    A. 5
    B. 10
    C. 20
    D. 30

References

1. Bernstein S, Heimler R, Sasidharan P: Approaching the management of the neonatal intensive care unit graduate through history and physical assessment, *Pediatr Clin North Am* 1998;45:97.

2. Wolkoff L, Davis J: Delivery room resuscitation of the newborn, *Clin Perinatol* 1999;26:641.

3. Kattwinkel J et al: 2005 American Heart Association (AHA) guidelines for cardiopulmonary resuscitation (CPR) and emergency cardiovascular care (ECC) of pediatric and neonatal patients: neonatal resuscitation guidelines, *Pediatrics* 2006;117:E1029.

4. Chahine A, Ricketts R: Resuscitation of the surgical neonate, *Clin Perinatol* 1999;26:693.

5. Kattwinkel J et al: An advisory statement from the Pediatric Working Group of the International Liaison Committee on Resuscitation, *Pediatrics* 1999;103:E56.

6. Narendran V, Hoath S: Thermal management of the low birth weight infant: a cornerstone of neonatology, *Pediatrics* 1999;134:E547.

7. Vohra S et al: Effect of polyethylene occlusive skin wrapping on heat loss in very low birth weight infants at delivery: a randomized trial, *J Pediatr* 1999;134:547.

8. Kattwinkel J et al: *Textbook of neonatal resuscitation*, ed 5, Dallas, Tex: American Academy of Pediatrics/American Heart Association; 2006.

9. Halbower A, Jones D: Physiologic reflexes and their impact on resuscitation of the newborn, *Clin Perinatol* 1999;26:621.

10. Vain NE et al: Oropharyngeal and nasopharyngeal suctioning of meconium-stained neonates before delivery of their shoulders: multicentre, randomized controlled trial, *Lancet* 2004;364:597.

11. Nadkarni V, Hazinski MF, Zideman D: Pediatric resuscitation: an advisory statement from the Pediatric Working Group of the International Liaison Committee on Resuscitation, *Circulation* 1997;95:2185.

12. Juretschke L: Apgar scoring: its use and meaning for today's newborn, *Neonatal Network* 2000;19:17.

13. Hegyi T, Carbone T, Anwar M: The Apgar score and its components in the preterm infant, *Pediatrics* 1998;101:77.

14. Weinberger B et al: Antecedents and neonatal consequences of low Apgar scores in preterm newborns: a population study, *Arch Pediatr Adolesc Med* 2000;154:294.

15. Jain L et al: Cardiopulmonary resuscitation of apparently stillborn infants: survival and long-term outcome, *J Pediatr* 1991;118:778.

16. Catlin E et al: The Apgar score revisited: influence of gestational age, *J Pediatr* 1986;109:865.

17. Lundstrom KE et al: Oxygen at birth and prolonged cerebral vasoconstriction in preterm infants, *Arch Dis Child Fetal Neonatal Ed* 1995;73:F81.

18. Tan A et al: Air versus oxygen for resuscitation of infants at birth, *Cochrane Database Syst Rev* 2005;2:CD002273.

19. Davis PG et al: Resuscitation of newborn infants with 100% oxygen or air: a systematic review and meta-analysis, *Lancet* 2004;364:1329.

20. Solas AB et al: Cerebral hypoxemia–ischemia and reoxygenation with 21% air or 100% oxygen in newborn piglets: effects on extracellular levels of excitatory amino acids and microcirculation, *Pediatr Crit Care Med* 2001;2:340.

21. Ginsberg H, Goldsmith J: Controversies in neonatal resuscitation, *Clin Perinatol* 1998;25:1.

22. Piazza A: Postasphyxial management of the newborn, *Clin Perinatol* 1999;26:749.

23. Verder H et al: Nasal continuous positive airway pressure and early surfactant therapy for respiratory distress syndrome in newborns of less than 30 weeks' gestation, *Pediatrics* 1999;103:E24.

24. Lindner W et al: Delivery room management of extremely low birth weight infants: spontaneous breathing or intubation? *Pediatrics* 1999;103:961.

25. Lacroze M et al: Early continuous positive pressure in the labor room [abstract], *Arch Pediatr* 1997;4:15.

26. Behar P, Todd N: Resuscitation of the newborn with airway compromise, *Clin Perinatol* 1999;26:717.

27. Martell RJ, Soder CM: Laerdal infant resuscitators are unreliable as free-flow oxygen delivery devices, *Am J Perinatol* 1997;14:347.

28. Kanter RK: Evaluation of mask-bag ventilation in resuscitation of infants, *Am J Dis Child* 1987;141:761.

29. Dockery WK et al: A comparison of manual and mechanical ventilation during pediatric transport, *Crit Care Med* 1999;27:802.

30. O'Donnell CP, Davis PG, Morley CJ: Positive pressure ventilation at neonatal resuscitation: review of equipment and international survey of practice, *Acta Paediatr* 2004;93:583.

31. Burchfield D: Medication use in neonatal resuscitation, *Clin Perinatol* 1999;26:683.

32. Gibbs J et al: Naloxone hazard in infant of opioid abuser, *Lancet* 1989;2:159.

33. Boyle R, Kattwinkel J: Ethical issues surrounding resuscitation, *Clin Perinatol* 1999;26:779.

34. Clark R: Support of gas exchange in the delivery room and beyond: how do we avoid hurting the baby we seek to save? *Clin Perinatol* 1999;26:669.

35. Haddad B et al: Outcome after successful resuscitation of babies born with Apgar scores of 0 at both 1 and 5 minutes, *Am J Obstet Gynecol* 2000;182:1210.

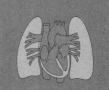

Chapter 5

Examination and Assessment of the Neonatal Patient

CRAIG PATRICK BLACK

OUTLINE

Gestational Age and Size Assessment
Physical Examination
  Vital Signs
  General Inspection
  Respiratory Function
  Chest and Cardiovascular System

Abdomen
Head and Neck
Musculoskeletal System, Spine, and Extremities
Cry
Neurologic Assessment
Laboratory Assessment

LEARNING OBJECTIVES

After reading this chapter the reader will be able to:
- Describe the factors that most influence neonatal outcome
- List criteria for determining whether an infant is large for gestational age, appropriate for gestational age, or small for gestational age
- List critical vital signs with normal values to be evaluated as part of the newborn's initial physical examination
- Describe criteria for determining whether an infant is displaying apneic spells
- Identify signs and symptoms of respiratory distress in the newborn
- Describe the technique for rapid identification of a pneumothorax in a newborn
- List the possible cardiovascular anomalies associated with different patterns of abnormal pulses

- List the elements of a normal abdominal examination and the significance of abnormal findings
- List the three types of scalp swelling observed in newborns and the characteristics and significance of each type
- List the most common structural abnormalities observed in the nose, lips, mouth, and oral cavity
- Describe the signs and symptoms of the most common types of birth injuries
- List the elements of a basic neurologic examination in the newborn
- Describe the signs and symptoms suggesting the presence of sepsis in the newborn
- List the laboratory tests most commonly done on the newborn and the range of normal values for each

Many factors, including size, weight, and gestational age, influence neonatal outcome. Therefore it is important to perform a newborn assessment early in the admission process.

GESTATIONAL AGE AND SIZE ASSESSMENT

Ideally, gestational age assessment is performed before the neonate is 12 hours old, to allow the greatest reliability for infants less than 26 weeks of gestational age.[1-3]

Evaluating gestational age requires consideration of several factors. The three main factors are as follows:
- Gestational duration based on the last menstrual cycle
- Prenatal ultrasound evaluation
- Postnatal findings based on physical and neurologic examinations

Postnatal examinations for determining gestational age include the Ballard score, which is based on external physical findings, and neurologic criteria (Figure 5-1).

Once gestational age is determined, weight, length, and head circumference are plotted on a standard newborn

Neuromuscular maturity

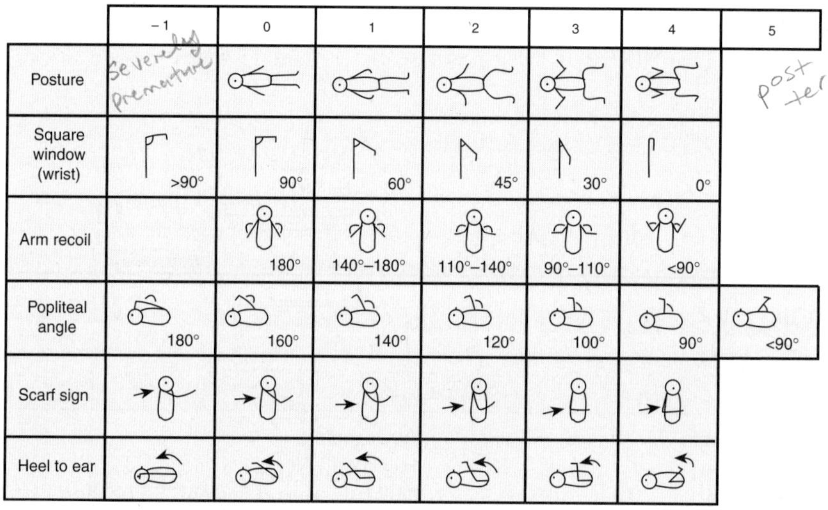

	−1	0	1	2	3	4	5
Posture							
Square window (wrist)	>90°	90°	60°	45°	30°	0°	
Arm recoil		180°	140°–180°	110°–140°	90°–110°	<90°	
Popliteal angle	180°	160°	140°	120°	100°	90°	<90°
Scarf sign							
Heel to ear							

Physical maturity

Skin	Sticky ?Friable Transparent	Gelatinous red, translucent	Smooth pink, visible veins	Superficial peeling &/or rash, few veins	Cracking pale areas, rare veins	Parchment, deep cracking, no vessels	Leathery, cracked, wrinkled
Lanugo	None	Sparse	Abundant	Thinning	Bald areas	Mostly bald	
Plantar surface	Heel-toe 40–50 mm: −1 <40 mm: −2	>50 mm no crease	Faint red marks	Anterior transverse crease only	Creases anterior 2/3	Creases over entire sole	
Breast	Imperceptible	Barely perceptible	Flat areola, no bud	Stippled areola, 1 - 2 mm bud	Raised areola, 3 - 4 mm bud	Full areola, 5-10 mm bud	
Eye/ear	Lids fused loosely: −1 tightly: −2	Lids open; pinna flat, stays folded	Sl. curved pinna; soft, slow recoil	Well-curved pinna; soft but ready recoil	Formed & firm; instant recoil	Thick cartilage; ear stiff	
Genitals (male)	Scrotum flat, smooth	Scrotum empty, faint rugae	Testes in upper canal, rare rugae	Testes descending, few rugae	Testes down, good rugae	Testes pendulous, deep rugae	
Genitals (female)	Clitoris prominent, labia flat	Prominent clitoris, small labia minora	Prominent clitoris, enlarging minora	Majora & minora equally prominent	Majora large, minora small	Majora cover clitoris & minora	

Maturity rating

score	weeks
−10	20
−5	22
0	24
5	26
10	28
15	30
20	32
25	34
30	36
35	38
40	40
45	42
50	44

FIGURE 5-1 Ballard examination for estimating gestational age, using scores determined on the basis of neurologic and physical signs.

grid. Any infant whose birth weight is less than the 10th percentile for gestational age is small for gestational age; similarly, an infant whose birth weight is more than the 90th percentile is large for gestational age. When using intrauterine growth curves, it may be necessary to consider specific charts that are race and gender specific.[4] Along with prematurity, abnormal gestational age and size for gestational age are associated with many neonatal disease processes (Figure 5-2).

PHYSICAL EXAMINATION

The physical examination of an adult is generally conducted in a rigid head-to-toe format. When examining an infant, however, the order of the examination is modified to establish critical information; for example, auscultation of the heart and lungs is done before the infant becomes agitated and begins to cry. However, the examiner must still completely examine the baby in an orderly and prioritized manner. As a general rule the following order works best, although this approach may require modification based on the clinical situation.

Vital Signs

Quickly assess the vital signs of the infant. Table 5-1 lists normal ranges for neonatal vital signs. Absolute numbers are not as important as the relative ranges when considering the clinical situation. As an example, the heart rate is normally 120 to 170 beats/minute. The heart rate of a term infant in deep sleep may decrease to 80 or 90 beats/minute. An infant undergoing a painful procedure or who is hungry may have a transient heart rate greater than 200 beats/minute. In comparison, a neonate older than 35 weeks of gestation has greater

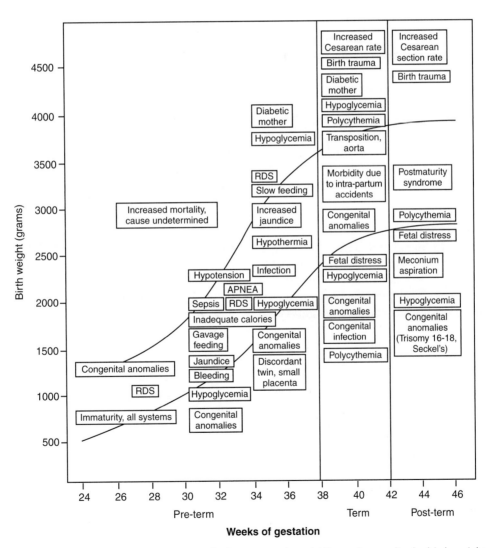

FIGURE 5-2 Overview of conditions producing neonatal morbidity and mortality by birth weight and gestational age. RDS, Respiratory distress syndrome.

TABLE 5-1

Normal Values for Vital Signs in the Neonatal Patient

Birth Weight (g)	Systolic/ Diastolic Blood Pressure (mm Hg)*	Mean Blood Pressure (mm Hg)
>600	45/20	25
>1000	48/25	35
>2000	50/30	40
>3000	50/35	45
>4000	65/40	50
Newborn older than 12 hr	75/50 60/40	60
Respiratory rate (30-60 breaths/min)		
Heart rate (120-170 beats/min)		

*From Versmold HT et al: Aortic blood pressure ranges during the first 12 hours of life in infants with birth weight 610 to 4220 grams, *Pediatrics* 1981;67:607.

variability in heart rate than an infant born at 27 to 35 weeks of gestation. Presumably, in the younger infant, parasympathetic–sympathetic interaction and function are less developed.[5]

Normal values for temperature are 97.6 ± 1 °F (axillary) and 99.6 ± 1 °F (rectal); however, temperature on arrival in the nursery may be lower if the delivery room was cold or may be higher if the radiant warmer was operating at a higher temperature due to incorrect probe position or warmer malfunction.

Record the respiratory rate and blood pressure when determining vital signs

General Inspection

Observing the infant's overall appearance is an important aspect of the physical examination. Ideally, examine the infant as it lies quietly and unclothed in a neutral thermal environment. Body position and symmetry, both at rest and during muscular activity, provide valuable information regarding possible birth trauma. For example, an infant who does not move its arms symmetrically could have a broken clavicle or an injury to the brachial plexus (Figure 5-3).

The infant's skin is an indicator of intravascular volume, perfusion status, or both. Both perfusion and underlying skin color affect the appearance of the skin. Capillary refill time should be less than 3 seconds. Assess refill by pressing the sole of the infant's foot or the palm of its hand with a finger. Perfusion should be good and skin color pink. Some infants have blue hands and feet with decreased perfusion, or *acrocyanosis*, in the immediate postnatal period. True cyanosis is associated with blue or dusky mucous membranes and circumoral area.

Observing skin and color often provides diagnostic clues. *Mottling* refers to irregular areas of dusky skin

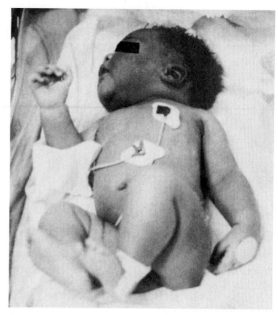

FIGURE 5-3 "Waiter's tip" positioning of the left arm of an infant with brachial plexus injury from a traumatic delivery.

alternating with areas of pale skin. An extremely pale or mottled infant suggests hypotension or anemia. A ruddy, reddish blue appearance is frequently associated with a high hematocrit value or polycythemia and neonatal hyperviscosity syndrome (hematocrit > 65%).[6] The yellow color associated with mild to moderate jaundice is common among newborns after the first day of life. Jaundice on the first day of life, however, is always an indication for immediate evaluation.[7]

Often a gray-white cheeselike substance, called *vernix caseosa*, is present in the skin folds of a term infant. However, vernix is even more abundant on a preterm infant and suggests an earlier gestational age. The presence of *lanugo*, the fine hair that covers premature infants mostly over the shoulders, back, forehead, and cheeks, indicates an even younger gestational age. An infant exposed to meconium-stained amniotic fluid in utero for more than a few hours frequently presents with yellow-green staining of the skin, nails, and umbilical cord. Irregular areas of pale blue-black pigmentation over the sacrum and buttocks (Mongolian spots) are often seen on black and Asian infants. These spots are frequently confused with bruising (Table 5-2).

Respiratory Function

The normal newborn respiratory rate is 40 to 60 breaths/minute but may vary depending on multiple factors. Watch the infant's respiratory effort closely and note irregular respirations. Respiratory rates that exceed 60 breaths/minute but normalize over the next several hours may indicate transient tachypnea of the newborn.

TABLE 5-2

Common Dermal Findings in the Neonatal Patient

Finding	Description	Condition
Jaundice	Yellowish skin	Hyperbilirubinemia
True cyanosis	Centrally blue or dusky skin	Hypoxia
Acrocyanosis	Bluish hands and feet	Cold stress, ↓ circulation; normal for first few hours
Petechiae	Pinpoint hemorrhagic areas	Birth trauma, thrombocytopenia
Telangiectatic nevi	"Stork bites": red, flat areas	Capillary dilation, benign
Subcutaneous fat necrosis	Discrete firm masses in subcutaneous tissue	Trauma
Lanugo	Fine hair	More noticeable in preterm infants, benign
Sclerema	Hardening of skin	Septicemia, shock, cold stress
Ruddy complexion	Deep reddish skin	Polycythemia or high hematocrit value
Ecchymoses	Bruising of various sizes	Birth trauma, disseminated intravascular coagulation
Mongolian spots	Irregular areas of pale blue over sacrum and buttocks	Benign, common in black and Asian infants
Strawberry hemangiomas	Bright red, flat spots 1-3 mm in diameter	Benign, usually resolve spontaneously
Milia	White papules <1 mm on forehead, chin, and nose	Distended sebaceous glands that disappear later
Erythema toxicum	Whitish pink papular rash	Cause unknown
Pallor	Pale or white skin	Blood loss or hypovolemia
Vernix caseosa	Whitish gray, cheeselike substance	More abundant on preterm infants
Mottled skin	Uneven color, blotchy	Decreased perfusion

All newborns display an irregular breathing pattern. The neonate normally breathes in the range of 70 to 80 breaths/minute for 10 to 20 seconds, slows to a rate of 20 or 30 breaths/minute for a short time, and then breathes at a faster rate again. The average respiratory rate over several minutes is 40 to 60 breaths/minute. *Periodic breathing*, a frequent finding among premature infants, is characterized by an irregular pattern of intermittent respiratory pauses longer than 5 seconds.

Apnea is a pathologic condition in which breathing ceases for longer than 20 seconds. Apnea may be associated with cyanosis, bradycardia, pallor, and hypotonia (abnormally low muscle tone). Frequently, apnea is associated with nonspecific symptoms of diseases seen with many neonatal conditions. All episodes of apnea must be investigated to establish the cause.[8]

It is important to note signs of respiratory distress. The Silverman scoring system considers multiple factors to quantify an infant's distress (Figure 5-4). Although not always used as a measure of respiratory distress, the Silverman system highlights important respiratory observations during a physical examination. Signs of distress include nasal flaring, expiratory grunting, tachypnea, and retractions. Nasal flaring, a sign of air hunger, occurs during inspiration as an effort to draw in more air through the nares. Partially closing the glottis during expiration causes grunting, apparently an attempt to maintain lung volume by increasing end-expiratory pressure.

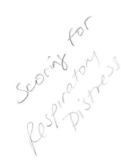
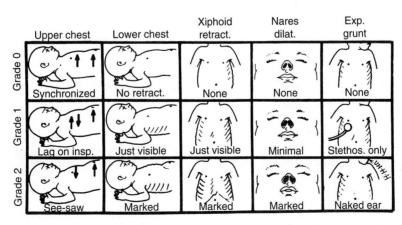

FIGURE 5-4 Silverman scoring system for assessing the magnitude of respiratory distress. Exp., Expiratory; insp., inspiratory; retract., retraction.

Retractions of the chest wall during inspiration may occur in the suprasternal, substernal, subcostal, and intercostal regions. Retractions usually indicate reduced lung compliance but are also associated with obstructive airway processes with normal lung compliance. Chest wall retractions are more prominent and easily observed in the neonate than in an older child or adult. The newborn musculature is relatively thin and weak, and the thoracic cage is not as rigid. The flexible chest wall and thoracic cage of the newborn exhibit noticeable retractions as lung compliance worsens. Abdominal and thoracic respiratory muscles normally move in parallel. Paradoxical respirations represent thoracic and abdominal respiratory efforts that are not synchronous. This "see-saw" effect frequently indicates severe respiratory distress (see Chapter 28, Congenital and Surgical Disorders That Affect Respiratory Care).

Auscultation of the newborn can sometimes prove difficult. The newborn chest is small, and sounds easily transmit from one lung region to another. Abdominal sounds may even transmit to the lungs, although bowel sounds heard from the chest in place of absent breath sounds may indicate a diaphragmatic hernia (see Chapter 28, Congenital and Surgical Disorders in Childhood That Affect Respiratory Care). Localizing auscultation findings in a preterm infant is frequently difficult or impossible with single-head stethoscopes. Auscultation with a double-head stethoscope has proved useful in some situations.[9] Comparison of the breath sounds from the right and left sides helps distinguish asymmetries. Asymmetric sounds may indicate unilateral disease such as pneumothorax or a malpositioned endotracheal tube.

Diminished breath sounds occur in neonates with respiratory distress syndrome, atelectasis, pulmonary interstitial emphysema, and shallow respirations. *Rhonchi,* coarse sounds similar to snoring, emanate from the large bronchi as air rushes through secretions contained within them. Suctioning with the endotracheal tube, if present, may eliminate the secretions responsible. *Wheezes* are commonly heard during expiration and represent turbulent air flow due to bronchoconstriction or the presence of secretions. Air rushing through fluid in the smaller airways and alveoli produce *rales* or *crackles.* Rales are heard in infants with respiratory distress syndrome, pneumonia, and pulmonary edema, as well as in normal infants soon after birth. Frequently, infants with large upper airway obstruction generate *stridor,* a high-pitched creaking or squeaking and primarily an inspiratory sound. To distinguish stridor from wheezing, place the head of the stethoscope over the neck area. If the sound is louder over the neck than over the chest, then it is most likely due to stridor rather than wheezing.

Other methods of respiratory assessment include chest radiography (see Chapter 8, Radiographic Assessment) and invasive or noninvasive blood gas analysis (see Chapter 10, Invasive Blood Gas Analysis and Monitoring; and Chapter 11, Noninvasive Monitoring in Neonatal and Pediatric Care). Frequently, chest radiographs and blood gas analysis assist in the interpretation of physical examination findings. Many pathologic processes, including pneumothorax and pleural effusion, may cause symptoms but may be difficult to diagnose on the basis of physical findings alone. Blood gas measurements supply additional information that facilitates the interpretation of physical findings. For example, an infant with severe tachypnea, normal chest examination, and normal chest radiograph has a blood gas diagnosis indicating severe metabolic acidosis. The tachypnea is not caused by a cardiopulmonary problem but rather by an effort to blow off carbon dioxide and increase the blood pH.

Table 5-3 summarizes signs of respiratory distress associated with several neonatal disorders.

Chest and Cardiovascular System

The circumference of a newborn's chest is equivalent to the head circumference. Inspection of the chest may reveal malformations such as *pectus carinatum* (protruding xiphisternum or xiphoid process, also called pigeon chest) or *pectus excavatum* (funnel chest). Bulging or asymmetry of the chest wall usually indicates an important pathologic condition, such as enlargement of the heart, pneumothorax, phrenic nerve damage, or diaphragmatic hernia.

The point of maximal cardiac impulse (PMI) is the position on the chest wall at which the cardiac impulse can be maximally seen. The PMI is usually seen in newborns because of the relatively thin and flexible chest wall. Typically, the PMI is relatively close to the sternal border because of the predominance of the right ventricle in the fetal period. A mediastinal shift due to a pneumothorax will move the PMI away from the affected side of the chest.

With suspected pneumothorax, perform transillumination of the chest wall, using a high-energy flashlight or fiberoptic device in a darkened room. Place the light source on the chest wall of the suspected side. A large pneumothorax will reveal an excessively pink and illuminated, usually irregular area of light, or "glowing" area, through the chest wall when compared with the contralateral side.

Heart rate variations from 120 to 170 beats/minute may be normal depending on gestational age, as discussed earlier. The rapid rate and rhythm of heart sounds make them difficult to determine. Neonates have a high incidence of arrhythmias in the first few days of life. From 1% to 5% of all newborns exhibit some disturbance in heart rate or rhythm.[10] Many demonstrate

TABLE 5-3

Signs of Respiratory Distress in the Neonatal Patient

	Apnea	Tachypnea	Refractions	Grunting	Nasal Flaring	Stridor	Cyanosis	Breath Sounds	Other Clinical Findings
Respiratory distress syndrome		++	++	++	++		+	Decreased, rales	Premature infants, infants of diabetic mothers
Pneumothorax		++	+	+	+		+	Decreased, asymmetric	Asymmetry of the chest, PMI shifted
Pneumonia	+	++	++	++	++		+	Rales and rhonchi	
Upper airway obstruction	+	±		++		++			Gasping or labored breathing
Diaphragmatic hernia		++		+	++		++	Bowel sounds in chest	Scaphoid abdomen, often associated with pneumothorax
Meconium aspiration	+	++	++	+	+		+	Decreased	Hyperexpansion of chest, atelectasis, pneumothorax
Transient tachypnea		++	+	+	+			Fine rales	Resolves in <24 hr
Apnea of prematurity	+++	±	±				±	Normal	Bradycardia

PMI, Point of maximal cardiac impulse.

"dropped beats," which on evaluation are premature atrial contractions. These episodes are usually benign, but any newborn with an irregular rhythm should have an electrocardiogram performed to assess the arrhythmia.

Cardiac murmurs are described as a soft to loud, harsh sound similar to a forcible exhalation with the mouth open. Many heart murmurs are transient and not associated with anomalies. Murmurs may be normal after birth and associated with the acute angle at the pulmonary artery bifurcation, patent ductus arteriosus, or tricuspid regurgitation. However, some murmurs are associated with congenital heart malformations and must be evaluated by chest radiography and echocardiography.

The heart size, shape, and thoracic positioning on chest X-ray film are often helpful in assessing infants with congenital heart disease. Investigate any uncertainty in the variations from a normal radiograph by using other diagnostic radiographic techniques. Other examination procedures, such as a four-limb blood pressure determination, may help to identify anomalies.[11]

Palpating the pulses of the quiet infant often provides important diagnostic information. Weak pulses suggest low cardiac output states such as shock and hypoplastic left-sided heart syndrome. Bounding pulses are seen in infants with patent ductus arteriosus and left-to-right shunt (see Chapter 31, Sudden Infant Death Syndrome and Sleep Disorders). The bounding characteristic of the pulse results from rapid runoff of the blood into the low-resistance pulmonary circulation. This lowers the systolic blood pressure and produces a wider pulse pressure. Brachial and femoral pulses should be equal in intensity and felt simultaneously. A delayed or weak femoral pulse can indicate coarctation of the aorta.

Comparison of upper and lower extremity blood pressures is frequently helpful in establishing this diagnosis. Normally, lower extremity blood pressure is slightly greater than the pressure in the upper extremities. The recognition and treatment of hypotension are particularly important to avoid complications, such as cerebral ischemic injury and intraventricular hemorrhage.[12] The range of normal blood pressures at various weights has been well established (see Table 5-1). In the absence of data, calculate an adequate mean blood pressure (MBP) as follows:

Adequate MBP = Gestational age (weeks) + 5

For example, an infant of 24 weeks of gestation should have an MBP of approximately 29 mm Hg, and a term newborn, 40 weeks of gestation, should have an MBP of approximately 45 mm Hg.

A pulse oximeter can provide valuable information in the evaluation of the cardiovascular system. Because the sensor of the pulse oximeter is applied to a distal extremity, the oximeter will display a low pulse rate and perfu-

sion signal as peripheral pulses and perfusion decrease. The cause of this poor perfusion must be determined. However, if the oximeter suggests decreased perfusion while central blood pressure remains normal, the cause may be volume depletion with compensatory peripheral vasoconstriction. In addition, placing pulse oximeters on preductal and postductal sites allows for assessing right-to-left ductal level shunting, as seen with persistent pulmonary hypertension of the newborn. In this case the right arm, or preductal site, will have a higher saturation, while the postductal site, or left arm and lower extremities, will have a lower saturation due to venous admixture occurring postductally.

Abdomen

Successful abdominal examination requires a calm and quiet infant. Observe the contour of the abdomen, and determine whether it is scaphoid (sunken anterior wall), flat, or distended. *Distention* is a significant finding characterized by tightly drawn skin through which engorged subcutaneous vessels can easily be seen. Distention can suggest a variety of pathologic conditions, including sepsis, obstruction, tumors, ascites, pneumoperitoneum, or necrotizing enterocolitis. *Enterocolitis* is a bowel infection characterized by sepsis, peritonitis, bowel perforation, and significant mortality.[13,14] Any of these conditions may cause elevation of the diaphragm and therefore compromise lung expansion.

A scaphoid, hollowed, or unusually flattened abdomen may be associated with congenital diaphragmatic hernia, in which abdominal contents are displaced into the chest through a defect in the muscular diaphragm.[15] More noticeable abnormalities of the abdomen include *prune-belly syndrome,* which is a congenital lack of abdominal musculature (Figure 5-5); *omphalocele,* a protrusion of the membranous sac that encloses abdominal contents through an opening in the abdominal wall

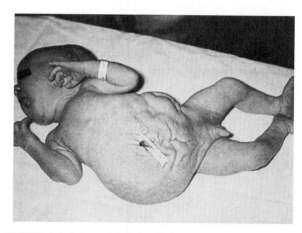

FIGURE 5-5 Infant with prune-belly syndrome.

into the umbilical cord; and *gastroschisis,* a defect in the abdominal wall lateral to the midline with protrusion of the intestines.[13,16]

When examining the abdomen, auscultate and palpate over all four quadrants. Bowel sounds are usually heard over the entire abdomen, generally described as a "tinkling" or "rumbling." Because bowel sounds are not continuous, it may take several seconds to hear them. Decreases or increases in the amount or changes in the characteristics of bowel sounds may indicate a pathologic abdominal condition.

The liver is usually felt as a rounded edge that rolls under the lightly palpating hand. Palpation should begin in the right lower quadrant so that an enlarged liver is not missed. The liver edge is usually easily defined 1 to 2 cm below the right costal margin in newborns. Hepatomegaly may be associated with congenital heart disease, infection, or hemolytic disease.[17] The spleen tip can sometimes be felt overlying the stomach. An easily palpable spleen more than 1 cm below the costal margin may indicate infection and requires further investigation. Abnormalities of the renal system are the most common cause of palpable abdominal masses in the newborn period. Normally the kidneys are felt on deep palpation.

The umbilical cord is yellowish white with three blood vessels. The two small and thick-walled arteries and one large and thin-walled vein are easily visible at the end of a freshly cut cord. Wharton's jelly surrounds the vessels. A single umbilical artery suggests congenital anomalies, especially those of the urinary tract. The presence of meconium in the amniotic fluid causes a greenish yellow staining of the umbilical cord. The umbilical cord of an infant who is large for gestational age and born to a diabetic mother is frequently large and fat. Conversely, infants with intrauterine growth retardation often have thin cords with little Wharton's jelly. With an umbilical hernia the intestinal muscles do not close around the umbilicus, and the intestines protrude into this weakened tissue. Such a defect may require surgery or may resolve without intervention as the muscles become stronger.

Head and Neck

The head is usually the presenting part and often shows evidence of bruising and molding as a result of pressures exerted during the birth process. Molding of the skull with overlapping cranial bones is common. In term infants the molding should resolve within a few days. The *fontanels* are the nonossified areas between the cranial bones that make up the skull. The fontanels and suture lines should be soft and should not bulge.[18] *Craniotabes* are soft skull areas that can be compressed like a ping-pong ball and may be a normal finding, especially in premature infants. However, congenital syphilis is also associated with craniotabes.

Any evidence of edema under the scalp should be examined carefully, especially in infants having vacuum or forceps-assisted delivery. Three different types of scalp edema occur. *Caput succedaneum,* the most common and least severe type, is an accumulation of serosanguineous fluid in the subcutaneous tissues just below the skin. It is movable across suture lines and generally resolves within 48 to 72 hours. The second type, *cephalhematoma,* is an accumulation of blood between the skull bone and the periosteum. It does not cross suture lines, bleeding is limited, and it resolves within 2 weeks to 3 months. The third type and most rare, *subgaleal hemorrhage,* occurs when the emissary veins that drain the scalp into the superior sagittal sinus are torn. A large amount of blood, potentially extending from the eyes to the nape of the neck, accumulates under the scalp. Blood loss may occur fairly rapidly after delivery and be sufficient to cause hypovolemic shock. Any infant suspected to have a subgaleal hemorrhage should have careful monitoring of head circumference and hemoglobin, hematocrit, and platelet measurements at least every 4 hours until values have stabilized. These infants may require fluid resuscitation and administration of blood products.[19,20]

More than 150,000 children are born with notable birth defects and syndromes in the United States each year.[21] Congenital anomalies are the leading cause of infant mortality in the postneonatal period. Unusual facies may suggest a number of distinct dysmorphic genetic syndromes. *Smith's Recognizable Patterns of Human Malformation* is an invaluable resource in the evaluation of infants with an unusual facies.[22] It also provides standard measurements for the newborn. Facial paralysis or an asymmetric facies is frequently noticed in the otherwise normal-appearing infant. Facial paralysis may be readily apparent only when the infant cries.

Unilateral facial paralysis is most commonly associated with birth trauma and forceps deliveries and occurs with an incidence of approximately 7.5 per 1000 live births.[23] This type of injury frequently resolves spontaneously, but until it does care must be taken to protect the eye on the affected side from desiccation.

The eyes are often swollen and edematous from the birth process. After resolution of the swelling, assess the eyes for excessive spacing and any unusual slant. Apply antibiotic ointment or silver nitrate to the eyes after delivery to prevent infection. In infants older than 28 weeks of gestation, the pupils should be round, regular, and should react to light. Examine the fundi of the eyes with an ophthalmoscope. In white infants the light ("cat's eye") reflex should be red. In Asian and black infants it is gray to yellow. A white reflex suggests cataracts or retinoblastoma, necessitating a complete ophthalmologic examination.

Examine the ears for placement and deformation. Deformed, posteriorly rotated, or low-set ears are associated with various genetic anomalies. Consider ears low set when the upper insertion of the ear is below the level of a line drawn through the corner of the orbits of the eyes. The ears are abnormally rotated if the slope of the auricle is greater than 10 degrees. The preauricular area frequently has tags containing cartilage. Although these tags are benign, they are a minor embryonic branchial cleft malformation. However, infants with preauricular tags have a higher incidence of additional branchial cleft abnormalities.

Newborns breathe preferentially through the nose; therefore alternately occlude each side and listen to breath sounds to assess the patency of each nostril. If the infant appears to be breathing comfortably, many nurseries no longer attempt to pass catheters because nasal trauma, obstruction, and edema are serious risks. An oral airway or endotracheal tube is often required if *bilateral choanal atresia,* the incomplete opening into the nasopharynx due to membranous or bony structures, is present.

Abnormalities of the mouth, lips, and oral cavity are seen in many infants. *Microstomia,* small mouth, is commonly seen in infants with the chromosomal defect trisomy 18, whereas midfacial clefts, cleft lip and palate, are frequently seen with trisomy 13. *Pierre Robin syndrome* is characterized by a cleft palate, posteriorly displaced tongue, and *micrognathia,* a small lower jaw. An artificial airway may be required in this condition to ensure an unobstructed airway. In previous years these infants were all thought to be congenitally mentally impaired. However, chronic hypoxia from airway obstruction has been recognized as a significant contributor to the retardation in these infants.[24]

Examination of the oral cavity and pharynx for less obvious palatal clefts, mucous cysts, Epstein's pearls, or natal teeth can be performed with a flashlight or laryngoscope blade light. A bifid uvula or no uvula can occur in normal infants but is often associated with a hidden cleft of the soft palate. A high-arched or cleft palate is associated with many syndromes. Excessive oral secretions may indicate the presence of a *tracheoesophageal fistula* (an abnormal connection between the trachea and the esophagus) or *esophageal atresia* (a blockage of the esophagus).

Examine the neck for obvious shortening, vertebral anomalies, or limitations in movement. A variety of cysts, *hygromas* (sacs of fluid resulting from a blockage in the lymphatic system), sinuses, and masses may be present laterally or at the midline. Large neck lesions may apply pressure to the trachea and impair breathing.

The clavicles are often broken during the delivery of large infants with *shoulder dystocia* (difficult delivery owing to the fact that the anterior shoulder of the infant cannot pass below the mother's hip bone) or in breech deliveries. Frequently the injury is noted when the infant refuses to move the affected shoulder. The break is usually easily palpable as an area of crepitus overlying the bone. Therapy is usually not necessary for fractured clavicles in the newborn because they heal without intervention.

Musculoskeletal System, Spine, and Extremities

The intrauterine environment frequently affects the extremities and musculoskeletal system. Many limb and other deformations in the fetus result from intrinsic (fetal) or extrinsic (uterine) factors.[22]

Extra digits may be familial or may be associated with a number of syndromes. They can be present on hands or feet, or both. The digits can vary from fully formed and articulated to simple skin tags. Variations in dermatoglyphic patterns, such as skin folds, palm print, and fingerprint, are frequently noted. The most widely known is the *simian crease,* a single transverse crease across the palm instead of the usual two creases. Simian creases are seen in several disorders, including Down syndrome, but are also found in 5% to 10% of normal individuals.

Joint contractures or abnormal positioning of one or more limbs may result from a fetal problem or intrauterine compression. Clubfoot, *talipes equinovarus,* is a typical example.[25,26] An isolated joint-extremity malformation suggests extrinsic factors, whereas multiple deformations are more often seen with primary fetal neurologic or muscular diseases.

The symmetry and bony structure of the spine are easily examined in the newborn. Suspend the infant in a prone position with one hand, then visually and digitally evaluate the structures. Many infants have a small indentation (sacral dimple) near the end of the spine. If the bottom of the dimple is easily seen without associated bony defects, no further evaluation is required. However, if the defect cannot be fully visualized or if there are bony defects, associated tufts of hair, or drainage of clear fluid, further evaluation is required. A few infants have the congenital malformations collectively called *spina bifida* (Figure 5-6). These defects result from failure of the embryonic neural tube to form correctly in the third to fifth week of gestation. The defects usually involve bone, skin, the covering of the central nervous system *(meninges),* and nerve tissue. Defects that occur over the spine are called *myelomeningoceles* (Figure 5-7), and those involving the brain are called *encephaloceles.*

It is important to evaluate the hips of all infants even if there is no evidence of asymmetry or other bone, joint, or muscular problems. Stabilize the pelvis on a flat

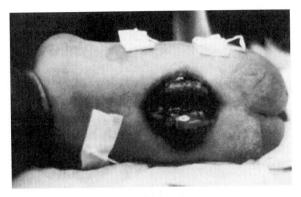

FIGURE 5-6 Infant with an open spinal defect.

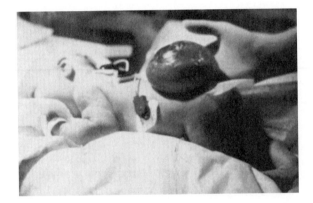

FIGURE 5-7 Infant with myelomeningocele.

surface while the joint is flexed and abducted to the surface. A telescoping feeling or the presence of a "clunk" suggests congenital laxity or dislocation of the hip.[26] Frequently, several days must pass before the hips of infants born in the breech position can be appropriately evaluated.

Cry

After the examiner has obtained some newborn experience, it is impressive how much information something as simple as a baby's cry can provide. A loud and vigorous cry is usually a sign of a healthy infant. A moaning, weak, or faint cry suggests serious illness. Frequently, an infant with respiratory distress syndrome strains with a grunting cry. An infant with a piercing, high-pitched cry often has a neurologic injury, drug withdrawal, or increased intracranial pressure. Hoarse crying can be associated with laryngeal edema, as in recently extubated infants. However, a hoarse cry may also be heard with congenital hypothyroidism, cretinism, or hypocalcemia with laryngospasm. Perhaps the most distinctive cry is associated with a deletion of the short arm of the fifth chromosome. The catlike cry of these infants gives the syndrome the name *cri du chat,* French for "cry of the cat."

NEUROLOGIC ASSESSMENT

The general neurologic state of the infant is assessed during much of the physical examination. Note whether the infant responds appropriately to its surroundings or is lethargic or overly irritable. It is also important to determine whether the infant moves all extremities and whether the movements are symmetric and smooth or jittery and jerky. Infants with evidence of difficult delivery may manifest signs of extremity weakness associated with trauma to the brachial plexus.

Pick the neonate up under the arms to assess muscle tone in the term infant. A normal infant will suspend well. An infant with decreased tone will noodle through the hands. Infants with normal tone will maintain their extremities in a flexed position at rest.

A number of reflexes are present in the newborn. Everyone has observed the *grasp reflex,* in which the newborn infant grasps a finger placed in the palm of the hand. A similar downward curving of the toes occurs if a finger is pressed against the sole of the foot; this is referred to as the *plantar grasp reflex.* The startle reaction to sound or touch is similar to the *Moro reflex,* which occurs when the head is allowed to fall back slightly. The normal term infant's extremities will extend rapidly with open hands. The neonate will then slowly flex them back toward the body. Infants will respond to a bright light by shutting their eyelids tight. They will often turn toward unique sounds or sights and may focus on objects, especially faces. Suspending the infant and touching the top of the foot against a surface can demonstrate the *stepping reflex*: the infant should lift the leg and then place it flat on the surface.[27]

Significant hearing loss at birth is common and if undetected can interfere with the development of speech and language. The American Academy of Pediatrics (Elk Grove Village, Ill) endorses hearing evaluation in the newborn period, using auditory-evoked brain wave responses or otoacoustic response.[28] Many physicians and hospitals routinely screen some or all infants before discharge.

LABORATORY ASSESSMENT

Routine laboratory studies play a limited but important role in the immediate newborn period. Most laboratory abnormalities seen in the first 24 hours of life result from sepsis, abnormally high or low levels of red blood cells, red blood cell isoimmunization, or temporary derangement in the regulation of glucose metabolism.

Infection is one of the most common problems in newborns. The diagnosis and initial therapy of neonatal sepsis are frequently based on clinical presentation and are seldom delayed until laboratory test results are available. The septic baby is often pale, mottled, or floppy. Some may lose interest in feeding, be slightly irritable, or even unresponsive. A typical sepsis evaluation includes blood cultures and a complete blood count. Many physicians also include lumbar puncture for cerebrospinal fluid and suprapubic aspiration for urine.[29] The advisability or necessity of these last two tests in the typical newborn is not clear.

The white blood cell (WBC) count of the newborn is usually significantly higher than pediatric or adult values. *Leukopenia*, WBCs less than 3500/mm³, and *leukocytosis*, WBCs greater than 25,000/mm³, suggest infection. WBCs greater than 25,000/mm³, however, are not unusual in the immediate newborn period. A number of investigators have studied ratios of immature to total granulocytes and have suggested that ratios greater than approximately 0.2:1 are predictive of infection. Similarly, the absolute number of platelets is associated with fetal/neonatal infection. A platelet count of less than 150,000 cells/mm³ is abnormally low and is usually seen with acute or chronic infections. Platelets are also decreased in a widespread disorder of the clotting system called *disseminated intravascular coagulation*. Overstimulation of the coagulation system leads to depletion of many coagulation factors and a generalized coagulation abnormality.

The newborn infant tends to have increased *hemoglobin* and *hematocrit* levels at birth. The fetus requires extra hemoglobin to maintain appropriate oxygen transport in the relatively low oxygen pressure of the fetal environment. The newborn's hematocrit is affected by many factors, including gestational age, the presence of placental abnormalities, the speed and mode of delivery, and the length of time after delivery that the infant remains attached to the placenta (with or without cord stripping by the obstetrician). Table 5-4 lists the range of normal values for newborns.

TABLE 5-4
Laboratory Values in the Neonatal Patient

Age	HGB (g/dl)	HCT (%)	WBCs (× 1000 cells/mm³)	PLATELETS (× 1000 cells/mm³)
28 wk of gestation	14.5	45	—	275
32 wk of gestation	15	47	—	290
Term newborn	16.5	51	18.1	310
1-3 days	18.5	56	18.9	300

Hgb, Hemoglobin; Hct, hematocrit; WBCs, white blood cells.
Data from Oski FA, Naiman JL: *Hematological problems in the newborn infant*, Philadelphia: WB Saunders; 1981.

Box 5-1 **"Red Flags" in Neonatal Patients**

RESPIRATORY
- Respiratory rate greater than 60 breaths/minute
- Grunting or retractions
- Cyanosis
- Apnea

CARDIAC
- Heart rate greater than 170 beats/minute, or less than 90 beats/minute
- New heart murmur
- Cyanosis
- Hypotension
- Decreased or no pulse

RENAL
- Edema
- Anuria (no urine)
- Oliguria (decreased urine output)
- No urine in first 24 hours

GASTROINTESTINAL
- Abdominal distention
- Bile-stained vomitus
- Abdominal mass
- Bloody stools
- Failure to pass stool in first 48 hours

METABOLIC
- Vomiting
- Diarrhea
- Jitteriness
- Seizures
- Jaundice on first day
- Hypoglycemia

GENERAL
- Lethargy
- Poor feeding
- "Not acting right"
- Floppy
- Cord blood pH less than 7.2
- Low Apgar score
- Small for gestational age
- Large for gestational age
- Minor congenital anomalies

Modified from Ackerman NB, Curran JS: The newborn. In Kaye R, Oski FA, Bainars LA, editors: *Textbook of pediatrics*, Philadelphia: Lippincott; 1988.

A number of biochemical and metabolic evaluations are performed in neonates. Electrolyte determinations, renal function tests, and calcium levels are typically measured after the first 12 to 24 hours of life in sick or at-risk neonates. There is little value in performing these measurements earlier because the infant's serum levels reflect those of the mother at birth. Conversely, glucose measurements are important for many infants in the first minutes to hours of life. Many newborns are at risk for hypoglycemia, and screening is performed routinely in most nurseries. Bilirubin should be measured in infants who are significantly jaundiced. Some hospitals routinely perform blood typing on cord blood and Coombs' tests to determine whether there is evidence of neonatal RBC hemolysis from maternal antibodies.

All states operate newborn programs that mandate mass screening of all newborns for uncommon metabolic diseases. These programs have proved effective in preventing mental retardation associated with unusual metabolic diseases such as congenital hypothyroidism.

Box 5-1 lists clinical symptoms, laboratory abnormalities, and physical signs that may be found in newborns. These "red flags" should alert the examiner and clinician to investigate further.

ASSESSMENT QUESTIONS

See Evolve Resources for answers

1. The ideal time to assess the gestational age of a newborn is
   A. Within the first 30 minutes after birth
   B. Within the first hour of life
   C. Within the first 12 hours of life
   D. Within the first 24 hours of life
2. Ideally, gestational age is evaluated on the basis of
   A. The gestational duration since the mother's last menstrual cycle
   B. Prenatal ultrasound evaluations
   C. The Ballard scoring system
   D. All of the above
3. Normal axillary temperature for a newborn is _____ ±1 °F.
   A. 95.6
   B. 96.6
   C. 97.6
   D. 99.6
4. Normal capillary refill time for a newborn should be less than _____ seconds.
   B. 1
   C. 3
   D. 5
   E. 10

ASSESSMENT QUESTIONS—cont'd

5. Choose the *incorrect* statement below:
   A. Mild to moderate jaundice that appears shortly after birth on the first day is considered normal.
   B. A central hematocrit of 65% or greater is diagnostic of polycythemia or neonatal hyperviscosity syndrome.
   C. Especially abundant vernix caseosa is suggestive of a preterm infant.
   D. Yellow-green staining of skin, nails, and umbilical cord is suggestive of prenatal exposure to meconium-stained amniotic fluid.
6. Apnea is a pathological condition in which breathing ceases for a period of _____ seconds or longer.
   A. 10
   B. 20
   C. 450
   D. 60
7. Signs of respiratory distress in a newborn include all of the following *except:*
   A. Vesicular breath sounds
   B. Grunting
   C. Nasal flaring
   D. Substernal retractions
8. An infant who shows femoral pulses that are significantly weaker than radial or brachial pulses should be evaluated for
   A. Patent ductus arteriosus
   B. Hypoplastic left heart syndrome
   C. Coarctation of the aorta
   D. Tetralogy of Fallot
9. Using the formula given in the text, the mean blood pressure of a 28-week gestation newborn should be at least _____ mm Hg.
   A. 28
   B. 33
   C. 40
   D. 50
10. Two pulse oximeter probes are placed on a newborn. One is on the right wrist and shows a reading of 95% on room air while the other one is placed on the left foot and shows a reading of 84% on room air. This is suggestive of
    A. Normal cardiopulmonary function
    B. Severe anemia
    C. Respiratory distress syndrome
    D. Significant shunting through a patent ductus arteriosus

Continued

ASSESSMENT QUESTIONS—cont'd

11. A full-term newborn infant demonstrates respiratory distress with breath sounds profoundly diminished on the left and a scaphoid or hollow appearance to the abdomen. This infant should immediately be evaluated for
  A. Diaphragmatic hernia
  B. Omphalocele
  C. Hypoplastic left heart syndrome
  D. Respiratory distress syndrome

12. The umbilical cord normally has _____ artery(ies) and _____ vein(s).
  A. 1 and 1
  B. 2 and 2
  C. 1 and 2
  D. 2 and 1

13. A newborn is observed to have a small, receding lower jaw, a tongue that seems large for the mouth, and a slight cleft palate, and is in respiratory distress. The most appropriate immediate action would be to
  A. Insert an appropriately sized oral airway
  B. Apply bag–mask ventilation with 100% O_2
  C. Continue to observe the infant, because there is little that can be done
  D. Place the infant in the prone position

14. The minimal platelet count for a newborn 24 hours old should be _____/mm³.
  A. 25,000
  B. 50,000
  C. 100,000
  D. 150,000

References

1. Donovan E et al: Inaccuracy of Ballard scores before 28 weeks' gestation, *J Pediatr* 1999;135:147.
2. Sanders M et al: Gestational age assessment in preterm neonates weighing less than 1500 grams, *Pediatrics* 1991;88:542.
3. Ballard JL et al: New Ballard score to include extremely premature infants, *J Pediatr* 1991;199:417.
4. Thomas P et al: A new look at intrauterine growth and the impact of race, altitude, and gender, *Pediatrics* 2000;106:e21.
5. Dunster K: Physiologic variability in the perinatal period, *Clin Perinatol* 1999;26:801.
6. Rosenkrantz T: Polycythemia and hyperviscosity in the newborn, *Semin Thromb Hemost* 2003;29:515.
7. Bhutani V et al: Noninvasive measurement of total serum bilirubin in a multiracial predischarge newborn population to assess the risk of severe hyperbilirubinemia, *Pediatrics* 2000;106:e17.
8. Rigatto H, Brady JP: Periodic breathing and apnea in preterm infants: hypoxia as a primary event, *Pediatrics* 1972;50:219.
9. Ackerman NB, Bell RE, DeLemos RA: Differential pulmonary auscultation in neonates, *Clin Pediatr* 1982;21:566.
10. Page J, Hosking M: An approach to the neonate with sudden dysrhythmia: diagnosis, mechanisms, and management, *Neonatal Network* 1997;16:7.
11. Monett ZJ, Moynihan PJ: Cardiovascular assessment of the neonatal heart, *J Perinat Neonatal Nurs* 1991;5:50.
12. Nuntnarumit P, Yang W, Bada-Ellzey H: Blood pressure measurements in the newborn, *Clin Perinatol* 1999;26:981.
13. Chahine A, Ricketts R: Resuscitation of the surgical neonate, *Clin Perinatol* 1999;26:693.
14. Reyes HM, Meller JL, Loeff D: Neonatal intestinal obstruction, *Clin Perinatol* 1989;16:85.
15. Thebaud B, Mercier JC, Dinh-Xuan AT: Congenital diaphragmatic hernia: a cause of persistent pulmonary hypertension of the newborn which lacks an effective therapy, *Biol Neonate* 1998;74:323.
16. Blakelock RT et al: Gastroschisis: can the mortality be avoided? *Pediatr Surg Int* 1997;12:276.
17. Thureen P et al: *Assessment and care of the well newborn*, Philadelphia: WB Saunders; 1999.
18. Popich GA, Smith DW: Fontanels: range of normal size, *J Pediatr* 1972;80:749.
19. Furdon S, Clark D: Differentiating scalp swelling in the newborn, *Adv Neonatal Care* 2001;1:22.
20. Davis DJ: Neonatal subgaleal hemorrhage: diagnosis and management, *Can Med Assoc J* 2001;164:1452.
21. Bodurtha J: Assessment of the newborn with dysmorphic features, *Neonatal Network* 1999;18:27.
22. Jones KL: *Smith's recognizable patterns of human malformation*, ed 4, Philadelphia: WB Saunders; 1988.
23. Levine MG et al: Birth trauma: incidence and predisposing factors, *Obstet Gynecol* 1984;63:792.
24. Dennison WM: The Pierre Robin syndrome, *Pediatrics* 1965;36:336.
25. Hashimoto BE, Filly RA, Callen PW: Sonographic diagnosis of clubfoot in utero, *J Ultrasound Med* 1986;5:81.
26. Fernach S: Common orthopedic problems of the newborn, *Nurs Clin North Am* 1998;33:583.
27. Majnemer A et al: A comparison of neurobehavioral performance of healthy term and low risk pre-term infants at term, *Dev Med Child Neurol* 1992;34:417.
28. Task Force on Newborn and Infant Screening, American Academy of Pediatrics: Newborn and infant hearing loss: detection and intervention, *Pediatrics* 1999;103:527.
29. Horns K: Neoteric, physiologic and immunologic methods for assessing early-onset neonatal sepsis, *J Perinat Neonatal Nurs* 2000;13:50.

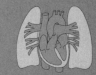

Chapter 6

Examination and Assessment of the Pediatric Patient

DENNIS E. SCHELLHAESE

OUTLINE

LEARNING OBJECTIVES

After reading this chapter the reader will be able to:
- Identify and use historical and physical findings to develop a differential diagnosis of a child's respiratory condition
- Determine the severity of a child's respiratory condition
- Communicate important historical and physical findings concerning a child's respiratory condition to the health care team in a timely manner
- Assist in planning and executing evaluation and management

PATIENT HISTORY

Despite numerous advances in laboratory testing, the ability to obtain a pediatric history and perform a physical examination well remains essential to the practice of pediatric respiratory care. Respiratory therapists (RTs) should be able to identify and use historical and physical findings to develop a differential diagnosis for a child with a respiratory condition, determine the severity of a child's respiratory condition, and communicate these findings to the health care team in a timely manner so that appropriate evaluation and management can be rapidly and effectively instituted. Input from the RT can be invaluable to the care of children in the intensive care unit, hospital ward, and outpatient clinic. In most encounters of children with respiratory conditions, the history provides the necessary information to formulate a differential diagnosis and suggest additional evaluation and management. Thus, the RT should spend considerable effort enhancing history-taking skills.

The history for a new patient can be divided into the following categories:

- Chief complaint or primary concern
- History of the present illness (HPI)
- Past medical history (PMH)
- Review of symptoms (ROS)
- Family history
- Social and environmental histories

The history for a follow-up or established patient can be modified to include interim health history and review of key components of the PMH, ROS, and social and environmental histories. A careful and detailed history often suggests further evaluation and management or results in changes in the course of therapy.

Chief Complaint

The *chief complaint* consists of the reason the child presents for health care. The chief complaint may simply be a symptom or sign observed by the child or caregivers and in need of further evaluation, as in the case of a new patient who presents for the evaluation of cough and/or chest pain. The chief complaint may also be a specific established diagnosis as in the case of a child admitted to the hospital for treatment of acute asthma or a pulmonary exacerbation of cystic fibrosis (CF). For a new patient, the initial step is to establish the chief complaint or primary concern. Additional information in the form of a medical history is then sought to further elucidate and clarify historical findings that point to either a specific diagnosis or set of diagnoses (differential diagnosis) that then leads to further evaluation (physical examination, laboratory testing).

New Patient History

For a new patient, the medical history consists of specific components including the HPI, PMH, ROS, family history, and social and environmental histories (Box 6-1). Important components of the HPI include duration, intensity or severity, and improvement or deterioration of symptoms. Knowledge of the following may help point to a specific disease or narrow the differential diagnosis:

- Triggers of symptoms
- Aggravating or alleviating factors
- Medications that have previously or are currently being used and whether or not these medications have been helpful
- Chronicity
- Recurrence or seasonality of symptoms

Review of current medications, including nonprescription and alternative medications, dosing, when and how taken, as well as what the medications are taken for, may provide useful information.

Important components of the PMH that may contribute to establishing a diagnosis include the following:

Box 6-1	New Patient History

CHIEF COMPLAINT OR PRIMARY REASON FOR VISIT

HISTORY OF PRESENT ILLNESS
- Duration
- Intensity or severity
- Improvement or deterioration
- Triggers
- Aggravating or alleviating factors
- Medications (past and current)
- Chronicity
- Seasonality

PAST MEDICAL HISTORY
- Perinatal history
- Acute care and emergency room visits
- Hospitalizations and surgeries
- Immunizations
- Previous evaluations

REVIEW OF SYMPTOMS
FAMILY HISTORY
SOCIAL AND ENVIRONMENTAL HISTORIES

- History of prematurity
- Birth weight
- Need for and duration of oxygen therapy, assisted ventilation, or both in the neonatal period
- Previous emergency room visits, hospitalizations, or both for respiratory disturbances (including intensive care unit admissions and any need for assisted ventilation)
- Previous surgeries
- Immunization history

Results of previous evaluations may also provide important diagnostic clues.

The ROS attempts to identify symptoms that were not identified in the HPI and that may be related or contribute to the child's underlying respiratory condition. A systematic review of symptoms in the following categories may suggest contributions of atopic diseases, gastroesophageal reflux, immunodeficiency, as well as thoracic cage, neurologic, and neuromuscular disorders to the presenting pulmonary complaint:

- Allergic
- Dermatologic
- Developmental
- Gastrointestinal
- Immunologic
- Otolaryngologic
- Musculoskeletal
- Neurologic
- Neuromuscular

The family history may also provide valuable information. Important conditions in the biological parents, siblings, and other close relatives to ask about include the following:

- Presence or absence of asthma
- Chronic or seasonal bronchitis
- Atopic diseases
- Recurrent pneumonia
- CF
- Immunodeficiency
- Infertile males (may suggest CF)
- Tuberculosis
- Hemoptysis
- Early childhood serious illnesses or deaths
- Congenital heart disease
- Dextrocardia (heart situated on the right side of the body)
- α_1-Antiprotease deficiency

Important components of the social and environmental histories include the following:

- Who the child lives with
- Who assists the child with medications and therapies
- Level of adherence to medications and therapies
- Occupations of the caregivers
- Housing conditions
- Environmental tobacco smoke exposure
- Personal smoking
- Presence of visible mold
- Pets in the home
- Other significant exposures
- Use of day care
- School grades and performance
- Participation in and any difficulties with extracurricular activities

Where the child lives, adult visitors from areas of endemic tuberculosis, and recent travel history may also suggest unsuspected exposures or diseases; for example, pulmonary blastomycosis should be included in the differential diagnosis of a child with unresolving pneumonia who is from southern Arkansas.[1]

Follow-up or Established Patient History

For a follow-up or established patient, the medical history is not usually focused on developing differential diagnoses or establishing a specific diagnosis, but rather on determining current lung health and whether there have been any changes since the last visit. In this situation, the medical history consists of an interim history and review of key components of the PMH, ROS, and social and environmental histories (Box 6-2). Questions are directed to determining whether there were any interim respiratory infections or exposures and whether these triggered exacerbation of the primary disease.[2] Exposure to environmental tobacco smoke should be asked about specifically.[3] If an exacerbation of the primary disease occurs, did this

Box 6-2	Follow-up or Established Patient History

CHIEF COMPLAINT AND/OR PREVIOUS DIAGNOSIS OR PROBLEM
INTERIM HISTORY
- Respiratory infections
- Exacerbations of primary disease
- Triggers and/or exposures
- Quality of life
- Medications

REVIEW OF KEY COMPONENTS
- Past medical history
- Review of symptoms
- Social and environmental histories

exacerbation lead to a clinic visit, emergency room visit, or hospitalization or were the caregivers able to manage the exacerbation at home? Information concerning the presence or absence of allergic, nasal, respiratory, or gastrointestinal symptoms is sought. If symptoms are present, are they better or worse than at the previous visit? Are new symptoms present and are these related to the primary disease? Quality of life issues should be explored. Missing school, inability to participate in normal daily and physical activities, or the caregiver(s) missing work because of an increase in the child's respiratory symptoms suggests that disease management is less than optimal. Review of current medications, including nonprescription and alternative medications; dosing; when and how taken; what the medications are taken for; and whether or not there have been changes in medications, dosing, or both since the previous visit, also yields important information. Adherence with and understanding of the treatment plan should be explored. Changes in school and family situations; exposure to environmental tobacco smoke, allergens, and airway irritants; as well as recent travel or exposure to sick adults may also yield clues to changes in status of the primary disease. If an explanation of worsening or less than optimal control of the primary disease is not forthcoming, then the RT should take a more detailed history similar to the initial medical history.

PULMONARY EXAMINATION

The RT should also be proficient at performing a pediatric pulmonary examination. The setting in which an examination occurs determines the pace of the examination as well as the information gained. A child with respiratory distress may require rapid physical assessment and immediate institution of therapy. A crying child is almost impossible to examine. Efforts should be made to perform an examination in a calm, expeditious, and professional manner as well as in such a manner as not to upset the child. Examination of the small child in the caregiver's lap may be particularly helpful in allaying the child's fears and keeping the child calm. In general, the pulmonary examination includes inspection, palpation, percussion, and auscultation (Box 6-3) and begins at the initiation of contact with the child. All components of the pulmonary examination yield valuable information and the impulse to primarily or only use one's stethoscope should be avoided. Establishing a specific examination routine is helpful in assisting in completion of all the evaluation components and in increasing one's comfort and expertise in physical assessment of the child with respiratory disease.

Box 6-3	Pulmonary Examination

1. Inspection
   a. Vital signs
      i. Heart rate
      ii. Respiratory rate
      iii. Temperature
      iv. Oxygen saturation
   b. Respiratory distress
      i. Tachypnea
      ii. Breathlessness
      iii. Head bobbing
      iv. Grunting
      v. Nasal flaring
      vi. Retractions
   c. Chest wall
      i. Shape
      ii. Muscle mass and strength
      iii. Adipose tissue
2. Palpation
   a. Neck
      i. Masses or adenopathy
      ii. Trachea
   b. Chest
      i. Fremitus
      ii. Motion with deep breathing
3. Percussion
   a. Hyperresonance
   b. Dullness
4. Auscultation
   a. Audible
      i. Grunting
      ii. Stridor
      iii. Stertor
   b. Breath sounds
      i. Symmetry
      ii. Intensity
      iii. Location: lobes and segments
      iv. Phases: inspiration, expiration, or both
   c. Adventitious sounds
      i. Crackles: fine or coarse
      ii. Wheezes: low or high-pitched
      iii. Monophonic or polyphonic

Inspection

Inspection begins at the bedside with review of the child's vital signs and first contact with the child and caregiver. Vital signs of importance to the RT include heart rate, respiratory rate, temperature, and, if available, pulse oximetry. Initial inspection is directed to determining whether the child is in respiratory distress. A child in respiratory distress may display both nonpulmonary and pulmonary signs. Nonpulmonary signs of respiratory distress include anxiety, fussiness, irritability, depressed level of consciousness or responsiveness, and tachycardia. Pulmonary signs include tachypnea, breathlessness, head bobbing, grunting, nasal flaring, retractions, oxygen saturation less than 95%, and/or cyanosis. A child in severe respiratory distress requires rapid assessment and immediate institution of appropriate therapy. Inspection of the chest wall is done to evaluate for chronic obstructive lung, neuromuscular, and musculoskeletal diseases. Inspection for respiratory distress and of the chest wall is best done with the child's upper torso unclothed.

The respiratory rate can be a sensitive indicator of the severity of underlying lung disease.[4-6] Normal respiratory rates vary on the basis of age and activity level (Table 6-1). In general, the respiratory rate is best determined when the child is asleep or resting quietly.[7,8] In the ill-appearing child, the presence of fever may be a confounding factor that results in tachypnea proportional to the degree of fever and the appearance of respiratory distress. In the child with no underlying lung disease, relief of fever should result in resolution of tachypnea and apparent respiratory distress.

Head bobbing, nasal flaring, and grunting are common signs of respiratory distress in infants and young children and are compensatory mechanisms to decrease the work of breathing. *Head bobbing* occurs when the *sternocleidomastoids* (neck muscles that serve to flex and rotate the head), in an attempt to overcome decreased lung compliance, increased airway resistance, or both, contract during inspiration, pulling the head down and the clavicles and rib cage up (Figure 6-1). This results in the head bobbing forward in synchrony with each inspiration. *Nasal flaring* occurs during inspiration when the muscles of the nasal passages contract, resulting in flaring of the *alae nasi*, widening of the nostrils, and reduction in airway resistance. *Grunting* is an audible expiratory noise caused by closure of the glottis during expiration in an attempt to provide increased positive end-expiratory pressure and to maintain lung volume. The presence of one or more of these signs typically indicates significant airway obstruction and/or lung disease.

Suprasternal, intercostal, and subcostal/substernal retractions and asynchronous chest and abdominal wall motion are common signs of respiratory distress in both younger and older children and may be due to

TABLE 6-1

Normal Respiratory Rates in Sleeping and Awake Pediatric Patients

	SLEEPING			AWAKE		
	BREATHS PER MINUTE			BREATHS PER MINUTE		
Age	Number Studied	Mean	Range	Number Studied	Mean	Range
6-12 mo	6	27	22-31	3	64	58-75
1-2 yr	6	19	17-23	4	35	30-40
2-4 yr	16	19	16-25	15	31	23-42
4-6 yr	23	18	14-23	22	26	19-36
6-8 yr	27	17	13-23	28	23	15-30
8-10 yr	19	18	14-23	19	21	15-31
10-12 yr	11	16	13-19	17	21	15-28
12-14 yr	6	16	15-18	7	22	18-26

From Iliff A, Lee VA: Pulse rate, respiratory rate, and body temperature of children between two months and eighteen years of age, *Child Dev* 1952;23:237.

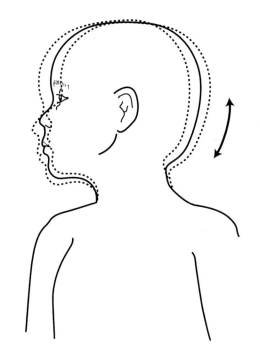

FIGURE 6-1 Head bobbing.

significant airway obstruction, lung disease, or both. *Retractions* result from the pulling in of the skin between and below the ribs, above the sternum in the suprasternal notch, or both, due to significant airway obstruction and/or lung disease (Figures 6-2, 6-3, and 6-4). Suprasternal retractions are also referred to as "tracheal tugging." In most circumstances, a direct correlation exists between the degree of retractions and the severity of respiratory distress. Infants, young children, and children with muscle weakness may develop paradoxical inward motion of the chest wall and concomitant outward movement of the abdominal wall (i.e., asynchrony of chest and abdominal wall, or "see-sawing"

motion) with increasing degrees of respiratory distress. In infants and young children this see-sawing motion occurs because of their compliant rib cage, whereas in older children with muscle disease it occurs because of weakness o f the abdominal wall musculature.

Inspection of the chest wall may reveal increased anteroposterior diameter, abnormal shape, muscular weakness, or obesity. Chest wall inspection should include anterior, posterior, and lateral examination. Chronic obstructive lung diseases such as severe asthma, advanced CF, and severe bronchopulmonary dysplasia may be associated with increased anteroposterior diameter of the chest, due to increased air trapping. The chest wall may be abnormally shaped such as in *pectus carinatum* ("pigeon breast"), *pectus excavatum* ("sunken chest"), *kyphosis* ("hunchback" appearance), and *scoliosis* (abnormal "sideways" spinal curvature). The chest wall may also be bell-shaped or have obvious rib abnormalities. Muscular weakness may result in decreased chest wall muscle mass, poor head control, or obvious weakness of the trunk, extremities, or both. Obesity may cause excessive deposition of adipose tissue around the neck, chest, and abdomen. Abnormal chest wall shape, muscular weakness, and obesity can result in significant restrictive lung dysfunction.

Palpation

Palpation of the chest wall and neck may be helpful in the physical examination of a child with respiratory disease. In infants and young children, palpation of the chest during quiet breathing may elicit *rhonchal* or *bronchial fremitus,* which are vibrations of the chest resulting from movement of air through airways partially obstructed by mucus. In an older child, palpation of the chest during normal speech may elicit *tactile fremitus,* vibrations of the chest produced by the spoken

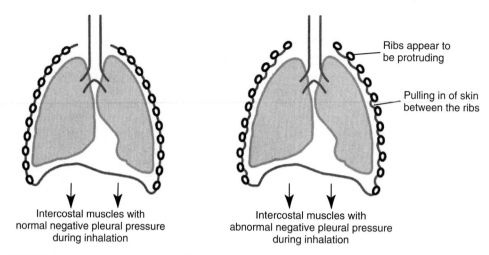

Ribs appear to be protruding

Pulling in of skin between the ribs

Intercostal muscles with normal negative pleural pressure during inhalation

Intercostal muscles with abnormal negative pleural pressure during inhalation

FIGURE 6-2 Intercostal retractions. Soft tissue between the ribs is pulled inward (retracted) because of the extremely high negative pleural pressure.

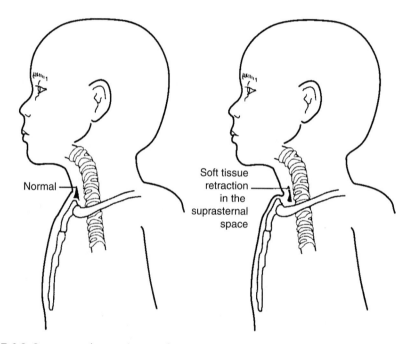

Normal

Soft tissue retraction in the suprasternal space

FIGURE 6-3 Suprasternal retractions. Soft tissue in the suprasternal space is retracted because of high negative pressure, most often caused by the patient's attempt to breathe against an airway obstruction.

voice. Tactile fremitus may be increased over areas of the chest wall corresponding to underlying pulmonary consolidation. In an older child, assessment of chest wall excursion can be accomplished by placement of the examiner's hands on both sides of the thoracic spine, with thumbs toward the spine, and observing the motion of the hands and patient's ribs during deep inspiration. Palpation of the anterior neck may be helpful in determining whether the trachea is in the midline (Figure 6-5) and whether there are masses or adenopathy compressing the trachea.

Percussion

Percussion of the chest wall may be helpful in the physical examination of an older child, but is typically unrewarding in the examination of an infant or younger child. Chest percussion is performed by tapping the finger of one hand with a finger of the other hand over corresponding areas of the patient's chest, usually while the patient is sitting upright. A relatively high-pitched percussion note, or *hyperresonance,* suggests focal or generalized air trapping or pneumothorax. A relatively dull percussion note indicates atelectasis, consolidation, or

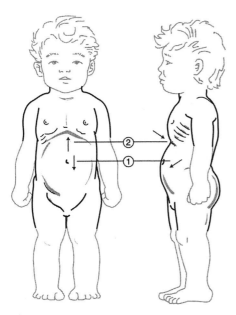

FIGURE 6-4 Subcostal/substernal retractions. Airway obstruction results in a pulling inward of the lower costal margins. The abdomen is protruding (*1*), and there is a sunken substernal notch (*2*). See-saw movement of the chest and stomach is also present.

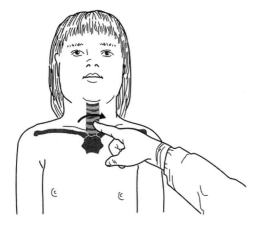

FIGURE 6-5 Technique for determining tracheal position in the older child.

pleural effusion. In the case of pleural effusion, changes in the level of the dull percussion note over time can be used to assess worsening or improvement.

Auscultation

Auscultation involves listening to the sounds of the heart, lungs, and gastrointestinal tract, sometimes with the ears alone but more generally with a stethoscope. Breathing is normally quiet, so that noises heard without the stethoscope or audible noises during "quiet" breathing are always abnormal. Grunting was previously discussed (see Inspection). Other audible noises include stridor, stertor,

and occasionally wheezing. Abnormal chest noises, or *adventitious sounds,* heard with the stethoscope include crackles and wheezes.[9-11] Stridor and wheezes are sometimes further described as *monophonic sounds*. Wheezes may also be described as *polyphonic sounds*. Monophonic sounds are usually associated with upper and central airway disorders and sound similarly throughout the chest. Polyphonic sounds are usually associated with small airway disorders and sound differently in different parts of the chest. Auscultation with the stethoscope should be done while the child is calm and quiet. Intensity and symmetry of breath sounds as well as duration of inspiration and expiration should be noted. Prolonged inspiration suggests extrathoracic (larynx and upper trachea) airway obstruction, whereas prolonged expiration suggests intrathoracic (lower trachea, mainstem bronchi, and smaller bronchi) airway obstruction.

Stridor is a high-pitched, monophonic, audible noise that may occur during inspiration or expiration, or may be biphasic.[12,13] Inspiratory stridor suggests extrathoracic airway obstruction, such as occurs in laryngomalacia, subglottic stenosis, and croup. Expiratory stridor suggests intrathoracic central airway obstruction, such as occurs in mass or vascular compression of the trachea, tracheomalacia, and bronchomalacia. Biphasic stridor typically indicates a more severe degree of laryngeal or central airway obstruction and may be associated with signs of respiratory distress. *Stertor* is a low-pitched, wet sound similar to snoring and suggests nasopharyngeal, oropharyngeal, and/or hypopharyngeal airway obstruction, such as occurs in adenotonsillar hypertrophy.[14] Audible wheezing may occur in asthma or in intrathoracic central airway obstruction and typically indicates a more severe degree of obstruction, and may be associated with signs of respiratory distress.

The classification of adventitious sounds is confusing. Most modern terminology primarily uses the terms *wheezes* for continuous sounds and *crackles* for discontinuous sounds.[9-11] Continuous sounds typically last for at least 250 milliseconds, whereas discontinuous sounds last for less than 20 milliseconds.[9] Wheezes can be further described as inspiratory, expiratory, monophonic, polyphonic, high-pitched, or low-pitched. Polyphonic high-pitched wheezes typically occur in asthma and as airway obstruction worsens wheezes tend to progress from end-expiratory, expiratory, to both expiratory and inspiratory sounds. The term *rhonchus* (plural, *rhonchi*) has also been used to describe a low-pitched wheeze and suggests movement of air through large airways partially obstructed by mucus. Crackles can be further described as inspiratory, expiratory, fine, and coarse. *Fine crackles* are less loud crackles with high-frequency components and short duration and are usually associated with distal small airway and/or alveolar diseases such as pneumonia or pulmonary edema. *Coarse crackles* are louder crackles with lower frequency and longer duration and are usually associated with medium and/or large airway disease such as bronchitis.[15] Where in the chest adventitious sounds are heard is also important to note and may suggest an etiology. Unilateral wheezes or wheezes heard over a specific segment or lobe suggest foreign body airway obstruction. Fine crackles heard over a specific segment or lobe suggest localized pneumonia.

NONPULMONARY EXAMINATION

In addition to examining the chest, a general examination should be done, including assessment of growth (weight, weight percentile, height, and height percentile) and examination of several other areas of the body including the eyes, ears, nose, throat, heart, abdomen, skin, and extremities for clues to underlying and/or contributing conditions (Box 6-4). Descriptions of many of the pathologic findings that may be found during a pediatric examination are outside the scope of this chapter and the interested reader is referred to other sources.[16] Conditions potentially associated with respiratory disease that can be detected during a general examination include significant poor growth, developmental delay, neurologic abnormalities or cerebral palsy, muscle weakness or atrophy, and adenopathy. Poor growth, manifested by weight, height, or both weight and height less than the 5th percentile for age, suggests a potentially serious chronic condition. Developmental delay, neurologic abnormalities, and muscle weakness or atrophy may result in ineffective cough, dysphagia with pulmonary aspiration, chest wall deformities, or restrictive lung dysfunction. Adenopathy may suggest immunodeficiency or an oncologic process.

Examination of the ears, eyes, nose, and throat, although usually performed by a physician, is part of the pulmonary examination and may reveal findings associated with a respiratory disease. Allergic disorders are suggested by the findings of serous otitis media; conjunctivitis; allergic shiners; Morgan-Dennie lines; nasal crease; nasal secretions; edematous, pale nasal mucosa; and posterior pharyngeal mucus (postnasal drip). Obstructive sleep apnea is suggested by severe tonsillar hypertrophy.

Cardiac dysfunction may contribute to or be the result of pulmonary dysfunction. Findings of an abnormal rhythm, murmur, gallop, and/or prominent second (pulmonic) heart sound during cardiac examination suggest cardiac dysfunction and should be noted.

Evaluation of the abdomen may reveal distention and/or hepatosplenomegaly that can be associated with CF or may result in impaired diaphragmatic excursion with resultant restrictive lung dysfunction.

Box 6-4 | Nonpulmonary Examination: Findings Possibly Associated With Pulmonary Disease

GENERAL
- Poor growth (weight, height, or both less than the 5th percentile for age)
- Developmental delay
- Neurologic abnormalities or cerebral palsy
- Muscle weakness or atrophy
- Adenopathy

EARS, EYES, NOSE, THROAT
- Serous otitis media
- Conjunctivitis
- Allergic shiners
- Morgan-Dennie lines
- Nasal crease
- Nasal secretions
- Edematous, pale nasal mucosa
- Tonsillar hypertrophy
- Posterior pharyngeal mucus (postnasal drip)

HEART
- Abnormal rhythm
- Murmurs or gallop
- Prominent second heart sound

ABDOMEN
- Distention
- Hepatosplenomegaly

SKIN
- Atopic dermatitis
- Urticaria
- Poor circulation
- Hemangiomas, telangiectasias
- Cyanosis

EXTREMITIES
- Digital clubbing
- Edema
- Arthritis

Inspection of the skin may reveal evidence of an allergic disorder such as atopic dermatitis and/or urticaria, cardiac dysfunction such as poor circulation and/or cyanosis, severe hypoxemia such as cyanosis, and/or lesions that suggest more generalized diseases with a pulmonary component such as hemangiomas (a benign tumor of blood vessel endothelial cells that may obstruct large airways or, if in the lung, result in right-to-left shunting of blood, causing hypoxemia) and/or telangiectasias (small dilated blood vessel malformations that if multiple or present in the nose may suggest hereditary hemorrhagic telangiectasia).

Inspection of the extremities may reveal evidence of cardiac dysfunction or hypoproteinemia, such as edema; immunologic disease, such as arthritis; or both. The

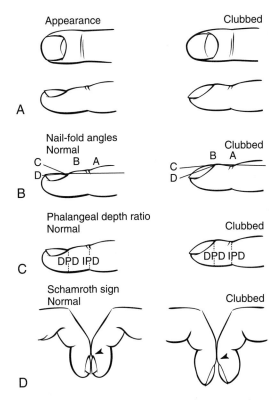

Appearance   Clubbed

A

Nail-fold angles
Normal   Clubbed
C   B   A   B   A
D   C
                                 D
B

Phalangeal depth ratio
Normal   Clubbed
DPD IPD   DPD IPD
C

Schamroth sign
Normal   Clubbed

D

FIGURE 6-6 A, Normal finger viewed from above and in profile, and the changes occurring in established clubbing, viewed from above and in profile. **B,** The finger on the left demonstrates normal profile (ABC) and normal hyponychial (ABD) nail-fold angles of 169 and 183 degrees, respectively. The clubbed finger on the right shows increased profile and hyponychial nail-fold angles of 191 and 203 degrees, respectively. **C,** Distal phalangeal finger depth (DPD)/interphalangeal finger depth (IPD) represents the phalangeal depth ratio. In normal fingers, the IPD is greater than the DPD. In clubbing, this relationship is reversed. **D,** Schamroth sign: in the absence of clubbing, opposition of the index fingers nail-to-nail creates a diamond-shaped window (arrowhead). In clubbed fingers, the loss of the profile angle due to an increase in tissue at the nail bed causes obliteration of this space (arrowhead).

finding of *digital clubbing* (Figure 6-6) in a child with any respiratory condition should strongly suggest chronic, potentially severe and life-threatening diseases such as CF, interstitial lung disorders, or other serious lung disorders. Although digital clubbing may be familial, it is also found in cyanotic congenital cardiac disease, infective endocarditis, cirrhosis, inflammatory bowel disease, and other infectious, neoplastic, inflammatory, and vascular disorders.[17] Thus, the finding of digital clubbing should always lead to additional laboratory evaluation.

LABORATORY TESTING

After completion of the history and physical examination, laboratory testing may be required for further diagnostic evaluation, objective quantification of

disease severity, assessment of previous management, or longitudinal follow-up (Box 6-5). Typically, diagnostic laboratory evaluation proceeds from noninvasive to invasive studies in a stepwise progression. Noninvasive diagnostic studies that may be considered for a child with a respiratory condition include chest radiography, pulmonary function testing (spirometry, lung volume determinations, DLCO [diffusing capacity of the lungs for carbon monoxide], bronchial challenge testing [exercise, cold air, and methacholine]), exercise desaturation testing, sweat chloride analysis, complete blood count, serum

---

Box 6-5   Laboratory Evaluation

1. Diagnostic
   a. Noninvasive
      i. Chest radiography
      ii. Pulmonary function testing (spirometry, lung volume determinations, DLCO, and bronchial challenge testing [exercise, cold air, and methacholine])
      iii. Exercise desaturation testing
      iv. Sweat chloride analysis
      v. Complete blood count
      vi. Serum immunoglobulins (IgG, IgA, IgM, and IgE)
      vii. Blood gas analysis (ABG, VBG, and CBG)
      viii. Allergy skin testing
      ix. Tuberculosis skin testing
      x. Sputum cultures (bacterial, fungal, mycobacterial, and viral)
      xi. Barium esophagography
      xii. Chest computed tomography
      xiii. Chest magnetic resonance imaging
      xiv. Overnight polysomnography
   b. Invasive
      i. Twenty-four–hour pH probe study
      ii. Rigid or flexible bronchoscopy
      iii. Lung biopsy (bronchoscopically directed, thoracoscopic, and open)
2. Assessment of disease severity, management, and follow-up
   a. Pulmonary function testing (spirometry, lung volume determinations, DLCO, and bronchial challenge testing [exercise, cold air, and methacholine])
   b. Exercise desaturation testing
   c. Sputum cultures (bacterial, fungal, mycobacterial, and viral)
   d. Chest radiography
   e. Chest computed tomography

ABG, Arterial blood gas; CBG, capillary blood gas; DLCO, diffusing capacity of the lungs for carbon monoxide; VBG, venous blood gas.

immunoglobulins (IgG, IgA, IgM, and IgE), blood gas analysis (arterial, venous, and capillary), allergy skin testing, tuberculosis skin testing, sputum cultures (bacterial, fungal, mycobacterial, and viral), barium esophagography, chest computed tomography, chest magnetic resonance imaging, overnight polysomnography, and so on. Invasive diagnostic studies that may be considered include a 24-hour pH probe study, rigid or flexible bronchoscopy, lung biopsy (bronchoscopically directed, thoracoscopic, and open), and others. Studies used to quantitate disease severity, to assess previous management, and/or for longitudinal follow-up include pulmonary function testing (spirometry, lung volume determinations, D$_{LCO}$, bronchial challenge testing [exercise, cold air, and methacholine]), exercise desaturation testing, sputum cultures (bacterial, fungal, mycobacterial, and viral), chest radiography, chest computed tomography, as well as others. Although pulse oximetry may be considered a laboratory evaluation in some clinical settings, because of its widespread availability it should be considered a vital sign.[18]

THE HEALTH CARE TEAM

Because of the complexity and severity of their respiratory disease and/or contributing disorders, many children with respiratory conditions require evaluation and management by a health care team, including the following:

- Physicians
- Nurses
- RTs
- Speech pathologists
- Physical and occupational therapists

The RT has unique opportunities during airway clearance, delivery of inhaled medications, or pulmonary function testing to contribute to the care of children with respiratory conditions by obtaining additional history and observing physical findings and then communicating these observations to the appropriate member of the health care team. Because children with respiratory conditions often have multiple encounters with the RT, the RT can make repeated observations of technique for delivery of inhaled medications and airway clearance and give encouragement to the child and caregiver for good technique or report any need for changes in technique to the appropriate member of the health care team. During the health care team's decision-making process regarding further evaluation and management, such information provided by an observant and caring RT often proves invaluable.

CASE STUDIES

CASE 1

A 6-year-old girl is brought by her mother to the pulmonary office because of recurrent pneumonia. This establishes the chief complaint. With only this information the RT faces an extensive differential diagnosis that might include CF, immunocompromise, aspiration, chronic infection, and asthma. Further questioning reveals that the child has had at least one episode of pneumonia in each of the last 4 years, usually in the winter months. Her symptoms during the acute illness include cough, fever, and dyspnea. Only one of the pneumonias resulted in hospitalization. The patient recovered completely between episodes.

At this point the RT needs to pursue additional history. The girl's growth has been good, and she does not have frequent gastrointestinal symptoms or greasy bowel movements, making CF less likely. Her mother is healthy and has no acquired immunodeficiency syndrome (AIDS) risk factors, making AIDS less likely. Each of the pneumonia episodes started with a common cold, often accompanied by wheezing. The patient has had occasional coughing when exposed to irritating smells such as cigarette smoke and cold air. During one emergency department visit, she received a nebulized medication, which greatly relieved her respiratory distress. These findings suggest that her primary disease might be asthma (Box 6-6).

The child has had no recognized exposure to tuberculosis and no foreign body aspiration history. She denies swallowing difficulty, frequent emesis (vomiting), or heartburn. She has had a red itchy rash in the elbow and knee regions in the past that her mother thinks is eczema. The patient has not had welts or hives (i.e., urticaria). The associated atopic history also points to asthma as the underlying explanation for the pneumonias.

Family History

The family history may also reveal valuable clues. In the case of this 6-year-old girl, her older brother was diagnosed with asthma as a young child; there was no recognized CF, infertile males, dextrocardia, immunodeficiency, or α$_1$-antiprotease deficiency. This further supports asthma as a potential cause of her recurrent pneumonia.

CASE 2

A 6-year-old patient with asthma was undergoing pulmonary function testing during a follow-up asthma clinic visit. She reported to the pulmonary nurse that her asthma had been under worse control over the past 2 months, especially during exercise and at night. The attending physician was prepared to prescribe a short course of oral prednisone and double the baseline dose of the inhaled corticosteroid. During administration of the inhaled bronchodilator as part of the pulmonary function test, the RT noticed that the metered-dose inhaler technique was quite poor (despite prior demonstration of correct technique). Further questioning identified that the spacing device prescribed to improve aerosol deposition had been "lost" several weeks ago. Neither the patient nor her family realized the significance of this loss. After discovering this, the RT told the asthma team about her concerns that neither the inhaled steroids nor the bronchodilators were likely to be optimally deposited in the lower airways. Rather than increase the patient's exposure to corticosteroids, inhaler technique was reviewed and another spacing device was prescribed. Both the patient and her mother were reeducated about the importance of adherence and the proper technique for use of a metered-dose inhaler and spacing device.

In this example, the RT's participation with the health care team helped avoid unnecessary additional medications.

CASE 3

A 28-month-old boy is admitted to the hospital for respiratory distress and pneumonia. During the initial assessment, the RT noted that the child is somewhat thin and anxious but sitting quietly in his mother's arms. The child's pulse is 140 beats/minute, respiratory rate is 52 breaths/minute, room air oxygen saturation is 91%, and he has mild intercostal retractions. Auscultation reveals diffuse fine crackles. The child does not have clubbing. The RT appropriately places the child on low-flow nasal cannula oxygen. Further history reveals that the boy has had recurrent cough since he was several months of age, several bouts of pneumonia, and recently has developed a productive cough and lost 3 pounds. The RT communicates these findings to the child's physician and asks if the child could have a chronic respiratory illness such as cystic fibrosis. After initiating appropriate immediate therapy, the physician obtains a sweat chloride analysis that is positive and refers the child to a nearby cystic fibrosis center for further evaluation and management.

In this example, the RT's brief assessment and recognition that the child not only had an acute respiratory illness but also a probable chronic pulmonary disease led to communication with the child's physician. This communication resulted in further diagnostic testing, leading to a diagnosis and referral to more specialized care.

Box 6-6 | **History Taking in the Pediatric Patient With Asthma**

MANIFESTATIONS
- Cough
- Wheeze
- Dyspnea
- Chest pain

AGGRAVATING FACTORS
- Upper respiratory tract infections
- Exercise or activity
- Allergens or exposures
- Irritants
- Emotions

ALLEVIATING FACTORS
- Bronchodilators
- Avoidance of aggravating factors

FAILED MEDICATION TRIALS (ANTIBIOTICS, DECONGESTANTS, HUMIDIFICATION, OTHER)

ASSOCIATED CONDITIONS (REVIEW OF SYMPTOMS)
- General: poor growth, activity intolerance
- Allergy/atopy: conjunctivitis, rhinitis, eczema, urticaria
- Gastrointestinal: dysphagia, dyspepsia, emesis, steatorrhea
- Pulmonary: recurrent pneumonia, foreign body aspiration
- Ear, nose, and throat: mouth breathing, snoring
- Exposure to infections: pertussis, tuberculosis, bronchiolitis, influenza, common cold

FAMILY HISTORY
- Allergic/atopic diseases: asthma, rhinitis, eczema, urticaria, food allergy
- Cystic fibrosis
- Infertile males (history of male infertility might suggest CF and need for further diagnostic testing)
- α_1-Antiprotease deficiency
- Dextrocardia
- Immunodeficiency states

ENVIRONMENTAL EXPOSURES
- Pets (cats, dogs, ferrets, hamsters, gerbils, birds, etc.)
- Tobacco smoke
- Visible household mold
- Areas of indoor dampness or water damage

ASSESSMENT QUESTIONS

See Evolve Resources for answers.

1. An 8 month old presents with head bobbing. The following is true about head bobbing:
   A. It usually suggests a brainstem lesion.

Continued

ASSESSMENT QUESTIONS—cont'd

   B. It is a voluntary action that can be stopped on command.

   C. It is best observed during crying.

   D. It usually suggests respiratory distress, airway obstruction, or decreased lung compliance.

   E. It is unrelated to cardiopulmonary disease.

2. Palpation of a patient's chest produces a vibration of the chest wall during quiet breathing *not* associated with the spoken voice. This suggests partial obstruction of the large airways by mucus. The name of this sign is:

   A. Fine crackles

   B. Rhonchal or bronchial fremitus

   C. Clubbing

   D. Pectus carinatum

   E. Stridor

3. An infant produces an audible noise that appears to be stridor. The following is true about stridor:

   A. It is a high-pitched, monophonic, audible noise.

   B. It may occur during inspiration or expiration, or may be biphasic.

   C. Patients with laryngomalacia or subglottic stenosis may have inspiratory stridor.

   D. Patients with a double aortic arch compressing the trachea, or tracheomalacia, may have expiratory stridor.

   E. All of the above.

4. A school-age child with acute asthma is undergoing examination. Auscultation should produce:

   A. Polyphonic, high-pitched inspiratory wheezes, expiratory wheezes, or both

   B. Fine crackles

   C. Stertor

   D. Inspiratory stridor

   E. Low-pitched wheezes or rhonchi

5. A teenager has a temperature of 38.5 °C, a respiratory rate of 28 breaths/minute, increased thoracic anteroposterior diameter, minimal subcostal retractions, and fine and coarse crackles heard over the right and left upper lobes. Further evaluation reveals mild digital clubbing of the fingers. This child probably has the following underlying disease:

   A. Asthma

   B. Gastroesophageal reflux

   C. Bilateral bronchomalacia

   D. Cystic fibrosis

   E. Acute respiratory distress syndrome

6. In the emergency room, the respiratory therapist is asked to give a 2 year old in respiratory distress an albuterol updraft. Prealbuterol assessment reveals a mildly uncomfortable afebrile child with a respiratory rate of 36 breaths/minute, mild subcostal retractions, and expiratory wheezes best heard over the right middle and lower lobes. Postalbuterol assessment is unchanged

ASSESSMENT QUESTIONS—cont'd

except that the respiratory rate is now 32 breaths/minute. A brief history reveals that coughing began abruptly several days ago and wheezing was noted this morning. The family has no history of atopic disease (allergic rhinitis, allergic conjunctivitis, asthma, or atopic dermatitis). This child was previously healthy with no history of chest disease. The respiratory therapist speaks with the attending physician and suggests that the child most likely has the following disorder/disease:

   A. Pneumonia

   B. Cystic fibrosis

   C. Foreign body aspiration

   D. Laryngeal cleft

   E. Double outlet right ventricle

References

1. Schutze GE et al: Blastomycosis in children, *Clin Infect Dis* 1996;22:496.
2. Glezen WP et al: Impact of respiratory virus infections on persons with chronic underlying conditions, *JAMA* 2000;283:499.
3. DiFranza JR, Aligne CA, Weitzman M: Prenatal and postnatal environmental tobacco smoke exposure and children's health, *Pediatrics* 2004;113:1007.
4. Morley CJ et al: Respiratory rate and severity of illness in babies under 6 months old, *Arch Dis Child* 1990;65:834.
5. Harari M et al: Clinical signs of pneumonia in children, *Lancet* 1991;338:928.
6. Margolis P, Gadomski A: Does this infant have pneumonia? *JAMA* 1998;279:308.
7. Iliff A, Lee VA: Pulse rate, respiratory rate, and body temperature of children between two months and eighteen years of age, *Child Dev* 1952;4:237.
8. Rusconi F et al: Reference values for respiratory rate in the first three years of life, *Pediatrics* 1994;94:350.
9. Loudon R, Murphy RL: State of the art: lung sounds, *Am Rev Respir Dis* 1984;130:663.
10. Mikami R et al: International symposium on lung sounds, *Chest* 1987;92:342.
11. Cugell DW: Lung sound nomenclature, *Am Rev Respir Dis* 1987;136:1016.
12. Eavey RD: A sound workup for evaluating airway obstructions, *Contemporary Pediatrics* 1986;3:78.
13. Tan HK, Holinger LD: How to evaluate and manage stridor in children, *J Respir Dis* 1994;15:245.
14. Cotton RT, Reilly JS: Stridor and airway obstruction. In Bluestone CD, Stool SE, Scheetz MD, editors: *Pediatric otolaryngology*, Philadelphia: WB Saunders; 1990, pp 1098-1111.
15. Piirila P, Sovijarvi AR: Crackles: recording, analysis and clinical significance, *Eur Respir J* 1995;8:2139.
16. Zitell BJ, Davis HW, editors: *Atlas of pediatric physical diagnosis*, Philadelphia: WB Saunders; 2002.
17. Myers KA, Farquhar DR: Does this patient have clubbing? *JAMA* 2001;286:341.
18. Mower WR et al: Pulse oximetry as a fifth pediatric vital sign, *Pediatrics* 1997;99:681.

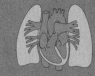

Chapter **7**

Pulmonary Function Testing and Bedside Pulmonary Mechanics

MICHAEL P. CZERVINSKE • MICHAEL A. GENTILE

OUTLINE

LEARNING OBJECTIVES

After reading this chapter the reader will be able to:

- Define the terminology and various abbreviations used in describing specific aspects of interpreting pulmonary function tests
- Describe the special considerations and limitations specific to neonates, infants, and children when performing pulmonary function tests or assessing respiratory function
- Appraise the standard and alternative instrumentation techniques available for pulmonary function testing of the newborn and the child
- Differentiate between the infant, child, and adult chest wall and pulmonary mechanics that affect correct interpretation of the pulmonary function data

- Compare the various techniques available for measuring airway function in both infants and children
- Compare the various techniques available for measuring lung volumes in both infants and children
- Explain the methods used to challenge, or provoke, the airways to assess more subtle lung function abnormalities or airway reactivity, and their role developing a treatment
- Describe the various tests and techniques used at the bedside to assess pulmonary function and lung mechanics in the spontaneously breathing and mechanically ventilated patient

Pulmonary function testing (PFT) is an objective measurement of the respiratory system under various conditions of normal, disease, and stress states. Pulmonary function measurements can be used as a primary diagnostic tool or, to frequently monitor disease progression by comparing previous or subsequent assessments.[1,2] PFT results corroborate a diagnosis suspected from the other components of the pulmonary assessment, primarily the patient history and physical examination.

The absolute values of PFT measurements change with growth and development of children; therefore using the percentage of predicted values best depicts pulmonary function over the long term.[3-5] Assessing whether a specific measurement is "normal" may be complex because of the wide range of variability in normal children and the relatively small number of children from whom the predicted norms have been gathered.[5-9] Despite these limitations, PFT measurements remain an integral component in evaluation and lengthy follow-up of children with pulmonary dysfunction over time. PFT measurements evaluate the degree of illness and quantitatively determine the efficacy of various therapeutic interventions.

The full range of pulmonary function tests includes assessing chest wall, lung, airway, and respiratory muscle performance, as well as gas exchange. These tests have traditionally been conducted in a laboratory setting with patient cooperation to determine maximal capability, for example, with physical exercise. Laboratory testing includes controlled measurement of lung compliance, airway resistance, and lung volumes and capacities.[5,6]

Bedside *pulmonary mechanics* (PM) studies apply PFT systems in the intensive care unit at the bedside to aid in mechanical ventilator management. Mechanical ventilators now provide the opportunity to measure and display airway graphics of pressure, flow, and volume on the ventilator screen. This provides real-time displays of PM studies and is useful when assessing the interaction between the ventilator and the patient. These measurements are used to optimize ventilator support and to reduce the potential complications of positive-pressure ventilation. Because of the differences in purpose, test conditions, and clinical application, PM studies at the bedside are differentiated from standard laboratory PFT studies.

DEFINITIONS

The terminology used to describe tests that are included in specific orders may vary across institutions. "Complete pulmonary function testing" may denote an extensive testing protocol at one institution or a more select group of tests at another. Similar variation exists for "lung function survey" and "pulmonary screening."

Therefore, clinicians need to be familiar with the specific testing protocols within their institution.

In this chapter, the term *spirometry* represents flow-volume or time–volume measurements. Spirometric measurements include forced vital capacity (FVC), forced expiratory volume in 1 second (FEV_1), the ratio of FEV_1 to FVC, forced expiratory flow at 25% to 75% of vital capacity (FEF_{25-75}), and forced expiratory flow at 50% of vital capacity (FEF_{50}). *Lung volume* describes the measurements of thoracic gas volume, functional residual capacity (FRC), residual volume (RV), total lung capacity (TLC), and the ratio of RV to TLC. Consider other measurements, such as carbon monoxide diffusing capacity, resistance or conductance, compliance, and maximal voluntary ventilation as separate tests. Sophisticated and seldom used tests are not addressed in this chapter, and more extensive texts for additional information are available.[1,2,9-13]

Bedside PFT refers to those tests often performed at the bedside, including tidal volume (V_T), vital capacity (VC), minute ventilation, peak expiratory flow rate (PEFR), and maximal inspiratory pressure. PM is the interaction of forces and physical principles that determine the characteristics of gas movement into and out of the lungs. Elasticity of the lung and chest wall, resistance to flow through the airways, and the action of the respiratory muscles (diaphragm, intercostal muscles, and accessory muscles) are measurable forces affecting ventilation. Volume, flow rate, duration, and frequency are characteristics of breathing. These measurements are typically performed at the bedside in the neonatal or pediatric intensive care unit.

SPECIAL CONSIDERATIONS

Neonatal Testing

A laboratory offering PFT for infants must be prepared to meet the special needs of these patients.[14] Infants, unlike older children and adults, are unable to voluntarily cooperate during PFT procedures. They may need to be lightly sedated in the laboratory for the 2 or 3 hours needed to complete a full set of studies. Some drugs may alter PM or the normal characteristics of breathing. Chloral hydrate is preferred by many laboratories because a dose of 50 to 75 mg/kg does not affect PM or respiratory pattern. Although normally a safe sedative for this purpose, using chloral hydrate when oxygen saturations are reduced increases the risk of respiratory distress.[15]

A face mask is required when testing neonates and infants. To ensure accurate testing, minimize both mask resistance and mask dead volume during measurement. Also exercise caution, because using a face mask can cause trigeminal nerve stimulation and induce vagal reflexes that may alter the pattern of heart or respiratory rhythm. All emergency supplies and equipment for infant resuscitation must be readily available in the laboratory area.

Pediatric Testing

The greatest obstacle to obtaining satisfactory pulmonary function measurements in children lies in enlisting their cooperation and effort. Clinicians who work predominantly with children develop their own unique systems for making children comfortable and eliciting an appropriate testing effort. Conversely, pulmonary function laboratories that have limited experience with children frequently do not obtain satisfactory cooperation, and therefore the test results are inconclusive and the information may not be useful.

There are several key factors common to successful approaches in performing PFT on children. The testing environment or laboratory should have a warm and friendly atmosphere with pediatric-oriented pictures and toys. Each portion of the testing procedure should be carefully explained at an age-appropriate level, and the child's participation should be elicited in a playful rather than a challenging fashion. For children undergoing their first PFT procedure, several efforts may be required before a satisfactory test is achieved. There is no substitute for patience and tolerance in this setting. Satisfactory performance can generally be achieved in the 5- or 6-year-old child, but some 8-, 9-, and 10-year-old children continue to have difficulty. Although uncommon, 3-year-old children may be able to do well, and good results have been reported more frequently among 4-year-old children. If the child is unable to perform satisfactorily at the first session, repeated attempts at subsequent visits should be encouraged, because most children learn quickly and frequently do much better at the next opportunity. Also, many software programs have visual aids to help make the breathing maneuvers a game, such as blowing out candles or blowing a boat across a lake.

Frequently, tests of younger children do not meet the American Thoracic Society (New York, NY) criteria for end of testing (a minim expiration time of 6 s with a volume change less than 30 ml over 1 s) and are discarded as clinically irrelevant. Although they may not be able to complete the end of testing criteria, small children can generate sufficiently reproducible results over multiple test efforts to guide clinical judgments and interpret the effectiveness of therapies.[16]

Instrumentation

Routine pediatric and infant PFT requires that certain technical obstacles be overcome. The use of computers and precision electronics surmounts many of these challenges, which include high respiratory rates, the need for low dead space in the airway connection, and accurate measurements of very small gas volumes. Current instrumentation employs rapid-response gas flow sensors that are easily calibrated, remain stable, and are accurate in a measurement range that extends to the gas volumes of the smallest newborns.[1,17]

The primary PFT measurements are gas volume and flow rates into and out of the lungs. A *pneumotachometer,* or "pneumotach," is a device that measures the rate of gas flow. Several types of pneumotachs are available as part of neonatal PFT systems. The most common type is called a *Fleisch pneumotach.* This device has been in use for many years with several variations, such as a fixed or variable orifice. However, all variations are based on the principle that an obstruction within a gas stream will cause a drop in pressure that is directly proportional to gas flow. Comparing gas pressure on both sides of the obstruction with a differential pressure transducer electronically converts the value to gas flow. Gas flow measured over a known time indicates *volume.* Importantly, with a pneumotach that uses a differential pressure transducer, any additional obstruction within the gas stream will cause a falsely high reading. Frequently, pneumotachs are internally heated to prevent water condensation when used for longer durations (Figure 7-1).

Another common type of flow measurement device is the *hot-wire anemometer.* This device incorporates a thin wire electrically heated to a high temperature, up to 400° F (204° C), and placed within a gas flow stream. As gas moves past the wire, it cools in proportion to the amount of gas in the stream and produces a flow reading that is converted electronically to volume. Some anemometers have two wires to determine the direction of gas flow.

Selection of Data for Analysis

Computerized infant PFT systems quickly provide a large amount of accurate data. However, not all information is clinically relevant. The clinician is still responsible for the ultimate task of deciding which information is valid and how to apply it in the care of the infant or child. Study results should be reproducible and consistent with other clinical data. Spontaneous and ventilator-assisted breaths have different mechanics and should not be included together in any study.

MECHANICS OF BREATHING IN NEWBORNS

With the first breaths of extrauterine life, a newborn must replace the in utero lung fluid with air. Surface tension forces in the fluid-filled lung require high negative pressure within the chest to establish normal

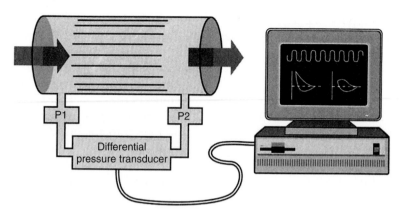

FIGURE 7-1 A pneumotachometer with a pulmonary function testing (PFT) computer system. As gas flow passes through the restrictive element, the difference in pressure between P1 and P2 is converted to a flow measurement. The flow rate over time is then converted to volume measurement.

air volume in the lungs. Newborns, particularly those born prematurely with respiratory distress syndrome, have low lung compliance. More pressure, or energy, is required to provide the normal amount of air volume brought into the baby's lungs with each breath. Because the newborn's ribs are mostly cartilage, the chest wall is flexible. With significant lung disease, the infant's chest wall may actually be more compliant than the lungs, causing *retractions,* in which the ribs and sternum distort inward during inspiration instead of expanding the lungs. The lung–thorax mechanical relationship is less of the traditional "bag in a box" analogy and more like a "bag in a bag."

The combination of *lung compliance* (C) and *airway resistance* (Raw) is the major force opposing inspiration, whereas *elastic recoil* is the force responsible for passive normal exhalation. When measured under static conditions (i.e., no gas flow into or out of the lungs), C is an assessment of the *elasticity (compliance) of the total respiratory system* (Crs).[18]

Lung Inflation and Transpulmonary Pressure

For both spontaneous and mechanically assisted breaths, the change in pressure within the airways is the driving force for gas movement into and out of the lungs. During spontaneous inspiration, moving the diaphragm and other muscles of ventilation expands the chest volume, which creates subatmospheric pressure in the thorax. During mechanically assisted breathing the ventilator applies positive pressure to the airways. Expiration is usually considered passive, but in fact the elastic recoil of the lungs and chest wall that causes gas movement out of the lungs requires energy.

Pulmonary mechanics are calculated by determining the change in pressure across the lung simultaneously with flow and volume measurements. During mechanically assisted ventilation, pressure in the airway is measured at the endotracheal tube. Gas flow and *airway pressure* are measured with a sealed face mask for spontaneous breathing studies. *Pleural pressure* may be approximated with a catheter placed in the esophagus.[18-20] The catheter is connected to a pressure transducer and either is filled with fluid or has an air-filled balloon at its tip.

Transpulmonary pressure is the pressure exerted on the lungs for gas movement; it is the difference between pleural and airway pressure. Pleural pressure measurements may not always be performed in assessing PM for ventilator–patient management. In general, under these circumstances, it is assumed that the pressure in the large airways equalizes to the distal airways in the lungs. In this case the compliance measurements are actually of the respiratory system, including the chest wall, rather than of the lungs alone.

NEONATAL PULMONARY FUNCTION TESTING IN THE LABORATORY

Measuring Static Compliance and Airway Resistance

Static compliance (Crs) describes the elastic properties of the total respiratory system. Crs is measured during no airflow, using the passive exhalation occlusion technique, and assesses elasticity of the respiratory system.[5,18,21] Volume and pressure are measured with a pneumotachometer at two points of a passive resting exhalation.

The airway is momentarily occluded at end inspiration by a shutter placed between the face mask and the pneumotachometer to stimulate the Hering-Breuer reflex. The occlusion creates an apneic pause and relaxes the respiratory muscles. Pressure is measured during the occlusion, and passive exhaled volume is measured after the shutter opens. Crs is calculated by dividing the total passive expiratory volume by the corresponding pressure change at the airway opening.

Airway resistance (Raw) reflects the nonelastic airway and tissue forces resisting gas flow. Raw is calculated from the ratio of airway occlusion pressure to expiratory flow. Raw is described in centimeters of water per liter per second (cm H_2O/L/s). Raw is dependent on the radius, length, and number of airways and varies with volume, flow, and respiratory frequency. The small diameters of an infant's tracheobronchial tree result in high resistance to gas flow. Airway irregularities; partial blocks caused by mucus, tumor, or foreign bodies; and partial closure of the glottis can also elevate Raw. The passive exhalation occlusion technique is noninvasive and can be performed with little disturbance to the infant.[22,23] However, infants with severe lung disease have an increased respiratory drive, and it may not be possible to induce a Hering-Breuer response.[5]

Raw measurements may be derived from body plethysmograph data, using a modified infant incubator as the enclosure. Since a pulmonary *plethysmograph* measures lung volumes, (FRC and TLC) measurements are acquired along with Raw.

Another method of determining Raw is to generate random noise signals at high frequencies at the mouth while the infant is breathing normal tidal breaths through a mouthpiece or mask. This technique is known as *forced oscillation* and measures the oscillation pressures compared with the flow and pressure measurements at the mouth. The forced oscillation technique is rapid, requires minimal patient cooperation, and helps optimize patient comfort.[23-25] As with the plethysmograph, forced oscillation also may be able to determine thoracic gas volume measurements, with minimal infant discomfort.

Crs and Raw measurements may be useful in patients
- Receiving diuretics for chronic lung disease such as bronchopulmonary dysplasia
- Undergoing high-frequency ventilation
- With meconium aspiration syndrome
- Subsequent to extracorporeal membrane oxygenation
- With respiratory syncytial virus infections and pneumonias
- With diaphragmatic hernia
- Receiving aerosolized bronchodilator therapy

Measuring Functional Residual Capacity

Functional residual capacity (FRC) is the resting volume of the lung at end expiration.[6] The chest wall of

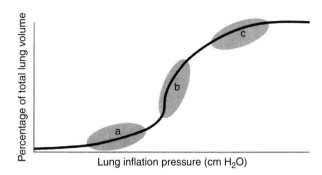

FIGURE 7-2 Volume–pressure loops of tidal breathing at various levels of functional residual capacity (FRC): *a,* low FRC; *b,* normal FRC; *c,* elevated FRC.

newborns is very compliant, and supine FRC values are lower than adult values, approximately 20% of total lung capacity. Preterm infants with respiratory distress syndrome have an abnormally low FRC because of alveolar collapse. This results in low lung volume, low compliance, and increased work of breathing to achieve adequate tidal volume. Figure 7-2 shows tidal volume–pressure loops at various FRC levels. Note that the slope of compliance is best, and thus work of breathing is least, at a normal FRC. Some infants maintain a dynamic FRC at this level by incorporating breathing strategies that limit the expiratory flow rate, such as expiratory grunting and increased postinspiratory diaphragmatic muscle tone. Neonates with severe respiratory distress syndrome need positive airway pressure during expiration to establish a normal FRC.

There are several methods for determining FRC.[26] Systems using helium dilution and nitrogen washout techniques are basically scaled-down versions of adult systems. Neonatal systems to determine FRC by plethysmography are also commercially available.

Helium Dilution Method

The helium dilution method of calculating FRC measures only the gas that is in direct communication with the central airways. This technique uses the principle that the concentration of a gas in one volume is proportional to the concentration of that same gas in another volume, provided there is no production or consumption of the measured gas. Therefore, knowing the concentration of the gas inside the lungs and outside, as well as knowing the external volume, allows calculation of the lung volume. The volume of gas in the lung at end expiration (FRC) mixes and equilibrates with a known amount and concentration of helium (usually 5% to 10%) in a closed breathing circuit. Applying petroleum jelly to the edges of a disposable mask is helpful for an airtight seal on the infant's face when connecting to the helium–oxygen rebreathing circuit. Soda lime in the circuit absorbs exhaled carbon dioxide. The infant breathes the helium–oxygen mixture while connected to a spirometer, until the helium concentration equilibrates between the circuit and lungs. The reduction in measured helium concentration in the circuit is equated to the FRC. Any gas leak in the circuit, which is often seen in intubated infants, must be corrected in FRC calculations. The helium dilution method may be used for very sick infants with a fraction of inspired oxygen as high as 0.95.[5,26]

Nitrogen Washout Method

The nitrogen washout method of calculating FRC also measures only the gas that is in direct communication with the central airways. With a sealed face mask in place, the infant breathes 100% oxygen in an open circuit, which displaces nitrogen in the lungs. The circuit must have no gas leaks. The system measures the volume of nitrogen washed out of the lungs. On the basis of the starting alveolar concentration of nitrogen, the computer uses a regression equation to calculate the volume of air in the lungs at end expiration, which is the FRC.[27] The nitrogen washout method cannot measure the FRC if the infant's fraction of inspired oxygen is greater than 0.65.[26] Atelectasis may result from washout of poorly ventilated and partially obstructed areas of the lung.

Plethysmography

The principle of body plethysmography is similar to that of the gas concentration techniques.[28] In a closed system the product of pressure and volume is constant (Boyle's law). The infant lies in an airtight incubator. Only *thoracic gas volume* (TGV) is actually derived; the other values are calculated. TGV is the total gas in the thorax and is measured at FRC because it is the easiest volume for the subject to reproduce consistently. In addition to measuring lung volumes, body plethysmography is used mainly to measure resistance and conductance.[5,29]

Measuring Maximal Expiratory Flow by Rapid Thoracic Compression Technique

Measuring gas flow during a forced expiratory maneuver is the conventional procedure used to evaluate airway obstruction in a cooperative infant. A relatively noninvasive technique to generate a *partial expiratory flow volume* (PEFV) curve in infants allows the measurement of expiratory flows during a forced maneuver in infants and small children.[28-30] A rapid thoracic compression or "hug" is delivered to the sleeping infant's chest and abdomen with an inflatable jacket

to produce a forced expiration. A pneumotachometer with sealed face mask measures exhaled gas flow. The flow at the end-expiratory point of a normal resting tidal breath (FRC) is measured on the PEFV curve. This flow value, the *maximal expiratory flow at FRC*, is reported as liters per second (Figure 7-3). Multiple tests at various jacket inflation pressures are conducted for a "best test" assessment.

The maximal expiratory flow test can demonstrate flow limitation in airway disease and is valuable for evaluating the response to bronchodilator therapy in infants.[31,32] PEFV studies are frequently performed before and after aerosolizing a bronchodilator. An increase in maximal expiratory flow at FRC by at least 20% demonstrates a positive response to bronchodilator therapy. A significant number of infants with chronic lung disease have a *negative* bronchodilator response.[33]

Problems with the "hug technique" occur infrequently in experienced hands. The clinician must avoid collapsing the upper airway due to hyperextending the neck, resulting in forced airflow limitation solely because of positioning. Other types of upper airway impedance may also affect the accuracy of the intrathoracic flow rates, and reflex glottic closure may complicate testing.[5]

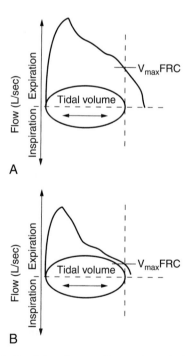

FIGURE 7-3 Partial expiratory flow–volume (PEFV) curves with identification of maximal expiratory flow at FRC (V_{max}FRC), demonstrating a normal resting tidal breath and one with flow limitation. **A,** Normal; **B,** abnormal (flow limited).

PEDIATRIC PULMONARY FUNCTION TESTING IN THE LABORATORY

Standard Spirometry

Standard spirometry is performed most often in PFT because of its relative ease and reproducibility.[5,13,34,35] It was traditionally carried out by time and volume measurements, using either a water seal spirometer or a wedge spirometer. This equipment required careful calibration, dedicated attention to technical detail during the performance of the test, and careful calculation of the reported values from the graph paper. Technological advances in the measurement of flow with a pneumotachograph and computing power have greatly simplified spirometry. This allows the clinician to focus on eliciting optimal patient cooperation and effort while the computer reports the predicted and measured values. However, improved technology does not allow clinicians to be naive concerning the basis of spirometry; it is their responsibility to guarantee that the reported values accurately reflect the testing situation.[5]

Figure 7-4 demonstrates traditional time–volume spirometry, indicating the various measurements available from this test. Integrating the flow signal with respect to time allows the calculation of volume and thus the time–volume curve.

Flow–Volume Loop

Figure 7-5 demonstrates the flow–volume loop and its specific measurements.[20,36] Interestingly, no FEV_1 is

clearly demonstrable on this visual representation, but the reported values include the FEV_1 as a key measurement. One advantage to the flow–volume representation is its clear depiction of whether subjects exhale to RV or whether they terminate their effort prematurely (Figure 7-6). "Early termination" is assessed by how gradual flow approaches zero and the duration of the exhalation effort

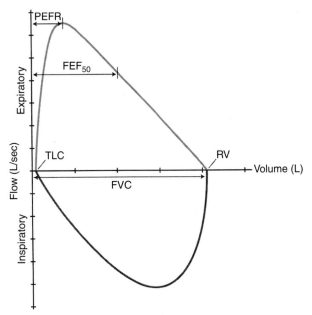

FIGURE 7-5 Normal flow–volume loop, showing both the expiratory and the inspiratory loops. The usual flow rates are identified. Note that no forced expiratory volume in 1 second (FEV_1) is evident because there is no time axis. FEF_{50}, Forced expiratory flow at 50% of vital capacity; FVC, forced vital capacity; PEFR, peak expiratory flow rate; RV, residual volume; TLC, total lung capacity.

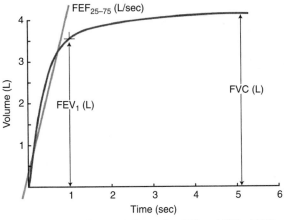

Calculation of FEF_{25-75}: 1. Determine 25% and 75% of FVC
2. Slope of line through 25% and 75% =
$$\frac{(V_{75}) - (V_{25})}{(T_{75}) - (T_{25})} \ (L/sec)$$

FIGURE 7-4 A normal standard time–volume spirometry graph, depicting the forced vital capacity (FVC), forced expiratory volume in 1 second (FEV_1), and forced expiratory flow between 25% and 75% of vital capacity (FEF_{25-75}).

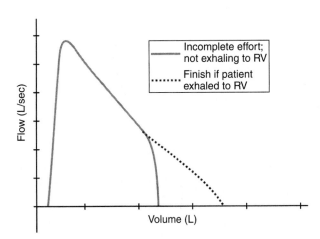

FIGURE 7-6 This expiratory flow–volume loop demonstrates the patient's failure to exhale completely to residual volume (RV). This will artificially decrease FVC and increase FEF_{50}.

displayed on the time–volume graph. This is less evident when using the time–volume plot alone. A disadvantage of the flow–volume method is that the computer automatically assigns the initiation of flow to TLC, whether or not subjects actually start with their lungs full (Figure 7-7). This is a particular problem with children, who may be apprehensive and therefore unable to fill their lungs completely before starting maximal exhalation. In this case the reported values will be artificially low, similar to those in restrictive disease. In addition, the shape of a flow–volume curve may also be of value in determining extrathoracic sources of airway obstruction.

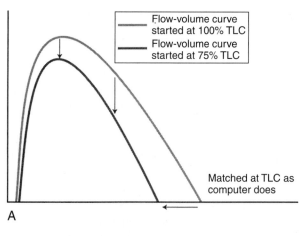

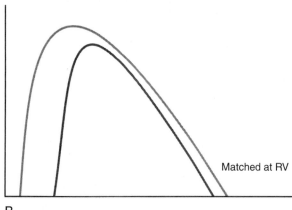

FIGURE 7-7 Comparison of a forced expiratory flow–volume curve starting from 100% of total lung capacity (TLC) with a curve starting at 75% of TLC. The computer software will have no way of knowing that the smaller curve was not started at 100% TLC and will start the smaller curve at zero volume. This artificially decreases FVC, PEFR, and FEF_{50}. **A,** Both curves start at TLC, as displayed by the computer. **B,** The curves, if matched at RV, would reflect that the smaller curve was not started at full lung volume. Clinicians must do their best to ensure that the patient starts the expiratory maneuver at 100% TLC.

Forced Vital Capacity, Forced Expiratory Volume, and Ratio of Forced Expiratory Volume to Forced Vital Capacity

The most common measurements from spirometry include the FVC, FEV_1, and FEV_1/FVC ratio. These measurements are reproducible for many disease states in adult patients, such as chronic obstructive pulmonary disease. Physiologists were concerned, however, that the FVC and FEV_1 might be relatively preserved despite the presence of moderately severe small airway disease, and thus significant lung disease might be missed by using only these measurements. Because small airways less than 2 mm in diameter contribute only a small part of the total lung resistance, 20% or less, these tiny airways have been described as the "silent zone" of the lung. In an effort to measure their function more independently, without the large airway functions obscuring the measurements, the "maximal mid-expiratory flow rates" were calculated. In current terminology, this is the FEF_{25-75} or the FEF_{50}.[5,37]

Forced Expiratory Flow at 25% to 75% and at 50% of Vital Capacity

Although the FEF_{25-75} and FEF_{50} reflect primarily the function of smaller airways, their measurement is considerably more variable than that of the FEV_1 or FVC.[6,14,38] This decreases their usefulness in distinguishing normal from abnormal and requires a considerably larger change to be considered physiologically significant, as opposed to just the normal variability found from one measurement to another.[39]

Table 7-1 demonstrates the variability, normal range, and clinically significant change for the most common spirometric and lung volume measurements in children.

TABLE 7-1

Pulmonary Function Measurements in Children

Measurement	Variability (%)	Normal Range (% Predicted)	Important Change (%)
FVC	5-7	80-120	>10
FEV_1	8	80-120	>15
FEV_1/FVC	—	*	—
FEF_{25-75}	15	60-140	>30
FEF_{50}	15	60-140	>30
TLC	7	80-120	>10
RV	7	80-120	>10
RV/TLC	7	†	—

*Absolute value is used; normal range for children is 82% to 95%.
†Absolute value is used; normal range for children is 20% to 30%.
FEF_{25-75}, Forced expiratory flow at 25% to 75% of vital capacity; FEF_{50}, forced expiratory flow at 50% of vital capacity; FEV_1, forced expiratory volume in 1 second; FVC, forced vital capacity; RV, residual volume; TLC, total lung capacity.

Furthermore, because many pulmonary diseases affect both the large and small airways, the FEF_{25-75} and FEV_1 often deteriorate in the same time frame, thus decreasing the usefulness of the FEF_{25-75} as an early detector of lung disease. However, because these measurements are often reported with standard spirometry, it is important that they be included in the analysis. Many childhood lung diseases, such as asthma and cystic fibrosis, have their roots in the tiny airways. Measurement of small airway function and attention to the results may enhance the overall interpretation of the tests. An abnormality isolated to the measurement of FEF_{25-75} or FEF_{50} is uncommon but more likely in children than in adults. Therefore, most pediatric PFT centers pay careful attention to small airway function. Figure 7-8 demonstrates the potential importance of these measurements in a child with asthma.

Spirometric Values

Spirometric values are frequently used to determine whether a disease has a restrictive or obstructive pattern. Table 7-2 demonstrates the expected changes with each pattern. The primary difference is whether the FEV_1/FVC ratio is decreased or preserved. The most common chronic diseases in children—asthma, cystic fibrosis, and bronchopulmonary dysplasia—

TABLE 7-2		
Characterization of Obstructive and Restrictive Patterns in Pulmonary Function Testing		
Measurement	**Obstructive**	**Restrictive**
FVC	Normal or decreased	Decreased
FEV_1	Decreased	Decreased
FEV_1/FVC	Decreased	Normal or increased
TLC	Normal or increased	Decreased
RV	Increased	Normal or decreased
RV/TLC	Increased	Normal or increased

FEV_1, Forced expiratory volume in 1 second; FVC, forced vital capacity; RV, residual volume; TLC, total lung capacity.

are *obstructive*. Most *restrictive* defects in children are related to an abnormal chest wall configuration or neuromuscular weakness rather than to interstitial fibrosis, as seen in adults. Caution must be used in describing restrictive lung disease on the basis of spirometry alone, because complete lung volumes are not measured. If the child did not start the expiratory maneuver from TLC, the FVC will be artificially decreased, and the reported values may appear restricted. Similarly, in a patient with severe obstructive disease in which the RV has expanded to encroach significantly on the FVC, the spirometric values may suggest a restrictive pattern. Therefore, if restrictive lung disease is a concern, consider performing one of the lung volume studies described in the next section. Figures 7-6 and 7-7 show examples of incomplete exhalation to RV and not starting at TLC, both of which produce artificially low spirometric values.

Lung Volumes

In contrast to the relative simplicity of spirometry, lung volume measurements are somewhat more involved and more difficult to perform. They include FRC, RV, TLC, RV/TLC ratio, and TGV. With the child sitting, the same techniques described earlier are used to measure lung volumes. These methods include helium dilution, nitrogen washout, body plethysmography, and forced oscillation.[24,40-42] Helium dilution or nitrogen washout techniques directly measure FRC.

Body plethysmography requires that the patient sit in an airtight box that looks similar to a telephone booth, commonly called a "body box" (Figure 7-9).[42] During constant-volume body plethysmography, the child voluntarily pants against a closed shutter. Using Boyle's law, the change in pressure against the closed shutter attached to a pneumotach is used to calculate a volume measurement, the TGV. TGV is measured at a known FRC value rather than on the basis of assumed values.

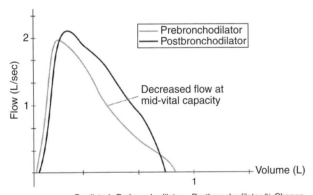

	Predicted	Prebronchodilator	Postbronchodilator	% Change
FVC (L)	0.89	0.81 (91)	0.78 (87)	−3
FEV_1 (L)	0.87	0.72 (83)	0.78 (89)	+8
FEV_1 : FVC (%)	95	88	100	
PEFR (L/sec)	2.13	1.78 (83)	2.18 (102)	+22
FEF_{50} (L/sec)	1.66	0.90 (54)	1.53 (92)	+70

FIGURE 7-8 Prebronchodilator and postbronchodilator expiratory loops produced by a 5-year-old patient with asthma. The prebronchodilator curve is slightly concave with respect to the volume axis, which is not evident on the postbronchodilator curve. The FEF_{50} is the only prebronchodilator measurement below the expected normal range of variability; it increased by 70% after bronchodilator therapy. FEF_{50}, Forced expiratory flow at 50% of vital capacity; FEV_1, forced expiratory volume in 1 second; FVC, forced vital capacity; PEFR, peak expiratory flow rate.

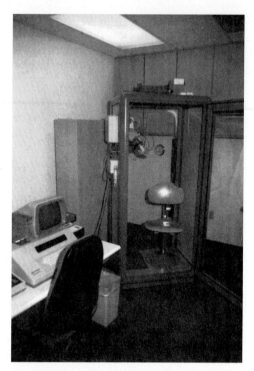

FIGURE 7-9 Body plethysmography "box."

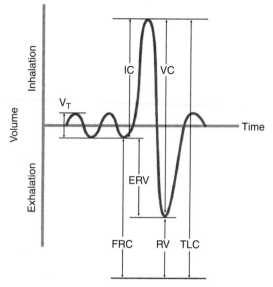

FIGURE 7-10 Graphic display of the subdivisions of total lung capacity (TLC), from quiet tidal breathing on the *left* to maximal inhalation and exhalation on the *right*. ERV, Expiratory reserve volume; FRC, functional residual capacity; IC, inspiratory capacity; RV, residual volume; VC, vital capacity; V_T, tidal volume.

TLC, the inspiratory capacity, is obtained by spirometry and added to the FRC. To calculate the RV, the expiratory reserve volume is subtracted from the FRC (Figure 7-10). In addition to measuring lung volumes, body plethysmography measures resistance and specific conductance. Using the attached pneumotach, voluntary spirometric measurements are acquired while the door is open, usually before volume testing to obtain the inspiratory capacity and expiratory reserve volume used in the FRC calculation.

Several potential errors are common when children perform these tests. If they are uncomfortable and anxious, pediatric patients may breathe at a slightly higher lung volume. If they are unable to start spirometry at TLC or exhale to RV, the values of inspiratory capacity and expiratory reserve volume will be incorrect. Therefore it is important to perform the test with the child completely relaxed and cooperative, and to record that this is the case, so that it is reflected in the interpretation.

Lung volume measurements are most useful in revealing restrictive lung diseases, in which they are decreased. It is critical to determine whether the lung volumes are smaller than expected because of a musculoskeletal problem (e.g., scoliosis and kyphosis), muscle weakness (e.g., Duchenne's muscular dystrophy and spinal muscular atrophy), or lung parenchymal disease (e.g., idiopathic pulmonary fibrosis). If it can be established that the patient's FVC as measured by spirometry correlates well with the TLC as measured on the basis

of lung volumes, spirometry may be sufficient for most patients' follow-up.

In addition to lung volumes, measuring maximal inspiratory and expiratory pressures helps assess overall respiratory muscle strength and augments volume measurements when assessing patients with muscle weakness.

Other measures of pulmonary function are seldom used in children for a variety of reasons. Some tests that have an invasive component, such as an esophageal balloon, are performed infrequently because of the perceived discomfort to the child. Other tests, such as diffusion capacity, are not often used because of uncertain predicted normal values and the infrequency of clinical diseases that make this a critical measurement in children. It is difficult to persuade a young child to cooperate with the maximal voluntary ventilation test and to provide a consistent maximal effort throughout the testing period. This raises uncertainty concerning whether the test is reliable in children.

Provocation Tests

Challenge testing, also known as *bronchial provocation,* may be used in documenting bronchial hyperreactivity.[5,43-45] This can help solidify the diagnosis of hyperreactive airway disease, or asthma, in a patient whose symptoms may not be typical of asthma. Alternatively, for the patient who has symptoms that might mimic asthma, the lack of bronchial oversensitivity may help initiate the search for an alternative explanation. Because the challenge tests are somewhat involved and time-consuming, they are not routinely used to document bronchial hyperreactivity. However, they are frequently used for research purposes to document a reversal of bronchial hyperreactivity in response to specific therapies.

Various techniques exist for challenging the airways, including administration of aerosolized medications, exercise, and hypertonic saline administration. Each institution typically develops expertise in one or two of these challenge techniques, using those that best fit patient needs. No standardized, universally acceptable protocol is in current use. Perhaps the most common testing method is to administer aerosolized medication designed to induce bronchoconstriction. *Methacholine* and *carbachol* are two cholinergic medications that induce nonspecific bronchoconstriction. *Histamine* is a by-product of mast cell degranulation and may play an important role in allergic responses. Histamine has also been used to induce bronchoconstriction during challenge testing. *Antigen inhalation* is infrequently used as a challenge because of the difficulty in quantifying the dose of antigen to administer. Furthermore, antigen inhalation carries the risk of a late-phase reaction 6 to 8 hours after the challenge, at which time the patient is unlikely to be near a medical facility for therapeutic intervention.

Many laboratories have used *exercise* as a challenge. Unfortunately, because the primary driving forces for bronchoconstriction appear to be lack of humidity and low air temperature, an exercise challenge in a comfortable pulmonary function laboratory may not be provocative. This has led some investigators to use *hyperventilation* while having the patient breathe cold air, without exercise, as the provocation test.

Provocation testing is usually considered positive if the FEV_1 falls more than 20% from baseline.[39,44,45] The concentration of the challenge drug is used as a marker of the degree of bronchial reactivity and is called the PD_{20}, the provocative dose that produces a 20% fall in FEV_1. For example, a patient with highly reactive asthma may have a fall in FEV_1 of 20% with a methacholine concentration of 0.25 mg/ml. A patient with mild asthma may experience a 20% fall in the FEV_1 at 10 mg/ml.

Table 7-3 shows a positive methacholine challenge test in a 7-year-old girl evaluated for a chronic cough. This positive study led to therapy for asthma, and her cough resolved. Interestingly, her previous spirometric measurements were normal and showed no improvement after bronchodilator therapy. The responses to exercise and cold air are measured by the duration of the challenge as well as the work performed during the exercise test. If other test parameters are used, such as the peak expiratory flow rate or specific Raw, different critical levels of positivity are used.

MEASURING PULMONARY MECHANICS AT THE BEDSIDE

Calculated Parameters

Tidal Volume

Tidal volume (V_T) is the gas volume (in milliliters) inhaled and exhaled during each resting breath. Frequently, V_T is indexed to body weight, and reported as milliliters per kilogram (ml/kg). Some PFT systems report inspired and expired V_T values separately, whereas some combine the two values. Infants in a neonatal intensive care unit may not normally inhale the same volume as they exhale for any given breath. This is visible as flow–volume (F–V) and pressure–volume (P–V) loops that are not closed. An average of at least 10 resting breaths is probably a better method of reporting V_T.[46]

TABLE 7-3

Positive Methacholine Challenge in a 7-year-old Girl With Chronic Cough*

METHACHOLINE		PULMONARY FUNCTION		
Concentration (mg/mL)	Cumulative Dose (mg/mL)	FVC (L)	FEV_1 (L)	Percent Change in FEV_1
Saline	0	1.51 (83%predicted)	1.4 (82%predicted)	—
Methacholine				
0.025	0.125	1.51	1.38	–1%
0.25	1.375	1.64	1.53	+9%
2.5	13.875	1.54	1.39	–1%
10	63.875	1.33	1.07	–24%
Albuterol	—	1.41	1.26	–10%

FEV_1, Forced expiratory volume in 1 second; FVC, forced vital capacity.

*In a methacholine challenge test, the patient first breathes aerosolized saline (as a baseline), followed by a breathing test. The subject then takes five breaths of methacholine at a low concentration, followed by another breathing test. The process continues with increasing concentrations of methacholine, until there is a 20% change in lung function or the maximal amount of methacholine has been inhaled. Albuterol, a bronchodilator, is then administered to help open the airways.

Infants receiving positive-pressure ventilation may have a gas leak around the uncuffed endotracheal tube. In this case, it is more accurate to report expired V_T. Some PFT systems report leakage as a percentage of exhaled to inhaled V_T, which is helpful in determining the delivered effective tidal volume. A system used for ventilator patient management should report V_T values for spontaneous and ventilator-delivered breaths separately.[47]

Respiratory Frequency

Most PFT systems report respiratory frequency, or rate, as breaths per minute. If the child or infant is intubated and receiving mechanical ventilation, the system should report spontaneous and ventilator breaths separately. Frequently, increased respiratory frequency is one of the first signs of reduced compliance, increased resistance, or fatigue.

Minute Ventilation

Minute ventilation is the volume of gas inspired and expired each minute by the infant. It is reported as liters per minute (L/min) or as liters per minute per kilogram (L/min/kg) of body weight and is the product of V_T and respiratory frequency. Viewing spontaneous and ventilator-delivered breathing separately or as a fraction of the total minute volume indicates the mechanical contribution of ventilation. This is helpful in assessing progress in weaning of a patient from assisted mechanical ventilation.

Rapid Shallow Breathing Index

The rapid shallow breathing index (RSBI) is a value that integrates two variables to determine the efficiency of tidal breathing. The RSBI is the ratio of spontaneous respiratory rate to V_T: divide the respiratory rate by V_T (in liters) to calculate the index. A calculated value less than 100 to 105 is predictive of a successful extubation in adults.[48,49] The RSBI has less predictive value when applied to children and infants.[50-52] Factors such as age, endotracheal tube size, agitation, sedation, and duration of mechanical ventilation all contribute to the success of extubation and the usefulness of the RSBI as a pediatric weaning tool. The RSBI can be a useful tool in evaluating relative increases or decreases in work of breathing and monitoring an infant before and after extubation. For infants and pediatrics, normalize the RSBI equation for infant size by dividing the V_T by weight. The resulting unit of measure becomes breaths per milliliter per kilogram and allows easier comparison among the various measurements.[49,52] Because of the range of normal respiratory rates and tidal volumes, no single RSBI value will predict extubation success in the pediatric population.

Inspiratory and Expiratory Times

PFT systems measure inspiratory and expiratory times (T_I and T_E) by gas flow. The reported values will be different from the set, or duty cycle, times of a mechanical ventilator. Some systems also calculate the inspiratory-to-expiratory T_I/T_E ratio or inspiratory time percent (T_I/T_{total}) from measured time.

Lung Compliance

At the bedside, compliance (C) is measured by the same technique as in the PFT laboratory.[18] When making bedside measurements, it is important to know the compliance test conditions to interpret the meaning of the reported value. Specific lung compliance describes compliance when it is measured at a known level of total lung volume. When measuring compliance under static conditions by airway occlusion, compliance is similar to the value derived in the laboratory and assesses Crs.[18] *Dynamic lung compliance* (C_{dyn}) is measured during resting tidal breathing and is affected by Raw.

There are some limitations to C_{dyn} measurement. This value reflects true compliance only when measuring transpulmonary pressure during spontaneous breathing with an esophageal catheter. Most centers do not routinely place an esophageal catheter for ventilator management studies. Instead, if the graph demonstrates that gas flow reaches zero at the end of inspiration and expiration, it is assumed that pressure has equalized from the proximal airway to the lungs. Compliance varies at different points of total lung volume, which is usually unknown during dynamic testing.

Airway Resistance

During bedside testing the best evaluation of Raw also uses transpulmonary pressure measurements. A high Raw value is visualized on the P–V loop, described later, as a bowing out of the curve from the line of idealized compliance, or slope of the curve. The presence of an endotracheal tube with a small inner diameter is an airway obstruction, and Raw will be high. Changes in mechanical ventilator settings greatly affect Raw values, as do airway impairments such as secretions, bronchospasm, and edema. Bedside measurements of Raw usually preclude techniques used in the laboratory and are derived from the passive occlusion technique.

Time Constants

Respiratory time constants, tau (τ), are the mathematical product of compliance and resistance expressed as seconds, because all the units of pressure and volume measurement cancel out except time. A time constant

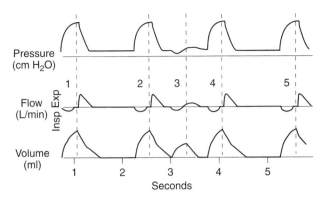

FIGURE 7-11 Tracing of pressure, flow, and volume over time (in seconds). Exp, Expiration; Insp, inspiration.

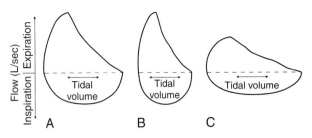

FIGURE 7-12 Patterns of flow–volume loops. **A,** Normal; **B,** restrictive; **C,** obstructive.

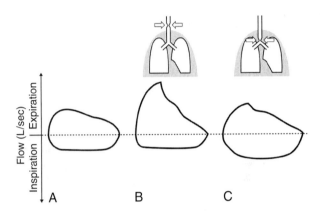

FIGURE 7-13 Flow–volume loops showing various forms of airway obstruction. **A,** Fixed obstruction; **B,** variable extrathoracic obstruction; **C,** variable intrathoracic obstruction.

is an interval over which a given change occurs, as a percentage of total change. Three time constants are required to reach 95% of inflation or exhalation. T_I, or inflation time, and T_E should be at least three times the respiratory time constants for optimal inspiration or expiration to occur.[53]

Pressure, Flow, and Volume Over Time

Most infant PFT systems graphically display measured airway (or transpulmonary) pressure, inspired and expired gas flow rates, and V_T on appropriate scales over a horizontal time axis "on screen" as the data are collected by the computer. This type of graphic display is also a component of most neonatal mechanical ventilators. Figure 7-11 shows a scalar tracing of pressure, flow, and volume over time. Pressure (Figure 7-11, top tracing) is either transpulmonary pressure or airway pressure measured at the endotracheal tube connection with the ventilator circuit. Gas flow at the airway (Figure 7-11, middle tracing) shows the inspiratory flow rate as a downward deflection and the expiratory flow rate as an upward deflection, with the center line being zero flow. V_T (Figure 7-11, bottom tracing) portrays inspiration as upward, with a return to the baseline as volume is exhaled. The vertical dashed lines delineate the change from inspiration to expiration for each breath. Breaths are numbered from left to right; *1, 2, 4,* and *5* are mechanically ventilated. Breath *3* is a spontaneous breath, with a lower V_T than the ventilator-delivered breaths.

Flow–Volume Loops

During bedside testing, F–V loops are typically generated during tidal breathing.[6,54] The peak of expiratory flow normally occurs within the first one third of expiratory volume. F–V loops that show decreased flow with relatively normal volume indicate an obstructive

process in the airways; loops with decreased volume and normal flow suggest a restrictive disorder (Figure 7-12).

Flow–volume loops demonstrate fixed airway obstruction, with flow limited during both inspiration and expiration. Figure 7-13 illustrates various types of obstruction. Flow limitation on the inspiratory portion of the loop is characteristic of an extrathoracic obstruction. Flow limitation on the expiratory part of the loop demonstrates an intrathoracic obstruction.[55] Some obstructions may also show a *flutter,* or irregular flow pattern, on either portion of the loop.

Pressure–Volume Loops

Graphically displaying a tidal breath with pressure change (airway or transpulmonary) on the horizontal axis and volume on the vertical axis also forms a loop. Spontaneous breathing is evidenced by a negative pressure change, and mechanical ventilator breaths display pressure in the positive direction. If the action of inhalation had only the elastic forces of lung tissue to overcome, the P–V graph would not be a loop but rather a straight line between the beginning and end points of

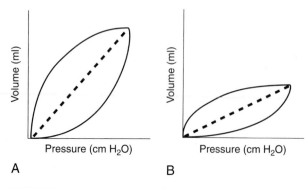

FIGURE 7-14 Pressure–volume loops demonstrating normal and decreased lung compliance. **A,** Normal lung compliance; **B,** decreased lung compliance.

inspiration (dashed line in Figure 7-14). The P–V loop bows out from that line of pure compliance, mostly because of pressure needed for gas flow through narrow, resistive airways. The loop meets the line of ideal compliance at the end points of a tidal breath, where gas flow is zero. The slope of the line, and of the loop as a whole, depends on compliance. The more compliant the lung, meaning less pressure needed for normal V_T, the more vertical the P–V loop appears.

Lung Overdistention

Ventilator-induced lung injury and pulmonary barotrauma are major complications of positive-pressure ventilation in all patient populations. Applying excessive distending airway pressures results in a characteristic distortion in the appearance of the normal P–V loop (Figure 7-15). To visualize this, imagine blowing up a balloon. At first it is necessary to blow hard (i.e., apply a large amount of pressure) to get any vol-

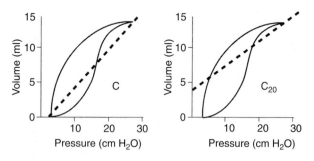

FIGURE 7-15 Pressure–volume loops demonstrating overdistention. Note the "penguin" or "bird's beak" appearance in the shape of the loops. These loops demonstrate idealized slopes *(dashed lines)* for change in compliance for the entire breath *(C)* and change in compliance in the last 20% of inspiratory pressure *(C_{20})*. The C_{20}/C ratio identifies lung overdistention.

ume into the balloon. It then seems easier to push additional volume into the balloon as it expands. Finally, as the balloon reaches its expansion limit, that is, starts to overdistend, it again becomes more difficult to blow up. In other words, the compliance of the balloon or lung changes with total volume.

Applying additional pressure to an overdistended lung produces little or no increase in delivered volume and is hazardous to the patient. Lung overdistention is quantified by comparing compliance change in the last 20% of inspiratory pressure (C_{20}) with compliance change for the entire breath (C), in the ratio C_{20}/C (see Figure 7-15). A C_{20}/C value less than 1.0 indicates lung overdistention during mechanical ventilation. Gas exchange can be improved in mechanically ventilated neonates with lung overdistention by reducing peak inspiratory pressure.[56]

Work of Breathing

The calculated work of breathing is determined as the integral of esophageal pressure for a given tidal volume and reflects the amount of energy required by the patient to breathe. Work of breathing is usually indexed to body weight, reported as grams-centimeters per kilogram (g-cm/kg) or as joules per liter (J/L). Work of breathing measurements have proven particularly useful when evaluating new ventilator techniques and response to various therapies.

Other Bedside Tests

Other common pulmonary function measurements performed at the bedside are vital capacity (VC), peak expiratory flow rate (PEFR), and maximal inspiratory pressure (MIP), often referred to as negative inspiratory force (NIF). These measurements require a respirometer or pneumotachometer, a peak flowmeter, and an NIF meter. The values are helpful in a variety of clinical situations, including weaning from mechanical ventilation, evaluating neuromuscular disorders such as myasthenia gravis or muscular dystrophy, and evaluating treatment for reactive airways.

Each of these measurements depends on patient cooperation and effort, which makes it challenging with children and prevents their use for infants. Pediatric patients may need to be more than 4 or 5 years of age to perform some of these tests because of equipment limitations. Also, the child must be able to understand the instructions and use the correct technique to perform the tests. Thoroughly explain the technique for each maneuver and provide a chance for practice before actually collecting the data. It is imperative that clinicians record their impression of the child's understanding and effort with the actual measurements.

Vital Capacity

VC is the maximal amount of gas that can be expired after a full inspiration. The patient inhales to TLC and then exhales completely through a respirometer or other measuring device. VC values are effort dependent, and the child must cooperate completely when asked to perform the maneuver. Incomplete effort will result in an artificially low value, which may lead to misdiagnosis. Forced vital capacity (FVC) differs from VC in that during the FVC maneuver the patient exhales as forcefully and rapidly as possible after a maximal inspiration. FVC is usually the same as a slow VC, except in patients who experience airway collapse with rapid, forceful expiration.

Peak Expiratory Flow Rate

PEFR is the maximal achievable flow during a rapid, forced expiration. The PEFR is used primarily to monitor patients with hyperreactive airways. It is generally measured with hand-held devices that sense flow against a turbine, through a variable orifice, or against a spring-loaded diaphragm. With increasing flow rates an indicator advances linearly on a scale that reveals the PEFR, usually as liters per minute. Note that the PEFR on the F–V loop measures the same function as the peak flowmeter, air flow in the large airways, but reported as liters per second. The PEFR measurement made during the recording of an F–V loop is an actual measurement of air flow. Because the hand-held peak flowmeter measures only the inertia from the initial blast of air, the value is not identical to the value reported during F–V loop measurement.

Portable peak flowmeters are used extensively in the study and management of patients with asthma. A significant decrease in the individual's baseline PEFR may indicate worsening asthma and the need for therapeutic interventions. In addition, measuring PEFR before and after bronchodilator administration evaluates the effectiveness of the therapy.[34]

Portable hand-held models are inexpensive and easy to use at home, at school, or in an office. When using hand-held peak flowmeters, care must be taken to avoid partial occlusion of the flow exit orifice during exhalation. Partial occlusion decreases the amount of flow required to raise the flow indicator, resulting in overestimation of PEFR. This measurement can also be erroneously high if the patient uses a "spitting" action during exhalation.[5,35]

Maximal Inspiratory Pressure

MIP, or NIF, is the maximal negative pressure, expressed as centimeters of water, generated during inspiration against an occlusion. Connect the patient's airway to an inspiratory pressure gauge with an adapter that allows occlusion of the airway during inspiration. Instruct the patient to exhale, and then occlude the airway while the patient inhales with maximal effort, which results in measuring the maximal negative pressure.

MIP is an important measure to help differentiate weakness from other causes of restrictive lung disease. It can be an important differentiating point for children and young adults with various neuromuscular diseases. These patients usually have a combination of scoliosis and muscle weakness, both of which might contribute to reduced lung volumes. Measuring MIP helps in determining how much reduction might be caused by weakness. Because many neuromuscular diseases are progressive, MIP helps to document this progression. MIP may also indicate the patient's physical ability to take a deep breath and is often measured when weaning a patient from mechanical ventilation is being considered.

Complex Bedside Measurements

Automated and computer monitors allow the measurement of more complex breathing variables at the bedside. Usually these measurements are useful for weaning a child from mechanical ventilation, but they may also be helpful when evaluating the pulmonary status of a neuromuscular patient.

An example of such a measurement is the $P_{0.1}$ pronounced "P one hundred." It is similar to MIP but measures the negative pressure generated in the first one hundred milliseconds. $P_{0.1}$ appears to be more indicative of the ability to sustain respiratory drive and predict successful extubation or weaning from mechanical ventilation.

Another such measure is the *tension time index* (TTI), which may assist in predicting successful weaning from mechanical ventilation. The TTI is essentially a measurement of the energy demand on the inspiratory muscles to tolerate the workload of breathing.[48] The TTI is the product of the inspiratory time-to-cycle time ratio and the integrated area under the pressure curve throughout the respiratory cycle. Unlike the adult measurement and similar to the RSBI, these advanced weaning predictors have no pediatric range that correlates with successful weaning.[48]

SUMMARY

Pulmonary function testing is a vital part of diagnosis and management of many respiratory diseases in both the intensive care unit and outpatient laboratory. Obtaining reliable pulmonary function information from infants may be challenging, but provides extremely valuable insight into respiratory mechanics. The use of improved technology by skilled clinicians has dramatically enhanced the accuracy of pulmonary function testing.

ASSESSMENT QUESTIONS

See Evolve Resources for answers.

1. When interpreting pulmonary function test results in children, assessing whether values are "normal" is complicated by:
   A. Applying the process of obligatory miniaturization
   B. The wide range of variability in normal children
   C. Relatively small sample sizes used in developing predicted normal values
   D. A and C
   E. B and C

2. Why do inspiratory retractions distort the ribs and sternum inward during distressed breathing in a premature newborn?
   A. Negative inspiratory pressures exceed transpulmonary pressure.
   B. The chest wall is compliant and does not expand the lungs.
   C. The specific conductance of the lungs is higher than the recoil of the chest wall.
   D. Time constant differences result in a lag between lung expansion and chest wall movement.
   E. None of the above.

3. Airway resistance (Raw) reflects the nonelastic airway and tissue forces resisting gas flow. How is Raw calculated?
   A. By dividing the peak ventilating pressures by the peak flow rate
   B. Using a modified Fick equation for gas flow
   C. From the ratio of airway occlusion pressure to expiratory flow
   D. Using a tonometer and paramagnetic analyzer
   E. By dividing the ratio of upper airway flow by lower airway compliance

4. Which of the following are possible tests that may be used to determine lung volume in an infant?
   I. Functional residual volume
   II. Helium dilution
   III. Plethysmography
   IV. Thoracic gas volume
   V. Nitrogen washout
   A. II, III, and V
   B. I, III, and V
   C. II and IV
   D. III and IV
   E. IV and V

5. What is the difference between pleural pressure and airway pressure?
   A. End-expiratory pressure
   B. Hyperinflation pressure
   C. PD_{20}
   D. Isovolume pressure
   E. Transpulmonary pressure

ASSESSMENT QUESTIONS—cont'd

6. Which of the following are considered a complication of using a face mask during infant pulmonary function tests?
   I. Trigeminal nerve damage
   II. Vagal reflex stimulation
   III. Increased lung compliance
   IV. Increased dead space volume
   V. Recurrent pharyngeal nerve damage
   A. I, II, and IV
   B. I, III, and IV
   C. II and IV
   D. II, III, and V
   E. III, IV, and V

7. What is one advantage to using a flow–volume loop instead of time–volume spirometry?
   A. A flow–volume loop is not dependent on patient cooperation or effort.
   B. Time–volume spirometry causes early fatigue in children.
   C. Flow–volume measurements are easier to record.
   D. A flow–volume loop displays early termination of the exhalation effort.
   E. Time–volume displays are not real time measurements.

8. How are spirometric values affected if a child fails to begin exhalation at 100% of total lung capacity?
   A. Reported tidal volume value is higher than the actual value.
   B. Reported FEF_{50} value is higher than the actual value.
   C. Reported FVC value is lower than the actual value.
   D. Reported PEFR value is higher than the actual value.
   E. All values are reported accurately.

9. Measuring flow from airways less than 2 mm in diameter is determined by evaluating
   A. The maximal midexpiratory flow rates
   B. The forced expiratory flow at 25% to 75% of exhalation
   C. The forced expiratory flow at 50% of exhalation
   D. B and C
   E. A, B, and C

10. When using a hand-held peak flowmeter, a 6-year-old patient with asthma partially occludes the exit orifice of the meter. On the basis of the flowmeter results, the physician may
   A. Erroneously prescribe the wrong medication dose, since the value reported is lower than the actual value.
   B. Prescribe the correct medication dose, since there is no effect on the actual value.
   C. Not prescribe medication, since the value reported is higher than the actual value.
   D. Prescribe a medication dose that is proportionate to the erroneous reduction in peak flow.
   E. None of the above.

References

1. Majaesic CM et al: Clinical correlations and pulmonary function at 8 years of age after severe neonatal respiratory failure, *Pediatr Pulmonol* 2007;42:829.
2. Hilman BC, Allen JL: Clinical application of pulmonary function testing in children and adolescents. In Hilman BC, editor: *Pediatric respiratory disease: diagnosis and treatment*, Philadelphia: WB Saunders; 1993, pp 98–107.
3. Wang X et al: Pulmonary function between 6 and 18 years of age, *Pediatr Pulmonol* 1993;15:75.
4. Robbins DR, Enright PL, Sherrill DL: Lung function development in young adults: is there a plateau phase? *Eur Respir J* 1995;8:768.
5. American Association for Respiratory Care: Clinical practice guideline: Infant/toddler pulmonary function tests, *Respir Care* 2008;53:929-945.
6. Brusasco V, Crapo R, Viegi G: General considerations for lung function testing, *Eur Respir J* 2005;26:153.
7. Hanrahan JP et al: Pulmonary function measures in healthy infants, *Am Rev Respir Dis* 1990;141:1127.
8. Rosenfeld M et al: Effect of choice of reference equation on analysis of pulmonary function in cystic fibrosis patients, *Pediatr Pulmonol* 2001;31:227.
9. Chatburn RL: Evaluation of pediatric pulmonary function theory and application, *Respir Care* 1989;34:597.
10. Hyatt RE: Expiratory flow limitation, *J Appl Physiol* 1983;55:1.
11. Gardner RM: Pulmonary function laboratory standards, *Respir Care* 1989;34:651.
12. Castile R. Novel techniques for assessing infant and pediatric lung function and structure. *Pediatr Infect Dis J* 2004;23: S246–S253.
13. Taussig LM et al: Standardization of lung function testing in children, *J Pediatr* 1980;97:668.
14. Blonshine SB: Pediatric pulmonary function testing, *Respir Care Clin North Am* 2000;6:27.
15. Mallol J, Sly PD: Effect of chloral hydrate on arterial oxygen saturation in wheezy infants, *Pediatr Pulmonol* 1988;5:96.
16. Desmond KJ et al: Redefining end of test (EOT) criteria for pulmonary function testing in children, *Am J Respir Crit Care Med* 1997;156:542.
17. Frey U et al: Specifications for equipment used for infant pulmonary function testing: ERS/ATS Task Force on Standards for Infant Respiratory Function Testing, European Respiratory Society/American Thoracic Society, *Eur Respir J* 2000;16:731.
18. Bhutani VK, Sivieri EM: Pulmonary function and graphics. In: Goldsmith JP, Karotkin EH, editors. *Assisted ventilation of the neonate*, 4th ed, Philadelphia: WB Saunders/Elsevier; 2003, pp 293–309.
19. Talmor D et al: Esophageal and transpulmonary pressures in acute respiratory failure, *Crit Care Med* 2006;34:1389.
20. Saslow JG et al: Work of breathing using high-flow nasal cannula in preterm infants, *J Perinatol* 2006;26:476.
21. Brar G et al: Respiratory mechanics in very low birth weight infants during continuous versus intermittent gavage feeds, *Pediatr Pulmonol* 2001;32:442.
22. Katier N et al: Passive respiratory mechanics measured during natural sleep in healthy term neonates and infants up to 8 weeks of life, *Pediatr Pulmonol* 2006;41:1058.
23. Katier N et al: Feasibility and variability of neonatal and infant lung function measurement using the single occlusion technique, *Chest* 2005;128:1822.
24. Gappa M et al: Lung function tests in neonates and infants with chronic lung disease: lung and chest-wall mechanics, *Pediatr Pulmonol* 2006;41:291.
25. Delacourt C et al: Use of the forced oscillation technique to assess airway obstruction and reversibility in children, *Am J Respir Crit Care Med* 2000;161:730.
26. Tepper RS, Asdell S: Comparison of helium dilution and nitrogen washout measurements of functional residual capacity in infants and very young children, *Pediatr Pulmonol* 1992;13:250.
27. Gerhardt T, Hehre D, Bancalari E: A simple method of measuring functional residual capacity in the newborn by N_2 washout, *Pediatr Res* 1985;19:1165.
28. Stocks J et al: European Respiratory Society/American Thoracic Society: Plethysmographic measurements of lung volume and airway resistance ERS/ATS task force on standards for infant respiratory function testing, *Eur Respir J* 2001;17:302.
29. Morgan WJ et al: Partial expiratory flow–volume curves in infants and young children, *Pediatr Pulmonol* 1988;5:232.
30. LeSouef PN, Hughes DM, Landau LI: Effect of compression pressure on forced expiratory flow in infants, *J Appl Physiol* 1986;61:1639.
31. Tepper RS et al: Use of maximal expiratory flows to evaluate central airways obstruction in infants, *Pediatr Pulmonol* 1989;6:272.
32. Maynard RC et al: Partial forced expiratory flow (PFEF) measurements in premature infants at discharge, *Pediatr Res* 1991;29:324A.
33. Becker MA, Donn SM: Real-time pulmonary graphic monitoring, *Clin Perinatol* 2007;34:1.
34. Slieker MG, van der Ent CK: The diagnostic and screening capacities of peak expiratory flow measurements in the assessment of airway obstruction and bronchodilator response in children with asthma, *Monaldi Arch Chest Dis* 2003;59:155.
35. Nair SJ, Daigle KL, DeCuir P, Lapin CD, Schramm CM. The influence of pulmonary function testing on the management of asthma in children. *J Pediatr*. 2005 Dec;147:797–801.
36. Davis S: Spirometry, *Pediatr Respir Rev* 2006;7:11.
37. Ciprandi G et al: Role of FEF_{25-75} as an early marker of bronchial impairment in patients with seasonal allergic rhinitis, *Am J Rhinol* 2006;20:641.
38. American Thoracic Society/European Respiratory Society Respiratory mechanics in infants; physiologic evaluation in health and disease, *Am Rev Respir Dis* 1993;147:474.
39. Beydon et al: An official American Thoracic Society/European Respiratory Society statement; pulmonary function testing in preschool children, *Am J Respir Crit Care Med* 2007;175:1304.
40. Wanger J et al: Standardization of the measurement of lung volumes, *Eur Respir J* 2005;26:511.
41. Snow MG: Determination of functional residual capacity, *Respir Care* 1989;34:586.
42. Pfaff JK, Morgan WJ: Pulmonary function in infants and children, *Pediatr Clin North Am* 1994;41:401.
43. Godfrey S et al: Timing and nature of wheezing at the endpoint of a bronchial challenge in preschool children, *Pediatr Pulmonol* 2005;39:262.

44. American Association for Respiratory Care: Clinical practice guideline for bronchial provocation, *Respir Care* 1992;37:902.

45. American Thoracic Society: Guidelines for methacholine and exercise challenge testing, 1999, *Am J Respir Crit Care Med* 2000;161:309.

46. Bhutani VK et al: Evaluation of neonatal pulmonary mechanics and energetics: a two factor least mean square analysis, *Pediatr Pulmonol* 1988;4:150.

47. Mammel MC et al: Effect of spontaneous and mechanical breathing on dynamic lung mechanics in hyaline membrane disease, *Pediatr Pulmonol* 1990;8:222.

48. Vassilakopoulos T, Spyros Z, Roussos C: The tension-time index and the frequency/tidal volume ratio are the major pathophysiologic determinants of weaning failure and success, *Am J Respir Crit Care Med* 1998;158:378.

49. Chatila W et al: The unassisted respiratory rate–tidal volume ratio accurately predicts weaning outcome, *Am J Med* 1996;101:61.

50. Venkataraman ST, Khan N, Brown A: Validation of predictors of extubation success and failure in mechanically ventilated infants and children, *Crit Care Med* 2000;28:2991.

51. Farias JA et al: Weaning from mechanical ventilation in pediatric intensive care patients, *Intensive Care Med* 1998;24:1070.

52. Thiagarajan RR et al: Predictors of successful extubation in children, *Am J Respir Crit Care Med* 1999;160:1562.

53. Hankinson JL, Crapo RO, Jensen RL. Spirometric reference values for the 6-s FVC maneuver. *Chest* 2003: 124:1805–1811.

54. Lucangelo U, Bernabe F, Blanch L: Respiratory mechanics derived from signals in the ventilator circuit, *Respir Care* 2005;50:55.

55. Blanch L, Bernabe F, Lucangelo U: Measurement of air trapping, intrinsic positive end-expiratory pressure, and dynamic hyperinflation in mechanically ventilated patients, *Respir Care* 2005;50:110.

56. Fisher JB et al: Identifying lung overdistention during mechanical ventilation by using volume–pressure loops, *Pediatr Pulmonol* 1988;5:10.

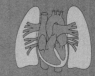

Chapter 8

Radiographic Assessment

J. DAVID INGRAM

OUTLINE

Radiographic Technique
Normal Chest Anatomy
Positioning of Lines and Tubes
Airway Obstruction
Respiratory Distress in the Newborn
Atelectasis

Pneumonia
Asthma
Cystic Fibrosis
Acute Respiratory Distress Syndrome
Chest Trauma

LEARNING OBJECTIVES

After reading this chapter the reader will be able to:

- Recognize differences in radiographic position that affect the appearance of the visualized anatomy
- Identify normal chest structures
- Examine the chest radiograph for proper placement of endotracheal tubes and vascular catheters
- Differentiate between the bacterial and viral infections responsible for acute upper airway symptoms
- List the most common causes that lead to radiographic evaluation of the newborn chest
- Describe how atelectasis affects the individual lobes of each lung

- Differentiate between the radiographic appearance of viral infections and bacterial pneumonias
- Explain the impact of acute viral or bacterial pneumonias on asthma symptoms
- Describe the hallmark radiographic appearance of cystic fibrosis
- Explain the implications of acute respiratory distress syndrome superimposed on underlying illnesses
- List the complications of chest trauma and identify the placement of support devices

Radiographic assessment of the chest and airway is often critical in patient evaluation by the respiratory care practitioner: the position of lines and tubes can be accurately determined; visualized lung fields on the radiographs can be correlated with the physical examination; and airways can be assessed for patency and abnormalities.

RADIOGRAPHIC TECHNIQUE

Radiographs are obtained with a portable x-ray machine at the patient's bedside or by using equipment in the radiology department. Because the quality of the examination is better when using the techniques and equipment available in the radiology department, portable radiographs should be used only when it is not safe or feasible to transport the patient. This is especially true for neonates, with almost all radiographs being obtained portably in the neonatal unit. Radiographs are increasingly being viewed as digital images either on a *picture-archiving and communication system* (PACS) monitor at the patient unit or with the radiologist in the radiology department.

The standard radiographic evaluation of the chest comprises both a *frontal view* and a *lateral view*. The frontal view shows the position of a structure in relation to right and left as well as to center. With the addition of the lateral view, the structure can also be positioned in an anterior-to-posterior plane, and a more three-dimensional representation can be surmised. *Posteroanterior* frontal views are obtained upright in the radiology department with the chest against the radiographic plate. The x-ray tube is placed behind the patient's back with the x-ray beam going through the patient in a posterior-to-anterior path. When the radiograph is performed portably, the plate is placed between the patient's back and the bed with the x-ray tube in front of the patient's chest. The *anteroposterior* technique, with the beam passing from anterior to posterior, causes magnification of structures such as the heart, located in the anterior half of the chest. Therefore knowledge of how the frontal film was obtained (anteroposterior vs. posteroanterior) is useful when deciding whether the heart size is different because of magnification or clinical change.

Although most chest radiographs are performed with frontal and lateral projections, other views may contribute additional information. The lateral decubitus view is a frontal projection performed with the patient lying on either the right side *(right-side down lateral decubitus)* or on the left side *(left-side down lateral decubitus)*. The down side can be evaluated for presence of a mobile pleural effusion, and the up side may better define a *pneumothorax* (air in the pleural cavity). These views may also be used if a foreign body is lodged in a bronchus, causing air trapping. The down-side lung normally loses volume but may remain expanded when a foreign body obstructs airflow out of the bronchus.

Forced expiratory films may also be used to evaluate for foreign body aspiration in small children. The technologist gently adds pressure to the abdomen during expiration. The obstructed lung will not decrease in size but remains normal to hyperexpanded (see Figure 8-1). In older and cooperative children the technologist can have the patient inspire and expire without assistance while the radiographs are obtained. *Oblique views* are typically used for rib fracture evaluations in the pediatric population.

Although the thoracic trachea and mainstem bronchi are demonstrated on chest radiographs, soft tissue

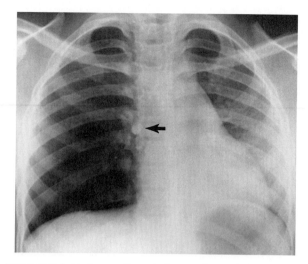

FIGURE 8-1 Expiratory frontal chest radiograph shows normal decrease in left lung volume. Tooth *(arrow)* obstructs the right mainstem bronchus and causes air trapping in the right lung.

frontal and lateral projections of the neck allow evaluation of the extrathoracic airway. These views may show *mass effect* on the airway from a retropharyngeal abscess or can show distortion of the tracheal caliber caused by croup and subglottic stenosis.

Real-time imaging of the airway by fluoroscopy will show the dynamic collapse of tracheal walls *(tracheomalacia)*. If a barium swallow *(esophagram)* is performed as well, the presence of a *vascular ring* (in which the trachea and esophagus are encircled by connected segments of the aortic arch and its branches) or *tracheoesophageal fistula* (an abnormal connection between the trachea and the esophagus) can be excluded. Swallowing studies are performed with the assistance of a speech therapist, using various consistencies of barium-impregnated food to determine which the patient is unlikely to aspirate.

NORMAL CHEST ANATOMY

The normal structures that are visualized on a chest radiograph are distinguishable because of differences in the absorption of the x-ray beam. Bone and metallic orthopedic hardware appear bright white because of greater x-ray absorption and less exposure of the film. In contrast, air has little beam absorption, and therefore well-expanded lungs appear relatively black. Soft tissue organs and fluid usually appear as shades of gray in between the white bones and black lungs. However, incorrect exposure of the film may alter the normal gray scale such that soft tissue organs can appear bright white in an underexposed film. Therefore the technical quality of the film must be considered when viewing.

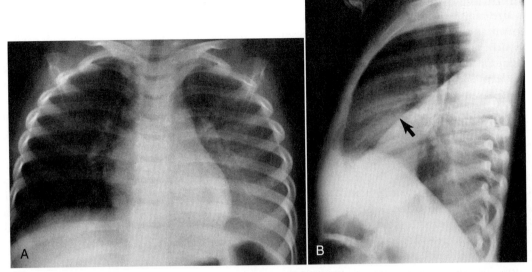

FIGURE 8-2 A, Left lower lobe pneumonia abuts the diaphragm, leading to nonvisualization of the normal edge of the diaphragm. The cardiac border is demarcated because the *lingula* (a segment of the upper lobe of the left lung) is normally aerated. **B,** Only the right hemidiaphragm is visualized because the left is obscured by the left lower lobe pneumonia. Major fissure appears as an edge *(arrow)*.

By using specialized tools available for adjusting images on a PACS monitor, the image may be manipulated to enhance visualization of the lung detail and to clarify the presence of abnormal collections of free air. Window level and zoom features are particularly useful. Inversion of the image sometimes will clarify the tip position of small catheters. Because of the complexity of image retrieval and portrayal with a PACS, instruction is usually provided to the clinicians by the PACS administrators from the radiology department.

A chest film is a two-dimensional representation of a three-dimensional object. When an x-ray beam passes through the chest, the densities of all the structures it encounters are summated. Thus a flat object such as platelike *atelectasis* (collapse of all or part of the lung) may add little to the opacity of the chest seen facing one projection but may appear opaque when viewed on edge in another projection. Pulmonary vessels appear as white dots when viewed in cross section but are fainter when viewed as tubes.

Differences in tissue density allow the viewer to discriminate between different structures. The heart, which is composed of soft tissue of waterlike density, is clearly demarcated by a distinct edge from the adjacent air-filled lung. However, if the lung becomes more waterlike in density from loss of air, as in atelectasis, or if the alveoli become filled with pus, as in pneumonia, the sharp edge between the heart and the lung is no longer apparent. The sign caused when two normal structures lose their distinct edge and blend imperceptibly is widely known as the *silhouette sign* (Figure 8-2).

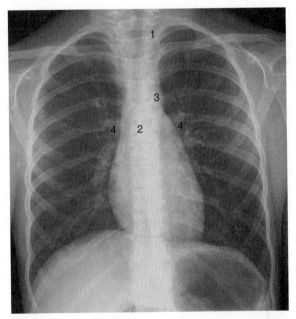

FIGURE 8-3 Normal frontal view of the chest demonstrating the thoracic inlet *(1)*, *carina* (the point at which the trachea splits into the two mainstem bronchi) *(2)*, the aortic arch *(3)*, and pulmonary hila *(4)*.

The normal structures that the respiratory care practitioner must evaluate on all chest films are the heart, lungs, and airways (Figure 8-3). Other structures that may be important in a specific patient include the diaphragm, bones, and organs in the upper abdomen. Although the heart is central in the chest, it normally projects more into the left hemithorax. Heart size may be accentuated by anteroposterior projection as well as decreased lung expansion. Pulmonary arteries and veins form confluent areas on either side of the heart called the right and left pulmonary *hila*. Enlargement of the hila may be caused by increased caliber of the pulmonary vessels or enlarged lymph nodes. The side of the aortic arch should also be noted. Normally the arch is on the left and causes a prominent bulge of the superior mediastinum and a mild indentation on the trachea.

The *mediastinum* is composed of the heart, aorta, main pulmonary artery and proximal branches, origins of the great vessels from the aorta, the superior vena cava, and thymus. Thymic tissue is usually prominent in the neonate and becomes less apparent with age because of regression of the thymus and growth of surrounding structures. Because it is an anterior mediastinal structure, the thymus in the small child fills the anterior clear space normally seen on the lateral view of a teenager or adult. On the frontal view it may only cause widening of the superior mediastinum. When the thymus projects away from the mediastinum, typically into the right upper lung, it appears as a "sail" with a sharp inferior margin. The lateral margins often have a characteristic wavy contour (Figure 8-4). Unlike a pathologic mass such as lymphoma, the normal thymus does not exert mass effect on the trachea.

The right lung is divided into three lobes and the left lung into two lobes. Both lungs have upper and lower lobes, but the right lung also has a middle lobe. The lingula of the left upper lobe may be thought of as corresponding to the right middle lobe, at least in location. Separating the upper and lower lobes, the *major fissures* (also called *oblique fissures*) extend diagonally on the lateral view in an anteroinferior-to-posterosuperior plane. Fluid in the fissures increases their visibility. The *minor*

fissure (also called the *horizontal fissure*) separates the middle lobe from the right upper lobe. It is horizontal in orientation on both frontal and lateral projections and terminates at the major fissure on lateral projection.

Lung density is greatly affected by the degree of inspiration. Poor inspiration will cause crowding of pulmonary vessels and airways, leading to an overall increase in lung density. When comparing the present chest radiograph with a prior film, the depth of inspiration should be taken into account and excluded as a cause of the change in appearance of both the lungs and size of the heart (Figure 8-5). When viewing infant and pediatric radiographs, body rotation may be difficult to avoid. Evaluating thoracic symmetry helps when interpreting the loss of lung volume or increased density in the rotated patient.

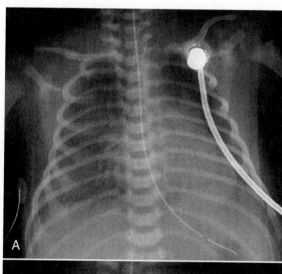

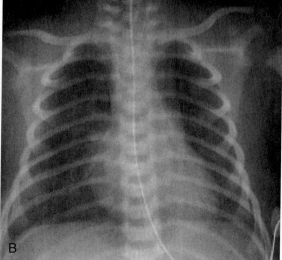

FIGURE 8-5 A, Infant with respiratory distress syndrome on lower ventilator setting. **B,** Same infant on higher ventilator setting.

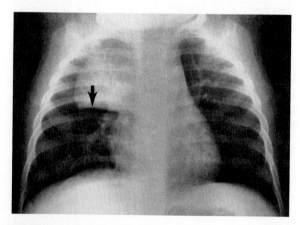

FIGURE 8-4 Normal thymus abuts the minor fissure *(arrow)* and has a curved lateral margin.

Evaluation of the trachea and mainstem bronchi should include the caliber as well as evidence of abnormal displacement or distortion by an adjacent mass. Truncation of a mainstem bronchus is often a sign of a mucous plug when the lung is collapsed. Although the right hemidiaphragm is usually slightly higher than the left because of the underlying liver, the position of the diaphragm may indicate hemidiaphragm paralysis or abdominal pathology. Congenital fusion anomalies may be seen in the neonatal rib cage, and rib fractures may contribute to difficult ventilation in a trauma patient.

POSITIONING OF LINES AND TUBES

The frontal chest radiograph can readily be used to assess the distance of the endotracheal tube to the carina. The tube should be located between the *thoracic inlet* (superior elliptical opening of the chest) and the carina. If the tube is at the carina or in one of the mainstem bronchi, overaeration of one lung and atelectasis of the opposite lung may result. The position of the head, especially in a neonate, may result in a significant change in position of the endotracheal tube tip: the tip will advance toward the carina when the head is flexed.

If a chest radiograph is obtained for suspected esophageal intubation, the stomach, small bowel, and esophagus will be distended with air while the lungs will be underinflated. Although usually not necessary, a lateral view would show the endotracheal tube in the more posterior esophagus. The lateral view may be more useful for showing adequate tracheal positioning and length in long-term placement of a tracheostomy tube.

The positions of vascular catheters should also be evaluated and repositioned if necessary. If the tip of the catheter is in the right atrium, arrhythmia may result. Pneumothorax and new ipsilateral pleural effusion could result from error in catheter placement.

AIRWAY OBSTRUCTION

The adenoids are posterior to the nasopharynx on the lateral neck radiograph. The palatine tonsils are best seen between the oropharynx and nasopharynx. Enlargement of these normal lymphoid structures is a major cause of sleep-related apnea. An acute infection can also cause adenoidal and tonsillar enlargement leading to airway obstruction (Figure 8-6).

Croup is the most common cause of upper airway obstruction in children, with a peak incidence in infants and children 6 months to 3 years of age. Most cases are virally induced (parainfluenza) and cause inspiratory stridor with a barking cough. Frontal and lateral neck radiographs may show the characteristic subglottic

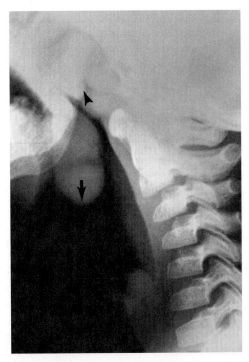

FIGURE 8-6 Enlarged tonsils *(arrow)* appear to hang down into the hypopharynx. The nasopharynx *(arrowhead)* is narrowed from enlarged adenoids located posterior and superior.

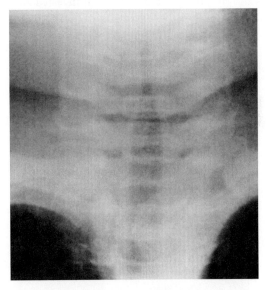

FIGURE 8-7 "Steepling" of the subglottic airway is caused by croup.

narrowing below the vocal cords with loss of the normal "shouldering" of the airway and resultant "church steeple" appearance. The hypopharynx usually appears overdistended (Figure 8-7).

Whereas croup usually improves within a few days of supportive therapy, *epiglottitis* is a life-threatening disease causing acute inspiratory stridor, fever, and *dysphasia* (speech impairment). The usual pathogen is *Haemophilus influenzae,* with the risk of infection now greatly reduced by immunization programs. The diagnosis should be made by physical examination or by direct visualization through a scope. If a lateral radiograph of the neck is obtained, the epiglottis is enlarged, and the aryepiglottic folds are thickened with overdistention of the hypopharynx. The radiograph is performed upright in the position most comfortable for the patient to breathe. Because safety of the child is of primary concern, the radiograph should be performed portably in the emergency department, where intubation can be performed quickly if necessary (Figure 8-8).

Retropharyngeal cellulitis and abscess are usually preceded by an upper respiratory infection, often with cervical adenopathy (enlargement of the cervical lymph nodes). Spread of infection along lymph channels leads to enlargement of the retropharyngeal (prevertebral) soft tissues on the lateral neck radiograph with forward displacement and bowing of the airway (Figure 8-9). Computed tomography (CT) is the modality of choice for distinguishing cellulitis from an abscess, which will appear as a walled-off fluid collection needing surgical drainage.

On occasion the child being evaluated for stridor has aspirated a foreign body such as a peanut into the bronchus and the airway is blocked, or has ingested an object such as a coin into the esophagus, causing compression of the trachea. If the child is suspected of ingesting a coin or other object, a lateral radiograph of the neck and frontal views of the chest and abdomen are usually obtained to locate the object (Figure 8-10). Nonradiopaque objects that are aspirated may be difficult to see unless outlined by air in the trachea or bronchi. Forced expiratory chest views, decubitus films, or

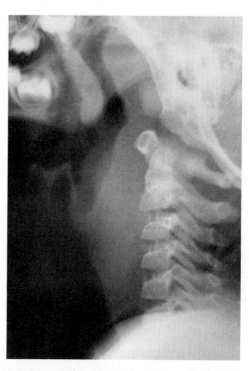

FIGURE 8-9 Hypopharynx and trachea are displaced away from the cervical spine by a retropharyngeal abscess.

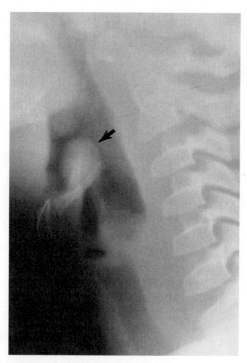

FIGURE 8-8 Enlarged epiglottis *(arrow)* appears as a "thumb" projecting into the airway.

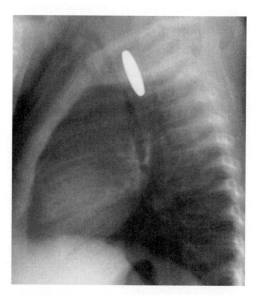

FIGURE 8-10 Edema from a coin in the upper esophagus causes marked narrowing of the adjacent trachea. The child presented with stridor and difficulty with swallowing.

fluoroscopy may be useful in showing the air trapping that may result when a foreign body is aspirated into a bronchus.

Tracheomalacia is diagnosed when the thoracic trachea abnormally collapses during expiration, leading to an expiratory wheeze. Although this may be seen in premature infants, other associations include tracheoesophageal fistula and vascular rings. The abnormal collapse may be easily demonstrated by airway fluoroscopy, which may be combined with a barium swallow to exclude a fistula or ring.[1,2]

RESPIRATORY DISTRESS IN THE NEWBORN

The various entities resulting in respiratory distress in the newborn may be combined under the mnemonic "CHAMPS" (Box 8-1).

One of the most common causes of respiratory distress in the newborn is transient tachypnea of the newborn. Conditions that decrease the thoracic squeeze to clear the lungs of fluid at delivery include cesarean section, mild or moderate prematurity, maternal diabetes, and precipitous delivery. The radiographic findings usually show mild vascular congestion with pulmonary edema and small pleural effusions. The chest film clears rapidly by 24 hours and is usually normal by 48 to 72 hours of age with conservative treatment.

Respiratory distress syndrome (RDS), or hyaline membrane disease, occurs in premature infants and is caused by a deficiency in pulmonary surfactant. By lowering the surface tension in the alveoli, surfactant prevents atelectasis. When surfactant is deficient, the chest radiograph shows the characteristic pattern of low lung volumes with a ground-glass or granular pattern of alveolar collapse surrounding *air bronchograms* (air-filled bronchus against surrounding opacified alveoli, indicating alveolar disease) (Figure 8-11).

Artificial surfactant given through the endotracheal tube may lead to rapid radiographic improvement, but it may also lead to asymmetric patterns of aeration if distributed unevenly. Gradual improvement over 1 week occurs with mild or moderate cases of RDS, but severe disease

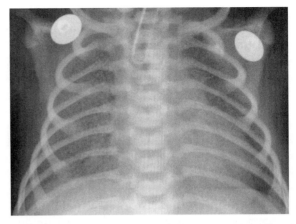

FIGURE 8-11 Even after intubation, the lungs are hypoinflated and have a granular pattern with faint air bronchograms in this infant with respiratory distress syndrome.

usually results in the chronic lung changes of bronchopulmonary dysplasia. This chronic disease is characterized by coarse, linear areas of scarring or atelectasis interspersed with areas of air trapping as well as shifting atelectasis. Both RDS and bronchopulmonary dysplasia may develop a variety of air leaks related to mechanical ventilation, including pneumothorax, pneumomediastinum, and pulmonary interstitial emphysema.

Pneumothoraces are the most common air leaks and are caused when air dissects in the pleural space surrounding the lung. On the frontal film of a supine patient, air is usually seen lateral to the lung but may be subpulmonic (between the lung and diaphragm) or medial (next to the heart), in the latter case mimicking a pneumomediastinum (Figure 8-12). If the hemithorax appears hyperlucent or the lateral costophrenic margin is too clearly visualized, a decubitus view or cross-table

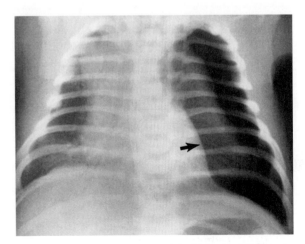

FIGURE 8-12 Large left pneumothorax appears black and outlines the partially collapsed left lung and left cardiac border *(arrow)*.

Box 8-1	Respiratory Distress in the Newborn
C: Cardiac, congenital anomalies	
H: Hyaline membrane disease	
A: Airway	
M: Meconium aspiration	
P: Pneumonia	
S: Surgical lesions	

lateral view (patient supine with x-ray beam parallel to the table and passing through the patient from one side to the other side) may be helpful to exclude a pneumothorax. The upright chest film is preferred in older children in whom the pneumothorax accumulates above the lung apex.

When air dissects into the mediastinal tissues, it is called a *pneumomediastinum*. This air elevates the thymus, producing a "spinnaker sail" appearance, and may dissect under the heart, leading to a continuous diaphragm appearance (Figure 8-13). A lateral decubitus film may cause a medial pneumothorax to shift to the elevated lateral pleural space, which distinguishes it from a pneumomediastinum. Air in a pneumopericardium surrounds only the heart and does not extend around other mediastinal structures such as the aorta. Neither a medial pneumothorax nor a pneumopericardium will elevate the thymus.

Pulmonary interstitial emphysema results from air dissecting within the interstitium of the lung. This condition appears as a diffuse pattern of random, small radiolucent bubbles combined with an irregular network of branching radiolucencies. Distribution is variable from entire lung to lobar to segmental. Interestingly, the pattern of involvement may shift from one lobe of one lung to another lobe in the other lung (Figure 8-14).

The radiographic appearance of RDS can also be complicated by the superimposition of a *patent ductus arteriosus* (in the newborn, a failure of the connection between the aorta and the pulmonary artery to close) or hemorrhage. The appearance of pleural effusions with increased heart size and edema several days after birth suggests patent ductus arteriosus. Whiteout of a lung or lobe without volume loss may result from pulmonary hemorrhage.

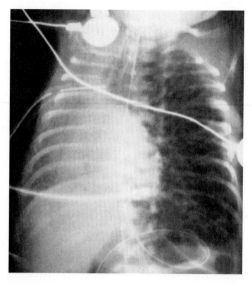

FIGURE 8-14 Massive pulmonary interstitial emphysema throughout the left lung causes shift of the mediastinum to the right and downward displacement of the left hemidiaphragm.

Although meconium staining of amniotic fluid occurs in 12% of deliveries, only 2% of these newborns develop meconium aspiration syndrome. Predisposing factors are postmaturity, intrauterine stress, and small size for gestational age. The aspirated meconium produced by the bowel plugs bronchi and produces a chemical pneumonitis. The chest radiograph is characterized by coarse, patchy opacities secondary to atelectasis from bronchial obstruction alternating with areas of hyperinflation (Figure 8-15). The severity of the radiographic abnormalities does not always correlate with the clinical severity of the disease. Likewise, an infant with

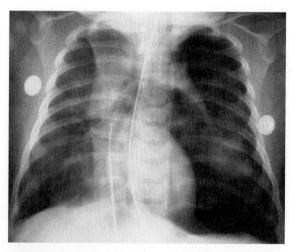

FIGURE 8-13 Pneumomediastinum elevates the left lobe of the thymus to produce a "spinnaker sail" in this child, who also has a large left pneumothorax.

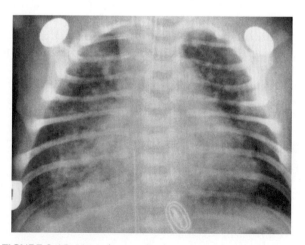

FIGURE 8-15 Meconium aspiration appears as a coarse asymmetric pattern. Enlargement of the heart may be secondary to fluid overload in this infant.

relatively mild radiographic findings may be worse clinically because of persistent pulmonary hypertension. Pneumothoraces and pneumomediastinum develop in about 25% of infants with meconium aspiration syndrome. Resolution of the radiographic findings may take several weeks.

Although a variety of organisms may cause neonatal pneumonia, the most common is group B *Streptococcus*, which is usually acquired transnatally. Premature rupture of the membranes and maternal infection are predisposing factors. The radiographic findings are variable and may mimic other disease entities. For example, pneumonia may have a pattern resembling RDS; however, the presence of pleural effusions is rare in RDS but common in neonatal pneumonia (Figure 8-16). Treatment is usually begun on the basis of the clinical assumption of pneumonia, with the radiographs used to monitor progress of the disease.[3]

Two surgical entities that may cause a cystic appearance in the lung are congenital diaphragmatic hernia and cystic adenomatoid malformation. In congenital diaphragmatic hernia, bowel herniates through the defect in the diaphragm, leading to a "cystic" appearance as the loops become air filled. If the stomach herniates as well, placement of a nasogastric tube may confirm the diagnosis. Because the bowel is in the chest, the abdomen will appear *scaphoid* (concave). Most of the hernias occur on the left. Patient outcome depends on the degree of pulmonary hypoplasia caused by compression of the developing lung tissue (Figure 8-17).

Cystic adenomatoid malformation is a derangement in normal pulmonary tissue development, leading to cysts ranging from millimeters to several centimeters in size. Initially the cysts are fluid filled but become air filled over the first day or two of life. A large dominant cyst could mimic congenital lobar overinflation,

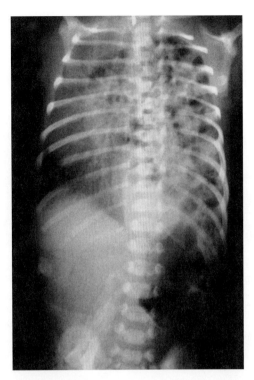

FIGURE 8-17 Multiple "cysts" in the left hemithorax are air-filled loops of bowel that herniated through a defect in the left hemidiaphragm. The abdomen is scaphoid from decreased bowel content.

whereas cysts appearing to fill one lung could mimic congenital diaphragmatic hernia. The presence of a normal amount of bowel in the abdomen would make a hernia unlikely.[4]

ATELECTASIS

Atelectasis is caused by an absence of air in the lung parenchyma from a myriad of causes, including bronchial obstruction or extrinsic compression. Most atelectasis is subsegmental in extent and appears as discoid or platelike opacities, often radiating from the hila or located just above the diaphragm. Segments, lobes, and entire lungs may be collapsed, or *atelectatic*. This loss of volume may shift fissures toward the area of atelectasis, cause mediastinal shift toward the affected side, and elevate the ipsilateral diaphragm. Crowding of the pulmonary vascular and interstitial markings in the affected region will occur. The other lung or adjacent lobes may become more lucent secondary to hyperexpansion.

When atelectasis occurs in the right upper lobe, the minor fissure and posterior half of the major fissure shift upward. The collapsed right upper lobe appears as a triangular wedge of opacity adjacent to the superior mediastinum in the frontal radiograph and as a

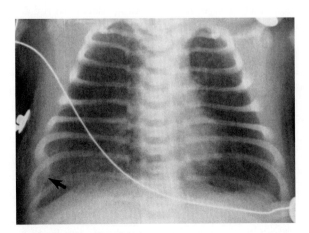

FIGURE 8-16 Group B streptococcal pneumonia presents in this infant with hyperinflation, small right pleural effusion *(arrow)*, and hazy infiltrative pattern.

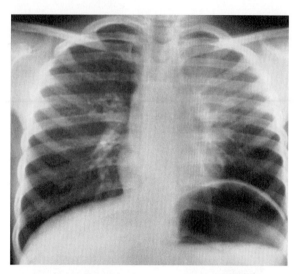

FIGURE 8-18 Left upper lobe collapse causes elevation of the left hemidiaphragm and crowding of the left ribs from volume loss. The cardiac and superior mediastinal borders are indistinct because of the "silhouette sign" while the diaphragm remains demarcated by the aerated left lower lobe.

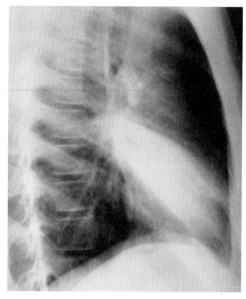

FIGURE 8-19 Collapsed right middle lobe appears as a triangular wedge of increased density extending anteriorly and inferiorly toward the anterior chest wall and diaphragm.

triangular wedge at the apex in the lateral radiograph. Because no minor fissure is present on the left, collapse of the left upper lobe appears different from the right, with the major fissure shifting in an anterior direction. The collapsed left upper lobe on frontal projection appears as an opacity in the upper two thirds of the lung that obscures superior mediastinal and left cardiac borders and lacks a sharply defined border with the aerated lower lobe (Figure 8-18). In lateral projection the left upper lobe collapses adjacent to the anterior chest wall, with the major fissure defining the edge against the lower lobe. Isolated lingular atelectasis obscures the left cardiac border.

Right middle lobe collapse is commonly seen in children with asthma and causes the major and minor fissures to approximate. The resultant triangular wedge or platelike opacity is most diagnostic in lateral projection and extends from the hilum to the anterior chest wall (Figure 8-19). It is less defined in frontal projection and may appear as a vague loss of the right cardiac border. A seldom used special view, called the *apical lordotic view*, rotates the right middle lobe collapse on the frontal projection so that it is better seen as a triangular opacity contiguous with the right cardiac border.

Both right and left lower lobe atelectasis cause downward and posterior displacement of the major fissure. The lower lobe collapses toward the posterior aspect of the diaphragm on the lateral view and retrocardiac adjacent to the spine on the frontal view. The sharp border of the adjacent diaphragm becomes

obscured in both projections. In the lateral radiograph the normally more lucent-appearing lower thoracic vertebral bodies appear denser than normal because the x-ray beam must penetrate through the adjacent collapsed lower lobe. This increased density of the lower thoracic vertebral bodies has been termed the "spine sign." Left lower lobe collapse is commonly seen in postoperative patients, especially those having undergone cardiothoracic surgery.

The previously described silhouette sign is useful in localizing suspected atelectasis. The right cardiac border loses its sharp definition with right middle lobe atelectasis, whereas the left border is associated with lingular pathology. The diaphragmatic border is lost when atelectasis or other pathology occurs in the adjacent lower lobe.[5]

PNEUMONIA

Viruses are the most common cause of pneumonia in children, especially in the outpatient population. Many bacterial pneumonias are superimposed over viral infections but may also be seen in hospitalized patients. Fungal and less common infections should be suspected in the immunocompromised patient.

Infections may involve primarily the airways, mainly the peripheral airspaces, or a combination of both. Bronchiolitis in the younger child and bronchitis in the older child are viral infections of the airways leading to a radiographic appearance of bronchial wall thickening. Hyperinflation of the lungs as well as linear areas of atelectasis secondary to airway plugging by mucus are often associated with airway inflammation.

Patchy areas of poorly defined parenchymal opacification characterize bronchopneumonia. The inflammation in the airways extends outward to involve the adjacent air spaces. The opacities may be caused by the air space inflammation as well as by atelectasis from associated mucous plugging of the peripheral airways. Air bronchograms occur when the open airways are surrounded by consolidated or collapsed air spaces. Both viral and bacterial pneumonias can cause a bronchopneumonia pattern. Although it may mimic other pulmonary diseases, *Mycoplasma* presents typically as a bronchopneumonia.

Filling of the peripheral air spaces with an infectious exudate causes a dense, consolidated appearance. The involvement may be limited to a segment of lung or spread to involve the entire lobe. Bacterial infections are usually the cause of consolidated, or lobar, pneumonia.

Pneumonia may be associated with hilar adenopathy and pleural effusions. When the pleura becomes infected, the resulting empyema may need to be surgically drained. Although decubitus films may be able to differentiate an uncomplicated mobile pleural effusion from loculated fluid or thickening, both ultrasound and CT can be used to better characterize the pleural fluid. Pulmonary abscesses are rare complications, but *pneumatoceles* (thin-walled, air-filled cavities in the lungs) may occur after staphylococcal pneumonia. Round pneumonias are usually of pneumococcal origin (Figure 8-20).[6-9]

ASTHMA

Asthma is caused by recurrent bronchospasm of the large intrathoracic airways, leading to wheezing and labored breathing. Chest radiographs are usually obtained to exclude the presence of pneumonia causing the acute episode. Typical findings are hyperinflation and bronchial wall thickening. Mucous plugging of the airways may lead to atelectasis and focal air trapping. Atelectasis is the usual cause of a focal opacity in the lung. Pneumomediastinum occurs in a small percentage of children evaluated for an acute asthma attack and is a cause of acute chest pain.[7,9]

CYSTIC FIBROSIS

Cystic fibrosis is a genetic disorder, more commonly found among white individuals, that causes increased viscosity of the respiratory mucus. This mucus is difficult to clear from the airways, leading to obstruction and promotion of bacterial infection. Early childhood radiographs may show nonspecific findings of airway disease with peribronchial thickening, atelectasis, and air trapping. These early changes are similar to the chest radiographs of a patient with asthma. As the disease progresses, fingerlike mucoid impaction of the airways may be demonstrated along with abnormal dilation of the airways, called *bronchiectasis*. Recurrent infections are common. Striking hyperinflation is seen in older patients, often with enlarged hila from pulmonary hypertension (Figure 8-21).[8]

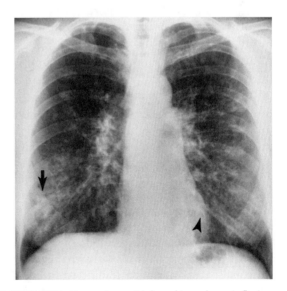

FIGURE 8-21 Coarse interstitial markings, hyperinflation, bronchiectasis, mucous plugging *(arrow)*, atelectasis *(arrowhead)*, and enlarged pulmonary hila are all demonstrated in this child with cystic fibrosis.

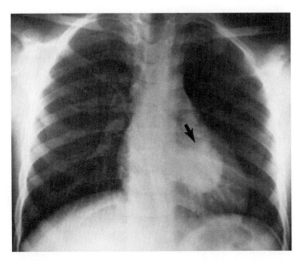

FIGURE 8-20 Round pneumonia *(arrow)* in the left lower lobe simulates a mass.

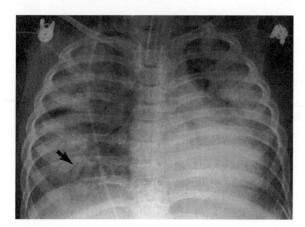

FIGURE 8-22 Pneumonia was the precipitating precursor to acute respiratory distress syndrome, with densely consolidated lungs and air bronchograms (*arrow*).

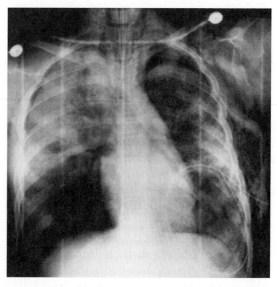

FIGURE 8-23 Trauma to the chest resulted in extensive bilateral air leaks and densely consolidated pulmonary contusions. Multiple rib fractures are present.

ACUTE RESPIRATORY DISTRESS SYNDROME

Although originally described in adults, acute respiratory distress syndrome may occur in children as well. These patients present initially with either sepsis, pneumonia, near drowning, inhalation injury, aspiration, or trauma. The acute lung insult can lead to increased capillary permeability, pulmonary edema, surfactant inactivation, alveolar filling, and reduced lung compliance. This leads to profound hypoxemia and acute respiratory distress syndrome. The disease passes through stages of acute lung injury, exudative alveolitis, fibroproliferative repair, and finally recovery if the patient survives. The mortality rate is high. Pneumothoraces and pneumomediastinum are common complications (Figure 8-22).[10]

CHEST TRAUMA

When an injured child is evaluated in the emergency department, initial radiographs to screen for trauma usually include a frontal view of the chest. Lines and tubes inserted at the accident site or on arrival in the emergency department should be assessed for position and effectiveness. A right mainstem intubation may lead to collapse of the left lung. The position of a chest tube may not be optimal for evacuating a pneumothorax, and the nasogastric tube may need to be advanced into the stomach.

Consolidation in the patient with blunt trauma may result from pulmonary contusion with hemorrhage into the air spaces. Aspiration leading to patchy consolidation in the upper lobes should be considered in the patient with loss of consciousness. Laceration of the lung may lead to cysts in the parenchyma as well as a pneumothorax. The rib cage should be evaluated for

fractures, especially adjacent to an area of lung injury. Multiple contiguous rib fractures may result in a flail chest (three or more rib fractures resulting in paradoxical motion of the chest wall with respiration) with associated ventilation difficulties (Figure 8-23).

Widening of the superior mediastinum suggests hemorrhage, which could be venous or related to aortic injury. Traumatic aortic rupture is rare in children as opposed to adults. Small children have prominent thymic tissue, so this should be excluded as the cause of mediastinal widening. Tracheal and bronchial fractures are rare but cause massive air leaks. Enlargement of the cardiac silhouette from a traumatic pericardial effusion is rare.

When significant chest injury is suspected clinically or demonstrated on chest radiographs, CT scans of the chest more clearly demonstrate the extent of the injury than plain radiographs. These are often rapidly performed in conjunction with imaging of the abdomen. Lung and mediastinal injury as well as placement of chest tubes can be further clarified. More injury is often shown by CT scans than was suspected on chest radiographs. Not uncommonly, small pneumothoraces are found by CT that cannot be seen even in retrospect on plain films. CT angiography of the chest has supplanted catheter aortography for exclusion of aortic injury. The need for CT is usually made clear after assessment of the previously obtained chest radiographs. Although CT scanning of the chest may provide additional information, routine scanning in children is discouraged because of the added radiation dose.[7,8]

ASSESSMENT QUESTIONS

See Evolve Resources for answers.

1. A mother states that she found her 18-month-old child choking near an open can of peanuts. Which set of chest radiographs would most likely suggest airway obstruction?
   A. Frontal and bilateral oblique
   B. Frontal inspiratory and forced expiratory
   C. Frontal and cross-table lateral
   D. Frontal and left-side down lateral decubitus

2. The normal thymus has a characteristic appearance with several radiographic findings *except:*
   A. Displacement of the trachea to the opposite side of the mediastinum
   B. Appearance of a sail
   C. Wavy margins
   D. Increased density in the anterior mediastinum on the lateral view

3. A pneumothorax is suspected on the left in a child's portable radiograph from the intensive care unit. Which of the following may better image and confirm a suspected pneumothorax?
   I. Cross-table lateral
   II. Upright frontal
   III. Left-side down decubitus
   IV. Right-side down decubitus
   A. I, II, and III only
   B. I, II, and IV only
   C. I, III, and IV only
   D. II, III, and IV only

4. Subglottic edema causing a "church steeple" appearance of the trachea on the frontal neck radiograph is characteristic of which infection?
   A. Retropharyngeal abscess
   B. Epiglottitis
   C. Adenoiditis
   D. Croup

5. Before intubation, the chest radiograph of a premature newborn reveals low lung volumes and diffuse ground-glass opacification of the lungs. These radiographic findings are most characteristic of
   A. Meconium aspiration
   B. Respiratory distress syndrome
   C. Bronchopulmonary dysplasia
   D. Transient tachypnea of the newborn

6. The initial chest radiograph of a neonate in severe respiratory distress and having a scaphoid abdomen reveals multiple round air-filled structures in the left chest, displacing the mediastinum to the right. The most likely etiology is
   A. Congenital adenomatoid malformation
   B. Pulmonary interstitial emphysema
   C. Congenital diaphragmatic hernia
   D. Staphylococcal pneumonia

ASSESSMENT QUESTIONS—cont'd

7. Left lower lobe collapse (atelectasis) is associated with the following radiographic findings:
   I. Loss of the left heart border
   II. Loss of the left hemidiaphragm border
   III. Increased retrocardiac density
   IV. "Spine sign"
   A. I, II, and III only
   B. I, II, and IV only
   C. I, III, and IV only
   D. II, III, and IV only

8. Pneumatoceles are occasionally seen as a complication of which of the following infections?
   A. Mycoplasmal
   B. Viral
   C. Streptococcal
   D. Staphylococcal

9. Which of the following is a hallmark of cystic fibrosis and is *not* also seen with asthma?
   A. Hyperinflation
   B. Atelectasis
   C. Bronchiectasis
   D. Airway disease

10. CT scans of the chest in a pediatric trauma patient are not routinely obtained because of
    A. Increased radiation
    B. Time consumption
    C. Intravenous contrast
    D. Atelectasis

References

1. Strife JL: Upper airway and tracheal obstruction in infants and children, *Radiol Clin North Am* 1988;26:309.
2. Griscom NT: Diseases of the trachea, bronchi and smaller airways, *Radiol Clin North Am* 1993;31:605.
3. Newman B, Bowen AD, Sang OK: A practical approach to the newborn chest, *Curr Probl Diagn Radiol* 1990;19:41.
4. Newman B, Sang OK: Abnormal pulmonary aeration in infants and children, *Radiol Clin North Am* 1988;26:323.
5. Paré JA, Fraser R: *Synopsis of diseases of the chest*, Philadelphia: WB Saunders; 1983.
6. Eggli KD, Newman B: Nodules, masses, and pseudomasses in the pediatric lung, *Radiol Clin North Am* 1993;31:651.
7. Hedlund GL, Kirks DR: Emergency radiology of the pediatric chest, *Curr Probl Diagn Radiol* 1990;19:133.
8. Kirks DR: Practical pediatric imaging. In *Diagnostic radiology of infants and children*, ed 3, Philadelphia: Lippincott-Raven; 1998.
9. Hilton SV, Edwards DK: *Practical pediatric radiology*, Philadelphia: WB Saunders; 1994.
10. Kuhn JP et al: *Caffey's pediatric diagnostic imaging*, ed 10, Philadelphia: Mosby; 2004.

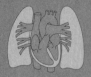

Chapter 9

Pediatric Flexible Bronchoscopy

KARL KALAVANTAVANICH • CRAIG M. SCHRAMM

OUTLINE

Indications
    Diagnostic Bronchoscopy
    Therapeutic Bronchoscopy
Contraindications
Equipment
    Flexible Bronchoscope
    Video Recording Equipment
Preparation
    Equipment and Supplies
    Patient
    Personnel

Procedure
    Conscious Sedation
    Topical Anesthesia
    Patient Monitoring
    Technique
Postprocedural Monitoring and Complications
Equipment Maintenance
Comparison With Rigid Bronchoscopy

LEARNING OBJECTIVES

After reading this chapter the reader will be able to:
- Identify common indications for bronchoscopy in infants and children and the differences between rigid and flexible bronchoscopy
- Prepare equipment and the patient for a flexible bronchoscopy procedure

- Monitor a patient during a flexible bronchoscopy, including what complications to watch for during and after the procedure
- Clean and disinfect bronchoscopes after procedures

Flexible fiberoptic bronchoscopy was first introduced for clinical practice in 1968, with the invention of flexible scopes containing fiberoptic bundles to illuminate and visualize the airways. The procedure was initially performed in adults because of the relatively large size of the fiberscopes, and most often by surgeons in operating suites. The development of smaller bronchoscopes in the late 1970s led to the widespread extension of this procedure to the pediatric population.[1] Pediatric flexible bronchoscopy is now performed by many medical specialists, including pediatric pulmonologists, otolaryngologists, surgeons, anesthesiologists, and pediatric intensivists. It is done in a variety of settings, including bronchoscopy suites, operating suites, intensive care units, and procedure rooms.[2-5] In the more recent past, direct visual inspection of the pediatric airways with or without bronchoalveolar lavage has become a major tool for the evaluation of several respiratory disorders.

INDICATIONS

Flexible bronchoscopy is indicated when (1) information valuable to the management of a patient cannot be obtained by less invasive techniques and (2) therapeutic interventions need to be directly administered to the airway (Box 9-1). As with any invasive procedure, the potential benefits to be gained in any given patient must be weighed against the risks of the procedure, even the most minor risk.

Diagnostic Bronchoscopy

For diagnostic purposes, persistent or recurrent respiratory symptoms are the most common indication for flexible bronchoscopy, including stridor and abnormal voice, wheeze, cough, and recurrent or persistent abnormalities on chest radiography.

Stridor

Stridor, a high-pitched sound produced by turbulent airflow through a partially obstructed airway, is the most common diagnostic indication for flexible bronchoscopy in infants. The possible causes of recurrent or persistent stridor include vocal cord dysfunction, laryngeal pathology, subglottic stenosis, mass or tumor, and extrinsic compression of the tracheobronchial tree.

Stridor often varies in intensity depending on the extent of a child's activity or agitation, which increases the child's minute ventilation. This increase in airflow will result in louder stridor. Thus, stridor is a dynamic process in children, and flexible bronchoscopy is ideally suited for its evaluation. Because flexible bronchoscopy can be performed on a sedated but spontaneously breathing patient, the dynamics of the airways are preserved, without disruption by general anesthesia, positive-pressure ventilation, or the oral approach of rigid bronchoscopy. Of all indications of diagnostic pediatric flexible bronchoscopy, stridor receives the highest diagnostic yield of the procedure, identifying specific lesions in more than 80% of patients.[6,7]

The most common cause of inspiratory stridor is *laryngomalacia,* which is a prolapse of the epiglottis or aryepiglottic folds into the supraglottic space during inspiration. Laryngomalacia is caused by a congenital weakness in cartilage stiffness and redundant aryepiglottic tissue. The condition occurs in three patterns:

- The prolapse of one or both arytenoids into the supraglottic space during inspiration
- The lateral infolding across the airway of a soft epiglottis that is more omega than crescent shaped in a young infant
- The anteroposterior bending of a soft epiglottis across the supraglottic space

Box 9-1	**Indications for Flexible Bronchoscopy**

DIAGNOSTIC

AIRWAY ANATOMY EVALUATION
- Fistulas
- Hemangiomas or tumors
- Stenoses or strictures
- Tracheal bronchus
- Tracheostomy evaluation
- Vascular rings

BRONCHOALVEOLAR LAVAGE AND BIOPSY
Cytopathology
- Lipid-laden macrophages
- Hemosiderin-stained macrophages
- Malignant cells

Microbiology
- Bacteria
- Fungi
- *Pneumocystis*
- *Mycobacterium tuberculosis*
- Viruses

FOREIGN BODY ASPIRATION

FUNCTIONAL AIRWAY EVALUATION
- Laryngo/tracheo/bronchomalacia
- Vocal cord dysfunction

HEMOPTYSIS

INHALATION INJURY

THERAPEUTIC
- Atelectasis
- Endotracheal intubation
- Foreign body aspiration
- Laser therapy

Other laryngeal lesions that can produce stridor include unilateral or bilateral abductor vocal cord paralysis from congenital lesions, birth trauma, or recurrent laryngeal nerve injury after thoracic surgery; laryngeal papillomatosis; and laryngeal webs. Inspiratory or biphasic stridor may also arise from subglottic lesions, such as congenital or acquired subglottic stenosis, subglottic edema resulting from infection or chronic acid aspiration, or subglottic hemangiomas.

Tracheomalacia, caused by a congenital or acquired weakness in tracheal cartilaginous support, may cause inspiratory stridor but is more often associated with biphasic or expiratory stridor. Tracheomalacia may be seen in up to one third of patients with laryngomalacia. It is also present when the cartilage is deformed by a tracheoesophageal fistula or a vascular ring, and it may develop with long-standing tracheal inflammation, as seen in infants with bronchopulmonary dysplasia. If the weakness in support extends into the mainstem bronchi, the condition is termed *bronchomalacia.*

Additional causes of expiratory stridor include extrinsic tracheal or bronchial obstruction from vascular rings or slings, anomalous arteries, congenital heart disease, hilar adenopathy, or mediastinal mass lesions.

Wheeze

Recurrent *wheezing,* a continuous, coarse, whistling sound, is another common respiratory symptom in the pediatric population. Wheezing usually results from a more distal site of airway obstruction than stridor. The most frequent cause of recurrent wheezing in children is asthma, and most patients with asthma do not require bronchoscopy as part of their evaluation. Exceptions to this rule include asthmatics with recurrent or persistent *atelectasis* (lung collapse, frequently of the right middle lobe) or asthmatics with gastroesophageal reflux, who may have chronic aspiration. A flexible bronchoscopic evaluation is often indicated to investigate other causes of wheezing, particularly when the wheezing is unilateral, is present at birth or at a young age, or is refractory to asthma medications. Nonasthmatic causes of wheezing include anatomic abnormalities of the airway (e.g., bronchomalacia, stenosis, and extrinsic compression of the left mainstem bronchus from a dilated heart), anomalies of the great vessels (vascular ring), recurrent aspiration, or foreign body aspiration.

Cough

Some disorders may produce chronic cough in addition to wheezing, and bronchoscopy is often indicated because of chronic refractory cough. This indication is particularly strong when there is radiographic indication of *bronchiectasis,* that is, chronic dilation of the bronchi and bronchioles associated with secondary infection, in an area of lung. There is little role for bronchoscopy in evaluating the cough that accompanies common childhood conditions such as upper and uncomplicated lower respiratory tract infections, sinusitis, postnasal drip syndrome, asthma, and exposure to environmental irritants. On the other hand, bronchoscopy should be considered to evaluate the possibilities of gastroesophageal reflux or aspiration, anatomic abnormalities of airways or large vessels, and any occult endobronchial lesions or foreign bodies, as well as to obtain culture specimens from children not responding to therapy.

Radiographic Abnormalities

Flexible bronchoscopy is indicated in the evaluation of a number of radiographic abnormalities in children, including recurrent or persistent atelectasis, localized pulmonary consolidation or hyperinflation, recurrent pneumonia, and focal atelectasis. Often, airway anatomic anomalies, mucous plugs, or unsuspected foreign body aspiration may be found. Children with lobar atelectasis or consolidation who have failed medical management may benefit from direct instillation of mucolytic agents and removal of mucous plugs via flexible bronchoscopy. Biopsies may also be obtained through the larger flexible bronchoscopes. These may include mucosal biopsies for the evaluation of ciliary motion and ultrastructure, as well as transbronchial biopsies for the diagnosis of certain pulmonary conditions, especially rejection or infection in lung transplant patients.

Foreign Body Aspiration

The flexible bronchoscope may be used to rule out the presence of a foreign body in the lower airways of children in whom the diagnosis is not strongly suspected. However, when the presence of a foreign body is confirmed or highly suspected either by radiographic evaluation or by history, the preferred approach is to identify and remove the foreign body by rigid bronchoscopy. Although some authors believe that the flexible bronchoscope can be used for the therapeutic purpose of foreign body removal, rigid bronchoscopy is a better and safer approach in children. It allows better ventilation of the patient under general anesthesia and facilitates safer delivery of large foreign bodies through the subglottic area and the larynx compared with the flexible bronchoscope.

Hemoptysis

Flexible bronchoscopy is sometimes indicated in selected pediatric patients with hemoptysis who need visual inspection of the airways for localization of their bleeding sites. It can be useful for therapeutic purposes as well, by removal of blood clots and placement of single-lumen or double-lumen endotracheal tubes and balloon catheters to tamponade (i.e., to exert direct pressure on) a bleeding site in the airway. In massive hemoptysis, however, the flexible bronchoscope is usually inadequate because of its limited visualization and suction capabilities compared with rigid bronchoscopy.

Inhalation Injury

In patients with acute inhalation of a toxic or heated gas, flexible bronchoscopic evaluation of the upper and lower airways can be helpful in judging the extent of injury and determining the therapy and level of respiratory support needed. The decision for elective intubation with the assistance of bronchoscopy may be made if significant laryngeal edema is visualized.

Therapeutic Bronchoscopy

The flexible bronchoscope is an excellent therapeutic tool. It is useful in placing an endotracheal tube in difficult intubation cases. The direct instillation of medications such as *N*-acetylcysteine (Mucomyst), dilute sodium bicarbonate, or recombinant human deoxyribonuclease I (DNase) can help dislodge retained secretions or mucous plugs before bronchoscopic suctioning. The flexible bronchoscope has also been used to administer surfactant in patients with acute respiratory distress syndrome. Laser surgery of airway lesions can be done through a flexible bronchoscope, but a rigid scope allows for mechanical as well as laser resection and for better control of bleeding complications.

CONTRAINDICATIONS

Flexible bronchoscopy has been shown to be a safe procedure, even when performed on ill pediatric patients. However, certain conditions can place a patient at risk for complications (Box 9-2). Most are relative contraindications. If, after careful evaluation, the possible benefit of bronchoscopy outweighs the risks, the procedure should be performed by an experienced bronchoscopist.

Flexible bronchoscopy frequently causes hypoxemia, most often due to occlusion of the airway by the bronchoscope during the procedure and hypoventilation or apnea from sedation. Pulse oximetry and cardiac and respiratory tracings should be continuously monitored during and after the procedure. Supplemental oxygen should be provided to maintain oxygen saturation, optimally above 95%. If the patient is already hypoxemic, flexible bronchoscopy can further worsen the hypoxemia and place the patient at serious risk. Patients with impending respiratory failure may be electively intubated before the bronchoscopy, in anticipation of worsening ventilation and oxygenation during and after the procedure.

Elective flexible bronchoscopy should not be performed in the patient who has cardiovascular instability, uncontrolled asthma, coagulopathy, pulmonary hypertension, severe upper airway obstruction, or superior vena cava obstruction, until these conditions are stabilized. It should be performed selectively and with great caution in patients with acute laryngotracheitis because of the risks of sudden laryngospasm during the procedure and additional postprocedural airway edema that may severely compromise an already swollen airway. The bronchoscope should never be inserted forcefully past any area of airway narrowing, to avoid further injury and compromise to that site. As noted earlier, the strong suspicion of foreign body aspiration is a relative contraindication to flexible bronchoscopy, and an indication for rigid bronchoscopy.

EQUIPMENT
Flexible Bronchoscope

The flexible bronchoscope may be divided into three sections: (1) the insertion tube, (2) the control head and eyepiece, and (3) the light source connector.

Insertion Tube

The insertion tube is the flexible portion of the bronchoscope that is inserted into the patient's airways. These tubes have the same working length of 55 cm, but they vary in outer diameter from less than 2.0 mm to 6.3 mm. The instruments most often used in pediatric patients are 2.2-mm-diameter scopes for neonates, 2.7- to 3.6-mm scopes for older children, and 4.9-mm scopes for adolescents (Figure 9-1). The composition of the tubes varies somewhat according to the diameter. All scopes contain one or two fiberoptic bundles for light transmission from the light source to the airway, as well as one fiberoptic cable for transmission of the airway image from the tip of the scope to the

Box 9-2	Contraindications to Flexible Bronchoscopy

ABSOLUTE CONTRAINDICATIONS
- Inability to oxygenate the patient adequately
- Cardiovascular instability
  - Hypotension
  - Malignant arrhythmias
  - Myocardial infarction

RELATIVE CONTRAINDICATIONS
- Coagulopathy
- Hypercapnia with acidosis
- Hypoxemia
- Severe pulmonary hypertension
- Severe upper airway obstruction
- Superior vena cava obstruction
- Uncooperative patient
- Uncontrolled asthma
- Uremia

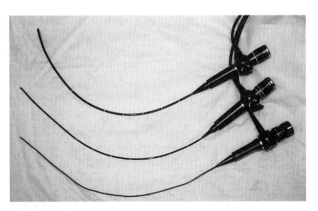

FIGURE 9-1 Three different sizes of pediatric flexible bronchoscopes. *Top to bottom*: 4.5-, 3.6-, and 2.2-mm outer diameter. Note that all scopes have similar working tube lengths.

eyepiece. These fiberoptic bundles consist of thousands of tiny (8-μm) glass fibers that are coated with a highly reflective glass material. These fibers transmit light and images by internal reflections at the core–coating interface. This arrangement of highly reflective, minute glass fibers accounts for the bronchoscope's flexibility and high image quality; however, it also imparts substantial fragility to the instrument. Efforts to miniaturize CCDs (charge-coupled devices) have led to the development of bronchoscopes with tiny CCDs in their tips that record an image and then transport it electronically to the recording device. The CCD bronchoscopes provide larger and clearer images, free of the dots characteristic of fiberoptic images. Previous size constraints have limited these scopes to adult patients, but a new 3.8-mm CCD bronchoscope promises to extend this technology to pediatric patients.

The insertion tubes of the thinnest bronchoscopes, those less than 2.0 mm in diameter, contain only light and image bundles. They are nondirectable because they lack the cables necessary to direct the distal section of the scope. Appropriately, they have been nicknamed "spaghetti scopes," and their use is limited to visualization of an airway via insertion down an endotracheal tube.

Larger, flexible bronchoscopes have two control cables aligned 180 degrees from each other that connect a hinged bending section at the distal tip of the tube to a control lever at the head of the scope. These cables allow the operator to flex and extend the distal tip of the bronchoscope, in order to direct the passage of the scope through the airways. The 2.2-mm scopes have this directable capability, but they lack the third major component of the insertion tube, a suction channel. The larger scopes contain suction channels, varying in diameter from 1.2 mm in the 3.5- to 3.7-mm scopes to 3.2 mm in the 4.5-mm scopes. These suction channels allow for the suction of airway secretions, the instillation of lavage fluids or medications into the airway, and the passage of brushes and biopsy instruments for obtaining airway cytology and pathology specimens. The channel, direction cables, and fiberoptic bundles are enmeshed in a woven metal sheath and then enclosed in a nonlatex flexible plastic membrane.

Control Head and Eyepiece

The control head directs the insertion tube and use of the bronchoscope and transmits its images to the operator. Transmission is accomplished with an eyepiece and focusing ring. The operator may look through the eyepiece directly at the distal image. Alternatively, the image is recorded by a camera attached to the eyepiece and displayed on a video monitor during the procedure. On directable bronchoscopes, the control head contains an angulation lever, which regulates

the cables attached to the bending tip of the scope. On the larger scopes there is also a channel port attached, or in addition to, a button that activates suction through the suction channel. Syringes attach to the port for airway lavage, and instruments may be passed through the port for the collection of airway specimens. A suction adapter extends at a right angle from the head of the bronchoscope and attaches to tubing connected to the suction source.

Light Source Connector

The control head is also attached to a cable. The other end of the cable contains the light source connector, for the transmission of light from a source to the fiberoptic cables in the insertion tube. The light source houses a bright halogen or xenon lamp, which provides adequate illumination via the fiberoptic cables.

Video Recording Equipment

Video recording has proven to be invaluable in flexible bronchoscopy procedures. Video allows the bronchoscopist to review the findings after the procedure, identifying or clarifying lesions missed during the actual procedure and at other times allowing for consultation with medical or surgical colleagues. Video of the recorded procedure may also be shown to the patient and family when discussing the pathology and treatment plan. The video also provides a record of the findings, which may be used for comparison with past or future bronchoscopies.

PREPARATION

To perform an efficient and safe procedure with minimal complications, the practitioner needs to fully prepare the bronchoscopy area and equipment, medications, the patient, and the bronchoscopist and assistants.

Equipment and Supplies

The proper selection and preparation of equipment are important to ensure a safe and effective procedure. The preparation of this equipment and certain medications is usually the responsibility of the respiratory therapist who will assist in the procedure.

Pediatric bronchoscopes come in many diameters, with the smaller ones used in patients who have small airways, such as neonatal patients or patients with airway obstruction. Smaller directable scopes do not have suction channels and are more difficult to handle because they are more rigid and less flexible. The larger bronchoscope has a suction channel and usually provides better visualization.

The light source, video recorder, and monitor are usually maintained on a portable bronchoscope cart.

Equipment, such as 1% to 2% lidocaine spray, 2% lidocaine jelly for lubricant, syringes containing aliquots of 1% to 2% lidocaine, a Lukens trap, 10-ml normal saline aliquots for lavage, and clean gauzes, may be placed on top of the cart for easy access (Figure 9-2). A cardiac monitor, pulse oximeter, noninvasive blood pressure monitor, and emergency resuscitation cart should also be placed at the bedside. The cart must contain an appropriately sized resuscitation bag and mask, laryngoscopes and endotracheal tubes, and resuscitation medications. Wall suction and oxygen should be connected and turned on for prompt access if needed. Two sources of wall suction are ideal: one connected to the bronchoscope to clear the field of vision and to obtain specimens, and the other connected to a suction catheter for use if the patient has excessive oropharyngeal secretions or vomits during the procedure. On certain occasions, special equipment or medications may be needed, such as a swivel adapter for an endotracheal tube, positive end-expiratory pressure valves, tracheostomy tubes, wire brushes for cytology, transbronchial needle catheters, sodium bicarbonate, *N*-acetylcysteine, and DNase (Box 9-3).

During the procedure, nearly all pediatric patients require some type of sedation. The most common approach is a conscious sedation. Intravenous drugs are preferable to intramuscular medications because of their quicker onset, shorter duration, and titratable

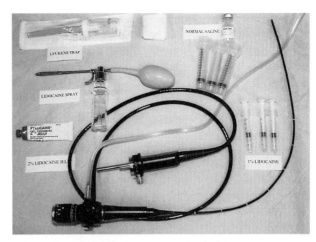

FIGURE 9-2 Necessary equipment for basic pediatric flexible bronchoscopy includes bronchoscope, attached suction tube, 2% lidocaine jelly, lidocaine spray, three 1-ml aliquots of 1% lidocaine solution, Luken trap, gauze pads, and three to five 10-ml aliquots of normal saline for bronchoalveolar lavage. These items are placed on a clean drape on top of a portable bronchoscopy cart.

dosage for optimal effects. Although various sedative agents are available, the combination of a benzodiazepine (e.g., midazolam) and a narcotic (e.g., fentanyl or morphine) is widely accepted. In addition to sedative

---

Box 9-3	Equipment and Supplies for Pediatric Flexible Bronchoscopy

Bronchoscope with light source
Endotracheal tube swivel adapter
Water-soluble lubricant
Monitoring equipment
- Cardiac monitor with electrode patches
- Pulse oximeter with probes
- Respiratory monitor
- Sphygmomanometer
- Stethoscope

Oxygen and aerosol equipment
- Aerosol mask
- Cannula with nasal prongs clipped
- Flowmeter
- Nebulizer
- Oxygen mask with nose cut out
- Oxygen source
- Oxygen tubing with connectors

Specimen collection equipment
- Biopsy forceps
- Channel brush
- Fixative
- Glass slides
- Luken trap
- Retrieval baskets and cages

- Syringes with nonbacteriostatic saline for bronchoalveolar lavage
- Transport media

Suction equipment
- Sterile gloves
- Suction canisters
- Suction catheters
- Suction tubing
- Tonsil-tip or Yankauer-type suction catheter
- Vacuum suction source

Intravenous equipment
- Isotonic saline
- Intravenous infusion sets
- Syringes with flush solution

Medications
- Topical anesthetics
  - Lidocaine solution (1% to 2%)
  - Lidocaine viscous (2%)
- Sedatives
  - Diazepam
  - Fentanyl
  - Meperidine
  - Midazolam
  - Morphine

Continued

Box 9-3	Equipment and Supplies for Pediatric Flexible Bronchoscopy—cont'd
Medications (cont'd)	**Resuscitation equipment**
• Aerosols	• Bite block
• Albuterol	• Endotracheal tubes
• Racemic epinephrine	• Laryngoscope with blades
• Emergency drugs	• Oral airways
• Atropine	• Resuscitation bag with oxygen tubing attached
• Bicarbonate	• Stylets
• Epinephrine (1:1000)	Extra batteries for laryngoscope
• Flumazenil	Extra light bulbs
• Furosemide	Face masks
• Intravenous corticosteroids	Video camera with recording equipment
• Naloxone	Bronchoscopist and assistant equipment
• Phenobarbital	• Eye protectors
• Succinylcholine	• Gloves
	• Gown
	• Mask
	• Scissors

effects, the narcotic provides analgesic and antitussive effects, and the benzodiazepine offers anxiolytic effects and antegrade amnesia. The most common side effect of this combination is respiratory depression. On occasion, benzodiazepines can induce cardiovascular depression, and narcotics can elicit muscular rigidity and impaired liver and kidney functions. Fortunately, if these complications occur, specific reversal agents, naloxone (0.01 mg/kg per dose) and flumazenil (0.2 mg/kg per dose), can be given to restore the patient's respiratory status. These antagonists, along with atropine and epinephrine for adverse cardiac events, should be immediately available.

Additional medications that should be available include aerosolized albuterol to treat any bronchospasm that may develop, aerosolized epinephrine for airway edema, and diphenhydramine and a corticosteroid to treat any potential anaphylactic reaction to the sedating medications.

Patient

Patient preparation includes a thorough history and physical examination before the procedure. Any radiographic studies are reviewed. Information regarding the child's current health status and drug allergies must be obtained. Elective bronchoscopic procedures should be postponed if the patient has a reversible condition or acute illness that may increase the risk for complications from the sedation or the procedure itself. After a thorough description of the procedure to the parents and to the patient, if the child is able to understand, written informed consent must be obtained. Patients must not take anything by mouth for 4 to 6 hours before the procedure, to ensure an empty stomach and minimize the risk of aspiration.

The need for intravenous access to the patient is somewhat controversial. Flexible laryngoscopy may be performed in infants and cooperative older children with only topical anesthesia because it causes no more trauma than nasopharyngeal suctioning and can be equally brief when done by an experienced operator. Many bronchoscopists require intravenous access in all young children in whom the scope will be passed below the glottis. Although sufficient conscious sedation can be achieved with oral, intranasal, and intramuscular agents in the absence of intravenous access, an intravenous line may prove lifesaving if rare complications arise.

For psychological support and patient comfort, parents should be allowed to stay with the patient as long as possible before starting the procedure. However, they should not overstimulate the patient, especially when conscious sedation is used. The importance of a calm, nonstimulating atmosphere in the bronchoscopy area cannot be overstated. This may be achieved by low-level lighting, calm and quiet actions by the bronchoscopist and support personnel, and a smooth prebronchoscopy routine. Premedication with a benzodiazepine 30 to 60 minutes before the procedure can help the patient relax before starting the procedure.

Personnel

In general, the flexible bronchoscopy team includes a bronchoscopist, a nurse, and a respiratory therapist. All team members should be informed of the patient's diagnosis, indication for bronchoscopy, allergies, and biologic risks to the patient and team members. In addition, the team should be fully informed of the planned procedures and any difficulties that may arise. Everyone should wear a clean protective gown, gloves, mask, and eye protection. All body fluids, including bronchoalveolar lavage specimens, should be handled carefully using universal precautions.

Personnel safety is increased by identifying patients with potentially transmissible pathogens, such as hepatitis viruses, human immunodeficiency virus, and *Mycobacterium tuberculosis*. Approved HEPA (high-efficiency particulate air) filter masks should be worn for all procedures involving patients with suspected *M. tuberculosis* infection, and the procedure should be performed in a room that meets ventilation requirements for tuberculosis. Patients with, or at risk of having, tuberculosis should be kept in a respiratory isolation room before and after the procedure.

PROCEDURE

Most pediatric flexible bronchoscopies are performed with the patient in a supine position on a bed. The height of the bed should be adjusted to the bronchoscopist's comfort level. When the patient and bronchoscopy team are ready and all preparations are completed, the selected sedation is initiated. Appropriate sedation will decrease the patient's anxiety, discomfort, and unwanted physiologic effects. Nevertheless, many younger patients may need a gentle restraining system even when sedated. General anesthesia is preferable in patients at risk of cardiorespiratory compromise with conscious sedation, along with an anesthesiologist to assist in patient monitoring, control of the airway, and assessment of additional risks.

Conscious Sedation

Several different conscious sedation regimens have been used safely and successfully for pediatric flexible bronchoscopy. As noted earlier, one of the most widely accepted is a combination of a benzodiazepine (e.g., midazolam) and a narcotic (e.g., fentanyl or meperidine) given intravenously. The usual pediatric dose of intravenous midazolam ranges from 0.05 to 0.3 mg/kg to a maximal total dose of 0.4 to 0.6 mg/kg (or 6 to 10 mg). Typically, sedation is begun with a small dose (0.05 to 0.1 mg/kg) and is then titrated upward every 5 minutes to achieve the optimal sedative effect. The same approach is also used for intravenous fentanyl, 1 to 3 µg/kg to a maximal total dose of 5 to 10 µg/kg, starting with a 1-µg/kg dose and titrating upward every 5 minutes. Some bronchoscopists prefer a stronger sedative, such as intravenous ketamine (1 mg/kg per dose) or intravenous propofol (1 to 2 mg/kg per dose).[5]

Other combinations of drugs are given intramuscularly and include meperidine, promethazine, and chlorpromazine and the combination of droperidol, promethazine, and thorazine. The disadvantages of intramuscular sedation include the inability to titrate the optimal dose of the medications and the lack of intravenous access in case of an emergency. However, the intramuscular approach is sometimes justified for short procedures in stable children with difficult intravenous access.

Intranasal midazolam has also been shown to induce adequate sedation for pediatric patients undergoing endoscopic procedures or imaging studies.[8] The usual dose of intranasal midazolam ranges from 0.2 to 0.5 mg/kg.

Regardless of the method, optimal sedation is achieved when the child is sleepy and has minimal reaction to noxious stimuli, while still maintaining adequate ventilation and protective airway reflexes.

Topical Anesthesia

Conscious sedation is augmented by application of the local anesthetic agent, 1% to 2% lidocaine, to the nasal cavity, posterior pharynx, vocal cords, and tracheobronchial tree. Another technique is to pretreat the subject with a lidocaine aerosol (4 to 8 mg/kg) given by nebulizer.[9] Lidocaine 2% jelly may also be applied to the nares with a cotton-tipped applicator or small syringe. With small infants, care should be taken that the total lidocaine dose does not exceed the maximal therapeutic range of 3 to 4 mg/kg. Toxic lidocaine levels have been reported with topical airway administration.

Patient Monitoring

Continuous cardiac, respiratory, and oximetry monitoring must be performed during and after the procedure. During the procedure the patient should be closely monitored for cardiac and respiratory rates and tracings, blood pressure, oxygen saturation, clinical airway obstruction, chest wall movement, peripheral perfusion, and cyanosis. Ideally, oxygen saturation should be maintained above 95% at all times, with supplemental oxygen delivered to the patient by mask or blow-by if necessary.

Technique

When the bronchoscope is balanced on the left hand, the left thumb controls the angulation lever on the control head, and the right thumb and index finger direct the insertion tube at the naris. Routes for bronchoscopic approaches include nasal, oral, and through endotracheal or tracheostomy tubes.

The most common route for pediatric patients is the transnasal approach. The flexible bronchoscope is lubricated with lidocaine jelly, or another sterile water–based lubricant, and then inserted through a nostril into the nasopharyngeal area. A topical decongestant (e.g., phenylephrine) may be administered to the nasal mucosa first to facilitate passage of the scope past edematous tissue and to reduce the risk of *epistaxis* (i.e., a nosebleed). The nasopharyngeal and laryngeal anatomy is visualized. The vocal cords are assessed for movement and then anesthetized with lidocaine sprayed through a suction channel of the bronchoscope. Adequate laryngeal anesthesia is critical to avoid sudden laryngospasm. The bronchoscope is then passed through the vocal cords into the tracheobronchial tree. Another dose of 1% to 2% lidocaine is usually applied to the carina to minimize a cough reflex. The tracheobronchial anatomy is then examined.

If bronchoalveolar lavage is performed, the bronchoscopist wedges the bronchoscope in the selected segmental or subsegmental bronchi, and normal saline is instilled in three to five aliquots of up to 1 ml/kg per aliquot. The saline is then suctioned back through the suction channel. Typically, one third to one half of the instilled volume is recovered with suctioning. A specimen is usually collected in a Lukens trap and sent for microbiology or pathology studies. Ideally, if a specimen is collected for microbiologic evaluation, suction should not be applied until the bronchoscope is inside the trachea, in order to minimize contamination of the channel with nasopharyngeal secretions. In special cases, consultation with the microbiologist or pathologist beforehand will ensure that the specimen is large enough for the requested study and is handled and sent appropriately.

During the bronchoscopy the respiratory therapist is often responsible for connecting and disconnecting suction, attaching normal saline syringes and traps for lavage, and giving certain transbronchoscopic medications. The therapist and assisting nurse may divide responsibility for monitoring the patient's oxygenation and respiratory status, stabilizing the patient's head and upper airway, and comforting the patient. Because the bronchoscopist is focused on the procedure, the therapist and nurse are responsible for detecting and promptly notifying the bronchoscopist of any untoward patient occurrence. The respiratory therapist is also responsible for assisting in emergency respiratory management, such as maintaining patency of the patient's airway, suctioning oropharyngeal secretions, handling emergency equipment, and giving certain respiratory medications.

When performing flexible bronchoscopy in a patient who is being mechanically ventilated, the risk of further compromise to the patient's respiratory condition is higher with a partially occluded endotracheal tube. Special considerations should be made for maximizing the patient's ventilation and oxygenation and compensating for air leaks that may occur. In this situation the respiratory therapist is responsible for ventilator adjustment and stabilization of the endotracheal tube.

POSTPROCEDURAL MONITORING AND COMPLICATIONS

Monitoring of the patient must continue after the procedure until the patient has fully awakened or has returned to preprocedural baseline status. Children, particularly anxious toddlers, often require large doses of medications, with the level of sedation increasing after the procedure, when the agents are still active and the child is no longer stimulated by the procedure. It is essential to continue to monitor the adequacy of the patient's oxygenation, ventilation, and airway patency until the sedation has completely resolved. Breath sounds should be monitored for the development of any stridor or wheezing after the procedure. To prevent aspiration, oral fluids are withheld until the patient is fully awake and the topical laryngeal anesthesia has worn off, usually about 1 hour after administering the topical anesthetic.

In general, flexible bronchoscopy is a safe and well-tolerated procedure in pediatric patients, especially when it is performed by an experienced bronchoscopy team that employs careful monitoring and takes appropriate precautions. Patient risk factors for adverse events include upper airway pathology, preprocedure hypoxemia, and weight less than 10 kg. The most common complications include transient cough, respiratory depression, hypoxemia, and bronchospasm during the procedure.[10] Cough is almost universally seen during and after the procedure, but it is usually self-limited and resolves within 24 hours. Minor epistaxis is common and does not require therapy. Respiratory depression is usually associated with oversedation and sometimes requires reversal agents. Any bronchospasm is relieved promptly in most patients by bronchodilator aerosol treatments.

A less common but potentially more serious complication is laryngospasm. This problem can be avoided by application of topical lidocaine to the vocal cords and minimal manipulation of the scope around the glottic area. If laryngospasm occurs, the bronchoscope must be withdrawn immediately and airway resuscitation initiated. These measures include jaw thrust, suction of secretions, and mask ventilation. Rarely, laryngospasm may become life threatening and require paralysis and endotracheal intubation.

Up to 20% of patients may have fever after bronchoalveolar lavage, but pneumonia is uncommon.[10] Other serious complications, including arrhythmias, pulmonary hemorrhage, and pneumothorax, are seldom encountered during pediatric flexible bronchoscopy. Deaths are extremely rare, with no bronchoscopy-related mortality reported in more than 3500 pediatric flexible bronchoscopy procedures.[10,11]

EQUIPMENT MAINTENANCE

Because the bronchoscope and its accessories are extremely fragile and expensive, special attention must be taken during care and cleaning and maintenance procedures. Proper care can increase the life span of the equipment, decrease repair and replacement costs, and reduce the potential risk of cross-contamination. Handling requires the avoidance of any excessive angulation or twisting of the scope, actions that can damage the quartz fiber bundles. Inadequate disinfection of a bronchoscope can result in serious outcome to a patient. The organisms most often responsible for cross-contamination between bronchoscopies are *Mycobacterium* and *Pseudomonas*.

The flexible bronchoscope should be cleaned immediately after each procedure. Dried secretions or blood will prevent penetration of the disinfecting agent. Therefore the exterior surface should be wiped or gently scrubbed with a soft cloth or brush. The suction channel and port should be irrigated and flushed with detergent solution and then scrubbed with a special brush. If the suction valve is not disposable, it should be disassembled and flushed thoroughly with a cleaning solution. The entire instrument is then rinsed copiously with tap water and immersed in a high-level disinfectant solution for 45 minutes.

Because flexible bronchoscopy is not a sterile procedure, cleaning a bronchoscope does not require routine sterilization, and high-level disinfection has been considered satisfactory. *High-level disinfection* is a cleaning method that inactivates all viruses, fungi, and vegetative microorganisms, but not necessarily all bacterial spores. The most common agent used is 2% alkaline glutaraldehyde. Immersion in glutaraldehyde for 20 minutes can destroy virtually all pathogens surviving on a well-cleaned bronchoscope.[12]

Because of increasing concern about more virulent and resistant microorganisms, many centers are adopting routine sterilization of their bronchoscopes. Two highly effective methods against all types of microorganisms are ethylene oxide gas sterilization and peracetic acid submersion. Ethylene oxide is noncorrosive and able to penetrate all portions of the bronchoscope without requiring high pressures. However, a venting cap must be placed to equalize the pressure between the interior and the exterior of the bronchoscope. The major disadvantage of ethylene oxide sterilization is that it is time-consuming, taking at least 12 to 16 hours to complete the process. An alternative method is the STERIS system (Figure 9-3), an automated, microprocessor-controlled device using a sterilant concentrate, peracetic acid, as the active biocidal agent. This chemical sterilization process requires only 25 minutes. Once the disinfection or sterilization process is completed, the bronchoscope is rinsed with tap water and may be wiped with alcohol before storage in a dry, clean cabinet.

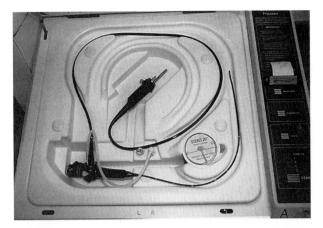

FIGURE 9-3 Correct placement of flexible bronchoscope in STERIS cleaning apparatus, used for chemical sterilization of the instrument.

COMPARISON WITH RIGID BRONCHOSCOPY

Rigid bronchoscopy is most often performed in the operating room by surgeons or otolaryngologists, with general anesthesia administered to the patient by an anesthesiologist. This procedure has some advantages over flexible bronchoscopy, including better control of the airway and ventilation and the ability to perform certain therapeutic maneuvers (e.g., foreign body removal, laser therapy). Relative disadvantages of rigid bronchoscopy include the inability to allow inspection of distal airways, the inability to assess the dynamic and natural state of the airways, and the complications associated with general anesthesia. Thus the risks and benefits of each procedure must be carefully considered for each patient before choosing the bronchoscopic method. On occasion the two procedures are coordinated and performed sequentially in the operating room for different diagnostic and therapeutic purposes in select patients.

ASSESSMENT QUESTIONS

See Evolve Resources for answers.

1. Flexible bronchoscopy is commonly performed in all the following settings, *except*:
   A. Operating rooms
   B. Bronchoscopy suites
   C. Pulmonary clinic rooms
   D. Intensive care units
   E. Procedure rooms

Continued

ASSESSMENT QUESTIONS—cont'd

2. The most common diagnostic indication for flexible bronchoscopy in infants is:
   A. Stridor
   B. Wheezing
   C. Hoarse voice
   D. Persistent atelectasis
   E. Difficult intubation
3. Which of the following disorders may cause *only* inspiratory stridor?
   A. Tonsillar hypertrophy
   B. Laryngomalacia
   C. Vascular ring
   D. Cardiomegaly
   E. Bronchial foreign body
4. Airway dynamics can be disrupted by:
   A. General anesthesia
   B. Conscious sedation
   C. Topical lidocaine
   D. Intranasal midazolam
   E. Sleep
5. Flexible bronchoscopy is indicated in the evaluation of wheezing in all the following settings, *except*:
   A. Wheezing that is unilateral
   B. Wheezing that has been present since birth
   C. Wheezing that is refractory to asthma therapy
   D. Wheezing that is triggered by viral infections
   E. Wheezing associated with persistent atelectasis
6. Bronchoalveolar lavage may be performed to look for:
   A. Infection
   B. Malignancy
   C. Bleeding
   D. Aspiration
   E. All of the above
7. The only absolute contraindication to flexible bronchoscopy is when:
   A. The diagnosis could be obtained by open lung biopsy.
   B. The patient is hypoxemic.
   C. The patient requires intubation and mechanical ventilation.
   D. The patient is febrile with acute pneumonia.
   E. The risks of bronchoscopy outweigh the potential benefits of the procedure.
8. A 3-year-old child is intubated with a 4.5-mm endotracheal tube and is mechanically ventilated for severe pneumonia. The respiratory therapist is asked to set up a bronchoscope for bronchoalveolar lavage to obtain microbiology specimens. The most appropriate-sized scope for this procedure would be a:
   A. 1.8-mm nondirectable "spaghetti" bronchoscope
   B. 2.2-mm directable flexible bronchoscope without suction channel
   C. 2.7-mm directable flexible bronchoscope with suction channel

ASSESSMENT QUESTIONS—cont'd

   D. 4.5-mm directable flexible bronchoscope with large suction channel
   E. 4.0-mm rigid bronchoscope
9. Topical anesthesia of the airway may be achieved by:
   A. Intranasal administration of midazolam
   B. Intravenous administration of fentanyl
   C. Intravenous administration of midazolam
   D. Airway instillation or nebulization of lidocaine
   E. Airway instillation or nebulization of a topical corticosteroid
10. During a bronchoscopy, the respiratory therapist may do each of the following *except*:
   A. Connect and disconnect suction and specimen traps
   B. Administer supplemental oxygen as needed
   C. Administer saline lavages or transbronchoscopic medications
   D. Administer conscious sedation medications
   E. Assist in emergency airway management
11. The commonest complication after flexible bronchoscopy is:
   A. Cough
   B. Wheezing
   C. Hemoptysis
   D. Fever
   E. Pneumothorax
12. Acceptable cleaning and decontamination of a flexible bronchoscope include all the following *except*:
   A. Washing the exterior and channel of the scope with a detergent solution
   B. Immersion in 70% ethanol solution
   C. Immersion in 2% alkaline glutaraldehyde solution
   D. Ethylene oxide gas sterilization
   E. Immersion in peracetic acid

References

1. Wood RE: Spelunking in the pediatric airways: explorations with the flexible fiberoptic bronchoscope, *Pediatr Clin North Am* 1984;31:785.
2. Wang KP, Mehta AC, editors: *Flexible bronchoscopy*, Cambridge, Mass: Blackwell Science; 1995.
3. Brutinel WM, Cortese DA: Fiberoptic bronchoscopy. In Burton GG, Hodgkin JE, Ward JJ, editors: *Respiratory care: a guide to clinical practice*, ed 4, Philadelphia: Lippincott; 1997. pp 281-294.
4. Hollinger LD, Lusk RP, Green CG, editors: *Pediatric laryngology and bronchoesophagology*, Philadelphia: Lippincott-Raven; 1997.
5. Midulla F et al; ERS Task Force: Flexible endoscopy of paediatric airways, *Eur Respir J* 2003;22:698.
6. Barbato A et al: Use of the pediatric bronchoscope, flexible and rigid, in 51 European centers, *Eur Respir J* 1997;10:1761.

7. Godfrey S et al: Yield from flexible bronchoscopy in children, *Pediatr Pulmonol* 1997;23:261.

8. Fishbein M et al: Evaluation of intranasal midazolam in children undergoing esophagogastroduodenoscopy, *J Pediatr Gastroenterol Nutr* 1997;25:261.

9. Gjonaj ST, Lowenthal DB, Dozor AJ: Nebulized lidocaine administered to infants and children undergoing flexible bronchoscopy, *Chest* 1997;112:1665.

10. de Blic J, Marchac V, Scheinmann P: Complications of flexible bronchoscopy in children; prospective study of 1,328 procedures, Eur Respir J 2002;20:1271.

11. Nussbaum E: Pediatric fiberoptic bronchoscopy, *Clin Pediatr* 1995;34:430.

12. Woodcock A et al: Bronchoscopy and infection control, *Lancet* 1989;ii:270.

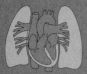
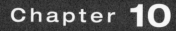

Chapter 10

Invasive Blood Gas Analysis and Cardiovascular Monitoring

ROBERT M. DiBLASI • MICHAEL P. CZERVINSKE

OUTLINE

LEARNING OBJECTIVES

After reading this chapter, the reader will be able to:
- Describe indications for obtaining blood gas samples
- Identify common anatomic sampling sites used to obtain blood gases
- Describe potential patient and caregiver complications associated with blood gas sampling
- Interpret a complete hemodynamic profile of a patient
- Illustrate the progression of blood pressure waveforms seen during the proper placement of a pulmonary artery catheter

- Describe invasive, semi-invasive, and noninvasive techniques for monitoring cardiac output and index in children
- Discuss various measurements that can be used to determine the adequacy of cellular oxygenation
- Identify variables that can shift the oxygen dissociation curve

Blood gases are considered the most effective test for evaluating the efficiency of gas exchange and cardio-pulmonary interaction. Evaluating an infant or child with respiratory impairment requires the analysis of blood gases in umbilical, arterial, capillary, or mixed venous blood samples. To interpret these blood gas values correctly, the clinician must understand acid–base balance and gas exchange and be able to recognize normal and abnormal blood gas values. The techniques of blood gas sampling can affect the results. This chapter reviews the procedures, indications, complications, and contraindications for each technique. It also reviews various clinical techniques that are used to monitor and evaluate cardiac performance in pediatrics. It is beyond the scope of this chapter to describe noninvasive methods to measure gas exchange. Chapter 11 (Noninvasive Monitoring in Neonatal and Pediatric Care) provides a complete overview of these concepts.

BLOOD GAS SAMPLING

Arterial blood gas (ABG) analysis is indicated when an accurate measurement of acid–base balance or pulmonary gas exchange is required.[1] This analysis may be needed for diagnosis or evaluation of response to therapy, and for patients with acute deterioration in clinical status (Box 10-1).[2] Figure 10-1 shows the various anatomic sites that provide access for percutaneous arterial puncture and catheterization.

Pain Control

Blood gas sampling is a painful procedure, but the resulting information is frequently a vital part of patient management. Because painful procedures do not always evoke vigorous pain responses in critically ill newborns,

Box 10-1	Indications for Blood Gas Analysis

- To evaluate ventilation (Pa_{CO_2})
- To evaluate acid–base balance (pH, Pa_{CO_2})
- To evaluate oxygenation (Pa_{O_2}, oxyhemoglobin)
- To evaluate the oxygen-carrying capacity (Pa_{O_2}, oxyhemoglobin, hemoglobin, dyshemoglobin)
- To evaluate intrapulmonary shunt
- To quantify response to therapy
  - Supplemental oxygen
  - Mechanical ventilation
- To assist in diagnosis
- To monitor the severity or progress of a disease

Pa_{CO_2}, Partial pressure of carbon dioxide in arterial blood; Pa_{O_2}, partial pressure of oxygen in arterial blood.

many believe that such newborns are not being affected by pain.[3] However, infants probably have a higher sensitivity to painful procedures than older age groups.[4,5] For infants more than 4 months of age and for children, anesthetic cream or a lidocaine injection may be used to control the pain felt during a blood gas procedure.[6] For nonintubated infants and premature newborns, a pacifier dipped in 24% sucrose is effective in helping to ameliorate the effects of pain. If the newborn is intubated, the sucrose can be administered as drops on the tongue or palate from an oral medication syringe.[7] Depending on the type and duration of procedure, more potent short-acting analgesic or anesthetic agents may be appropriate.[8]

Arterial Sampling Sites

Figure 10-1 illustrates potential sites for arterial puncture or catheterization in infants or children. Arterial

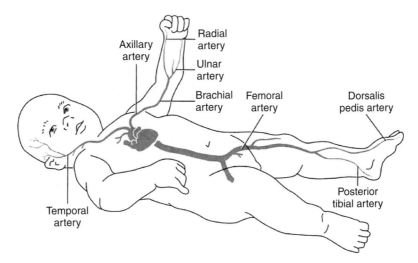

FIGURE 10-1 Arterial sites that may be used for peripheral artery puncture in infants and children.

sampling sites provide the most accurate blood gas results. The brachial and femoral sites are usually avoided because both feed large distal networks, and neither has collateral circulation. Also, the brachial pulse is difficult to palpate in infants and small children because of the naturally large fat pad located in that area of the arm. Injury to the brachial nerve can also result in serious complications. Only a highly skilled clinician should perform a brachial artery puncture if necessary.

In a child, the femoral artery is reserved for an emergency, and then only as a last resort. In the neonate or infant, the femoral artery lies close to the femoral vein, nerve, and hip joint and because of their proximity, damage inflicted on any one of these structures by femoral puncture is likely to cause severe complications and is thus not indicated for this population.[9]

The preferred site in both neonatal and pediatric populations is the radial artery. The radial artery provides good access as well as collateral circulation to the hand by the ulnar artery. There are no nerves or veins directly adjacent to the radial artery, and the patient's wrist is easier to manipulate than other body parts. The bone and firm ligaments of the wrist make it easy to palpate, stabilize, and compress the radial artery.[1,7] A modified Allen's test (described in the next section) is performed to ensure collateral circulation around the radial artery and to avoid complications. The ulnar artery should be avoided because it runs adjacent to the ulnar nerve.

The dorsalis pedis or posterior tibial artery is considered if the radial artery shows signs of poor collateral circulation. In addition, the temporal artery provides an alternative site for the premature or newborn infant. Access is generally good because two branches are close to the scalp. In most premature and neonatal patients, the temporal artery branches are larger than the radial artery.

Modified Allen's Test

The modified Allen's test is used to verify the presence of collateral circulation to the hand and should be performed in order to confirm whether poor circulation exists prior to puncturing the radial, posterior tibial, or dorsalis pedis artery. To assess blood flow to the hand, hold the child's wrist with both hands, thumbs on top. Ask the child to make a tight fist, and then occlude the radial and ulnar arteries by pressing down on them with the thumbs, one on each artery. Keeping both arteries occluded, ask the child to unclench the fist and note whether the palm is blanched, which indicates impaired blood flow. Then remove the pressure from the ulnar artery. The palm will become pink within 5 seconds if the ulnar artery is patent and able to provide collateral circulation.[7]

The passive method for performing the modified Allen's test, used on an infant or child who cannot follow commands, is performed by gently squeezing or elevating the hand while occluding both arteries. Once the ulnar artery is released, the results are interpreted as previously described.[1] Allen's test can also be used to verify collateral circulation when using one of the arteries of the foot as a puncture site, by elevating the foot and compressing the dorsalis pedis and posterior tibial arteries. Collateral circulation is confirmed by releasing pressure from the artery that will not be punctured, and assessing the nail beds and sole of the foot for return of blood flow.[1,7]

ARTERIAL PUNCTURE

When infrequent sampling is required, ABG samples are obtained by percutaneously puncturing one of the aforementioned peripheral artery sites. Obtaining a blood gas sample from an infant or child is generally more difficult than in an adult and requires more patience, skill, and time. However, an experienced clinician using proper technique can quickly obtain a sample that yields accurate results. Two individuals are helpful when performing an arterial puncture on a child who is too young to understand the need for the test but strong enough to react to the procedure. On a small infant or neonate, a transilluminating light placed behind the wrist may help visualize the location of the radial artery.[1,7]

Procedure

Performing a successful arterial puncture requires knowledge of the anatomy involved and proficient technical skills. Collect the equipment required for the arterial puncture (Box 10-2). Use the following sequence of technical steps as a guideline for performing the puncture.[1,7]

1. Wash hands and adhere to universal precautions for blood-borne pathogens, using proper-fitting examination gloves, along with eye and splash protection.[10-12]
2. Palpate the pulse at various sites (see Figure 10-1) to determine the best site for testing.

Box 10-2	Equipment for Arterial Puncture and Blood Gas Collection

- 1-ml preheparinized* tuberculin syringe
- 25-gauge needle *or* preheparinized* 25-gauge butterfly needle infusion kit
- Correctly fitting examination gloves
- Povidone-iodine and alcohol wipes
- Sterile gauze
- Needle-capping and protection device
- Eye and splash shield
- Patient label

---

* Use dry heparin or expel liquid heparin from the syringe and needle hub or butterfly set before starting the procedure.

3. Perform the modified Allen's test if appropriate for the artery being sampled.

4. Use an assistant to help restrain the child and immobilize the limb if required.

5. Scrub the puncture site with an approved antiseptic swab and allow to air dry, or use a sterile gauze pad. Do not blow on the site to dry it.

6. Palpate the artery again, and position the index and middle finger of the nondominant hand to stabilize the artery.

7. Maintain a clean field around the syringe and syringe kit while opening it. Prepare the kit for use, and heparinize the syringe if required. Remember to expel the heparin completely from the barrel of the syringe and hub of the needle.

8. Insert the needle of the syringe or butterfly catheter into the artery at a 35- to 45-degree angle with the bevel up, and advance it gently. Enter the artery from the direction opposite, or against, the blood flow. A flash in the hub of the syringe or butterfly catheter verifies that the needle penetrated the artery and is located in the lumen. In the small pediatric patient it is quite easy to pass through the artery with the needle. If a good pulse is palpated and no blood return occurs after the needle is inserted, pull the needle back incrementally and continue to watch for a flash of blood. If resistance is met when inserting the needle, slowly withdraw it immediately and change direction because it has most likely touched the bone.

9. Obtain the required amount of blood. Because the arterial pressure is usually high enough, manual aspiration is not required. If manual aspiration is required, however, the barrel of the syringe is withdrawn slowly. When using a butterfly catheter, attach the syringe to the catheter and slowly aspirate the correct amount of blood into the syringe. Maintain the sample amount as close to the technically feasible minimal volume as possible.[2,7]

10. After obtaining the sample, withdraw the needle and immediately apply firm pressure to the puncture site with a sterile gauze pad for at least 5 minutes. Apply pressure for a longer period if the patient has a coagulopathy or is receiving anticoagulation therapy (e.g., heparin). Avoid using pressure dressings. Patients should not apply the pressure because they may not press hard or long enough.

11. While holding the site, gently remove air bubbles from the sample. If using a butterfly catheter, remove it from the syringe.

12. Continue compressing the site, and seal the syringe with a one-handed safety cover device to prevent exposure of the sample to air. Gently roll the syringe between the hands or fingers to mix the heparin with the specimen.[3]

13. Immediately apply the proper patient label to the specimen according to institutional policy.

14. For accurate results, analyze the sample immediately, or analyze room temperature samples within 10 to 15 minutes after they are drawn. Samples placed on ice should be analyzed within 1 hour.[13]

Contraindications

The major contraindication to an arterial puncture is lack of collateral circulation. Punctures should not be performed at sites where the extremity has previously blanched, which may result from arterial obstruction or spasm. Punctures should not be performed through a site distal to or through a surgical shunt, as in a dialysis patient. If a limb is infected or shows evidence of peripheral vascular disease, an alternative sight should be selected.[11]

Complications

Hematoma formation is the most common complication during arterial puncture and is seen more often in brachial than in radial artery punctures. Complication can be minimized by immediately applying adequate pressure to the puncture site after the needle is withdrawn. As with any invasive procedure, infection is a possible complication but is relatively low with aseptic technique. Scarring, laceration of the artery, and hematoma formation are more likely to occur with repeated puncture of an artery.[8] Alternating puncture sites decreases this risk. Other complications associated with arterial punctures in infants and children include nerve damage, bleeding, obstruction of the artery by clots or spasms, trauma to the artery, and pain.

Because the median nerve is close to the brachial artery, the nerve may be punctured as well during the procedure, which will cause intense pain down the arm. Because the posterior tibial artery and nerve are also close to one another, special care should also be taken to avoid nerve damage during puncture of this artery. Although the femoral artery is much easier to puncture, complications in infants tend to occur more frequently, including thrombosis, nerve damage, and necrosis of the head of the femoral bone.[7]

Although gloves are worn and universal precautions applied during all arterial punctures, needle sticks remain a risk to the clinician and are the most frequent source of transmission of blood-borne pathogens to health care workers.[2,8-10] Most of these complications are avoided by having only thoroughly trained and highly skilled clinicians perform a puncture.

CAPILLARY BLOOD GAS SAMPLES

Capillary blood gas (CBG) sampling provides a frequent alternative to ABG analysis in the infant or child. Punctures for capillary samples are less invasive than arterial punctures, are easier and quicker to perform, and can be used when there is no arterial catheter for drawing ABG samples.[14,15] Drawing a CBG sample is usually less painful, but local anesthetic application helps alleviate pain associated with the procedure.[6,7,16]

In general, a CBG sample correlates best with arterial pH and carbon dioxide tension ($Paco_2$) values. Correlation of capillary samples with arterial samples varies depending on the parameters measured.[11,17,18] When a capillary sample site is adequately "arterialized" and puncture and sampling procedures are performed correctly, the pH and carbon dioxide partial pressure (Pco_2) of capillary samples can accurately reflect those of arterial samples. Frequently, capillary Po_2 is lower than arterial values; however, given a clinically acceptable difference between capillary Po_2 and Pao_2, the capillary Po_2 may trend with increases and decreases in arterial values.[11,16] Although infrequent, capillary oxygen partial pressure (Po_2) may correlate with arterial pressure (Pao_2) in isolated cases and must be assessed on an individual basis before using the capillary Po_2 to monitor oxygenation in lieu of the PaO_2.

The accuracy of capillary blood gas values is severely attenuated by the presence of hypotension, hypothermia, hypovolemia, and lack of perfusion.[11] Conversely, correlation of capillary and arterial blood gas values improves with hypoxemia, as venous and arterial Po_2 converge. Special consideration should be given to patients with circulatory defects. Decreased venous return, secondary to cor pulmonale or decreased cardiac output, leads to venous congestion and peripheral pooling, which may result in an increase in Pco_2. Conversely, increased blood flow may result in decreased capillary Pco_2.[14]

Although capillary punctures are less invasive, it is necessary to obtain an arterial sample at some point to ensure correlation and accuracy. Using noninvasive monitors such as pulse oximeters or transcutaneous oxygen monitors to monitor oxygenation and ventilation when arterial samples are not obtained is an effective way to eliminate the need for frequent CBGs.[13] However, many factors that lead to inaccurate CBG sampling may also affect the accuracy of monitoring (see Chapter 11, Noninvasive Monitoring in Neonatal and Pediatric Care).[1]

Puncture Sites

The least hazardous puncture site for infants is the posterolateral foot, just anterior to the heel (Figure 10-2).[1,12]

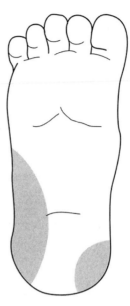

FIGURE 10-2 Recommended puncture sites *(shaded areas)* in infant's heel to obtain capillary blood for analysis.

The posterior heel curvature and back of the heel must be avoided because the lancet could puncture the bone and result in calcaneous osteomyelitis. Do not perform a capillary puncture on the medial aspect of the heel, which is the location of the posterior tibial artery. For children and some infants, use the palmar or fleshy surface of the distal aspects of the fingers (middle or ring) and toes (Figure 10-3).[11,12,14] The earlobes are a secondary site for puncture in children. In general, avoid punctures on the fingers and toes of neonates because of

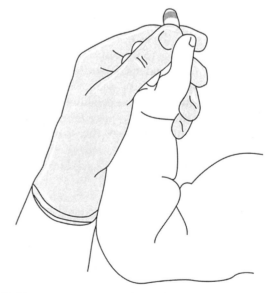

FIGURE 10-3 Technique for grasping the finger for a capillary puncture, with recommended site for puncture indicated *(shaded area).*

the higher risk of nerve damage in this area.[12] Previous puncture sites or inflamed areas with an apparent or possible infection should not be used. As previously discussed, extremities with localized swelling or edema should be avoided because of the effect of extracellular or interstitial fluid on sample accuracy. Cyanotic areas should also be avoided.[11]

Procedure

Successful capillary puncture is not complicated, but it does require proficient technical skill. Collect the equipment required (Box 10-3), and use the following sequence of steps as a guide to collect a CBG sample.[1,7,12]

1. Select a puncture site and warm the area for 5 to 10 minutes. Use a warm (less than 42° to 45° C) wet cloth or disposable warming pack, and apply with caution.[1,7]
2. Give a 12% to 24% sucrose solution pacifier 2 minutes before the procedure, or apply an anesthetic cream or subcutaneous injection for pain control.[3,5-7]
3. Wash hands and adhere to universal precautions for blood-borne pathogens, using proper-fitting examination gloves, along with splash protection.[8,9]
4. Remove the warming device. Clean the site with an antiseptic, and dry with a sterile gauze pad; alcohol will hemolyze the blood.
5. Immobilize the area by properly grasping the hand or foot (see Figure 10-3 and Figure 10-4) and stabilize the area by anchoring the hand or foot on a hard surface. Use an assistant to help restrain a child and immobilize the limb if required. Restrain infants by swaddling them in a blanket.[7]
6. Finger or toe stick: Hold the digit (patient's finger or toe) with the thumb and forefinger, supporting the digit behind or close to the nail (see Figure 10-3). Keep fingertips well away from the puncture site.

Box 10-3	Equipment for Capillary Puncture and Blood Gas Collection

- Warming device or warm damp cloth
- Lancet and mechanical puncture device
- Lancet disposal system
- Correctly fitting examination gloves
- Alcohol wipes
- Sterile gauze
- Adhesive bandage
- Eye and splash shield
- Preheparinized capillary tubes
- Metal "flea," magnet, and capillary tube caps (if required)
- Patient label

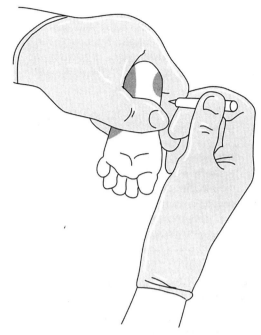

FIGURE 10-4 Technique for stabilizing the heel for a capillary puncture.

7. Heel stick: Consider using venipuncture or a digit first, because either may be less painful and require less resampling.[3-7] Hold the heel gently but firmly. Wrap the forefinger around the infant's upper heel and ankle while holding the arch of the foot with the thumb (see Figure 10-4).
8. Position the lancet.
   a. For a finger or toe stick, hold the lancet at a 10- to 20-degree angle to the longitudinal axis of the phalangeal bone. Do not direct it into the bone.
   b. For a heel stick, hold the lancet between the thumb and index finger of the opposite hand, perpendicular to the puncture site.
9. Poke the point of the lancet into the skin with one continuous, deliberate motion. Correct depth depends on the infant, but 1 to 2 mm is generally sufficient to produce a free-flowing drop of blood.[7,17] Use a mechanical puncture when available because most produce consistent results with less need for resampling.[7,16] Avoid superficial punctures and the need to repeat the puncture. Do not slice, dig, or make multiple punctures.[1,6,7,17]
10. Ease thumb pressure after the lancet is removed.
11. Wipe away the first drop of blood, which may be contaminated with intracellular, interstitial, or lymphatic fluids, with a dry sterile gauze pad.
12. Apply moderate pressure to the heel or digit, without massaging or squeezing, until a free-flowing drop of blood appears. Squeezing or

"milking" the sample may cause red blood cell hemolysis, especially in newborns, because their hematocrit levels are higher and their red blood cells more fragile. Squeezing also results in bruising and contamination of the specimen with lymphatic and venous drainage.

13. Collect the blood by placing the tip of the capillary tube into the blood droplet without touching the puncture wound. Hold the capillary tube angled horizontally, or slightly downward, with the colored ring away from the infant. Keep the tube in contact with the blood droplet until the required amount of blood fills the tube, usually 40 to 125 μl.[7] Maintaining contact with the droplet limits unnecessary exposure to air and reduces the incidence of air bubbles in the sample. Do not scrape blood that has smeared onto the skin surface into the capillary tube. Scraping from the skin surface increases exposure to air and alters the partial pressure of the gases being measured.[1,7,12]

14. Apply pressure to the puncture site with a sterile gauze pad until the bleeding stops. Use an adhesive bandage only on children old enough not to place it in their mouth and possibly aspirate it.

15. Label the tube with the proper patient information.

16. If the sample cannot be analyzed immediately after collection, insert a metal mixing "flea" into the capillary tube and seal it. Mix the sample by running a magnet gently back and forth along the tube, and place the sample on ice; this decreases the incidence of sample clotting. Remove the metal flea before analyzing the blood.

Contraindications

CBG sampling should not be performed when accurate assessment of oxygenation or ABG values is necessary. CBGs should not be used for routine blood gas monitoring when less painful or noninvasive measurements provide results that are more accurate.

Capillary puncture is contraindicated in neonates less than 24 hours old. A newborn has a low systemic output, and vasoconstriction tends to be maximal during this stage secondary to a decrease in environmental temperature and an increase in circulating catecholamines.[12,17,20,21] CBG sampling is not recommended in a patient with decreased peripheral blood flow, especially in the case of hypotension.[12,17,19] CBG sampling may be difficult to perform on a patient with polycythemia (hematocrit greater than 70%) because of the short clotting time. Do not use areas that are edematous, inflamed, or infected, or other areas previously mentioned. Avoid heel samples from ambulatory children who have formed calluses on the soles of their feet.[7,22]

Complications

Serious complications may result in medical management if capillary results do not accurately reflect the patient's condition. Consider potential errors in correlation with arterial values before deciding on a clinical course of action based on CBG values.[12,14,19]

Although capillary puncture is a relatively safe procedure, complications have been observed. Burns have been reported secondary to heel warming, but using a prepackaged warming kit that does not require an external heat source minimizes this problem. Other complications include infection, scarring, calcaneous osteomyelitis, calcifications, nerve damage, arterial laceration, bruising, cellulitis, hematoma, and bleeding.[1,11,12] Some of these complications may seem benign at first but lead to developmental delays in such milestones as grasping and walking.

ARTERIAL CATHETERS

For frequent blood gas sampling, an umbilical artery catheter (UAC) in the newborn and a peripheral artery catheter or arterial line in the older infant or child is used for critically ill patients (Figure 10-5). Arterial catheters provide access for arterial blood pressure analysis and ABG sampling. UACs and arterial catheters also allow blood pressure monitoring in patients who are hemodynamically unstable.

Umbilical Artery Catheterization

In the infant the umbilicus provides ready access to two arteries. Facing the child, the two umbilical arteries are located at about the 5 and 7 o'clock positions. Prompt catheterization is essential in neonates because these vessels will undergo arterial spasm in the presence of increased arterial oxygen, making cannulation difficult if not impossible.[7]

Two positions are typically used to place the tip of the UAC. In the *high position* the catheter overlies the sixth through eighth thoracic vertebrae (T6 to T8); this position avoids major tributaries of the aorta because it is below the ductus arteriosus and above the celiac access. The *low position* is usually at the third to fourth lumbar (L3 to L4) space, between the renal artery and aortic intersection and above the takeoff of the inferior mesenteric artery. The UAC is placed to avoid the large tributaries supplied by these vessels to minimize trauma and hemodynamic disturbances of vital organs.[23]

The choice of high or low catheter placement is empiric. Hospitals tend to favor one site or the other; both are associated with their own set of complications related to hypoglycemia, hypotension, vasospasm, and embolic disturbances of organs distal to the catheter tip. A meta-analysis and literature reviews demonstrate

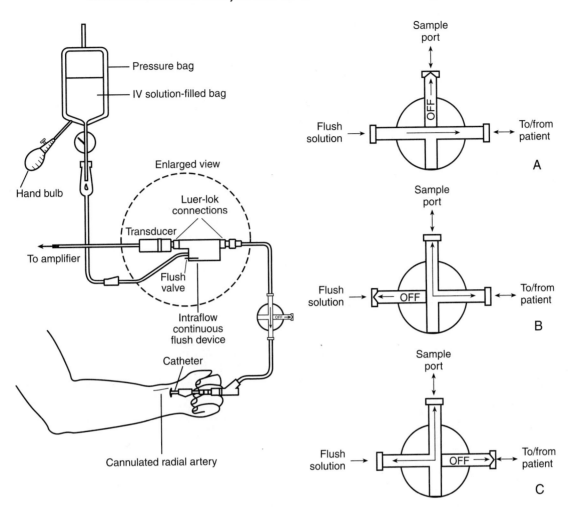

FIGURE 10-5 An indwelling arterial line and continuous infusion/flush system used to monitor blood pressure and obtain blood gas samples. Exploded view shows a three-way stop-cock system. **A,** Normal position with stop-cock off to sampling port allows continuous monitoring of blood pressure and flushing of the line if using a (pig tail) flush system. **B,** Position to draw blood or inject flush solution to the patient with stop-cock turned off to flush solution. **C,** Position to flush sample port with stop-cock off to patient. All ports are closed at all intermediary positions

a small advantage when using the high position over the low position.[24]

The starting point for how far a catheter should be inserted is determined by first measuring the distance from the umbilicus to the shoulder. This measurement is then looked up on a *nomogram* (a diagram allowing computation of a function) to determine the correct catheter insertion distance.[25-29]

Using sterile technique, insert the catheter into one of the arteries. The artery that is less tortuous upon initial insertion will be easier to cannulate. Direct the tip toward the ipsilateral groin. The catheter is advanced with a gentle downward pressure, using a rotating motion to allow the catheter to seek the arterial lumen. Advance to a distance one third the infant's body length plus 1 cm for the high position. Patency is confirmed by

the ease of blood flow. Connect the UAC to a prepared fluid pressure–transducing system (Figure 10-5).[7,21]

The catheter is secured by suturing it into the umbilical artery, and taping it to the abdomen. Chest and abdominal radiographs help to confirm placement. A UAC may remain in place for several days to weeks as indicated by patient need.[1,21,26]

Peripheral Artery Catheterization

The clinician must rely on peripheral arterial catheterization in the pediatric patient. An arterial line is also used for blood gas monitoring in an infant or a newborn without umbilical artery access.

Arterial line placement is accomplished by using either a *percutaneous* method (through the skin) or a *cutdown* method (a small surgical stoma that allows direct visualization and cannulation of the isolated vessels). As previously noted, the most commonly used site is the radial artery; the posterior tibial and dorsalis pedis arteries are occasionally used. Other monitoring sites, such as the brachial artery, superficial temporal artery, and femoral artery, are rarely used because of the increased risk of complications. Arterial catheter sizes range from 22 to 24 gauge for a neonate and from 20 to 22 gauge for a pediatric patient.[26]

Before placing an arterial catheter, the modified Allen's test previously described can be performed to observe collateral blood flow to the hand or foot being punctured.[1,7] When performing a radial artery puncture in small children and infants, the use of a transilluminating light to locate the radial artery is helpful.[27]

Procedure for Sampling

Use the following procedure as a guideline for drawing a blood sample from an arterial or umbilical artery catheter.[1,27] Both catheters are connected to a heparinized normal saline continuous infusion/flush source and blood pressure–monitoring transducer (Figure 10-5).

1. Wash hands and adhere to universal precautions for blood-borne pathogens, using proper-fitting examination gloves, along with eye and splash protection.[8,9]
2. Uncap the locking port of the three-way stopcock. Apply appropriate antibacterial solution to the stopcock port or rubber infusion port, depending on institutional procedures, and allow to dry.[1] Because multiple syringes are required, maintain a clean field around the site and a place to set the syringes that are not in use.
3. Attach a 3-ml syringe to the stopcock, or attach a syringe with a 25-gauge needle to the infusion port (Figure 10-5, A).
4. Turn the stopcock off to continuous infusion/flush line, aspirate 1.25 to 2.0 ml of blood diluted with the infusion fluid, and remove the syringe. Do not discard this sample, and keep the tip sterile because it must be reinfused after the blood sample is acquired.
5. Close the stopcock by making a one-quarter turn between the syringe and the line to the continuous infusion/flush line.
6. Attach a sterile preheparinized syringe to the port. Switch the stopcock back one-quarter turn toward the continuous infusion/flush line to the off position.
7. Aspirate 0.25 to 1.0 ml of blood into the sampling syringe, depending on the volume required by the blood gas analyzer.

8. Close the stopcock by making a one-quarter turn back toward the syringe, and remove the sample (Figure 10-5, A).
9. Reattach the syringe with the aspirated infusion volume, and switch the stopcock back turn toward the infusion line (Figure 10-5, B) to the off position and toward the sampling syringe to the on position. Slowly reinfuse the solution from the syringe.
10. Repeat the procedure for turning the stopcock off to the continuous infusion/flush line, remove the syringe, and attach a syringe prefilled with flush solution.
11. Open the stopcock back to the flush syringe, and infuse 0.5 to 1.5 ml of solution to flush blood from the line. Turn the stopcock off to the sampling port, and remove the flush syringe. Return the stopcock cap to its position.
12. If using a flush device (pigtail) instead of a flush syringe then turn the stop-cock off to the patient (Figure 10-5, C) and open to the continuous infusion/flush line, then flush solution through the sample port and then turn stop-cock off to the sample port to flush blood through the line to the patient.
13. Record the amount of blood sampled and flush solution infused to keep accurate input and output records.
14. Immediately apply the proper patient label to the specimen according to institutional policy.
15. For accurate results, analyze the sample immediately, or analyze room-temperature samples within 10 to 15 minutes after they are drawn. Samples placed on ice should be analyzed within 1 hour.[11]

When infusing or reinfusing solution into the umbilical or arterial line, tapping the syringe while holding it upward releases bubbles to the surface, where they can be expelled before attaching the syringe to the stopcock. When infusing, keep the syringe in a perpendicular position to allow air bubbles to rise toward the plunger. If bubbles form, tap them so they rise toward the plunger. Continue infusing the solution, but do not infuse air bubbles into the arterial line.

Complications

As with any invasive method of monitoring, peripheral artery catheterization carries an increased risk of infection.[26,28] The risk is greater when a catheter has been in place for longer than 72 hours. Some complications associated with the use of arterial catheters are related to thrombotic phenomena, either at the site of the catheter tip or distal to catheter placement.

The risk of thrombosis tends to depend on the size of the catheter and the duration of placement.

Children younger than 5 years are at greater risk. Once significant perfusion or thrombotic problems are identified, remove the catheter as soon as possible, and manage the affected extremity to improve perfusion.

The circulating blood volume in a neonate is approximately 85 to 90 ml/kg; it is 70 to 75 ml/kg in children.[29] Therefore it is important to record and limit the amount of blood drawn from these patients. Hemorrhage may occur during insertion, from frequent or excessive blood sampling and if the catheter tubing is inadvertently disconnected. Blood transfusions are given to replace the blood volume lost due to these factors. Pallor, decreased pulses, and poor capillary refill are all signs of ischemia. Injection of even a small amount of air into the arterial system can result in rapid and devastating air embolism to the brain.

UAC complications may also include intraventricular hemorrhage, altered mesenteric blood flow, and necrotizing enterocolitis.[26,30] These and other complications, such as misplacement into the iliac artery or infarction of various organ systems, including the kidney, liver, and spinal cord,[31,32] may result in life-threatening or prolonged severe disability.

Measurements

The placement of arterial catheters allows direct measurement of arterial blood pressure values: the systolic and diastolic pressures. Monitoring arterial pressure waveforms helps to determine the patency of the arterial line and the quality of the pulse pressure and to calculate the mean arterial pressure (MAP). The arterial line monitor calculates MAP internally. However, use the following formula to obtain an indirect measurement of MAP with a sphygmomanometer:

$$MAP = \frac{[(2 \times diastolic) + systolic]}{3}$$

MAP is often used as an indication of left ventricular afterload, thus representing the resistance against which the left ventricle must pump. The pulse pressure is the difference between the systolic and the diastolic blood pressure. A decreasing pulse pressure may indicate hypovolemia, and an increasing pulse pressure may indicate a restoration of normal volume status.

CONTINUOUS INVASIVE BLOOD GAS MONITORING

In-line continuous infant blood gas monitors can be used as an alternative strategy for patients requiring frequent blood gas analysis. These devices are specifically designed for small patients with low blood volumes and volume restriction. The monitor is placed directly in-line with an arterial or umbilical catheter (Figure 10-6). Using a closed loop system, it obtains a 1.5-ml sample

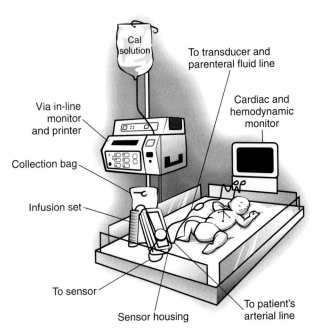

FIGURE 10-6 An ex vivo in-line continuous blood gas monitor designed for use in critically ill newborn infants.

of arterial blood, measures the blood gases via an in-line microelectrochemical sensor, and reinfuses the blood back into the patient. Clinical trials using in-line monitors in neonates found that this method provided frequent, reliable results in a short amount of time, while substantially reducing the amount of blood loss and less exposure to health care providers.[33]

CENTRAL VENOUS CATHETERS

Indications for a central venous catheter are as follows:
- Cardiovascular instability
- Intravascular volume disturbances (e.g., extreme dehydration, hemorrhage, increased intracranial pressure, renal failure, and diabetic ketoacidosis)
- Administration of drugs, fluids, or nutritional support to the central circulation
- The need for central venous pressure (CVP) monitoring[34]

Central venous catheterization is also indicated when other peripheral access sites have been exhausted. Placing a CVP line allows measurement of right atrial pressure (RAP) to assist in:
- Managing fluid volume
- Infusing fluid volumes larger than a peripheral intravenous catheter can accommodate
- Administering total parenteral nutrition, and providing a secure long-term venous site in a chronically ill child[33,35,36]

Monitoring Sites

Techniques for central line placement in infants and children vary according to the patient's age and condition. *Monitoring sites* for central venous catheterization are locations where a peripheral vein can be cannulated by either the percutaneous or the cutdown method and the catheter can be advanced to a central location in the vena cava. The percutaneous technique is relatively safe and easy, with many potential sites.

The cutdown method, or surgical cannulation, reduces the risk of trauma to the vein and adjacent tissue. Cutdown also provides additional sites for patients with poor peripheral perfusion or lack of percutaneous sites. Cutdown locations include the internal and external jugular veins, common facial vein, brachial vessels, saphenous vein, and femoral veins. The cutdown technique requires experience to avoid surgical complications such as bleeding, inadvertent interruption of arterial flow, and dissection through vital structures such as muscles and nerves.

Common vessels used for percutaneous approaches are the external and internal jugular veins (the right is preferred over the left vein), subclavian vein, brachial veins, and saphenous vessels.[37,38]

The umbilicus offers a unique site in the newborn because the umbilical vein is available for placement of a central catheter.[36]

Procedure

Placement of the catheter is performed under sterile conditions with the child sedated and in accordance with the recommendations for pain control.[6] The site is usually anesthetized with lidocaine before the catheter is placed in the vein. Advance the catheter until an RAP waveform appears on the monitor. Connect a flush line and pressure transducer as with any indwelling catheter used for pressure monitoring. Confirm catheter placement with a chest radiograph.

Complications

The major complication of venous catheter use in general is catheter-related *sepsis*, especially when the catheter is in place longer than 72 hours.[33] Fungal sepsis is especially significant in the neonatal population.[39,40] In older children the additional complication of *pulmonary embolism* is significant.[41] Embolism appears to be an unrecognized clinical entity in the neonate.

The percutaneous approach may be difficult in patients with poor peripheral perfusion and in those with chronic disease who require many venous catheters. The cutdown method requires a higher degree of skill and training than the percutaneous approach to avoid complications. Dysrhythmias may occur if the catheter tip slips into the right ventricle. Inadvertent placement of the catheter tip in the left atrium is possible if the patient has a patent foramen ovale or atrial septal defect. Perforation of the trachea is rare but has occurred with insertion into the jugular vein. Saphenous and femoral vein sites tend to be at higher risk for thrombosis. Air embolus may occur during insertion and when tubing is disconnected.[41]

Catheterization should be discontinued at the first sign of inflammation or when the patient's condition no longer requires its use. Percutaneous sites should be rotated on a regular basis. Any vein may be safely reused after 4 to 7 days.

Measurements

The placement of a central venous catheter allows measurement of the RAP, which represents the filling pressure of the right atrium. Systemic venous return, intravascular volume, tricuspid valve performance, myocardial function, and right ventricular pressure all affect the RAP. Normal values for RAP range from 2 to 7 cm H_2O but must be interpreted cautiously, because filling pressures vary with changes in thoracic and intrapleural pressure, such as during mechanical ventilation. The value of the RAP measurement is useful in monitoring trends and after changes in therapy.

Blood samples taken from the right atrium may be similar to mixed venous samples; however, the "gold standard" for measuring mixed venous oxygenation is obtained by using a pulmonary artery catheter. This approach demands caution because catheter tip placement may be influenced by venous return from one portion of the body rather than the whole body. Analyzing mixed venous oxygen saturation ($S\bar{v}o_2$) and Po_2 in mixed venous blood provides information about overall tissue oxygenation and can be compared with arterial samples to monitor changes in oxygen consumption. The use of a catheter with light-transmitting fiberoptics allows continuous measurement of oxygen saturation.

Decreased CVP values usually indicate hypovolemia. Reduced CVP values occur during fluid imbalance, hemorrhage, extreme vasodilation, and shock. Increased CVP values may result from the following:

- Hypervolemia, as with sudden fluid shifts or volume overload
- Interference with the right ventricle's ability to pump blood, such as tricuspid valve regurgitation or stenosis, right ventricular failure or infarction, increased pulmonary vascular resistance, or cardiac tamponade
- Increased systemic vasoconstriction
- Left ventricular failure[38]

PULMONARY ARTERY CATHETERIZATION

The pulmonary artery catheter provides important physiologic information about the cardiopulmonary vascular system (not attainable with other catheters), intravascular volume status, and the effects of various pharmacologic therapies.[42] The pulmonary artery catheter is often referred to as a "Swan-Ganz" catheter and is indicated for critically ill patients with respiratory failure or profound shock requiring vasoactive drugs. It is used to assess left ventricular function, guide fluid management, and aid in diagnosing and managing pulmonary disease and cardiac dysfunction. Direct intracardiac and pulmonary pressure monitoring, along with cardiac output measurement and mixed venous oxygen monitoring, can be accomplished with a pulmonary artery catheter.[43,44]

Pulmonary artery catheters are used less frequently in pediatrics and are generally reserved for the sickest of patients. The standard use of pulmonary artery catheters is divergent and its implementation varies from hospital to hospital. An analysis of risk versus benefit should be considered before using pulmonary artery catheters.

Pulmonary artery catheters contain quadruple lumens and come in 5-French (for patients less than 18 kg) and 7-French outer diameters. They are marked in 10-cm increments along the outside, and a balloon is fastened 1 to 2 mm from the tip. A four-lumen catheter has the following ports (Figure 10-7):

- Proximal port for placement in the right atrium; this port terminates in an opening at the tip of the catheter and is used to measure RAP
- Distal port for placement in the pulmonary artery; this lumen terminates in an opening at the tip of the catheter and lies in the pulmonary artery. It is used to measure pulmonary artery pressure (PAP) and pulmonary capillary wedge pressure (PCWP) and to sample mixed venous blood
- Port for inflation of the balloon at the catheter tip; when inflated, the balloon should surround but not cover the tip of the catheter.
- Port for the temperature-measuring thermistor; this port connects to the cardiac output monitor. The thermistor wires transmit the temperature of the blood flowing over them to the cardiac output monitor.[45]

Procedure

If tolerable, the patient is placed in a Trendelenburg's position to prevent air embolism and to enhance neck vein filling. The catheter is primed with intravenous flush solution, and the integrity of the balloon is evaluated by injecting air into it. The catheter is placed in a large vessel, using a cutdown or percutaneous approach, and advanced until an RAP tracing appears on the monitor. The balloon is inflated with air, and floated through the tricuspid valve into the right ventricle. The catheter is advanced into the pulmonary artery and then into a wedged position, where the catheter occludes the artery. As the catheter is advanced, characteristic waveforms are observed for each heart and vessel location, which assists with placement (Figures 10-8 and 10-9). Once the catheter is wedged, the balloon is deflated and the pulmonary artery waveform is confirmed on the monitor.

Inflating and deflating the balloon demonstrates the ability to acquire a PCWP and a PAP. The catheter is then sutured in place, and the length of the catheter is recorded at the insertion site. The catheter should never be inserted to a length greater than that measured before placement. This avoids complications, such as knotting or unintentional wedging of the catheter without balloon inflation. A chest radiograph can be obtained immediately to rule out a pneumothorax and to verify the catheter's position.

Continuous monitoring of the catheter waveforms and pressures is necessary. On the monitor, the catheter position is maintained to produce a PAP waveform, except for those brief intervals when PCWP readings are obtained. To obtain a PCWP reading, a syringe is attached to the balloon port and aspirated to ensure complete emptying of the balloon, which avoids overinflation and rupture. Normally, when inflating the balloon, there is some initial resistance. If there is no resistance, the integrity of the balloon should be evaluated and inflation should be discontinued.[38,46]

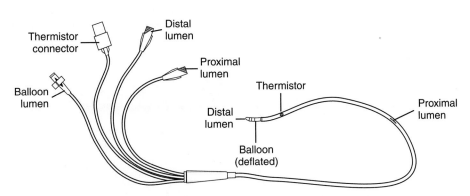

FIGURE 10-7 Conventional pulmonary artery (Swan-Ganz) thermodilution catheter.

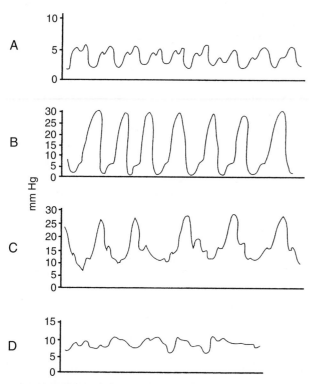

FIGURE 10-8 Examples of pressure waveform patterns at various locations in and around the heart. **A,** Central venous pressure; **B,** right ventricular pressure; **C,** pulmonary artery pressure; **D,** pulmonary capillary wedge pressure.

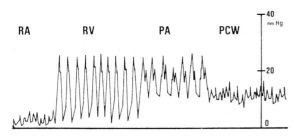

FIGURE 10-9 Pressure waveforms as the catheter travels through the right atrium (RA), right ventricle (RV), and pulmonary artery (PA), becoming wedged (pulmonary capillary wedge pressure [PCWP]).

Complications

At insertion, complications include bleeding, pneumothorax, tricuspid or pulmonic valve damage, right atrium or right ventricle perforation, and arrhythmias resulting from the catheter traversing the right ventricle. The most frequently observed arrhythmias are premature ventricular contractions and ventricular tachycardia. Overinflation of the balloon may result in rupture of the pulmonary artery, pulmonic valve obstruction, and air embolization. Pulmonary infarction may occur if the catheter is left in the wedge position for extended periods. The major complications remain catheter-induced thrombosis and sepsis.[46-54]

Positive-pressure ventilation affects PCWP measurements. Erroneous measurements may result from changes in baseline during the inspiratory and expiratory phases. Other sources of measurement error are failure to zero-set or calibrate the transducer properly, misalignment of the transducer with the tip of the catheter in the pulmonary artery, and dampening of the waveform secondary to thrombus formation.[28] Accurate hemodynamic values can be difficult to obtain in children with intracardiac shunts and tricuspid regurgitation.

Measurements

The proximal port measures the RAP and the distal port the PAP (Box 10-4). A decrease in PAP usually indicates hypovolemia or pulmonary vasodilation. An increase in PAP may indicate an increase in pulmonary vascular resistance, mitral stenosis, left ventricular failure, or hypervolemia. Increased PAP also may result from pulmonary edema or an increase in pulmonary blood flow, as with left-to-right shunts in congenital heart defects.

The PCWP reflects downstream pressures in the left side of the heart under conditions of absent flow in the pulmonary capillary bed. Variations in airway pressures, such as during mechanical ventilation, with positive end-expiratory pressure (PEEP), can influence PCWP. The degree to which ventilation affects the relationship between PCWP and left atrial pressure depends on lung compliance. Under normal conditions, only 50% of the alveolar pressure is transmitted to the intrapleural space. Patients with low lung compliance, and hence low lung volumes, experience a negligible effect from variations in positive pressure on the PCWP. Higher compliance results in larger lung volumes and higher alveolar pressures. Therefore, higher intrapleural pressure is transmitted to the adjacent cardiovascular structures. PCWP should be measured at end expiration and without PEEP if tolerated by the patient. Measuring the PCWP with PEEP to establish trends in changes in clinical conditions is common. If not caused by PEEP, increased PCWP usually indicates left ventricular failure, hypervolemia, or intravascular fluid overload. Pulmonary artery catheters can have an additional fiberoptic lumen that provides continuous measurement of $S\bar{v}o_2$ from the pulmonary artery.[45,48]

Box 10-4	Normal Pressure Values From Pulmonary Artery Catheters	
Mean right atrial pressure		2-7 mm Hg
Pulmonary artery systolic pressure		15-30 mm Hg
Pulmonary artery diastolic pressure		5-15 mm Hg
Mean pulmonary artery pressure		10-20 mm Hg
Pulmonary capillary wedge pressure		5-15 mm Hg

Cardiac Output

The cardiac output is the single most important hemodynamic measurement used to evaluate cardiac function and to determine the therapeutic effects of various treatments in critically ill pediatric patients. Cardiac output is the amount of blood ejected from the heart over the course of 1 minute. It is the product of stroke volume and heart rate. At birth, a newborn's cardiac output is approximately 0.6 L/minute and increases to 6 L/minute in an adolescent male.[30] Cardiac output is referenced to the body surface area as the *cardiac index*. The cardiac index is normally 3 to 4.5 L/minute/m² throughout childhood.[30] Traditionally, cardiac output measurements use the thermodilution technique. Measurements are derived from injecting a known volume of liquid at a set temperature, 22° to 24° C, or iced, 0° to 4° C, into the right atrium through the right atrial port of the catheter. The solution is injected with a rapid and constant motion. The exact temperature and amount of liquid is entered into the cardiac output computer. As the liquid mixes with the blood and passes through the right ventricle into the pulmonary artery, the thermistor measures the rate of change in blood temperature from the value entered into the computer. The computer calculates the rate at which the blood warms the liquid, which is proportional to blood flow, and yields cardiac output.

By using the cardiac output and pressure measurements from the pulmonary and peripheral artery catheters clinicians can construct a complete hemodynamic profile of a patient (Table 10-1).[28,49,50]

The injectate volume used with pediatric patients is smaller than that used with adults. However, it is important to limit excessive fluid administration by reducing the number of tests being done.

Pulmonary artery catheters are now available that do not require a cold injectate bolus to determine the cardiac output. Thermodilution is applied by using a thermal element on the catheter that warms up the surrounding blood, making it a warm bolus with a known temperature. Cardiac output is calculated, as the area under the curve, on the basis of the temperature change of the blood bolus as measured by a downstream thermistor.

Pulse contour analysis offers a minimally invasive technique that uses measurements obtained from arterial and central venous catheters to continuously calculate cardiac output. This method analyzes variations in the arterial pressure waveform during ventilation to determine stroke volume and hence cardiac index.[52] In addition, this method integrates a thermal dilution technique, using a central venous catheter, for initial and periodic system calibrations.

TABLE 10-1

Normal Ranges of Derived Hemodynamic Parameters

Parameter	Formula	Range
Cardiac index	CO/BSA	3.0-4.5 L/min/m²
Stroke volume	CO/HR	50-80 ml/beat
Stroke volume index	SV/BSA	30-65 ml/beat/m²
Systemic vascular resistance	MAP – LAP/CO	11-18 mm Hg/L/min
Pulmonary vascular resistance	PAP – PCWP/CO	1.5-3.0 mm Hg/L/min
Shunt fraction	$(Cc_{O_2} - Ca_{O_2})/$ $(Cc_{O_2} - C\bar{v}_{O_2})$	Less than 5%

BSA, Body surface area; Ca_{O_2}, arterial oxygen content; Cc_{O_2}, pulmonary end-capillary oxygen content; CO, cardiac output; $C\bar{v}_{O_2}$, mixed venous oxygen content; HR, heart rate; LAP, left atrial pressure; MAP, mean arterial pressure; PAP, pulmonary artery pressure; PCWP, pulmonary capillary wedge pressure; SV, stroke volume.

Pulse contour analysis has been shown to be an effective way to measure cardiac index in pediatric patients without using a pulmonary artery catheter or subjecting small patients to excessive fluid boluses.[51]

NONINVASIVE MEASUREMENT OF CARDIAC OUTPUT AND PERFUSION

Because of the inherent risks and limitations associated with pulmonary artery catheters, trends favoring noninvasive techniques to accurately measure cardiac output and tissue perfusion have resulted in new technologies.

A noninvasive cardiac output monitor that uses partial rebreathing of CO_2 to determine cardiac output via the Fick principle can now be used in mechanically ventilated children. A study has shown that this method correlates well with simultaneous cardiac output measurements obtained from a pulmonary artery catheter in patients with a body surface area of at least 0.6 m² and a tidal volume of at least 300 ml.[52]

Signal extraction pulse oximetry, which uses signal extraction software to analyze the plethysmographic waveform to determine pulsatile strength, is now being used to provide continuous noninvasive measurements of peripheral perfusion.[53] "The perfusion index (PI) is the ratio of the pulsatile blood flow to the nonpulsatile or static blood in peripheral tissue."[54] The (PI) has been used as an objective parameter to evaluate perfusion and determine severity of illness in critically ill neonates.[55] The pulse variability index (PVI) continuously detects the cyclic changes of the perfusion index signal caused by variations in the intrathoracic pressure during a complete respiratory cycle. The PVI value has been shown to reliably predict fluid responsiveness in mechanically ventilated patients.[56]

PATIENT INFORMATION

It is important to monitor and record several parameters when taking a blood gas sample. Documenting the specific puncture or sample site and whether it is arterial, venous, mixed venous, or capillary is essential. The caregiver should also record the date and time at which the sample was taken, along with the patient's respiratory variables. Important respiratory variables include respiratory frequency, temperature, fraction of inspired oxygen (FIO_2), and specific oxygen device used. If the patient is mechanically ventilated, include the type of ventilator, mode of ventilation, tidal volume, peak inflation pressure, PEEP, and other relevant settings. Note the patient's position (e.g., upright in an infant seat), activity level (e.g., whether crying or breath holding), clinical appearance, and other signs of respiratory distress. Be sure to document any adverse reactions, along with the corrective action taken.

FREQUENCY

The clinical status of the patient, rather than an arbitrarily set time or frequency, should dictate the need for arterial and capillary punctures.[2,10,12] It is also important to understand that an infant, especially a premature neonate, has a much smaller quantity of blood. Frequent blood sampling results in hypovolemia and anemia in these patients. During mechanical ventilation, wait 10 minutes after changing the FIO_2 in a patient without chronic pulmonary disease to take an ABG sample.[57] Samples should not be drawn until 20 to 30 minutes after changing the FIO_2 of a spontaneously breathing patient without chronic pulmonary disease. Patients with chronic pulmonary disease should not have samples drawn for at least 30 minutes after an FIO_2 change.[2]

BLOOD GAS INTERPRETATION

Although a thorough discussion of blood gas interpretation is beyond the scope of this chapter, using the blood gas result requires some explanation of acid-base balance and gas exchange. *Gas exchange* refers to the exchange of oxygen and carbon dioxide between air and blood and then between blood and tissue. Proper gas exchange depends on many factors, such as blood flow, cardiac output, metabolic rate, diffusion, shunting, and gas concentration of the inspired air. An abnormality in any of these factors will result in a change in blood gas values and possibly an increase in the work of the cardiopulmonary system. Usually, only three values are measured during blood gas analysis: pH, PCO_2, and PO_2. Bicarbonate (HCO_3^-) and oxygen saturation are also usually calculated. On occasion, other non–blood gas values may be measured simultaneously, depending on the analyzer in use at the time.

Typically, interpretation of blood gas values involves acid-base interpretation, to evaluate the pH and PCO_2 values, and evaluation of oxygenation, or PO_2, separately. Normal PaO_2 and $PaCO_2$ values reflect normal gas exchange, whereas an abnormality in gas exchange results in abnormal values. Normal values can vary considerably, based on patient age. Some mechanical ventilator strategies that use a lung-protective strategy have redefined normal ranges in acid-base status, especially in premature infants. Recognizing normal and abnormal values helps to understand more completely, and to interpret, blood gas values (Table 10-2).

TABLE 10-2

Approximate Normal Range of Arterial Blood Gas Values

Parameter	ELBW Premature Infant	VLBW Premature Infant to Near-term Infant	Term Infant to Toddler	Child to Adult
	(<28 wk of GA)	(28-40 wk of GA)	(Up to 2 yr)	(>2 yr)
pH	≥7.25 (≥7.20)*	≥7.25 (≥7.20)*	7.3-7.4	7.35-7.45
Arterial carbon dioxide tension ($PaCO_2$, mm Hg)	45-55 (60)	45-55 (60)	30-40	35-45
Arterial oxygen tension (PaO_2, mm Hg)	45-65	50-70	80-100	80-100
Bicarbonate (HCO_3^-) (mEq/L)	15-18	18-20	20-22	22-24

ELBW, Extremely low birth weight; GA, gestational age; VLBW, very low birth weight.
* Values in parentheses may be accepted for certain lung protection ventilator strategies.
Modified from Pagtakhan RD, Pasterkamp H: Intensive care for respiratory disorders. In Chernick V, editor: *Kendig's disorders of the respiratory tract in children*, ed 5, Philadelphia: WB Saunders; 1990. pp 205-224; and Durand DJ, Philips P, Boloker J: Blood gases: technical aspects and interpretation. In Goldsmith JP, Karotkin EH, editors: *Assisted ventilation of the neonate*, ed 4, Philadelphia: WB Saunders/Elsevier Science; 2003.

Acid–Base Balance

Assessing acid–base balance is accomplished by evaluating the pH, $Paco_2$, and HCO_3^- values for acidosis or alkalosis and the degree of compensation present (Table 10-3). $Paco_2$ is directly proportional to the adequacy of alveolar ventilation. Thus acid–base abnormalities are classified as primarily respiratory or metabolic. The amount to which the pH is balanced by the metabolic or respiratory processes determines the degree of compensation. Boxes 10-5 to 10-8 list common causes of metabolic acidosis/alkalosis and respiratory acidosis/alkalosis.

Oxygenation

The arterial partial pressure of oxygen (Pao_2) reflects exchange of oxygen, or oxygenation. Oxygen moves into the airway and the alveolus, at which point a pressure gradient causes it to diffuse across the alveolar–capillary membrane into the pulmonary capillary blood. It is then carried in the blood to the tissues in two forms: (1) dissolved in plasma and (2) bound to hemoglobin. Although the amount of oxygen dissolved in plasma is small, it is critical because it determines the pressure gradients among the inspired air, the blood, and the tissues. Hemoglobin carries the majority of the oxygen as oxyhemoglobin.

The amount of oxygen bound to hemoglobin is expressed as *arterial oxygen* saturation (Sao_2) or % O2 Hb saturation. The oxyhemoglobin dissociation curve illustrates the relationship between Pao_2 and Sao_2 regarding the loading and unloading of oxygen by the hemoglobin molecule (Figure 10-10). The sigmoid shape of the curve shows that the hemoglobin loads and unloads oxygen differently at various PaO_2s. The PaO_2 at which the $SaO2$ is 50% saturated is known as the P_{50} value. Under normal conditions, the P_{50} is approximately

Box 10-5 Causes of Metabolic Acidosis

Diarrhea
Small bowel, biliary, or pancreatic tube or fistula drainage
Hyperalimentation
Ingestion of chloride-containing compounds
- Calcium chloride
- Magnesium chloride
- Ammonium chloride
- Hydrochloric acid
Renal tubular acidosis
Renal failure
Carbonic anhydrase deficiency
Lactic acidosis
- Tissue hypoxia
- Sepsis
- Neonatal cold stress
Ketoacidosis
- Diabetes mellitus
- Starvation
Ingestion of toxins
- Salicylate poisoning
- Methanol poisoning
- Ethylene glycol poisoning
- Prolonged use of paraldehyde
Inborn errors of metabolism

Modified from Brewer ED: Disorders of acid–base balance, *Pediatr Clin North Am* 1990;37:429.

Box 10-6 Causes of Metabolic Alkalosis

Vomiting
Nasogastric suctioning
Congenital chloride-wasting diarrhea
Dehydration
Drugs
- Diuretics
- Steroids
- Sodium bicarbonate
Cushing's syndrome
Bartter's syndrome
Hypokalemia
Hypochloremia
Chewing tobacco
Massive blood transfusion
Infants with cystic fibrosis fed regular formula or breast milk (low in sodium)

Modified from Brewer ED: Disorders of acid–base balance, *Pediatr Clin North Am* 1990;37:429.

TABLE 10-3

Laboratory Values for Acid–base Disturbances

Disease	pH	$Paco_2$	HCO_3^-
Metabolic acidosis			
Uncompensated	↓	N	↓
Partially compensated	↓	↓	↓
Compensated	N	↓	↓
Metabolic alkalosis			
Uncompensated	↑	N	↑
Partially compensated	↑	↑	↑
Compensated	N	↑*	↑
Respiratory acidosis			
Uncompensated	↓	↑	N
Partially compensated	↓	↑	↑
Compensated	N	↑	↑
Respiratory alkalosis			
Uncompensated	↑	↓	N
Partially compensated	↑	↓	↓
Uncompensated	N	↓	↓
Mixed acidosis	↓	↑	↓
Mixed alkalosis	↑	↓	↑

HCO_3^-, Bicarbonate; N, normal; $Paco_2$, arterial carbon dioxide tension.
*Compensation of metabolic alkalosis by hypoventilation is limited by the physiologic response to hypoxic hypoxia due to the elevated $Paco_2$.

Box 10-7	Causes of Respiratory Acidosis

LUNG DISEASE
Upper airway obstruction
- Laryngotracheobronchitis (croup)
- Epiglottitis
- Foreign body

Small airway obstruction
- Asthma
- Bronchiolitis

Chronic obstructive pulmonary disease
- Cystic fibrosis
- Bronchopulmonary dysplasia
- Bronchiectasis

Pneumonia
Pulmonary edema
Respiratory distress syndrome
Aspiration
- Meconium
- Foreign body

Pulmonary hypoplasia

IMPAIRED LUNG MOTION
Pleural effusion
Pneumothorax
Thoracic cage abnormalities
- Flail chest
- Scoliosis
- Osteogenesis imperfecta
- Thoracic dystrophy

APNEA

NEUROMUSCULAR DISORDERS
Brainstem/spinal cord injury or tumor
Paralysis of diaphragm
Drug overdose/oversedation
Muscular dystrophy
Guillain-Barré syndrome
Myasthenia gravis
Poliomyelitis

OTHER
Botulism
Extreme obesity

Modified from Brewer ED: Disorders of acid–base balance, *Pediatr Clin North Am* 1990;37:429.

Box 10-8	Causes of Respiratory Alkalosis

Anxiety
Fever
Sepsis
Hypoxemia
- Pneumonia
- Atelectasis
- Pulmonary emboli
- Congestive heart failure
- Asthma

Central nervous system disorders
- Head injury
- Brain tumor
- Infection
- Cerebrovascular accident
- High altitude

Liver failure
Reye's syndrome
Hyperthyroidism
Salicylate poisoning
Mechanical ventilation

Modified from Brewer ED: Disorders of acid–base balance, *Pediatr Clin North Am* 1990;37:429.

The oxygen content of the blood, expressed as a percentage, is the sum of the oxygen dissolved in the plasma and the oxygen in combination with hemoglobin (Hb, g/dl). Oxygen content accurately reflects the amount of oxygen in the blood, as follows:

$$O_2 \text{ content} = (Hb \times 1.34 \times Sao_2) + (Pao_2 \times 0.003)$$

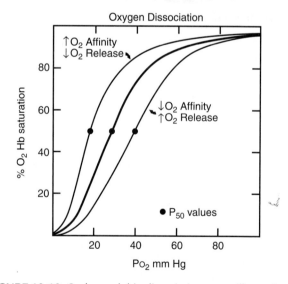

FIGURE 10-10 Oxyhemoglobin dissociation curve, illustrating the P_{50} value (Po_2 at 50% saturation) with the effects of right and left shifts of the curve. As the curve shifts to the right, the oxygen affinity of hemoglobin decreases, more oxygen is released at a given Po_2, and the P_{50} value increases. When the curve shifts to the left, there is increased oxygen affinity, less oxygen is released at a given Po_2, and the P_{50} value decreases.

26.5 mmHg; however, this value can change depending on conditions that cause shifts in the oxyhemoglobin dissociation curve. The oxyhemoglobin dissociation curve is affected by several factors and may shift left or right (Table 10-4). A shift to the *right* results in a decrease in oxygen affinity, decrease in oxyhemoglobin and an increase the unloading of oxygen at the cellular level. A shift to the *left* increases oxygen affinity, increases oxyhemoglobin and a decrease in the unloading of oxygen at the cellular level.

TABLE 10-4	
Factors That May Shift Oxyhemoglobin Dissociation Curve	
Increased Affinity (Shift to Right)	**Decreased Affinity (Shift to Left)**
Increased pH	Decreased pH
Decreased P_{CO_2}	Increased P_{CO_2}
Decreased temperature	Increased temperature
Decreased 2,3-DPG	Increased 2,3-DPG
Fetal hemoglobin	
Carboxyhemoglobin	
Methemoglobin	

2,3-DPG, 2,3-diphosphoglycerate; P_{CO_2}, partial pressure (tension) of carbon dioxide.

Oxygen delivery, expressed as milliliters per minute, is the product of the O_2 content of the arterial blood and the cardiac output (Figure 10-11). Oxygen delivery reflects the total oxygen available at the cellular level in 1 minute as follows:

$$O_2 \text{delivery} = O_2 \text{ content} \times \text{cardiac output} \times 10$$

Normal oxygen delivery ranges from 133-200 ml/minute in newborns and from 200-400 ml/minute during infancy, and 460-1200 ml/minute during childhood.[30]

Determining serum lactate in a blood sample provides important information about oxygenation. Lactic acid is commonly the by-product of anaerobic metabolism, which results from hypoxia at the cellular level. Higher lactate levels are indicative of decreased O_2 delivery. Normal values for serum lactate typically range from 0.7 to 1.3 mmol/L.[58] A serum lactate concentration of 4.8 mmol/L and greater has been associated with increases in morbidity and mortality in children.[59]

ABNORMAL HEMOGLOBIN

Abnormal hemoglobin may also have an effect on the capacity of hemoglobin to combine with oxygen. The following hemoglobins are sometimes encountered in the infant and pediatric population. Fetal hemoglobin accounts for approximately 85% of the hemoglobin in the full-term infant. It causes a shift to the left of the oxyhemoglobin dissociation curve and consequently an increased affinity of hemoglobin for oxygen. In utero, this compensates for the low fetal Pa_{O_2} and causes more oxygen to be picked up in the placenta. At about 6 months to 1 year of age, all fetal hemoglobin should be converted to normal hemoglobin.

Methemoglobin forms when hemoglobin is oxidized to the ferric state. It causes the oxyhemoglobin dissociation curve to shift to the left, resulting in a decrease in hemoglobin's ability to combine with oxygen. Nitrate-containing molecules in medications and therapeutic gases may cause methemoglobinemia.

Carboxyhemoglobin forms when carbon monoxide combines with hemoglobin, which reduces the amount of oxygen that can attach to the hemoglobin. In carbon monoxide poisoning the patient has reduced oxygen content even though the Pa_{O_2} may be normal (see Chapter 39, Head Injury and Cerebral Disorders). A left-shifted oxyhemoglobin dissociation curve compounds the tissue hypoxia further.

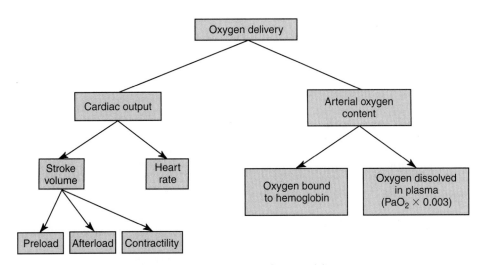

FIGURE 10-11 Components of oxygen delivery.

ASSESSMENT QUESTIONS

See Evolve Resources for answers.

1. The most accurate way to detect changes in oxygenation in the blood is by obtaining the following:
   A. Capillary blood gas
   B. Mixed venous blood gas
   C. Arterial blood gas
   D. Pulse oximetry
2. What method for obtaining blood gases should be tried initially in a neonate?
   A. Capillary blood gas determination
   B. Pulmonary artery catheterization
   C. Umbilical artery catheterization
   D. Femoral artery puncture
3. The high placement of an umbilical artery catheter should be visually confirmed at which anatomic landmark, using an X-ray?
   A. T6-T8
   B. T3-T4
   C. L1-L2
   D. T1-T3
4. The most important advantage of continuous in-line blood gas sampling compared with umbilical blood gas sampling in neonates is:
   A. Lower risk of infection
   B. Lower incidence of clot formation
   C. Decrease in the amount of blood wasted
   D. The advantage of also being able to measure the cardiac index
5. The cardiac index is calculated by the following equation:
   A. $Cao_2/Spo_2 \times 100$
   B. Stroke volume/cardiac output
   C. $Cao_2 \times CO$
   D. Cardiac output/BSA
6. Common factors that can reduce pulmonary vascular resistance include:
   A. Hypoxemia and acidosis
   B. High mean airway pressure
   C. Fluid resuscitation
   D. Nitric oxide
7. Which of the following may be used to clinically measure the cardiac index and tissue perfusion *without* a pulmonary (Swan-Ganz) artery catheter?
   A. Pulse variability index
   B. Pulse contour analysis
   C. Partial CO_2 rebreathing, using the Fick method
   D. All of the above
8. Complications associated with indwelling vascular catheters include:
   A. Infection
   B. Air embolism
   C. Periventricular leukomalacia
   D. Both A and B

ASSESSMENT QUESTIONS—cont'd

9. Which of the following statement(s) is correct regarding the affects of positive pressure on the measurement of pulmonary capillary wedge pressure?
   A. PCWP is higher when lung compliance is low.
   B. PCWP is lower when lung compliance is high.
   C. PCWP is higher when lung compliance in high.
   D. There are no affects from positive pressure on PCWP
10. Oxygen delivery is comprised of all of the following, Except:
    A. Cardiac Index
    B. Cardiac output
    C. Hemoglobin
    D. CaO_2
    E. A and C
    F. A, C, and D

References

1. Czervinske MP: Arterial blood gas analysis and other cardiopulmonary monitoring. In Koff PB, Eitzman DV, Neu J, editors: *Neonatal and pediatric respiratory care*, St. Louis: Mosby, 1988.
2. American Association for Respiratory Care: Clinical practice guideline: blood gas analysis and hemoximetry, 2001 revision and update, *Respir Care* 2001; 46:498.
3. Johnston CC et al: Factors explaining lack of response to heel stick in preterm newborns, *J Obstet Gynecol Neonat Nurs* 1999;28:587.
4. Anand KJS: Clinical importance of pain and stress in preterm newborn infants, *Biol Neonate* 1998;73:1.
5. Johnston CC et al: Differential response to pain by very premature neonates, *Pain* 1995;61:471.
6. Stevens B, Yamada J, Ohlsson A: Sucrose for analgesia in newborn infants undergoing painful procedures, *Cochrane Database Syst Rev* 2004;3:CD001069.
7. Lefrak L, Burch K, Caravantes R: Sucrose analgesia: identifying potentially better practice, *Pediatrics* 2006;118;S197.
8. Anand KJS; International Evidence-Based Group for Neonatal Pain: Consensus statement for the prevention and management of pain in the newborn, *Arch Pediatr Adolesc Med* 2001;155:173.
9. National Committee for Clinical Laboratory Standards (Clinical and Laboratory Standards Institute): Procedures for the collection of arterial blood specimens, ed 4. NCCLS document no. H11-A3. Wayne, Pa: Clinical and Laboratory Standards Institute; 2004.
10. American Association for Respiratory Care: Clinical practice guideline: sampling for arterial blood gas analysis, *Respir Care* 1992;37:913.
11. Centers for Disease Control and Prevention: Update: universal precautions for prevention of transmission of human immunodeficiency virus, hepatitis B virus, and other blood borne pathogens in health

care settings, *MMWR Morb Mortal Wkly Rep* 1988;37: 377-388.

12. U.S. Occupational Safety and Health Administration: Occupational exposure to bloodborne pathogens—OSHA. Final rule [29 CFR 1910.1030], *Fed Regist* 1991;56:64004. Available at http://www.osha.gov/pls/oshaweb/owadisp.show_document?p_table=STANDARDS&p_id=10051. Retrieved August 2008.

13. Escalante-Kanashiro R, Tantalean Da Fieno J: Capillary blood gases in a pediatric intensive care unit, *Crit Care Med* 2000;28:224.

14. American Association for Respiratory Care: Clinical practice guideline: capillary blood gas sampling for neonatal and pediatric patients, *Respir Care* 1994;39: 1180.

15. McLain BI, Evans J, Dear PFR: Comparison of capillary and arterial blood gas measurements in neonates, *Arch Dis Child* 1988;63:743.

16. Johnson KJ et al: Neonatal laboratory blood sampling: comparison of results from arterial catheters with those from an automated capillary device, *Neonatal Network* 2000;19:27.

17. Courtney SE et al: Capillary blood gases in the neonate: a reassessment and review of the literature, *Am J Dis Child* 1990;144:168.

18. Yildizdas D et al: Correlation of simultaneously obtained capillary, venous, and arterial blood gases of patients in a paediatric intensive care unit, *Arch Dis Child* 2004;89:176.

19. Ueta I, Jacobs BR: Capillary and arterial blood gases in hemorrhagic shock: a comparative study, *Pediatr Crit Care Med* 2002;3:375.

20. Cousineau J et al: Neonate capillary blood gas reference values, *Clin Biochem* 2005;38:905.

21. Koch G, Wendel H: Comparison of pH, carbon dioxide tension, standard bicarbonate, and oxygen tension in capillary blood and in arterial blood during neonatal period, *Acta Paediatr Scand* 1967;56:14.

22. Sell EJ, Hansen RC, Struck-Pierce S: Calcified nodules on the heel: a complication of neonatal intensive care, *J Pediatr* 1980;96:473.

23. Symansky MR, Fox HA: Umbilical vessel catheterization: indications, management and evaluation of the technique, *J Pediatr* 1972;80:820.

24. Barrington KJ: Umbilical artery catheters in the newborn: effects of position of the catheter tip, *Cochrane Database Syst Rev* 2000;2:CD000505.

25. MacDonald MG: Umbilical artery catheterization. In Avery GB, Fletcher MA, MacDonald MG, editors: *Neonatology: pathophysiology and management of the newborn*, Philadelphia: Lippincott Williams & Wilkins; 1999. p 1338.

26. Cole FS, Todres ID, Shannon DC: Technique for percutaneous cannulation of the radial artery in the newborn infant, *J Pediatr* 1978;92:105.

27. Tibby SM, Murdoch IA: Monitoring cardiac function in intensive care, *Arch Dis Child* 2003;88:46.

28. Eshali H et al: Septicaemia with coagulase negative staphylococci in a neonatal intensive care unit: risk factors for infection, and antimicrobial susceptibility of the bacterial strains, *Acta Paediatr Scand Suppl* 1989;360:127.

29. Hazinski MF: Hemodynamic monitoring of children. In Daily EK, Schroeder JS, editors: *Techniques in bedside hemodynamic monitoring*, ed 5, St. Louis: Mosby; 1994. pp 275-341.

30. Lott JW, Conner GK, Phillips JB: Umbilical artery catheter blood sampling alters cerebral blood flow velocity in preterm infants, *J Perinatol* 1996;16:341.

31. Cumming WA, Burchfield DJ: Accidental catheterization of internal iliac artery branches: a serious complication of umbilical artery catheterization, *J Perinatol* 1994;14:304.

32. Brown MS, Phibbs RH: Spinal cord injury in newborns from use of umbilical artery catheters: report of two cases and a review of the literature, *J Perinatol* 1988;8:105.

33. Widness JA et al: Clinical performance of an in-line point-of-care monitor in neonates, *Pediatrics* 2000;106;497.

34. Duck S: Neonatal intravenous therapy, *Neonatal Intensive Care* 1998;11:36.

35. Chiang VW, Baskin MN: Uses and complications of central venous catheters inserted in a pediatric emergency department, *Pediatr Emerg Care* 2000;16:230.

36. Hamilton H, Fermo K: Clinical assessment of patients requiring IV therapy via a central venous route, *Br J Nurs* 1998;7:451.

37. MacDonald MG: Umbilical vein catheterization. In Avery GB, Fletcher MA, MacDonald MG, editors: *Neonatology: pathophysiology and management of the newborn*, Philadelphia: Lippincott Williams & Wilkins; 1999. p 148.

38. Jordan W: Arterial catheters. In Blumer JL, editor: *A practical guide to pediatric intensive care*, St. Louis: Mosby; 1990. p 825.

39. Green C, Yohannan MD: Umbilical arterial and venous catheters: placement, use, and complications, *Neonatal Network* 1998;17:23.

40. Trotter CW: Percutaneous central venous catheter-related sepsis in the neonate: an analysis of the literature from 1990 to 1994, *Neonatal Network* 1996;15:15.

41. Wynsma LA: Negative outcomes of intravascular therapy in infants and children, *AACN Clin Issues* 1998;9:49.

42. Osgood CF, Watson MH, Slaughter MS: Hemodynamic monitoring in respiratory care, *Respir Care* 1984;29:25.

43. Abou-Khalil B: Hemodynamic responses to shock in young trauma patients: need for invasive monitoring, *Crit Care Med* 1994;22:633.

44. Katz RW, Pollack MM, Weibley RE: Pulmonary artery catheterization in pediatric intensive care, *Adv Pediatr* 1983;30:169.

45. Marini JJ: Obtaining meaningful data from the Swan-Ganz catheter, *Respir Care* 1985;30:572.

46. Pollack MM et al: Bedside pulmonary artery catheterization in pediatrics, *J Pediatr* 1980;96:274.

47. Perloff WH: Invasive measurements in the PICU. In Fuhrman BP, Zimmerman JJ, editors: *Pediatric critical care*, ed 2, St. Louis: Mosby; 1998. pp 70-86.

48. White KM: Completing the hemodynamic picture: $S\bar{v}o_2$, *Heart Lung* 1985;14:272.

49. Moodie DS et al: Measurement of cardiac output by thermodilution: development of accurate measurements at flows applicable to the pediatric patient, *J Surg Res* 1978;25:305.

50. Koppl J et al: Hemodynamic monitoring using a PiCCO in a ten month old infant suffering from serious burn injury, *Bratisl Lek Listy* 2000;108:359.

51. Fakler U et al: Cardiac index monitoring by pulse contour analysis and thermodilution after pediatric cardiac surgery, *J Thorac Cardiovasc Surg* 2007;133:224.

52. Levy RJ et al: An evaluation of a noninvasive cardiac output measurement using partial carbon dioxide rebreathing in children, *Anesth Analg* 2004;99:1642.

53. Goldman JM et al: Masimo signal extraction pulse oximetry, *J Clin Monit Comput* 2000;16:475.

54. Masimo Corporation: *Clinical applications of perfusion index.* Available at http://www.masimo.com/pdf/whitepaper/LAB3410E.pdf. Retrieved August 2008.

55. De Felice C et al: The pulse oximeter perfusion index as a predictor for high illness severity in neonates, *Eur J Pediatr* 2002;161:561.

56. Cannesson M et al: The ability of a novel algorithm for automatic estimation the respiratory variations in arterial pulse pressure to monitor fluid responsiveness in the operating room, *Anesth Analg* 2008;106:1195.

57. Hess D et al: The validity of assessing arterial blood gases 10 minutes after an F_{IO_2} change in mechanically ventilated patients without chronic pulmonary disease, *Respir Care* 1985;30:1037.

58. Vincent JL: Lactate and biochemical indexes of oxygenation. In Tobin MJ, editor: *Principles and practices of intensive care monitoring*, New York: McGraw-Hill; 1998. pp 369-375.

59. Basaran M et al: Serum lactate level has prognostic significance after pediatric cardiac surgery, *J Cardiothorac Vasc Anesth* 2006;20:43.

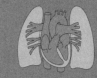

Chapter **11**

Noninvasive Monitoring in Neonatal and Pediatric Care

CYNTHIA JACOBUS

OUTLINE

Pulse Oximetry
Principles of Operation
Application
Disadvantages
Transcutaneous Monitoring
Principles of Operation
Application
Disadvantages
New Technology
Capnometry
Principles of Operation

Interpretation of Capnogram
Detection of Ventilation Problems
Impedance Pneumography
Principles of Operation
Application
Disadvantages
Electrocardiography
Calorimetry
Principles of Operation
Disadvantages

LEARNING OBJECTIVES

After reading this chapter the reader will be able to:
- Recognize the principles of operation of pulse oximetry
- Identify three ways to confirm proper application of pulse oximeter sensors
- Explain the importance of proper transcutaneous site selection and application
- List two problems associated with transcutaneous monitoring
- Interpret specific abnormalities associated with capnograms

- Detect ventilation problems in neonatal and pediatric patients by capnogram
- Discuss the principles of operation of impedance pneumography
- Recognize limitations of impedance pneumography
- Understand challenges associated with infant electrocardiograms
- State the objective of indirect calorimetry
- Identify three disadvantages of indirect calorimetry

Cardiorespiratory alterations are the most frequent problems encountered in sick neonatal or pediatric patients. Poor gas exchange and acid–base disturbances are characteristic of pediatric patients with cardiopulmonary failure. Respiratory failure can occur quite suddenly or over a period of time. As a result, continuous monitoring equipment available to caregivers is essential in the clinical setting and can prove to be lifesaving.[1] Noninvasive monitoring provides the bedside clinician with the ability to monitor the patient's cardiopulmonary status continuously. These machines can detect subtle changes in patient condition before the appearance of clinical symptoms. Monitors also have the ability to acquire data and display this information as a trend over several hours, which may lead to improved patient outcomes. Continuous noninvasive monitoring can not only help improve patient outcomes, but is generally more cost-effective than serial laboratory testing. Furthermore, some types of noninvasive monitors are available for home use, enabling the caregiver in the home setting to benefit from this technology as well.

PULSE OXIMETRY

The monitoring of oxygenation in the pediatric patient is critical to patient outcomes. *Hypoxemia* is one of the major causes of morbidity and mortality. *Hyperoxemia* can lead to lung damage and retinopathy of prematurity. Even skilled caregivers cannot always detect hypoxemia when oxygen saturation levels drop below 80%. Pulse oximetry provides a useful means of monitoring oxygenation levels as well as trends in oxygenation. Numerous studies have found pulse oximetry to provide a reasonable degree of accuracy. This, as well as the ease of use of most of the instruments, has led to the widespread use of pulse oximetry for monitoring patients.[2]

Principles of Operation

Oxygen is carried in the blood in two forms: bound and dissolved. Approximately 98% of the oxygen is bound to hemoglobin, and the other 2% is dissolved in the plasma.[3] The hemoglobin binds with oxygen in the pulmonary circulation and then releases oxygen at the tissue level. The relationship between the arterial oxygen bound to hemoglobin, that is, oxygen saturation (SaO_2), and the oxygen dissolved in the plasma (PaO_2) is displayed as the oxyhemoglobin dissociation curve. Pulse oximeters transcutaneously measure the pulsatile arterial oxygen saturation (SpO_2), which is physiologically related to arterial oxygen tension (PaO_2) according to the oxyhemoglobin dissociation curve described above.[2]

A pulse oximeter sensor has two light-emitting diodes (LEDs) that function as light sources and one photodiode

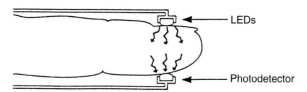

FIGURE 11-1 Proper alignment of light-emitting diodes (LEDs) opposite the photodetector in a sensor applied to a patient's finger.

acting as a light receiver (Figure 11-1). One LED emits red light, and the other diode emits infrared light. As the light from the diodes passes through the blood and tissue, some of the light from both the red and the infrared diodes is absorbed. The photodiode then measures the amount of light that passes through the body without being absorbed. By knowing the amount of light that is entering the body and the amount of light leaving the body, the amount of light absorbed is easily determined. This absorption of both the red and infrared light is used to determine the percentage of functional hemoglobin that is saturated with oxygen (Figure 11-2). To measure arterial blood, the sensor detects pulsatile blood as it enters the tissue. SaO_2 is measured in both nonpulsatile and pulsatile states, and the ratio is corrected to determine functional saturation.

Application

Pulse oximeters are precalibrated. The calibration is built into the instrument's algorithm. Each sensor is calibrated during manufacture. The wavelength of the sensor diodes is checked and then coded into a calibration resistor. The instrument decodes the resistor each time it is turned on, at periodic intervals during use, or when a new sensor is used.

Various sensors are available for different clinical settings. The disposable bandage type for wrapping around a finger or toe is used most often for neonates and infants (Figure 11-3). Application of the sensor is crucial to the quality of readings from the pulse oximeter. The sensor should be placed over a vascular area with the diodes and the photodiode directly opposite each other and in good contact with the skin. The sensors should be placed firmly to avoid falling off or motion artifact, but care should be taken to avoid overtightening and compromising the circulation.[4] The sensor sites should be changed routinely and the monitoring sites assessed for tissue injury. Finger and ear clips are also available for larger patients. Care must be taken with the clip type of sensors because the clinician has no control over the spring tension and the pressure created on the extremity.

Arterial blood gases can be used to diagnose blood oxygenation. The fear and stress involved with an arterial

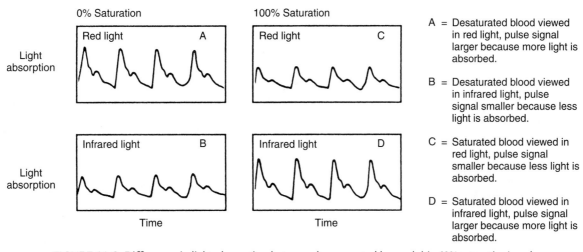

A = Desaturated blood viewed in red light, pulse signal larger because more light is absorbed.

B = Desaturated blood viewed in infrared light, pulse signal smaller because less light is absorbed.

C = Saturated blood viewed in red light, pulse signal smaller because less light is absorbed.

D = Saturated blood viewed in infrared light, pulse signal larger because more light is absorbed.

FIGURE 11-2 Differences in light absorption between deoxygenated hemoglobin (0% saturation) and oxygenated hemoglobin (100% saturation) during pulsatile signals.

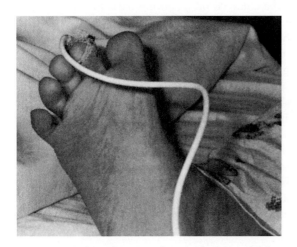

FIGURE 11-3 Pulse oximeter probe attached to a child's toe.

stick can change a patient's breathing pattern, increase agitation, and lead to deterioration in clinical status, particularly in the pediatric population, thus rendering the arterial blood gas useless for diagnosis. Because pulse oximetry is noninvasive and much less of a discomfort to the patient, it has become the standard for assessing hypoxemia in the pediatric population.[5]

Disadvantages

Pulse oximetry was originally developed by anesthesiologists for use in the operating room. In this well-controlled environment the patient is warm, still, and well perfused. As use of the pulse oximeter expanded to other areas of the hospital, the well-controlled environment was lost, and problems with artifacts causing oximetry alarms arose. False alarms occurred more often because patients could be awake and moving and may poorly perfuse. Artifact can occur in two ways. First, if

misinterpreted by the machine as a pulse wave, the artifact can corrupt the measurement and set off an alarm limit. Second, if the artifact obscures the pulse, the "loss of pulse" alarm could be triggered. Patient movement, electrical noise, and rapidly changing ambient light (e.g., fluorescent) can produce artifacts that affect pulse oximeters.[4] In addition, at arterial oxygen saturation levels below 80%, accuracy of the pulse oximeter deteriorates. When using a finger probe, some nail polishes can affect Sao_2 accuracy, causing the value reflected to be falsely low. Acrylic nails do not appear to interfere with pulse oximetry readings.[2] Impaired peripheral perfusion can affect the Spo_2. Conditions such as low cardiac output, vasoconstriction, vasoactive therapy, and hypothermia can all cause the oximetry to have difficulty detecting pulse waves.[6]

Some studies are questioning the correlation of pulse oximeters and arterial blood gases in the neonate.[3] Neonatal patients with hyperbilirubinemia or anemia and those receiving hyperalimentation, total parenteral nutrition (TPN), or inotropic infusions may not yield comparable data between pulse oximeters and arterial blood gases. Even when properly functioning, the pulse oximeter does not provide good information regarding hyperoxia in the neonatal patient. If the oximeter is reading an Sao_2 of 100%, the arterial oxygen tension (Pao_2) could be between 90 and 250 mm Hg. Proper site selection, understanding the principles of operation, and routinely assessing the patient to correlate the Sao_2 with other vital signs will help to minimize these problems and make the pulse oximeter a valuable clinical tool.[7-9]

Newer technology has been developed in an effort to combat difficulties in achieving accurate Spo_2 measurements when less than optimal conditions are present, for example, patient movement and poor tissue perfusion, both prevalent in the neonatal and pediatric populations. Signal Extraction Technology (SET) pulse oximetry combines the traditional method based on red and infrared pulse oximeter signals with advanced techniques allowing signal "noise" produced by venous blood movement during motion to be filtered out, producing more accurate measurements of the arterial oxygenation of patients who are moving or with poor tissue perfusion.[10]

TRANSCUTANEOUS MONITORING

In the hands of an experienced and trained clinician, a well-maintained and properly calibrated transcutaneous monitor will provide accurate information regarding the pediatric patient's oxygenation status.[11] Transcutaneous measurement of Po_2 and carbon dioxide tension (Pco_2) provides continuous information about the body's ability to deliver oxygen to the tissues and to remove carbon dioxide by way of the cardiopulmonary system. An important consideration to bear in mind is that the electrode is actually measuring the gas tension of the underlying tissue, *not* the arterial gas tension. When hemodynamic conditions are stable, transcutaneous measurements correlate well with arterial values, but this correlation does not necessarily mean that the measured values will be identical.

Principles of Operation

Transcutaneous measurements of Po_2 and Pco_2 are based on the principle that a heating element in the sensor elevates the temperature in the underlying tissue. Increasing the skin's temperature increases capillary blood flow to the tissues and makes the skin more permeable to gas diffusion. Because metabolism in the tissue consumes oxygen and produces carbon dioxide, transcutaneous values differ from arterial values.[12] Usually the Po_2 is slightly lower than in the arteries, and the Pco_2 is slightly higher, when measured transcutaneously.

Application

The most critical aspect of transcutaneous monitoring is site selection and the application of the sensor (Figure 11-4). The site should be a highly vascular area such as the upper chest, abdomen, and thighs, or the lower back if the patient is supine. Bony areas over the spine should be avoided. Another consideration when selecting a site is that the right side of the upper chest will give preductal oxygenation values, whereas the left side of the chest and the lower parts of the body will give postductal values.

Selecting a sensor temperature is important to proper operation.[13] The temperature range is usually

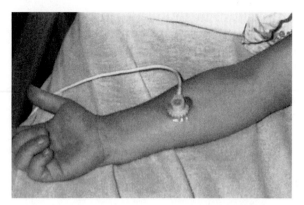

FIGURE 11-4 Transcutaneous oxygen monitor electrode placed on a child's arm.

43° to 44° C, with thicker skin requiring the higher temperature. Heating of the sensor requires that the site be changed on a routine basis to prevent thermal injuries. The frequency of site changes ranges from 3 to 4 hours and can be increased to 2 or 3 hours if the skin at the site has a reaction or if the sensor is operated at higher temperatures.

Meticulously following the manufacturer's membrane-changing procedure and calibration instructions will result in the most accurate readings. Once the machine has been prepared and the site selected, the skin must be cleaned to wipe away dead skin, oils, and medications. The accuracy of the sensor is improved by using 1 or 2 drops of contact gel. This liquid-to-liquid medium makes the diffusion of gases more efficient. The sensor is then attached to the skin with a fixation ring. This ring must seal the ambient air from the sensor and the skin.

Disadvantages

Transcutaneous monitoring provides a noninvasive, simple means of continuously monitoring ventilation. However, it is labor intensive, involving sensor preparation, frequent site and membrane changes, and calibration.[14]

The main physiologic factor relating to good correlation is good peripheral blood perfusion. The skin reacts to cold, shock, and certain drugs by contracting the superficial blood vessels and by opening the larger, deeper lying arterioles to achieve a shunting effect. On exposure to cold, capillary blood flow is stopped to reduce the loss of body heat. Shock and certain cardiopulmonary medications will dilate the blood vessels, causing the blood pressure in the body to drop. In response to this drop in blood pressure, the body will shunt blood from the skin and toward major organs. If the blood flow in the capillary bed is reduced, the capillary blood rapidly becomes more or less venous, with a considerably lower Po_2 and higher Pco_2. Therefore, in patients with impaired peripheral blood perfusion, large deviations may occur between central Po_2/Pco_2 and the transcutaneous values.[15] If a patient has poor skin integrity, transcutaneous monitoring may also be contraindicated.

New Technology

For newborns, noninvasive methods available to measure oxygen saturation and arterial carbon dioxide partial pressure are helpful in quickly detecting respiratory deterioration. Frequently repeated blood gas draws can be decreased, reducing blood loss and other potential complications associated with invasive procedures.

New technology has been introduced that combines arterial oxygen saturation (Sao_2) and transcutaneous carbon dioxide ($Pcco_2$) measurements in a single ear sensor. The sensor is heated to 42° C to produce localized hyperanemia, which maximizes capillary blood flow. The location of the sensor on the ear could mean a decrease in motion artifact because less head movement occurs in neonates. This type of sensor reduces the number of wires attached to the patient and the sensor would not have to be removed for chest X-rays.[14] When the $ETco_2$ (the end-tidal carbon dioxide partial pressure in exhaled gases) is unreliable, that is, newborns with large air leaks or with continuous positive airway pressure, this ear sensor could also be beneficial.[16] Combined Spo_2 and $Pcco_2$ ear sensors appear to be promising, given the benefit of quickly and reliably monitoring patient's oxygenation and ventilation status with a single, noninvasive probe.[17]

CAPNOMETRY

Measurement of oxygenation saturation with a pulse oximeter has revolutionized the assessment of oxygenation in patients with respiratory failure. Techniques are also available to assess ventilatory status by measuring carbon dioxide from exhaled breaths in a noninvasive manner. Known as *capnometry*, this technique is especially useful in pediatric settings, because of the large number of this population having respiratory disorders.

Principles of Operation

The most common methods used to continuously measure carbon dioxide concentration in an exhaled gas employ infrared spectrometry and mass spectrometry. Infrared spectrometry operates under the concept that carbon dioxide is strongly absorbed by infrared light. Mass spectrometry involves an electronic beam that ionizes gases. The resulting particles are then deflected emitting a specific wavelength by which the concentration of the gas can be determined. Infrared spectrometry allows for real-time, continuous measurement and display of Pco_2 with a delay time of about 0.25 second. Mass spectrometry is also accurate but has a delay time of 0.1 to 80 seconds, it is expensive, and not as portable.[18]

Gases from an exhaled breath can reach the sample chamber in one of two ways. Mainstream capnographs are used in ventilated patients, with placement at the proximal end of an endotracheal tube (Figure 11-5). This method generally employs infrared spectrometers. Caution must be taken because the analyzer can be a heavy addition to an infant or pediatric circuit

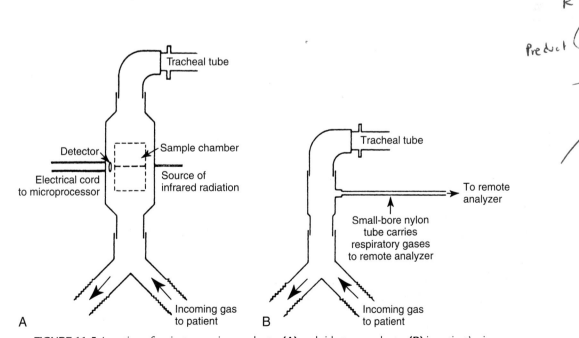

FIGURE 11-5 Location of mainstream airway adapter **(A)** and sidestream adapter **(B)** in patient's airway.

and can cause kinking or disconnection of the endotracheal tube. Sidestream analyzers continuously aspirate a sample of gas through a small tube to the analyzer. This method is used primarily with mass spectrometry and some infrared analyzers. It is advantageous in that it does not add much weight to the breathing circuit. However, the narrow tubing can become occluded with mucus or water, causing inaccuracies. In addition, infants with small tidal volumes can contaminate the sample line with fresh gases.[6]

Interpretation of Capnogram

Trending $ETco_2$ will give the bedside clinician a good sense of the adequacy of ventilation for the patient. An increase in $ETco_2$ from previous levels might indicate hypoventilation. The possibility of decreased tidal volume or respiratory rate should be investigated. A decrease in $ETco_2$ from previous levels might indicate hyperventilation. Interpretation of the capnogram (waveform display of the exhaled carbon dioxide) can also help the clinician detect other ventilatory abnormalities.

The normal capnogram can be divided into four phases (Figure 11-6):

Phase A-B: The inspiratory phase, during which the sensor detects no carbon dioxide

Phase B-C: The initial expiratory phase, during which carbon dioxide rapidly increases as the alveoli begin to empty

Phase C-D: The completion of expiration as the alveoli empty (alveolar plateau) and shows a slight increase in carbon dioxide

Phase D-E: The beginning of inspiration as the waveform returns to zero

Detection of Ventilation Problems

The clinician can use the capnogram to detect important ventilation problems in neonatal and pediatric patients.

Endotracheal Tube in Esophagus

A normal capnogram provides evidence that the endotracheal tube is in the proper position and that alveolar ventilation is occurring. When the endotracheal tube is placed incorrectly in the esophagus, no carbon dioxide will be detected, or only small transient capnograms will be present.

Rebreathing

Rebreathing is characterized by an elevation in the A-B phase of the capnogram, with a corresponding increase in $ETco_2$. It indicates the rebreathing of previously exhaled carbon dioxide. Rebreathing can be caused by allowing an insufficient expiratory time or by inadequate inspiratory flow (Figure 11-7).

Obstructed Airway

Obstruction of the expiratory flow of gas will be noted as a change in the slope of the B-C phase of the capnogram. The B-C phase may diminish without a plateau. Obstruction can be caused by a foreign body in the upper airway, increased secretions in the airways, the patient having bronchospasms, or partial obstruction of the ventilator circuit (Figure 11-8).

Paralyzed Patients

Patients who are paralyzed and receiving mechanical ventilation may develop a cleft in the C-D phase of the capnogram. The cleft may indicate a return in diaphragmatic activity and the need for additional paralytic agents (Figure 11-9).

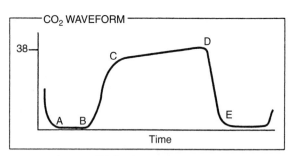

A–B:	Exhalation of CO_2 free gas from dead space.
B–C:	Combination of dead space and alveolar gas.
C–D:	Exhalation of mostly alveolar gas (alveolar plateau).
D:	"End-tidal" point—CO_2 exhalation at maximum point.
D–E:	Inhalation of CO_2 free gas.

FIGURE 11-6 Normal capnogram.

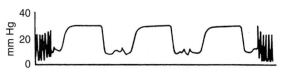

FIGURE 11-7 Effect of rebreathing carbon dioxide on the capnogram. Note that the inspiratory level does not return to zero.

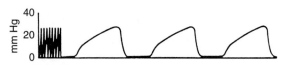

FIGURE 11-8 Capnogram with sloping alveolar plateau representative of airway obstruction.

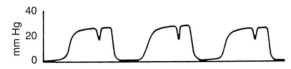

FIGURE 11-9 Curare cleft in the alveolar plateau.

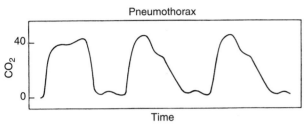

FIGURE 11-10 Stair effect on the descending limb of the capnogram indicating a potential pneumothorax.

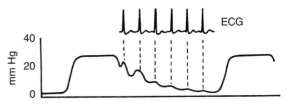

FIGURE 11-11 Cardiogenic oscillations in synchrony with the ECG signal.

Pneumothorax

A stair-stepping of the D-E phase of the capnogram, caused by unequal and incomplete emptying of the lungs, and a failure to return to baseline may suggest a pneumothorax (Figure 11-10).

Cardiogenic Oscillations

Cardiogenic oscillations may be seen in patients with long expiratory times and slow respiratory rates. The oscillations will be seen in the D-E phase of the capnogram and are caused as the heart contracts and moves the lungs, causing gas flow (Figure 11-11).

IMPEDANCE PNEUMOGRAPHY

Measuring the respiratory rate and assessing the breathing patterns are critical to the care of neonatal and pediatric patients, especially those susceptible to apnea. The incidence and number of apneic events or fluctuations in respiratory condition may suggest a changing respiratory status or alterations in central nervous system function. Rate counts—by observation, by placing a hand on the patient, or by auscultation—may be grossly inaccurate because of the time required for the measurement as well as the result of tactile stimulation, which may alter breathing patterns.

Advances in technology have resulted in increased survival rates of more and more premature infants. Oftentimes, these patients are being discharged home, and as a result of potential apneic episodes, have the need to be monitored. Impedance pneumography provides an easy-to-perform continuous, noninvasive monitoring of respiration. One set of electrodes for both electrocardiographic and respiratory monitoring makes the application simple. Keep in mind that the monitor functions only as a warning device that sounds when breathing or heart rate (or both) is outside the set alarm limits. The monitor will not prevent any abnormal episodes from occurring.

Principles of Operation

Impedance pneumography is based on the principle of transthoracic impedance combined with electrocardiogram (ECG) monitoring. The monitor passes an electric current between two standard ECG electrodes placed on the patient's chest along the midaxillary line. Thoracic impedance can then be calculated. Impedance is a function of the distance between electrodes, which increases with inspiration and decreases during expiration. The electric current will change as the chest expands and contracts. The monitor interprets these data and, via an algorithm, calculates a respiratory rate. This value is displayed on the monitor.[19]

Application

The patient's chest should be washed to remove all soap, oil, powder, and lotion before the electrode pads are applied. The electrode pads are secured by a foam belt placed under the patient's back and wrapped around the patient's chest, with the top of the belt usually at the patient's nipple line and held snugly with adhesive strips (Figure 11-12). The electrode pads are placed under each armpit, with the wires directed down toward the lower ribs. Correctly sized and placed electrodes are critical to obtaining a reliable signal. The belt should be snug, but with enough room to allow one finger to slide under it after it is closed. The electrode pads are connected to the monitor via lead wires. These wires carry the electric signals back to the monitor through a patient cable. The monitors have an alarm system that warns of problems with both the patient and the equipment.

The monitor is generally portable and relatively small, having high and low alarm limits for apnea and heart rate. The monitor is powered by electricity, with some having a battery source available.[18] Monitors can detect slow, fast, or absent respiratory and heart rate in the neonatal or pediatric patient. Most monitors can detect equipment problems involving the battery functions, lead wire, electrode pad, patient cable, and monitor.

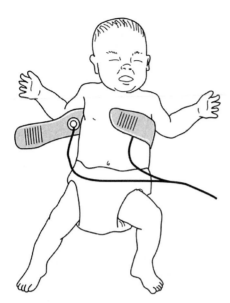

FIGURE 11-12 Neonatal impedance pneumography. With the infant on a flat surface, the belt is positioned in line with the nipples. After the electrodes are placed, the belt is wrapped snugly around the infant's chest.

An event log should be placed near the monitor if an impedance pneumograph is used in a home care situation. Events logged may include alarms sounded, changes in the monitor controls and alarm settings, and times when the monitor is turned on and off.

Disadvantages

Changes in body position or postural changes can cause the results of impedance pneumography to be erroneous. The monitor may also incorrectly detect cardiogenic oscillations as respiration and cause an incorrect interpretation of the respiratory rate. Obstructive apneas cannot be determined by impedance pneumography because the monitor bases respirations on changes in thoracic impedance. Respiratory rates may be displayed on the monitor, but are not indicative of the patient's effectiveness of ventilation. The caregiver must also be mindful when placing leads. If the leads are too near the abdomen, the monitor could incorrectly read interference from the abdomen as a respiration. If the leads are placed too high, the monitor may miss abdominal movements used in respiration and cause a false apnea alarm to sound. Because of the frequency of false alarms, newer documentation-type monitors have been developed. The newer generation monitors not only record the apnea event, but events before and after the apnea episode as well. This information can include changes in heart rate and oxygen saturation levels. New versions of the impedance pneumography monitors can also store data such as ECG and respiratory effort waveforms, oxygen saturations,

and trends in heart rate that can be downloaded to a computer for interpretation.[18]

ELECTROCARDIOGRAPHY

The ECG is a recording of body surface electric potentials generated by the heart. It is easy to perform and noninvasive and has been used for many years to provide important information about cardiac anatomy and pathology.

In the intensive care unit the primary reasons for continuous monitoring of the ECG are to ensure an adequate heart rate and to sound an alarm if the heart rate drops below a set limit. To detect and record the electric potential created by the heart's activity, electrodes are attached to the patient on the left arm, right arm, and left leg for typical six-lead intensive care monitoring. Careful attention should be paid to electrode placement on infants and small children; pediatric-sized electrodes should be used to guarantee recording from the proper area without overlapping the electrodes.

The quality of ECG recordings can be influenced by a number of technical problems that lead to artifact. Common sources are patient movement, shaking due to tremulousness, and interference from another electric source causing a fuzzy baseline.

Infant electrocardiographs present extra challenges caused by rapidly changing hemodynamics. A full-term infant will have a different ECG than a premature baby (34 wk of gestation or less). In addition, the ECG of a normal infant will undergo rapid changes during the baby's first few weeks of life. Not until a child is approximately 3 years of age will the ECG start to resemble that of an adult, although still with considerable differences.[20]

CALORIMETRY

Ensuring that nutritional requirements are correctly met for critically ill neonatal and pediatric patients can be a daunting task. A neonate's energy expenditure, when expressed per unit of body weight, is higher than at any other time in life.[21] By correctly assessing nutritional needs and tracking adequate nutritional intake, complications can potentially be avoided. Determining a patient's resting energy expenditure (REE) helps reduce overfeeding and underfeeding. Formulas are available to predict the REE of neonatal, pediatric, and adult patients. However, measuring the REE by a process known as calorimetry has been shown to be more accurate than published formulas.[23] Two methods exist for measuring calorimetry: direct and indirect. *Direct calorimetry* directly measures heat produced and lost from the body. *Indirect calorimetry* measures oxygen consumption and carbon dioxide production. From the rate of oxygen consumed and carbon dioxide produced, the clinician can calculate the corresponding energy expenditure.[22]

Principles of Operation

The indirect calorimeters most often used are open-circuit systems. The patient inspires room air, and the expired air is then collected and analyzed for oxygen and carbon dioxide content. Normally, room air contains 20.93% oxygen and 0.003% carbon dioxide. The difference in oxygen and carbon dioxide partial pressures of the control (inspired air) and the sample (expired air) is assumed to be the result of the patient's metabolism, that is, the patient's consumption of oxygen and production of carbon dioxide. Newer systems are computerized and can perform the calculations quickly.

Disadvantages

Direct calorimetry is cost prohibitive, equilibration and measurement are time consuming, and few exist in the United States. Indirect calorimetry is not without its limitations: expense, requirement for trained personnel, and the potential for significant errors at higher inspired oxygen concentrations. Unstable hemodynamic conditions and agitation may also preclude the use of indirect calorimetry.[24] In addition, a particular problem with the neonatal (and some pediatric) populations is that uncuffed endotracheal tubes are generally used for these patients receiving mechanical ventilation. Leakage around the tube can result in false REE values.[22] Understanding and weighing the advantages and limitations of indirect calorimetry can help to decide whether indirect calorimetry is a valid clinical tool to aid the clinician in determining proper nutritional support of the critically ill neonatal or pediatric patient.

ASSESSMENT QUESTIONS

See Evolve Resources for answers.

1. Which of the following demonstrates *incorrect* application of the pulse oximeter sensor?
   A. Tight placement over a bony area
   B. Placement over a vascular area
   C. Diodes and photodiode directly opposite each other and in good contact with the skin
   D. Firm placement to help avoid motion artifact
2. The following choices are all disadvantages of a pulse oximeter *except:*
   A. Ease of use
   B. Artifact
   C. Poor tissue perfusion
   D. Hypothermia

ASSESSMENT QUESTIONS—cont'd

3. Which of the following measurements is obtained via transcutaneous monitoring in the neonatal and pediatric population?
   A. P_{O_2}, P_{CO_2}
   B. Hemoglobin
   C. pH, bicarbonate ion
   D. Oxygen saturation
4. The following are all important aspects to consider when choosing transcutaneous monitoring *except:*
   A. Application and site selection of the sensor
   B. Selection of proper sensor temperature
   C. The patient's weight, age, and sex
   D. Correct procedure when changing the membrane and calibrating
5. The following choices are all disadvantages of transcutaneous monitoring *except:*
   A. Use is labor intensive because of required frequent site and membrane changes and calibration requirements.
   B. Good correlation requires good peripheral blood perfusion.
   C. Use requires the patient to be paralyzed and sedated.
6. Trending ET_{CO_2} via capnometry enables the clinician to have a good sense of the adequacy of _____ for the patient.
   A. Oxygenation
   B. Ventilation
   C. Perfusion
   D. Saturation
7. The normal capnogram can be divided into four phases. Phase B-C, as illustrated below, is indicative of which phase?
   A. The completion of expiration as the alveoli empty (alveolar plateau)
   B. The initial expiratory phase, during which carbon dioxide rapidly increases as the alveoli begin to empty

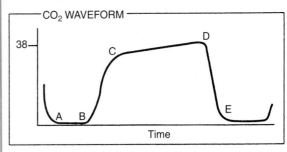

C. The inspiratory phase, during which the sensor detects no carbon dioxide
D. The beginning of inspiration as the waveform returns to zero

Continued

ASSESSMENT QUESTIONS—cont'd

8. A cleft in phase C-D of the capnogram in the figure accompanying question 7 may indicate:
   A. An obstruction in the airway, possibly caused by a foreign body in the upper airway, increased secretions in the airways, bronchospasms, or partial obstruction of the ventilator circuit
   B. Medication used to paralyze the infant is wearing off.
   C. Pneumothorax
   D. Rebreathing of the previously exhaled carbon dioxide
9. Impedance pneumography is an important tool used for neonatal and pediatric patients who:
   A. Are susceptible to apnea
   B. Require evaluation of arrhythmias
   C. Are experiencing recurring fevers of unknown origin
   D. Are having an asthma attack
10. Limitations of impedance pneumography include all the following *except:*
   A. Sensitivity to body movement and postural changes causing false alarms.
   B. Cardiogenic oscillations may be detected as respirations.
   C. Measurement of changes in chest wall configuration does not allow for measurement of the effectiveness of ventilation.
   D. The sensor temperature must be maintained between 43° and 44° C.

References

1. Folke M et al: Critical review of non-invasive respiratory monitoring in medical care, *Med Biol Eng Comput* 2003;41:377.
2. Jubran A: Pulse oximetry, *Critical Care* 1999;3:R11.
3. Gibson LY: Pulse oximeter in the neonatal ICU: a correlational analysis, *Pediatr Nurs* 1996;22:511.
4. Barker SJ, Shah NK: The effects of motion on the performance of pulse oximeters in volunteers, *Anesthesiology* 1997;86:101.
5. Pulse Oximetry FORUM: The FORUM offers recommendations on best practices in pediatric pulse oximetry, *AARC Times* 2000;April:36.
6. Soubani AO: Noninvasive monitoring of oxygen and carbon dioxide, *Am J Emerg Med* 2001;19:141.
7. Wipperman CF et al: Continuous measurement of cardiac output by the Fick principle in infants and children: comparison with the thermodilution method, *Intensive Care Med* 1996;22:467.
8. Tallon RW: Oximetry: state of the art, *Nurs Manage* 1996;27:43.
9. Trivedi NS et al: Pulse oximeter performance during desaturation and resaturation: a comparison of seven models, *J Clin Anesth* 1997;9:184.
10. Goldman JM et al: Masimo signal extraction pulse oximetry, *J Clin Monit Comput* 2000;16:475.
11. Lewer BMF et al: Accuracy of transcutaneous carbon dioxide measurement, *Can J Anaesth* 1998;45:186.
12. Carter B et al: A comparison of two transcutaneous monitors for the measurement of arterial Po_2 and Pco_2 in neonates, *Anaesth Intensive Care* 1995;23:708.
13. Talbot A et al: Dynamic model of oxygen transport for transcutaneous Po_2 analysis, *Ann Biomed Eng* 1996;24:294.
14. Bernet-Buettiker V et al: Evaluation of a new combined transcutaneous measurement of Pco_2/pulse oximetry oxygen saturation ear sensor in newborn patients, *Pediatrics* 2005;115:e64.
15. Tobias JD, Meyer DJ: Noninvasive monitoring of carbon dioxide during respiratory failure in toddlers and infants: end-tidal versus transcutaneous carbon dioxide, *Anesth Analg* 1997;85:55.
16. Dullenkopf A et al: Evaluation of a new combined Spo_2/$Ptcco_2$ sensor in anaesthetized paediatric patients, *Paediatr Anaesth* 2003;13:777.
17. Kocher S, Rohling R, Tschupp A: Performance of a digital PCO_2/SpO_2 ear sensor, *J Clin Monit Comput* 2004;18:75.
18. Stock C. Nonivasive carbon dioxide monitoring. *Crit Care Clin* 1988;4:511.
19. Sittig SE: Transitional technology from NICU to home, *AARC Times* 2000;September:37.
20. Tipple M: Interpretation of electrocardiograms in infants and children, *Images Paediatr Cardiol* 1999;1:3.
21. Pencharz P: A new approach to measure energy expenditure in the neonate, *Pediatr Res* 2000;47:707.
22. Flancbaum L et al: Comparison of indirect calorimetry, the Fick method, and prediction equations in estimating the energy requirements of critically ill patients, *Am J Clin Nutr* 1999;69:461.
23. Coss-Bu JA et al: Resting energy expenditure in children in a pediatric intensive care unit: comparison of Harris-Benedict and Talbot predictions with indirect calorimetry values, *Am J Clin Nutr* 1998;67:74.
24. O'Leary-Kelley CM et al: Nutritional adequacy in patients receiving mechanical ventilation who are fed enterally, *Am J Crit Care* 2005;14:222.

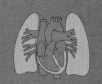

Chapter **12**

Oxygen Administration

SHERRY L. BARNHART

OUTLINE

Indications
    Documented or Suspected Hypoxemia
    Evidence of Hypoxemia
Complications
Oxygen Administration

Variable-performance Oxygen Delivery Systems
Fixed-performance Oxygen Delivery Systems
Enclosures
Manual Resuscitation Systems

LEARNING OBJECTIVES

After reading this chapter the reader will be able to:
- Discuss causes, clinical signs and symptoms, and evidence of hypoxemia
- Identify adverse physiologic effects and equipment-related complications associated with oxygen administration to neonates, infants, and children
- Differentiate between variable-performance and fixed-performance oxygen delivery systems and provide examples of each

- Discuss the indications and contraindications for use of oxygen delivery devices in the neonatal and pediatric populations
- Describe the methods used to apply devices to deliver oxygen to neonates, infants, and children
- Compare and contrast self-inflating and non–self-inflating resuscitation systems

In 1774, Joseph Priestley was credited with discovering the colorless, odorless, tasteless gas that Antoine Lavoisier 1 year later named *oxygen*.[1] Nearly 150 years would pass before the Finnish pediatrician Arvo Ylppö recommended the intragastric administration of this gas to infants.[2] It was not until 1934 that Dr. Julius Hess, chief of pediatrics at the Michael Reese Hospital in Chicago, created the first inhaled oxygen delivery device for a premature infant. His "oxygen box," which consisted of a metal hood with a small window, was the first

oxygen chamber used within an incubator.[3] Although the device was criticized both for making it difficult to view the infant and for its inability to maintain high oxygen concentrations, it led the way in the development of oxygen administration devices for premature infants and children.[4] Further development and use of these delivery devices has resulted in significant health care benefits including a reduction in mortality. Today the administration of oxygen by inhalation continues to play an essential role in the survival of infants and children.

The goal of oxygen administration is to achieve adequate tissue oxygenation. The system used to provide supplemental oxygen must be appropriate to the patient's size, gestational and postnatal age, and clinical condition. Selection of the oxygen delivery device and flow rate is targeted to meet the specific physiologic needs and therapeutic goals of each patient.[5] Unfortunately, adverse reactions from the therapeutic use of oxygen are well documented in neonatal and pediatric patients. Therefore it is imperative that oxygen therapy be provided at accurate and safe levels with the lowest fractional concentration of inspired oxygen (FIO_2) possible.

INDICATIONS

Documented or Suspected Hypoxemia

A need to correct hypoxemia (low oxygen content in the blood) is the most common indication for oxygen therapy.[6] Left untreated, hypoxemia progresses to hypoxia (low tissue oxygen) and possibly anoxia (absent tissue oxygen), which if severe enough, leads to metabolic abnormalities and the development of acidosis.

Hypoxemia occurs as a result of decreased alveolar ventilation, decreased inspired oxygen, poor ventilation–perfusion relationships, intrapulmonary or cardiac shunting, diffusion defects, or short red blood cell transit times. In conditions such as anemia or carbon monoxide poisoning, the oxygen-carrying capacity of the blood is reduced despite the presence of normal arterial oxygen tension (PaO_2). Bradycardia, cardiac failure, hypotension, and hypothermia leave the circulatory system unable to provide adequate tissue oxygen. In rare cases, such as cyanide poisoning, the tissue is unable to accept and use oxygen, despite adequate oxygen delivery.[7] The documentation of hypoxemia through arterial blood gas sampling or pulse oximetry provides the most definitive evidence of actual or impending tissue hypoxia.

Administration of oxygen is also appropriate if hypoxia is strongly suspected on clinical grounds. However, substantiation of either the PaO_2 or the percentage of oxygen saturation (SpO_2) is required within an appropriate period after administration.[6,7] In emergency situations, such as severe respiratory distress, shock, or cardiopulmonary arrest, oxygen therapy is never withheld even if laboratory test results are unavailable.

Evidence of Hypoxemia
Measurement of Oxygen Tension and Saturation

In the child, a PaO_2 less than 80 mm Hg and an SpO_2 less than 95% usually indicate hypoxemia. Because fetal hemoglobin has a much greater affinity for oxygen, the oxygen dissociation curve is shifted to the left, allowing a higher saturation for any given PaO_2. The normal immediate postnatal PaO_2 of 60 mm Hg corresponds closely with an SpO_2 of 90%. For this reason, it is generally agreed that a PaO_2 less than 60 mm Hg and an SpO_2 less than 90% in the newborn indicate hypoxemia and necessitate initiation of oxygen therapy. The PaO_2 and the SpO_2 are the principal clinical indicators used to begin, monitor, adjust, and terminate oxygen administration.

Clinical Signs and Symptoms

In the infant and child the earliest clinical manifestations of hypoxia are tachycardia and tachypnea. Worsening hypoxia results in decreased ventilation, apnea, and bradycardia. This is especially true in both the neonate and the term infant. Other physical signs of hypoxia include grunting, nasal flaring, retractions, paradoxical breathing, cyanosis, irritability, and increased restlessness.[8] Often the neonate or infant becomes lethargic and flaccid, with arms and legs extended in a "frog leg" position.

The presence of cyanosis has often been used to determine inadequate oxygenation. Although this clinical sign is somewhat useful in the pediatric and adult patient, its presence in infants is often a late sign of severe hypoxia. Peripheral cyanosis (acrocyanosis) is the bluish discoloration of the skin or extremities. It occurs when a decrease in body temperature results in poor peripheral circulation or vasoconstriction. Central cyanosis involves the warm and well-perfused areas of the tongue and mucous membranes. It does not occur until reduced hemoglobin reaches 4 to 6 g/dl in arterial blood. In the child and adult the reduced hemoglobin concentration at which cyanosis occurs corresponds to a PaO_2 of approximately 50 to 60 mm Hg and an SpO_2 of 85% to 90%. In the infant, the stronger affinity of fetal hemoglobin for oxygen results in the PaO_2 falling to a significantly lower level before reduced hemoglobin is present at 5 g/dl in arterial blood. In fact, by the time central cyanosis is present in the infant, oxygen delivery to the tissues is grossly insufficient. For this reason central cyanosis is considered an unreliable indicator of the degree of tissue hypoxia. The clinical impression of cyanosis in the infant must be confirmed by arterial blood gas analysis or pulse oximetry.

COMPLICATIONS

Complications of therapeutic oxygen administration are separated into two categories: adverse physiologic effects and equipment-related complications. Adverse reactions that result directly from using a specific oxygen delivery device are discussed in later sections describing that device. Although potential risks are present whenever oxygen is administered, the consequences of hypoxia are more severe.

In certain chronic lung disorders, including cystic fibrosis and bronchopulmonary dysplasia, the normal response to ventilation is blunted because of chronic carbon dioxide retention. Abrupt and excessive increases in supplemental oxygen decrease the respiratory drive and result in *hypoventilation* and respiratory acidosis that may lead to respiratory arrest.[9] The goal of oxygen therapy in patients with this degree of chronic lung disease is to correct the hypoxemia without decreasing the pH. Supplemental oxygen should be initiated at a low F_{IO_2} and increased on the basis of the results of Pa_{O_2} or Sp_{O_2} monitoring.

The role of oxygen in the development of retinopathy of prematurity (ROP) is controversial. It is believed to cause constriction of retinal and cerebral vessels in neonates and infants, which can lead to ischemia, varying degrees of retinal scarring, and retinal detachment. Formerly referred to as "retrolental fibroplasia," ROP may resolve spontaneously or result in permanent visual impairment, including blindness. In the 1940s and 1950s when oxygen was administered to premature infants without blood gas monitoring, ROP reached epidemic proportions.[10,11] Many other factors, in addition to oxygen, appear to correlate with the development of ROP, including gestational age, intraventricular hemorrhage, sepsis, and low birth weight.[12] Evidence now exists that supports targeting Sp_{O_2} levels at 89% to 90% and maintaining a Pa_{O_2} value of 50 to 80 mm Hg in infants weighing less than 1500 g. Studies that have examined the relationship between hospital policies concerning Sp_{O_2} limits, and the survival and ophthalmic and developmental outcome of premature infants who have received supplemental oxygen, have concluded that vigilance concerning oxygen management, without adversely affecting death and disability, was in some part responsible for the current decline in severe ROP.[13-16] But despite the knowledge that hyperoxia (high levels of oxygen in the blood) can be detrimental to the premature infant, there remains a challenge in establishing limits for the rational use of supplemental oxygen in the extremely premature infant. The optimal range of oxygenation that can balance the risks of mortality, ROP blindness, chronic lung disease, and brain damage continues to be studied.[17]

High concentrations of oxygen have been linked to atelectasis, pulmonary vasodilation, and pulmonary fibrosis. In the face of high oxygen levels, the alveolar oxygen tension (Pa_{O_2}) may increase and the alveolar nitrogen decrease, resulting in absorption atelectasis. As the nitrogen is replaced by oxygen, the blood rapidly absorbs the oxygen, gas volume decreases, and atelectasis develops. High F_{IO_2} levels may also result in pulmonary vasodilation. As the pulmonary vasculature dilates and alveolar volumes decrease, areas of ventilation–perfusion mismatch occur with increased intrapulmonary shunting and worsening of arterial oxygen delivery. In patients with a hypoplastic left ventricle or a single ventricle, the increased Pa_{O_2} that occurs with oxygen therapy has been reported to compromise the balance between pulmonary and systemic blood flow.[18] There are also reports of pulmonary fibrosis occurring after oxygen administration to patients with Paraquat poisoning and to those receiving the chemotherapeutic agent bleomycin.[19,20]

OXYGEN ADMINISTRATION

Many of the devices used to deliver supplemental oxygen to neonatal and pediatric patients are simply smaller versions of the adult devices. They are similarly classified in the same manner as either variable-performance oxygen delivery systems (low-flow and reservoir systems) or fixed-performance oxygen delivery systems (high-flow systems).[5]

Variable-performance oxygen delivery systems include devices that are not capable of meeting the patient's inspiratory demand and therefore provide a fractional concentration of delivered oxygen ($F_{D_{O_2}}$) that varies with the patient's rate and depth of ventilation and the flow rate of the gas. These devices include low-flow nasal cannulas, nasopharyngeal catheters, tracheostomy oxygen adapters, simple oxygen masks, partial-rebreathing masks, and nonrebreathing masks.

Fixed-performance oxygen delivery systems include devices that can meet or exceed the patient's inspiratory demand and thereby provide an accurate $F_{D_{O_2}}$ that is not affected by changes in the ventilatory pattern. These devices include high-flow nasal cannulas, air-entrainment masks, air-entrainment nebulizer systems, and oxygen blender systems. The last category of oxygen delivery devices includes enclosure systems that provide some means of controlling oxygen concentration, temperature, and humidity. These devices include oxygen hoods, oxygen tents, and closed incubators.[5]

Variable-performance Oxygen Delivery Systems
Nasopharyngeal Catheter

The nasopharyngeal catheter is a soft plastic tube with several holes at its distal tip. Oxygen flows from the catheter into the patient's oropharynx, which acts as an anatomic reservoir. The nasopharyngeal catheter comes in a variety of sizes, with the smallest size having an 8-French outer diameter. Flow rates from 0.25 to 1 L/minute on 100% oxygen provide a variable F_{IO_2} of approximately 0.24 to 0.35, depending on the patient's inspiratory flow rate.[5,21,22] However, with the increase in variety of nasal cannula sizes available as well as the nasal cannula fixation devices, selection of a nasopharyngeal catheter to deliver oxygen to a child is rarely indicated today and is not appropriate for oxygen administration in the neonatal population.[5]

Indications and Contraindications. Because the catheter can be firmly secured in position, it does not impose a barrier between the infant and caregivers. Feeding, bathing, and other activities are accomplished without interrupting oxygen delivery. Infants can be placed in a sitting position and can roll over, reach for objects, and even crawl while oxygen delivery is maintained. Catheters are not used in patients with maxillofacial trauma, nasal obstruction such as choanal atresia and nasal polyps, and existing or suspected basilar skull fracture.[5,23] Catheter use may be limited by excessive mucus drainage, mucosal edema, or a deviated septum.[24]

Application. After the tip is lubricated with a sterile, water-soluble material, insert the catheter through the patient's nose into the oropharynx. Determine the proper distance to insert the catheter by gently advancing the catheter until the tip rests slightly above the uvula or by inserting the catheter to a depth equal to the distance from the ala nasi (tip of the nose) to the tragus (earlobe).[22,24] Take care during insertion so that nasal turbinates are not damaged and excessive nasal bleeding does not occur. After verifying the correct position of the catheter, tape the catheter to the patient's face. Using small-bore oxygen supply tubing, connect the catheter to a bubble humidifier and low-flow flowmeter (less than 3 L/min). An 8-French catheter may be too large for the premature or very small infant. In this case, insert a 5-French feeding tube in the same manner, and connect it to the small-bore oxygen supply tubing. However, the smaller 5-French feeding tube is less effective in oxygen delivery than the 8-French catheter.[22]

Hazards and Complications. Major problems associated with nasopharyngeal catheters involve the insertion and removal process, correct catheter positioning, and obstruction of the catheter end. Nasal trauma and bleeding may occur if the catheter is forced into small or obstructed nasal passages. If the catheter is not secured properly and slips past the oropharynx, gagging may occur and lead to vomiting and aspiration.[24] Excessive flow can produce pain in the frontal sinuses as well as gastric distention and impaired diaphragm movement.[22]

Pneumocephalus is also a rare but possible complication.[25] The catheter can become blocked with mucus or blood, obstructing the flow of oxygen to the patient. Accumulation of mucus can also result in upper airway obstruction.[26] For this reason, frequently clear the catheter to prevent occlusion of the distal holes. Observe the patient for evidence of catheter occlusion, and alternate the catheter between nares every 8 to 12 hours, replacing it every 24 hours.[21,27,28] Effective humidification is necessary to prevent drying of the pharyngeal mucosa and to reduce the accumulation of mucus.[29] If an infant receiving oxygen by nasopharyngeal catheter becomes cyanotic and agitated, shows a decrease in food intake, or if there is a profound change in the ventilatory pattern, remove the catheter and initiate an alternative method of oxygen delivery.

Nasal Cannula

The nasal cannula consists of flexible small-bore tubing ending in two soft prongs that are about 1 cm in length (Figure 12-1). Oxygen flows from the cannula into the patient's nasopharynx, which acts as an anatomic reservoir. For many years, the cannula was used only in pediatric and adult patients. It was not until the 1980s that it was proposed for use in infants as well.[30] Today its ease of administration makes it the preferred and most commonly used device for oxygen delivery to neonates, infants, and children. As with the nasopharyngeal catheter, the cannula is designed to provide low oxygen concentrations from approximately 24% to 45%, with the F_{IO_2} varying with the patient's inspiratory flow.[31,32]

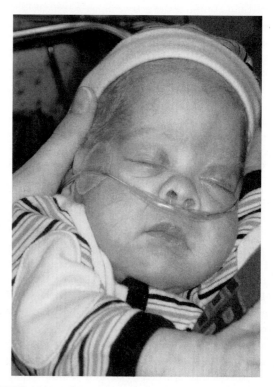

FIGURE 12-1 Infant with a neonatal nasal cannula.

Indications and Contraindications. Caregivers are able to feed and provide for the patient without interrupting the delivery of oxygen. When compared with an oxygen hood, the nasal cannula allows the patient greater mobility, which may increase interactions with the patient's caregivers and environment.[33] Nasal cannulas are contraindicated in patients with nasal obstruction, such as facial trauma and choanal atresia.[5]

Application. Select the appropriate size cannula and insert the prongs into the patient's nares, making sure that the nares are not completely occluded. Wrap the lightweight tubing around the ears, and hold it under the chin with an adjustable plastic notch. In the very small or active infant, secure the cannula to the face to prevent dislodgment, and position the tubing past the ears, securing it behind the head, instead of under the chin, to prevent airway obstruction. Oxygen is delivered from a flowmeter and bubble humidifier through the small-bore oxygen tubing.

When adhesive tape is used to secure the cannula to the fragile skin of the neonatal patient, epidermal stripping can result each time the tape is moved to readjust the tubing. Skin irritation can also occur from a local allergic reaction to polyvinyl chloride.[5] Popular alternatives to using adhesive tape or stoma adhesive are the NeoHold cannula/tubing holder (Neotech Products, Valencia, CA) (Figure 12-2) and the Tender Grip skin fixation system (Salter Labs, Arvin, CA) (Figure 12-3). These commercially available devices consist of a latex-free base with an adhesive backing of tinted microporous tape that is applied to the skin, usually on the patient's cheek. On top of this base is a clear tab with an adhesive backing. The tab folds over the cannula tubing and secures the cannula in place (cannula lies between the base and the tab). To reposition the cannula simply peel back the tab, adjust the tubing, and reapply the tab. The microporous tape allows the skin to breathe and

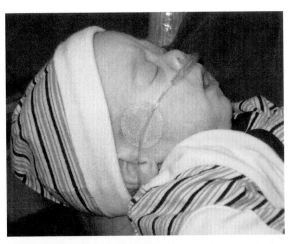

FIGURE 12-3 Tender Grip skin fixation pad. A round base of microporous tape is applied to the infant's skin. The flap on top of the base is designed to position and secure the tubing in place.

the tab makes it easy to adjust the cannula without irritating the skin. The devices usually adhere to the skin for 1 to 3 weeks, staying in place even during baths.

Blenders and Low-flow Flowmeters. Two methods of providing oxygen at low flows through a nasal cannula are common in neonatal and pediatric units. The first method entails connecting the cannula to a flowmeter attached to an air–oxygen blender. The second method consists of simply connecting the cannula to a low-flow flowmeter attached to a 100% oxygen source.

Oxygen blenders set at specific oxygen concentrations can be used to regulate the FIO_2 to infants receiving oxygen with nasal cannulas. Using this method, adjust both the oxygen concentration and the flow rate of the gas to achieve the appropriate FD_{O_2}. With a cannula connected to the flowmeter on the blender, set the oxygen concentration at 100% and the flow rate at the lowest possible flow. Many protocols begin the flow rate at 1 L/minute. Adjust the flow rate, decreasing it in small increments until reaching the flow necessary to maintain adequate SpO_2 levels. Continue weaning by decreasing the flow rate until reaching the minimal flow setting of the flowmeter. Proceed with weaning by decreasing the oxygen concentration setting on the blender to maintain adequate SpO_2 levels, or until oxygen is no longer required. Although some centers lower the oxygen concentration first, a lower flow rate may maximize the stability of delivered oxygen over time, as well as minimize the degree of change in FIO_2 during the weaning process.[34,35] Tables have been constructed to estimate hypopharyngeal oxygen concentrations at various settings, but reproducibility is affected by the range of infant sizes and variable breathing patterns.[35-37]

Because hypopharyngeal oxygen concentrations tend to be more stable when using lower flows, the use of a

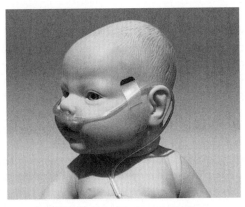

FIGURE 12-2 NeoHold cannula/tubing holder. The 4-cm-long strip attaches to the skin with hydrocolloid while the flap on top positions and secures the tubing in place. The clear flap allows visualization of the tubing.

low-flow flowmeter helps to optimize continuous oxygen administration in the infant population. Depending on the flowmeter, the flow rates range from 0.1 to 3.0 L/minute, with some adjustable in increments of less than 0.125 L/minute.[5] Using this method, connect the cannula to a low-flow flowmeter receiving 100% oxygen. Set an appropriate flow rate, as determined by the Spo_2, and wean the oxygen by decreasing the flow rate in small increments of 0.1 to 0.2 L/minute. Continue weaning in small increments until the minimal desired Spo_2 is reached, or until oxygen is no longer required.

Inspired Oxygen Determination. In the infant and child, Fio_2 provided with a nasal cannula is controlled primarily by varying the flow rate of the gas or the oxygen concentration of the blender. At low flow rates, Fio_2 also varies with the patient's minute ventilation and the relative duration of inspiration and expiration.[35] Fio_2 may decrease as a result of room-air entrainment that occurs during the patient's inspiration. In the small or premature infant, inspiratory flow rates are quite small and result in less room-air entrainment during inspiration. On the other hand, sedated infants may have decreased minute ventilation resulting in an increase in the actual Fio_2.[38] The Fio_2 is higher in infants receiving oxygen via nasal cannula than in adults and can exceed potentially toxic levels.[39] Several studies have documented high Fio_2 when supplemental oxygen is supplied to neonates via nasal cannula, ranging from 22% to 95% on various flows of 100% oxygen.[34,36,40]

Oxygen delivered by nasal cannula is measured in liters per minute (L/min) rather than Fio_2. Translating a flow rate into an approximate Fio_2 is helpful in gauging the degree of respiratory compromise and comparing oxygen conditions in clinical studies. Tables and equations are available for this purpose and in fact were distributed in the multicenter STOP-ROP (Supplemental Therapeutic Oxygen for Pre-threshold Retinopathy of Prematurity) study on the safety of oxygen use and the progression of ROP.[13,35] Although it potentially provides a more rational basis for oxygen prescription through a nasal cannula, the calculation and subsequent documentation of the effective Fio_2 is rarely implemented in clinical practice. Perhaps this is because the calculations are too cumbersome to undertake during routine clinical care.[33]

Because the concentration of oxygen inhaled into the lungs varies according to respiratory rate, tidal volume, inspiratory flow, and other factors such as ratio of mouth to nose breathing, it is difficult to determine the Fio_2 with certainty.[35,41,42] When compared with the adult patient, an infant can experience a substantial difference in Fio_2 when there is just a fraction of a change in the flow rate. An approximation of Fio_2 at low flows can be determined using the regression equation (Box 12-1).[34] This equation incorporates minute ventilation,

---

Box 12-1	Regression Equation for Estimating Nasal Cannula Fio_2 at Low Flow Rates

$$\text{Approximate } Fio_2 = (O_2 \text{ flow} \times 0.79)[(0.21 \times \dot{V}_E)/(\dot{V}_E \times 100)]$$

This equation is most predictive with an assumed tidal volume of 5.5 ml/kg for infants less than 1500 g.
Fio_2, fractional concentration of inspired oxygen; O_2 flow, expressed as milliliters per minute; $\dot{V}_E$ (minute ventilation) = tidal volume × respiratory rate.

---

but it does not account for changes in respiratory pattern and is more accurate for infants weighing less than 1500 g. Use such an equation only as a comparative estimate, and do not rely on it as an accurate determination of breath-to-breath Fio_2. During most routine clinical situations, approximating the Fio_2 from cannula flow is unnecessary. However, when weaning a patient from a cannula, the clinician can determine the measure of improvement by monitoring the incremental decreases in oxygen flow rate.

Hazards and Complications. Depending on the type of nasal cannula, the flow rate, and the infant's anatomy, an increase in exhaled resistance can result in substantial inadvertent continuous positive airway pressure (CPAP) being delivered to an infant's airway.[5,43] This occurs when using either the blender or the low-flow flowmeter to deliver supplemental oxygen. Significant CPAP tends to occur more often when the cannula has large-diameter prong tips and when flow rates are set above 2 L/minute.[40, 43-46] CPAP may precipitate intraventricular hemorrhage in neonates and can be detrimental to an infant with obstructive pulmonary disease.[39] It also carries the potential risk of pneumothorax, pulmonary interstitial emphysema, and pneumopericardium. Although the amount and certainty of CPAP may not be determined, keep in mind the possibility of such complications when improvement in response to nasal oxygen is less than expected.

Although the nasal cannula is relatively comfortable, lightweight, and easy to apply, the prongs are difficult to keep in the nares of active infants, often becoming displaced and resulting in loss of oxygen delivery.[47] Prongs that are too large can occlude the nares and increase the patient's work of breathing. An improperly sized cannula can cause irritation. Excessive flows may result in drying of the nasal mucosa as well as mucosal irritation. It is recommended that maximal flow be limited to 2 L/minute in infants and newborns.[5] There is a slight risk of airway obstruction caused by mucus, especially in the low birth weight infant. Therefore it is important to inspect and clean the nostrils daily.[26] Keep the nose clean and free of mucus by gently cleaning the nostril areas with a soft, moist cloth, being careful to avoid causing irritation and swelling of the nasal mucosa. Also, monitor the skin around the patient's ears and face for irritation as well as proper fit and placement of the cannula and tubing.

Disadvantages to using a nasal cannula to deliver oxygen include the instability of oxygen administration in transitions between oral and nasal breathing and the lack of precise knowledge concerning the delivered oxygen concentration. Unknown F_{IO_2} values may contribute to inconsistent weaning practices that could potentially result in unnecessary days of supplemental oxygen, delays in hospital discharge, and high costs of care.[33]

Simple Oxygen Mask

The simple oxygen mask is a lightweight plastic reservoir designed to fit over the patient's nose and mouth and is secured by an elastic strap around the patient's head (Figure 12-4). Open ports on both sides of the mask allow exhalation, and also allow the patient to draw in room air during inspiration. F_{IO_2} varies with the patient's inspiratory flow and the oxygen flow into the mask.[48] Room air is entrained through the exhalation ports in the mask if the patient's inspiratory flow rate exceeds the oxygen flow rate. Flow rates from 6 to 10 L/ minute provide a variable F_{IO_2} of 0.35 to 0.5; however there are no data concerning newborns and infants to predict the effective F_{IO_2}.[49]

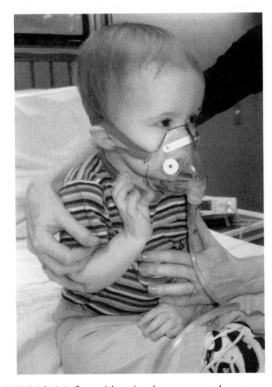

FIGURE 12-4 Infant with a simple oxygen mask.

Indications and Contraindications. Administration of oxygen with a simple mask is reserved for infants and children who need moderate concentrations of supplemental oxygen for short periods. Such situations include medical transport, emergency stabilization, postanesthesia recovery, and during medical procedures. The oxygen concentrations may be higher in patients with small tidal volumes, and therefore simple masks are not suitable for infants and small children who require low or precise concentrations of oxygen.[5,6]

Application. The mask is secured around the patient's head by a strap, and oxygen is delivered to the mask from a flowmeter and bubble humidifier through small-bore tubing. The cone shape of the simple mask may act as a reservoir for accumulated exhaled carbon dioxide if a minimal flow of gas is not maintained. In older children and adults, 6 L/minute is the recommended minimal flow rate to flush accumulated carbon dioxide.

Hazards and Complications. Because this mask is strapped to the face, infants and small children often refuse to keep the mask on. In addition, the confinement of the mask interferes with speech, eating and breast or bottle feeding, and may increase the risk for aspiration of vomitus. The elastic strap is often uncomfortable and can cause skin irritation with prolonged use.

Reservoir Masks

A reservoir mask consists of a soft lightweight mask with a plastic reservoir bag attached to its front (Figure 12-5). Oxygen source gas flows directly into the neck of the mask and is directed into the bag during exhalation. When the patient inhales, high concentrations of oxygen can be delivered from the bag through the mask. Currently, there are two types of reservoir masks: partial-rebreathing and nonrebreathing masks.

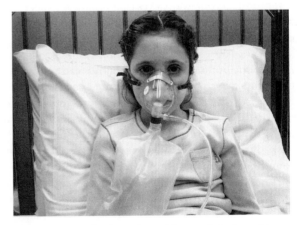

FIGURE 12-5 Pediatric patient with a partial-rebreathing mask, a type of reservoir mask.

If functioning properly, reservoir masks have the advantage of providing high concentrations of oxygen. However, the tight fit necessary to achieve optimal performance makes the masks impractical for long-term therapy. As with the simple oxygen mask, the elastic straps may cause the reservoir masks to be uncomfortable, confining, and not well tolerated by infants and children. The use of reservoir masks is limited to short-term situations requiring high F_{IO_2} administration or specific gas mixture therapy. Reservoir masks are not recommended for use in the neonatal population.[5]

Partial-rebreathing Mask. The partial-rebreathing mask is similar to a simple oxygen mask but contains a reservoir bag at the base of the mask. It is designed to conserve oxygen by receiving 100% oxygen along with a small portion of the patient's exhaled volume (approximately equal to the volume of the patient's "anatomic dead space"). The oxygen concentration of the exhaled gases combined with the supply of fresh oxygen permits the use of oxygen flows lower than those necessary for other devices, potentially conserving oxygen use. The remaining portion of the patient's exhaled volume is vented through open exhalation ports located on the sides of the mask.

Fit the mask securely to the patient's face to minimize the amount of room air entrained during inspiration. Adjust the oxygen flow rate to a level sufficient to keep the bag partially inflated during inspiration; usually 6 to 15 L/minute is sufficient. If the reservoir bag becomes totally deflated when the patient inspires, increase the flow rate. When there is an adequate seal around the mask and an appropriate flow rate is maintained, an F_{IO_2} of up to 0.6 is delivered to the patient.[5,48] However, this F_{IO_2}, as in other variable performance devices, is also influenced by the patient's ventilatory pattern.

Nonrebreathing Mask. The nonrebreathing mask is similar in design to the partial-rebreathing mask but in addition has one-way valves that function to keep the patient from rebreathing any exhaled gas.[48] A one-way valve located between the face mask and the reservoir bag allows 100% source gas to enter the mask during inspiration, but unlike the partial-rebreathing mask, it prevents any of the patient's exhaled gas from entering the bag. Instead of entering the reservoir bag, the exhaled gas is directed through one-way leaflet valves located over the exhalation ports on the sides of the mask. The leaflet valves also ensure minimal dilution from the entrainment of room air.

The nonrebreathing mask is designed to provide a higher F_{IO_2} than the simple and partial-rebreathing masks and the nasal delivery devices.[31] If there is an adequate seal around the mask and the flow rate is sufficient to keep the bag partially inflated during inspiration, oxygen concentrations can conceivably reach greater than 90%. Because it is designed to provide almost 100% source gas, the nonrebreathing mask is the recommended device to deliver specific gas mixtures, as in helium–oxygen therapy, or specific concentrations from a blender.[6,49]

Fixed-performance Oxygen Delivery Systems
Air-entrainment Mask

Air-entrainment masks, or Venturi masks, are examples of high-flow systems that provide the patient's entire inspiratory requirements while delivering predetermined, precise oxygen concentrations (Figure 12-6). This is accomplished by providing a total flow of gas that exceeds the patient's ventilatory demands, thus eliminating dilution of the oxygen concentration with room air, as occurs in low-flow devices.

The performance of the mask is based on principles described by Bernoulli.[50] As 100% oxygen under pressure flows through a small jet orifice entering the mask, the velocity increases, creating viscous shearing forces. As a result, room air is entrained through open ports located at the base of a reservoir tube attached to the front of the mask. By varying either the diameter of the jet orifice or the size of the entrainment ports, the amount of room air entrained can be proportionally changed, resulting in higher total flows and specific concentrations delivered to the patient's proximal airway.

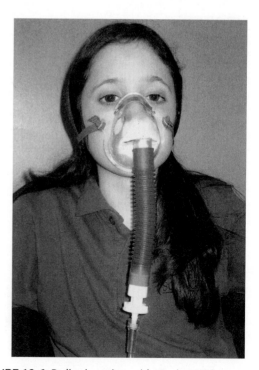

FIGURE 12-6 Pediatric patient with an air-entrainment mask.

Indications and Contraindications. The air-entrainment mask is indicated for patients who require a controlled F_{IO_2} at either low or moderate levels. The commercially available masks are capable of providing oxygen concentrations ranging from 24% to 50%. In the hypoxic child with increased respiratory rates and tidal volumes, the air-entrainment mask is the preferred oxygen delivery system because it is capable of maintaining total flows in excess of the patient's inspiratory flow rate. For pediatric patients with chronic carbon dioxide retention who have the potential to hypoventilate with increased oxygen concentrations, the air-entrainment mask is ideal because it maintains a constant F_{IO_2} even at low concentrations.

Application. An air-entrainment mask is designed to fit over the patient's nose and mouth and contains a short corrugated hose with a jet orifice that is connected to oxygen supply tubing. Because the high total flows produced by this system can be quite drying, humidification is provided with a bubble-diffusion humidifier. At the lower concentrations of 24% and 28%, oxygen flow through the small, restricted orifice creates excessive back pressure in the humidifier. For these levels of oxygen concentration, an alternative method may be used in which a bland aerosol is applied through a 22-mm cuplike collar attached to the base of the corrugated hose at the air-entrainment ports. This collar is often placed on the hose even when no aerosol is applied, simply to act as a shield to prevent the accidental occlusion of the air-entrainment ports with bed linens.

Hazards and Complications. Correct performance of the air-entrainment mask can be altered by resistance to the flow of gas that may occur distal to the restricted orifice. The resistance to flow at this particular point creates back pressure, resulting in less air entrainment. As a result, higher oxygen concentrations and lower total flows are delivered to the patient. If total flow decreases significantly, room air may be inhaled around and through the mask ports. This same phenomenon will occur if the entrainment ports are partially or completely obstructed. Also, at the 50% oxygen setting, total gas flow delivered by the device is less than that at the lower concentrations. Because of this, there is the potential for the patient with an increased inspiratory flow requirement to receive an oxygen concentration less than 50%.

Air-entrainment Nebulizer

The gas-powered, large-volume or all-purpose nebulizer is another fixed-performance system that provides particulate water and contains an adjustable air-entrainment port that controls oxygen concentrations.[51] The addition of heat gives this type of system the advantage of providing 100% body humidity when clinically indicated. The nebulizer provides oxygen at fixed concentrations by adjusting the size of the air-entrainment port located at the top of the nebulizer lid. The small size of the nebulizer jet restricts maximal flow to 15 L/minute from any 50-psi gas source.

Indications and Contraindications. Air-entrainment nebulizers are used when high levels of humidity or aerosol are desired. Patient application devices used with the nebulizers include a tracheostomy collar, face tent, aerosol mask, and blow-by arrangement (Figure 12-7).[5]

Application. Each patient application device is attached to the nebulizer unit with 4 to 6 ft of large-bore corrugated tubing that allows high gas flows and maximal aerosol delivery to the patient. Both the aerosol mask and the face tent apparatus are indicated primarily for short-term administration of oxygen with high humidity, as in postextubation or postanesthesia hypoxemia. In the immediate postoperative recovery period, a blow-by method of oxygen administration set close to the patient's face may be more easily tolerated and thus more effective (Figure 12-8).[52]

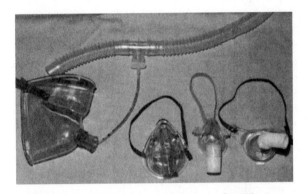

FIGURE 12-7 Various aerosol attachments. *Left to right:* Face tent, T-piece attached to an endotracheal tube, pediatric aerosol mask, infant aerosol mask, and tracheostomy mask (collar).

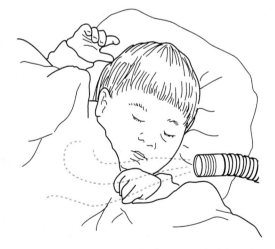

FIGURE 12-8 Blow-by method of oxygen administration used in postanesthesia recovery rooms.

When used to deliver oxygen to the older patient with an artificial airway, the aerosol is heated and the temperature of the gas–aerosol mixture is monitored. A tracheostomy collar is recommended for use with a tracheostomy; however, if a precise F_{IO_2} is required, a T-piece device may ensure delivery of a more exact F_{IO_2} because of its close fit on the tracheostomy tube. Provided that the gas flow from the nebulizer exceeds the patient's inspiratory flow rate, room-air entrainment is limited and the delivered F_{IO_2} is stable.

An air-entrainment nebulizer used with a collar or T-piece is not appropriate for oxygen delivery to infants and young children with a tracheostomy. Instead, a heated humidifier is recommended along with an oxygen blender used to regulate the F_{IO_2}. Using small-bore oxygen supply tubing attached to the flowmeter on the blender, the oxygen is directed through the humidifier where large-bore corrugated tubing is connected to the tracheostomy collar.

Hazards and Complications. As with all masks used to deliver oxygen therapy to the infant or pediatric patient, the aerosol mask and face tent frequently provoke unnecessary agitation and anxiety, especially in the treatment of postanesthesia hypoxemia. Infants and young children often find it difficult to keep the masks in place. Nebulizers are susceptible to bacterial contamination and require replacement according to hospital policy. Condensate in the aerosol tubing is considered infectious waste and should never be drained back into the nebulizer.[5] The condensate can completely obstruct gas flow or cause increased resistance to flow, which may increase the F_{IO_2} above the desired setting.

The weight of the T-piece and tubing assembly often creates torque on the endotracheal or tracheostomy tube, causing tracheal irritation and possible displacement. The tracheostomy collar may cause skin irritation around the patient's neck and condensate in the aerosol tubing may result in inadvertent tracheal lavage.[5]

A cool mist is not recommended for newborns because of the potential to induce cold stress.[53] If the gas flow from the oxygen source is cool and is directed toward the infant's face, stimulation of the trigeminal nerves may cause alterations in the respiratory pattern and lead to apnea.[54]

High-flow Nasal Cannula

In the past the nasal cannula has always been classified as a low-flow, variable-performance oxygen delivery system, with recommendations that no more than 6-L/minute gas flows be used with adults and that the maximal flow to newborn infants not exceed 2 L/minute.[5,6,31] Flow limitations have largely been due to the airway cooling and drying that occur at higher flows. Using a bubble humidifier to humidify oxygen with a nasal cannula does not provide adequate humidification to premature infants and has been associated with decreased airway patency, nasal mucosal injury, and coagulase-negative staphylococcal sepsis in extremely low birth weight infants.[55-57] Although face masks can safely deliver oxygen at higher flows, these devices are confining and often poorly tolerated by infants and children.

Using a nasal cannula at high flows is still a relatively new means to deliver oxygen to infants and children. It has been used only a few years more in the adult population. However, studies with adults have been favorable, with data showing the high flows providing moderate-to-high F_{IO_2} values and possibly providing a cost-efficient alternative for patients who require this level of oxygen concentration.[58] One study indicated that when the oxygen delivered through a high-flow nasal cannula is warmed and humidified, adult patients with advanced obstructive airway disease experience an increase in oxygenation. The warm humidification may have likely contributed to the improvement of airway function by maximizing mucociliary clearance and preventing inflammatory reactions. Also, nasal breathing of warm, humidified gas tends to inhibit the bronchoconstrictor reflex, which in turn prevents the increase in airway resistance that is often triggered by cold air.[59]

Approval by the U.S. Food and Drug Administration of commercially available humidification systems and nasal cannulas specifically designed for use at high flow rates has changed the way the nasal cannula is used and how it is classified. The present ability to provide high flows with optimal humidification has led to an increase in use of the high-flow nasal cannula in the neonatal and pediatric population.[60]

Indications and Contraindications. Oxygen delivery with a high-flow nasal cannula is most often indicated for use in patients with hypoxemia who have not responded to oxygen administered with a low-flow nasal cannula. It may also be indicated for use in infants and children with lung disorders who require improved oxygenation or a reduction in work of breathing. The high-flow nasal cannula has also been recommended for infants in the management of apnea of prematurity.[44] As a less intrusive method to deliver high flows of oxygen, its use may reduce the potential risk of the iatrogenic injuries associated with nasal CPAP and mechanical ventilation.[61] Contraindications for use of the high-flow nasal cannula may include suspected or confirmed pneumothorax, severe upper airway obstruction, and absence of spontaneous ventilation.

Application. To provide optimal humidification, the high-flow nasal cannula must be used with a hydration system. The Vapotherm 2000i (Vapotherm, Stevensville, Md) is one system that is used in the neonatal, infant, and pediatric population. In 2004, it was approved by the U.S. Food and Drug Administration to humidify and deliver high-flow air or oxygen by nasal cannula and other patient interfaces. It is not approved, nor is it recommended for use, as a CPAP delivery system.[43,44,46] The system can provide oxygen flow at a relative humidity of 99.9% with a temperature setting of 37° C.[62] Oxygen is supplied to the unit from an air–oxygen blender. The flow rate of the gas is controlled by the flowmeter on the blender. The oxygen travels through a vapor exchange cartridge, where it is separated from the water by a microporous membrane material with a pore size less than 0.01 µm.[63] The membrane allows water vapor to pass into the flow of gas, but the small pore size of the membrane prevents direct contact between the water source and the oxygen, effectively serving as a filter.[62] After it is warmed and humidified, the oxygen flows through a water-heated delivery tube that is connected to the nasal cannula. This tubing maintains the temperature of the gas and minimizes condensation in the cannula.

The Vapotherm system has cannulas available in six sizes:

- Premature
- Neonatal
- Infant
- Intermediate infant
- Pediatric
- Adult

It also has two vapor transfer cartridges: a low-flow cartridge that is used to deliver flows of 1 to 8 L/minute and a high-flow cartridge that is used to deliver flows of 5 to 40 L/minute. The temperature range is selectable from 33 to 43° C. The unit will shut down if temperature safety limits are exceeded or if the water level is low; however, the gas flow will continue. The unit will also shut down if the gas supply is interrupted. Disinfection and sterilization are performed according to the manufacturer's recommendations.

Select the cannula that is most appropriate for the size of the patient, making sure that the prongs do not occlude the patient's nares. Attach the high-flow nasal cannula to the patient in the same manner as one would a low-flow nasal cannula. Adjust the oxygen concentration with the blender and set the flow rate on the flowmeter. Increase or decrease the flow in small increments. Assess the patient's breathing pattern, breath sounds, and vital signs. Also monitor the Spo_2 and chest radiographs to determine appropriate flow rates. The high-flow nasal cannula and the delivery tubing are single-patient disposables and are discarded after each patient's use.

Hazards and Complications. To a greater extent than with the low-flow nasal cannula, there is considerable concern as to the lack of knowledge of the actual amount of positive pressure generated when

using a high-flow nasal cannula. A critical issue is the inability of current systems to prevent the occurrence of excessive pressures being delivered to a patient's airways. Without a pressure pop-off within the system, the actual airway pressure delivered when using a high-flow gas source depends on the presence of leaks within the airway. Unless there is a means to regulate the pressure, the development of gastric distension or lung overexpansion is a dangerous possibility.[64]

More data are needed to support the clinical efficacy of using the nasal cannula at high flows and to determine safety hazards, including the amount of positive pressure delivered. Evaluating the nasopharyngeal and esophageal pressure generated by the high-flow nasal cannula, as well as assessing work of breathing and patient comfort, will assist in finding the safest and most cost-effective means to deliver high flows to the neonatal and pediatric population.

Enclosures
Oxygen Tent
In the past, oxygen tents were one of the primary methods of oxygen administration for both adults and children. At present, however, their use is limited. Tents are designed to provide a cool, oxygen-enriched environment with high humidity. A high-output aerosol generator or large-volume nebulizer powered by oxygen or compressed air (with oxygen titrated into the system) produces a dense mist. The mist is cooled and circulated by a refrigerator unit and connected to a transparent canopy placed over the patient and secured under the mattress of the crib or bed (Figure 12-9).[65]

Oxygen concentrations are quite variable and seldom reach greater than 50%, even with flow rates greater than 10 L/minute and 100% oxygen source gas. This is due

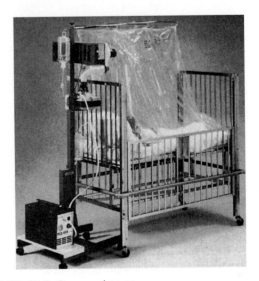

FIGURE 12-9 Oxygen mist tent.

primarily to leaks that occur when the tent is opened or inadequately sealed around the patient's bed. Because of variation in F_{IO_2}, the oxygen concentration is monitored with an oxygen analyzer, with the analyzer sensor placed near the patient's face.

Indications and Contraindications. Tents are used most often to deliver supplemental oxygen and cool, high-humidity gas mixtures to pediatric patients with laryngotracheobronchitis,[66] to those with artificial airways in whom direct attachment of a device to the airway is contraindicated, or to patients who are too large for hoods.[5] Only low to moderate oxygen concentrations less than 40% can be achieved in a tent.

Hazards and Complications. Electric shock or fire can result from sparks generated by nurse call devices, electric and battery-operated toys, vibrators, percussors, and static electricity. These devices are not allowed under the tent canopy when in use. A dense fog or excessive condensation can develop inside the tent, which is frightening to a child and makes it difficult for the child to be observed. Loss of air in the circulation system may result in failure to cool the tent.[5] Check the tent frequently to ensure proper cooling and circulation and to empty the condensate collection bottle. Opening the tent decreases the oxygen concentration, and therefore a nasal cannula may be indicated during feeding and nursing care. Close monitoring of the patient is necessary because of the potential for asphyxiation if the patient becomes lodged between the mattress and the tent.[5]

Oxygen Hood

The oxygen hood is a transparent enclosure constructed of clear plastic material in a cylinder or boxlike design (Figure 12-10). Oxygen is administered through large-bore corrugated tubing attached to the back of the hood. The hood surrounds the infant's head, leaving the body accessible for nursing care. This design also allows the infant to be placed in a neutral thermal environment, such as an incubator, and still receive controlled oxygen concentrations. Variations in hood design allow access to the infant's head by removing the top lid or by opening large ports on the sides or top of the hood.

Indications and Contraindications. Hoods are indicated most often for neonates, infants, and small children who require supplemental oxygen with heated humidity. Hoods are used to provide a controlled F_{IO_2} and increased heated humidity to patients who are unable to tolerate other oxygen or humidification devices. An oxygen hood can also be used to perform an oxygen challenge (hyperoxia) test in a spontaneously breathing neonate. Oxygen concentration in a hood can be varied from 21% to 100% and is more stable than that provided by a tent.[5]

Application. Oxygen is delivered to the hood with heated humidification by means of an oxygen blender, dual air and oxygen flowmeters, or a heated air-entrainment nebulizer. When using the heated air-entrainment nebulizer, power the nebulizer with compressed air, setting the oxygen concentration dial at 100% and bleeding

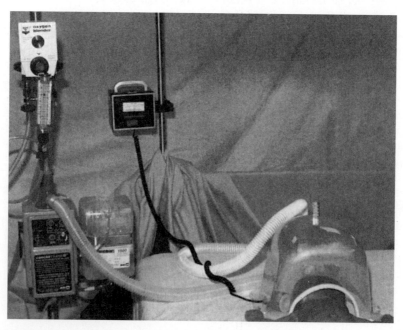

FIGURE 12-10 Infant oxygen hood with gas delivered through an oxygen blender system with heated humidification. The oxygen analyzer sensor is placed inside the hood close to the infant's head.

oxygen into the nebulizer. In this way, oxygen concentrations are more easily regulated and noise levels are reduced.[67]

The oxygen blender system premixes oxygen concentrations and passes the blended gas through a heated humidifier before entering the hood. This allows more precise control over both oxygen concentration and temperature and virtually eliminates noise inside the hood. With dual air and oxygen flowmeters, both air and oxygen are titrated through the heated humidifier and tubing into the hood and analyzed until accurate prescribed oxygen concentrations are obtained. Regardless of which system is used, oxygen is analyzed on a continuous basis to ensure accurate concentrations.

When high oxygen concentrations are used, a layering effect occurs inside the hood, with the highest oxygen concentrations settling toward the bottom. For this reason, place the oxygen analyzer sensor as close to the infant's head as possible. It is also important that an adequate flow of gas be delivered to wash out any carbon dioxide that may accumulate inside the hood. In general, flow rates should be greater than 7 L/minute.[5] Flows of 10 to 15 L/minute are adequate for most infants and children.

It is important that adequate heat and humidity be maintained inside the hood. Administration of cool, dry gas induces cold stress in infants, resulting in increased oxygen consumption. Likewise, delivery of overheated gases induces apnea.[54] Temperature is maintained at or near body temperature with a thermometer placed inside the hood for continuous monitoring.

Oxygen hoods come in a variety of sizes to fit the very small neonate and very large infant. For patients too large for neonatal-size hoods, there are transparent enclosures in larger sizes called tent houses or huts (Figures 12-11 and 12-12). For optimal temperature,

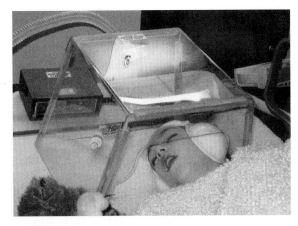

FIGURE 12-12 Older pediatric patient requiring low oxygen concentration after surgical repair of earlobes. Because use of a face mask or cannula would require straps or tubing placed around the patient's ears, a hood is used.

flow, and oxygen control, choosing the proper-sized hood is imperative.

Hazards and Complications. Limited mobility may be an issue with the oxygen hood if the infant requires oxygen for a prolonged period. Opening the hood decreases the oxygen concentration and can result in hypoxia. If the hood is opened for an extended period, such as during feeding and nursing procedures, it is appropriate to provide nasal oxygen with a cannula while the patient is eating or until the procedure is completed. Just as a loss of gas flow to the hood can result in hypoxia, hypercapnia, and even death, excessive oxygen concentrations can lead to irreversible complications. For these reasons, use an oxygen analyzer to continuously monitor the oxygen concentration in the hood, maintaining high and low alarms on the analyzer at all times. Although the oxygen hood is usually well tolerated, irritation to the infant's skin, especially around the neck, may occur because of pressure from an improperly sized hood or active movement of the patient. Cutaneous fungal infections have been associated with prolonged exposure to humidified oxygen in hoods.[68] High gas flow into the hood may produce noise levels that induce hearing impairment.[67]

Incubators

In 1893, Thomas Morgan Rotch presented a wooden box with hot water bottles, known as a "brooder," that was to provide technology's answer to the uterus in the case of the premature infant.[69] Since that time, incubators have enjoyed both favorable and unfavorable status in the care of infants. An incubator is a clear Plexiglas enclosure that controls temperature and humidity and has the ability to deliver supplemental oxygen.

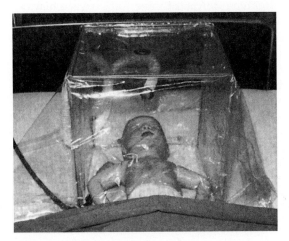

FIGURE 12-11 Tent house for oxygen administration to larger infants.

Indications and Contraindications. In the past, incubators were used frequently as a primary mode of delivering oxygen to the premature infant.[70] At present, however, the primary purpose of an incubator is to provide a temperature-controlled environment to small infants with temperature instability.[5,65] Precise oxygen delivery is more effectively administered with the oxygen hood, which can be set up within the incubator, or with a nasal cannula.

Application. The temperature of the incubator is servo-controlled and maintained with a skin probe attached to the infant. Humidity is provided either by using a baffled blow-over water reservoir within the unit itself or by attaching an alternative humidification system.[65] Oxygen is provided by attaching small-bore tubing to a flowmeter and an inlet nipple connection to the incubator. Some units have two oxygen connections, one for low to moderate oxygen concentrations (approximately 40%) and one for high oxygen concentrations (nearly 100%). In some models, oxygen analyzers are incorporated with flow-controlling solenoids. When oxygen levels decrease to less than preset values, solenoids open and increase the oxygen flow rate until the analyzed value of oxygen equals the preset value on the controller.

Hazards and Complications. The greatest disadvantage of using an incubator to administer oxygen is the inability to stabilize and maintain the FIO_2, regardless of whether the unit has flow-controlling solenoids or conventional methods of oxygenation. This drawback results from the large open space within the incubator and the inherent leaks that occur.

Manual Resuscitation Systems

Neonatal and pediatric manual resuscitators are used most often to support ventilation in emergency situations. They are also used to hyperoxygenate patients intermittently before or during invasive procedures and during periods of apnea or bradycardia. Effective use of these devices depends not only on their physical structure and performance characteristics, but also on the knowledge and skill of the clinician. Two types of manual resuscitation systems are available for use in the neonatal and pediatric patient: the self-inflating system and the non–self-inflating system.

Self-inflating Resuscitation System

The self-inflating systems for neonatal and pediatric use are similar in design and function to those used in adult resuscitation bags (Figure 12-13). They consist of a self-inflating compressible bag that has a tidal volume range of 200 to 300 ml for neonates and 400 to 500 ml for pediatric patients.[71] One-way valves pre-

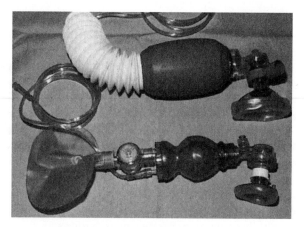

FIGURE 12-13 Pediatric *(top)* and neonatal *(bottom)* self-inflating manual resuscitation bags.

vent the rebreathing of exhaled gas and allow source gas to be directed into the bag during inflation, which in some models may prevent free flow of oxygen to the patient. Self-inflating systems are also equipped with pressure-relief valves that prevent the administration of excessive pressures. Most models have reservoirs that help to achieve high oxygen concentrations.

Although the self-inflating systems are the most frequently used devices for resuscitation efforts, there have been reports of failure to meet one or more of the ASTM International (West Conshohocken, Pa) standards for safety.[72,73] First, pressure-relief valves within a system may activate over a wide range of pressures rather than the manufacturer's stated limits, which are usually 30 to 40 cm H_2O. In addition, activation of the pressure-relief valve may cause a significant reduction in the delivered oxygen concentration from a unit, even when a reservoir system is in place. Second, although the addition of a reservoir system increases the delivered oxygen concentrations, 100% oxygen may not be readily achievable. Finally, the patient valve assembly may crack or break when dropped on hard surfaces, rendering the unit useless. The clinician should be aware of these potential problems when selecting a self-inflating resuscitation bag. Because the key to successful use of a resuscitation bag is effective ventilation, it is just as imperative that an appropriately sized face mask be used. Leaks around the mask may result in less than adequate volumes delivered during the positive pressure ventilation.[74]

Non–self-inflating Resuscitation System

The non–self-inflating, or *flow-inflating*, manual resuscitation system consists of an anesthesia reservoir bag

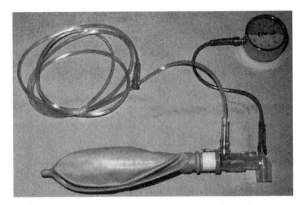

FIGURE 12-14 Neonatal non–self-inflating manual resuscitation bag with in-line pressure manometer.

connected either to a T-piece adapter and corrugated reservoir tube or to a patient adapter with a pressure-relief valve (Figure 12-14). The gas source is connected to an oxygen nipple adapter in front of the bag, and a pressure manometer is connected in-line between the patient adapter and gas source inlet.

A flow rate of gas at least two to three times the patient's minute ventilation (ranging from 3 to 15 L/min) is sufficient to fill the bag and flush the reservoir tube, allowing exhaled gas to be continuously flushed out of the system.[71] During inspiration, fresh gas is delivered to the patient by compressing the bag. As the bag is compressed, excess gas exits simultaneously through the pressure-relief valve and prevents excessive ventilating pressures and volumes. The in-line pressure manometer is a critical component of the non–self-inflating bag and is used to monitor the peak inspiratory pressures and the positive end-expiratory pressure maintained during ventilation.[75] In intensive care settings, it is helpful to have large manometers permanently mounted on the patient bed columns.

The non–self-inflating systems have the advantage of allowing more control over delivery pressures, inspiratory time, the addition of positive end-expiratory pressure, and the assurance of delivering 100% oxygen or exact oxygen concentrations from an air–oxygen blender. Unfortunately, many clinicians are not adequately skilled in the operation of non–self-inflating bags. Although the bags can deliver prolonged inflations, difficulty may arise in maintaining an adequate seal with the face mask or selecting the proper flow rate, often resulting in collapse of the anesthesia bag and reduced levels of ventilation.[76, 77] For these reasons, the use of non–self-inflating resuscitation bags should be reserved for clinicians who are adequately trained and proficient in using such systems.

ASSESSMENT QUESTIONS

See Evolve Resources for answers.

1. Bedside evaluation of the degree of hypoxemia may best be accomplished by which of the following?
   A. Auscultation
   B. Pulse oximetry
   C. Capillary blood gas analysis
   D. Capillary refill time
2. Which of the following are potential complications associated with the use of nasopharyngeal catheters in infants?
     I. Nasal polyps
    II. Epistaxis
   III. Pneumothorax
    IV. Gastric distention
   A. I and III only
   B. II and III only
   C. I and IV only
   D. II and IV only
3. A 5-year-old patient with a history of asthma is admitted to the emergency department after complaining of chest tightness and wheezing. The pulse oximeter reading drops from 95% to 91%. Which of the following devices should be selected to deliver oxygen to this patient?
   A. Nasal cannula
   B. Oxygen hood
   C. Oxygen mist tent
   D. Non-rebreathing mask
4. What is the minimal flow rate that should be used to deliver oxygen through a hood to an infant?
   A. 5 L/minute
   B. 7 L/minute
   C. 10 L/minute
   D. 15 L/minute
5. The physician orders 32% oxygen for a 12-year-old patient with cystic fibrosis. Which of the following oxygen delivery devices would best ensure this oxygen concentration?
   A. Low-flow nasal cannula
   B. Simple mask
   C. Non-rebreathing mask
   D. Air-entrainment mask
6. Which of the following statements is true regarding the use of a self-inflating resuscitation system?
   A. A pressure-relief valve is an optional component of the system.
   B. The neonatal compressible bag can deliver a maximal tidal volume of 100 ml.
   C. It allows for more control over the delivered pressure than the non–self-inflating system.
   D. Most models have reservoirs that help to achieve high oxygen concentrations.

Continued

ASSESSMENT QUESTIONS—cont'd

7. A 9-year-old patient is admitted to the hospital after smoke inhalation. While receiving oxygen with a nonrebreathing mask, it is noted that the reservoir bag becomes totally deflated when the patient inspires. Which of the following should be recommended?
   A. Increase the oxygen flow rate.
   B. Decrease the oxygen flow rate.
   C. Change to a nasal cannula.
   D. Change to a partial rebreathing mask.

8. A premature infant is receiving oxygen by nasal cannula at 1.5 L/minute. The following capillary blood gas and pulse oximetry values are obtained:

pH	7.37
P_{CCO_2}	41 mm Hg
P_{CO_2}	43 mm Hg
HCO_3^-	23 mEq/L
BE	–1 mEq/L
Sp_{O_2}	98%

BE, Base excess in blood; HCO_3^-, bicarbonate; P_{CCO_2}, partial pressure of carbon dioxide, determined transcutaneously; P_{CO_2}, partial pressure of oxygen, determined transcutaneously; Sp_{O_2}, percentage of oxygen saturation.

Which of the following should be recommended?
   A. Replace the nasal cannula with an oxygen hood.
   B. Decrease the nasal cannula flow to 1 L/minute.
   C. Increase the nasal cannula flow to 2 L/minute.
   D. Discontinue the nasal cannula.

9. All of the following statements are true regarding an incubator *except*:
   A. Oxygen may be provided through a nipple connection on the incubator.
   B. An advantage of using an incubator is its ability to stabilize and maintain the F_{IO_2}.
   C. A nasal cannula or an oxygen hood may be used to deliver oxygen to an infant in an incubator.
   D. An incubator is used primarily to provide a temperature-controlled environment to small infants.

10. What is the greatest concern when using a high-flow nasal cannula?
   A. An inability to obtain an oxygen flowmeter that can provide the high flows
   B. An increased risk of developing chronic lung disease
   C. A lack of knowledge concerning the actual amount of positive pressure applied to the patient's airways
   D. The high cost of nasal cannulas that can accommodate high gas flows

References

1. Partington JR, editor: *A short history of chemistry*, ed 3, New York: Dover; 1989. pp 110–152.
2. Saugstad OD: Oxygen toxicity in the neonatal period, *Acta Pediatr Scand* 1990;79:881.
3. Hess JH: Oxygen unit for premature and very young infants, *Am J Dis Child* 1934;47:916.
4. Baker JP, editor: *The machine in the nursery: premature technology and the origins of newborn intensive care*, Baltimore, Md: Johns Hopkins University Press; 1996. pp 152–174.
5. American Association for Respiratory Care: Clinical practice guideline: selection of an oxygen delivery device for neonatal and pediatric patients: 2002 revision and update, *Respir Care* 2002;47:707.
6. American Association for Respiratory Care: Clinical practice guideline: oxygen therapy for adults in the acute care facility: 2002 revision and update, *Respir Care* 2002;47:717.
7. Fulmer JD, Snider GL; American College of Chest Physicians; National Heart, Lung, and Blood Institute: National conference on oxygen therapy, *Chest* 1984; 86:234 [concurrent publication in *Respir Care* 1984; 29:922].
8. Bonadio W: The history and physical assessments of the febrile infant, *Pediatr Clin North Am* 1998;45:65.
9. Fisher AB: Oxygen therapy: side effects and toxicity, *Am Rev Respir Dis* 1980;122:61.
10. Lanman JT et al: Retrolental fibroplasia and oxygen therapy, *JAMA* 1954;155:223.
11. Patz A: The role of oxygen in retrolental fibroplasia, *Pediatrics* 1957;19:504.
12. George DS et al: The latest on retinopathy of prematurity, *Maternal Child Nurs* 1988;13:254.
13. STOP-ROP Multicenter Study Group: Supplemental Therapeutic Oxygen for Pre-threshold Retinopathy of Prematurity (STOP-ROP), a randomized, controlled, trial: primary outcomes, *Pediatrics* 2000;105:295.
14. Tin W et al: Pulse oximetry, severe retinopathy, and outcome at one year in babies of less than 28 weeks gestation, *Arch Dis Child Fetal Neonatal Ed* 2001;84:F106.
15. Askie LM et al: Oxygen-saturation targets and outcomes in extremely preterm infants, *N Engl J Med* 2003;349:959.
16. Chow LC et al: Can changes in clinical practice decrease the incidence of severe retinopathy of prematurity in very low birth weight infants? *Pediatrics* 2003;111:339.
17. Silverman WA: A cautionary tale about supplemental oxygen: the albatross of neonatal medicine, *Pediatrics* 2004;113:394.
18. El-Lessy HN: Pulmonary vascular control in hypoplastic left-heart syndrome: hypoxic- and hypercarbic-gas therapy, *Respir Care* 1995;40:737.
19. Fairshter RD et al: Paraquat poisoning: new aspects of therapy, *Q J Med* 1976;45:551.
20. Ingrassia TS et al: Oxygen-exacerbated bleomycin pulmonary toxicity, *Mayo Clin Proc* 1991;66:173.
21. Coffman JA, McManus KP: Oxygen therapy via nasal catheter for infants with bronchopulmonary dysplasia, *Crit Care Nurs* 1984;4:22.
22. Shann F et al: Nasopharyngeal oxygen in children, *Lancet* 1988;2:1238.

23. Fremstad JD, Martin SH: Lethal complication from insertion of nasogastric tube after severe basilar skull fracture, *J Trauma* 1978;18:820.
24. Guilfoile T, Dabe K: Nasal catheter oxygen therapy for infants, *Respir Care* 1981;26:35.
25. Frenckner B et al: Pneumocephalus caused by a nasopharyngeal oxygen catheter, *Crit Care Med* 1990;18:1287.
26. Weber MW et al: Comparison of nasal prongs and nasopharyngeal catheter for the delivery of oxygen in children with hypoxemia because of a lower respiratory tract infection, *J Pediatr* 1995;127:378.
27. Givan DC, Wylie P: Home oxygen therapy for infants and children, *Indiana Med* 1986;45:849.
28. Shann F: Nasopharyngeal oxygen in children [letter], *Lancet* 1989;1:1077.
29. Klein M, Reynolds LG: Nasopharyngeal oxygen in children [letter], *Lancet* 1989;1:493.
30. Kloor TH Jr, Carbajal D: Infant oxygen administration by modified nasal cannula, *Clin Pediatr* 1984;23:447.
31. Leigh JM: Variation in performance of oxygen therapy devices, *Anaesthesia* 1970;25:210.
32. Ooi R et al: An evaluation of oxygen delivery using nasal prongs, *Anaesthesia* 1992;47:591.
33. Walsh M et al: Oxygen delivery through nasal cannulae to preterm infants: can practice be improved? *Pediatrics* 2005;116:857.
34. Finer NN et al: Low flow oxygen delivery via nasal cannula to neonates, *Pediatr Pulmonol* 1996;21:48.
35. Benaron DA, Benitz WE: Maximizing the stability of oxygen delivered via nasal cannula, *Arch Pediatr Adolesc Med* 1994;148:294.
36. Vain NE et al: Regulation of oxygen concentration delivered to infants via nasal cannulas, *Am J Dis Child* 1989;143:1458.
37. Stevens DP et al: Hypopharyngeal O_2 concentration in infants breathing O_2 by nasal cannula [abstract], *Respir Care* 1986;31:988.
38. Hammer J et al: Effect of jaw-thrust and continuous positive airway pressure on tidal breathing in deeply sedated infants, *J Pediatr* 2001;138:826.
39. Kuluz JW et al: The fraction of inspired oxygen in infants receiving oxygen via nasal cannula often exceeds safe levels, *Respir Care* 2001;46:897.
40. Fan LL, Voyles JB: Determination of inspired oxygen delivered by nasal cannula in infants with chronic lung disease, *J Pediatr* 1983;103:923.
41. Miller MJ et al: Oral breathing in newborn infants, *J Pediatr* 1985;107:465.
42. Miller MJ et al: Effect of maturation on oral breathing in sleeping premature infants, *J Pediatr* 1986;109:515.
43. Locke RG et al: Inadvertent administration of positive end-distending pressure during nasal cannula flow, *Pediatrics* 1993;91:135.
44. Sreenan C et al: High-flow nasal cannula in the management of apnea of prematurity: a comparison with conventional nasal continuous positive airway pressure, *Pediatrics* 2001;107:1080.
45. Frey B et al: Nasopharyngeal oxygen therapy produces positive end-expiratory pressure in infants, *Eur J Pediatr* 2001;160:556.
46. Courtney SE et al: Lung recruitment and breathing pattern during variable versus continuous flow nasal continuous positive airway pressure in premature infants: an evaluation of three devices, *Pediatrics* 2001;107:304.
47. Thilo EH et al: Home oxygen therapy in the newborn: costs and parental acceptance, *Am J Dis Child* 1987;141:766.
48. Cairo JM, Pilbeam SP: Administering medical gases: regulators, flowmeters, and controlling devices. In *Mosby's respiratory care equipment*, ed 7, St. Louis: Mosby; 2004. pp 71–72.
49. Redding JS et al: Oxygen concentrations received from commonly used delivery systems, *South Med J* 1978;71:169.
50. Scacci R: Air entrainment masks: jet mixing is how they work; the Bernoulli and Venturi principles are how they don't, *Respir Care* 1979;24:928.
51. Cairo JM, Pilbeam SP: Humidity and aerosol therapy. In *Mosby's respiratory care equipment*, ed 7, St. Louis: Mosby; 2004. pp 73–74.
52. Amar D et al: An alternative oxygen delivery system for infants and children in the post-anesthesia care unit, *Can J Anaesth* 1991;38:49.
53. Scopes JW, Ahmed I: Ranges of critical temperatures in sick and premature newborn babies, *Arch Dis Child* 1966;41:417.
54. Daily WJR et al: Apnea in premature infants: monitoring, incidence, heart rate changes, and an effect of environmental temperature, *Pediatrics* 1969;43:510.
55. Walsh B: Comparison of Vapotherm™ 2000i with a bubble humidifier for humidifying flow through an infant nasal cannula, *Respir Care* 2003;48:1086.
56. Kopelman AE, Holbert D: Use of oxygen cannulas in extremely low birthweight infants is associated with mucosal trauma and bleeding and possibly with coagulase-negative staphylococcal sepsis, *J Perinatol* 2003;23:94.
57. Kopelman AE: Airway obstruction in two extremely low birthweight infants treated with oxygen cannulas, *J Perinatol* 2003;23:164.
58. Wettstein RB et al: Delivered oxygen concentration using low-flow and high-flow nasal cannulas, *Respir Care* 2005;50:604.
59. Chatila W et al: The effects of high-flow versus low-flow oxygen on exercise in advanced obstructive airways disease, *Chest* 2004;126:1108.
60. Waugh JB, Granger WB: An evaluation of 2 new devices for nasal high-flow gas therapy, *Respir Care* 2004;49:902.
61. Juretschke R, Spoula R: High flow nasal cannula in the neonatal population, *Neonatal Intensive Care* 2004;17:20.
62. Waugh JB, Lain DC: Evaluation of a new high flow gas humidification device [abstract], *Am J Respir Crit Care Med* 2003;167:A996.
63. 2000i Operating instruction manual. Vapotherm, Inc. Stevensville, MD.
64. Finer NN: Nasal cannula use in the preterm infant: oxygen or pressure? [commentary], *Pediatrics* 2005;116:1216.
65. Thalken FR: Medical gas therapy. In Scanlan CL, Spearman CB, Sheldon RL, editors: *Egan's fundamentals of respiratory care*, St. Louis: Mosby; 1990. pp 606–632.
66. Skolnik NS: Treatment of croup, *Am J Dis Child* 1989;143:1045.

67. Beckham RW, Mishoe SC: Sound levels inside incubators and oxygen hoods used with nebulizers and humidifiers, *Respir Care* 1982;27:33.

68. Lanska MJ et al: Cutaneous fungal infections associated with prolonged treatment in humidified oxygen hoods [letter], *Pediatr Dermatol* 1987;4:346.

69. Baker JP: The incubator controversy: pediatricians and the origins of premature infant technology in the United States, 1890 to 1910, *Pediatrics* 1991;87:654.

70. Simpson H, Russell DJ. Oxygen concentrations in tents and incubators in paediatric practice. *Br Med J.* 1967;4:201.

71. Thompson JE et al: Neonatal and pediatric airway emergencies, *Respir Care* 1992;37:582.

72. Barnes TA, McGarry WP: Evaluation of ten disposable manual resuscitators, *Respir Care* 1990;35:960.

73. Finer NN et al: Limitations of self inflating resuscitators, *Pediatrics* 1986;77:417.

74. O'Donnell CPF et al: Neonatal resuscitation. 2. An evaluation of manual ventilation devices and face masks, *Arch Dis Child Fetal Neonatal Ed* 2005;90:392.

75. Zmora E, Merritt TA: Control of peak inspiratory pressure during manual ventilation: a controlled study, *Am J Dis Child* 1982;136:46.

76. Kanter RK: Evaluation of mask-bag ventilation in resuscitation of infants, *Am J Dis Child* 1987;141:761.

77. Colm PF et al: Resuscitation of premature infants: what are we doing wrong and can we do better? *Biol Neonate* 2003;84:76.

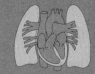

Chapter 13

Aerosols and Administration of Medication

JAMES B. FINK • BRUCE K. RUBIN

LEARNING OBJECTIVES

After reading this chapter the reader will be able to:
- Describe impact of differences in patient size and age
  on aerosol delivery
- Understand the basic mechanisms of operation of
  nebulizer, pressurized metered-dose inhalers, and dry
  powder inhalers

- Select the best device for a pediatric patient for
  specific clinical applications
- Initiate and modify aerosol therapy
- Discuss the range of medications available for
  administration via aerosol

ecades of research have established the scientific principles underlying the use of therapeutic aerosols. In general, the advantages of aerosol therapy include a smaller but targeted dose, lower cost, fewer side effects, efficacy comparable to or better than that observed with systemic administration of the drug, and usually a more rapid onset of action.[1] When inhaled drugs are delivered directly to the conducting airways, their systemic absorption is limited and systemic side effects are minimized, providing a high therapeutic index.[2] On the other hand, peptides and other macromolecules can be targeted to the terminal airways and alveoli for systemic administration across the pulmonary vascular bed. This is an exciting and evolving use for therapeutic aerosols.

The uses for aerosol devices vary widely, ranging from bronchodilation to insulin administration; and the range of uses for aerosol devices continues to increase. Nebulizers, pressurized metered-dose inhalers (pMDIs), and dry powder inhalers (DPIs) are often used as aerosol generators because they produce respirable particles with a mass median aerodynamic diameter (MMAD) of 0.5 to 5.0 μm.[3] Other types of nonpressurized metered dose inhalers, such as nasal sprays, produce particles in the 10- to 100-μm range, too large for pulmonary delivery Although pMDIs and DPIs are used chiefly to deliver bronchodilators and steroids, nebulizers can be used to administer antibiotics, mucoactive agents, and other drugs.[4] Given the appropriate formulation, even complex molecules can potentially be delivered by aerosol. The operating characteristics and limitations of aerosol-generating devices, how they are matched to the needs of specific patients, and how they are used largely determine the efficacy of aerosol therapy. This chapter reviews the key principles of how aerosols are generated, deposited, and administered in the neonatal and pediatric patient.

NEONATAL AND PEDIATRIC MEDICATION DELIVERY

Compared with adults, infants and children have smaller airway diameters, higher and irregular breathing rates, engage in nose breathing (which filters out large particles), and often have difficulty with mouthpiece administration. Cooperation and ability to perform aerosol inhalation techniques effectively vary with the child's age and developmental ability.

The size of the airways changes dramatically in the first years of life. Breathing patterns, flows, and volumes all change with growth and development. The resting respiratory rate decreases with age as tidal volume and minute ventilation increase. Tidal volume is approximately 7 ml/kg in the newborn, with a 300% increase

Box 13-1	Factors That Reduce Rate and Depth of Aerosol Particle Deposition in Neonatal and Pediatric Patients

- Large tongue in proportion to oral airway
- Nose breathing
- Narrow airway diameter
- Fewer and larger alveoli
- Fewer generations of airway
- More rapid respiratory rate
- Small tidal volume
- Inability to hold breath and coordinate inspiration
- High inspiratory flow rate during respiratory distress and crying

in tidal volume in the first year. Inspiratory flow also increases with vital capacity. The low tidal volume, vital capacity, functional residual capacity, and short respiratory cycles of infants result in a low residence time for small particles, resulting in a further decrease in pulmonary deposition (Box 13-1).[5]

Direct information regarding inhaled particle mass, lung deposition, and regional distribution of aerosols is limited concerning neonates, infants, and young children. Nevertheless, the data suggest that aerosol delivery is substantially less efficient for this population. Pulmonary deposition of aerosol to neonates may be less than 1% of the nominal dose being nebulized, compared with 8 to 22% in an adult.[5]

This reduced efficiency may result in infants receiving weight-appropriate dosing compared with adults. For example, the deposition efficiency of 0.5% of a standard dose of albuterol sulfate (2500 μg) would result in a lung dose of 12.5 μg, or 6.25 μg/kg for a 2-kg infant, whereas a 70-kg adult with 10% deposition has a lung dose of 250 μg, equivalent to 3.6 μg/kg. In this example, the infant actually receives a similar but slightly greater dose per unit weight. To some extent, the reduced deposition of aerosolized bronchodilators results in safety and efficacy profiles for infants and children similar to those reported for adults. Extrapolation of data from Wildhaber and colleagues[6] (Figure 13-1) demonstrates that whereas deposition from a pMDI with nonelectrostatic valved holding chamber varies with child age, the amount of drug per kilogram of body weight is consistent across ages. This suggests that the same dose that is effective for an adult will probably be safe in infants. In contrast, rationales to reduce drug doses for infants and small children have not been well substantiated in the literature.

Figure 13-2 illustrates the impact of changes in breathing patterns in the transition from infant to child to adult, with a lung simulator inhaling aerosolized drug

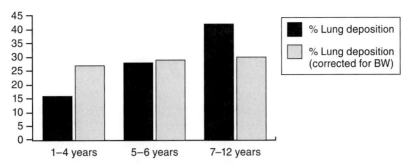

FIGURE 13-1 Although the percentage of drug deposited in the lung varies with age *(darker columns),* the percentage of lung deposition corrected for body weight *(lighter columns)* is consistent across age groups.

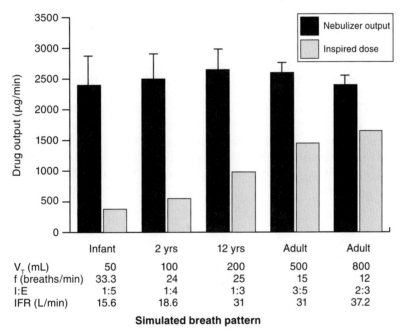

	Infant	2 yrs	12 yrs	Adult	Adult
V_T (mL)	50	100	200	500	800
f (breaths/min)	33.3	24	25	15	12
I:E	1:5	1:4	1:3	3:5	2:3
IFR (L/min)	15.6	18.6	31	31	37.2

Simulated breath pattern

FIGURE 13-2 Assessing nebulizer performance. F, frequency; I:E, ratio of inspiratory to expiratory time; IFR, inspiratory flow rate; V_T, tidal volume.

from a continuous breath enhanced nebulizer (PARI LC Star; PARI, Starnberg, Germany) producing a relatively consistent output.[7] The drug inhaled at the "mouth" of this in vitro model varies with the different simulated breath patterns, so that the infant and small child are apt to inhale less of the aerosol emitted from the nebulizer than the larger adult. Tidal volume, inspiratory-to-expiratory (I/E) ratio, and inspiratory flow rates are key to the ability to efficiently inhale output from a nebulizer. In infants less than 6 months of age, reduced inspiratory flow rates and broad I/E ratios result in less aerosol inhaled than by a larger child or adult.

These factors may decrease the rate and depth of aerosol deposition to the respiratory tract to as little as 0.1% to 1% of the medication dose placed in a nebulizer, or the dose emitted from a pMDI, regardless of whether the infant is breathing spontaneously or is intubated.[8]

AEROSOL ADMINISTRATION IN NONINTUBATED INFANTS AND CHILDREN

Limited studies are available that directly quantify deposition of aerosols in nonintubated infants and children.

Wildhaber and colleagues[9] studied children, 2 to 9 years of age, with stable asthma inhaling radiolabeled salbutamol from a nebulizer and a pMDI through a nonstatic holding chamber. Mean (absolute dose) total lung deposition expressed as a percentage of the nebulized dose was 5.4% (108 µg) in younger children (<4 yr) and 11.1% (222 µg) in older children (>4 yr). Mean (absolute dose) total lung deposition expressed as a percentage of the metered dose was 5.4% (21.6 µg) in younger children and 9.6% (38.4 µg) in older children. The authors reported equivalent percentages of total lung deposition of radiolabeled salbutamol aerosolized by either a nebulizer or a pMDI/holding chamber within each age group. However, the delivery rate per minute and the total dose of salbutamol deposited were significantly higher for the nebulizer.

DEPOSITION IN INTUBATED INFANTS

Fok and colleagues[8] measured radioaerosol deposition of salbutamol by jet nebulizer and pMDIs in ventilated and nonventilated infants with bronchopulmonary dysplasia, finding less than 1% of dose delivered to the lung in all cases (Figure 13-3). Delivery of aerosol was low for all delivery systems, and similar whether or not subjects were intubated, with considerable variability across patients. Lung deposition in the ventilated infants was similar to those obtained from previous in vitro, in vivo animal, and indirect human studies.

AEROSOL CHARACTERISTICS
Deposition of Particles

An *aerosol* is a group of particles that remain suspended in air for a relatively long time because of low terminal settling velocity. The *terminal settling velocity* of a particle is the velocity at which the particle will fall, due to gravity, through the air; it is related to the size and density of the particle. For a spherical particle, MMAD = $\delta \times \rho^{(1/2)}$, where δ is the particle diameter and ρ is the particle density.[9] Aerosols are also described by their geometric standard deviation (GSD), a measure of the particle size distribution. A *monodisperse aerosol* has a GSD less than 1.22, and a *heterodisperse aerosol* has a GSD greater than 1.22. Monodisperse aerosols are used for diagnostic and research purposes. Most therapeutic aerosols are heterodisperse, which means they contain a wider range of particle sizes. The greater the MMAD, the larger the median particle size, the greater the GSD, and the more heterodisperse is the aerosol. The particle size and size distribution of an aerosol are the major factors determining deposition efficiency and distribution in the lung.[10]

Gravitational sedimentation occurs when the aerosol particles lose inertia and settle onto the airway as a result of gravitational forces. The greater the mass of the particle, the faster it settles, affecting particles with

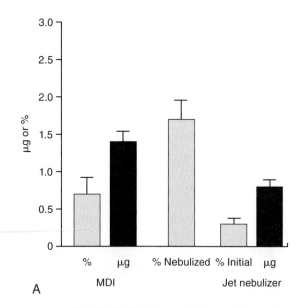
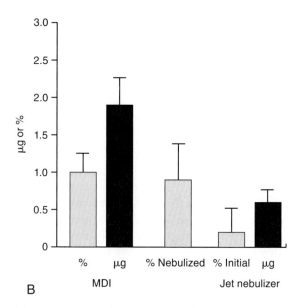

FIGURE 13-3 A dose of 200 µg of albuterol was administered by jet nebulizer or metered dose inhaler (MDI) with chamber to infants with bronchopulmonary dysplasia, between 1 and 4 kg in size, and either ventilated or nonventilated. Mean (SEM) values for lung deposition are shown in **A,** nonventilated infants (n = 13) and **B,** ventilated infants (n = 10). Values are given as the percentage of the amount delivered to the infants and, for nebulizers, also as the percentage of the initial nebulizer dose. The absolute amount (µg) of salbutamol deposited in the lungs *(solid columns)* is given for reference.

diameters of 0.5 μm or less. Breath holding for 4 to 10 seconds increases the residence time for particles in the lung, extending the time allowed for deposition through gravitational sedimentation, especially in the last six generations of the airway.[11] A breath hold can increase deposition of an aerosol by up to 10%, and is associated with a shift of deposition from the central to peripheral airways. This marginal increase in deposition may explain why breath holding has not been demonstrated to significantly improve the clinical response to aerosolized medications. Breath holding after inhalation does not appear to influence the response to administration of a bronchodilator given by DPI to children with asthma.[12]

Inertial impaction is the primary mechanism for deposition of particles with diameters of 5 μm or greater and an important mechanism for particles as small as 2 μm in diameter. A particle traveling in a stream of gas that is diverted by a turn in the airway tends to continue on its initial path, impacting with and depositing on the surface of the airway. This tendency increases with the velocity and mass of the particle. The higher the inspiratory flow of gas, such as during crying, the greater the velocity and inertia of the particles, which increase the tendency for even smaller particles to impact and deposit in large airways. Common factors that increase the rate of inertial impaction of particles larger than 2 μm include turbulent flow, bifurcations, complex passageways, narrow or obstructed airways, and inspiratory flows greater than 30 L/minute.

Diffusion, also known as brownian movement, is the primary mechanism for deposition of particles less than 3 μm in diameter in the airway. As gas reaches the more distal regions of the lung, gas flow ceases. Aerosol particles bounce against air molecules and each other and deposit on contact with the airway surfaces. Particle deposition in the particle size range of 0.5 to 3.0 μm is reported to be divided between the central and peripheral airways.[10]

Aerosol droplets in the respirable range (MMAD, 0.5 to 5.0 μm) have a better chance to deposit in the lower respiratory tract than larger or smaller particles.[10, 11] For particles greater than 0.5 μm, the depth of penetration into the lung is inversely proportional to the size of the particles, whereas particles less than 0.5 μm are so small, light, and stable that a significant proportion entering the lung do not deposit and are exhaled. Very large particles may go into suspension as an aerosol or may "rain out" before reaching the airway.

Translocation of Aerosols

To be effective as a therapeutic agent, an aerosol medication first must efficiently deposit in the airway and then must translocate across the mucous barrier, retaining bioactivity in this process. The optimal site of action depends on the agent administered. Bronchodilators and steroids need to reach the epithelium to be effective. Aerosolized antibiotics and mucolytics are most effective when dispersed in infected airway secretions at sites of maximal airway obstruction. Gene transfer therapy must not only access the epithelium through the mucous barrier but must then gain access to the submucous glands or basal progenitor cells of the epithelium.

Particle size, charge, and solubility, and the biophysical properties of secretions, all affect the ability of an aerosol to penetrate the mucous barrier. A consistent inverse relationship exists between molecular mass and particle diffusion through mucus, especially at molecular masses greater than 30 kD.[13] Turbulent flow and airway obstruction can affect the airway deposition pattern. Other factors limiting efficacy, especially of macromolecules, include binding to constituents of mucus, including mucin and DNA, and the breakdown of bioactive molecules by proteases and other enzymes. Translocation of macromolecules can be further compromised by the hypersecretion that accompanies inflammation and chronic pulmonary disease. These secretions can be a barrier to the penetration of any aerosol.[14,15]

The antibiotic diffusion barrier represented by mucin may be significant in vitro, particularly for nebulized antibiotics.[16] Some antibiotics bind to whole cystic fibrosis sputum, with the degree of binding dependent on the DNA concentration and the presence of acidic mucins.[17] Mucolytic agents might be able to increase diffusion and increase antibiotic levels in the sputum.[18] Similarly, treatment of the sputum-covered cells with recombinant human deoxyribonuclease at 50 μg/ml significantly improved gene transfer in patients with cystic fibrosis (CF).[19]

Factors promoting translocation include an effective surfactant layer and increased particle retention time. Discontinuity of mucus in the airway may assist deposition and translocation. The translocation of particles through the mucous layer is likely to depend partly on the presence of bronchial surfactant. In vitro experiments have shown that pulmonary surfactant promotes the displacement of some particles from air to the aqueous phase and that the extent of particle immersion depends on the surface tension of the surface-active film.[20,21]

Drug Dose Distribution

Dosing of aerosolized medication is an imprecise science. It is unclear how much, if any, drug is delivered to targeted areas of the lung with progressive disease states or during acute exacerbations. All the factors previously discussed decrease the rate and depth of aerosol deposition to the respiratory tract to as little as 0.5% of the medication dose placed in a nebulizer, regardless of whether the patient is breathing spontaneously or intubated. High flow increases aerosol impaction in larger airways, whereas lower inspiratory flow with high-resistance DPIs can reduce the amount of medication inhaled.

Humidity also influences medication delivery, especially for DPIs and in ventilator circuits. Droplets of solution may evaporate or grow, depending on the water content and temperature of the gas, and powder can clump or aggregate in high humidity. High ambient humidity can also result from a child exhaling into a DPI or from a DPI being brought into a warm indoor environment from the cold outdoors (or from inside a car on a very cold day), with condensation forming inside the device.[22]

Drug formulations dictate in part which aerosol options are available for medication delivery. Most solutions can be nebulized if the medication is soluble (corticosteroids are a notable exception), but the physical characteristics of the solution (or suspension) can affect particle size and nebulizer output. Furthermore, some macromolecules may not enter suspension well and can shatter into nonbioactive forms with the force of air required to generate an aerosol. Because of development costs, many aerosol medications are initially developed as nebulizer solutions and later reformulated for DPI or pMDI delivery.

Theoretically, if a particle can be milled to a respirable size while retaining bioactivity, it can be delivered by DPI or pMDI. However, development costs are greater for these devices than for nebulizer solutions. At present, DPI formulations are limited to only a few preparations. With more effective DPI devices being developed and the need to eliminate chlorofluorocarbon (CFC)–based propellants in accordance with the Montreal Protocol on Substances that Deplete the Ozone Layer (see http://www.unep.org/OZONE/pdfs/Montreal-Protocol2000.pdf), it is anticipated that a greater variety of DPI medications and devices will soon be commercially available. A greater variety of formulations are available for pMDIs, and more are being developed for the newer hydrofluoroalkane (HFA)–based pMDIs.

AEROSOL DELIVERY

The most common methods of generating therapeutic aerosols are with nebulizers (jet pneumatic, ultrasonic [USN], and vibrating mesh [VMN]) and inhalers (pMDIs and DPIs). Older methods based on the spray "atomizer" or the addition of medications to room humidifiers are ineffective, and their use should be discouraged.

Pneumatic Nebulizers

Pneumatic nebulizers use the Bernoulli principle to drive a high-pressure gas through a restricted orifice and draw the fluid into the gas stream from a capillary tube immersed in the solution. Shearing of the fluid stream in the jet forms the aerosol stream that impacts against a baffle removing larger particles that may return to the reservoir.

An effective pneumatic nebulizer should deliver more than 50% of its total dose as aerosol in the respirable range in 10 minutes or less of nebulization time. Performance varies with diluent volume, operating flow, pressures, gas density, and manufacturer.[23] The amount of drug that is nebulized increases as the volume of diluent is increased. The residual volume of medicine that remains in commercial small-volume nebulizers (SVNs) varies from 0.5 to 2.0 ml depending on the specific device; thus increasing the fill volume allows a greater proportion of the active medication to be nebulized. For example, with a residual volume of 1 ml, a fill of 2 ml would leave only 50% of the nebulizer charge available for nebulization, whereas a fill of 4 ml would make 3 ml, or 75%, of the medication available for nebulization. No significant difference in clinical response has been shown with varying diluent volumes and flow rates.[24]

Droplet size and nebulization times are both inversely proportional to gas flow through the jet. Proper operating gas flow varies with each model of nebulizer, from 2 L/minute (MiniHEART; Westmed Inc., Tucson, AZ) to 10 L/minute (Misty Max: Cardinal Health, Dublin, OH). For any given nebulizer, the higher the flow to the nebulizer, the smaller the particle size generated and the shorter the time required to nebulize the full dose.[25, 26] Nebulizers that produce smaller particle sizes by use of baffles such as one-way valves may have a lower total drug output per minute than the same nebulizer without baffling, requiring more time to deliver a standard dose of medication.

Gas density affects both aerosol generation and delivery of aerosol to the lungs, especially with low-density helium–oxygen mixtures. The lower the density of a carrier gas, the less turbulent the flow, which theoretically decreases aerosol impaction, allowing more aerosol to pass beyond an obstructed airway.[27] This is true with virtually any aerosol, with high-concentration heliox increasing aerosol delivery by as much as 50%. Heliox concentrations as low as 40% can improve aerosol delivery. When using heliox to drive a jet nebulizer, the aerosol output is much less than with air or oxygen, requiring double the flow to produce a comparable output of respirable aerosol per minute. Thus, although helium can increase the amount of aerosol reaching the lungs, it impairs the production of aerosol from jet nebulizers.[28]

Humidity and temperature affect the particle size and the concentration of drug remaining in the nebulizer. Evaporation of water and adiabatic expansion of gas can reduce the temperature of the aerosol to as much as 5° C below ambient temperature. Aerosol particles entrained into a warm and fully saturated gas stream increase in size. These particles can also stick together, further increasing the MMAD, and with a DPI this can severely compromise the output of respirable particles.

With three different fill volumes, albuterol delivery from a nebulizer was found to cease after the onset of inconsistent nebulization (sputtering).[29] Aerosol output declined by one half within 20 seconds of the onset of sputtering. The concentration of albuterol in the nebulizer cup increased significantly once the aerosol output declined, and further weight loss in the nebulizer was caused primarily by evaporation. The conclusion was that aerosolization past the point of initial jet nebulizer sputter is ineffective.

Nebulizer selection affects aerosol delivery. Only nebulizers that have been shown to work reliably under specific conditions, with specific medications, and with specific compressors should be used.[30] When used to treat small children or during mechanical ventilation, nebulizers producing aerosols with an MMAD of 0.5 to 3.0 μm are more likely to achieve greater deposition in the lower respiratory tract.[5]

Continuous aerosol generation wastes medication because the aerosol is produced throughout the respiratory cycle and is largely lost to the atmosphere (Figure 13-4, A). Patients with an I/E ratio of 1:3 lose a minimum of 75% of the aerosol generated to the atmosphere. If only 50% of the dose is available from the nebulizer as aerosol in the respiratory range and only 25% of that is inhaled by the patient, it is clear that less than 10% deposition is typically measured with nebulizer therapy.

A reservoir on the expiratory limb of the nebulizer conserves drug aerosol.[30] A simple approach is to place 6 in. of aerosol tubing on the expiratory side of the nebulizer T-tube device. Alternatively, select a commercial device such as the Piper (Piper Medical Products) or Circulaire (Westmed, Tucson, Ariz) system. These simple bag reservoirs hold the aerosol generated during exhalation, allowing the small particles to remain in suspension for inhalation with the next breath while larger particles rain out.

As another alternative to continuous nebulization, the thumb control port allows the patient to direct gas to the nebulizer only on inspiration. This improves efficiency only if there is good hand–breath coordination. Rather than having the patient control when nebulization occurs, a one-way valve system can be used to reduce aerosol waste.[31] Breath-enhanced nebulizers may increase inhaled dose by as much as 50% (see Figure 13-4, B).

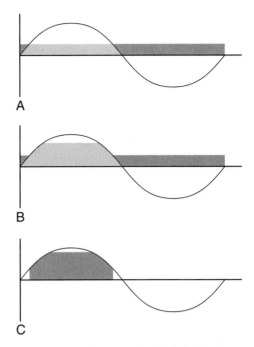

FIGURE 13-4 Aerosol generated and inhaled during nebulization therapy. **A,** Continuous nebulization; **B,** breath-enhanced nebulization; **C,** breath-actuated nebulization.

Breath-actuated nebulization occurs by generating aerosol in synchrony with inspiration. Nebulizing only during inspiration is more efficient than continuous or vented systems (see Figure 13-4, C). Breath-actuated nebulizers deliver the same or greater dose in the same amount of time as the continuous nebulizer. However, to nebulize the same total dose placed in the nebulizer, the breath-actuated system may take four times longer (delivering four times more drug) than the continuous nebulizer. The most primitive method of synchronization is the use of a thumb port control, requiring the operator to cover the port during inspiration. On the other extreme, the HaloLite and Prodose AAD (adaptive aerosol delivery) systems (Philips Respironics, Murrysville, Pa) use a microprocessor and pressure transducer to regulate nebulization during the first half of inspiration. The AeroEclipse (Monaghan Medical, Plattsburgh, NY) is a purely pneumatic device that nebulizes only during inspiration.

A typical dose of albuterol sulfate solution is 2.5 mg (2500 μg). If only 34% (850 μg) leaves the nebulizer and is inhaled by the patient, and some of that drug deposits in the upper airways (50 μg) and is exhaled (500 μg), it should not be surprising that 12% deposition of the nominal dose, typical of ambulatory adult patients, would be 300 μg (Figure 13-5). In small children and infants, deposition can be less than 1%, representing less than 25 μg delivered to the lung.

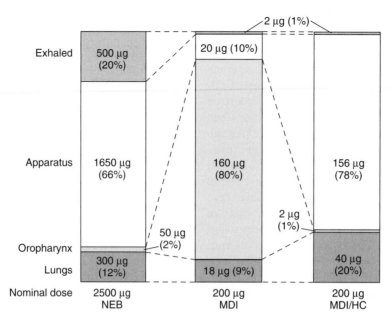

FIGURE 13-5 Distribution of albuterol delivered via nebulizer (NEB), pressurized metered-dose inhaler (MDI), and pressurized metered-dose inhaler with holding chamber (MDI/HC).

Gas pressure and flow affect particle size distribution and output. A nebulizer that produces an MMAD of 2.5 μm when driven by a gas source at 50 psi with a flow rate of 6 to 10 L/minute may produce an MMAD greater than 8 μm when used with a home compressor (or ventilator) providing only 10 psi. Insufficient flow can result in negligible respirable nebulizer output. As a consequence, nebulizers used for home care should be matched to the compressor on the basis of data supplied by the manufacturer so that the specific combination of equipment will efficiently nebulize the desired medications prescribed. European standards require equipment manufacturers to demonstrate that their nebulizer and compressor combination can nebulize the appropriate fill volume of drug within 10 minutes, deliver more than 50% of the drug in the nebulizer as respirable particles, and identify all medications with which the nebulizer and compressor might reliably meet these two criteria.[32] Until such time that standards are required in the United States, clinicians should ascertain that patients are prescribed only systems that have been demonstrated to meet these criteria.

Repeated use of a nebulizer will not alter the MMAD, or output, as long as it is properly cleaned (rinsed and dried between treatments). Failure to clean the nebulizer properly results in degradation of performance from clogging the jet (Venturi) nebulizer to increasing bacterial contamination, and buildup of electrostatic charge in the device.[33] The Centers for Disease Control and Prevention (CDC, Atlanta, Ga) recommend cleaning and disinfecting nebulizers or rinsing with sterile water between uses, and then air drying.[34] Storage of multidose solutions at room temperature and reuse of syringes to measure the solution represent the main sources of nebulizer microbial contamination.[35] Refrigerating the solution and disposing of syringes every 24 hours help to eliminate bacterial contamination.

Large-volume Nebulizer

The large-volume pneumatic nebulizer (LVN) has a reservoir volume greater than 100 ml and can be used to administer an aerosol solution over a prolonged time. Indications for using an LVN to administer a bland solution (i.e., sterile water or saline) include the need to humidify medical gases when the upper airway is bypassed, control stridor with a cold aerosol, and induce sputum. Because nebulizers provide a route of transmission for pathogens, pass-over humidifiers and heater wire humidifiers are preferable.

LVNs work on the same principles as SVNs, except that the residual volume is greater and the effects of evaporation, changing the concentration of medication over time, are more profound.

Caution should be exercised when using LVNs with incubators or hoods because of the noise produced. The American Academy of Pediatrics recommends a sound level less than 58 dB to avoid hearing loss in patients in incubators and hoods. Many LVNs are designed to deliver controlled concentrations of oxygen and use a Venturi system to entrain air into the stream of gas administered to the patient. Standard entrainment nebulizers may deliver a fractional concentration of delivered oxygen approaching 1.00 but cannot provide a fractional concentration of inspired oxygen (F_{IO_2}) greater than 0.40. High-flow nebulizers are designed to deliver high flow rates of oxygen, bringing the F_{IO_2} up to 0.60 to 0.80. Closed dilution and gas injection nebulizers provide high-flow access to the nebulizer from two gas sources, allowing gas to mix without compromising F_{IO_2}.

Small-particle Aerosol Generator

The small-particle aerosol generator (SPAG; Valeant Pharmaceuticals International, Aliso Viejo, Calif) is a jet aerosol generator used to nebulize the antiviral agent ribavirin (Figure 13-6). The SPAG incorporates a secondary drying chamber that reduces the MMAD to 1.2 μm, with a GSD of 1.4 and relatively high output. The SPAG reduces the 50 psi of line pressure medical gas to 26 psi, which supplies gas to separate flowmeters controlling flow to the nebulizer and the drying chamber. As the aerosol leaves the medication reservoir, it enters the long cylindrical drying chamber, where additional flow of dry gas reduces the size of the aerosol particles through evaporation. The nebulizer flow is adjusted to maximum, approximately 7 L/minute, with a total flow from both flowmeters equal to at least 15 L/minute.

Ribavirin is an expensive antiviral agent that has been used to treat high-risk infants and children with severe respiratory syncytial viral infections. The effectiveness of ribavirin is poor, with few data to support its use for such a broad population. In addition, concerns about the second-hand exposure of health care workers to ribavirin have resulted in recommendations to avoid open-air administration, use specific room filtration techniques, and use personal protective equipment for staff and visitors.[36] Ribavirin tends to precipitate into a thick powder that forms on the surfaces of tubing and tents. Recommendations for ribavirin use are now limited to treatment of patients who have severe respiratory syncytial virus infection and require mechanical ventilation.[37] Risks of using ribavirin during mechanical ventilation include delivering excessive volume and pressure, so that care should be taken to place and frequently change filters in the expiratory limb of the circuit.[38]

Ultrasonic Nebulizers

The ultrasonic nebulizer (USN) uses a piezoelectric crystal vibrating at a high frequency (1.3 to 1.4 mHz) to create an aerosol. The crystal transducer converts electricity to sound waves, which creates motion and standing waves in the liquid immediately above the transducer, forming a geyser of droplets (Figure 13-7). USNs are capable of a broader range of aerosol output (0.5 to 7.0 ml/min) and higher aerosol densities than most conventional jet nebulizers. Particle size is affected by frequency, whereas output is affected by the amplitude of the signal. Particle size is inversely proportional to the frequency of vibrations. Frequency is

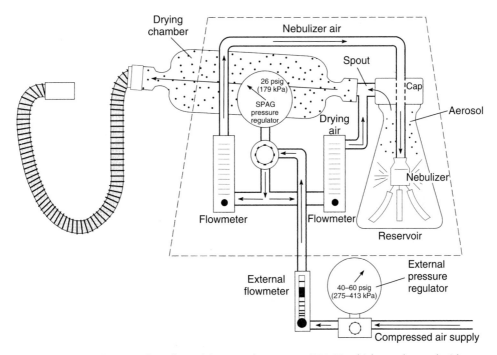

FIGURE 13-6 Diagram of small-particle aerosol generator (SPAG), which may be used with a hood, tent, mask, or ventilator. psig, Pounds-force per square inch gauge.

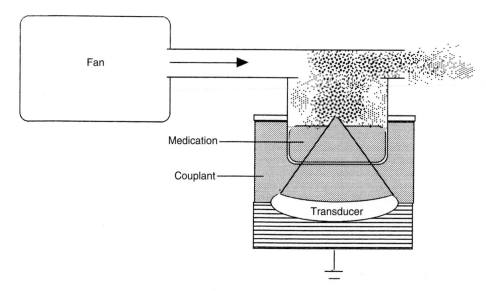

FIGURE 13-7 Aerosol is produced in an ultrasonic nebulizer by focusing sound waves, which disrupt the surface of the fluid, creating a standing wave that produces droplets. Flow from a fan pushes the aerosol out of the chamber.

device specific and is not user adjustable. For example, the DeVilbiss Porta-Sonic (DeVilbiss Healthcare, Somerset, Pa) operates at a frequency of 2.25 MHz and produces a MMAD of 2.5 μm, and the DeVilbiss Pulmo-Sonic operates at 1.25 MHz and produces particles in the 4- to 6-μm range. Large-volume USNs, used mainly for bland aerosol therapy or sputum induction, incorporate air blowers to carry the mist to the patient. Low flow rates of gas through the nebulizer are associated with higher mist density. Unlike jet nebulizers, which cool through evaporation, USNs increase the temperature of the drug during use, which is associated with increased concentration; however, some medications may be denatured by the increased operating temperature.[39]

A number of small-volume USNs are available for aerosol drug delivery.[40] Unlike the larger reservoir USNs, these systems do not always use a water-filled couplant compartment; instead, medication is placed directly into the manifold on top of the transducer connected to a battery power source. The patient's inspiratory flow draws the aerosol from the nebulizer into the lungs. As the USN operates, the aerosol remains in the medication cup/chamber until a flow of gas draws the aerosol from the nebulizer. Thus, during exhalation, aerosol generated by the USN remains in the chamber, awaiting the next breath.

Small-volume USNs may have less residual drug volume than SVNs, reducing the need for a large quantity of diluent to ensure delivery of drugs. The contained portable power source provides convenience and mobility. These advantages of USNs may be outweighed by

their high cost, however, which can be several orders of magnitude greater than that of pMDI therapy. USNs have been promoted for administration of a wide variety of formulations, ranging from bronchodilators to antiinflammatory agents and antibiotics.[41] In general, however, USNs have been shown to be less effective than other aerosol delivery devices.[42] This is particularly true with suspensions.

Several hazards, in addition to bacterial contamination, are associated with using a USN. The high-density aerosol from USNs has been associated with bronchospasm, increased airway resistance, and irritability in a substantial portion of the population.[43] Overhydration may occur when using a USN for prolonged treatment of a neonate, small child, or patients with renal insufficiency. The structure of the medication may be disrupted by acoustic power output rated greater than 50 W/cm[2].[44,45] Several ventilator manufacturers have provided USNs for administration of aerosols during mechanical ventilation. The advantage of the USN during ventilation is that no driving gas flow is added to the circuit, changing ventilator parameters and alarm settings.[46] Disadvantages may be the weight of the USN in the ventilator circuit, a tendency to heat up over time, and the potential for reduced therapeutic efficacy of medications.

Vibrating Mesh Nebulizers

Vibrating mesh nebulizers (VMNs) use electricity to stimulate a piezo element to vibrate a ceramic or metal disk, which in turn presses or pumps medication through multiple orifices. Particle size is dependent on the diameter of the orifices through which the medication passes, and VMNs can be manufactured to produce specific MMADs between 2 and 6 μm. VMNs typically operate at one tenth the frequency and consume less than one tenth the power of a USN, so medications are not heated or reconcentrated. This class of nebulizer can efficiently nebulize suspensions, with mean particle sizes that are smaller than the diameter of the apertures. These nebulizers are quite efficient, having residual drug volumes of medication ranging from 1 to 100 μl. Because the VMN does not add gas to the patient airway or ventilator circuit, greater aerosol concentrations can be reached than with jet nebulizers. VMNs produce the same size aerosol particles with air, oxygen or helium. Handheld VMN nebulizers tend to be much more efficient than continuous jet nebulizers or USNs, with inhaled mass ranging from 25 to 55%. When used with mechanical ventilators, VMNs do not change volumes or flows.

Pressurized Metered-dose Inhalers

The pressurized metered-dose inhaler (pMDI) is the most frequently prescribed device for aerosol delivery. pMDIs are used to administer bronchodilators, anticholinergics, and antiinflammatory agents. More drug formulations are available for administration by pMDIs than by any other nebulization system. Properly used, pMDIs are at least as effective as other nebulizers for drug delivery.[47] Therefore pMDIs are often the preferred method for delivering bronchodilators to spontaneously breathing, as well as intubated, ventilated patients.[48]

A pMDI is a pressurized canister containing a drug in the form of a micronized powder or solution that is suspended with a mixture of propellants along with a surfactant or a dispersal agent (Figure 13-8).[5] Dispersing agents are present in concentrations equal to or greater than that of the medication. In some patients these agents may be associated with coughing and wheezing.[49] The bulk of the spray, up to 80% by weight, is composed of a propellant, typically a CFC such as Freon. Adverse reactions to CFCs are extremely rare.[50-52] Because of international agreements to ban CFCs (Montreal Protocol on Substances that Deplete the Ozone Layer), new pMDIs are being developed to use more environmentally safe propellants such as HFA-134a. The U.S. Food and Drug Administration has mandated transition from CFC pMDIs by December 31, 2008. As HFA pMDIs are introduced, they represent newer technologies with potentially improved performance.

The output volume of the pMDI varies from 30 to 100 μl and contains 20 μg to 5 mg of drug. Lung deposition is estimated as between 10% and 25% in adults, with high intersubject variability largely dependent on

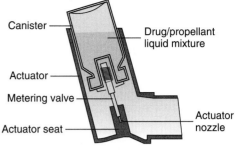
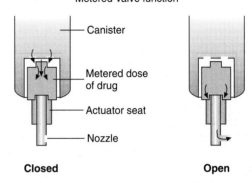

FIGURE 13-8 Cross-sectional diagrams of a pressurized metered-dose inhaler.

user technique. When proper technique is used, the pMDI delivers as much or more of the dose of medication to the lung than an SVN.

The pMDI canister contains a pressurized mixture containing propellants, surfactants, preservatives, and sometimes flavoring agents, with approximately 1% of the total contents being active drug. This mixture is released from the canister through a metering valve and stem that fits into an actuator boot, designed and tested by the manufacturer to work with the specific formulation. Small changes in actuator design can change the characteristics and output of the aerosol from a pMDI.

Up to 80% of the emitted dose from a pMDI impacts in the oropharynx. Actuation of a pMDI into a valved holding chamber decreases impaction losses by reducing the velocity of the aerosol jet,[5] allowing time for evaporation of the propellants and for the particles to "age" before impacting on a surface. The nominal dose of medication with a pMDI is much smaller than with a nebulizer. The quantity of albuterol exiting the actuator nozzle of a pMDI is 100 μg with each actuation, or 90 μg from the opening of the actuator boot; this is how pMDI aerosol actuations are characterized in the United States. Thus a dose of 2 to 4 actuations (200- to 400-μg nominal dose) is typically used. In ambulatory patients, 10% deposition may deliver a dose of 20 to 40 µg for an effective bronchodilator response.

Technique

Effective use of a pMDI is technique dependent. Up to two thirds of patients who use pMDIs and health professionals who prescribe pMDIs do not perform the procedure well enough to derive benefit from the medication.[53,54] Box 13-2 outlines the recommended steps for self-administering a bronchodilator with a pMDI.[55] Good patient instruction can take 10 to 30 minutes and should include demonstration, return demonstration, practice, and confirmation of patient performance (demonstration placebo units should be available for this purpose). Repeated instruction with every visit improves performance.[56]

All pMDIs require priming, firing one to four actuations, before first use, and after the device has not been used for a prolonged period of time (1 to 4 d). The HFA pMDIs require less frequent priming than CFC devices (check the label for each specific device).

Problems with home use of pMDI devices include not only poor technique but also poor storage. The pMDI should always be stored with cap on, both to prevent foreign objects from entering the boot and to reduce humidity and microbial contamination.[56]

Each type of pMDI contains a specific number of actuations (between 60 and 400 actuations). After those doses have been administered the pMDI will continue to actuate, with or without medication emitted (tailing-off effect), placing the patient at risk of not receiving prescribed medication. Pressurized MDIs should always be discarded when empty to avoid administering propellant without medication. The suggestion that pMDIs can be tested for drug remaining by floating the canister in water has proven not to be accurate and to compromise performance for the pMDI.

It is more accurate for the patient or parent to note when the medication was started, the number of doses to be taken each day, and the number of doses in the canister, and from this information to calculate a discard date. For example, if 200 actuations are in a canister (information always indicated on the canister label) and 4 "puffs" are taken per day, the canister should be discarded 50 days, or 7 weeks, after the start date. This discard date should be written on the canister label on the day the new canister is started. A more user-friendly alternative is to attach a dose counter to the pMDI. In the near future, the U.S. Food and Drug Administration will require new pMDIs to be manufactured with dose counters. Because pMDIs deposit up to 80% of their emitted dose in the oro- and hypopharynx, patients should "rinse and spit" to remove excess drug from the mouth and back of the throat.

Infants, young children up to age 3 years, and patients in acute distress may not be able to use a pMDI effectively. A "cold Freon effect" can occur when the aerosol plume reaches the back of the mouth and the patient stops inhaling. These problems can be corrected by using the proper pMDI accessory device (see the next section).

Accessory Devices

Various pMDI accessory devices have been developed to overcome the primary limitations of pMDI administration: hand–breath coordination problems, high oropharyngeal deposition, and difficulty in tracking doses. Accessory devices include flow-triggered pMDIs, spacers, valved holding chambers, and dose counters.

Flow-triggered Device. The Maxair Autohaler (Graceway Pharmaceuticals, Bristol, Tenn) and Easyhaler (Orion Pharma, Espoo, Finland) are flow-triggered pMDIs designed to reduce the need for hand–breath coordination by firing in response to the patient's inspiratory effort.[57] To use the Autohaler, the patient cocks a lever on the top of the unit that spring-loads the canister against a vane mechanism. When the patient's inspiratory flow exceeds 30 L/minute, the vane moves, allowing the canister to be pressed into the actuator, firing the pMDI. This device is available only with the

Box 13-2	Optimal Self-administration Technique for Using Pressurized Metered-dose Inhaler

1. Warm pMDI canister to hand or body temperature.
2. Shake the canister vigorously.
3. Assemble the apparatus, and uncap the mouthpiece.
4. Ensure that no loose objects are in the device that could be aspirated or could obstruct outflow.
5. Open the mouth wide.
6. Keep the tongue from obstructing the mouthpiece.
7. Hold the pMDI vertically with the outlet aimed at the mouth.
8. Place the canister outlet between the lips, or position the pMDI 4 cm (two fingers) away from the mouth.*
9. Breathe out normally.
10. Begin to breathe in slowly (less than 0.5 L/s).
11. Squeeze and actuate ("fire") the pMDI.
12. Continue to inhale to total lung capacity.
13. Hold breath for 4 to 10 seconds.
14. Wait 30 seconds between inhalations (actuations).
15. Disassemble the apparatus, and recap the mouthpiece.

pMDI, Pressurized metered-dose inhaler.
*Open mouth technique is not recommended with ipratropium bromide.

β-agonist pirbuterol in the United States, but other formulations are in development. The Easyhaler has been introduced in Europe with several medications, and may soon be available in North America The flow required to actuate these devices may be too great for some children to generate, especially during acute exacerbations of disease.

Spacers and Holding Chambers. When properly designed, spacers and valved holding chambers do the following:

- Reduce oropharyngeal deposition of drug
- Relieve the bad taste of some medications by reducing oral deposition
- Eliminate the cold Freon effect
- Decrease aerosol MMAD
- Increase respirable particle mass
- Improve lower respiratory tract deposition
- Significantly improve therapeutic effects[40,56,58]

Spacers should be differentiated from valved holding chambers. A spacer device is a simple open-ended tube, chamber, or bag that has sufficiently large volume to provide space for the pMDI plume to expand by allowing the propellant to evaporate. To perform this function, a spacer device must have an internal volume greater than 100 ml and must provide a distance of 10 to 13 cm between the pMDI nozzle and the first wall or baffle. Smaller, inefficient spacers can reduce respiratory dose by 60% and offer no protection against poor coordination between actuation and breathing pattern. Spacers with internal volumes greater than 100 ml generally provide some protection against early firing of the pMDI, although exhaling immediately after the actuation clears most of the aerosol from the device, wasting the dose.

The valved holding chamber, usually 140 to 750 ml in volume, allows the plume from the pMDI to expand. It incorporates a one-way valve that permits the aerosol to be drawn from the chamber during inhalation only, diverting the exhaled gas to the atmosphere and not disturbing the remaining aerosol suspended in the chamber (Figure 13-9). Patients with small tidal volumes may empty the aerosol from the chamber with five to six breaths, except when there is a large dead space. A valved holding chamber can also incorporate a mask for use by an infant or child. These devices allow effective pMDI administration in a patient who is unable to use a mouthpiece because of size, age, coordination, or mental status.[59] With infants these masks should have minimal dead space, should be comfortable on the child's face, and should have a valved chamber that will open and close with the low inspiratory flow and volume generated by the patient. Box 13-3 describes the correct technique for using a pMDI with a holding chamber.

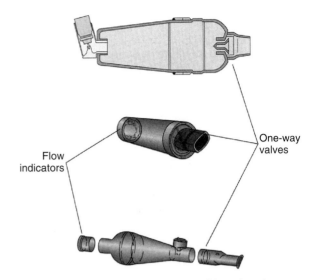

FIGURE 13-9 Metered dose inhaler holding chambers are spacers with one-way valves that allow the chamber to be emptied only when the patient inhales, by preventing the exhaled gas from re-entering the chamber.

Valved holding chambers, which reduce the need to coordinate breathing with actuation, should be used with infants, small children, and any child taking steroids. In addition, the chambers reduce the pharyngeal dose of aerosol from the pMDI 10- to 15-fold over administration without a holding chamber. This decreases the total body dose from swallowed medications, which is an important consideration with steroid administration.[58,60,61]

Box 13-3	Optimal Technique for Using Pressurized Metered-dose Inhaler With Valved Holding Chamber

1. Warm the pMDI to hand or body temperature.
2. Shake the canister vigorously, holding it vertically.
3. Assemble the apparatus.
4. Ensure that no loose objects are in the device that could be aspirated or could obstruct outflow.
5. Place the holding chamber in the mouth (or place the mask completely over the nose and mouth), encouraging the patient to breathe through the mouth.
6. Have the patient breathe normally, and actuate at the beginning of inspiration.
7. For small children and infants, have them continue to breathe through the device for five or six breaths.
8. For patients who can cooperate and clear the chamber with one breath, encourage larger breaths with breath holding.
9. Allow 30 seconds between actuations.

pMDI, Pressurized metered-dose inhaler.

The high percentage of oropharyngeal drug deposition with steroid pMDIs can increase the risk of oral yeast infections (thrush). Rinsing the mouth after steroid can reduce this problem, but most pMDI steroid aerosol impaction occurs deeper in the pharynx, which is not easily rinsed. For this reason, steroid MDIs should always be used in combination with a valved holding chamber.

Wheezing Infants

Valved holding chambers make pMDIs as reliable as SVNs for aerosol administration. In one study, 34 infants between 1 and 24 months of age and with acute asthma received two doses of terbutaline, 20 minutes apart, as either 2 mg/dose in 2.8 ml of 0.9% saline by nebulizer or as 0.5 mg/dose (5 puffs) by pMDI with a valved holding chamber.[62] No difference was found in the rate of improvement or clinical score, and both devices were reported equally effective. Similarly, 60 children 6 years of age or less who had an acute asthma exacerbation were randomized to receive albuterol through a nebulizer or pMDI with valved holding chamber for three treatments over 1 hour.[63] All patients showed improvement over baseline, with no difference between treatment groups.

In another study, 84 children were enrolled in the emergency department to receive inhaled medication with or without a valved holding chamber to determine whether a single brief demonstration of the proper use of a valved holding chamber would result in improved outcomes.[64] The valved holding chamber group reported significantly faster resolution of wheezing, fewer days of cough, and fewer missed days of school.

Evidence-based research does not support the belief that an SVN is better than a pMDI if the patient is not able to inhale with optimal technique. In fact, if unable to perform an optimal maneuver with a pMDI, the patient cannot perform an optimal maneuver with an SVN. Although optimal technique is always preferred, it is often difficult to attain with an infant, small child, or severely dyspneic patient. For such patients, an alternative may be to increase the pMDI or nebulizer dose (see later discussion).

Care and Cleaning

Particles containing drug settle and deposit within these devices, causing a whitish buildup on the inner chamber walls. This residual drug poses no risk to the patient but should be rinsed out periodically. After washing a plastic chamber or spacer with tap water, it is less effective for the next 10 to 15 puffs, until the static charge in the chamber (which attracts small particles) is once again reduced. Use of regular dish soap to wash the chamber reduces or eliminates this static charge. Metal and non-electrostatic plastic spacers should be cleaned as recommended by their manufacturers.

Accessory devices either use the manufacturer-designed boot that comes with the pMDI or incorporate a "universal canister adapter" to fire the pMDI canister. Different formulations of pMDI drugs operate at different pressures, and devices have different orifice sizes in the boot specifically designed for use exclusively with the specific pMDI. Output characteristics of pMDIs will change when using an adapter with a different-size orifice; therefore spacers or holding chambers with universal canister adapters should be avoided. Devices that include the manufacturer's boot with the pMDI should be used, when available.

Dry Powder Inhalers

Dry powder inhalers (DPIs) create aerosols by drawing air through a dose of dry powder medication. The powder contains micronized drug particles (MMAD less than 5 μm) with larger lactose or glucose particles (greater than 30 to 100 μm in diameter), or it contains micronized drug particles bound into loose aggregates.[65] Micronized particles adhere strongly to each other and to most surfaces. Addition of the larger particles of the carrier decreases cohesive forces in the micronized drug powder so that separation into individual respirable particles (deaggregation) occurs more readily. Thus the carrier particles aid the flow of the drug powder from the device. These carriers also act as "fillers" by adding bulk to the powder when the unit dose of a drug is small. Usually the drug particles are loosely bound to the carrier,[66] and they are stripped from the carrier by the energy provided by the patient's inhalation (Figure 13-10). The release of respirable particles of the drug requires inspiration at relatively high flow (30 to 120 L/min).[67,68] A high inspiratory flow results in pharyngeal impaction of the larger carrier particles that comprise the bulk of the aerosol and, as with pMDIs, results in up to 80% of the drug dose being deposited in the oro- and hypopharynx. Impaction of lactose carrier particles gives the patient the sensation of having inhaled a dose. Like with pMDIs, patients should rinse and spit after inhalation of steroid preparations from a DPI.

The internal geometry of the DPI device influences the resistance offered to inspiration and the inspiratory flow required to deaggregate and aerosolize the medication. Devices with higher resistance require a higher inspiratory flow to produce a dose. Inhalation through high-resistance DPIs may improve drug delivery to the lower respiratory tract compared with pMDIs as long as the patient can reliably generate the required flow rate.[50,69] High-resistance devices have not been shown to improve either deposition or bronchodilation compared with low-resistance DPIs. DPIs with multiple components require correct assembly of the apparatus and priming of the device to ensure aerosolization of

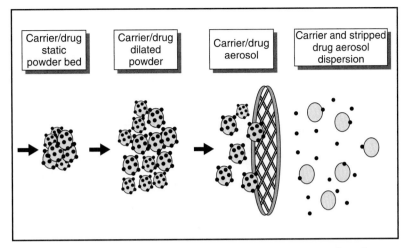

FIGURE 13-10 As patient inhales through a dry powder inhaler, inspiratory flow deaggregates particles from the powder bed or capsule and is drawn through a screen that strips the small drug particles from the larger carrier particles, creating an aerosol dispersion.

the dry powder. Periodic brushing is needed to remove any residual powder accumulated within some DPIs.

DPIs produce aerosols in which most of the drug particles are in the respirable range, with distribution of particle sizes (GSD) differing significantly among various DPIs.[51] High ambient humidity produces clumping of the dry powder, creating larger particles that are not as effectively aerosolized.[52] Air with a high moisture content is less efficient at deaggregating particles of dry powder than dry air, such that high ambient humidity increases the size of drug particles in the aerosol and may reduce drug delivery to the lung. Newer DPI devices contain individual doses more protected from humidity. Humidity can accumulate once the device is opened, or if the DPI is stored with the cap off, or by condensation when the device is brought from a very cold environment into a warmer area.

Because the energy from the patient's inspiratory flow disperses the drug powder, the magnitude and duration of the patient's inspiratory effort influence aerosol generation from a DPI.[70] Failure to perform inhalation at a sufficiently fast inspiratory flow reduces the dose of the drug emitted from DPIs and increases the distribution of particle sizes within the aerosol with a variety of devices.[71,72] For example, the Advair Diskus (GlaxoSmithKline, London, UK) delivers approximately 90% of the labeled dose at an inspiratory flow ranging from 30 to 90 L/minute, whereas the dose delivered by the high-resistance Pulmicort Turbuhaler (AstraZeneca, Lund, Sweden) is significantly lower at an inspiratory flow of 30 L/minute compared with the dose delivered at 90 L/minute. The variability between doses at different inspiratory flows is higher with the Turbuhaler.[73,74] Figure 13-11 shows the effect of two inspiratory flows

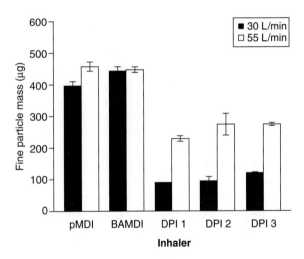

FIGURE 13-11 Fine particle mass delivered from a 100-μg target dose (±SD) as a function of flow rate. pMDI, Pressurized metered-dose inhaler; BAMDI, breath-actuated MDI (Autohaler); DPI 1, Rotahaler; DPI 2, Turbuhaler; DPI 3, Diskhaler.

(30 and 55 L/min) when using a pMDI, a breath-actuated MDI (Autohaler), a Rotahaler (previously GlaxoSmithKline) (DPI 1), a Turbuhaler (DPI 2), and a Diskhaler (GlaxoSmithKline) (DPI 3).[75] The peak inspiratory flow rate of children is limited and associated with age, making it unlikely that a child less than 6 years old could reliably empty a DPI requiring greater than 50 L/minute (Figure 13-12).[75]

Active DPI devices such as the Exubera inhaler (Pfizer, New York, NY) use compressed gas to disperse the powder into a reservoir chamber from which it can be inhaled. Aerosol production and airway deposition, when using these devices, are influenced by the patient's

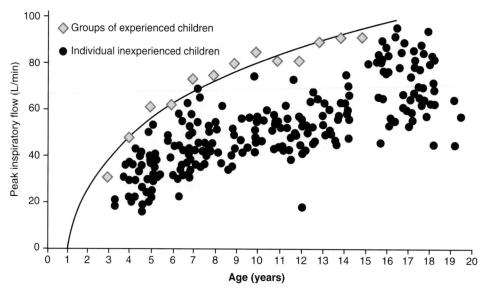

FIGURE 13-12 Peak inspiratory flows in individual inexperienced children and in groups of experienced children.

inspiratory flow to a lesser extent than with DPIs that rely solely on patient effort for aerosol production.

Breath coordination is also important when using DPIs. Exhalation into a DPI blows out the powder from the device and reduces drug delivery. Moreover, the humidity in the exhaled air reduces subsequent aerosol generation from the DPI. Therefore patients must be instructed not to exhale into a DPI.

DPIs are breath actuated and reduce the problem of coordinating inspiration with actuation. The technique of using DPIs differs in important respects from the technique employed to inhale drugs from a pMDI (Table 13-1). Although DPIs are easier to use than pMDIs, up to 25% of patients may use DPIs improperly.[75] DPIs are critically dependent on inspiratory airflow to generate

the aerosol. Thus they should be used with caution, if at all, in the very young or ill child, weak patients, elderly persons, and those with altered mental status. Patients may need repeated instruction before they can master the technique of using DPIs, and periodic assessment is necessary to ensure that patients continue to use an optimal technique.[75] Clinicians must also learn the correct technique of using DPIs to train their patients in the proper use of these devices.

DEVICE SELECTION AND COMPLIANCE

Whenever possible, patients should use only one type of aerosol-generating device for inhalation therapy. Each type requires a different technique, and repeated instruction is necessary to ensure that the patient uses a device appropriately. The use of different devices for inhalation can be confusing for patients and may decrease their compliance with therapy. This has been referred to as "device dementia."[56]

At present, DPIs may be considered alternatives to pMDIs for patients who can generate inspiratory flow rates greater than 30 to 60 L/minute but who are unable to use pMDIs effectively. DPIs are recommended for therapy for patients with stable asthma and chronic obstructive pulmonary disease, but not for patients with acute bronchoconstriction or children less than 6 years of age. Therefore one drawback of DPIs is that they do not substitute for pMDIs in all clinical situations. Moreover, dose adjustment may be needed when the same drug is administered by a DPI instead of a pMDI. Table 13-2 compares DPIs, pMDIs, and nebulizers. Deciding on

---

TABLE 13-1

Differences in Inhalation Technique Between Pressurized Metered-dose Inhaler With Holding Chamber and Dry Powder Inhaler

Step	pMDI/HC	DPI
Shaking the inhaler	Yes	No
Actuation with inspiration	Optional	Essential
Inspiration	Slow, deep; improves deposition	Fast, prolonged; required for deposition
Interval between doses	30–60 s	20-30 s
Exhalation into device	Small decrease in dose	Large decrease in dose

DPI, Dry powder inhaler; pMDI/HC, pressurized metered-dose inhaler with holding chamber.

TABLE 13-2

Comparison of Pressurized Metered-dose Inhaler With Holding Chamber, Dry Powder Inhaler, and Nebulizer as Aerosol Delivery Device

Factor	pMDI/HC	DPI	Nebulizer
Performance			
Most aerosol particles <5 µm in size	+	+	±
High pulmonary deposition	+	±	±
Low mouth deposition	+	±	−
Reliability of dose	+	±	±
Influenced by humidity	−	+	−
Physical and chemical stability	+	+	+
Breath actuated	−	+	−
Risk of contamination	−	−	+
Convenience			
Lightweight, compact	+	+	−
Multiple doses	+	+	−
Dose indicator	−	+	−
Inexpensive	+	+	−
Easy and quick operation	±	±	−
Suitable for all ages	+	−	+
Suitable for multiple clinical situations	+	±	+

DPI, Dry powder inhaler; pMDI/HC, pressurized metered-dose inhaler with holding chamber.

the appropriate dose of inhaled corticosteroids may be a particularly vexing problem because it is difficult to determine bioequivalence with these agents. Further research is needed to determine equivalent doses when both the drug and the device used for inhalation therapy are altered.[76,77]

Infants and small children, under the age of 4 years, may not be able to use a mouthpiece, requiring a mask for administration. Because some children may cry when a mask is applied, some clinicians have recommended the use of blow-by, that is, directing a stream of aerosol from a nebulizer toward the mouth and nose of an infant, often from up to 6 in. away. Just as crying greatly reduces lung delivery of aerosol, so does blow-by. Aerosol administration with a mask with a leak or distance between mask and face of as little as 2 mm can reduce the inhaled dose by 80%.[5] Therefore use of blow-by should be discouraged. Infants need to be taught to play with their mask and learn to tolerate it being placed on the face. This takes some time but with a little patience from the care provider, can greatly enhance the efficacy of the aerosol therapy.

To improve compliance, aerosol therapy should be administered along with some easily remembered activity of daily living. For twice-daily administration, medications can be kept with the toothbrush and inhaled just before brushing teeth. This approach also reduces aerosol corticosteroid deposition in the oral pharynx. It is always best to avoid the regular use of medication at school because the inconvenience can significantly reduce compliance and may embarrass some children. However, the availability of rescue medication at school (or day care or other caregiver's home) must be ensured. It helps to prepare written guidelines for medication use. Distribute these guidelines to all the places where the child stays, such as home, school, or the residence of each parent if divorced or separated.[78]

It is helpful, at least initially, to keep a diary of medication use. Lack of response to inhaled asthma medication can be related to a number of factors, including incorrect technique of inhalation; inhalation from depleted canisters of medications, thinking that they still contain active drug; not taking preventive medications as prescribed; change in the child's environment; or misdiagnosis. For example, children with aspirated foreign body, gastroesophageal reflux disease, or psychogenic wheeze will have a poor response to asthma therapy. Infants with tracheomalacia or bronchopulmonary dysplasia may even become much worse after inhaling a bronchodilator aerosol because of increased dynamic airway collapse.[79]

EMERGENCY BRONCHODILATOR RESUSCITATION

When a patient comes to the emergency department with an acute exacerbation of asthma, the onset of the exacerbation was often 12 to 36 hours earlier. These children have often taken rescue medications without obtaining sufficient relief. They, and their parents, are anxious, uncomfortable, and exhausted. The goal is to provide relief as soon as possible and to decrease the work of breathing until antiinflammatory medications take effect. Administration of selective β_2-agonists and anticholinergics such as ipratropium (Atrovent) by aerosol is usually the first therapy given. Albuterol (salbutamol outside the United States) reaches 85% of bronchodilator effect in the first 5 minutes after administration. The national asthma guidelines recommend albuterol administration with either 2.5 or 5.0 mg by jet nebulizer, or 4 to 8 puffs of albuterol by pMDI with valved holding chamber at 20-minute intervals for the first hour.[80,81]

Intermittent versus Continuous Therapy

If the patient does not experience relief of symptoms with standard dosing, frequency of administration is often increased to hourly, or even every 15 to 20 minutes, in the emergency department. Treatments can be continued at this frequency until symptoms are relieved. The standard SVN treatment takes 10 to 15 minutes and requires that a clinician be at the bedside constantly. An alternative to intermittent treatments is continuous nebulization delivering at a controlled rate of medication over an extended period of time, with the patient monitored for rapid identification of increases in heart rate. Doses of albuterol between 7.5 and 15 mg/hour have been shown to be effective in treating acute exacerbation of asthma in adults and children.[82-85]

One strategy for continuous nebulization is to use an intravenous infusion pump to drip a premixed bronchodilator solution through a port into the reservoir of a standard SVN (operating at 6 to 8 L/min) or specialty nebulizer such as the MiniHEART nebulizer (Westmed) (operating at 2 L/min). More recently a VMN, the Aeroneb Solo (Aerogen, Dangan, Galway, Ireland), with a port for drip feed and continuous operation has been introduced. Another solution is to use an LVN that produces an MMAD in the respirable range and that is known to deliver a consistent output of medication at a specific flow. Albuterol solution and normal saline are mixed in the reservoir, and the LVN is operated at a specific flow, identified by the manufacturer, to deliver the desired dose. Several LVNs are now commercially available for continuous administration of bronchodilators. The HEART™ High Output nebulizer (Westmed) has an output of approximately 30 ml/hour at a flow of 10 L/minute for up to 6 or 8 hours. The HOPE nebulizer (B&B Medical Technologies, Loomis, Calif) is a closed dilution nebulizer that allows drug output and oxygen or heliox administration. The medication can be delivered through an aerosol mouthpiece or mask or in-line with a ventilator circuit. For patients with moderately severe asthma, continuous therapy and intermittent therapy have similar effects with either low-dose or high-dose β-agonists. For patients with a severe asthma exacerbation, or forced expiratory volume in 1 second (FEV_1) less than 40% of predicted values, continuous therapy may work more rapidly.[85]

Although β$_2$-agonists are the first-line agents for acute exacerbation of asthma, data from both adults and children suggest that ipratropium bromide is synergistic with β-agonists for the therapy of acute asthma.[86-91] Combination bronchodilator therapy using albuterol and ipratropium in patients with severe asthma significantly reduced the percentage of patients hospitalized (Figure 13-13).[92] It is important to remember that poor relief of acute asthma with bronchodilators may signify a nonasthmatic cause of wheezing, such as foreign body aspiration or tracheitis. Infants with bronchiolitis respond poorly to bronchodilator

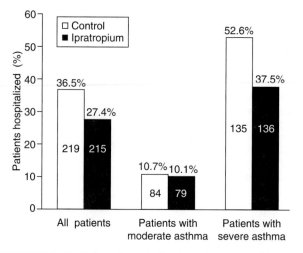

FIGURE 13-13 Rates of hospitalization of patients with asthma from the emergency department after treatment with albuterol (*control*) or with albuterol and ipratropium (*ipratropium*). *Numbers in columns,* number of children tested. In patients with moderate asthma, no difference was seen in hospitalization rate. In patients with severe asthma, the benefits of combined therapy were significant.

medications, which are therefore not recommended for this condition.

Undiluted Bronchodilator

A faster method of administering albuterol is achieved by placing undiluted medication into the nebulizer. Diluent is typically added to medication in the nebulizer to reduce the fraction of the dose that is trapped as residual volume. With undiluted administration, enough medication must be added to the nebulizer to exceed the residual volume of the nebulizer and to allow 1.0 to 2.0 ml of albuterol solution (5 to 10 mg) to be nebulized. Patients should be monitored closely during administration, and the treatment should be terminated if the patient has significant reduction of symptoms and begins to develop tremor or other side effect. Undiluted albuterol administered with specialty nebulizers achieves similar improvements in clinical status in less time. The osmolarity of undiluted medication may be a problem for some patients, especially children less than 2 years old.[93]

MECHANICAL VENTILATION

In the past the consensus was that the efficiency of aerosol delivery to the lower respiratory tract in mechanically ventilated patients was much lower that that in ambulatory patients.[93] Data suggest that this might be overly pessimistic, however, because a number of variables affect aerosol delivery during mechanical ventilation (Box 13-4).

Box 13-4	Variables That Affect Aerosol Delivery and Deposition During Mechanical Ventilation

VENTILATOR RELATED
- Mode
- Tidal volume
- Respiratory frequency
- Duty cycle
- Inspiratory flow waveform
- Trigger mechanism

DEVICE RELATED
METERED-DOSE INHALER
- Type of spacer or adapter
- Position of spacer in circuit
- Timing of actuation

NEBULIZER
- Type of nebulizer
- Fill volume
- Gas flow
- Cycling: inspiration versus continuous
- Duration of nebulization
- Position in circuit

CIRCUIT RELATED
- Endotracheal tube
- Inhaled gas humidity
- Inhaled gas density

DRUG RELATED
- Dose
- Formulation
- Aerosol particle size
- Targeted site for delivery
- Duration of action

PATIENT RELATED
- Severity of airway obstruction
- Mechanism of airway obstruction
- Presence of dynamic hyperinflation
- Patient–ventilator synchrony

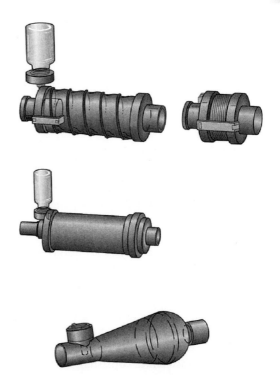

FIGURE 13-14 MDI holding chambers to use in-line with mechanical ventilator circuits or in intubated patients or those with tracheostomies.

Factors Affecting Aerosol Delivery
Ventilator–Patient Interface

The ventilator circuit is typically a closed system that is pressurized during operation, requiring the nebulizer or pMDI to be attached with connectors that maintain the integrity of the circuit during operation. The pMDI cannot be used with the actuator designed by the manufacturer, and use of a third-party actuator is required (Figure 13-14). The size, shape, and design of these actuators greatly affect respirable drug available to the patient and may vary with different pMDI formulations.[94]

Breath Configuration

During controlled mechanical ventilation (CMV) the pattern and rate of inspiratory gas flow and breathing differ from spontaneous respiration. Ambulatory adult patients under normal stable conditions tend to have sinusoidal inspiratory flow patterns of about 30 L/minute, whereas ventilators may use square or decelerating waves with considerably higher flow. Also, the airways are pressurized on inhalation when using CMV, whereas spontaneous inspiration is generated by negative airway pressure drawing gas deep into the lungs. All these factors influence aerosol delivery to the lung.

Airway

In the mechanically ventilated patient, the conduit between the aerosol device and lower respiratory tract is narrower than the oropharynx and trachea. Although the endotracheal tube (ETT) is narrower than the trachea, its smooth interior surface may create a more laminar flow path than the structures of the glottis and larynx and may be less of a barrier to aerosol delivery than the ventilator circuit. In vitro studies demonstrate that three times more aerosol from the pMDI is delivered past the ETT during CMV under dry condition than deposits in the lung through an intact upper airway, raising some doubt that the ETT is the primary barrier to aerosol.[95]

Environment

Ventilator circuits are typically designed to provide heat and humidity for inspired gas to compensate for bypassing the normal airway. Humidity can increase particle size and reduce deposition during CMV, but no data suggest that this reduction is unique to the ventilated patient. The ambulatory patient receiving aerosol, from either an inhaler or nebulizer, in a hot, high-humidity climate may experience a similar reduction in delivered dose.

Response Assessment

The most common method by which to assess patient response to bronchodilator administration is through changes in expiratory flow. During mechanical ventilation forced expiratory maneuvers are impractical, poorly reproducible, and rarely performed, requiring other, less sensitive methods such as monitoring pressure changes (peak and plateau) during ventilator-generated breaths (e.g., passive inspiration). Fok and colleagues demonstrated differences in the response in a rabbit model of ventilated infants, and found that a pMDI was more effective than a jet nebulizer, and that a USN was more effective than either (Figure 13-15).[96] Other changes in mechanics consistent with bronchodilator therapy include decreasing the pressure needed to deliver a set tidal volume during volume ventilation, decreasing the mean airway pressure (now continuously monitored electronically by most mechanical ventilators), and decreasing the requirement for supplemental oxygen. Flow–volume loops have been used to demonstrate bronchodilator response in infants, but unless the patient is sedated and paralyzed, respiratory efforts can provide misleading differences pre- and postbronchodilator administration. Chest auscultation to detect changes in wheezing is notoriously inaccurate and should *never* be used as the sole criterion for evaluating the effect of inhaled bronchodilators.

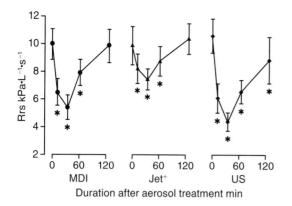

FIGURE 13-15 Measurements of respiratory system resistance (Rrs) before, and 15, 30, 60 and 120 min after, salbutamol treatment via a metered dose inhaler (MDI), a jet nebulizer (Jet: Sidestream), and an ultrasonic nebulizer (US). *Posttreatment values were significantly lower than the pretreatment Rrs, $P < 0.0001$.

For example, wheezing may become more prominent as severe bronchospasm is relaxed and the lungs begin to open up.

Nebulizer Placement

Placement of a continuous jet nebulizer 30 cm from the ETT is more efficient than placement between the patient Y-device and the ETT because the inspiratory ventilator tubing acts as a spacer for the aerosol to accumulate between inspirations.[97] Addition of a spacer device between the nebulizer and ETT modestly increases aerosol delivery.[98] Placement of an ultrasonic or vibrating mesh nebulizer near the patient Y-device is more efficient than placement near the ventilator, unless bias flow exceeds 2 L/minute. Operating the nebulizer only during inspiration is marginally more efficient for aerosol delivery compared with continuous aerosol generation.[97]

Inhaler Adapters

Several types of commercial adapters are available to connect the pMDI canister to the ventilator circuit. Pressurized MDIs can be used with adapters that attach directly to the ETT, with in-line chamber or nonchamber adapters placed in the inspiratory limb of the ventilator circuit. In vitro and in vivo studies have shown that the combination of a pMDI and an accessory device with a chamber results in a four- to sixfold greater delivery of aerosol than pMDI actuation into a connector attached directly to the ETT or into an in-line device that lacks a chamber.[59,97-101] When using the elbow adapter connected to the ETT, actuation of the pMDI out of synchrony with inspiratory airflow delivers little aerosol to the lower respiratory tract. This observation may explain the lack of therapeutic effect with this type of adapter after administration of high doses (100 puffs, 1.0 mg of albuterol) of aerosol from a pMDI in some studies.[102]

Aerosol Particle Size

In mechanically ventilated patients the ventilator circuit and ETT act as baffles that trap particles with larger diameter en route to the bronchi, and hygroscopic particles might increase further in size in the ventilator circuit. Wide variability exists in the MMAD of aerosol particles produced by different brands of nebulizers. Nebulizers producing smaller aerosol particles (MMAD, <2 μm) are likely to produce greater deposition in the lower respiratory tract of ventilator-supported patients.[103]

Endotracheal Tube

Aerosol impaction in the ETT can reduce the efficiency of aerosol delivery in mechanically ventilated patients. The efficacy of aerosol delivery decreases when narrow

ETTs are used in pediatric ventilator circuits.[103,104] The efficiency with which various nebulizers deliver aerosols beyond the ETT did not vary among tube sizes ranging in internal diameter from 7 to 9 mm.[99]

Heating and Humidification

Humidification of inhaled gas decreases aerosol deposition with pMDIs and nebulizers by approximately 40% using in vitro models, probably because of increased particle loss in the ventilator circuit.[59,103-105] More recently, evidence suggests that models that exhale humidity, more accurately simulating patient conditions, show little to no difference in delivered aerosol with passive or active humidity. This would eliminate any benefit of turning off active humidification before administration of aerosol. Absence of humidification may not pose problems during the brief period required to administer a bronchodilator with a pMDI; however, inhalation of dry gas for more than a few minutes can damage the airway.[59] In addition, the disconnection of the ventilator circuit required to bypass the humidifier interrupts ventilation and may increase the risk of ventilator-associated pneumonia. For routine bronchodilator treatment, we recommend using either a pMDI or a nebulizer with a humidified ventilator circuit.

Density of Inhaled Gas

High inspiratory flow with air or oxygen produces turbulence, and increased aerosol impaction. Breathing less dense gas such as helium–oxygen improves aerosol deposition. Studies in ambulatory patients with airway obstruction reveal higher aerosol retention when breathing helium–oxygen compared with air.[106,107] The effects of helium–oxygen mixtures on aerosol deposition during mechanical ventilation demonstrated an up to 50% increase in deposition of albuterol from a pMDI or SVN during CMV of a simulated adult patient.[108]

Ventilator Mode and Settings

The ventilator mode and settings of tidal volume, flow, and respiratory rate influence the characteristics of the airflow used to deliver aerosol in mechanically ventilated patients. For optimal aerosol delivery, actuation of a pMDI into a spacer needs to be synchronized with the onset of inspiratory airflow. Actuation of a pMDI into a cylindrical spacer synchronized with inspiration results in approximately 30% greater efficiency of aerosol delivery compared with actuation during exhalation.[59] When using an elbow adapter, actuation of a pMDI that is not synchronized with inspiratory airflow achieves negligible aerosol delivery to the lower respiratory tract. Aerosol can be delivered during assisted modes of ventilation, provided that the patient is breathing in synchrony with the ventilator. Albuterol

deposition may be up to 23% higher during simulated spontaneous breaths than with controlled breaths of equivalent tidal volume.[105] For efficient aerosol delivery to the lower respiratory tract, the tidal volume of the ventilator-delivered breath must be larger than the volume of the ventilator tubing and ETT. Tidal volumes of 500 ml or greater in adults are associated with adequate aerosol delivery, but the higher pressures required to deliver larger tidal volumes can be detrimental to the lungs. For infants and small children, volumes that exceed the mechanical dead space of the circuit and airway help to optimize delivery.

Aerosol delivery directly correlates with longer inflation times.[103,105] Because nebulizers generate aerosol over several minutes, longer inspiratory times have a cumulative effect in improving aerosol delivery. However, pMDIs produce aerosol only over a portion of a single inspiration, and the mechanism by which longer inspiratory times increase aerosol delivery is unclear. Aerosol particles that deposit in the ventilator tubing may be swept off the walls and entrained by longer periods of inspiratory flow.

In addition, the diluent volume and the duration of treatment influence nebulizer efficiency.[102] Approximately 5% of the nominal dose of albuterol administered by a pMDI is exhaled in mechanically ventilated patients, whereas less than 1% is exhaled with the use of pMDIs in ambulatory patients.[108,109] The mean exhaled fraction (7%) with the use of nebulizers in mechanically ventilated patients is similar to that with MDIs, but considerable variability exists between patients (coefficient of variation, 74%).[110]

Technique of Aerosol Administration in Critical Care

Deposition of aerosol during mechanical ventilation varies with the type of aerosol generator used. During mechanical ventilation of adult patients under standard conditions (humidity on; I/E ratio, 1:2), 1% to 3% of the dose is delivered to the lungs.[111] Under similar conditions, a pMDI, with proper spacer and synchronized actuation, can deliver 11% of an emitted dose to the lungs. Both ultrasonic and vibrating mesh nebulizers may deliver up to 10% to 15% of a dose.[112,113]

In the infant, the deposition is considerably less (0.2% to 1.0%) with jet nebulizers and pMDIs, whereas the vibrating mesh nebulizer appears to be an order of magnitude more efficient (9% to 12.9%).[113]

In both adults and infants, the gas driving the jet nebulizer enters the ventilator circuit, with the potential for changing delivered volumes, pressures, and parameters; this can set off alarms. Because of the relatively low flow rates used in infant ventilator circuits, the addition of 2 to 6 L/minute of gas can more than double the delivered volume. With other aerosol generators such as pMDIs and ultrasonic and vibrating mesh nebulizers, there is no substantial increase in gas volume and ventilator parameters remain consistent.

Specific techniques can improve the efficiency of every ventilator circuit. In vitro the best delivery with a jet nebulizer during CMV (15% to 35%) was accomplished with a nebulizer (e.g., AeroTech II; Biodex Medical Systems, Shirley, NY) that produces particles with an MMAD less than 2 μm, but it can take 35 minutes to administer a 3 mL dose of medication. This dose was nebulized into a dry ventilator circuit, with a duty cycle of 0.5 at inverse-ratio ventilation.[110] Admittedly, this approach might be difficult to tolerate for a patient requiring mechanical ventilation. A common nebulizer that generates particles with an MMAD of 3.5 μm takes half the time but may reduce the dose to the lung by up to 50%, reducing total deposition to 7.5%. Keeping the humidifier on during administration reduces delivery by another 40% (decreasing total deposition to 4%), and reducing the duty cycle to a normal 0.25 reduces deposition to 2%.[102]

Studies on the dose response to bronchodilators in mechanically ventilated patients have not been done in children and infants. This requires us to extrapolate data from adult ventilated patients, in whom bronchodilator effects were observed with the administration of a 3 mL unit dose containing 2.5 mg of albuterol with a JN, or 4 actuations (400 μg) with a pMDI.[114] The pMDI was administered to stable patients through a humidified ventilator circuit, with a chamber-style adapter placed in the inspiratory limb at the Y-piece. Actuations were synchronized to inspiration, with a pause of 20 to 30 seconds between actuations. Minimal therapeutic advantage was gained by administering higher doses, but the potential for side effects was increased.[113,114] In the routine clinical setting, higher doses of bronchodilators may be needed for patients with severe airway obstruction or if the technique of administration is not optimal. Because these results were observed with humidified ventilator circuits, we do not recommend bypassing the humidifier for routine bronchodilator therapy. In summary, when the technique of administration is carefully executed, most stable mechanically ventilated patients achieve near maximal bronchodilation after administration of 4 puffs of albuterol with a pMDI or 2.5 mg with a nebulizer. Dosing requirements for infants and small children during mechanical ventilation have not been established and should be titrated to effect. In this case, to a decrease in airway resistance, or an increase in tachycardia or tremor. Some authors have recommended that flow–volume loops be monitored before and after bronchodilator administration to quantify changes in airway resistance. In patients who are not totally sedated these loops can change with patient inspiratory efforts and may be misleading.

Single-dose ampoules of drug are preferred to multidose containers or bottles, which are more easily contaminated. Similarly, when the chamber spacer remains in the ventilator circuit between treatments, condensate collects inside. Using a heated wire circuit can reduce the formation of condensate within the spacer. Care must be taken to prevent the condensate in the spacer from being washed into the patient's respiratory tract when the spacer is pulled open during use. When a noncollapsible spacer chamber is used to actuate a pMDI, it should be removed from the ventilator circuit between treatments. No studies demonstrate contamination problems with administration of aerosol from a pMDI during CMV.

The administration of medication by pMDI to the mechanically ventilated neonate may not be well tolerated. Leaving a chamber device in-line is not practical because of the increased compressible volume incorporated into the ventilator circuit. Depending on the F_{IO_2} and the propellant gas volume, an in-line pMDI actuation theoretically may result in the delivery of a hypoxic gas mixture to an infant receiving a tidal volume less than 100 ml. It is possible to deliver a pMDI aerosol medication to the intubated neonate, especially for medications available only in pMDI preparations. However, it may be preferable to hand-ventilate the pMDI delivery of medication to the patient. If a chamber adapter is used, the infant must be removed from the circuit, the chamber placed in-line, and the infant reattached to the circuit before the pMDI is administered. The large dead space volume caused by placing a spacer or chamber at the end of the ETT must also be considered when administering pMDI medications to an infant.

BRONCHODILATOR ADMINISTRATION

Inhaler versus Nebulizer

Nebulizers and pMDIs are equally effective in the treatment of airway obstruction in ambulatory children.[115] Similarly, nebulizers and pMDIs produce similar therapeutic effects in mechanically ventilated patients. In 1- to 4-kg infants, Fok and colleagues[8] demonstrated less than 1% deposition with jet nebulizers and pMDIs with spacers during mechanical ventilation and spontaneous breathing.

The use of pMDIs for routine bronchodilator therapy in ventilator-supported patients is preferred because of several problems associated with the use of jet nebulizers. The rate of aerosol production by nebulizers is highly variable, not only in nebulizers from different manufacturers, but also in different batches of the same brand. Furthermore, the nature of the aerosol produced, especially the particle size, is also highly variable among different nebulizers. The issue is further complicated because the operating efficiency of a nebulizer changes with the pressure of the driving gas and with different fill volumes. Because the pressure of the gas supplied by a ventilator to drive the nebulizer during inspiration is lower than that supplied by a tank/air compressor unit, the efficiency of some nebulizers can be drastically decreased in a ventilator circuit. The gas flow driving the nebulizer produces additional airflow in the ventilator circuit, necessitating adjustment of tidal volume and inspiratory flow when the nebulizer is in use. When patients are unable to trigger the ventilator during assisted modes of mechanical ventilation because of the additional nebulizer gas flow, hypoventilation can result.[114] Therefore, before using a jet nebulizer to treat a ventilator-supported patient, it is imperative to characterize its efficiency in a ventilator circuit under the typical clinical conditions in which it will be used.

Box 13-5 outlines a modification of the technique of aerosol administration with jet nebulizers to mechanically ventilated patients. Box 13-6 provides another strategy for bronchodilator therapy using a pMDI.[5]

Care of Accessory Devices and Nebulizers

For intubated infants or children with increased work of breathing or poor I/E ratios and for those in whom intubation is imminent, a nebulizer or pMDI adapted to a resuscitation bag can be used. The same F_{IO_2} is used with the jet nebulizer and the resuscitation bag. Flow to the nebulizer should be optimal for the nebulizer used, and flow to the bag should be reduced to compensate for the flow from the nebulizer. When using a bag and mask to deliver medication, care must be taken to avoid gastric insufflation, pulmonary hyperinflation, and hyperventilation or hypoventilation. The mask is used to create a good seal, and attempts must be made to time the inflation with the inspiratory effort. Care must be taken to stabilize the ETT to prevent accidental extubation with the added weight of the equipment. The patient is ventilated using the same pressures and rate as with the mechanical ventilator. It is theoretically helpful to deliver an occasional sigh by providing a slight inspiratory hold at the peak inspiratory pressure, thereby enhancing the volume and depth of medication delivered while providing additional time for deposition to occur in the airways.

Box 13-5 Technique for Using Nebulizers to Treat Mechanically Ventilated Patients

1. Place drug solution in the nebulizer to the optimal fill volume (2 to 6 ml).*
2. Place the nebulizer in the inspiratory line, about 30 cm from the patient Y-piece.
3. Ensure sufficient airflow (6 to 8 L/min) to operate the nebulizer.†
4. Ensure adequate tidal volume (about 500 ml in adults, 7 mg/kg for infants and children). Attempt to use a duty cycle greater than 0.3, if possible.
5. Adjust the minute volume, sensitivity trigger, and alarms to compensate for additional airflow through the nebulizer, if required.
6. Turn off flow-by or continuous-flow mode on the ventilator and remove the heat moisture exchanger (if present) from between the nebulizer and the patient.
7. Observe the nebulizer for adequate aerosol generation throughout use.
8. Disconnect the nebulizer when no more aerosol is being produced.
9. Rinse with sterile water or air-dry between uses. Store the nebulizer under aseptic conditions.
10. Reconnect the ventilator circuit, and return to original ventilator and alarm settings. Confirm proper operation with no leaks in circuit.

*The volume of solution associated with maximal efficiency varies with different nebulizers and should be determined before using any nebulizer.
†The nebulizer may be operated continuously or only during inspiration; the latter method is more efficient for aerosol delivery. Some ventilators provide inspiratory gas flow to the nebulizer. Continuous gas flow from an external source can also be used to power the nebulizer.

HOME CARE AND MONITORING COMPLIANCE

With most therapeutic aerosols being administered in the home, patient education and adherence with written medicine and action plans are critical. Standard nebulizers and pMDIs have no intrinsic mechanism for tracking use or compliance. The pMDI also has no mechanism to track how many doses remain in the canister. If accurately completed, medication diaries can help to track medication use and the use of rescue medications while monitoring prescription refill records.

Several aerosol delivery devices entering the market can directly track use and monitor compliance. These devices range from electronic models integrated with the nebulizer that track number of breaths taken, size of breaths, and duration and frequency of treatment, to simple counting devices attached to the pMDI actuator boot. More sophisticated devices allow monitoring

Box 13-6	Technique for Using Pressurized Metered-dose Inhalers to Treat Mechanically Ventilated Patients

1. Minimize the inspiratory flow rate during administration.
2. Aim for an inspiratory:expiratory ratio (excluding the inspiratory pause) greater than 0.3 of total breath duration.
3. Ensure that the ventilator breath is synchronized with the patient's inspiration.
4. Shake the pMDI vigorously.
5. Place the canister in the actuator of a cylindrical spacer situated in the inspiratory limb of the ventilator circuit.*
6. Actuate the pMDI to synchronize with precise onset of inspiration by the ventilator.†
7. Allow passive exhalation.
8. Repeat actuations after 20 to 30 seconds until total dose is delivered.‡

pMDI, Pressurized metered-dose inhaler.
*With pMDIs, it is preferable to use a spacer that remains in the ventilator circuit so that disconnection of the ventilator circuit can be avoided at the time of each bronchodilator treatment. Although bypassing the humidifier can increase aerosol delivery, it prolongs the time for each treatment and requires disconnection of the ventilator circuit.
†In ambulatory patients with the pMDI placed inside the mouth, actuation is recommended briefly after initiation of inspiratory airflow. In mechanically ventilated patients in whom a pMDI and spacer combination is used, actuation should be synchronized with onset of inspiration.
‡The manufacturer recommends repeating the dose after 1 minute. However, pMDI actuation within 20 to 30 seconds after the prior dose does not compromise drug delivery.

of both pMDI use and expiratory maneuvers for later transmission to the care provider's office. Some newer DPI devices contain a built-in counter that advances each time a dose is loaded. These devices also give a visual signal when only a few doses remain in the device.

OTHER MEDICATIONS FOR AEROSOL DELIVERY

Antibiotics

Aerosol antibiotics can deliver high concentrations of antibiotics to the airway with low systemic bioavailability, thus reducing toxicity. This approach is of particular importance in patients with cystic fibrosis (CF), who frequently require courses of antibiotic therapy.[116] In a phase 3 registration study, 468 patients with CF were enrolled in a 6-month masked, placebo-controlled trial of preservative-free, nonpyrogenic tobramycin solution for inhalation (TOBI; Novartis, Emeryville, CA),

alternating between 4-week courses of tobramycin and placebo. During treatment the patients received 300 mg of tobramycin in 5 ml of ¼ strength saline. The FEV_1 increased by more than 10% by the end of 6 months, with patients receiving tobramycin 26% less likely to be hospitalized and 36% less likely to require IV antipsuedomonal antibiotics and a > 10-fold reduction in sputum bacterial density.[117] Follow-up studies in CF and non-CF bronchiectasis have generally been consistent with these earlier results.[118]

Other antibiotics are being prepared for aerosol delivery including colistin, gentamicin, ciprofloxacin, and aztreonam. As this chapter is being prepared, the latter has completed phase 3 trials in CF by Gilead Sciences (Foster City, Calif) using a novel vibrating mesh aerosol delivery device (eFlow; PARI Pharma, Midlothian, Va). Although aerosolized antibiotics may find a role in the therapy of patients with severe BPD or those with chronic tracheostomies, the emergence of bacterial resistance to these antibiotics is a real risk and must be closely monitored.[119]

Mucoactive Agents

Sputum is expectorated mucus mixed with inflammatory cells, cellular debris, polymers of DNA and F-actin, as well as bacteria. Mucus is usually cleared by airflow and ciliary movement, and sputum is cleared by cough.[120] Dornase alfa (Pulmozyme; Genentech, South San Francisco, Calif) was the first approved mucoactive agent for the treatment of CF.[9] Dornase alfa is safe and effective, even in patients with more severe pulmonary disease defined as a forced vital capacity less than 40% of the predicted value.[121] Efficacy has not yet been demonstrated for the therapy of acute exacerbations of CF lung disease or for the treatment of other chronic airway diseases.[122] A small phase 1 study in non-CF bronchiectasis demonstrated no efficacy in non-CF bronchiectasis, and there was a suggestion that the use of dornase worsened disease in this adult population.[123] This may be due to the fact that secretions in bronchiectasis and chronic obstructive pulmonary disease are composed primarily of mucin and related proteins, thus constituting true mucous hypersecretion,[124] whereas in the CF airway there is significantly decreased mucin and mucus, the CF secretions being almost entirely neutrophil-derived pus.[125]

Other mucoactive agents under development include mucolytics such as Nacystelyn (acetylcysteine lysinate),[126] thymosin β_4, and low molecular weight dextran[127]; mucokinetic agents such as surfactant; and $P2Y_2$ chloride channel activators.[128] The use of hyperosmolar saline or mannitol to improve secretion clearance in CF is discussed in a following section (see Hyperosmolar Aerosols).

Surfactant

There is profound loss of surfactant in the inflamed airway with bronchitis or cystic fibrosis.[129] Randomized, masked, placebo-controlled studies demonstrate that surfactant aerosol improves pulmonary function and sputum transportability in patients with chronic bronchitis and that this effect is dose dependent with no significant side effects.[130] As a wetting and spreading agent, the surfactant also has the ability to increase the lower airway deposition of other aerosol medications, such as dornase alfa or gene therapy vectors, and may increase small particle translocation through the mucous layer.[20]

Hyperosmolar Aerosols

For many years, sputum induction by hyperosmolar saline inhalation has been used to obtain specimens for the diagnosis of pneumonia. In a pilot study, 58 patients with CF were randomly assigned to receive 10 ml of either 0.9% normal saline or 6% hypertonic saline twice daily by ultrasonic nebulization.[131] Spirometry was measured for 2 weeks during therapy and for 2 weeks after therapy. At 2 weeks there was a significant increase in the FEV_1 in the hypertonic saline group, with a return to baseline by 28 days. Despite pretreatment with 600 μg of inhaled albuterol, several patients had an acute decrease in FEV_1 after inhaling hypertonic saline. Similarly, hyperosmolar dry powder mannitol improves quality of life and pulmonary function in adult subjects with non-CF bronchiectasis and significantly improves the surface adhesivity and cough clearability of expectorated sputum.[132]

Subsequent studies, as reviewed in the *Cochrane Database of Systematic Reviews,* tend to confirm that the long-term use of inhaled hyperosmolar saline improves pulmonary function in patients with CF[133] and that inhaled hyperosmolar saline or mannitol is beneficial in non-CF bronchiectasis.[134] Although this therapy is readily available and inexpensive, it has been reported that hypertonic saline aerosol is not as effective as dornase alfa in the therapy of CF lung disease.[135]

Gene Transfer Therapy

Gene transfer therapy represents a novel use for aerosols. Efforts in this arena have centered largely on complementary (copy) DNA transfer of the normal CF transmembrane regulator (CFTR) gene to patients with CF. Gene transfer was first attempted by inserting the normal CFTR gene into a replication-defective adenovirus vector with bolus bronchoscopic delivery of the vector. An unanticipated host immune response to the vector led to re-evaluation of this strategy.[136]

For gene transfer to be effective, the vector and its package must be nonimmunogenic, stable to shear forces during aerosolization, and safe to transfected cells. The vector should not increase cell turnover. It should either stably integrate into the progenitor (basal) cell genome or be safe and effective with repeated administration and should be able to reach the cellular target of relevance. Part of the difficulty with CF is that this cellular target has not been clearly identified as epithelial cell, goblet cell, submucous gland, or all of these. The amount of gene and vector and persistence in the airway must also be determined for each vector and delivery system.[137]

Viral vectors that have been studied include adenovirus, adeno-associated virus, and lentivirus. Adenovirus naturally targets the airway epithelium. Adeno-associated virus is a small organisms that requires a "helper" virus to replicate. These viruses are capable of site-directed insertion into DNA, reducing the risk of insertional mutagenesis (initiating cancer by activation of an oncogene or inactivation of an oncogene suppressor). Gene therapy with adeno-associated virus appears to be especially promising.[138] Lentiviruses are retroviruses such as human immunodeficiency virus. They are able to transfect cells that are not terminally differentiated, such as the basal or airway progenitor cell, but insertional mutagenesis is a substantial risk.

The primary nonviral vectors studied to date have been cationic liposomes. These lipid capsules are able to form complexes with DNA and then enter cells. With the first generation of liposome vectors, the efficiency of gene transfer was poor; however, this has improved dramatically with newer systems.[139] The development of this technology will result in revolutionary aerosol generators.[140]

Aerosols for Systemic Administration

Aerosols can be targeted to different sites in the airway. Depending on the intrapulmonary behavior of each molecule, the aerosol mode of administration allows airway/secretion delivery, cellular delivery, or systemic delivery. Most medications are targeted to the airway epithelium, including the neuromuscular plexus (bronchodilators) and inflammatory cells (corticosteroids). Epithelial agents such as the $P2Y_2$ ion channel activators are targeted directly to the ciliated epithelium. Mucolytics, proteases, and antibiotics are targeted to secretions in the airway rather than to the epithelial cells.

Small particles targeted to the alveolus can be effective for systemic delivery of macromolecules through the extensive pulmonary vascular bed. Insulin is likely to be the first such medication introduced for systemic administration through aerosol administration, but other peptides and macromolecules are under development. Considerations for systemic administration include cost, convenience, efficacy, and safety. The pulmonary behavior of an inhaled molecule is not predictable and must be studied individually.[141]

Insulin

Insulin was one of the first medications to be administered by aerosol. Because of the nebulizer and insulin formulation available at that time, absorption and efficacy were highly unpredictable. This has changed dramatically with the development of ultrafine particles and aerosol devices that can efficiently and reliably target the alveolar space.

With a rapid and smooth onset of action and elimination of the necessity for injections with their attendant risks and discomfort, inhaled insulin has great potential for clinical use. Intrapulmonary insulin administration to healthy subjects can induce significant hypoglycemia and a clinically relevant increase in serum insulin concentrations.[142] Once plasma glucose levels are normalized, postprandial glucose levels can be maintained below diabetic levels by delivering insulin into the lungs 5 minutes before ingestion of a meal.[143,144]

Studies have confirmed that inhaled insulin is safe and effective for the therapy of type 2 diabetes even when this is not controlled by diet[145,146] and that the addition of inhaled insulin or oral therapy with hypoglycemic agents improves glycemic control.[147]

With the success of inhaled insulin demonstrating the safe and effective systemic administration of complex peptides via the pulmonary bed, it is highly probable that we will see the development of other aerosol therapies that could revolutionize fields as diverse as endocrinology, critical care, immunology, and genetics.[148,149] As the respiratory therapist will be at the front line for teaching and administering these novel therapies this will greatly expand the role of the respiratory therapist in the future.

SUMMARY

The use of therapeutic aerosol medications is evolving from a basis of optimizing the delivery of asthma medications to the airway to understanding how the extensive pulmonary vascular bed can be used for the systemic administration of a variety of macromolecules. Evolving and novel uses of therapeutic aerosols will require an understanding of aerosol generation, deposition, and translocation, as well as target organ physiology and pharmacology.

ASSESSMENT QUESTIONS

See Evolve Resources for answers.

1. Which of the following is true when a standard unit dose is nebulized to patients of different size/age?
   A. Smaller percentage of dose delivered to bigger patients
   B. Larger percentage of dose delivered to smaller patients
   C. Similar inhaled dose per kilogram of body weight
   D. Similar total inhaled dose
   E. No dose is delivered to infants
2. In infants between 1 and 4 kg, deposition of aerosol with a pMDI or jet nebulizer is:
   A. Similar whether intubated and mechanically ventilated or spontaneously breathing with a normal airway
   B. Less than 1% in all cases
   C. Slightly greater with a pMDI than with a jet nebulizer
   D. All of the above
   E. None of the above
3. What should the operator do when operating a jet nebulizer with a mixture of helium–oxygen?
   A. Provide the same total flow of gas to the nebulizer as with air or oxygen.
   B. Increase the flow of gas to the nebulizer by two- or threefold.
   C. Reduce the flow of gas to the nebulizer by one half.
   D. Never use heliox to drive a nebulizer.
   E. Never use an air or oxygen flowmeter.
4. Which of the following statements is true about the SPAG aerosol generator?
   A. It makes very small particles.
   B. It uses a secondary chamber to dry particles.
   C. It is used to administer ribavirin.
   D. It is often used with double containment systems.
   E. All of the above
5. What is the most reliable way to determine how many actuations are left in a pMDI?
   A. Float the canister in water.
   B. Count the number of doses.
   C. Actuate until it is empty.
   D. Use it for only 1 month.
   E. All of the above
6. Why are DPIs not recommended for children less than 5 years of age?
   A. They are not big enough to generate sufficient inspiratory flow.
   B. They cannot use a mouthpiece.
   C. DPIs make them cough.
   D. They cannot coordinate actuation with inspiration.
   E. None of the above

Continued

ASSESSMENT QUESTIONS—cont'd

7. Which of the following choices is/are true about a large proportion of patients and their caregivers?
   A. They do not know how to properly use a DPI.
   B. They do not know how to properly use a pMDI.
   C. They do not know how to properly clean and assemble a nebulizer.
   D. They misuse their inhaler to the point of not benefiting from their medication.
   E. All of the above
8. During bronchodilator administration in severe airway obstruction:
   A. An increased dose may be more effective than increased frequency.
   B. Undiluted bronchodilator may be substituted for diluted bronchodilator.
   C. Continuous nebulization may work better than intermittent nebulizations.
   D. Patients who do not respond to initial high doses more often are admitted to hospital.
   E. All of the above
9. What is the most practical way to improve aerosol deposition during mechanical ventilation?
   A. Use a nebulizer with a small particle size.
   B. Use a ramp versus square-wave pattern.
   C. Minimize inspiratory flow rates.
   D. Use a pMDI instead of a nebulizer.
   E. All of the above
10. Which drug was one of the first to be administered by aerosol?
   A. Mucolytics
   B. Antibiotics
   C. Gene therapy
   D. Surfactant
   E. Insulin

References

1. Newhouse MT, Dolovich MB: Control of asthma by aerosols, *N Engl J Med* 1986;315:870.
2. Janson C: Plasma levels and effects of salbutamol after inhaled or i.v. administration in stable asthma, *Eur Respir J* 1991;4:544.
3. Brain JD, Valberg PA: Deposition of aerosol in the respiratory tract, *Am Rev Respir Dis* 1979;120:1325.
4. Gross NJ, Jenne JW, Hess D: Bronchodilator therapy. In Tobin MJ, editor: *Principles and practice of mechanical ventilation*, New York: McGraw-Hill; 1994. pp 1077-1123.
5. Rubin BK, Fink JB: Aerosol therapy for children, *Respir Care Clin N Am* 2001;7:175.
6. Wildhaber JH et al: High percentage lung delivery in children from detergent-treated spacers, *Pediatr Pulmonol* 2000;29:389.
7. Dolovich MB: Assessing nebulizer performance, *Respir Care* 2002;47:1290.
8. Fok TF et al: Efficient of aerosol medication delivery from a metered dose inhaler versus jet nebulizer in infants with bronchopulmonary dysplasia, *Pediatr Pulmonol* 1996;21:301.
9. Wildhaber JH et al: Inhalation therapy in asthma: nebulizer or pressurized metered-dose inhaler with holding chamber: in vivo comparison of lung deposition in children, *J Pediatr* 1999;135:28.
10. Fink JB, Dhand R: Aerosol therapy. In Fink JB, Hunt G, editors: *Clinical practice in respiratory care*, Philadelphia: Lippincott-Raven; 1998.
11. Dolovich M: Physical principles underlying aerosol therapy, *J Aerosol Med* 1989;2:171.
12. Pedersen S: Delivery systems in children. In Barnes PJ, Grunstein MM, Leff AR, Woolcock AJ, editors: *Asthma*, Philadelphia: Lippincott-Raven; 1997. pp 1915-1929.
13. Desai MA, Mutlu M, Vadgama P: A study of macromolecular diffusion through native porcine mucus, *Experientia* 1992;48:22.
14. Bolister N et al: The diffusion of β-lactam antibiotics through mixed gels of cystic fibrosis–derived mucin and *Pseudomonas aeruginosa* alginate, *J Antimicrob Chemother* 1991;27:285.
15. King M, Kelly S, Cosio M: Alteration of airway reactivity by mucus, *Respir Physiol* 1985;62:47.
16. De Sanctis GT et al: Hyporesponsiveness to aerosolized but not to infused methacholine in cigarette-smoking dogs, *Am Rev Respir Dis* 1987;135:338.
17. Bataillon V et al: The binding of amikacin to macromolecules from the sputum of patients suffering from respiratory diseases, *J Antimicrob Chemother* 1992;29:499.
18. Taskar VS et al: Effect of bromhexeine on sputum amoxicillin levels in lower respiratory infections, *Respir Med* 1992;86:157.
19. Stern M et al: The effect of mucolytic agents on gene transfer across a CF sputum barrier in vitro, *Gene Ther* 1998;5:91.
20. Schürch S et al: Surfactant displaces particles toward the epithelium in airways and alveoli, *Respir Physiol* 1990;80:17.
21. Kharasch VS et al: Pulmonary surfactant as a vehicle for intratracheal delivery of technetium sulfur colloid and pentamidine in hamster lungs, *Am Rev Respir Dis* 1991;144:909.
22. Newhouse MT, Kennedy A: Rapid temperature change from 25° C to 15° C impairs powder deaggregation in Bricanyl Turbuhaler, *J Aerosol Med* 1999;12:113.
23. Hess D et al: Medication nebulizer performance effects: of diluent volume, nebulizer flow, and nebulizer brand, *Chest* 1996;110:498.
24. Johnson MA et al: Delivery of albuterol and ipratropium bromide from two nebulizer systems in chronic stable asthma: efficacy and pulmonary deposition, *Chest* 1989;96:1.
25. Hadfield JW, Windebank WJ, Bateman JRM: Is driving gas flow clinically important for nebulizer therapy? *Br J Dis* 1986;80:550.
26. Douglas JG et al: A comparative study of two doses of salbutamol nebulized at 4 and 8 L/min in patients with chronic asthma, *Br J Dis* 1986;80:55.
27. Hess DR et al: The effect of heliox on nebulizer function using a β-agonist bronchodilator. *Chest* 1999;115:184.

28. Goode ML et al: Improvement in aerosol delivery with helium–oxygen mixtures during mechanical ventilation, *Am J Respir Crit Care Med* 2001;163:109.

29. Malone RA et al: Optimal duration of nebulized albuterol therapy, *Chest* 1993;104:1114.

30. Thomas SH et al: Improving the efficiency of drug administration with jet nebulisers, *Lancet* 1988;1:126.

31. Newnham DM, Lipworth BJ: Nebulizer performance, pharmacokinetics, airways and systemic effects of salbutamol given via a novel nebulizer system (Ventstream), *Thorax* 1994;49:762.

32. Nebuliser Project Group of the British Thoracic Society Standards of Care Committee: Current best practice for nebuliser treatment, *Thorax* 1997;52:S4.

33. Standaert TA et al: Effects of repetitive use and cleaning techniques of disposable jet nebulizers on aerosol generation, *Chest* 1998;114:577.

34. Centers for Disease Control and Prevention: Guideline for prevention of nosocomial pneumonia, *Respir Care* 1994;39:1191.

35. Oie S, Kamiya A: Bacterial contamination of aerosol solutions containing antibiotics, *Microbios* 1995;82:109.

36. Kacmarek RM, Kratohvil J: Evaluation of a double-enclosure double-vacuum unit scavenging system for ribavirin administration, *Respir Care* 1992;37:37.

37. Adderley RJ: Safety of ribavirin with mechanical ventilation, *Pediatr Infect Dis J* 1990;9:S112.

38. Committee on Infectious Diseases, American Academy of Pediatrics: Reassessment of the indications for ribavirin therapy in respiratory syncytial virus infections, *Pediatrics* 1996;97:137.

39. Phillips GD, Millard FJL: The therapeutic use of ultrasonic nebulizers in acute asthma, *Respir Med* 1994;88:387.

40. Summer W et al: Aerosol bronchodilator delivery methods' relative impact on pulmonary function and cost of respiratory care, *Arch Intern Med* 1989;149:618.

41. Yuksel B, Greenough A: Comparison of the effects on lung function of two methods of bronchodilator administration, *Respir Med* 1994;88:229.

42. Nakanishi AK et al: Ultrasonic nebulization of albuterol is no more effective than jet nebulization for the treatment of acute asthma in children, *Chest* 1997;97:1505.

43. Lewis RA et al: Ultrasonic and jet nebulizers: differences in the physical properties and fractional deposition on the airway responses to nebulized water and saline aerosols [abstract], *Thorax* 1984;39:712.

44. Doershuk CF et al: Evaluation of jet type and ultrasonic nebulizers in mist tent therapy for cystic fibrosis, *Pediatrics* 1968;41:723.

45. Boucher RM, Kreuter J: The fundamentals of the ultrasonic atomization of medicated solutions, *Ann Allergy* 1968;26:591.

46. Thomas SH et al: Delivery of ultrasonic nebulized aerosols to a lung model during mechanical ventilation, *Am Rev Respir Dis* 1993;148:872.

47. Lin YZ, Hsieh KH: Metered dose inhaler and nebulizer in acute asthma, *Arch Dis Child* 1995;72:214.

48. American Association for Respiratory Care: Clinical practice guideline: selection of aerosol delivery device, *Respir Care* 1992;37:891.

49. Newhouse MT, Dolovich M: *Aerosol therapy in children: basic mechanisms of pediatric respiratory disease, cellular and integrative*, New York: Marcel Dekker; 1991.

50. Svartengren K et al: Added external resistance reduces oropharyngeal deposition and increases lung deposition of aerosol particles in asthmatics, *Am J Respir Crit Care Med* 1995;152:32.

51. Hill LS, Slater AL: A comparison of the performance of two modern multidose dry powder asthma inhalers, *Respir Med* 1998;92:105.

52. Rajkumari NJ, Byron PR, Dalby RN: Testing of dry powder aerosol formulations in different environmental conditions, *Int J Pharmacol* 1995;113:123.

53. Larsen JS et al: Evaluation of conventional press-and-breathe metered-dose inhaler technique in 501 patients, *J Asthma* 1994;31:193.

54. Guidry GG et al: Incorrect use of metered dose inhalers by medical personnel, *Chest* 1992;101:31.

55. Newman SP, Pavia D, Clarke SW: Simple instructions for using pressurized aerosol bronchodilators, *J R Soc Med* 1980;73:776.

56. Fink J, Rubin B: Problems with inhaler use: a call for improved clinician and patient education, *Respir Care* 2005;50:1.

57. Hampson NB, Mueller MP: Reduction in patient timing errors using a breath-activated metered dose inhaler, *Chest* 1994;106:462.

58. Toogood JH et al: Use of spacer to facilitate inhaled corticosteroid treatment of asthma, *Am Rev Respir Dis* 1984;129:723.

59. Diot P, Morra L, Smaldone GC: Albuterol delivery in a model of mechanical ventilation: comparison of metered-dose inhaler and nebulizer efficiency, *Am J Respir Crit Care Med* 1995;152:1391.

60. Salzman GA, Pyszczynski DR: Oropharyngeal candidiasis in patients treated with beclomethasone dipropionate delivered by metered-dose inhaler alone and with Aerochamber, *J Allergy Clin Immunol* 1988;81:424.

61. Rubin BK: Pressurized metered-dose inhalers and holding chambers for inhaled glucocorticoid therapy in childhood asthma, *J Allergy Clin Immunol* 1999;103:1224.

62. Closa RM et al: Efficacy of bronchodilators administered by nebulizers versus spacer devices in infants with acute wheezing, *Pediatr Pulmonol* 1998;26:344.

63. Williams JR, Bothner JP, Swanton RD: Delivery of albuterol in a pediatric emergency department, *Pediatr Emerg Care* 1996;12:263.

64. Cunningham SJ, Crain EF: Reduction of morbidity in asthmatic children given a spacer device, *Chest* 1994;106:753.

65. Ganderton D: The generation of respirable clouds from coarse powder aggregates, *J Biopharm Sci* 1992;3:101.

66. Dolovich M et al: Measurement of the particle size and dosing characteristics of a radiolabelled albuterol-sulphate lactose blend used in the SPIROS dry powder inhaler. In Dalby RN, Byron P, Farr SY, editors: *Respiratory drug delivery*, Buffalo Grove, NY: Interpharm Press; 1996. pp 332-335.

67. Engel T et al: Peak inspiratory flow rate and inspiratory vital capacity of patients with asthma measured with and without a new dry powder inhaler device (Turbuhaler), *Eur Respir J* 1990;3:1037.

68. Pederson S, Hansen OR, Fuglsang G: Influence of inspiratory flow rate on the effect of a Turbuhaler, *Arch Dis Child* 1990;65:308.

69. Thorsson L, Edsbacke S, Conradson TB: Lung deposition from Turbuhaler is twice that from a pressurized metered-dose inhaler (pMDI), *Eur Respir J* 1994;7:1839.

70. Timsina MP et al: The effect of inhalation flow on the performance of a dry powder inhalation system, *Int J Pharm* 1992;81:199.

71. Hindle M, Byron PR: Dose emissions from marketed dry powder inhalers, *Int J Pharm* 1995;116:169.

72. Gansslen M: Uber inhalation von insulin, *Klin Wochenschr* 1925;4:71.

73. Bisgaard H et al: Inspiratory flow rate through the Diskus/Accuhaler inhaler and Turbuhaler inhaler in children with asthma, *J Aerosol Med* 1995;8:100.

74. Smith KJ, Chan H-K, Brown KF: Influence of flow rate on particle size distributions from pressurised and breath actuated inhalers, *J Aerosol Med* 1998;11:231.

75. Pederson S: Delivery options for the inhaled therapy in children over the age of 6 years, *J Aerosol Med* 1997;10:41.

76. Fok TF et al: Aerosol delivery to non-ventilated infants by metered dose inhaler: should a valved spacer be used? *Pediatr Pulmonol* 1997;24:204.

77. Kesten S et al: Patient handling of a multidose dry powder inhalation device for albuterol, *Chest* 1994;105:1077.

78. Rubin BK, Newhouse MH, Barnes PJ: *Conquering childhood asthma: an illustrated guide to the understanding and control of childhood asthma*, Hamilton, ON, Canada: BC Decker; 1998.

79. Rubin BK: Tracheomalacia as a cause of respiratory compromise in infants, *Clin Pulm Med* 1999;6:195.

80. National Asthma Education and Prevention Program, National Heart, Lung, and Blood Institute; National Institutes of Health: *Expert Panel Report 2: guidelines for the diagnosis and management of asthma*. NIH Publication No. 97-4051. Bethesda, Md: National Institutes of Health; 1997.

81. Schuh S et al: High- versus low-dose, frequently administered nebulized albuterol in children with severe acute asthma, *Pediatrics* 1989;83:513.

82. Colacone A et al: Continuous nebulization of albuterol (salbutamol) in acute asthma, *Chest* 1990;97:693.

83. Portnoy J, Aggarwal J: Continuous terbutaline nebulization for the treatment of severe exacerbations of asthma in children, *Ann Allergy* 1988;60:368.

84. Rebuck AS et al: Nebulized anticholinergic and sympathomimetic treatment of asthma and chronic obstructive airways disease in the emergency room, *Am J Med* 1987;82:59.

85. Amado M, Portnoy J: A comparison of low and high doses of continuously nebulized terbutaline for treatment of severe exacerbations of asthma [abstract], *Ann Allergy* 1988;60:165.

86. Rubin BK, Albers GM: Use of anticholinergic bronchodilation in children, *Am J Med* 1996;100:49S.

87. Zorc JJ et al: Ipratropium added to asthma treatment in the pediatric emergency department, *Pediatrics* 1999;103:748.

88. Lanes SF et al: The effect of adding ipratropium to salbutamol in the treatment of acute asthma: a pooled analysis of three trials, *Chest* 1998;114:365.

89. Lin RY et al: Superiority of ipratropium plus albuterol over albuterol alone in the emergency department management of adults asthma: a randomized clinical trial, *Ann Emerg Med* 1998;31:208.

90. Qureshi F et al: Effect of nebulized ipratropium on the hospitalization rates of children with asthma, *N Engl J Med* 1998;339:1030.

91. Schuh S et al: Efficacy of frequent nebulized ipratropium bromide added to frequent high-dose albuterol therapy in severe childhood asthma, *J Pediatr* 1995;127:842.

92. Qureshi F et al: Effect of nebulized ipratropium on the hospitalization rates of children with asthma, *N Engl J Med* 1998;339:1030.

93. American Association for Respiratory Care: Aerosol consensus statement, *Chest* 1991;100:1106.

94. Fink JB, Dhand R: Bronchodilator therapy in mechanically ventilated patients, *Respir Care* 1999;44:53.

95. Fink JB et al: Reconciling in vitro and in vivo measurements of aerosol delivery from a metered-dose inhaler during mechanical ventilation and defining efficiency-enhancing factors, *Am J Respir Crit Care Med* 1999;159:63.

96. Fok TF, al-Essa M, Monkman S, Dolovich M, Girard L, Coates G, Kirpalani H. Pulmonary deposition of salbutamol aerosol delivered by metered dose inhaler, jet nebulizer, and ultrasonic nebulizer in mechanically ventilated rabbits. *Pediatr Res.* 1997; 42(5):721-7.

97. Hughes JM, Saez J: Effects of nebulizer mode and position in a mechanical ventilator circuit on dose efficiency, *Respir Care* 1987;32:1131.

98. Harvey CJ et al: Effect of a spacer on pulmonary aerosol deposition from a jet nebulizer during mechanical ventilation, *Thorax* 1995;50:50.

99. Rau JL, Harwood RJ, Groff JL: Evaluation of a reservoir device for metered-dose bronchodilator delivery to intubated adults: an in vitro study, *Chest* 1992;102:924.

100. Bishop MJ, Larson RP, Buschman DL: Metered dose inhaler aerosol characteristics are affected by the endotracheal tube actuator/adapter used, *Anesthesiology* 1990;73:1263.

101. Fuller HD et al: Efficiency of bronchodilator aerosol delivery to the lungs from the metered dose inhaler in mechanically ventilated patients: a study comparing four different actuator devices, *Chest* 1994;105:214.

102. Manthous CA et al: Metered-dose inhaler versus nebulized albuterol in mechanically ventilated patients, *Am Rev Respir Dis* 1993;148:1567.

103. O'Riordan TG et al: Nebulizer function during mechanical ventilation, *Am Rev Respir Dis* 1992;145:1117.

104. Garner SS, Wiest DB, Bradley JW: Albuterol delivery by metered-dose inhaler with a pediatric mechanical ventilatory circuit model, *Pharmacotherapy* 1994; 14:210.

105. Fink JB et al: Deposition of aerosol from metered-dose inhaler during mechanical ventilation: an in vitro model, *Am J Respir Crit Care Med* 1996;154:382.

106. Svartengren M et al: Human lung deposition of particles suspended in air or in helium/oxygen mixture, *Exp Lung Res* 1989;15:575.

107. Anderson M et al: Deposition in asthmatics of particles inhaled in air or in helium–oxygen, *Am J Respir Crit Care Med* 1993;147:524.

108. Goode ML, Fink JB, Dhand R, Tobin MJ. Improvement in aerosol delivery with helium-oxygen mixtures during mechanical ventilation. *Am J Respir Crit Care Med.* 2001; 163(1):109–114.

109. Moren F, Andersson J: Fraction of dose exhaled after administration of pressurized inhalation aerosols, *Int J Pharm* 1980;6:295.

110. O'Riordan TG, Palmer LB, Smaldone GC: Aerosol deposition in mechanically ventilated patients: optimizing nebulizer delivery, *Am J Respir Crit Care Med* 1994;149:214.

111. Thomas SHL et al: Pulmonary deposition of a nebulized aerosol during mechanical ventilation, *Thorax* 1993;48:154.

112. Dubus JC et al: Aerosol deposition in neonatal ventilation, *Pediatric Res* 2005;58:10.

113. Fink JB: Aerosol delivery to ventilated infant and pediatric patients, *Respir Care* 2004;49:653.

114. Dhand R et al: Dose response to bronchodilator delivered by metered-dose inhaler in ventilator-supported patients, *Am J Respir Crit Care Med* 1996;154:388.

115. Dolovich MB et al: American College of Chest Physicians; American College of Asthma, Allergy, and Immunology: Device selection and outcomes of aerosol therapy: evidence-based guidelines, *Chest* 2005;127:335.

116. Rubin BK: Emerging therapies for cystic fibrosis lung disease, *Chest* 1999;115:1120.

117. Ramsey BW et al: Efficacy of aerosolized tobramycin in patients with cystic fibrosis, *N Engl J Med* 1993;328:1740.

118. Sexauer WP, Fiel SB: Aerosolized antibiotics in cystic fibrosis, *Semin Respir Crit Care Med* 2003;24:717.

119. Ryan G, Mukhopadhyay S, Singh M: Nebulized antipseudomonal antibiotics for cystic fibrosis, *Cochrane Database Syst Rev* 2003;3:CD001021.

120. Rubin BK, van der Schans CP, editors: *Lung Biology in Health and Disease*, Vol 188: *Therapy for mucus-clearance disorders*, Boca Raton, Fla: CRC Press/Taylor & Francis; 2004.

121. McCoy K, Hamilton S, Johnson C: Effects of 12-week administration of dornase alfa in patients with advanced cystic fibrosis lung disease, *Chest* 1996;110:889.

122. Wilmott RW et al: Aerosolized recombinant human DNase in hospitalized cystic fibrosis patients with acute pulmonary exacerbations, *Am J Respir Crit Care Med* 1996;153:1914.

123. O'Donnell AE et al; rhDNase Study Group: Treatment of idiopathic bronchiectasis with aerosolized recombinant human DNase I, *Chest* 1998;113:1329.

124. Henke MO, Shah SA, Rubin BK: The role of airway secretions in COPD: clinical applications. *J COPD* 2005;3:377.

125. Henke MO et al: MUC5AC and MUC5B mucins are decreased in cystic fibrosis airway secretions, *Am J Respir Cell Mol Biol* 2004;31:86.

126. App EM et al: Dose-finding and 24-h monitoring for efficacy and safety of aerosolized Nacystelyn in cystic fibrosis, *Eur Respir J* 2002;19:294.

127. Feng W et al: Improved clearability of cystic fibrosis sputum with dextran treatment in vitro, *Am J Respir Crit Care Med* 1998;157:710.

128. Deterding R et al; Cystic Fibrosis Foundation Therapeutics Development Network: Safety and tolerability of denufosol tetrasodium inhalation solution, a novel P2Y$_2$ receptor agonist: results of a phase 1/phase 2 multicenter study in mild to moderate cystic fibrosis, *Pediatr Pulmonol* 2005;39:339.

129. Griese M et al: Sequential analysis of surfactant, lung function and inflammation in cystic fibrosis patients, *Respir Res* 2005;6:133.

130. Anzueto A et al: Effects of aerosolized surfactant in patient with stable chronic bronchitis: a prospective randomized controlled trial, *JAMA* 1997;278:1426.

131. Eng PA et al: Short-term efficacy of ultrasonically nebulized hypertonic saline in cystic fibrosis, *Pediatr Pulmonol* 1996;21:77.

132. Daviskas E et al: Inhaled mannitol for the treatment of mucociliary dysfunction in patients with bronchiectasis: effect on lung function, health status and sputum, *Respirology* 2005;10:46.

133. Wark PA, McDonald V, Jones AP: Nebulised hypertonic saline for cystic fibrosis, *Cochrane Database Syst Rev* 2005;3:CD001506.

134. Wills P, Greenstone M: Inhaled hyperosmolar agents for bronchiectasis, *Cochrane Database Syst Rev* 2002;1:CD002996.

135. Suri R et al: Comparison of hypertonic saline and alternate-day or daily recombinant human deoxyribonuclease in children with cystic fibrosis: a randomised trial, *Lancet* 2001;358:1316.

136. Knowles MR et al: A controlled study of adenovirus-vector-mediated gene transfer in the nasal epithelium of patients with cystic fibrosis, *N Engl J Med* 1995;333:823.

137. Rochat T, Morris MA: Gene therapy for cystic fibrosis by means of aerosol, *J Aerosol Med* 2002;15:229.

138. Moss RB et al: Repeated adeno-associated virus serotype 2 aerosol-mediated cystic fibrosis transmembrane regulator gene transfer to the lungs of patients with cystic fibrosis: a multicenter, double-blind, placebo-controlled trial, *Chest* 2004;125:509.

139. Eastman SJ, Scheule RK: Cationic lipid: pDNA complexes for the treatment of cystic fibrosis, *Curr Opin Mol Ther* 1999;1:186.

140. Flotte TR, Carter BJ: In vivo gene therapy with adeno-associated virus vectors for cystic fibrosis, *Adv Pharmacol* 1997;4:199.

141. Mallet JP, Diot P, Lemarie E: Inhalation route for administration of systemic drugs, *Rev Malad Respir* 1997;14:257.

142. Heinemann L, Traut T, Heise T: Time–action profile of inhaled insulin, *Diabet Med* 1997;14:63.

143. Jedle JH, Karlberg BE: Intrapulmonary administration of insulin to healthy volunteers, *J Int Med* 1996;240:93.

144. Laube BL, Benedict GW, Dobs AS: The lung as an alternative route for delivery for insulin in controlling postprandial glucose levels in patients with diabetes, *Chest* 1998;114:1734.

145. DeFronzo RA et al; Exubera Phase III Study Group: Efficacy of inhaled insulin in patients with type 2 diabetes not controlled with diet and exercise: a 12-week, randomized, comparative trial, *Diabetes Care* 2005;28:1922.

146. Dawson M, Wirtz D, Hanes J: Enhanced viscoelasticity of human cystic fibrotic sputum correlates with increasing microheterogeneity in particle transport, *J Biol Chem* 2003;278:50393.

147. Rosenstock J et al: Inhaled insulin improves glycemic control when substituted for or added to oral combination therapy in type 2 diabetes: a randomized, controlled trial, *Ann Intern Med* 2005;143:549.

148. Laube BL: The expanding role of aerosols in systemic drug delivery, gene therapy, and vaccination, *Respir Care* 2005;50:1161.

149. Edwards DA, Dunbar C: Bioengineering of therapeutic aerosols, *Annu Rev Biomed Eng* 2002;4:93.

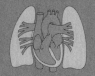

Chapter 14

Airway Clearance Techniques and Lung Volume Expansion

BRIAN K. WALSH

LEARNING OBJECTIVES

After reading this chapter the reader will be able to:
- Explain the indications and risks of airway clearance techniques

- Apply the various techniques of airway clearance
- Understand how to avoid complications associated with airway clearance techniques

Classic airway clearance techniques are designed to remove secretions from the lungs and include postural drainage, percussion, chest wall vibration, and coughing. Newer techniques considered part of chest physical therapy (CPT) are maneuvers to improve the efficacy of cough, such as the following:

- The forced expiration technique (FET)
- Positive expiratory pressure (PEP) therapy
- High-frequency chest compression (HFCC)
- Specialized breathing techniques, such as autogenic drainage (AD)

Because all of these techniques share the same goal—removal of bronchial secretions—the term *bronchial drainage* is often employed to describe them collectively. This term may be preferable to CPT because it highlights the aims, rather than the means, of treatment. This chapter is devoted to describing and analyzing bronchial drainage techniques and how they should be applied to the infant or pediatric patient with lung disease or respiratory impairment.

HISTORY AND CURRENT STATUS OF AIRWAY CLEARANCE TECHNIQUES

Postural drainage was used as early as 1901 in the treatment of bronchiectasis.[1] In the 1960s and 1970s we saw an increase in the use of CPT.[2] It was introduced in many U.S. hospitals concurrent with a wave of mounting criticism of intermittent positive-pressure breathing (IPPB) therapy. Many institutions found that the routine use of IPPB was replaced with the routine use of CPT. Beginning in the late 1970s, experts in the field began to point to the lack of evidence to support the routine use of CPT in pulmonary disorders such as pneumonia and chronic bronchitis.[3] However, despite a steady stream of criticism, the use of CPT appears to have increased dramatically.[4-12]

CHEST PHYSICAL THERAPY TECHNIQUES

Classic CPT has four components: (1) postural drainage, (2) percussion, (3) vibration of the chest wall, and (4) coughing.

Postural Drainage

Postural drainage attempts to use gravity to move secretions from peripheral airways to the larger bronchi, from which they are more easily expectorated. The patient is placed in various positions, each designed to drain specific segments of the lung, and may be supported by rolled towels, blankets, or pillows. Figures 14-1 and 14-2 illustrate postural drainage positions used in infants and children.[13] Other versions incorporating minor variations have also been published.[2,14,15] Postural drainage can be performed with or without percussion or vibration. When accompanied by percussion or vibration, each position is maintained for 1 to 5 minutes, depending on the severity of the patient's condition. When percussion or vibration is omitted, longer periods of simple postural drainage can be performed.

Percussion

Percussion is believed to loosen secretions from the bronchial walls. While the patient is in the various postural drainage positions, the clinician percusses the chest wall, using a cupped hand (Figure 14-3). The areas to be percussed are illustrated in Figures 14-1 and 14-2. Clinicians should not percuss over bony prominences; over the spine, sternum, abdomen, last few ribs, sutured areas, drainage tubes, kidneys, or liver; or below the rib cage. The ideal frequency of percussion is unknown; however, some reports recommend a frequency of 5 to 6 Hz (300 to 360 blows/min), whereas others recommend slow, rhythmic clapping.[14,16] Several devices can be used for percussion, including soft face masks as well as those commercially designed, such as "palm cups" and mechanical percussors (Figure 14-4). Infants and children may have CPT performed in the lap of the clinician. However, if the patient is mechanically ventilated or has multiple tubes and intravenous lines in place, it may be preferable to perform therapy with the patient in the bed. Catheters, tubes, and indwelling lines are easily dislodged in infants and young children, and appropriate care must be taken.

Postural Drainage and Percussion

Many investigations have been conducted to determine the relative importance of percussion, vibration, and postural drainage. In a study designed to determine the contribution of these maneuvers to clearance of mucus, there was no demonstration of improvement in clearance of mucus from the lung when percussion, vibration, or breathing exercises were added to postural drainage.[17] These investigators also showed that FET was superior to simple coughing and when combined with postural drainage was the most effective form of treatment.[18] Other studies[19-21] have reported that:

1. Percussion without postural drainage or cough produced minimal change in the clearance of mucus.
2. When compared with simple postural drainage, chest percussion actually reduced the amount of sputum mobilized.
3. Manual self-percussion did not increase the amount of sputum expectorated compared with simple postural drainage in a group of patients with cystic fibrosis (CF).

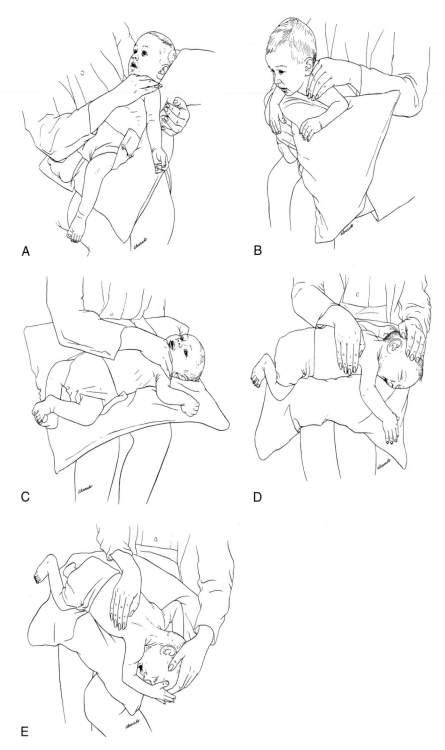

A

B

C

D

E

FIGURE 14-1 Postural drainage positions for infants. **A,** Apical segment of the right upper lobe and apical subsegment of the apical–posterior segment of the left upper lobe. **B,** Posterior segment of the right upper lobe and posterior subsegment of the apical–posterior segment of the left upper lobe. **C,** Anterior segments of right and left upper lobes. **D,** Superior segments of both lower lobes. **E,** Posterior basal segments of both lower lobes.

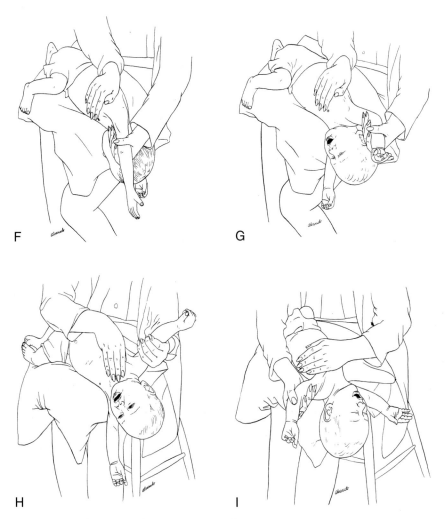

FIGURE 14-1—cont'd Postural drainage positions for infants. **F,** Lateral basal segment of the right lower lobe. Lateral basal segment of the left lower lobe is drained in a similar fashion but with the right side down. **G,** Anterior basal segment of the right lower lobe. The segments on the left side are drained in a similar fashion but with the right side down. **H,** Right middle lobe. **I,** Left lingular segment of lower lobe.

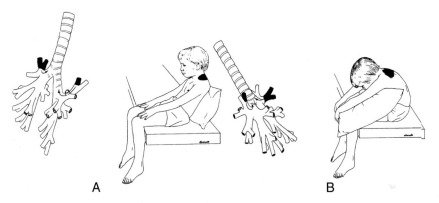

FIGURE 14-2 Postural drainage positions for the child or adult. The model of the tracheobronchial tree next to or above the child illustrates the segmental bronchi being drained. The *stippled area* on the child's chest illustrates the area to be percussed or vibrated. **A,** Apical segment of right upper lobe and apical subsegment of apical-posterior segment of left upper lobe (area between the clavicle and top of the scapula). **B,** Posterior segment of right upper lobe and posterior subsegment of apical-posterior segment of left upper lobe (area over the upper back).

Continued

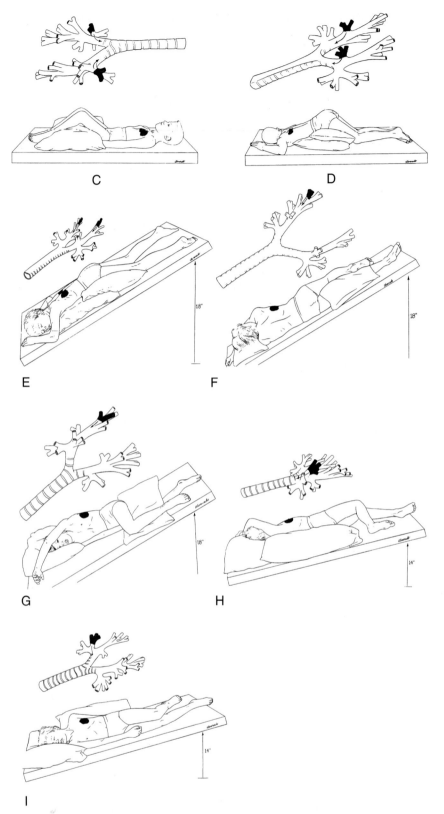

FIGURE 14-2—cont'd Postural drainage positions for the child or adult. The model of the tracheobronchial tree next to or above the child illustrates the segmental bronchi being drained. The *stippled area* on the child's chest illustrates the area to be percussed or vibrated. **C,** Anterior segments of right and left upper lobes (area between clavicle and nipple). **D,** Superior segments of both lower lobes (area over middle of back at tip of scapula, beside spine). **E,** Posterior basal segments of both lower lobes (area over lower rib cage, beside spine). **F,** Lateral basal segment of right lower lobe. Segment on left is drained in a similar fashion but with the right side down (area over middle portion of rib cage). **G,** Anterior basal segment of left lower lobe. Segment on right is drained in a similar fashion but with the left side down (area over lower ribs, below the armpit). **H,** Right middle lobe (area over right nipple; below breast in developing females). **I,** Left lingular segment of lower lobe (area over left nipple; below breast in developing females).

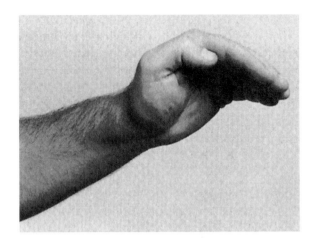

FIGURE 14-3 Proper cupping of hand for percussion.

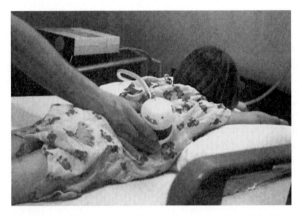

FIGURE 14-4 Percussion being performed on a child with a manual percussor.

Vibration of the Chest Wall

Vibrations represent an additional method of transmitting energy through the chest wall to loosen or move bronchial secretions. Unlike in percussion, the clinician's hand does not lose contact with the chest wall during the procedure. Vibrations are performed by placing both hands (one over the other) over the area to be vibrated and tensing and contracting the shoulder and arm muscles while the patient exhales. To prolong exhalation, the patient may be asked to breathe through pursed lips or make a "hissing" sound. As with percussion, the ideal frequency is unknown, although some recommend 10 to 15 Hz.[22] It is unclear how well clinicians are able to perform vibrations at this frequency. Several mechanical vibrators are commercially available. An electric toothbrush with foam padding covering the bristle or a padded syringe barrel attached to the handle of the toothbrush can be used with an infant. Some models of mechanical percussors or vibrators are appropriate only for the newborn or premature infant, whereas other models are appropriate for the larger child. When evaluating such devices, the clinician should consider whether the appearance and sound of the device will be frightening and whether the amount of force is appropriate for the size of the patient. All percussion and vibration devices should be cleaned after each use.

CHEST PHYSICAL THERAPY IN THE NEWBORN

Collapse of the right upper lobe after extubation is a common complication in the premature infant, and routine treatment of premature infants after extubation is common.[23,24] Treatment may be given to the right upper lobe only and need not be prolonged, nor does it require the routine use of percussion. A treatment length of 5 minutes is sufficient, and vibration is applied to the right upper lobe in one of the three standard drainage positions every 1 to 3 hours for 24 to 48 hours.[24]

Patients with esophageal atresia and tracheoesophageal fistula often require assistance in mobilizing thick secretions. Aspiration of oropharyngeal secretions, leading to atelectasis or pneumonia, is common. If surgical repair has been performed, deep endotracheal suctioning (beyond the tip of the endotracheal tube) is contraindicated because the suction catheter may reopen the closed fistula. Likewise, nonintubated patients should rarely have the catheter advanced more than 7 cm because this makes removal of secretions more difficult. On occasion, tracheal suction under direct vision with a laryngoscope is necessary. If the fistula has been closed, Trendelenburg (head-down) positioning may be used. This is especially helpful if the patient has difficulty clearing oral secretions by swallowing. These patients should not be routinely placed flat on their backs because this promotes aspiration of oral secretions. Given that a thoracotomy has been performed to repair the defect, use of a small mechanical vibrator may be preferable to chest percussion.

The clinician must be careful to avoid excessive movement (extension or extreme turning) while treating the infant. Esophageal atresia is repaired by performing an anastomosis of the distal and proximal esophagus. Excessive head movement may result in its disruption. Many other patients often require CPT in the neonatal intensive care unit. Usually, such patients have been intubated for some time and have responded to prolonged intubation with excessive production of secretions.

CHEST PHYSICAL THERAPY IN YOUNG CHILDREN

When performing CPT on young children, the clinician must make a special effort to secure the patient's confidence and cooperation. Some children may have seen

CPT performed on other patients and may conclude that it is a painful procedure. Spending a few moments to gain the child's confidence is well worth the effort. Assigning the same clinician to treat the child as often as is practical may be useful in establishing a rapport. Likewise, allowing the child as much control over the situation as possible, such as deciding which lobes will be treated first, may increase the child's sense of control and reduce hospitalization-related anxiety. Having a parent available during therapy, especially when the child is unfamiliar with CPT, is useful as well.

CPT may be extremely uncomfortable for the postoperative patient, and routine use of CPT in these patients may actually promote atelectasis. Some patients, however, suffer from excessive secretions or mucous plugging and atelectasis. Performing CPT in these patients can be difficult. Adequate analgesia is essential, and attempts should be made to schedule CPT shortly after pain medication is administered. Coughing is also a considerable source of discomfort in pediatric patients postoperatively. Cough efficacy can be improved if the patient is taught to splint the wounds when coughing. Holding a pillow over the incision may also be useful in minimizing movement of the incision when coughing.

Adverse Consequences

Several conditions common to the full-term or preterm newborn suggest that these infants may be at risk for ncreased complications from CPT; therefore modification of routine CPT procedures is advisable. Because the newborn has high chest wall compliance, the loss of lung volume due to chest wall compression (e.g., from percussion) may be greater in the infant than in the adult.[25] For this reason, some institutions routinely omit chest wall percussion in neonatal CPT treatments, opting instead for the use of small vibrators. Because an infant's chest wall is not as thick as an adult's, and the infant's ribs are more cartilaginous, a gentler touch is required during therapy.[26] Hypoxemia has been reported after CPT in the newborn.[27-30] Handling infants, for whatever reason, frequently results in hypoxemia. It is therefore essential that oxygenation be monitored during CPT in infants.

Routine application of CPT in the preterm infant has been associated with an increased risk of intraventricular hemorrhage (IVH).[31] The preterm infant is unable to adequately regulate cerebral blood flow, and changes in blood pressure often lead to increased intracranial pressure and volume, with rupture of immature blood vessels. Trendelenburg positioning and chest wall percussion would seem likely to increase cerebral blood flow and to reduce venous return, further increasing the risk of IVH. Therefore

these procedures should be used sparingly, if at all, in infants at risk. If possible, CPT should be withheld from infants at high risk for IVH (i.e., very premature infants in the first few days of life).

Critically ill newborns are unable to adequately maintain body temperature and are therefore routinely placed in incubators or under radiant warmers. Caregiver interventions of any kind, including CPT, interfere with maintaining temperature stability, especially for infants in closed incubators. Treatment time with these patients should be kept to a minimum, usually between 5 and 10 minutes. If a patient is in a temperature-regulated environment, special attention must be given to preventing heat loss during therapy.

The trachea and bronchi of the newborn appear especially vulnerable to damaging effects from endotracheal tubes and suction catheters. Consequences of deep endotracheal suctioning include the development of bronchial stenosis and granulomas. Avoiding deep endotracheal suctioning minimizes risks.[32] Therefore, when suctioning intubated infants after CPT, the suction catheter should not be routinely advanced beyond the end of the endotracheal tube. If there is evidence of persistent secretion retention despite adequate suction of the endotracheal tube, the suction catheter can be carefully and slowly advanced 1 or 2 cm beyond the tip of the endotracheal tube.

Many infants in the neonatal intensive care unit are sensitive to handling. This is especially true of the preterm infant as well as the full-term infant with pulmonary hypertension, who may develop hypoxemia or bradycardia in response to excessive stimulation. Many clinicians believe that the adverse consequences of handling can be minimized by clustering as many caregiver interventions as possible, thereby leaving the infant undisturbed for longer periods. Minimizing excessive light and sound associated with therapy is also desirable.

Cough

All CPT sessions should end with a period of coughing. Patients with minimal lung disease should be able to clear the lungs after one or two attempts. Those with severe lung disease may need more prolonged coughing periods. Prolonged periods of unproductive coughing should be avoided because they may tire the patient. The clinician should emphasize effective, productive coughing. Infants may require nasopharyngeal suction to stimulate a cough, whereas patients with artificial airways may require endotracheal suctioning.

The following procedures are sometimes incorporated into CPT treatments, or used independently, with the aim of promoting bronchial drainage: (1) FET, (2) PEP therapy, (3) AD, and (4) automatic HFCC.

Forced Expiration Technique

FET is also known as "huff" coughing. This maneuver requires the patient to forcibly exhale, from a middle to low lung volume, with an open glottis, but cannot be performed on infants or young children. This is repeated several times, after which the patient coughs to remove any loosened mucus.[33] FET can be used alone or in conjunction with other forms of therapy. It is designed to prevent dynamic airway collapse by preventing the explosive pressure changes associated with coughing.[8,33] Studies have documented that patients with long-standing lung disorders characterized by destruction or weakening of the bronchial wall, such as CF and bronchiectasis, have ineffective coughing secondary to dynamic airway compression while coughing.[34] The developers of this technique now use the term *active cycle of breathing* to refer to FET. They emphasize the importance of interspersing "huff" coughs with periods of deep, relaxed breathing. This helps prevent bronchospasm and ensures sufficient lung volume to promote an effective cough.

Coughing and Forced Expiration Technique

Over the years, a number of investigators have demonstrated that the single most important component of CPT is vigorous coughing.[35-39] Simple postural drainage has been reported to improve secretion clearance, whereas the addition of percussion did not.[36] Several other studies in patients with CF and other chronic lung diseases likewise support the notion that vigorous coughing, especially when used in conjunction with FET, may be as effective as postural drainage and percussion.[37,38,40]

Many clinicians, however, are reluctant to abandon postural drainage, percussion, or vibration in favor of simple FET, especially in patients needing life-long assistance with secretion removal, such as those with CF. A 3-year prospective study in children with CF demonstrated that conventional CPT, performed twice a day, was more effective than FET used at the same frequency.[41] Patients performing FET in this study had an average age of slightly younger than 12 years. In contrast, patients in studies that showed FET to be successful were older.[38,40] This suggests that forms of self-care may be more effective in adolescents than in younger children, who perhaps require more supervision. Likewise, comparison of studies on the efficacy of exercise as pulmonary therapy in CF suggests that self-therapy is more effective in older patients.[42,43]

Positive Expiratory Pressure Therapy

PEP therapy uses an expiratory resistor, coupled with the patient's active expiration, to generate positive airway pressure throughout expiration. This prevents dynamic airway collapse and improves clearance of mucus.[44] It is widely used in Europe, and increasingly in the United States, as an adjunct or substitute for conventional CPT in the treatment of CF or bronchiectasis, and to a lesser extent in postoperative patients. Various devices are available to serve as expiratory resistors: anything from simple high-resistance 2.5 ETT adapters attached to a mask or mouthpiece to a Flutter (Axcan Pharma, Mont-Saint-Hilaire, PQ, Canada), acapella (blue; Smiths Medical, Weston, Mass), or Quake device (Thayer Medical, Tucson, Ariz) that requires hand motion and breathing coordination. PEP therapy is essentially the same as the "blow bottles" that have been used to prevent postoperative atelectasis.[45] Both PEP therapy and FET are advocated as forms of simple, self-treatment for patients with CF. PEP therapy is better tolerated by children than conventional IPPB.

Autogenic Drainage

AD is a series of breathing exercises designed to mobilize secretions in patients with bronchiectasis or CF.[46-48] To loosen secretions from the smallest airways, the patient begins breathing in a slow, controlled manner, first at the expiratory reserve volume level. The volume of ventilation is then increased, with the patient breathing in the normal tidal volume range but exhaling approximately halfway into the expiratory reserve volume. This moves secretions from the peripheral to the middle airways. Finally, the depth of inspiration is increased, with the patient inhaling maximally to total lung capacity and exhaling as before about halfway into the expiratory reserve volume. Figure 14-5 graphically illustrates the autogenic drainage technique. Advocates of AD claim that its simplicity (no devices or clinicians are needed) and efficacy make it an ideal form of self-treatment for patients with CF.

Positive Expiratory Pressure Therapy and Autogenic Drainage

PEP therapy, AD, and HFCC have been shown to be highly effective. PEP therapy, especially, has been shown by a number of researchers to be beneficial in mobilizing secretions and preserving pulmonary function in patients with CF, and with FET it was marginally superior to simple FET and postural drainage.[49-56] Less information is available on AD, although a few reports indicate it is highly effective and that compliance is improved.[46-48,57]

High-frequency Chest Compression

A commercially available device (The Vest [ThAIRapy] bronchial drainage system; Hill-Rom, St. Paul, Minn) has been developed that compresses the entire chest wall at high frequencies by means of a snug-fitting inflatable

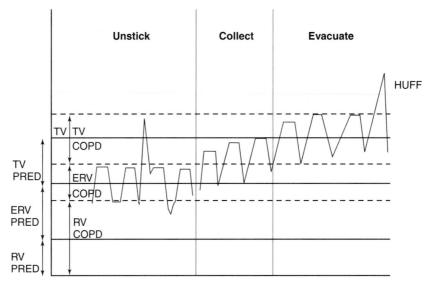

FIGURE 14-5 Graphic illustration of the depth of successive breaths by lung volumes, using the autogenic drainage technique. COPD, Chronic obstructive pulmonary disease; ERV, expiratory reserve volume; HUFF, huff maneuver; PRED, predicted; RV, residual volume; TV, tidal volume.

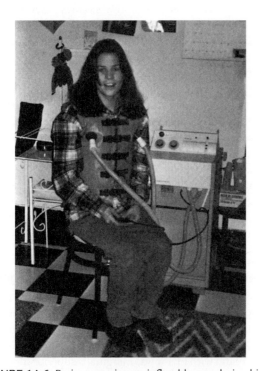

FIGURE 14-6 Patient wearing an inflatable vest during high-frequency chest compression therapy in the home.

vest connected to a high-performance air compressor (Figure 14-6). Intermittent chest wall compression produces brief periods of high expiratory air flow, which loosens and mobilizes mucus from bronchial walls.[58] The device is widely used in patients with CF (see Chapter 32, Acute Respiratory Distress Syndrome).

HFCC has also been evaluated in a long-term study. After a 22-month period of using HFCC as the sole form of CPT, patients experienced a small but significant improvement in pulmonary function. In contrast, after a similar period on conventional manual CPT, pulmonary function declined somewhat.[58] HFCC does not require the patient to perform postural drainage (known to be effective for sputum mobilization) and incorporates rapid percussion (generally demonstrated to be ineffective). What accounts for this seeming paradox? HFCC compresses the chest at frequencies up to 22 Hz, which is much higher than can be generated by manual percussion (5 to 8 Hz). Furthermore, compression is usually applied only on exhalation. In the initial studies with HFCC, the developers of this device measured expiratory volumes and flows and selected the frequencies that resulted in the highest values for these variables. High expiratory air flow is maintained with HFCC, even at low lung volumes. The result is multiple, brief periods of high expiratory air flow (or more precisely air velocity), similar to "huff" coughing or FET.[59]

High expiratory air velocity at low lung volumes produces the greatest air–mucus interaction and hence mucous mobilization. HFCC does not directly dislodge mucus from the bronchial wall, as conventional percussion is thought to do, but instead simulates multiple coughs or FETs by generating high expiratory air velocities. Because the compressive phase of HFCC is brief (as short as 0.02 s at a frequency of 22 Hz) and the glottis remains open during therapy, it is unlikely that dynamic airway collapse occurs, as happens with natural coughing in patients with bronchiectasis or CF.

Manual percussion bears little resemblance to HFCC. In contrast to HFCC, manual percussion is rarely, if ever, adjusted to produce optimal expiratory air flow to simulate cough or FET. In addition, it is given during inspiration as well as expiration, which may limit the deep breathing that is essential for producing high expiratory air velocities. Finally, manual percussion is applied only to a small portion of the chest wall at one time, which may be insufficient to generate adequate expiratory flows.

Effectiveness of Techniques

Proponents of conventional CPT techniques often describe the problem that CPT aims to treat as abnormal (excessive, thick, tenacious) secretions. Although this is partially correct, therapies that would seem to attack this problem directly have proved disappointing. Manual, low-frequency chest percussion does not seem to jar mucus loose from the airways, nor does chest wall vibration. Of the therapies that do work—postural drainage, PEP, AD, FET, and the HFCC system—all attempt to prevent or compensate for dynamic airway collapse. Postural drainage attempts to move mucus passively, by force of gravity, past the damaged, collapsible portions of the airways and toward less diseased, more rigid central airways. The remaining therapies attempt to prevent dynamic airway collapse while at the same time producing high expiratory air velocity at low lung volumes. This develops the shearing forces required to mobilize sputum.[4] A novel explanation for the efficacy of simple postural drainage is suggested by Lannefors and Wollmer,[60] who demonstrated improved mucous clearance in the dependent lung of patients undergoing postural drainage. For most patients, lung volumes and airway diameter are reduced in the dependent lung but ventilation is increased. These factors result in increased air movement at high velocity, which increases turbulence and shearing in small airways and results in greater mobilization of mucus.

Deep breathing associated with vigorous exercise has also been shown to be an effective technique for mobilization of secretions in patients with CF.[61,62] To accommodate the increased ventilatory demands of exercise, rate and depth of breathing are increased and active exhalation may occur. Hence, vigorous exercise produces a ventilatory pattern that, like AD or FET, increases air velocity at low lung volumes and promotes sputum mobilization.

"Take a deep breath and you'll feel better." This is a sound piece of advice that was given long before the advent of incentive spirometry or IPPB. Taking a deep breath to total lung capacity, either by sighing or yawning, is a normal, unconscious maneuver performed periodically to keep the lungs inflated and to avoid ventilation–perfusion mismatch.[63] When the breathing pattern becomes one of tidal ventilation without periodic maximal inflation, atelectasis ensues within a few hours.[64] Variations in the normal pattern of breathing may result in respiratory complications and an increase in postoperative morbidity and mortality. Changes in the breathing patterns of pediatric patients are most often caused by increased sedation, narcotics, pain, fluid overload, parenchymal lung damage, fear and anxiety, and abdominal or thoracic surgery. It has been estimated that 10% to 40% and even as many as 70% of patients undergoing abdominal or thoracic surgery experience postoperative pulmonary complications,[65,66] consisting of atelectasis, pneumonia, pulmonary embolism, and hypoxemia. These conditions are believed to be caused by reduced diaphragmatic movement (especially after upper abdominal surgery), changes in chest wall muscle tone, and secretion retention, all of which result in decreased lung volumes.[67]

The modalities and methods used to increase a child's lung volume can be classified as (1) voluntary—using the patient's own effort and initiative to sustain a deep breath (incentive spirometry) and (2) applied—providing the patient with a positive-pressure-generated breath to achieve an increase in lung volume (IPPB). In this chapter these methods of lung volume expansion therapy are discussed as they relate to the pediatric patient.

COMPLICATIONS OF CHEST PHYSICAL THERAPY

Numerous studies have demonstrated that CPT can be detrimental, especially when applied in patients with little or no sputum production. Reported complications of CPT range from rare reports of complete airway obstruction and respiratory arrest to bronchospasm and hypoxemia.

Hypoxemia

The most commonly cited adverse effect of CPT is hypoxemia. Several studies have reported hypoxemia in infants receiving CPT.[27-30] Hypoxemia has also been documented in studies of adolescent and adult patients receiving CPT and was reported to occur more often in patients with preexisting cardiovascular complications, with minimal sputum production, and when mucoid rather than mucopurulent secretions were present. It occurred in patients with good pulmonary function and also when supplemental oxygen was being used.[68-73] Tachypnea and tachycardia may occur in patients who experience hypoxemia during CPT.

There may be a variety of reasons why CPT often causes hypoxemia. Among the proposed mechanisms are ventilation–perfusion ($\dot{V}/\dot{Q}$) abnormalities caused by postural changes, atelectasis, bronchospasm, alterations in cardiac output and oxygen consumption, and incomplete expectoration of mobilized secretions. In addition, each of the CPT techniques may contribute to hypoxemia to differing degrees.

Position

Most studies of the effects of posture on oxygenation in adults would suggest that putting the diseased portion of the lung uppermost, as in postural drainage therapy, improves oxygenation.[74-76] This is a consequence of improved perfusion of the healthy, dependent lung tissue at the expense of the diseased, elevated lung segments. Thus, at least for patients with localized, unilateral lung disease, $\dot{V}/\dot{Q}$ abnormalities secondary to postural changes are an unlikely explanation for CPT-associated hypoxemia in patients outside of infancy. Infants, however, have better oxygenation when the affected side is dependent (i.e., the good lung is up).[77] This may in part be the result of higher baseline pulmonary artery pressures, which would mitigate the effects of gravity on pulmonary blood flow. Hence, alterations in $\dot{V}/\dot{Q}$ relationships as a direct result of postural changes are a possible explanation for CPT-associated hypoxemia in infants. Patients with generalized lung disease may respond differently to postural changes, however, and careful monitoring of oxygenation with position changes may be warranted. Positional changes during CPT may also result in hypotension or hypertension.

Percussion

Several studies report that chest percussion, rather than postural changes, is responsible for CPT-associated hypoxemia.[29,68-70] These studies suggest that chest percussion causes significant $\dot{V}/\dot{Q}$ abnormalities, and unless counterbalanced by removal of a substantial quantity of mucus and improvement in $\dot{V}/\dot{Q}$ ratios, the net change will be a deterioration in $\dot{V}/\dot{Q}$ relationships and hypoxemia.

Atelectasis

Both human and animal studies have shown an increase in atelectasis when CPT was given.[67,78] Vigorous chest percussion has been noted to produce pressure swings in the chest of up to 30 cm H_2O. Such pressures generated by intermittent compression or percussion of the chest wall would seem sufficient to expel appreciable quantities of air from the lung, especially if chest wall compliance is high. Chest wall vibration, in contrast to percussion, has been associated with hypoxemia in some studies.[28-30,79,80] This reflects the fact that vibration may or may not be associated with chest wall compression, depending on the techniques or equipment used, whereas chest percussion invariably causes chest wall compression.

Bronchospasm

An additional explanation for the association of chest percussion with hypoxemia is the observation that chest percussion can cause bronchospasm in susceptible patients, especially when sputum production is minimal. Administering bronchodilators before therapy may be desirable, especially when CPT is applied in patients with reactive airway disease.

Increased Oxygen Consumption

Oxygen consumption is increased during CPT.[81,82] If significant shunting is present, or if an increase in cardiac output is not produced, increased oxygen consumption can be manifested by decreased Pao_2 (partial pressure of oxygen in the arterial blood).

Gastroesophageal Reflux

Gastroesophageal reflux (GER) is a common cause of respiratory problems in infants and children, and CPT is often ordered for patients who have GER. One study found that in patients with GER, CPT resulted in a fivefold increase in reflux episodes, compared with periods when CPT was not given.[83] This increase in GER was seen even though treatments were withheld up to 3.5 hours after the infant's last feeding. The study did not link the increase in reflux episodes to any particular aspect of CPT, such as head-down positioning. GER may cause severe esophagitis, bronchospasm, or pneumonia and has been linked to apnea and sudden infant death syndrome.[84] Therefore CPT should be given only when the benefits of treatment clearly outweigh the risks of aggravated GER. Although withholding treatment as long as possible after an infant's feeding is advisable, it clearly will not eliminate the risks involved.

Airway Obstruction and Respiratory Arrest

Although CPT can be an effective means of removing bronchial foreign bodies in children, it may also result in acute upper airway obstruction and death.[85] This is especially true when the foreign body consists of organic material, such as seeds or nuts, that may increase in size (secondary to water absorption) after a period of time in the lung. Vomiting and aspiration may also occur during CPT, especially if therapy is given soon after the patient has eaten. Therefore at least 1 hour should be allowed after the last meal or feeding before beginning CPT. Patients receiving continuous feedings through gastric tubes should have the feedings turned off at least 30 minutes before therapy. More time may be needed in patients with a history of vomiting or reflux. For patients in whom feedings cannot be interrupted, Trendelenburg (head-down) positioning should not be used.

Intracranial Complications

Studies in preterm infants have reported that certain positions of the infant's head may increase intracranial pressure and that routine application of CPT, especially in the first few days of life, can significantly increase the risk of IVH.[31,86] CPT procedures in the child or adult with a recent head injury can also increase intracranial pressure.[87] Because of these concerns, many institutions do not place premature infants or patients with head injuries in the Trendelenburg position during CPT.

Rib Fractures and Bruising

Rib fractures have been reported as a complication of chest percussion in preterm infants with bronchopulmonary dysplasia.[88] The infants in this study suffered from rickets secondary to long-term parenteral nutrition. Improvement in nutritional therapy for preterm infants, however, should make rickets a rare finding in the infant with bronchopulmonary dysplasia. Infants with the rare condition of osteogenesis imperfecta are also at high risk of rib fractures. Bruising may occur in some patients, especially in the very small premature infant and the child with vitamin K deficiency. Most patients are more comfortable if percussion or vibration is performed with the skin covered by a pajama top or T-shirt. If the patient is not wearing pajamas or clothing, a lightweight blanket or towel should be placed on the chest and back. Excessive padding, however, should be avoided.

Airway Trauma

In all patients, extreme care must be taken to maintain a proper airway. Infants and children with artificial airways in place can be accidentally extubated during CPT, especially if they are being mechanically ventilated. The ventilator tubing or endotracheal tube, or both, are easily pulled during position changes, and extubation may result. When turning the patient, condensation in the ventilator tubing can be inadvertently drained into the patient's airway, which may result in bronchospasm and respiratory distress. Special attention should also be given to patients who receive CPT during the first 24 hours after a tracheostomy because hemorrhage may occur if therapy is given too vigorously.[26] Therefore, for patients in intensive care units or those with artificial airways in place, suction equipment as well as a manual resuscitator and mask should be readily available, preferably at the patient's bedside.

SELECTION OF PATIENTS FOR CHEST PHYSICAL THERAPY

CPT is ordered for a multiplicity of conditions, including acute respiratory infections, postoperative complications, CF, and asthma, to name a few. Evidence is increasing, however, that CPT is required in only a limited number of conditions, all of which are characterized by chronic, excessive sputum production.

Conditions in Which Chest Physical Therapy May Not Be Beneficial

Various studies in children and adults have demonstrated that CPT may not be beneficial in certain conditions.

In studies of the effects of CPT in children hospitalized with severe exacerbation of asthma, no difference was found in the rate of improvement of pulmonary function, even in the most severe cases.[89] Other studies in adults with reactive airway disease have shown that chest percussion can cause bronchospasm and hypoxemia.[70,90,91] Selected patients with asthma may benefit from CPT, especially when copious secretions or obstructive atelectasis are present. However, bronchospasm and hypoxemia should be well controlled before treatment. CPT is no substitute for adequate treatment with bronchodilating agents. It is also essential that a patient with asthma be well hydrated before CPT is begun.

Although bronchiolitis is characterized by increased secretions, studies have reported CPT to be of minimal value. CPT made no difference in the length of hospital stay or the severity or duration of symptoms in patients with bronchiolitis, even when associated pneumonia or atelectasis was present.[92] It also produced no beneficial changes in lung mechanics or work of breathing in patients with bronchiolitis.[93] The failure of CPT to produce an effect in bronchiolitis most likely results from the fact that the disease affects the smaller, peripheral airways, where CPT techniques are generally not effective.[8]

Several studies have evaluated the role of CPT in pneumonia and have reported that CPT either had no effect or actually delayed resolution, especially in young adults.[92,94,95]

In a study of a group of closely matched pediatric cardiac surgery patients, Reines and colleagues[96] reported that those treated with CPT had twice the incidence of atelectasis as did the control group (68% vs. 32%), which received deep-breathing instruction, coughing, or suction as appropriate. Moreover, atelectasis was more severe and the duration of hospitalization was prolonged in the CPT group.

CPT to the right upper lobe every 1 to 2 hours for 24 hours after extubation is a common practice in many neonatal intensive care units. This practice is based on a report by Finer and associates[95] that claimed a dramatic reduction in the risk of right upper lobe atelectasis after extubation when CPT was given. However, it is unclear from the study if suctioning alone or CPT was responsible for the results.

Conditions in Which Chest Physical Therapy May Be Beneficial

In contrast to the reports criticizing its effectiveness, CPT has been shown to be beneficial in patients with acute and chronic conditions characterized by excessive secretion production or mucous plugging of large airways that does not clear with coughing or suction. "Excessive secretions" usually means 30 ml of sputum per day in adults. Obviously, lesser amounts would qualify as excessive secretions in children. CPT is also useful in the treatment of obstructive atelectasis. Figure 14-7 illustrates the process of evaluation of the pediatric patient for CPT.

Acute Lobar Atelectasis

The majority of patients with acute atelectasis secondary to mucous plugs respond with one CPT treatment.[23,98,99] If patients fail to respond to several CPT treatments, the atelectasis most likely is caused by conditions not amenable to CPT, and therapy should be discontinued. The presence of an air bronchogram,

suggesting no mucous obstruction of the airways, has been shown to predict a poor response to CPT.[23,99] Although a period of CPT after resolution of the atelectasis may be warranted, prolonged CPT should not be necessary. As discussed earlier, CPT is not useful in preventing the return of atelectasis, except in patients with large amounts of secretions.

Cystic Fibrosis

CPT has been widely employed as a mainstay of treatment for the pulmonary complications of CF. In fact, much of our knowledge of CPT comes from studies conducted in patients with CF.[41,97,99] Current issues in the application of CPT in these patients include the following questions: (1) Which techniques are most effective? (2) How can self-care be promoted? and (3) How can compliance with therapy be improved?

Effective techniques are those that foster high expiratory air velocity at low lung volume, such as FET, PEP therapy, HFCC, vigorous exercise, and AD. Postural drainage is also a useful adjunct to PEP therapy or FET. Although little evidence is available to support the routine use of manual chest percussion in the treatment of CF, and although some CF centers (especially in Europe) have abandoned the routine use of manual chest percussion, most CF treatment centers in the United States still consider it an integral component of CPT. Many patients will expect percussion to be a part of their CPT treatments, especially when hospitalized. Therefore elimination of chest percussion from routine CPT treatments should not be carried out arbitrarily. Radical changes in CPT practice for patients facing a lifelong battle with excessive pulmonary secretions should be made only after careful deliberation and consultation with the pulmonary physicians responsible for their care.

The issue of promoting self-care is especially important when dealing with patients with CF and their families. Patients with CF differ from most patients receiving CPT in that they need to employ some technique or techniques for removal of bronchial secretions on a daily basis for the rest of their lives. Current practices, especially those that require the routine application of chest percussion by a second person, often give the message that CPT is a passive technique; that it is something that is done "to" rather than "by" the patient. This may promote passivity and dependence on parents or other caregivers. As a result, compliance is often poor, and treatments become a frequent source of arguments in families of patients with CF, with difficulties increasing as the patients grow older.[40,100] Also, because CPT must be administered by a parent two or more times a day, it may interfere with normal adolescent developmental processes, such as increasing autonomy and separation

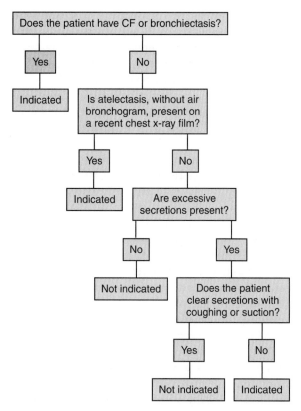

FIGURE 14-7 Algorithm for evaluating patients for chest physical therapy.

from parents. Therefore increasing the patient's ability to perform self-care is essential. All patients with CF, especially as they approach adolescence, should be well instructed in one of the forms of self-care, such as PEP, AD, FET with or without postural drainage, or HFCC. Vigorous exercise, such as running or swimming, is also an effective form of self-therapy in well-motivated patients. The techniques selected will depend on patient preference and learning ability, the preferences of the attending physician and, in the case of HFCC, the ability to arrange financing. Patients and their families often report improved compliance with self-care over parent-administered CPT, and treatment-related conflicts are minimized.[40]

Follow-up and consistency are essential when teaching bronchial drainage techniques. Reteaching may be necessary at intervals, and most patients with CF and their families are interested in learning new developments in CPT. Families often need assistance in adapting CPT practices to changing life circumstances, such as the patient entering school, traveling, entering college, and leaving home.

Patients with advanced CF often have hemoptysis. CPT is usually withheld until the bleeding is controlled because vigorous coughing may aggravate the bleeding or dislodge clots. Likewise, CPT may need to be withheld in patients with pneumothorax, another common complication of advanced CF. Patients with end-stage disease may be especially reluctant to cooperate with CPT, especially the Trendelenburg positioning that is required. Supplemental oxygen may allow some patients with advanced disease to tolerate postural drainage. Withholding percussion may also improve the patient's ability to maintain the Trendelenburg position. Some investigators have reported that PEP therapy is better tolerated than postural drainage and percussion in patients with end-stage disease.[44]

Neuromuscular Disease or Injury

CPT is often used in many patients with neuromuscular injury or disease, and survival is often improved when CPT, coughing, turning, and deep breathing are incorporated into routine care (see Chapter 44, Neurological and Neuromuscular Disorders).[10,101-103] Prolonged postural drainage is often especially helpful. However, patients with acute head injury should have well-controlled intracranial pressures before CPT is initiated.

Lung Abscess

Some patients with lung abscesses, especially older children, may be successfully treated with CPT.[104] Fearing that discharge of large amounts of infected material may spread the infection and lead to acute respiratory distress, some clinicians are reluctant to use CPT in the

treatment of lung abscess.[22] Likewise, hemoptysis is a common complication in patients with lung abscess, and CPT may increase this risk. These concerns must be balanced against the knowledge that alternative treatments for lung abscess, such as lung resections, are also risky.

CONTRAINDICATIONS

Frank hemoptysis, empyema, foreign body aspiration, and untreated pneumothorax are often considered contraindications to all components of CPT. Withholding CPT, especially percussion, is sometimes recommended when the platelet count is low (less than 50,000 cells/mm³). CPT is also usually withheld in the immediate postoperative period after tracheostomy, tracheobronchial reconstruction, and selected other conditions in which postoperative movement is extremely dangerous. Chest percussion should not be performed directly over fractured ribs, areas of subcutaneous emphysema, or recently burned or grafted skin. Some conditions may require modification of therapy or omission of certain components of CPT.

LENGTH AND FREQUENCY OF THERAPY

Treatments for patients with CF or bronchiectasis should be performed for at least 30 minutes, with many patients benefiting from therapy lasting 45 minutes or longer. Patients with severe dyspnea may require rest periods, which will further prolong therapy. Most pediatric respiratory care departments limit routine CPT treatments to 15 to 20 minutes.[105] CPT is rarely needed more than every 4 hours, although selected patients may benefit from more frequent suctioning or coughing. CPT orders should be evaluated at least every 48 hours for patients in intensive care units, at least every 72 hours for acute care patients, or whenever there is a change in a patient's status.[106]

THERAPY MODIFICATION

Many patients require modification of therapy because of medical or surgical procedures. Percussion may be extremely painful for patients postoperatively, and the use of manual vibration or mechanical vibrators is sometimes better tolerated. Also, clinicians should be careful to avoid percussion over implanted devices, such as ventricular–peritoneal shunts or implantable venous access devices (often used in patients with CF). Percussion is also omitted in patients with brittle bones, for example, in those with rickets or osteogenesis imperfecta.

Many patients may not tolerate Trendelenburg positioning. Included in this group are those with severe GER, recent intracranial trauma or surgery, increased intracranial pressure, abdominal distention or ascites, compromised diaphragm movement, uncontrolled hypertension, and severe cardiopulmonary failure.[106] With careful monitoring, simple side-to-side positioning may be attempted in these patients. The patient with a gastrostomy tube or chest tube, or both, may also require modifications in drainage positions.

Patients receiving CPT often have a disorder affecting only one lobe. These patients do not need CPT in all 11 positions but rather an abbreviated CPT treatment that uses postural drainage positions for the affected lobe only.

Infants and small children are unable to perform maneuvers such as FET or AD. Some clinicians have attempted to mimic these techniques with gentle chest wall compression during the expiratory phase, allowing the child to exhale to less than functional residual capacity. Like AD or FET performed in cooperative older patients, this technique results in increased expiratory air velocity at low lung volumes, improving mucous mobilization.

MONITORING DURING THERAPY

Patients in an intensive care unit who require CPT should have continuous monitoring of arterial oxygen saturation (Sao_2), heart rate, and respiratory rate. Breathing pattern, skin color, and breath sounds should also be noted.[106] Patients not in an intensive care unit who require high oxygen concentrations or who have a condition presenting a high risk of respiratory or cardiac failure should also have these variables monitored. Other patients with mild respiratory distress should have pulse and respiratory rate as well as breathing pattern, skin color, and breath sounds measured before and after therapy. This is especially true for younger patients who cannot verbalize complaints of distress. Routine monitoring of heart rate and respiratory rate for patients with chronic respiratory disorders, such as CF, is probably not warranted and may inadvertently give the message that CPT is harmful. When performing percussion or vibration on patients who are connected to cardiopulmonary monitors, the alarm on the monitor may become activated because of interference from the percussion or vibration. It is best to refrain from turning the monitor alarms completely off.

EVALUATION OF THERAPY

Because the goal of CPT is to promote the removal of excessive bronchial secretions, the single most important variable in evaluating the effectiveness of CPT is

the amount of secretions expectorated with therapy; however, this cannot be done in a vacuum and the basics should not be forgotten. The hydration status of the patient, and whether or not the patient's lungs are acidic, can play a huge role in the success of airway clearance.[107,108] Mucus changes from sol to gel if the lungs are acidic. Changes in sputum production, breath sounds, vital signs, chest radiographic findings, blood gas values, and lung mechanics may indicate a positive response to the therapy.[106] The removal of excessive bronchial secretions is not always associated with an immediate change in blood gases, breath sounds, or lung mechanics. Patients with advanced CF, for example, almost always have audible rales before and after therapy, whereas pulmonary function and blood gas determinations change little.

Patients undergoing mechanical ventilation may have measurements of lung mechanics as well as noninvasive blood gas monitoring data readily available. If so, the clinician should note any changes associated with therapy. Deterioration in these variables, especially if unaccompanied by removal of secretions, suggests that therapy should be modified or discontinued.

DOCUMENTATION OF THERAPY

When charting CPT treatments, the clinician should describe the techniques used (e.g., postural drainage, percussion, and AD), which lobes were treated, and what positions the patient was placed in. If certain segments or positions are omitted, this should be documented as well as the reason why this was done. The clinician should also note if suctioning was performed. To document the response to therapy, pretreatment and posttreatment breath sounds, vital signs, and the amount and quality of sputum expectorated should be noted.

INCENTIVE SPIROMETRY

Incentive spirometry, also referred to as *sustained maximal inspiration,* was introduced in the early 1970s in an effort to prevent postoperative pulmonary complications.[78,109] It was designed to encourage patients to improve their inspiratory volumes while visualizing their inspiratory effort. Forced expiratory maneuvers using devices such as blow bottles, blow gloves, and balloons have been prescribed in the past to prevent postoperative complications; however, they have been associated with the development of atelectasis and do not result in the same physiologic effects as incentive spirometry.[110-112] Although it is still debated which methods are most effective for the prevention and management of postoperative pulmonary complications, it is estimated that incentive spirometry is prescribed in 95% of all U.S. hospitals for prophylaxis and treatment of postoperative atelectasis.[113-117] The objectives of incentive spirometry are to prevent or reverse atelectasis, improve lung volumes, and improve inspiratory muscle performance (including use of the diaphragm).[110]

Indications, Contraindications, and Complications

Clinical conditions that may benefit from incentive spirometry are listed in Box 14-1.[110] Clinical symptoms often include fever, increased work of breathing, tachypnea, hypoxia, and evidence of atelectasis on the chest radiograph. For incentive spirometry to be effective in the pediatric patient, he or she must be able to cooperate and understand the procedure and to be able to breathe volumes exceeding his or her normal tidal volume.

Incentive spirometry is contraindicated in patients who cannot cooperate or follow instructions concerning the proper use of the device. The child may be uncooperative, physically disabled, or simply too young to effectively perform the maneuvers. Alternative methods to improve lung volumes should then be considered.[118,119]

The majority of problems that patients experience with incentive spirometry are the result of inadequate supervision or instruction, or both. These two factors account for a large number of ineffective treatments.[120] Hyperventilation may occur in the patient who performs the maneuvers too rapidly, and he or she may complain of lightheadedness or tingling in the fingers. The patient may also complain of fatigue during the procedure. These complaints can be alleviated by coaching the patient to slow down and rest between each maneuver. Pain from surgical incisions is frequently encountered postoperatively and can be decreased by splinting the surgical area with a pillow during deep breathing and coughing. Airway closure and bronchospasm may occur if the patient exhales forcefully to less than functional residual capacity before taking a deep inspiration. Again, this can be avoided with proper coaching by the clinician. Hypoxia may develop if the patient's oxygen

therapy is interrupted, especially when a mask is used. This can be prevented by using a nasal cannula during therapy.

Devices

The original Bartlett-Edwards incentive spirometer operated on a piston–bellows principle and was designed to fall open by gravity at a preset volume. A battery-operated light was activated when the patient inhaled from the spirometer and the preset volume was reached. To keep the light on, the patient had to continue to inhale. The light went off when the patient's glottis closed or total lung capacity was reached.[121] There are many different types and brands of incentive spirometers, including disposable and nondisposable devices. They are classified according to how inhalation is activated: (1) volume oriented or (2) flow oriented.

Most of the current volume-oriented incentive spirometers are based on the original Bartlett-Edwards spirometer. A volume is preset as a goal, and the patient is instructed to inhale until the preset goal is reached. The spirometer volume is measured according to the amount of volume displaced during the inhalation. Flow-oriented spirometers operate by using a floating ball or bar that is raised by the negative flow generated with inspiration. The more rapid and forceful the inspiratory flow, the higher the ball rises. Although differences in the inspiratory work of breathing among the various incentive spirometers have been reported, in terms of clinical outcome the differences among the devices appear to be negligible.[122,123] The device used will vary from one institution to another and may even vary among patients within the institution. Regardless of the type, the operator's instructions should be read and universal precautions followed.[124]

Procedure

Because the effectiveness of incentive spirometry relies mainly on the patient's effort and cooperation, it is essential that the procedure be understood. Even though incentive spirometry is routine to the clinician, it is not routine to the patient, and its importance, as well as its technique, should be thoroughly explained.

- The teaching session should be conducted preoperatively, before the child experiences the pain and trauma of surgery.
- The parents should be involved in the teaching process whenever possible, because they eventually assume the role of coach.
- The explanation should include the reason for therapy, how to use the incentive spirometry device, the goals of therapy, what is expected postoperatively, the importance of an effective cough, and how the patient may feel after surgery.

Box 14-1	Indications for Incentive Spirometry

- Abdominal surgery
- Thoracic surgery
- Surgery in patients with pulmonary disease
- Atelectasis
- Restrictive lung defects associated with quadriplegia
- Restrictive lung defects associated with a dysfunctional diaphragm

- The use of charts and pictures is especially effective with young patients.
- Explaining to the older patient that he or she normally sighs every 6 to 10 minutes and that the spirometer helps to make up for this is a simple way to emphasize the reason for the therapy.
- The specific incentive spirometer used should be shown to the child and family. A demonstration unit can be used to show the child exactly how to breathe and how the spirometer functions. The patient should then demonstrate its use. It may take several attempts before the patient can effectively use the device.

If the patient cannot be instructed preoperatively, the postoperative teaching should be carried out only after the patient is awake and alert enough to follow instructions. If preoperative instruction has taken place, the postoperative teaching should briefly review the procedure and specifically convey to the patient the frequency and duration prescribed by the physician (Figure 14-8).

Application

- The patient should be positioned in an upright sitting position or a semi-Fowler position so that there is minimal restriction to chest expansion. This may not be possible depending on the type of surgery or injuries that the patient might have received.
- The chest should be auscultated and the volume goal on the incentive spirometer preset. In the postoperative patient, the goal should begin with 75% of the preoperative volume and be increased or decreased according to the patient's ability.

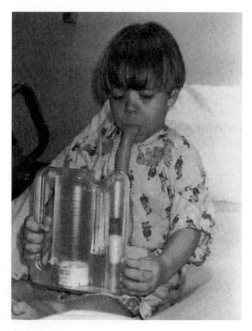

FIGURE 14-8 Child using incentive spirometry device.

- The patient should be instructed to exhale normally and then to place the mouth tightly around the mouthpiece and to inhale as slowly and deeply as possible through the mouth. Inspiring slowly will assist in even distribution of air to the alveoli. The breath should be held at end inspiration for 3 to 5 seconds and followed by a normal exhalation.[110]
- The patient should then remove the mouthpiece and exhale slowly.
- The patient should be allowed a short time to rest between maneuvers to help prevent fatigue and dizziness.
- A nose clip can be used for the patient who continues to inhale through the nose.
- The maximal volume of air the patient inhales is noted. (When teaching the use of this device preoperatively, the volume obtained should be recorded and used postoperatively as a baseline.)

The number of maneuvers to be performed per session should be either prescribed by the physician or set by departmental policy. Several sources have suggested 5 to 10 *effective* breaths per treatment as an adequate frequency.[110] The patient should cough during the session whenever it is felt necessary and then again when the maneuvers have been completed. The postoperative patient may need assistance with splinting of the incision during coughing as well as during deep breathing. A pillow or folded blanket can be placed over the incision area. The inspiratory volume goal may be increased when the patient reaches the preset goal repeatedly. Breath sounds should be assessed after coughing, and the incentive spirometer should be left within the patient's reach before the clinician leaves the room. The patient should be encouraged to perform the maneuvers independently between scheduled sessions. The frequency of sessions varies with the patient and may be prescribed as often and specifically as once per hour or as variably as three times per day.[16,17]

Assessment of Therapy

Documentation of the patient's response during therapy should include the following:

- Heart rate
- Respiratory rate
- Breath sounds
- Inspiratory volume or flow achieved
- Number of goals achieved
- Description of cough and sputum production
- Patient effort and tolerance
- How many maneuvers the family has tried/agreed to get the patient to do per hour
- Any patient complaints or adverse reactions, or both, and the corrective action taken

Therapy is considered effective if atelectasis is prevented or resolved and inspiratory muscle performance is improved.[110] Clinical signs of this would include a decreased respiratory rate, normal temperature, normal pulse rate, normal or improved breath sounds that were previously absent or diminished, a normal chest radiograph, improved oxygenation, and increased vital capacity and peak expiratory flows.[110]

Although there have been numerous studies evaluating the therapeutic value of incentive spirometry, it is difficult to compare them because of the variation in patients and study design.[125] However, a number of studies have indicated that incentive spirometry, along with other deep breathing maneuvers, is effective in reducing pulmonary complications when used correctly.[115,117,126-128] A study comparing the efficacy of postoperative incentive spirometry between children and adults concluded that incentive spirometry is as effective in reducing the incidence of atelectasis in children who have undergone cardiac surgery.[129]

INTERMITTENT POSITIVE-PRESSURE BREATHING

IPPB is the intermittent, short-term delivery of positive pressure to a patient for the purpose of improving lung expansion, delivering aerosolized medications, and assisting ventilation.[130] Since its inception in 1947 and its introduction into the medical arena in 1948, IPPB has been one of the most controversial topics in respiratory care.[131] It was one of the most popular therapeutic modalities prescribed in the 1960s and 1970s and was regarded as the panacea to all pulmonary ailments. Not until the American College of Chest Physicians' conference on oxygen therapy in September 1983, when both its overuse and its doubtful efficacy were discussed, did IPPB decline as a treatment modality.[132] Today newly practiced modalities, such as bilevel positive airway pressure and incentive spirometry, have rendered the prescription of IPPB more selective than in the past.[133,134]

Indications, Contraindications, and Complications

Clinically, IPPB is given to provide a significantly larger inhaled volume at a physiologically advantageous inspiratory to expiratory pattern than the patient can produce with spontaneous ventilation. If this goal is met, there should be improvement in the cough mechanism, distribution of ventilation, and delivery of medication.[135] In the pediatric population, however, the hazards and potential complications that can result from its use render it unpopular and ineffective among infants and children.[136] It is indicated most often in the older patient who needs increased lung expansion but has failed to respond to other modes of treatment, such as incentive spirometry, chest physiotherapy, deep-breathing exercises, and bilevel positive airway pressure. This includes patients with neuromuscular disease or chest wall deformity that inhibits maximal inspiratory efforts. Medication can also be delivered via IPPB to these patients. However, studies have continued to report that the delivery of medications via IPPB depends on the technique and that the first mode of choice for aerosolized medication therapy should be a small-volume nebulizer or metered-dose inhaler.[137-139]

The absolute contraindication to IPPB is a tension pneumothorax; however, there are other factors that should be considered carefully before IPPB therapy is recommended. Because the effectiveness of applying IPPB therapy hinges on the cooperation of the patient, any infant or child who most likely would not cooperate and who has difficulty coordinating deep breathing should not be considered for this therapy. (Asynchronous breathing as well as breathing against the high positive pressure could result in increased work of breathing.) According to the American Association for Respiratory Care's clinical practice guideline for IPPB, other clinical contraindications include increased intracranial pressures (greater than 15 mm Hg); recent facial, oral, or skull surgery; tracheoesophageal fistula; recent esophageal surgery; active hemoptysis; active, untreated tuberculosis; radiographic evidence of blebs; hemodynamic instability; nausea; and swallowing of air.[130] Because IPPB is so rarely used in pediatrics, it is possible that the clinician may be inexperienced in administering the therapy and unable to provide optimal respiratory care. When this situation arises, the objective of providing a safe, effective treatment may be unattainable, and it is in the patient's best interest not to have the treatment administered.

Complications associated with IPPB therapy are listed in Box 14-2.[130,140,141] This list demonstrates the need for an experienced clinician to administer the therapy and to monitor the patient and the equipment closely. Should adverse reactions occur, the treatment should be discontinued and the physician notified of the situation.

Equipment

The equipment used during an IPPB treatment includes the IPPB device, the circuit, the patient application device, and the volume measuring device. Although the addition of a humidifier is not essential, it is recommended in patients with mucus retention. The most popular IPPB devices used in pediatric patients are the Bird series (Cardinal Health, Dublin, Ohio), the Puritan Bennett series (Puritan Bennett, Boulder, Colo), and the Monaghan 515 (Monaghan Medical, Plattsburgh, NY).

Box 14-2	Complications Associated With Intermittent Positive-Pressure Breathing

- Bronchospasm
- Gastric distention and ileus
- Nosocomial infection
- Decreased venous return
- Hyperventilation
- Hypoventilation
- Impaction of secretions
- Fatigue
- Air trapping
- Volutrauma, pneumothorax
- Hemoptysis
- Reduction of respiratory drive in patients with chronic hypercarbia

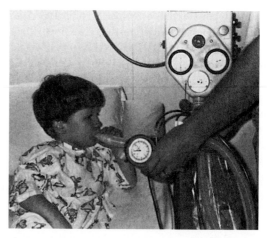

FIGURE 14-9 Intermittent positive-pressure breathing (IPPB) therapy being administered to a child, with a respirometer attached to the exhalation valve for exhaled volume monitoring.

The devices vary in design and in flow, volume, and pressure capabilities.[142] The patient application devices are dependent on the patient's needs and include a mouthpiece, lip–mouth seal, mask, or endotracheal tube/tracheostomy adapter. A nose clip should be available for the patient who uses either a mouthpiece or lip seal. The volume measuring can be obtain by a spirometer. Suctioning equipment should be available, as should containers for collecting or disposing of sputum.[130]

Procedure

An explanation of the equipment and the procedure should be given to the patient. The equipment may be frightening, and the clinician should soothe and encourage the patient by explaining exactly what the patient will feel and how the IPPB machine will perform. Manually cycling the machine on and listening to the gas flow may be helpful in alleviating some of the patient's fears. Allowing the patient to examine the mouthpiece (lip seal, mask, or adapter) and circuit before therapy begins may also help. A thorough explanation of the proper breathing pattern is essential *before* therapy begins. The patient should be encouraged to inhale slowly with the machine and to exhale passively, not forcefully.

Application

The patient should be placed in a sitting position if possible and therapy initiated at low pressures (10 cm H_2O). The pressure can be gradually increased until one of the following conditions is met:

1. The pressure provides the set volume goal.
2. Further increase in pressure provides a minimal increase in volume.
3. The patient becomes intolerant of the pressure increase.

The gas flow rate should be set by the clinician and will vary depending on the individual patient (Figure 14-9).

Monitoring

The patient and equipment should be monitored closely during therapy. The heart rate and respiratory rate should be obtained before, during, and after each treatment. Breath sounds should be assessed before and after each treatment and any time the patient complains of respiratory difficulty or chest pains. With the goal of therapy being to generate a tidal volume during IPPB that is at least 15 ml/kg or to exceed one third of inspiratory capacity, it is essential that tidal volume be monitored.[143] To determine whether lung volume is being augmented, the patient's tidal volume should be monitored before (spontaneous breathing) and several times during therapy. The exhaled gas is measured during therapy at the exhalation valve with either a respirometer or spirometer. If the tidal volume delivered during IPPB therapy is not greater than that during spontaneous breathing, the therapy is of little, if any, value to the patient. The patient's peak flow should also be monitored before and after treatment.

Assessment of Therapy

Document the following with each IPPB treatment:

- Heart rate
- Respiratory rate
- Breath sounds
- Pressure used (beginning and end of therapy)
- Tidal volume obtained (before and during therapy)

- Machine controls used (i.e., sensitivity, flow)
- Fraction of inspired oxygen (FI_{O_2}) values
- Medication aerosolized
- Peak flow
- Description of cough and sputum production
- Patient cooperation and tolerance
- Duration of therapy
- Any patient complaints or adverse reactions and the corrective action taken

IPPB therapy is believed to be effective if the therapeutic goals are met, including:

- An augmented tidal volume during IPPB (15 ml/kg or more than one third of the inspiratory capacity)
- An increase in peak flow or forced expiratory volume in 1 second (FEV_1)
- A more effective cough
- Secretion clearance
- Improved breath sounds
- An improved chest radiograph[130]

When compared with other aerosol delivery devices, IPPB in the pediatric patient is both equipment and labor intensive.[91] With this in mind, perhaps thought should be given *not* to whether IPPB is effective in delivering aerosols but rather to whether IPPB is the most effective method of delivery.[105] However, although there are other less expensive and less invasive lung expansion maneuvers, there remain patients who fail to respond to these maneuvers but who do benefit from IPPB. If there are no observable benefits from the therapy, however, its use cannot be justified.

FUTURE OF AIRWAY CLEARANCE THERAPY

The future of airway clearance will center on normalization of physiologic airway clearance mechanisms. This will be accomplished by new and novel drug therapies such as hypertonic saline or such simple devices as the Cough Assist (Emerson) which helps neuromuscular patients mimic a stronger cough. Due to the understood benefits of the cough paralytics in acute lung injury are no longer common practice. Gene therapy for CF is just around the corner. Advances in technology will continue to give us tools that allow us to accomplish the basics while reducing the overall physical size and power consumption. Many of these new devices will provide a user-friendly interface that can be utilized by non-healthcare providers in the home care setting. This will allow us to customize our therapy for the best outcome depending on the social, economic, and educational needs of the patient and family.

ASSESSMENT QUESTIONS

See Evolve Resources for answers.

1. Many institutions found that the routine use of IPPB was replaced with routine use of CPT in what two decades?
   A. 1900s and 1910s
   B. 1920s and 1930s
   C. 1960s and 1970s
   D. 1980s and 1990s
2. Postural drainage was used as early as
   A. 1901
   B. 1911
   C. 1940
   D. 1953
3. When doing percussion therapy, what is the recommended frequency?
   A. 1-2 Hz
   B. 3-4 Hz
   C. 5-6 Hz
   D. 7-8 Hz
4. When providing vibration chest physiotherapy, what is the recommended frequency?
   A. 6-7 Hz
   B. 8-9 Hz
   C. 10-15 Hz
   D. >20 Hz
5. The four components of *classical* CPT are
   A. Postural drainage, percussion, vibration, and coughing
   B. FET, IS, IPPB, and HFFC
   C. PEP, position, AD, and resistance
   D. Hydration, percussion, deep breathing, and FET
6. Premature infants may be at risk for increased complications from CPT. Why?
   A. The high chest wall compliance of premature infants can cause loss of lung volume.
   B. CPT is associated with IVH.
   C. Prolonged handling can interfere with the temperature-regulated environment of these patients.
   D. A, B, and C are correct
7. What airway clearance technique was introduced in the 1970s to prevent postoperative pulmonary complications?
   A. Deep breath and cough
   B. Incentive spirometry
   C. CPT
   D. PEP

Continued

ASSESSMENT QUESTIONS—cont'd

8. CPT is required in only a limited number of conditions, all of which are characterized by which of the following?
   A. Chronic, excessive sputum production
   B. Disease state
   C. Patient age and disease state
   D. None of the above
9. Treatments for patients with CF or bronchiectasis should be performed for at least _____ and re-evaluated every _____ for acute care?
   A. 10 minutes, 24 hours
   B. 15 minutes, 48 hours
   C. 20 minutes, 96 hours
   D. 30 minutes, 72 hours
10. What are the contraindications for CPT?
    A. Frank hemoptysis
    B. Empyema
    C. Foreign body aspiration
    D. All of the above

References

1. Ewart W: The treatment of bronchiectasis and of chronic bronchial affections by posture and respiratory exercises, *Lancet* 1901;2:70.
2. Gaskell DV, Webber BA: *The Brompton Hospital guide to chest physiotherapy*, Oxford: Blackwell Scientific Publications; 1973.
3. Murray JF: The ketchup-bottle method, *N Engl J Med* 1979;300:1155.
4. Sutton PP et al: Chest physiotherapy: a review, *Eur J Respir Dis* 1982;63:188.
5. Kirilloff LH et al: Does chest physical therapy work? *Chest* 1985;88:436.
6. Sutton P: Chest physiotherapy: time for a reappraisal, *Br J Dis Chest* 1988;82:127.
7. Selsby D: Chest physiotherapy may be harmful in some patients, *BMJ* 1989;298:541.
8. Selsby D, Jones JG: Chest physiotherapy: physiological and clinical aspects, *Br J Anaesth* 1990;64:621.
9. Pavia D: The role of chest physiotherapy in mucus hypersecretion, *Lung* 1990;168(suppl):614.
10. Stiller KR: Chest physiotherapy for the medical patient: are current practices effective? *Aust N Z J Med* 1990;20:183.
11. Eid N et al: Chest physiotherapy in review, *Respir Care* 1991;36:270.
12. Lewis RM: Chest physical therapy: time for a redefinition and a renaming, *Respir Care* 1992;37:419.
13. Waring WW: Diagnostic and therapeutic procedures. In Chernick V, editor: *Kendig's disorders of the respiratory tract in children*, ed 5, Philadelphia: WB Saunders; 1990. pp 77-95.
14. Hough A: *Physiotherapy in respiratory care: a problem solving approach*, London: Chapman & Hall; 1991.
15. Cystic Fibrosis Foundation: *Consumer fact sheet: an introduction to chest physical therapy*, Bethesda, Md: Cystic Fibrosis Foundation; 1992.
16. Mellins RB: Pulmonary physiotherapy in the pediatric age group, *Am Rev Respir Dis* 1974;110 (2, suppl):137.
17. Sutton PP et al: Assessment of percussion, vibratory shaking, and breathing exercises in chest physiotherapy, *Eur J Respir Dis* 1985;66:147.
18. Sutton PP, Parker RA, Webber BA: Assessment of the forced expiration technique, postural drainage and directed coughing in chest physiotherapy, *Eur J Respir Dis* 1983;64:62.
19. van der Schans CP, Piers DA, Postma DS: Effect of manual percussion on tracheobronchial clearance in patients with chronic airflow obstruction and excessive tracheobronchial secretion, *Thorax* 1986;41:448.
20. Murphy MB, Concannon D, FitzGerald M: Chest percussion: help or hindrance to postural drainage, *Ir Med J* 1983;76:189.
21. Webber B et al: Evaluation of self-percussion during postural drainage using the forced expiration technique, *Physiother Pract* 1985;1:42.
22. Faling LJ: Chest physical therapy. In Burton GG, Gee GN, Hodgkin JE, editors: *Respiratory care: a guide to clinical practice*, ed 3, Philadelphia: JB Lippincott; 1991. pp 625-654.
23. Marini JJ, Pierson DJ, Hudson LD: Acute lobar atelectasis: a prospective comparison of fiberoptic bronchoscopy and respiratory therapy, *Am Rev Respir Dis* 1979;19: 971.
24. Finer NN, Boyd J: Chest physiotherapy in the neonate: a controlled study, *Pediatrics* 1978;61:282.
25. O'Bradovich HM, Chernick V: The functional basis of respiratory pathology. In Chernick V, editor: *Kendig's disorders of the respiratory tract in children*, ed 5, Philadelphia: WB Saunders; 1990. pp 3-47.
26. Walters P: Chest physiotherapy. In Levin DL, Morris FC, Moore GC, editors: *A practical guide to pediatric intensive care*, St. Louis: Mosby; 1979. pp 395-403.
27. Holloway R et al: Effect of chest physiotherapy on blood gases of neonates treated by intermittent positive pressure respiration, *Thorax* 1969;24:421.
28. Fox WW, Schwartz JG, Schaffer TH: Pulmonary physiotherapy in neonates: physiologic changes and respiratory management, *J Pediatr* 1978;92:977.
29. Curran CL, Kachoyeanos MK: The effects on neonates of two methods of chest physical therapy, *MCN Am J Matern Child Nurs* 1979;4:309.
30. Walsh CM et al: Controlled supplemental oxygenation during tracheobronchial hygiene, *Nurs Res* 1987;36:211.
31. Raval D et al: Chest physiotherapy in preterm infants with RDS in the first 24 hours of life, *J Perinatol* 1987;7:301.
32. Green CG: Assessment of the pediatric airway by flexible bronchoscopy, *Respir Care* 1991;36:555.
33. Pryor JA: The forced expiration technique. In Pryor JA, editor: *International perspectives in physical therapy*, Vol 7: *Respiratory care*, Edinburgh: Churchill Livingstone; 1991. pp 79-100.
34. Zapletal A et al: Chest physiotherapy and airway obstruction in patients with cystic fibrosis: a negative report, *Eur J Respir Dis* 1983;64:426.

35. Oldenburg FA et al: Effects of postural drainage, exercise, and cough on mucus clearance in chronic bronchitis, *Am Rev Respir Dis* 1979;120:739.

36. Rossman C et al: Effect of chest physiotherapy on the removal of mucus in patients with cystic fibrosis, *Am Rev Respir Dis* 1982;126:131.

37. DeBoeck C, Zinman R: Cough versus chest physiotherapy, *Am Rev Respir Dis* 1984;129:132.

38. Bain J, Bishop J, Olinsky A: Evaluation of directed coughing in cystic fibrosis, *Br J Dis Chest* 1988;82:138.

39. van Hengstum M et al: Conventional physiotherapy and forced expiratory manoeuvres have similar effects on tracheobronchial clearance, *Eur Respir J* 1988;1:758.

40. Klig S et al: A biopsychosocial examination of two methods of pulmonary therapy [abstract], *Pediatr Pulmonol* 1989;4(suppl):145.

41. Reisman J et al: Role of conventional physiotherapy in cystic fibrosis, *J Pediatr* 1988;113:632.

42. Holzer FJ, Schnall R, Landau LI: The effect of a home exercise programme in children with cystic fibrosis, *Aust Paediatr J* 1984;20:297.

43. Blomquist M et al: Physical activity and self treatment in cystic fibrosis, *Arch Dis Child* 1986;61:362.

44. Mahlmeister MJ et al: Positive-expiratory-pressure mask therapy: theoretical and practical considerations and a review of the literature, *Respir Care* 1991;36:1218.

45. Iverson LIG et al: Comparative study of IPPB, the incentive spirometer and blow bottles: the prevention of atelectasis following cardiac surgery, *Ann Thorac Surg* 1978;25:197.

46. Schoni MH: Autogenic drainage: a modern approach to physiotherapy in cystic fibrosis, *J R Soc Med* 1989;82(16, suppl):32.

47. David A: Autogenic drainage—the German approach. In Pryor JA, editor: *International perspectives in physical therapy*, Vol 7: *Respiratory care*, Edinburgh: Churchill Livingstone; 1991. pp 65-78.

48. Davidson AGF et al: Long-term comparison of conventional percussion and drainage physiotherapy versus autogenic drainage in cystic fibrosis [abstract], *Pediatr Pulmonol* 1992;8(suppl):298.

49. Falk M et al: Improving the ketchup bottle method with positive expiratory pressure, PEP, in cystic fibrosis, *Eur J Respir Dis* 1984;65:423.

50. Tonnesen P, Stovring S: Positive expiratory pressure (PEP) as lung physiotherapy in cystic fibrosis: a pilot study, *Eur J Respir Dis* 1984;65:419.

51. Tyrell JC, Hiller EJ, Martin J: Face mask physiotherapy in cystic fibrosis, *Arch Dis Child* 1986;61:598.

52. Oberwaldner B, Evans JC, Zach MS: Forced expirations against a variable resistance: a new chest physiotherapy method in cystic fibrosis, *Pediatr Pulmonol* 1986;2:358.

53. Van Asperen PP et al: Comparison of a positive expiratory pressure (PEP) mask with postural drainage in patients with cystic fibrosis, *Aust Paediatr J* 1987;23:283.

54. Falk M, Andersen JB: Positive expiratory pressure (PEP) mask. In Pryor JA, editor: *International perspectives in physical therapy*, Vol 7: *Respiratory care*, Edinburgh: Churchill Livingstone; 1991. pp 51-63.

55. Oberwaldner B et al: Chest physiotherapy in hospitalized patients with cystic fibrosis: a study of lung function effects and sputum production, *Eur Respir J* 1991;4:152.

56. Mortensen J et al: The effects of postural drainage and positive expiratory pressure physiotherapy on tracheobronchial clearance in cystic fibrosis, *Chest* 1991;100:1350.

57. Lindemann H et al: Autogenic drainage: efficacy of a simplified method, *Acta Univ Carol* 1990;36:210.

58. Warwick WJ, Hansen LG: The long-term efficacy of high-frequency chest compression on pulmonary complications of cystic fibrosis, *Pediatr Pulmonol* 1991;11:265.

59. Warwick WJ: High frequency chest compression moves mucus by means of sustained staccato coughs [abstract], *Pediatr Pulmonol* 1991;6(suppl):283.

60. Lannefors L, Wollmer P: Mucus clearance with three chest physiotherapy regimes in cystic fibrosis: a comparison between postural drainage, PEP, and physical exercise, *Eur Respir J* 1992;5:748.

61. Zach M et al: Cystic fibrosis: physical exercise versus chest physiotherapy, *Arch Dis Child* 1982;57:587.

62. Andreasson B et al: Long-term effects of physical exercise on working capacity and pulmonary function in cystic fibrosis, *Acta Paediatr Scand* 1987;76:70.

63. Bartlett RH et al: Physiology of yawning and its application to postoperative care, *Surg Forum* 1970;21:223.

64. Bartlett RH: Incentive spirometry. In Kacmarek R, Stoller J, editors: *Current respiratory care: techniques and therapy*, St. Louis: Mosby; 1988.

65. Bartlett RH: Post-traumatic pulmonary insufficiency. In Cooper P, Nyhus L, editors: *Surgery annual*, New York: Appleton-Century-Crofts; 1971.

66. Ali J et al: Consequences of postoperative alterations in respiratory mechanics, *Am J Surg* 1974;128:376.

67. Meyers JR et al: Changes in residual capacity of the lung after operation, *Arch Surg* 1975;110:567.

68. McDonnell T, McNicholas WT, Fitzgerald MX: Hypoxaemia during chest physiotherapy in patients with cystic fibrosis, *Ir J Med Sci* 1986;155:345.

69. Gormezano J, Branthwaite MA: Pulmonary physiotherapy with assisted ventilation, *Anaesthesia* 1972;27:249.

70. Gormezano J, Branthwaite MA: Effects of physiotherapy during intermittent positive pressure ventilation, *Anaesthesia* 1972;27:258.

71. Huseby J et al: Oxygenation during chest physiotherapy [abstract], *Chest* 1976;70:430.

72. Tyler ML et al: Prediction of oxygenation during chest physiotherapy in critically ill patients [abstract], *Am Rev Respir Dis* 1980;121:218.

73. Dhainaut JF, Bons J, Bricard C: Improved oxygenation in patients with extensive unilateral pneumonia using the lateral decubitus position, *Thorax* 1980;35:792.

74. Emolina C et al: Positional hypoxemia in unilateral lung disease, *N Engl J Med* 1981;304:523.

75. Rivara D: Positional hypoxemia during artificial ventilation, *Crit Care Med* 1984;12:436.

76. Heaf DP et al: Postural effects on gas exchange in infants, *N Engl J Med* 1983;308:1505.

77. Holody B, Goldberg HS: The effect of mechanical vibration physiotherapy on arterial oxygenation in acutely ill patients with atelectasis or pneumonia, *Am Rev Respir Dis* 1981;124:372.

78. Mohsenifar Z et al: Mechanical vibration and conventional chest physiotherapy in outpatients with stable chronic obstructive lung disease, *Chest* 1985;87:463.

79. Weissman C et al: Effect of routine intensive care interactions on metabolic rate, *Chest* 1984;86:815.
80. Weissman C, Kemper M: The oxygen uptake–oxygen delivery relationship during ICU interventions, *Chest* 1991;99:430.
81. Vandenplas Y et al: Esophageal pH monitoring data during chest physiotherapy, *J Pediatr Gastroenterol Nutr* 1991;13:23.
82. Orenstein SR, Orenstein DM: Gastroesophageal reflux and respiratory disease in children, *J Pediatr* 1988;112:847.
83. Kosloske A: Tracheobronchial foreign bodies in children: back to the bronchoscope and a balloon, *Pediatrics* 1980;66:321.
84. Emery JR, Peabody JL: Head position affects intracranial pressure in newborn infants, *J Pediatr* 1983;103:950.
85. Ersson U et al: Observations on intracranial dynamics during respiratory physiotherapy in unconscious neurosurgical patients, *Acta Anaesth Scand* 1990;343:99.
86. Purohit DM, Caldwell C, Levkoff AH: Multiple rib fractures due to physiotherapy in a neonate with hyaline membrane disease, *Am J Dis Child* 1975;129:1103.
87. Asher MI et al: Effects of chest physical therapy on lung function in children recovering from acute severe asthma, *Pediatr Pulmonol* 1990;9:146.
88. Campbell AH, O'Connell JM, Wilson F: The effects of chest physiotherapy upon the FEV$_1$ in chronic bronchitis, *Med J Aust* 1975;1:33.
89. Wollmer P et al: Inefficiency of chest percussion in the physical therapy of chronic bronchitis, *Eur J Respir Dis* 1985;66:233.
90. Webb MSC et al: Chest physiotherapy in acute bronchiolitis, *Arch Dis Child* 1985;60:1078.
91. Quittell LM et al: The effectiveness of chest physical therapy (CPT) in infants with bronchiolitis [abstract], *Am Rev Respir Dis* 1988;137:406.
92. Graham WGB, Bradley DA: Efficacy of chest physiotherapy and intermittent positive-pressure breathing in the resolution of pneumonia, *N Engl J Med* 1978;299:624.
93. Britton S, Bejstedt M, Vedin L: Chest physiotherapy in primary pneumonia, *BMJ* 1985;290:1703.
94. Reines HD et al: Chest physiotherapy fails to prevent postoperative atelectasis in children after cardiac surgery, *Ann Surg* 1982;195:451.
95. Finer NN et al: Postextubation atelectasis: a retrospective review and a prospective controlled study, *J Pediatr* 1979;94:110.
96. Stiller K et al: Acute lobar atelectasis: a comparison of two chest physiotherapy regimens, *Chest* 1990;98:1336.
97. Desmond J et al: Immediate and long-term effects of chest physiotherapy in patients with cystic fibrosis, *J Pediatr* 1983;103:538.
98. Currie DC et al: Practice, problems and compliance with postural drainage: a survey of chronic sputum producers, *Br J Dis Chest* 1986;80:249.
99. Hammon W, Martin RJ: Chest physiotherapy for acute atelectasis, *Phys Ther* 1981;61:217.
100. MacKenzie CF, Shing B, McAslun TC: Chest physiotherapy: the effect on arterial oxygenation, *Anesth Analg* 1978;57:28.
101. Connors AF et al: Chest physical therapy: the immediate effect on oxygenation in acutely ill patients, *Chest* 1980;79:559.
102. McMichan JC, Michel L, Westbrook PR: Pulmonary dysfunction following traumatic quadriplegia, *JAMA* 1980;243:528.
103. Kosloske A et al: Drainage of pediatric lung abscess by cough, catheter, or complete resection, *J Pediatr Surg* 1986;21:596.
104. Lewis R: Chest physical therapy in pediatrics: a national survey [abstract], *Respir Care* 1991;36:1307.
105. American Association for Respiratory Care: Clinical practice guideline: postural drainage therapy, *Respir Care* 1991;36:1418.
106. Holma B, Hegg PO: pH- and protein-dependent buffer capacity and viscosity of respiratory mucus: their interrelationships and influence on health, *Sci Total Environ* 1989;84:71.
107. Zelenina M et al: Nickel and extracellular acidification inhibit the water permeability of human aquaporin-3 in lung epithelial cells, *J Biol Chem* 2003;278:30037.
108. Bartlett RH, Gazzaniga AB, Geraghty TR: Respiratory maneuvers to prevent postoperative pulmonary complications: a critical review, *JAMA* 1973;224:1017.
109. Bakow ED: Sustained maximal inspiration: a rationale for its use, *Respir Care* 1977;22:379.
110. American Association for Respiratory Care: Clinical practice guideline: incentive spirometry, *Respir Care* 1991;36:1402.
111. Harken DE: A review of the activities of the thoracic center for the III and IV hospital groups, 160th general hospital European theater of operations, June 10, 1944 to Jan 1, 1945, *J Thoracic Cardiovasc Surg* 1946;15:31.
112. Iverson LIG et al: A comparative study of IPPB, the incentive spirometer and blow bottles: the prevention of atelectasis following cardiac surgery, *Ann Thoracic Surg* 1978;35:197.
113. O'Donohue WJ: National survey of the usage of lung expansion modalities for the prevention and treatment of postoperative atelectasis following abdominal and thoracic surgery, *Chest* 1985;87:76.
114. Oikkonen M et al: Comparison of incentive spirometry and intermittent positive pressure breathing after coronary artery bypass graft, *Chest* 1991;99:60.
115. Stock MC et al: Prevention of postoperative pulmonary complications with CPAP, incentive spirometry, and conservative therapy, *Chest* 1985;87:151.
116. Stock MC et al: Comparison of continuous positive airway pressure, incentive spirometry, and conservative therapy after cardiac operations, *Crit Care Med* 1984;12:969.
117. Celli BR, Rodriguez KS, Snider GL: A controlled trial of intermittent positive pressure breathing, incentive spirometry, and deep breathing exercises in preventing pulmonary complications after abdominal surgery, *Am Rev Respir Dis* 1984;130:12.
118. Craven JL et al: The evaluation of incentive spirometry in the management of postoperative pulmonary complications, *Br J Surg* 1974;61:793.
119. Bartlett RH: Respiratory therapy to prevent pulmonary complications of surgery, *Respir Care* 1984;29:667.

120. Scuderi J, Olsen GN: Respiratory therapy in the management of postoperative complications, *Respir Care* 1989;34:281.

121. Bartlett RH et al: Studies on the pathogenesis and prevention of postoperative pulmonary complications, *Surg Gynecol Obstet* 1973;137:925.

122. Mang H, Obermayer A: Imposed work of breathing during sustained maximal inspiration: comparison of six incentive spirometers, *Respir Care* 1989;34:1122.

123. Lederer DH, Van de Water JM, Indech RB: Which deep breathing device should the postoperative patient use? *Chest* 1980;77:610.

124. Centers for Disease Control and Prevention: Update: universal precautions for prevention of transmission of human immunodeficiency virus, hepatitis B virus, and other bloodborne pathogens in health care settings, *MMWR Morb Mortal Wkly Rep* 1988;37:377.

125. Schwieger I et al: Absence of benefit of incentive spirometry in low-risk patients undergoing elective cholecystectomy, *Chest* 1986;89:652.

126. Davies BL, Macleod JP, Ogilvie HM: The efficacy of incentive spirometers in postoperative protocols for low-risk patients, *Can J Nurs Res* 1990;22:19.

127. Gale GD, Sanders DE: Incentive spirometry: its value after cardiac surgery, *Can Anaesth Soc J* 1980;27:475.

128. Jung R et al: Comparison of three methods of respiratory care following upper abdominal surgery, *Chest* 1980;78:31.

129. Gooding JM et al: Is incentive spirometry valuable as an addition to traditional respiratory maneuvers? [abstract], *Respir Care* 1977;22:414.

130. Krastins I et al: An evaluation of incentive spirometry in the management of pulmonary complications after cardiac surgery in the pediatric population, *Crit Care Med* 1982;10:525.

131. American Association for Respiratory Care: : Clinical practice guideline: intermittent positive pressure breathing, *Respir Care* 2003;48:540.

132. Motley HL et al: Use of intermittent positive pressure breathing combined with nebulization in pulmonary disease, *Am J Med* 1948;5:853.

133. Eubank DH, Bone RC: Intermittent positive pressure breathing. In Eubank DH, Bone RC, editors: *Comprehensive respiratory care: a learning system module*, St. Louis: Mosby; 1985. pp 430-450.

134. Chang N, Levison H: The effect of nebulized bronchodilator administration with or without IPPB on ventilatory function in children with cystic fibrosis and asthma, *Am Rev Respir Dis* 1972;106:867.

135. Baker JP: Magnitude of usage of intermittent positive pressure breathing, *Am Rev Respir Dis* 1974;110S:170.

136. Handelsman H; Agency for Health Care Policy and Research: Health technology reports: intermittent positive pressure breathing (IPPB) therapy. AHCPR Pub. No. 92-0013. Rockville, Md: Office of Health Technology, U.S. Department of Health and Human Services Public Health Service; 1991.

137. Burgess WR, Chernick V: Humidity and aerosol therapy. In Burger WR, Chernick V, editors: *Respiratory therapy in newborn infants and children*, New York: Thieme-Stratton; 1982. pp 74-84.

138. Jasper AC et al: Cost-benefit comparison of aerosol bronchodilator delivery methods in hospitalized patients, *Chest* 1987;91:614.

139. Summer W et al: Aerosol bronchodilator delivery methods: relative impact on pulmonary function and cost of respiratory care, *Arch Intern Med* 1989;149:618.

140. American Association for Respiratory Care: Clinical practice guideline: selection of a device for delivery of aerosol to the lung parenchyma, *Respir Care* 1996;41:647.

141. Bierman CW: Pneumomediastinum and pneumothorax complicating asthma in children, *Am J Dis Child* 1967;114:43.

142. Moore RB, Cotton EK, Dinnery MA: The effect of IPPB on airway resistance in normal and asthmatic children, *J Allergy Clin Immunol* 1972;49:137.

143. McPherson SP: *Respiratory therapy equipment*, ed 7, St. Louis: Mosby; 2004.

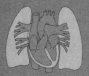

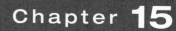

Chapter 15

Airway Management

IAN N. JACOBS • MARY M. PETTIGNANO • ROBERT PETTIGNANO

OUTLINE

LEARNING OBJECTIVES

After reading this chapter the reader will be able to:

- Identify four general indications for intubation
- Explain how to perform orotracheal intubation
- Explain how to perform nasotracheal intubation
- Select the correctly sized endotracheal tube for patients of different ages
- Describe the complications of intubation
- Explain the criteria for extubation

- Appraise the reasons for failed extubation and treatment strategies
- List the indications for tracheotomy
- Describe the major complications of tracheotomy
- List the criteria for decannulation
- Compare the three approaches for decannulation
- Describe the setup and list the equipment needed for tracheotomy tube changes

Recognizing the child who is in respiratory distress or failure is an integral step in caring for the critically ill child. Ensuring adequate oxygenation and ventilation is a major goal in managing any ill child. In the acute setting this is best accomplished by using a bag and mask in patients of all ages. Establishing and maintaining a patent airway is a crucial part of this effort. It is one of the unique and challenging procedures associated with pediatric acute and critical care that has a profound impact on life and death.

INTUBATION

Rapid and unencumbered intubation of the trachea depends on knowledge of the upper airway anatomy, the indications for intubation, the appropriate use of airway equipment, and the medications available to facilitate translaryngeal intubation. There must be an appreciation for the potentially difficult airway and preparations made so in the event standard methods of maintaining a patent airway go awry, a backup plan is available. The ability to perform safe and rapid laryngoscopy and endotracheal tube (ETT) placement enables the clinician to immediately manage and secure the airway in any emergency.

Indications

The specific indications for translaryngeal intubation are numerous; however, all can be placed in one of four broad categories, which can be defined by the four "Ps":

- *P*ulmonary function
- *P*rovide an airway
- *P*rotect the airway
- *P*ulmonary hygiene

The need for translaryngeal intubation, due to a lack of pulmonary function, results from deficits in oxygenation, ventilation, or both taken in concert with the patient's clinical condition. Acute ventilatory dysfunction can be defined as an arterial partial pressure of carbon dioxide ($Paco_2$) greater than 50 to 60 mm Hg with a pH less than 7.3. Pulmonary dysfunction due to hypoxemia is defined as an arterial partial pressure of oxygen (Pao_2) less than 60 mm Hg with a fraction of inspired oxygen (Fio_2) greater than or equal to 0.60. These standards may be different for neonates, especially the extremely low birth weight infants. These definitions assume there is no intracardiac shunt resulting from an underlying cardiac abnormality. The definitions have been established as indicators of severe oxygenation or ventilation failure based on the fact that acidosis with a pH less than 7.2 may result in myocardial irritability and calcium and potassium disturbances.

It is difficult to reliably administer an Fio_2 greater than 0.8, using traditional devices for the administration of supplemental oxygen. Therefore a patient with decreasing oxygen saturation that is unresponsive to increases in oxygen concentration is a candidate for an escalation of care that may include both noninvasive and invasive methods of providing support, such as noninvasive positive pressure or intubation and mechanical ventilation. Disease processes that fall into the pulmonary function category as an etiology for intervention include apnea requiring mechanical ventilation, central nervous system disease requiring respiratory support, and other forms of respiratory distress or failure.

Upper airway obstruction may also require an artificial airway. Examples that are included in this category are diseases such as laryngotracheobronchitis, epiglottitis, subglottic stenosis, and anatomic abnormalities such as craniofacial syndromes and laryngomalacia. Head and neck trauma is also a consideration for intubation; however, it requires a specialized approach that depends on the nature of the injury.

Intubation to protect the airway is most commonly performed when there is loss of protective airway reflexes such as gag, cough, and swallowing. Intubation in this scenario is necessary to minimize aspiration of oropharyngeal or gastric secretions that may lead to aspiration pneumonitis. Patients at risk include those with neuromuscular disturbances, such as Guillain-Barré syndrome and Werdnig-Hoffman disease, or after intracranial injuries leading to depressed airway reflexes. More commonly, patients requiring airway protection are those who are comatose secondary to drug or alcohol ingestion.

Finally, patients with persistent, recurring lobar or whole-lung atelectasis with an inability to clear secretions are candidates for endotracheal intubation to provide pulmonary hygiene. These patients usually have inadequate ventilatory reserve, as evidenced by a vital capacity less than 20 ml/kg, a negative inspiratory force of less than –20 cm H_2O, the need for supplemental oxygen, and increased work of breathing.

Equipment

Anticipating and preparing for intubation by collecting the proper equipment is an essential component of a successful translaryngeal intubation. The equipment necessary for intubation is listed in Table 15-1. Using the mnemonic "MSMAID" facilitates preintubation preparation so that essential equipment is not inadvertently omitted.

Endotracheal Tubes

Once a decision has been made to undertake translaryngeal intubation, the appropriate size and type of ETT must be identified. The ETTs most commonly used are sterile, disposable, and made of clear nontoxic plastic or polyvinyl chloride. The tubes have markings placed longitudinally 1 cm apart and can be used as reference points for proper placement once endotracheal intubation is accomplished (Figure 15-1). The distal end of the ETT should contain a side port, termed the *Murphy eye,* to prevent complete obstruction of the ETT if mucoid secretions occlude the end hole. The appropriate ETT size is determined by the patient's age and size. Suggested ETT diameters based on age and size are listed in Table 15-2. The appropriate ETT for any child 1 year of age or older may be determined by the following formula[1]:

$$Internal\ diameter(mm) = (age[yr] \div 4) + 4$$

TABLE 15-1

Essential Equipment for Intubation

Mnemonic	Equipment
Monitors	ECG, pulse oximeter, BP, ETco$_2$ detector, stethoscope
Suction	Apparatus, Yankauer, catheters without relief valve, sterile catheter to fit ETT
Machine	Bag and mask, ventilator
Airway	Masks, oronasal airways, endotracheal tubes, stylet, laryngoscopes (handles, curved and straight blades, bulbs, batteries), McGill or Kolodny forceps, alligator forceps (infant), 1-in. tape, benzoin
Intravenous	Two patent intravenous lines
Drugs	Anesthetic and resuscitative agents

BP, Blood pressure; ECG, electrocardiogram; ETco$_2$, end-tidal carbon dioxide; ETT, endotracheal tube.

TABLE 15-2

Neonatal Resuscitation Program Guidelines for Pediatric Endotracheal Tube Size

Child's Age	Internal Diameter (mm)
Premature	
Less than 1000 g	2.5
1000-2000 g	3.0
2000-3000 g	3.5
Normal newborns	
3000-4000 g	3.5-4.0
Infants and children less than 12 yr old	
6-12 mo	4.0-4.5
1-2 yr	4.5
4 yr	5.0
6 yr	5.5
8 yr	6.0
10 yr	6.5
Children 12 yr of age and older	
Female	7.0-8.5
Male	8.0-10.0

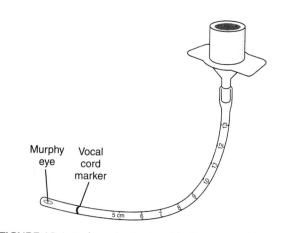

FIGURE 15-1 Endotracheal tube with distance markings.

Accurate selection of an ETT takes into consideration the child's size and length.[2-4] Comparing the size of the pinky of the patient with the size of the ETT is a method that can be used to approximate the appropriate size ETT for a child. In addition, the appropriate size ETT can be determined by using a Broselow pediatric emergency tape, which measures the child's length to estimate their weight, drug doses, and equipment needs. So that the laryngoscopist is prepared for any emergency, ETTs one-half size smaller and one-half size larger than the estimated or calculated size should always be available. The trachea becomes adult in size at approximately 12 to 14 years of age. The appropriate ETT size for adult females is between 7 and 8.5 mm; for adult males, it is between 8 and 10 mm[5] (see Table 15-2).

Cuffed and Uncuffed Tubes

Because the cricoid cartilage is the narrowest portion of the pediatric airway until about 8 years of age, use of an uncuffed ETT was traditionally recommended until that time. In 2005, the American Heart Association's Pediatric Advance Life Support program (PALS) stopped recommending uncuffed tubes as there was no evidence to support one over the other. Today it is left up to the clinician to determine whether a cuff is needed for patients less than 8 years of age. As a child grows, the airway becomes more adult-like and tubular, with the vocal cords, not the subglottic space, becoming the smallest cross-sectional area of the airway.[6] A cuffed ETT helps create a seal to occlude unwanted air leaks during positive pressure ventilation. The cuff also reduces the likelihood of pulmonary aspiration, although this not guaranteed simply by placing a cuffed ETT. However, with the advent of low profile cuffs in smaller endotracheal tubes (as low as 3.0 mm) more anesthesiologists at children's hospitals are using low profile cuffs in the operating room in small children and infants. The deflated cuff on the distal end of the ETT increases the outer diameter of the tube by approximately 0.5 mm when compared with uncuffed tubes. To compensate for the increased diameter of the cuff on the ETT, a smaller sized tube, 0.5 to 1 mm, is inserted when the cuff is present.

Laryngoscope Blades and Handles

The laryngoscope is the instrument used to expose the glottic opening during intubation. It consists of two parts: a handle and a blade. The handle is available in two sizes: large and small. The handle also contains batteries that power a light source incorporated into the blade. The large handle is recommended for an adult, but it may also be suitable for an infant, child, or adolescent depending on operator preference and patient characteristics. Because of its size and ease of manipulation, the small handle should be used for a premature infant or newborn. Before commencing the process of intubation, the blade and handle should be tested to ensure they fit together properly and lock in place. This will also allow testing of the integrity of the light source.

Although many types of laryngoscope blades are available, the curved (MacIntosh) and straight (Miller) blades are most common. The straight blade is preferred for an infant or small child, and the curved blade is most commonly used when intubating an adult. Each blade requires a different technique for exposing the glottis. When a straight blade is used, the epiglottis is lifted with the tip of the blade and pressed against the base of the tongue (Figure 15-2). The advantage of this technique is the ability to elevate the floppy infantile epiglottis. In contrast, for the adult the tip of the curved blade is placed in the vallecula, the space between the epiglottis and the base of the tongue. As the laryngoscope is pulled forward, it elevates the epiglottis and exposes the glottis (Figure 15-3).[7] This method may also be helpful to visualize the cords when using a straight blade during intubation of a small newborn.[1] Although different blades and handles are recommended for intubation, ease of use, comfort with a particular instrument, and personal preference are the important guides to determin-

ing which technique to use. The MacIntosh curved blade, for example, has a wider flange, which provides better control of the tongue. This may be helpful in intubation of a small infant or child, whose anatomy is such that the tongue can be a major obstacle to success.

Laryngeal Mask Airway

The laryngeal mask airway (LMA) is a useful alternative in maintaining the airway with a bag–valve–mask setup (Figure 15-4).[8] Today, the laryngeal mask airway may be used in the unconscious patient to maintain an airway without having to intubate. It may be useful as part of a backup plan in the event that endotracheal intubation is difficult or hazardous. However, the LMA does not

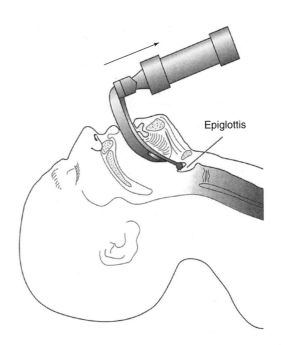

Epiglottis

FIGURE 15-3 Direct laryngoscopy using a curved (MacIntosh) blade and demonstrating proper lifting technique. Note the upward and forward lift while the wrist is held straight.

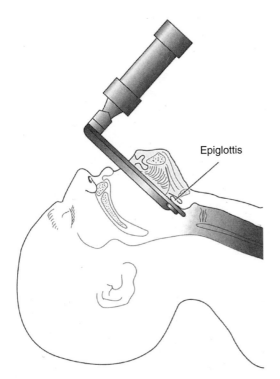

Epiglottis

FIGURE 15-2 Direct laryngoscopy using a straight (Miller) blade.

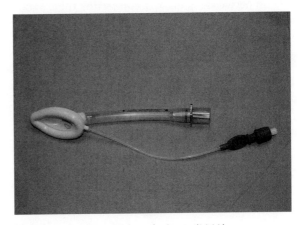

FIGURE 15-4 A laryngeal mask airway (LMA).

provide a barrier between the esophagus and the trachea and therefore the potential for aspiration is greater than with translaryngeal intubation.

There is a learning curve for LMA insertion that must be overcome to be able to place it in the proper position within the airway. However, one study by Pennant and White showed that in a 90-minute didactic session, medical students, paramedics, and respiratory therapists with no prior experience inserted the LMA correctly 71% of the time on the first attempt.[9] In addition, first-attempt success has been reported as higher with pediatricians inserting LMAs rather than ETTs.[10] Studies of its use by various medical personnel reveal an ease of use and lack of significant complications.[11,12]

The LMA is placed by itself into the pharynx above the epiglottis and can be used for gentle positive-pressure ventilation. The deflated mask is manually inserted into the patient's mouth and guided blindly along the hard palate by hand (feel). It is advanced until resistance is encountered and the distal tip of the device rests against the upper esophageal sphincter. The balloon is inflated with 2 to 4 ml of saline to form a seal in the pharynx. LMAs can be used in the operating room for short procedures and may be useful in operative patients with subglottic stenosis or other airway problems that make it difficult to intubate. The LMAs come in different sizes including 1, 1.5, 2, 2.5, 3, 4, and 5. Every emergency airway cart should have all sizes of LMAs available (Table 15-3).

Suction Equipment

Suctioning both the upper and lower airway will contribute to both successful intubation and maintenance of a patent airway. Suctioning equipment should always be immediately accessible in anticipation of airway problems in any intensive care unit or operating room suite. Portable suction devices are available for use during the transportation of intubated patients or in those who may require airway intervention. In addition to the vacuum device, a regulator, a connecting tube, a tonsillar tip suction handle, such as a Yankauer, and several

standard sterile suction catheters, with and without a control port, are required to address the need for suctioning in a multitude of situations.

The suction device should be located at the head of the bed, and the regulator set at a medium setting, between 80 and 120 mm Hg suction.[13] The tonsillar tip handle is used to quickly clear the upper airway of large amounts of liquid or particulate matter. Using the suction catheter without a control port provides continuous suction. During intubation this allows the clinician to continuously visualize the glottic opening without stopping to occlude the control port. Finally, once the intubation is successful, the sterile suction catheter with a control port can be placed through the ETT to suction pulmonary secretions. Suctioning is indicated for pulmonary hygiene and to obtain secretions for possible diagnostic purposes, such as a Gram's stain or culture.

INTUBATION PROCEDURE

The indication for translaryngeal intubation will determine the most appropriate technique to use during the process of providing an airway for the patient. The options available to the clinician are orotracheal intubation, nasal or blind nasal intubation, awake intubation, or anesthetized intubation using neuromuscular blockers, sedatives to provide anxiolysis and/or amnesia agents, and opioids for pain. Universal precautions, such as the wearing of gloves and eye protection, should be observed with all intubation procedures to reduce the risk of transmitting infectious diseases.

Orotracheal Intubation

In the great majority of cases, translaryngeal intubation takes place with the patient supine. The height of the bed, stretcher, or operating room table should be such that the patient's head is level with the laryngoscopist's xiphoid process. This will allow direct visualization of the airway without putting undue physical stress or strain on the clinician. The larynx in the pediatric patient is anterior and cephalad, and therefore placing a small towel or roll underneath the patient's occiput optimally aligns the axes of the mouth, pharynx, and larynx. Flexing the neck forward and the head backward maintains the "sniffing" position.[14] The infant's or small child's occiput is more prominent than in the older child. The occipital prominence may naturally place the patient in the sniffing position without the use of head elevation. Head elevation in these patients may push the airway farther anterior, making translaryngeal intubation more difficult. Instead, it may be necessary to place a towel under the shoulders to properly align the airway.

TABLE 15-3	
Suggested Laryngeal Mask Airway Size Based on Weight	
Size	**Weight (kg)**
0.5	Infants up to 2.5
1	2.5-5
1.5	5-10
2	10-20
2.5	20-30
3	30-50
4	>50
5	>70

If the patient is breathing spontaneously, the application of 100% oxygen for 3 to 5 minutes with a bag and mask with or without applying positive pressure is sufficient to fully oxygenate and denitrogenate the lungs. In the event that there are no spontaneous respirations, three to five maximal breaths of 100% oxygen over 30 seconds accomplishes the same goal. Because of the risk of retinopathy of prematurity, providing oxygen at about 95% to optimize oxygen saturation is an acceptable practice. Adjuvant agents, such as sedatives, amnesic agents, or neuromuscular blockers, are administered at this point to facilitate airway exposure. If the patient is at risk for regurgitation and aspiration, cricoid pressure is applied to compress the esophagus against the cervical vertebrae (Sellick's maneuver).[15] Sellick's maneuver is used to prevent passive regurgitation and should not be maintained if the patient begins to actively regurgitate. The cricoid pressure is not withdrawn until a secure airway is assured. Cricoid pressure may also help prevent the gastric distention associated with bag-and-mask ventilation of the pediatric airway.[16]

Once the patient is fully oxygenated, the mouth is opened wide, using the forefinger and thumb in a scissoring motion. This is accomplished by depressing the mandible with the thumb of the right hand and applying pressure on the upper teeth with the index finger of the same hand. Once the mouth has been opened, the upper airway is suctioned as necessary. If and when the airway is deemed clear, laryngoscopy can be initiated.

Before commencing the process of intubation, the blade and handle should be tested to ensure they fit together properly and lock in place. This will also allow testing of the integrity of the light source. To use the laryngoscope, the handle is grasped midshaft with the left hand and the blade is inserted on the right side of the patient's mouth, sweeping the tongue toward the left. The laryngoscope is advanced forward in the midline while a forward and upward motion is exerted, as shown in Figure 15-3. Individual blade preference determines whether the epiglottis is lifted with the tip of a straight blade or exposed by placing the tip of the curved blade in the vallecula. It is important to remember that throughout this portion of the technique the wrist cannot be flexed or rotated. Remember: "Never lever." A levering motion causes undue pressure on the upper teeth and can chip or dislodge them if present. Pressure on the maxillary ridge in the small infant or child can cause hematoma and damage to unerupted teeth.

Figure 15-5 illustrates the glottic structures as viewed through the laryngoscope. After visualizing the glottic opening, the appropriate-sized ETT is held in the right hand and is introduced into the right side of the patient's mouth to avoid obstructing the view of the glottic opening while placing the ETT. The tip of the ETT

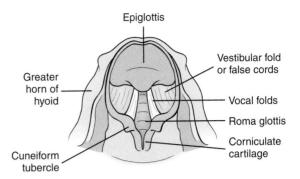

FIGURE 15-5 Glottic structures viewed through the laryngoscope.

is advanced through the glottic opening so that the single black ring, the cord guide, lies just distal to the opening of the glottis. Fogging in the endotracheal tube is immediately noted after starting ventilation. The presence of vapor in the ETT, however, is not an accurate or confirmatory test for proper ETT placement. If the ETT is marked with three rings, it should be inserted until the double black ring is distal to the glottic opening. In the event of inserting a cuffed ETT, the tube is advanced until the cuff is distal to the vocal cords.

The proper ETT position is in the midtrachea, or about 2 cm above the carina. In an adult, this is at the 21- to 23-cm mark. For the toddler or small child, correct ETT placement for oral intubation is estimated by using the following "lip-to-tip" formula[17]:

Pediatric ETT position (cm) = 12 + (age [yr] ÷ 2)

The depth needed for proper positioning of the ETT can also be estimated by multiplying the internal diameter by three and taping the ETT at that centimeter mark at the lip until a chest radiograph can be obtained to ascertain position. There is a six plus weight in kilograms formula (e.g., 6 + 1 kg = 7 at the lip for a 1-kg infant) used in the neonatal patient population to more accurately place an ETT. Any single attempt at intubation should not exceed 30 seconds. In the event that the glottic opening cannot be visualized or the ETT cannot be placed in that time period, the attempt should be aborted. The patient's airway should be reestablished by bag-and-mask ventilation to ensure adequate oxygenation before another attempt at intubation is made.

The chest is auscultated after intubation as a method for assessing whether the ETT is in the trachea. Breath sounds should be heard bilaterally over the lateral chest wall. Auscultating over the anterior chest wall of an infant or neonate can cause gastric sounds from an esophageal intubation to be mistaken for adequate breath sounds. It should be noted that auscultation is not the most accurate method of assessing proper ETT placement. The most accurate assessment of whether

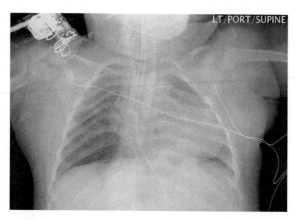

FIGURE 15-6 Anterior–posterior chest radiograph of right main bronchus intubation of a toddler.

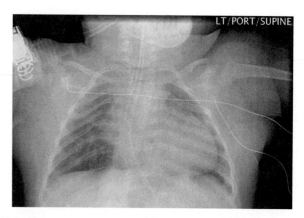

FIGURE 15-7 Anterior–posterior chest radiograph of properly positioned endotracheal tube.

the ETT has passed into the trachea is direct visualization. This can be done during laryngoscopy or after placing the ETT, using a fiberoptic scope. After visualization, obtaining carbon dioxide as measured with disposable end-tidal carbon dioxide ($ETCO_2$) detectors or by capnography is the next most accurate method and should be done after every intubation. A pediatric disposable colorimetric $ETCO_2$ detector (Pedi-Cap; Nellcor, Boulder, Colo) can easily detect carbon dioxide concentrations as low as 0.5%. The device, which is placed between the endotracheal tube and the anesthesia bag, will fluctuate in color from purple (<0.03%) to yellow (5%) after six breaths. This confirms the proper placement of the endotracheal tube.[18]

Ultimately capnometry may be more helpful because esophageal intubation can cause an initial observation of carbon dioxide, but within one or two breaths a negligible amount of carbon dioxide is observed.[19,20] In poor pulmonary perfusion situations (i.e., cardiac arrest) the lack of carbon dioxide can lead to a false-negative result. Proper tube position can be further assessed by one of several other methods, such as observing chest wall movement, observing condensation in the ETT during exhalation, palpating the ETT in the suprasternal notch, flexible tracheoscopy, improving color, improving heart rate, improving oxygen saturations, and chest radiograph (Figures 15-6 and 15-7). A chest radiograph is the most common method of assessing tube position, although the delay associated with the procedure and processing of the radiograph does not allow the results to be immediately available.

Each of the methods suggested for assessing proper ETT placement has some potential for a false-positive result.

The ETT is secured by preparing the skin with tincture of benzoin. Two strips of tape are cut long enough to reach from the lateral aspect of the right eye to the lateral aspect of the left eye. Each piece is split into a Y shape with the arms of the Y two-thirds the length of the tape. The tape should have a width that will easily fit on the upper lip and around the ETT. One end of the tape is secured to the cheek and wrapped around the tube in "barber pole" fashion (Figure 15-8). The necessary equipment (Box 15-1) for securing the ETT is assembled before attempting intubation. Other taping methods may be used to secure the ETT, as long as the method can be performed by all personnel involved in airway care and is fast and secure. The centimeter mark at which the ETT is secured must be recorded to allow assessment of proper position at a later time if needed.

There are various devices available to secure the ETT as an alternative to using tape. Figure 15-9 illustrates an example of one of these devices. When selecting a device to secure the tube it is important that it does not occlude access to the mouth, provides minimal tube movement when the head moves, and secures without creating decubitus ulcers at pressure points. In addition, the same rules apply as with taping methods: fast, easy, and can be applied by all personnel. Evidence that these devices help reduce the incidence of accidental extubations is inconclusive. However, it does suggest that the devices may be more effective on a small infant than on a larger infant or child.[21,22]

Nasotracheal Intubation

Once a patent and stable airway has been established by the orotracheal route, switching to a nasal tube can follow. The patient's nares are prepared by spraying a vasoconstrictive agent, such as phenylephrine, into the opening. Alternatively, the nose may be decongested with oxymetalozine. These drugs decrease mucosal swelling and inflammation. An ETT of a size that will pass easily through the nares is used. Depending on the patient's anatomy, this may be the same size as the tube selected for orotracheal intubation or, as is usually the case, approximately one size smaller.

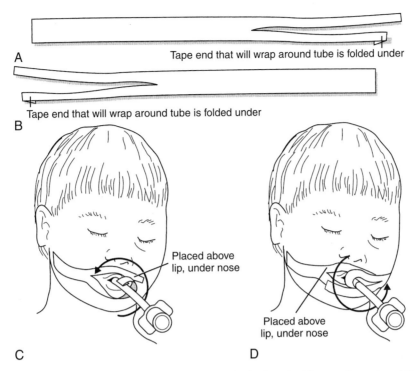

A — Tape end that will wrap around tube is folded under

B — Tape end that will wrap around tube is folded under

C — Placed above lip, under nose

D — Placed above lip, under nose

FIGURE 15-8 Steps used to secure an endotracheal tube (ETT) with tape. Steps **A** and **B,** Slit two pieces of tape, making a Y on one end of each piece (as shown). Turn under the end of the tape that will be wrapped around the ETT. This will make tape removal easier. Step **C,** Apply benzoin to the area below the nose and across the cheeks (where tape will be placed). Attach one piece of tape to the cheek and below the nose, wrapping the bottom of the Y around the ETT. The tape should be placed under the tube (chin side) first, and then wrapped around the top of the tube. Step **D,** Repeat step **C** on the other side of the face.

Box 15-1	Equipment for Endotracheal Tube Stabilization

- Alcohol
- Tincture of benzoin
- Scissors
- Adhesive tape
- Two precut Y-shaped pieces

The tube is lubricated with either petroleum jelly or 2% lidocaine jelly. The tube is then inserted into the nares until approximately one half of it has passed through the nose. While an assistant holds the existing oral ETT in the left corner of the mouth, the glottis is exposed in the same manner as for orotracheal intubation. Once the nasal tube is visualized in the hypopharynx, the tip of the tube is grabbed with McGill forceps held in the right hand and the nasal tube is lifted up and in front of the opening to the larynx. In small infants, otologic alligator forceps may be used in place of the previously mentioned forceps. When direct visualization of the glottic opening is ensured, the assistant is asked to remove the orotracheal tube while the nasotracheal tube

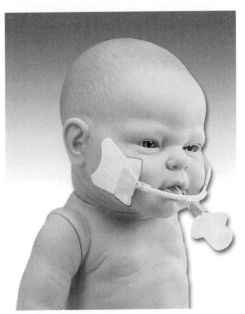

FIGURE 15-9 The NeoBar. A commercial adaptation of the Logan bow for stabilizing an infant endotracheal tube.

is simultaneously advanced into the trachea. Difficulty in passing the tube through the cords may be encountered because of the upward curve of the ETT and the limited mobility of the forceps in the small pharyngeal opening. Gentle rotation of the tube to the right or left may allow easier passage. In addition, the assistant may gently advance the tube from above while the clinician guides the ETT through the glottic opening. On occasion the bend of the tube at the end of the nasopharynx may occlude the tube and make suctioning and ventilation difficult. In this situation the ETT should be removed and the patient reintubated orally. Proper tube position is assessed by the methods described in the section Orotracheal Intubation. For the proper ETT depth after nasal intubation, the following formula is used:

$$ETT\ depth(cm) = 15 + (age[yr] \div 3)$$

The centimeter mark at the nares is noted and the ETT is taped securely in place. The major contraindications to nasotracheal intubation are a bleeding diathesis, such as thrombocytopenia, abnormal clotting times, facial trauma, suspected basilar skull fracture, and abnormal anatomy such as choanal atresia. In this author's experience, with the proliferation of pediatric intensive care units and the staff trained in the care of the critically ill pediatric patient, the need to switch to nasal intubation on a routine basis in mechanically ventilated patients in the pediatric intensive care unit has decreased significantly.

Blind Nasal Intubation

The larynx of an infant or small child is anterior and cephalad, making intubation more difficult in general. This anatomic difference between adults and children makes attempts at blind nasal intubation almost uniformly unsuccessful. Wisdom dictates that attempts at a blind nasal intubation be vigorously discouraged, because of the potential for damaging the airway. Mechanically generated damage and subsequent bleeding would make further intervention and attempts at intubation more difficult and dangerous.

Oral versus Nasal Intubation

One of the most frequently used arguments for nasal over oral intubation is patient comfort. Although it is believed that a nasal tube is more comfortable than an oral tube, evidence may dispute this and, in fact, there may be no difference between the two.[23] In the small infant and pediatric population, there is less effort in securing and maintaining a nasotracheal tube in the proper position when the patient is nasally intubated. Because the ETT is in the nares, salivation, which interferes with the adhesiveness of the tape, is not stimulated, so the ETT does not slip out of position as readily as with oral intubation. Paying particular attention to the method used to tape the ETT in place during oral intubation and regularly assessing how well the tape is

adhering to the ETT alleviate this problem significantly. Another reason why nasal intubation is preferred is that patients with teeth can bite the ETT, producing a hole or occluding it. Careful adherence to standard methods of sedation and analgesia used in the pediatric intensive care unit can alleviate this problem also. Although oral hygiene is facilitated, the trade-off is that endotracheal suctioning may be more difficult.

Disadvantages to nasal intubation include a predisposition to sinusitis, pressure necrosis of the nares, and bleeding complications associated with passing the ETT through the nares and upper airway. Another disadvantage is that a higher incidence of postextubation atelectasis among very low birth weight infants has been reported.[23]

Neonatal Intubation

The current recommendation for ETT placement for neonates is the "lip-to-tip" formula (see the earlier section, Orotracheal Intubation), which requires the addition of 6 to the infant's weight in kilograms and finding this number on the ETT. For example, for a 2-kg infant: 6 + 2 = 8 cm. The number should be viewed on the ETT at the patient's lip and then secured with tape.[24] The correct ETT size for infants is given by the Neonatal Resuscitation Program, described in Chapter 26 (Assessment and Monitoring of the Neonatal and Pediatric Patient). The Neonatal Resuscitation Program guidelines from the American Academy of Pediatrics recommend a 2.5 ETT for less than 1000 g, a 3.0 ETT for 1000 to 2000 g, a 3.5 ETT for 2000 to 3000 g, and a 3.5 or 4.0 ETT for greater than 3000 g.[25] Although in the past cuffed ETTs were not often used in children less than 8 years of age, softer and low-profile cuffs are now available in sizes down to 3.0 and may be considered in specific situations, such as when the leak around an ETT interferes with ventilation during a surgical procedure requiring positive pressure ventilation.

Approaches to the Difficult Airway

Some children may present challenging anatomic or physiologic problems that may make intubation difficult or impossible. These problems include patients with craniofacial syndromes, orofacial trauma, airway infections, and complete laryngeal obstruction. The clinician should always have additional options available to secure the airway in the event that orotracheal intubation is not successful. Other methods of securing an airway include anterior commissure intubation, flexible fiberoptic intubation, or emergency tracheotomy.

Anterior Commissure Intubation

Children with craniofacial malformations may present a significant challenge to what would normally be

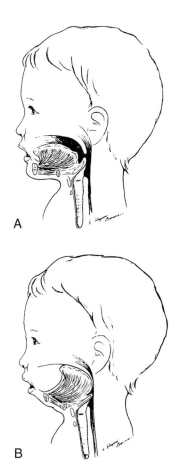

FIGURE 15-10 Anatomic features of the normal larynx **(A)**, and of the larynx in the presence of mandibular hypoplasia **(B)** In the presence of mandibular hypoplasia, the posterior displacement of the tongue makes the larynx appear more anteriorly situated than normal.

considered a straightforward intubation. In addition to the reasons cited previously, many of these children require intubation for plastic reconstructive surgery. The child with the hypoplastic mandible presents an extremely challenging situation. These patients include children with Pierre Robin sequence (retrognathia, glossoptosis, and cleft palate), Treacher Collins syndrome, and hemifacial microsomia. A young patient with the Pierre Robin sequence has a larynx that is exceedingly difficult to expose. In such cases, the larynx is high, anterior, and concealed by the tongue base (Figure 15-10). During intubation the clinician may be able to visualize only the tips of the arytenoid cartilage. Handler[26] described a technique known as *anterior commissure intubation*, using the Holinger anterior commissure laryngoscope. This rigid and tubular style laryngoscope offers excellent exposure of the endolarynx (Figure 15-11). The narrow end of the laryngoscope is placed into the laryngeal inlet, and the ETT can be passed directly into the scope with long alligator forceps

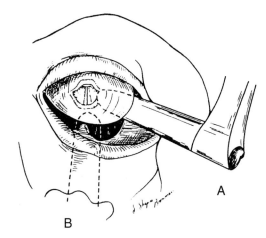

FIGURE 15-11 Laryngoscope placed laterally in the right oral commissure **(A)**, permitting more complete visualization of the larynx than when the instrument is passed in the standard midline position **(B)**.

and advanced as the laryngoscope is withdrawn (Figure 15-12). This technique may be useful to intubate a child who cannot be intubated with a standard laryngoscope and thus avoid an emergency tracheotomy without an airway.

Flexible Fiberoptic Intubation

When the larynx cannot be visualized with a rigid endoscope, the flexible fiberoptic bronchoscope offers several advantages for intubation. First, the flexible scope can navigate into an endolarynx that is impossible or difficult to expose with the rigid scope. This enables the clinician to pass an ETT previously placed over the flexible scope into the trachea once the flexible scope is through the cords. Second, the flexible scope facilitates nasotracheal intubation, which may be a more secure airway in certain clinical situations, such as hypopharyngeal masses, craniofacial anomalies, and muscular dystrophy. Older children or young adults with certain muscular dystrophies may have such severe contractures that it is impossible to expose with the anterior commissure laryngoscope. In such cases the best option for a controlled intubation is with the flexible fiberoptic scope.

Although beyond the scope of this chapter, there are several other methods of orotracheal intubation worth mentioning. These include finger intubation of the trachea, retrograde tracheal intubation, intubation with the laryngeal mask airway, and several new fiberoptic laryngoscopes such the Bullard and Neustein laryngoscopes.[9,27-31]

Emergency Tracheotomy

In the infant and small child it is preferred to perform a tracheotomy after the airway has been secured. In

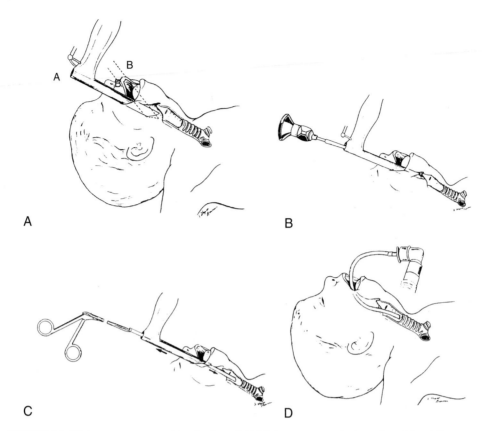

FIGURE 15-12 Laryngoscopy and intubation. **A,** With laryngoscope in lateral position (*A*), approximately 30 degrees of anterior angulation is gained over the standard midline position (*B*), thus permitting more complete visualization of the larynx. **B,** Endotracheal tube (without 15-mm anesthetic adapter) is inserted into the barrel of the laryngoscope under direct visualization. In this example, an optical stylet is used. **C,** The endotracheal tube is grasped with alligator forceps and advanced slightly (*small arrow*) as the laryngoscope is withdrawn (*large arrow*). **D,** Anesthetic adapter (15 mm) is replaced, and ventilation is begun.

most cases endotracheal intubation is preferred yet not always possible. Circumstances under which endotracheal intubation may be difficult or impossible include severe trauma or hemorrhage, craniofacial problems, and the newborn with complete laryngeal obstruction. Alternative approaches to securing the airway are dictated by the urgency of the clinical situation and the age of the patient. These include tracheotomy under local anesthesia, mask ventilation, or cricothyroidotomy. If at all possible it is better to have an airway in place while doing a tracheotomy in infants and small children. In certain situations, a rigid ventilating bronchoscope may be used to visualize and secure the laryngotracheal airway before tracheotomy.

In an older patient with airway obstruction who can cooperate, a tracheotomy under local anesthesia is preferred. The infant with near-total laryngeal obstruction may require facemask or laryngeal mask airway ventilation during tracheotomy. In the emergency setting, an option in older children and adolescents is a cricothyroidotomy in which the tracheotomy tube is inserted into the cricothyroid membrane. This is a relatively expeditious way of placing an emergency tracheostomy tube in older patients.[32] In infants and small children, an emergency cricothyroidotomy may be difficult to perform and other options are less difficult and safer.

Epiglottitis

Since the *Haemophilus influenzae* type B (Hib) vaccine was introduced in the United States in 1988, the frequency of epiglottitis has decreased dramatically. The incidence of Hib disease in children less than 5 years of age between the years 1987 and 1995 decreased by 96%.[33] Today epiglottitis is a rare disorder and experience with its emergency management is declining. Epiglottitis is a true pediatric emergency. It is important to follow the same basic airway management principles and to be fully prepared if adherence to basic principles cannot be maintained.

The child with clinical manifestations of epiglottitis should not undergo a visual examination in the emergency department (see Chapter 32, Asthma). The child should not be stimulated and should be kept as calm as possible.

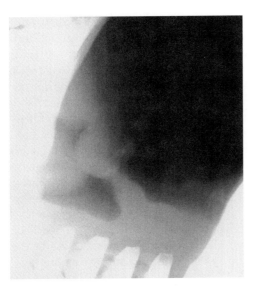

FIGURE 15-13 Lateral soft tissue neck radiograph revealing epiglottitis.

The patient should be accompanied by medical personnel, with the appropriate airway skills to accomplish emergency intubation, to an area where diagnosis can be confirmed by a soft tissue lateral neck radiograph (Figure 15-13). Radiologic findings include thickening of the epiglottis and aryepiglottic folds and the classic "thumbprint" sign. Once the diagnosis has been established, arrangements should be made for immediate transport to the operating room for intubation by an anesthesiologist, with backup by an otorhinolaryngologist in the event an emergency tracheotomy is required. An emergency tracheotomy set and bronchoscope should be available and ready for use. Intubation is done by the anesthesiologist after a slow mask induction with continuous spontaneous ventilation. A vallecular laryngoscope is then used to expose the epiglottis and endolarynx. This confirms the diagnosis and exposes the airway for intubation. The larynx is orally intubated, and then a nasotracheal tube is placed. Check the leak pressure daily and attempt extubation when there is a leak of less than 20 cm H_2O around an age-appropriate ETT. In general, 48 to 56 hours of intubation and intravenous antibiotics is needed before extubation is successful.

Laryngotracheal Stenosis

Children with laryngotracheal stenosis who do not have a tracheotomy may require intubation. The severity of the stenosis may dictate the approach used to access the airway. Plain magnified soft tissue radiographs may show subglottic narrowing or long segment tracheal stenosis. In cases of mild subglottic stenosis the patient may be intubated orally, but it would be essential to start with an endotracheal tube size at least one smaller than the age-appropriate tube and air leakage must be checked. A leak between 10 and 20 cm H_2O during the time of intubation

is necessary so that further damage is not incurred. If the air leak is greater than 20 cm H_2O a smaller tube should be placed. In cases of severe laryngotracheal stenosis an LMA may be used, or occasionally an emergency tracheotomy may be performed, as an alternative.

Artificial Airway Cuff Management

If a cuffed ETT or tracheostomy is used the cuff is inflated once proper placement of the artificial airway is ensured. If the patient has a large leak with the cuff deflated, then the cuff is inflated to minimal leak (see the next paragraph). To inflate the cuff, a 5- or 10-ml syringe is attached to the pilot balloon and gradually air is added to the cuff. Positive pressure applied through the ETT should produce an audible escape of air, or leak, at less than or equal to 20 cm H_2O. The larynx should be auscultated to confirm the leak. Intracuff pressures are maintained at less than 20 to 25 cm H_2O because higher pressures are associated with ischemia and necrosis of the tracheal mucosa and can lead to tracheal stenosis.

Cuff pressures should be checked approximately every 8 hours to guarantee that the pressure does not exceed the recommended levels. If a cuff pressure–measuring device is not available, the minimal leak test can be performed. To inflate the cuff to minimal leak, the cuff is inflated until no air leak is noted during the application of positive pressure. Then a small amount of air is withdrawn from the cuff until a slight leak is auscultated. During certain positive-pressure applications, the minimal occlusion technique may be necessary. The procedure is the same as that just described, with the exception that enough air is left in the cuff to prevent a leak.

If large amounts of air are required in the cuff and a leak persists, one of two possibilities exists: (1) The cuff is damaged or (2) it has not been completely advanced through the cords. The latter problem can be identified by direct laryngoscopy. In patients younger than 8 years, the cricoid cartilage, the narrowest portion of the airway, serves as a functional cuff. Once again, the clinical situation may direct the clinician to use a cuffed or uncuffed ETT depending on need. In the neonate, the leak pressure should be kept at less than or equal to 10 cm H_2O if possible to prevent tracheal damage.

Patient Monitoring

Continuously evaluating the patient undergoing intubation is essential to ensure a safe and effective outcome. Before the airway is manipulated, the heart rate, capillary refill, blood pressure, and oxygen saturation should be monitored and recorded. Under ideal circumstances, a precordial stethoscope is used to continuously monitor heart tones and breath sounds. At a minimum, the patient's heart rate, blood pressure, and oxygen saturation should be monitored continuously. A continuous electrocardiogram monitors the heart for dysrhythmias. Noninvasive means of monitoring blood pressure include palpation, auscultation, and automated devices. Pulse oximetry and patient color best indicate oxygen saturation during intubation. A single individual should be made responsible for the task of monitoring the patient continuously during the procedure. If, at any time, acceptable values or rhythms are breached, the clinician should be warned and attempts at intubation stopped. The airway should be re-established without delay, using a bag and mask.

Complications

Serious complications from endotracheal intubation may occur at any time during or after the intubation procedure. The immediate complications encountered during intubation include both mechanical processes caused by the laryngoscopist and reflex reactions of the patient. Immediate mechanical complications include tissue trauma, perforation or laceration of the pharynx or larynx, esophageal intubation, and pneumothorax. Risks involving autonomic reflexes include laryngospasm and bronchospasm, resulting in hypoxia, cardiac dysrhythmias, and hypotension. Stimulation of the vagal reflex leads to severe bradycardia and arterial hypotension.

The spectrum of complications changes after intubation is completed. Endotracheal tube obstruction secondary to kinking, biting, blood, and secretions becomes more common. Cuff ruptures are also prominent when using cuffed tubes. The incidence of accidental extubation has been reported to be between 3% and 13% and appears to be more common in infants younger than 1 year of age. Aspiration, endobronchial intubation, and atelectasis are not uncommon. Laryngeal edema is a common complication associated with intubation. The edema may be glottic, supraglottic, or subglottic. Subglottic edema is more common because of the infant's small airway; it can cause narrowing of the trachea and may require urgent reintubation. The incidence of clinically significant subglottic stenosis has been reported to be 2% to 6% of the pediatric population. Endotracheal tube cuff injuries may cause tracheal stenosis and require intervention. Maxillary sinusitis and nosocomial pneumonia are long-term infectious complications associated with significant mortality and morbidity.

EXTUBATION

The most important question to consider when evaluating a patient for extubation is whether there has been improvement or reversal of the disease process that initially mandated the intubation. Before extubation, the patient must be hemodynamically stable, must be able to breathe spontaneously with an adequate tidal volume and respiratory pattern, and must have adequate neurologic integrity to protect the airway.

Hemodynamic stability is manifested by normal cardiac output, capillary refill, urine output, and blood pressure. The patient should be alert and awake with evidence of adequate muscle strength. In older children, muscle strength is evaluated by measuring maximal inspiratory pressure during airway occlusion and vital capacity. In an adult, a negative inspiratory force greater than -20 cm H_2O and a vital capacity greater than 20 ml/kg correlate with successful extubation. It is important to point out that these tests, although used in the pediatric population, have not been validated by prospective trials. In addition, adequate airway protective reflexes include being able to gag, swallow, and cough. The gag reflex can be stimulated by placing a tongue blade in the posterior pharynx, and a cough reflex can be evaluated as the trachea is stimulated during suctioning.

Accidental Extubation

The reported incidence of accidental extubation in the pediatric and neonatal intensive care population is between 3% and 13%. Other methodologies for reporting the number of accidental extubations have focused on accidental extubation per 100 intubated days. This rate varies from 0.72 per 100 intubated days in the neonatal intensive care unit to 1.1 per 100 intubated days in the pediatric intensive care unit.[34] Risk factors associated with accidental extubation include failure to secure the ETT properly, lack of adequate sedation, failure to provide adequate restraint, and the performance of a procedure, such as chest radiography, on a patient. In the adult population, deliberate self-extubation despite sedation and restraints also contributes to unplanned extubations. Although death can result from self-extubation in any population, it is an infrequent complication. Despite its potential for adverse outcome, self-extubation is usually well tolerated by most patient populations.

Equipment

As with the intubation procedure, anticipation and preparation are essential in accomplishing a smooth extubation. The equipment necessary for extubation includes a bag-and-mask setup, suction equipment, adhesive remover, and all the equipment previously listed for intubation (see Table 15-1). This ensures a proactive approach to patient care in the event that the patient does not tolerate extubation and requires reintubation.

Procedure

Pulmonary function is optimized by administering aerosolized β-agonists as needed and suctioning the oropharynx and trachea before extubation. If the patient has been receiving enteral feedings, the feedings are discontinued for approximately 6 hours before the planned extubation. Although this allows gastric emptying, it does not guarantee that the aspiration of gastric contents will not occur.

If a cuffed tube is in place, the cuff should be deflated. While the ETT is held in place, the tape is removed from the face and tube with an adhesive remover. One large breath is administered and the ETT is withdrawn from the trachea near peak inflation. The majority of patients will then cough and begin to breathe spontaneously. It is not unusual, especially in small children, for a short interval of breath holding to occur. However, this must be distinguished from the more severe complication of laryngospasm. Oxygen is administered by the most appropriate delivery device, such as a nasal cannula, face tent, facemask, or oxyhood. The oxygen concentration is titrated to maintain an oxygen saturation level that is clinically indicated.

The ETT should not be removed during a cough or at end expiration. During a cough, the tissues of the trachea are collapsed into the air column and tighten around the ETT. If the patient is extubated at this point, he or she will not have sufficient lung inflation for an effective cough and may aspirate oral secretions.

Explanation to Patient and Parent

Before extubation of any patient, the extubation procedure and possible complications should be explained to the patient if he or she is old enough to understand; if not, the parents should be informed. Guidelines regarding the need for reintubation should be discussed in depth with either the patient or the patient's family. The first two topics are delineated in detail in other sections of this chapter. It is essential that any explanation be clear, using a vocabulary easily understood by the patient and parents. The patient and parents must be made aware that every effort has been made to adequately evaluate the patient's readiness for extubation, but that there is a possibility that reintubation may be required. A review of possible scenarios requiring reintubation may help alleviate the parental disappointment associated with this apparent setback. Common scenarios include, but are not limited to, laryngospasm that will not respond to conservative therapy, the development of postextubation stridor that is not amenable to therapy, and hypoxemia or hypercarbia associated with a patient's inability to maintain adequate oxygenation and ventilation. It is important to relieve patient or parental anxiety as much as possible. Reassurances that the procedure will be as painless and effortless, and done as smoothly as possible, aid in a successful and atraumatic extubation for both the patient and family.

Complications

Sore throat and hoarseness are common complaints after extubation. The presence of an ETT may cause edema of the laryngeal structures. Once extubation is successfully accomplished, postextubation stridor can develop within minutes and usually peaks within 8 hours. This condition has been well described and occurs frequently in the pediatric population. Corticosteroids, aerosolized racemic epinephrine, and helium–oxygen mixtures have all been used to treat this complication.[35,36] A meta-analysis of the use of corticosteroids in the prevention of reintubation and postextubation stridor did not show any statistically significant difference in reintubation rates, but there was a significant decrease in stridor.[35] Laryngospasm, another known complication postextubation, is caused by stimulating the larynx when removing the ETT or from pooled secretions that may drain into the airway. Treatment for this complication is by the application of basic airway maneuvers and positive pressure through a bag-and-mask setup connected to 100% oxygen. If laryngospasm persists in concert with arterial desaturation, a short-acting neuromuscular blocker should be administered while the patient is supported with the bag and mask or reintubated.

Difficulty with extubation can be associated with poor pulmonary function or can occur secondary to mechanical complications. Patients who have not been adequately assessed regarding their pulmonary status may not tolerate extubation. An ineffective cough and gag reflex will predispose the patient to aspiration of secretions or gastric contents, possibly leading to alveolar collapse and pneumonitis. A mechanical problem related to extubation is failure to deflate the ETT cuff, resulting in direct trauma and the potential for laryngeal edema.

Extubation Failure

A child may fail one or more controlled attempts at extubation for any number of reasons. These include pathologic processes of both the upper and lower airway as well as the general medical and neurologic condition of the patient. In the premature infant the lungs may not be developed enough for the child to breathe without ventilatory support or positive pressure. In these cases the infant may need time for further pulmonary development. In addition, the child who is neurologically compromised or oversedated may not be able to breathe spontaneously and protect the airway. One must wait for the child's neurologic status to improve to its former baseline or until the child has the neuromuscular competence to breathe adequately and protect the airway.

Some children may have congenital or acquired causes for obstruction of the upper airway that will prevent successful extubation. These include choanal atresia, severe laryngomalacia, vocal cord paralysis, laryngeal edema, stenosis (congenital or acquired), subglottic cysts, hemangiomas, and tracheomalacia. In these situations the child does well with minimal or no ventilator support but develops a problem as soon as the ETT is removed.

Treatment Strategies

First, the reason for extubation failure and/or the site of obstruction must be determined. It is important to know the degree of ventilatory support that is required before extubation. Children who cannot be weaned from mechanical ventilation may have underlying pulmonary or central neurologic pathology. In such cases, long-term ventilation may need to be considered. In contrast, the child who easily weans from mechanical ventilation but cannot be extubated may have significant upper airway obstruction. In such a case, endoscopy may be useful in determining the site and cause of the problem. The child should undergo rigid laryngoscopy and bronchoscopy in the operating room to localize the site of obstruction. Treatment then depends on the specific pathology. The child with subglottic stenosis may need surgical intervention and may be considered for laryngotracheal reconstruction (LTR) to achieve extubation. The patient with a subglottic cyst or hemangioma may require laser ablation of the lesion. The infant with bilateral choanal atresia requires immediate surgical repair with stenting. The child with distal tracheomalacia may have a vascular compression and will require additional tests such as magnetic resonance angiography to define the vascular pathology. When there are vascular anomalies, cardiovascular intervention may be necessary.

Nasal Mask Ventilation, Heliox

To ease the transition to spontaneous ventilation or when there is residual upper airway obstruction, noninvasive positive-pressure mask ventilation may be helpful. A nasal facemask that fits over the nose and mouth is used to deliver both inspiratory and expiratory pressure. The so-called BiPAP (bilevel positive airway pressure) system may be a useful method to transition the patient to spontaneous respiration after extubation. In the event that a fixed narrow opening such as in subglottic stenosis or laryngeal edema is the cause of difficulty, a helium-oxygen mixture (heliox) may be beneficial. Its lower density may reduce the viscosity of airflow and decrease airway resistance. Mixtures of helium to oxygen are available as 80% helium–20% oxygen and 70% helium–30% oxygen. Additional oxygen can be titrated into these mixtures; however, as the concentration of oxygen increases, the density of the gas decreases, and so does the agent's efficacy. When the upper airway obstruction has resolved, one can then gradually wean the heliox.[36]

Laryngotracheal Reconstruction

The child with critical subglottic stenosis and adequate pulmonary function may be a good candidate for LTR.

This involves expansion of the airway with cartilage grafts or resection of the stenotic portion of the airway. In a child without a tracheotomy LTR may be performed in a single-stage fashion. The child may be kept intubated nasally for 3 to 10 days, depending on the type of repair. Repeat endoscopy confirms successful healing of the repair and extubation may be attempted in the intensive care unit or operating room when extubation parameters have been met. Heliox may be necessary immediately after extubation in case edema and secretions are an issue.

TRACHEOTOMY

The child who is not a candidate for extubation or LTR may require a tracheotomy. The decision to perform a tracheotomy is based on the future airway prognosis, as well as on the family's ability to care for an artificial airway at home. Before proceeding with a tracheotomy the risks as well as the significant burden for the family must be considered.

Tracheotomy Indications

The three main indications for tracheotomy in infants and children are for airway obstruction, long-term ventilation, and pulmonary hygiene. Children with congenital or acquired upper airway obstruction may require a tracheotomy at an early age if extubation cannot be accomplished. Congenital laryngeal stenosis, which varies in severity, may require a tracheotomy at an early age or even in the delivery room. Bilateral vocal cord paralysis, usually secondary to central neurologic causes such as Arnold-Chiari malformation, results in severe airway obstruction. Tracheotomy may be required in approximately 66% of these cases.[37] In many cases the vocal cord paralysis resolves within several years of the initial insult. Acquired laryngeal stenosis is related to prematurity, prolonged intubation, traumatic intubation sepsis, and a host of other factors. Premature children with bronchopulmonary dysplasia may require a tracheotomy for long-term ventilation. In addition, children with neurologic problems, especially if they have impairment of brainstem function, may develop difficulties with pulmonary hygiene because of their inability to clear secretions, causing aspiration. This situation will predispose the patient to recurrent hospitalizations and intubations, further limiting their quality of life. A tracheotomy will allow for improved pulmonary hygiene and potentially an improved lifestyle.

Tracheotomy Tubes

Tracheotomy tubes come in various dimensions and materials, and selecting an appropriately sized tracheotomy tube is an important issue before placement. The age, size, and medical condition of the patient determine the type of tracheotomy tube selected. Tracheotomy tubes come in various sizes, which are usually chosen on the basis of age (Table 15-4). Tracheotomy tubes have three dimensions: inner diameter, outer diameter, and length. The depth of the tube from the flange is usually

TABLE 15-4

Age and Tracheotomy Tube Size*

Age	Size	Inner Diameter (mm)	Outer Diameter (mm)	Overall Length (mm)	Length (mm)
Shiley†					
Premature	00	3.1	4.5	14	30, 39
Newborn	0	3.4	5.0	15	32, 40
3-10 mo	1	3.7	5.5	17	34, 41
10-12 mo	2	4.1	6.0	18	42
13-24 mo	3	4.8	7.0	21	44
2-9 yr	4	5.5	8.0	24	46
9 yr+	4 adult	5.0	8.5	26	67
	6 adult	7.0	10.0	30	78
	8 adult	8.5	12.0	36	84
	10 adult	9.0	13.0	39	84
Holinger‡					
Premature	000	13	2.1	4.1	26, 30, 33, 36, 40, 46
Premature	00	13	2.4	4.5	26, 30, 33, 36, 40, 46
Newborn	0	15	2.9	5.0	26, 30, 33, 36, 40, 46
Newborn-3 mo	1	17	3.0	5.5	30, 33, 36, 40, 46
3-10 mo	2	18	3.3	6.0	30, 33, 40, 46
10-24 mo	3	21	4.4	7.0	33, 40, 50, 55, 60
2-7 yr	4	24-25	5.3	8.0	50, 55, 60
8-9 yr	5	27	6.1	9.0	63, 68
10 yr+	6	30	7.1	10.0	63, 68, 73
Portex§					
Newborn	0	15	3.0	5.0	36
Newborn-3 mo	1	16	3.5	5.5	40
3-10 mo	2	18	4.0	6.0	44
10-12 mo	—	19	4.5	6.5	48
2-7 yr	3	21	5.0	7.0	48.5
8-11 yr	4 adult	24	6.0	8.1	55
12 yr+	6 adult	30	7.0	9.7	75
	7 adult	33	8.0	11.0	82
	8 adult	36	9.0	12.1	87
	9 adult	40	10.0	13.5	98
Argyll‖					
Premature	000	2.5	4.0	34.4	
Premature	00	3.0	4.7	35.9	
Newborn-3 mo	0	3.5	5.4	38.5	
3-10 mo	1	4.0	6.0	41	
10-12 mo	2	4.5	6.6	45.5	
2.7 yr-3 adult	22	5.0	7.3	52.1	
2-9 yr	4	5.5	7.8	56.5	
9 yr + 5 adult	26	6.0	8.5	61.6	
9 yr +	Adult	30	7.0	10.0	
Adult	33	8.0	11.0		
Adult	37	9.0	12.3		
Adult	40	9.5	13.3		

* Ages adapted from Bluestone CD, Stool SE, editors: Pediatric otolaryngology, Vol 2, Philadelphia: WB Saunders; 1983. This information is only a guide; individual adaptation may be necessary.
† From Covidien (Mansfield, MA).
‡ From Pilling-Weck (Research Triangle Park, NC), 1986. Sizes may vary with Holinger tubes manufactured by other companies.
§ From Concord Portex (Keene, NH).
‖ From Sherwood Medical (St. Louis, Mo). Formerly Dover brand.
From Myer CM, Cotton RT, Shott SR, editors: *Pediatric airway: an interdisciplinary approach.* Philadelphia. Lippincott-Raven, 1995; p 165.

related to the length of the tube. The dimensions of three common brands of tracheotomy tubes are compared in Table 15-5. Customized tracheotomy tubes may be needed in certain situations.

When selecting a tube, in addition to the size, the shape and composition must be considered. Some tubes are made of polyvinyl chloride, which is rigid, whereas other brands are made of silicone and require wire reinforcement. Softer does not always equal better. Whereas softer tube composition may be used to overcome pressure ulcerations, it does not aid in healing ulcerations caused by friction forces. Most of the time, patient comfort will dictate which material to use in any given clinical situation.

An arched tube is curved in the shape of one fourth of a circle and is short. An angled tube is curved into a 90-degree bend and slightly longer than the arched tube. Each tube must be positioned correctly in the airway to optimize performance. Malpositioning of these tubes may result in kinking, mainstem intubation, or occluding on the anterior or posterior wall of the trachea (Figure 15-14).[34] However, once the tube warms to body temperature, it usually conforms to the shape of the airway. Sometimes changing the tube to a different shape may overcome a stoma track that is difficult to cannulate.

A cuffed tracheotomy tube may be needed for a child requiring higher ventilatory pressures for chronic lung disease. There are three basic types of cuff: high-volume low-pressure, foam cuff, and tight-to-shaft. The first two are inflated with air, whereas the last requires saline. The type of cuff to be used is decided by the team and ordered specifically for each patient. It is important to avoid overinflation of the cuff. This may lead to problems with tracheal erosion and stenosis. It is essential to visualize the tracheotomy endoscopically with the cuff inflated with the usual amount of saline or air. The cuff should not be causing pressure necrosis on the distal tracheal mucosa. If the cuff appears tight, then less air or saline should be used. The technique for determining minimal leak or minimal occlusion pressures for tracheotomy tube cuffs is the same as described for ETT cuffs.

There are several types of tracheotomy ties that caregivers may use. These include tracheotomy string or twill tape, felt with a Velcro fastener (Figure 15-15), and metal chain. Each has its advantages and disadvantages and depends on the individual preference of the caregivers. The latter two facilitate cleaning and are easier to remove in an emergency.

TABLE 15-5

Dimensions of Three Commonly Used Brands of Tracheotomy Tube

Cannula	Inner Diameter (mm)	Outer Diameter (mm)	Length of Cannula (mm)
Shiley			
3.0 Neonatal	3.0	4.5	30
3.5 Neonatal	3.5	5.2	32
4.0 Neonatal	4.0	5.9	34
3.0 Pediatric	3.0	4.5	39
3.5 Pediatric	3.5	5.2	40
4.0 Pediatric	4.0	5.9	41
4.5 Pediatric	4.5	6.0	42
5.0 Pediatric	5.0	7.1	44
5.5 Pediatric	5.5	7.7	46
Portex			
3.0	3.0	5.0	36
3.5	3.5	5.8	40
4.0	4.0	6.5	44
4.5	4.5	7.1	48
5.0	5.0	7.7	50
5.5	5.5	8.3	52
Bivona Neonatal Cuffless*			
2.5	2.5	4.0	30
3.0	3.0	4.7	32
3.5	3.5	5.3	34
4.0	4.0	6.0	36
Bivona Pediatric*			
2.5	2.5	4.0	38
3.0	3.0	4.7	39
3.5	3.5	5.3	40
4.0	4.0	6.0	41
4.5	4.5	6.7	42
5.0	5.0	7.3	44
5.5	5.5	8.0	46

* From Smiths Medical (St. Paul, Minn).

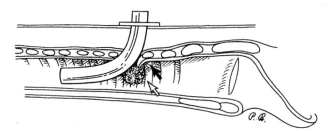

FIGURE 15-14 Midsagittal section of a trachea with tracheotomy tube in position. This reveals two common problems: suprastomal granulation tissue *(open arrow)* and suprastomal collapse *(solid arrow)*.

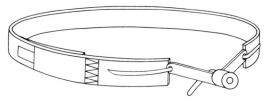

FIGURE 15-15 Diagram of a tracheostomy securing system with Velcro ties.

Procedure and Technique

There are special concerns with respect to tracheotomy in the infant and small child. First, the anatomic characteristics of this population make it more difficult to localize the trachea than in adults. The major landmarks, including the cricoid and thyroid cartilage, are not prominent. The trachea is smaller and not as superficial, and it is more mobile and easier to push over to one side. Furthermore, the rapid placement of a tracheotomy tube in the cricothyroid membrane (cricothyroidotomy) is contraindicated in an infant or small child but may be performed in an emergent situation in an older child or adolescent.

Routine tracheotomy for infants and small children requires careful dissection while having an already established airway such as an orotracheal tube. If the airway is not already established, then the child may undergo bronchoscopy or intubation before tracheotomy. On occasion, a tracheotomy is performed in older children or adolescents with the use of local anesthesia, but this should be avoided if possible in small children. The airway is usually managed by mask ventilation or by using a laryngeal mask airway when performing the procedure on difficult airways, such as in patients with the Pierre Robin sequence.

Once the airway is established, the child is positioned for tracheotomy (Figure 15-16). All indwelling feeding tubes are removed from the esophagus. A shoulder roll is used for hyperextension. The anesthesiologist is at the patient's head and has access to the airway at all times. A transverse incision is made through the skin and subcutaneous tissue. The strap muscles are separated to identify the midline, and careful midline dissection is performed to avoid pneumothorax. The upper tracheal cartilages are identified. On occasion, the isthmus of the thyroid gland must be divided to expose the upper tracheal rings. The tracheotomy tube is usually placed between the second and third tracheal rings. One surgeon holds the tracheotomy tube while an assistant secures the tube. Two stay sutures, which are removed after the first tracheotomy tube change, are placed on either side of the midline (Figure 15-17). These sutures are used to access the airway in the case of accidental decannulation and before the site has had time to mature. A vertical midline incision is made, and the tracheotomy tube is inserted. If a cuff tracheotomy is used, then the cuff is inflated with saline or air.

Complications

In the 1970s, the mortality rate from tracheotomy was reported to be as high as 24%.[38] More recent reports indicate mortality rates ranging from 0.5% to 3%.[39-43] This may be attributed to improvements in monitoring techniques such as pulse oximetry as well as frequency

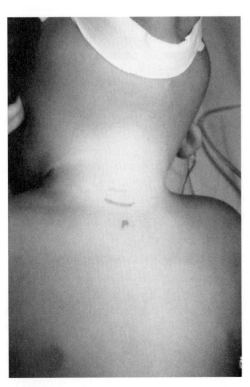

FIGURE 15-16 An infant in a hyperextended position for tracheotomy.

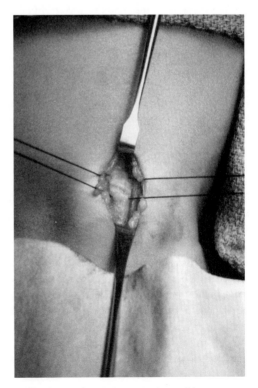

FIGURE 15-17 Tracheotomy procedure with two stay sutures placed on either side of the tracheotomy incision.

of medical follow-up visits and heightened vigilance. Avoidable deaths can be prevented by a thorough education program for all persons caring for a child in the hospital and the home. The ability to recannulate in case of accidental decannulation, proper airway assessment, good hygiene, and adequate systemic hydration and nutrition are important factors for a successful long-term outcome for a tracheotomized infant or child. Teaching the parents or caregivers to teach others caring for the child how to care for the tracheotomy site is a critical component of this training.[44]

The two most common reasons for death of a tracheotomy tube–dependent child are plugging of the tube with mucus and accidental decannulation. Plugging with mucus occurs when thick, viscous mucus obstructs the lumen of the tracheotomy tube. Several factors that lead to this problem include dehydration, infection, and lack of humidity. Many children with bronchopulmonary dysplasia develop frequent exacerbations of mucous plugging with increased bronchorrhea. Tracheitis, either viral or bacterial, may also lead to an increase in thick secretions. These problems can be avoided with appropriate hydration, chest physiotherapy, and frequent suctioning. Antibiotic therapy is necessary in the case of infection. Sometimes the use of a humidifier or passive humidification device may help alleviate thick secretions. A new device (Vapotherm 2000i; Vapotherm, Stevensville, Md) may help to deliver high-flow humidified oxygen to patients requiring supplemental oxygen. At this time there are, however, insufficient data to support its use. Acute mucous plugging requires emergency suctioning. The tube is changed immediately if suctioning does not relieve the obstruction. Once the obstruction is relieved and the patient is out of danger, the previously mentioned treatments are initiated to help prevent a recurrence of the problem.

Another serious complication is accidental dislodgment of the tracheotomy tube. This accounts for most tracheotomy-related deaths. Accidental dislodgment may occur during play activity or tracheotomy care or when the child is alone. Immediate reinsertion is required. This may be difficult during an emergency situation. If the same size of tracheotomy tube cannot be inserted, then an attempt should be made to insert a tube that is one size smaller. If this is unsuccessful, the patient should be ventilated with a bag and mask until additional medical help arrives. Parents are usually sent home with a mask and bag for use in case of an emergency. When there is a critical airway and there is no reserve airway around the tracheotomy tube, such as total laryngeal stenosis, then insertion of an ETT into the tracheotomy site is an acceptable alternative option in securing the airway.

Other complications associated with tracheostomy use include bleeding, stomal and suprastomal granulation tissue, tracheal erosion, and suprastomal tracheomalacia. External granulations may be removed or cauterized. Suprastomal granulation is not routinely removed during endoscopy unless there is bleeding or obstruction beyond the distal end of the tracheotomy tube. Suprastomal granulation is also removed just before decannulation. Tracheal granulation usually recurs if the tracheotomy tube is left in place. In contrast, obstructive granulation tissue in the distal airway should be removed early. Suprastomal tracheomalacia may also be repaired at the time of decannulation.

Bleeding from the tracheotomy tube is usually related to tracheitis, but on occasion it may be caused by granulation polyps or even erosion into a major vessel such the innominate artery. Innominate arterial bleeding may require intervention by a thoracic surgeon. In addition, suction trauma causes bleeding; however, that is usually self-limited. Suctioning beyond the end of the tracheotomy tube should not be done so as to avoid direct tracheal trauma and bleeding. Routine care of a tracheostomy includes interval bronchoscopies every 6 months to ensure there are no major problems developing with the tracheotomy site.

Other problems encountered with a chronic tracheotomy include speech delay and difficulty with phonation. The underlying airway lesion may limit phonation, such as in the child with total laryngeal stenosis. In addition, the ventilator or the tracheotomy tube itself may block the flow of air. Unless there is a critical airway, the child with a tracheotomy may be fitted for a Passy-Muir speech valve. This valve allows one-way flow of air up through the glottis to allow phonation (Figure 15-18).[42]

Moreover, many tracheotomized children have significant swallowing difficulties and problems with certain food textures. These problems may be related to the tracheotomy tethering the airway and preventing elevation of the larynx during deglutition or to actual food aversion by the child, who may be protecting the airway. Finally, the sense of smell and taste may be altered in a child who is bypassing the nasal airway. Close work with a speech and swallowing therapist is essential for the young child or infant with a tracheotomy.[42]

Tracheotomy Tube Changes

Safe tracheotomy tube changes are an important part of routine tracheotomy care. It is essential that the child's parents or caregivers learn proper tracheotomy tube care before the child is discharged.[44] Preparation is the key to safety. It is always imperative to have proper equipment around for the tracheotomy change, as listed in Box 15-2. It is also important to perform routine tracheotomy tube changes during daytime hours when everyone is alert and a "partner" is available. It is best to perform a routine

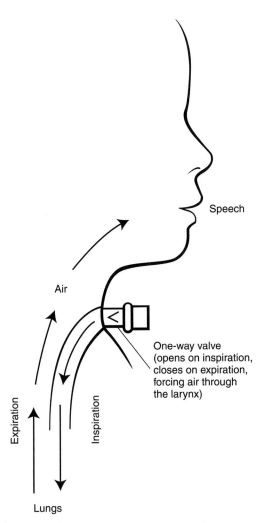

FIGURE 15-18 Passy-Muir tracheostomy speaking valve enabled by redirecting exhaled air around the tracheostomy tube and through the larynx and upper airway.

Box 15-2	Equipment Needed for Tracheotomy Tube Changes

- Correct size tracheotomy tube and obturator
- Smaller size tracheotomy tube
- Blanket roll
- Lubricant
- Tracheotomy ties
- Scissors
- Clean wet and dry gauze
- Stethoscope
- Resuscitation bag with mask
- Oxygen source

tracheotomy tube change with two people. Proper lighting and position are essential. One must always communicate with the helper, be prepared for the worst, and remain calm, especially during an emergency.

At least 2 hours should have passed after the last feeding before the tracheotomy tube is changed. All supplies and emergency equipment are assembled. The role of the partner is determined and then the child is positioned on a shoulder roll with the neck hyperextended to make tube insertion easier. It is important to be prepared for any emergency such as a difficult cannulation, inability to reaccess the airway, significant bradycardia, or desaturation.

First, the child is adequately hyperoxygenated. During the routine tube change, the person inserting the tracheotomy tube takes charge. On this person's count, the "partner" removes the old tracheotomy tube and the person changing the tracheotomy tube places it at a right angle into the stoma and quickly advances it into the airway. The partner listens for breath sounds and then reattaches the ventilator if required. After the change, the stoma is cleaned and dressed with gauze to protect the skin. The tracheotomy ties are threaded and secured, and then checked for correct tension: The ties should be tight enough to hold the tube in place without movement yet not bind or pinch the neck.[44]

Tracheotomy Home Care

Many of the complications of tracheotomy take place in the home. Therefore, an optimal home-care environment is essential. Parents and caregivers should be able to smoothly and quickly perform tracheotomy tube changes even in an urgent situation and should be trained in cardiopulmonary resuscitation. They must be able to perform routine functions such as suctioning and cleaning. Adequate tracheotomy equipment should always be available. Suctioning should be performed just beyond the length of the tracheotomy tube to avoid suction trauma to the carina. This includes such items as spare tracheotomy tubes, smaller size tracheotomy tubes, tracheotomy ties, dressing, suction catheters, suction machine, humidity devices, and monitors (Box 15-3). For monitoring, a pulse oximeter is preferred over an apnea monitor, because the apnea monitor will not detect an obstructed tracheotomy tube. Home nursing care is also required, the amount depending on the clinical and family situation. In general, for a child who is tracheotomy and ventilator dependent, a parent can be expected to manage at least 8 hours of care alone and have up to 16 hours of nursing care per day.[44] However, each family has unique needs, resources, and capabilities. In addition, different insurance companies allow various amounts of home nursing support.

Decannulation

Using a standard approach to routine decannulation in children promotes safe and expeditious removal of the tracheotomy tube once it is no longer required. Three conditions must be met before decannulation. First, the

Box 15-3	Equipment Needed for Tracheotomy Tube Care

- Correct size tracheotomy tube and obturator
- Smaller size tracheotomy tube
- Pipe cleaners
- Container for sterile water
- Sterile water
- Gauze
- Portable suction machine
- Long flexible suction catheters
- Humidity valves
- Gauze tracheotomy dressing
- Oxygen
- Tracheotomy collar

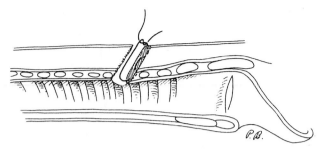

FIGURE 15-19 Repair of suprastomal collapse, using absorbable sutures placed on the collapsing suprastomal cartilage and tied to the stomal skin.

original condition requiring the tracheotomy must be resolved or improved, and there should be no comorbid condition that would impact the success of decannulation. For instance, has the child's cardiac or pulmonary status improved? In addition, one might postpone decannulation if there is upcoming surgery that affects the airway.[45] Second, the airway must be adequate to handle the respiratory requirements of the patient. The entire airway should be evaluated endoscopically before decannulation to determine patency. Last, the child must be able to protect the airway with adequate cough and gag reflexes.

The airway is evaluated by both flexible and rigid laryngoscopy and bronchoscopy in the operating room with the patient under general anesthesia. A pediatric flexible fiberoptic scope is passed through the nose to rule out choanal atresia, septal deformities, adenotonsillar obstruction, or laryngeal stenosis. Esophageal reflux may be inferred in the presence of supraglottic edema or laryngotracheal cobblestoning. The dynamic characteristics of the larynx, such as supraglottic collapse and vocal fold mobility, are evaluated. Normal laryngeal reflexes and mobility are important to demonstrate before decannulation. Airway patency is assessed by rigid laryngoscopy and bronchoscopy. Immobile vocal cords are palpated to rule out glottic fixation. Suprastomal and other obstructing granulation polyps are excised with forceps or a laser, and bleeding is controlled by cautery or vasoconstrictive solutions, such as oxymetazoline. Suprastomal collapse is repaired surgically by hooking the collapsing segment and passing a suture from the cartilage to the tracheostoma skin (Figure 15-19). In some cases, tracheal collapse may be severe enough to require an open tracheoplasty. After the procedure, the same size tracheotomy tube is inserted and decannulation is deferred until later that day, or the next day, when the patient has recovered from anesthesia.[45]

There are several reasons why a child may not be ready for decannulation. First, the original condition may not

have resolved. If the child had a tracheotomy tube in place for upper airway obstruction, then there may still be some degree of dynamic collapse while asleep, leading to sleep apnea. A monitored sleep study in a laboratory may help determine whether the obstruction has resolved.[46] Other examples of reasons to delay decannulation are diminished vocal cord abduction from posterior glottic stenosis or vocal cord paralysis and may require reconstructive surgery.

Decannulation Methods

There are three methods of decannulation:
1. Immediately remove the tube.
2. Downsize and cap the tube.
3. Extubate after single-stage laryngotracheal reconstruction.

All three methods are performed in a carefully monitored environment. The clinical situation as well as the preference of the clinician determines which method to use.

Once the airway is deemed adequate, the first method is to remove the tracheotomy tube in a monitored environment, such as the postanesthesia care unit. This is scheduled for a time when the child is fully awake and alert. The child is monitored by pulse oximetry and kept calm in a parent's arms. Then the tube is gently removed. The stoma may be covered with gauze. The child is discharged to the floor once the criteria are met for discharge from the postanesthesia care unit. On occasion an insecure child may develop decannulation panic and may need the tracheotomy tube replaced.

The other common method involves downsizing the tracheotomy with a significantly smaller tube. Then, while monitoring the patient, the tube is capped or plugged and the child is allowed to breathe around it. If the child has normal gas exchange without tachypnea or respiratory distress for at least 24 hours, then the tracheotomy tube can be removed. The child is observed for at least another 24 hours. The disadvantage to this technique is with the borderline airway; the small tracheotomy tube may lead to airway obstruction, whereas complete removal would not.

Airway Reconstruction

When there is acquired or congenital laryngeal or tracheal stenosis, the child may require laryngotracheal reconstruction (LTR) before decannulation. Acquired subglottic stenosis is usually related to endotracheal intubation. The treatment depends on the patient's age, the severity and location of stenosis. The infant with subglottic stenosis may present with failure of extubation, or an older child may present with a tracheotomy tube in place and mature stenosis. The challenge becomes repairing the stenosis so the child may safely undergo decannulation.

The first step in evaluating a tracheotomy-dependent child with subglottic stenosis is a comprehensive history to determine if the child is ready for decannulation (Box 15-4). The airway is fully evaluated endoscopically as previously described. Oral intubation is performed with various-sized ETTs and the leak test is performed on each tube. One can infer the caliber of the airway and degree of stenosis from age if the tube size leaks at 10 to 15 cm H_2O (Figure 15-20).[47] There are a number of approaches depending on the age, medical condition, and degree of stenosis. In some cases of mild stenosis the airway may grow as the child matures.[48] Laser treatment may be useful for thin webs or mild stenosis; however, most cases of severe subglottic stenosis require open reconstructive surgery.

There are many surgical approaches to LTR, again depending on the situation.[48,49] For circumferential stenosis with good cartilaginous support, an anterior costal (rib) cartilage graft without stenting will be adequate (Figure 15-21). When there is posterior glottic stenosis or severe loss of cartilaginous support, then a

Box 15-4	Evaluation for Decannulation

- Prematurity and gestational age
- Birth weight
- Number of intubations and duration
- Traumatic intubations
- Voice
- What happens when the tracheotomy tube is removed during tube changes?
- Mechanical ventilation and how long?
- Continuous positive airway pressure or oxygen?
- Cyanotic events or blue spells with the tracheotomy tube in position?
- Recent hospitalizations for respiratory events?
- Oral feedings? Aspiration?
- Weight gain or failure to thrive?
- Overall medical status?
- Upcoming surgeries?

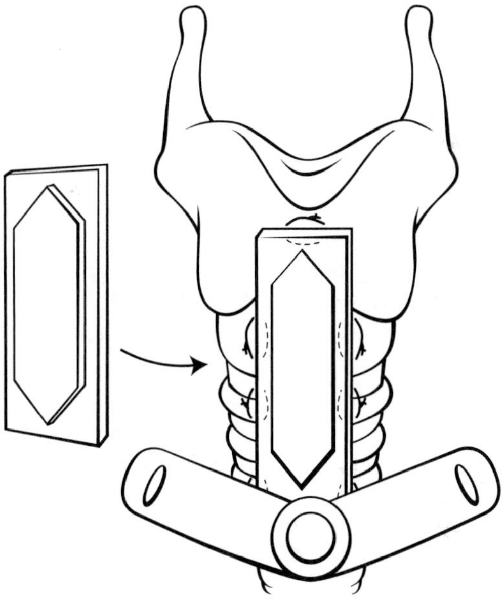

FIGURE 15-21 Laryngotracheoplasty using an anteriorly placed costal cartilage graft.

Classification of Stenosis With Actual Endotracheal Tube Size:		ID 2.0	ID 2.5	ID 3.0	ID 3.5	ID 4.0	ID 4.5	ID 5.0	ID 5.5	ID 6.0
Patient age										
Premature	No detectable lumen	NO								
		40	NO							
		58	30	NO						
0-3/12		68	48	26	NO					
3/12-9/12		75	59	41	22	NO				
9/12-2		80	67	53	38	20	NO			
2		84	74	62	50	35	19	NO		
4		86	78	68	57	45	32	17	NO	
6		89	81	73	64	54	43	30	16	NO
	Grade IV	Grade III			Grade II			Grade I		

FIGURE 15-20 Proposed grading system for subglottic stenosis based on endotracheal tube size. ID, inner diameter; NO, no obstruction.

posterior split with costal cartilage grafting and a short stenting period may be required (Figure 15-22). For severe or total stenosis of the high trachea or subglottis, then a partial cricotracheal resection (PCTR) rather than a traditional LTR would be indicated (Figure 15-23).[50]

Stenting and postoperative care depend on the situation. If the patient requires a short period of stenting, the procedure may be accomplished in a single-stage manner and the tracheotomy tube removed at the time of surgery. With PCTR the child may be left intubated nasally after the resection if the child has excellent pulmonary status. For longer periods of stenting, staged LTR may be used with synthetic stents secured into the airway for various periods of time.

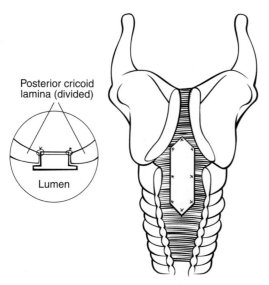

FIGURE 15-22 A posteriorly placed costal cartilage graft maintains excellent expansion of the cricoid and glottis.

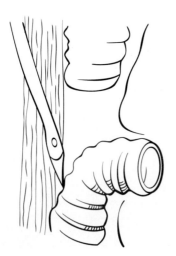

FIGURE 15-23 Partial cricotracheal resection. Dissection of the stenotic trachea away from the esophagus.

Providing a safe and adequate airway while preserving or improving normal laryngeal functions, such as voice and protection during swallowing, is the goal of LTR or PCTR. However, voice and swallowing functions may be impaired by the surgery. An absolute contraindication to LTR or PCTR is gross impairment in the swallow mechanism because the stenosis is actually protecting against chronic aspiration. As our understanding of wound healing, swallowing, and laryngeal biomechanics improves, so will the outcome for LTR and PCTR.

SUCTIONING

Suctioning secretions from the airway or ETT maintains patency, prevents aspiration, assists an ineffective cough, and can be used to obtain specimens for diagnostic purposes. Because suctioning is not a benign procedure, recognizing when it is or is not indicated is important. Some specific indications include auscultating decreased breath sounds, implicating a possible mucous plug, difficulty during mechanical ventilation possibly resulting from ETT occlusion or airway secretions, decreasing oxygen saturation, and the visible presence of secretions.[51] Although there are no absolute contraindications to suctioning, relative contraindications include patients with thrombocytopenia, epiglottitis, an unsecured airway, and labile cardiovascular or respiratory conditions. It is best to suction only when required and to avoid potential complications by repeatedly suctioning without indication.

Procedure

The necessary equipment for suctioning is gathered before initiating the procedure. This includes oxygen, a resuscitation bag and mask, suction catheters, sterile gloves, lavage fluid, a stethoscope, and a suction regulator to set the appropriate vacuum pressure. The vacuum pressure is set at 60 to 80 mm Hg for a neonate and at 80 to 100 mm Hg for a pediatric patient. The appropriate catheter length is determined by measuring the length of the ETT or tracheotomy tube against the suction catheter. The proper length should pass the end of the tube but not touch the carina.[52] Optimally, the catheter should be less than one half the size of the internal diameter of the ETT to avoid total obstruction of the tube.

The patient's breath sounds, heart rate and pattern, respiratory rate and pattern, arterial oxygen saturation, and excessive ventilator pressures are monitored continuously. As with all procedures, an adequate explanation of the process must be provided to the patient and family before the procedure. The patient is ventilated with an FIO_2 of at least 0.1 to 0.2 greater than the oxygen being delivered at the time of the intervention, or an FIO_2 of 1.0 when necessary. The same peak inspiratory pressures and positive end-expiratory pressure as set on the ventilator are used.

To suction, the catheter is moistened with sterile water or saline and, without applying suction, inserted into the airway to the predetermined length, or until resistance is met. It is pulled back 0.5 to 1.5 cm, and intermittent suction is applied, using the thumb port, while withdrawing and rotating the catheter. Hypoxemia and atelectasis are avoided by keeping the duration of suctioning to less than 10 seconds per pass, and less than 5 seconds when applying the vacuum. The patient is oxygenated and ventilated between passes while observing the patient's vital signs on the monitors. Breath sounds are checked to evaluate the need for repeating the procedure. The need for further suctioning is re-evaluated on the basis of the patient's clinical status. Potentially, rotating the head to the right facilitates entry into the left mainstem bronchus, whereas turning the head to the left facilitates entering the right mainstem bronchus.

Although not always required and somewhat controversial,[51-53] instilling a lavage solution may be necessary to remove mucous plugs or thick, tenacious secretions. Lavage or irrigating solutions include wetting agents such as normal saline, detergents such as sodium bicarbonate, and mucolytics such as N-acetylcysteine. For the neonatal patient, small incremental amounts are instilled to a volume of 0.5 to 1 ml. In the older child, 2 to 5 ml is instilled. Lavage is followed by manual ventilation and subsequent suctioning. Bagging the instilled solution into the ETT allows it to disperse throughout the lung fields to help liquefy and loosen secretions. Before instilling any solution, it is important to know the patient's pertinent clinical history. Careful attention must be paid to the amount of solution instilled in the patient who is salt or fluid restricted. Certain types of wetting agents, such as sterile water or hypertonic saline solution, cause mucosal irritation, bronchospasm, and overhydration.

Nasotracheal Suction

Blind nasotracheal suctioning requires that all of the previously mentioned equipment used for ETT suctioning be readily available.[44] The procedure for blind nasotracheal suctioning differs in that an ETT is not present. An infant is placed in the sniffing position, and the head and neck of an older child are slightly hyperextended. The suction catheter is lubricated with water or soluble jelly and placed in the nares. With the clinician facing the patient, the catheter is inserted slightly medial to the septum. The natural curve of the catheter is used as a guide to advance it over the top of the palate. When the catheter reaches the oropharynx, it is advanced into the tracheobronchial tree during inspiration. The catheter is pulled back 0.5 to 1.0 cm once resistance is felt, and suction is intermittently applied as previously described.

Hypoxemia, bradycardia with resultant hypotension, bronchospasm, laryngospasm, airway trauma, hemorrhage, infection, and aspiration are all potential complications of blind nasotracheal suctioning. The most frequent complication in the neonatal patient is hypoxemia and subsequent bradycardia. The incidence of this complication can be reduced by frequent bagging between suctioning, limiting suction time, and increasing the F_{IO_2}. Before the procedure is begun in the premature infant and unstable neonate, careful monitoring of the blood pressure is performed because hypertension associated with the procedure predisposes the patient to intracranial hemorrhage.

Bulb Suction

The bulb syringe is a manually operated device for use in the home or hospital. It is important to be gentle when using it because vigorous suctioning can lead to bleeding and airway damage. The bulb syringe is squeezed gently and held down. It is inserted in the area of mucus, and the pressure on the bulb is released to suction the mucus. Once the syringe is removed from the nasal passage, secretions are removed with a combination of squeezes, and the syringe is cleansed with water and wiped with gauze pads. The bulb syringe should be cleansed thoroughly after each use and allowed to air dry.

Closed Tracheal Suction Systems

As the frequency of suctioning increases, the need for a closed tracheal suction system or special suctioning adapter becomes imperative. These systems are necessary to prevent alveolar collapse associated with the loss of distention from positive end-expiratory pressure during suctioning and to reduce suction-related pulmonary complications. Closed tracheal suction systems are designed to allow minimal disruption with mechanical ventilation, to prevent the loss of positive end-expiratory pressure, and to avoid hypoxia. This system is added to an adapter, as well as an irrigation port, protective sleeve, closed lock, and control valve, and markings on the suction catheter to help determine the approximate depth of suctioning. Additional advantages include less contamination of the sheathed catheter, a decrease in airborne particles being introduced into the ETT, and a faster return to the preoxygenation baseline.

There are some disadvantages with these systems. Bacterial growth can occur if the catheter is not changed in a timely manner, but this is no different than with the ETT itself. Failure to pull the catheter back fully into the correct position can cause damage to or occlude the airway. Other disadvantages may be the possibility of leaving the continuous suction in the "on" position, causing hypoxemia, and causing increased dead space if an inappropriate adapter size is used.

ASSESSMENT QUESTIONS

See Evolve Resources for answers.

1. Which is *not* a reason for intubation?
   A. Pulmonary function
   B. Central apnea
   C. Upper airway obstruction
   D. Pulmonary hygiene
2. What is the age-appropriate ETT for a 1 year old? A 2 year old? A 4 year old? A 6 year old?
   A. 4.0, 4.5, 5, 5.5
   B. 3.5, 5, 5.5, 6
   C. 4.0, 5, 6, 7
   D. 4.5, 5.5, 6.5, 7
3. When would one consider an LMA instead of intubation?
   A. Awake, short-term ventilation
   B. To protect against aspiration
   C. To protect the vocal cords
   D. Unconscious, backup to intubation
4. What are the disadvantages of nasotracheal intubation?
   A. Sinusitis
   B. Pressure necrosis, bleeding
   C. Postextubation atelectasis
   D. All of the above
5. What intubation approach would one use in a larynx that is difficult or impossible to expose with a standard rigid laryngoscope?
   A. LMA
   B. Cricothyroidotomy
   C. Flexible fiberoptic intubation
   D. Tracheotomy
6. Which of the following choices may be used/performed to treat extubation failure?
   A. Reintubation
   B. Steroids
   C. Heliox
   D. Tracheotomy
   E. All of the above
7. The following is *not* an indication for a tracheotomy:
   A. Severe subglottic stenosis
   B. Mild laryngomalacia
   C. Chronic ventilation
   D. Poor pulmonary hygiene
8. Which method of decannulation would be most appropriate for a child with resolved chronic lung disease and stenosis just above and close to the tracheotomy site?
   A. Removal of tracheotomy
   B. Downsizing and capping trial
   C. Partial cricotracheal resection
   D. Single-stage laryngotracheal reconstruction

ASSESSMENT QUESTIONS—cont'd

9. What is the difference between the outside diameter of a tracheotomy tube and an endotracheal tube?
   A. The tracheotomy tube has a larger outside diameter.
   B. They have the same outside diameter.
   C. The endotracheal tube has a much larger outside diameter.
   D. It depends on the manufacturer.
10. Which tracheotomy complication is most likely to be lethal?
    A. Mucous plugging or accidental dislodgement
    B. Bleeding
    C. Distal granulation
    D. Tracheal–esophageal fistula

References

1. International Guidelines for Neonatal Resuscitation: An Excerpt from the Guidelines 2005 for Cardiopulmonary Resuscitation and Emergency Cardiovascular Care: International Consensus on Science, *Pediatrics* 2005.
2. Keep PJ, Manford ML: Endotracheal tube sizes for children, *Anaesthesia* 1974;29:181.
3. Hinkle AJ: A rapid and reliable method of selecting endotracheal tube size in children [abstract], *Anesth Analg* 1988;67:S592.
4. Luten RC et al: Length-based endotracheal tube and emergency equipment selection in pediatrics, *Ann Emerg Med* 1992;21:900.
5. Brunel W et al: Assessment of routine chest roentgenograms and physical examination to confirm endotracheal tube position, *Chest* 1989;96:1043.
6. Berry FA, Yemen TA: Pediatric airway in health and disease, *Pediatr Clin North Am* 1994;41:153.
7. Behar PM, Todd NW: Resuscitation of the newborn with airway compromise, *Clin Perinatol* 1999;26:717.
8. Brain AIJ: The laryngeal mask: a new concept in airway management, *Br J Anaesth* 1983;55:801.
9. Pennant JH, White PF: The laryngeal mask airway: its uses in anesthesiology, *Anesthesiology* 1993;79:144.
10. Mora EU, Weiner GM: Alternative ventilation strategies: laryngeal masks, *Clin Perinatol* 2006;33:99.
11. Lopez-Gil M, Brimacombe J, Alvarez M: Safety and efficacy of the laryngeal mask airway: a prospective study of 1400 children, *Anesthesia* 1996;51:969.
12. Lopez-Gil M et al: Laryngeal mask airway in pediatric practice: a prospective study of skill acquisition by anesthesia residents, *Anesthesiology* 1996;84:807.
13. Zander J, Hazinski MF: Pulmonary disorders: airway obstruction. In Hazinski MF, editor: *Nursing care of the critically ill child*, ed 2, St. Louis: Mosby-Year Book; 1992.
14. Westhorpe RN: The position of the larynx in children and its relationship to the ease of intubation, *Anaesth Intensive Care* 1987;15:384.

15. Sellick BA: Cricoid pressure to control regurgitation of stomach contents during induction of anesthesia, *Lancet* 1961;2:404.
16. Moynihan RJ et al: The effect of cricoid pressure on preventing gastric insufflation in infants and children, *Anesthesiology* 1993;78:652.
17. Tochen ML: Orotracheal intubation in the newborn infant: a method for determining depth of tube insertion, *J Pediatr* 1979;95:1050.
18. Aziz HF, Martin JB, Moore JJ: The pediatric disposable end-tidal carbon dioxide detectors role in endotracheal intubation in newborns, *J Perinatol* 1999;19:110.
19. MacLeod BA et al: Verification of endotracheal tube placement with colorimetric end-tidal CO_2 detection, *Ann Emerg Med* 1991;20:267.
20. Sum-Ping ST, Mehta PA, Anderton JM: A comparative study of methods of detection of esophageal intubation, *Anesth Analg* 1989;69:627.
21. Brown MS: Prevention of accidental extubation in newborns, *Am J Dis Child* 1988;142:1240.
22. Volsko TA, Chatburn RL: Comparison of two methods for securing the endotracheal tube in neonates, *Respir Care* 1997;42:288.
23. Spence K, Barr P: Nasal versus oral intubation for mechanical ventilation of newborn infants, *Cochrane Database Syst Rev* 2000;2:CD000948.
24. Kattwinkel J: *Textbook of neonatal resuscitation*, ed 5, Elk Grove Village, Ill: American Academy of Pediatrics; 2006.
25. Zaickin J: NRP 2006: what you should know, *Neonatal Networks* 2006:25:145.
26. Handler SD: Craniofacial surgery: otolaryngologic concerns, *Int Anesthesiol Clin* 1988;26:61.
27. Hancock PJ, Peterson G: Finger intubation of the trachea in newborns, *Pediatrics* 1992;89:325.
28. Fontarosa PB et al: Sitting oral-tracheal intubation, *Ann Emerg Med* 1988;17:336.
29. Barriot P, Riou B: Retrograde technique for tracheal intubation in trauma patients, *Crit Care Med* 1988;16:712.
30. Neustein S: The Neustein laryngoscope: a new solution to the difficult intubation, *Anesthesiol Rev* 1992;19:54.
31. Verdile VP et al: Nasotracheal intubation using a flexible lighted stylet, *Ann Emerg Med* 1990;19:506.
32. Peak DA, Roy S: Needle cricothyroidotomy revisited, *Pediatr Emerg Care* 1999;15:224.
33. Lee AK, Crutcher JM: Oklahoma notes decline in *Haemophilus influenzae*: invasive *Haemophilus influenzae* disease among children aged < 5 years in Oklahoma, 1990-1997, *J Oklahoma State Med Assoc* 1999;92:276.
34. Kallstrom TJ, Salyer JW: The incidence of accidental extubations in the neonatal intensive care unit, *Respir Care* 1989;34:1006.
35. Markovitz BP, Randolph AG: Corticosteriods for the prevention of reintubation and postextubation stridor in pediatric patients: a meta analysis, *Pediatr Crit Care* 2002;3:223.
36. Duncan PG: Efficacy of helium-oxygen mixtures in the management of severe viral and postintubation croup, *Can Anaesth Soc J* 1979;26:206.
37. Rosin DF et al: Vocal cord paralysis in children, *Laryngoscope* 1990;100:1174.
38. Fearon B, Cotton RT: Surgical correction of subglottic stenosis of the larynx in infants and children: a progress report, *Ann Otol Rhinol Laryngol* 1974;83:428.
39. Wetmore RF, Handler SD, Potsic WP: Pediatric tracheostomy: experience during the past decade, *Ann Otol Rhinol Laryngol* 1982;91:628.
40. Kenna MA, Reilly JS, Stool SE: Tracheotomy in the preterm infant, *Ann Otol Rhinol Laryngol* 1987;96:68.
41. Crysdale WS, Feldman RI, Nabtio K: Tracheotomies: a 10-year experience in 319 children, *Ann Otol Rhinol Laryngol* 1998;97:439.
42. Orringer MK: The effects of tracheostomy tube placement on communication and swallowing, *Respir Care* 1999;44:845.
43. Czervinske MP: Pediatric tracheostomy: clinical perspectives, part I, *AARC Times* 1999;23:31.
44. Panitch HB et al: Guidelines for home care of children with chronic respirator insufficiency, *Pediatr Pulmonol* 1996;21:52.
45. Gray RF, Todd NW, Jacobs IN: Tracheostomy decannulation in children: approaches and techniques, *Laryngoscope* 1998;108:8.
46. Tunkel DE et al: Polysomnography in the evaluation of readiness for decannulation in children, *Arch Otolaryngol Head Neck Surg* 1996;122:721.
47. Myer CM, O'Conner DM, Cotton RT: A proposed laryngotracheal stenosis grading system based on endotracheal tube size, *Ann Otol Rhinol Laryngol* 1994;103:319.
48. Cotton RT, Gray SD, Miller RP: Update of the Cincinnati experience in pediatric laryngotracheal reconstruction, *Laryngoscope* 1989;99:1111.
49. Holinger LD: Treatment of severe subglottic stenosis without tracheotomy, *Ann Otol Laryngol Rhinol* 1982;91:407.
50. Monnier P, Lang F, Savary M: Partial cricotracheal resection for severe pediatric subglottic stenosis: update of the Lausanne experience, *Ann Otol Laryngol Rhinol* 1998;107:961.
51. Ridling DA, Martin LD, Bratton SL: Endotracheal suctioning with or without instillation of isotonic sodium chloride solution in critically ill children, *Am J Crit Care* 2003;12:212.
52. Hagler DA, Traver GA: Endotrsacheal saline and suction catheters: sources of lower airway contamination, *Am J Crit Care* 1994;3:444.
53. Raymond SJ: Normal saline instillation before suctioning: helpful or harmful? A review of the literature, *Am J Crit Care* 1995;4:267.

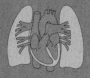

Chapter **16**

Surfactant Replacement Therapy

SANTINA A. ZANELLI ● DAVID KAUFMAN

OUTLINE

LEARNING OBJECTIVES

After reading this chapter the reader will be able to:
- Explain how surfactant affects surface tension and improves lung function
- Identify disease processes associated with surfactant deficiency, dysfunction, or inactivation
- Discuss the delivery, benefits, and adverse effects of surfactant replacement

The successful introduction of surfactant therapy into clinical care is one of the best examples of how discoveries in the laboratory can be directly translated into improved patient care. Basic science research linked relative or total lack of surfactant secondary to decreased production and/or inactivation to respiratory distress syndrome (RDS) in preterm infants. The phenomenal success of surfactant replacement in RDS has prompted investigation into the possible role of surfactant therapy in other types of acute lung injury, including acute RDS (ARDS).[1,2] It is clear that qualitative and quantitative surfactant abnormalities are present in many non-RDS types of acute lung injury and that the expanding role of surfactant replacement must be explored.

THE DISCOVERY OF SURFACTANT

The seeds were sown in the early nineteenth century with the observations of Pierre Simon Laplace and Thomas Young.[3] In his theory of capillary action he described the relationship of transsurface pressure and surface tension at a gas–fluid interface in a sphere as $P = 2 \times ST/R$ (where P is the transsurface or distending pressure, ST is surface tension, and R is the radius of the sphere). More than a century later, in 1929, the Swedish physiologist Kurt von Neergaard,[4] while studying respiratory mechanics, discovered that the retractile force of the lung was dependent on the surface tension

246

in the alveoli (Figure 16-1). Twenty years later, Macklin[5] postulated the existence of a "mucoprotein" lining in the lung that had the surface tension–lowering properties observed by von Neergaard. In the 1950s, Mead and co-workers[6] at the Harvard School of Public Health discovered that surface forces at the lung's air–liquid interface contributed to elastic recoil, especially at large lung volumes. Simultaneously, Clements[7] discovered the role of the alveolar lining layer in mediating surface tension changes with area, thereby stabilizing air-filled spaces at low lung volumes and augmenting elastic recoil at large lung volumes. He named the material "pulmonary surfactant" and established its role as an antiatelectasis factor. In 1955, Pattle[8] discovered that bubbles expressed from the lungs of fetal guinea pigs did not have the stability of those found in term mammalian lungs, stating that the immature lung of the premature baby may have increased surface forces. In 1959, Avery and Mead[9] noted from autopsies that the lungs of infants who died of hyaline membrane disease never had foam in their airways. They lacked foam because they lacked surfactant and therefore the capacity to reduce surface tension when surface area is reduced during exhalation. These findings identified surfactant deficiency as the cause of RDS. Finally, in 1980, Fujiwara and colleagues reported success in producing and using surfactant replacement for preterm infants with RDS.[10] The release of surfactant for clinical use in the United States by the U.S. Food and Drug Administration in 1990 resulted in a measurable reduction in perinatal mortality and morbidity. The use of exogenous surfactants for treatment of lung injury beyond the neonatal period is only now being studied but may offer similar promise.[11-13]

SURFACTANT PHYSIOLOGY

Function

A surfactant is any molecule that localizes on aqueous surfaces. In the lung, alveolar surfaces are lined by a layer of fluid, called *surfactant,* that creates an air–liquid interface and reduces surface tension. Surface tension is created by the attraction of water molecules to one another. This is best illustrated by observing that water placed on a flat surface coalesces to form a droplet. During respiration, carbon dioxide and water are exhaled at the surface of the alveoli, creating a liquid interface with inhaled air. As indicated by the Laplace law, this attraction would lead to the collapse of alveoli as each alveolus becomes smaller. However, in the presence of surfactant, water molecules are pushed apart in the alveolus and prevent alveolar collapse during exhalation. Surface tension is reduced in proportion to the number of surfactant molecules per surface area. Surfactant displaces water from the air–liquid surface and lowers the surface tension from 75 to 25 dyn/cm (during inflation).[14]

The lung can be thought of as a large number of interconnected bubbles that form the interface between the gaseous environment and the wet alveolar surface. If this interface were without surfactant, two consequences would ensue: (1) every breath would take a considerable amount of pressure to expand the lung, comparable to the 80 to 90 cm H_2O of pressure required for a newborn's first breath, and (2) the lung would rapidly collapse during exhalation.

Pulmonary surfactant not only lowers surface tension at all lung volumes but, more importantly, also decreases surface tension as alveolar surface decreases (Figure 16-2). If surface tension did not decrease with decreasing lung volume, alveoli of different sizes would require different distending pressures. Small alveoli would empty into large ones and there would be an overall tendency for the lung to coalesce into a smaller number of large alveoli as lung volume diminished. This would significantly decrease the surface area for gas exchange as well. Surfactant not only decreases surface tension but also reduces it to a greater degree at low lung volume and counteracts the effect of decreasing alveolar size.

Functionally, surfactant increases lung compliance, promotes homogeneous gas distribution during inhalation, and allows a residual volume of gas to be evenly distributed throughout the lung during exhalation; that is, it maintains functional residual capacity. In the absence of surfactant, distribution of ventilation

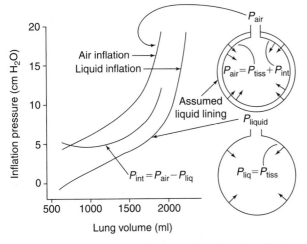

FIGURE 16-1 A, Pressure–volume relationship of air-filled versus liquid-filled lung from von Neergaard's original data (1929). **B,** The difference in recoil attributed to a liquid–air interface (i.e., "bubble lining") that is eliminated by a liquid-only interface. P, Pressure; tiss, tissue; int, air–liquid interface; liq, liquid.

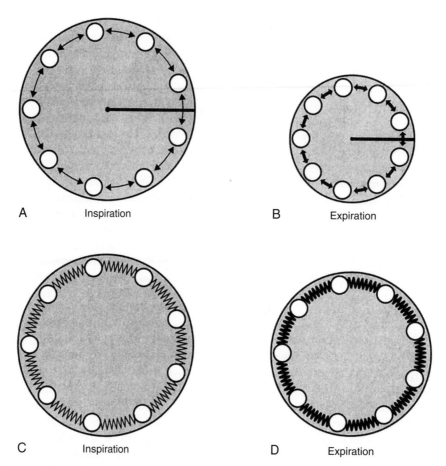

FIGURE 16-2 A, Alveolar surface tension is a manifestation of the strong attraction between molecules that are aligned on the surface of the alveoli. **B,** During expiration, when the alveolar radius is smaller, attraction between the molecules is stronger and there is a greater tendency to collapse. **C,** When surfactant is present, it spreads over the alveolus and dilutes the molecules. **D,** During expiration, the surfactant is compressed and the alveolar surface tension is lowered. This stabilizes the alveoli and prevents collapse of those with smaller radii.

Box 16-1	Surfactant Function

- Prevents collapse of lung during deflation (expiration)
- Lessens work of breathing (oxygen consumption)
- Optimizes surface area for gas exchange and ventilation–perfusion matching
- Optimizes lung compliance (high at low lung volumes and low at high lung volumes)
- Protects the lung epithelium and facilitates clearance of foreign material
- Prevents capillary leakage of fluid into alveoli
- Defends against microorganisms (infection)

becomes uneven, the lungs become stiff, and atelectasis ensues during exhalation. The result is increased work of breathing, hypoxia, and respiratory failure, the clinical picture exemplified by preterm infants with RDS. Surfactant functions are summarized in Box 16-1.

Surfactant Metabolism and Composition

Surfactant is produced by type II alveolar epithelial cells (pneumatocytes) in the lung (Figure 16-3). After synthesis, the surfactant components are packaged in the form of lamellar bodies and secreted into the fluid layer lining the alveoli in response to a variety of stimuli including mechanical stretch (Figure 16-4). After secretion into the alveolar space, surfactant is transformed into tubular myelin, a highly organized lipid-rich monolayer responsible for reducing surface tension. The half-time for turnover of human surfactant is not known, but in animals such as rats and rabbits it is 5 to 10 hours.[15] Secretion and clearance are balanced, with 90% of the surfactant being recycled by the type II pneumatocytes. Studies using labeled surfactant introduced into the airways have shown the majority being taken up directly

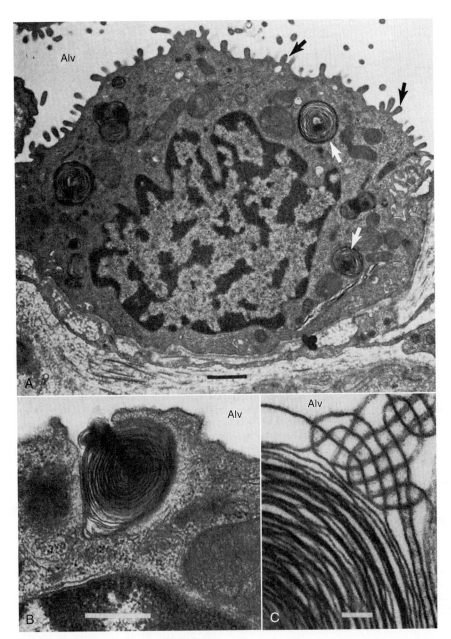

FIGURE 16-3 **A,** Type II cell from a human lung, showing characteristic lamellar inclusion bodies *(open arrows)* within the cell, which are the storage sites of intracellular surfactant. Microvilli *(solid arrows)* are projecting into the alveolus (Alv). **B,** Beginning exocytosis of a lamellar body into the alveolar space of a human lung. **C,** Secreted lamellar body and newly formed tubular myelin (appearing as a lattice) in the alveolar liquid in a fetal rat lung. Membrane continuities between outer lamellar bodies and adjacent tubular myelin provide evidence of intraalveolar tubular myelin formation.

by the pneumatocytes and being repackaged in lamellar bodies and eventually resecreted.[16] The remaining 10% are cleared by alveolar macrophages.

Surfactant composition is fairly constant among mammalian species. Surfactant is composed mainly of lipids (phospholipids, neutral lipids, and cholesterol; >90%), with only approximately 5% to 10% proteins (Table 16-1). Phosphatidylcholine (PC) is the most

abundant phospholipid (85%) and is mostly saturated (40% to 55%) in the form of dipalmitoyl phosphatidylcholine (DPPC), the most important surfactant component in reducing surface tension. DPPC consists of two molecules of palmitic acid and one molecule of phosphatidylcholine attached to a glycerol backbone. DPPC has a hydrophobic end (fatty acids) and a hydrophilic end (nitrogenous base) and aligns itself in the air–liquid

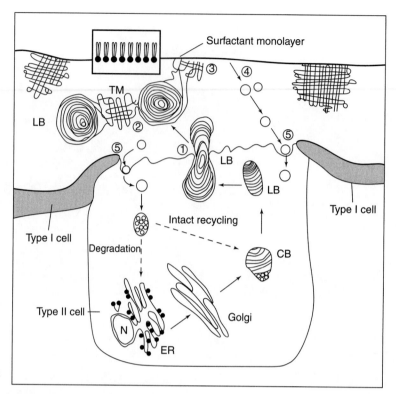

FIGURE 16-4 Schematic diagram of surfactant metabolism. *1,* secretion of LB; *2,* conversion of LB into TM; *3,* generation of monolayer from TM material; *4,* formation of small aggregate material from monolayer; *5,* reuptake of surfactant material. In general, *solid arrows* indicate accepted pathways. Probable pathways are indicated by *dashed arrows*. N, nucleus; ER, endoplasmic reticulum; CB, composite body; LB, lamellar body; TM, tubular myelin.

TABLE 16-1	
Components of Pulmonary Surfactant	
Component	**Amount (%)**
Lipids	90-95
Phospholipids	
Saturated phosphatidylcholine	45
Unsaturated phosphatidylcholine	20
Phosphatidylglycerol	8
Other phospholipids	5
Neutral lipids	10
Other lipids	2
Proteins	5-10
Loosely associated (mainly serum)	0-5
Surfactant apoproteins	
Hydrophilic proteins, SP-A, SP-D*	2-4
Hydrophobic proteins, SP-B, SP-C*	1-2

SP-A, SP-B, SP-C, SP-D, surfactant proteins A, B, C, and D.
*Data from Young SL et al: Pulmonary surfactant lipid production in oxygen-exposed rat lungs, *Lab Invest* 1982;46:570.
Modified from Rooney SA: The surfactant system and lung phospholipid biochemistry, *Am Rev Respir Dis* 1985;131:439.

interface with the hydrophobic end toward the gas phase and the hydrophilic end toward the liquid phase (Figure 16-5). This configuration aligns negative charges in the gas phase and positive charges in the liquid phase, allowing like charges to repel each other, displacing water, and creating the pressure required to keep alveoli expanded during expiration. This alignment of DPPC is critical to the ability of surfactant to lower surface tension, and surfactant proteins B and C appear vital for this process. If proper alignment does not occur, positive and negative ends of DPPC attract and cause surfactant to clump together, rendering it ineffective and actually resulting in atelectasis.

Surfactant protein (SP)-A, SP-B, SP-C, and SP-D are the known proteins associated with surfactant.[12,17] SP-A and SP-D are hydrophilic (water soluble) and SP-B and SP-C are hydrophobic (lipid soluble and positively charged).

SP-A is a calcium-dependent collectin (*coll*agen-like *lectin*). Collectins bind to the surface of microorganisms via polysaccharides, phospholipids and glycolipids-dependent interactions and lead to aggregation, opsonization, and clearance of the organisms by alveolar macrophages in the lung. SP-A is the most abundant of the surfactant-associated proteins. It is thought to be important in the regulation of surfactant metabolism, as well as in tubular myelin formation.[18] The most important role of SP-A, however, is in innate host

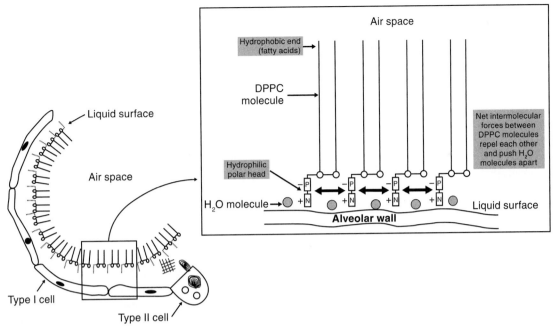

FIGURE 16-5 A cross-section of an alveolus wall is shown. In the presence of surfactant protein B (not shown), dipalmitoylphosphatidylcholine (DPPC) aligns in the air–liquid interface with the hydrophobic end toward the gas phase (air space) and hydrophilic end toward the liquid phase (liquid surface). Strong molecular interactions occur between the polar heads of the hydrophobic end. Note that the polar head has a positive charge associated with its nitrogenous base (N) and a negative charge associated with its phosphate group (P). This alignment creates electrostatic forces of repulsion, pushing water molecules apart, preventing atelectasis, and holding the airway open during exhalation.

defense of the lung. SP-A functions as an opsonin for bacteria, fungi, and viruses. In SP-A–deficient mice tubular myelin is absent, but surfactant processing and function are intact. Despite relatively normal lung function, SP-A–deficient mice are highly susceptible to infections.

SP-D is also a collectin and enhances the binding, phagocytosis, and killing of microbes by alveolar macrophages. In addition, SP-D has a role in the suppression of proinflammatory responses. Lack of SP-D in transgenic mice leads to emphysema, macrophage activation, accumulation of oxygen reactive species, and increased surfactant alveolar pools. So, SP-D also plays a key role in surfactant homeostasis. Polymorphisms of the human genes for SP-A and SP-D have been documented and result in increased susceptibility to infections with respiratory syncytial virus and *Mycobacterium tuberculosis*.

SP-B is a membrane-associated protein that binds to the surface of lipid bilayers. SP-B, as discussed previously, is critical for alignment of surfactant at the air–liquid interface and for the formation of surfactant storage lamellar bodies in type II cells. SP-B is the only surfactant protein that humans cannot live without. SP-B protein deficiency is fatal in infancy without lung transplantation.

SP-C is necessary for the stability of the surfactant phospholipid film and for stability during dynamic compression in the respiratory cycle.[19] SP-C–deficient mice develop interstitial lung disease with emphysema, epithelial cell dysplasia, and inflammation. Infants with SP-C deficiency have RDS and pulmonary fibrosis. SP-C is not required for the formation of lamellar bodies or tubular myelin.

There are other alveolar proteins that are important in host defense: SP-D and SP-A as mentioned, fibronectin, lysozyme, antiproteases, immunoglobulins (IgA), defensins, mucins, and Clara cell proteins. Excluding nonsurfactant proteins from the alveolus is critical to surfactant function and processing as surfactant homeostasis may be disrupted by blood proteins, albumin, fibrin, edema, as well as other substances.

Hormonal Effects on Surfactant Production

Antenatal steroids have been extensively studied and have been shown to decrease RDS in infants between 24 and 34 weeks of gestation. There is no increased infection risk with rupture of membranes, prolonged rupture of membranes, or chorioamnionitis. A single course (two doses 24 h apart) is recommended at this time, as multiple courses have not demonstrated any benefit and may be associated with poorer outcomes.[20,21]

There is an increase in RNA within 2 hours of the first dose and an increase in protein secretion within 12 hours.[22] The full effect on surfactant production is present by 48 hours after the first dose. Antenatal steroid use in infants with less than 24 weeks of gestation has not been studied prospectively, but its use may be beneficial if resuscitation is planned.

Thyroid hormones, in addition to other hormones, are also important for lung development. Because thyroid hormones do not cross the placenta several investigators examined antenatal thyrotropin-releasing hormone for the prevention of RDS in preterm infants. Unfortunately, no benefit was demonstrated in multicenter clinical trials.[23,24]

Fetal Lung Maturity Testing

Measurement of phospholipids in the amniotic fluid can be used to determine fetal lung maturity, as phosphatidylglycerol (PG) and phosphatidylcholine (lecithin) increase while sphingomyelin decreases during gestation. Available tests include quantification of phospholipids present in the amniotic fluid as well as measurement of surfactant characteristics, and function and number of lamellar bodies (Table 16-2).[25] The first test used for this purpose was based on the lecithin-to-sphingomyelin ratio. This has been replaced by PG measurement in the amniotic fluid. PG is produced by type II pneumatocytes and is nearly undetectable until 35 weeks of gestation. Interestingly, PG is not required for surfactant function but correlates with pulmonary maturity. PG measurement is a more accurate test than previously used lecithin-to-sphingomyelin ratios. PG is now the basis of a rapid and inexpensive slide agglutination test (Amniostat-FLM-PG; Irvine Scientific, Santa Ana, Calif) with 90% sensitivity. PG can be used for both amniotic fluid and vaginal pool samples in infants with premature rupture of membranes. False positives can occur if the samples are contaminated by bacteria containing PG in their cell wall. Another rapid and widely used test is TDx-FLM (Abbott Diagnostics, Abbott Park, Ill). It detects the presence of phospholipids per gram of albumin, using a fluorescent dye. Specific clinical settings need to be considered, as gestationnal diabetes delays maturation and PG is the preferred test. Fetal lung maturity may be accelerated in some but not all pregnancies with pregnancy-induced hypertension, intrauterine growth restriction, and in utero exposure to maternal smoking and cocaine.

TABLE 16-2

Fetal Lung Maturity Testing*

Quantification of Surfactant Components	Mature	Transitional	Immature
Phospholipid measurement			
Lecithin-to-sphingomyelin ratio	>2.0	1.5-2.0	<1.5
Phosphatidylglycerol	Present	Trace	Absent
Desaturated phosphatidylcholine	>70	50-70	<50
Fluorescence detection	>50,000	15,000-70,000	<15,000
Microviscometer assay			
TDx-FLM assay (mg/g albumin)			
Lamellar bodies			
Lamellar body count			
Surfactant characteristics			
Surfactant function			
Foam stability index	>48%	47%	<47%
Shake test			
Tap test			
Amniotic fluid turbidity			
Optical density			
Visual inspection			

From Geary CA, Whitsett JA: Amniotic fluid markers of fetal lung maturity. In Spitzer AR, editor: *Intensive care of the fetus and neonate*, ed 2, St. Louis: Elsevier Mosby; 2005. pp 122-132.

TDx-FLM, Fetal lung maturity test using a TDx analyzer (Abbott Diagnostics, Abbott Park, Ill).

*Includes testing values for the five most common tests.

SURFACTANT DYSFUNCTION IN ACUTE LUNG INJURY

Abnormalities in surfactant (quantity or pool size, function, composition, and metabolism), destruction and/or inactivation of surfactant, and direct type II cell damage have been described in ARDS and other types of acute lung injury (Box 16-2).[26]

Altered Surfactant Quantity

The evidence related to altered surfactant pool size in acute lung injury is variable. Decreases, increases, and no changes in pool size have all been reported.[27-30] This confusion reflects the difficulty in quantifying surfactant material obtained from bronchoalveolar lavage. Different clinical factors or types of lung injury may affect the lung and surfactant function differently. For example, prolonged exposure to 85% oxygen results in type II alveolar cell hyperplasia and increased surfactant secretion, whereas 100% exposure decreases alveolar cell numbers and surfactant secretion.[31,32] Direct type II cell injury or necrosis will result in a decreased surfactant pool. At present, no firm conclusions can be drawn regarding the effects of acute lung injury on the quantity of surfactant.

Altered Surfactant Composition

A consistent finding in studies of acute lung injury is that alterations in the composition of surfactant

Box 16-2	Diseases That Affect Surfactant	
Surfactant Deficiency	**Surfactant Inactivation or Destruction**	
Respiratory distress syndrome	Aspiration syndromes	
SP-B deficiency	• Meconium	
SP-C deficiency	• Blood	
	• Amniotic fluid	
	Pulmonary hemorrhage	
	Infections	
	• Pneumonia	
	• Respiratory syncytial virus	
	• Sepsis	
	Pulmonary diseases	
	• Asthma	
	• Cystic fibrosis	
	Shock	
	Near drowning	
	Smoke inhalation	
	Transfusions	
	Trauma	
	Lung transplantation	

SP-B, Surfactant protein B; SP-C, surfactant protein C.

occur. These findings include a decrease in surfactant-associated proteins in patients with ARDS and decreases in the quantities of phosphatidylcholine and phosphatidylglycerol along with an increase in sphingomyelin and other phospholipids.[29,33] Furthermore, these abnormalities appear to reverse with recovery from acute lung injury.[34] The relationship of these abnormalities in surfactant composition to lung dysfunction is unknown, but surfactant isolated from animal models of lung injury has abnormal surface activity in vitro.[35,36]

Altered Surfactant Metabolism

Studies indicate that surfactant metabolism may be altered in acute lung injury. Animals injured by hyperoxia have decreased incorporation of surfactant precursors into lung tissue that reverses with recovery.[37] Other animal models show more rapid conversion of large to small surfactant forms that have poor surface tension–lowering properties. Bronchoalveolar lavage specimens from patients with ARDS also support evidence of altered surfactant metabolism, showing increased levels of proteases and alterations in the density profiles of surfactant.[38]

Surfactant Inactivation

Inactivation by proteins is the most common surfactant abnormality seen in acute lung injury. These proteins competitively displace surfactant phospholipid from the alveolar monolayer and are less surface-active

molecules than surfactant; this results in a decreased capacity to reduce surface tension.

Many etiologies are associated with increased capillary permeability leading to pulmonary edema and resulting in surfactant inactivation. Albumin, hemoglobin, fibrin, complement, blood, meconium, and other proteins may gain access to the alveolar space secondary to alveolar–capillary membrane damage and have been shown in vitro to diminish the surface tension–reducing properties of surfactant.[38-40] Proteins compete with surfactant for the air–fluid interface and interfere with monolayer formation.[41] Several blood components are strong inactivators of surfactant including hemoglobin, fibrin, fibrinogen, red blood cell membrane lipids, immunoglobulins, and plasma proteins. Similarly, several substances in meconium inactivate or alter surfactant function including proteolytic enzymes, free fatty acids, phospholipases, bile salts, lanugo, squamous cells, bilirubin, steroid compounds, cholesterol, and triglycerides.[11] Regardless of the etiology, surfactant inactivation leads to diminished lung compliance, increased intrapulmonary shunting, and atelectasis characteristic of ARDS (Figure 16-6).[42]

CLINICAL APPLICATIONS AND REPLACEMENT

The typical clinical presentation of surfactant deficiency is summarized in Table 16-3. At present, exogenous surfactant administration is most commonly used for prophylaxis or treatment of preterm infants with RDS. It is also increasingly used in neonates as well as pediatric and adult patients with diseases associated with or leading to surfactant inactivation.

Respiratory Distress Syndrome
Incidence

Typically, RDS affects premature infants of less than 35 weeks gestation. Its incidence increases with lower gestational ages. RDS affects 86% of infants weighing 501 to 750 g at birth, 79% of infants weighing 751 to 1000 g, 48% of infants at 1000 to 1250 g, and 27% between 1251 and 1500 g.[43] Typical chest radiographs of a premature infant with RDS before and after surfactant administration as well as typical pathology findings in RDS are presented in Figure 16-7.

Treatment

Early experimental animal studies with administration of phospholipid mixtures showed some effect, but more dramatic and sustained improvements in oxygenation could be demonstrated only with natural surfactant complexes, harvested from the lavage of adult rabbit lungs, and later obtained from cows, pigs,

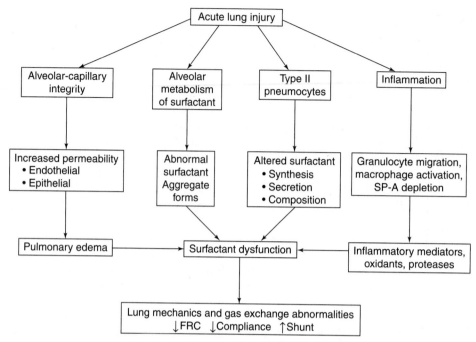

FIGURE 16-6 Four pathways that contribute to surfactant dysfunction during acute lung injury. FRC, functional residual capacity; SP-A, surfactant protein A.

TABLE 16-3

Clinical Presentation of Surfactant Deficiency RDS and ARDS

Pathophysiology	Laboratory Changes	Physical Examination	Radiographic Changes
Atelectasis ↓ FRC Ventilation–perfusion mismatch	↓ Po_2 ↑ Carbon dioxide Metabolic acidosis	Lung • Tachypnea • Apnea • Nasal flaring • Retractions • Grunting Auscultation • ↓ Breath sounds • Poor air entry Cardiovascular • Cyanosis (oxygen requirement) • Pale • Poor perfusion	Diffuse reticular granular pattern Air bronchograms Atelectasis

ARDS, Acute respiratory distress syndrome; FRC, functional residual capacity; Po_2, oxygen pressure; RDS, respiratory distress syndrome.

and human amniotic fluid. Bioactivity of the synthetic preparations was improved with the addition of alcohols such as hexadecanol as well as tyloxapol (a formaldehyde polymer) to enhance dispersion and spread in the aqueous phase.

The first human trial in 1980 by Fujiwara and colleagues showed that natural animal-derived surfactant was effective in treating 10 premature infants with RDS.[44] The investigators instilled 3 to 5 ml of surfactant (from minced bovine extract and containing DPPC) directly to the trachea and enhanced distribution by changing the position of the infant. They demonstrated a prompt increase in oxygenation after one dose that was sustained for 2 to 3 days in some infants. This represented a marked improvement when compared with results obtained with synthetic DPPC.

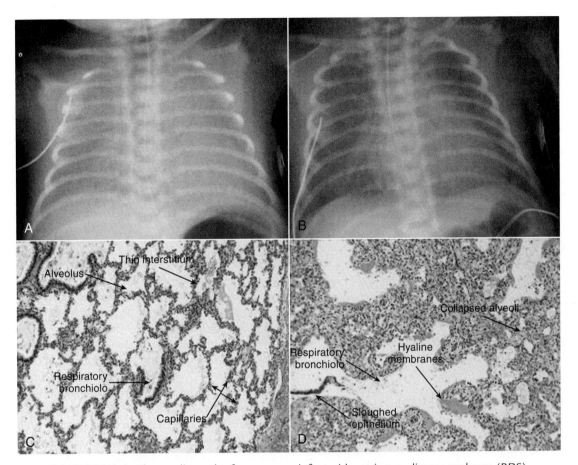

FIGURE 16-7 A, Chest radiograph of a premature infant with respiratory distress syndrome (RDS) demonstrating diffuse reticulogranular pattern (ground-glass appearance), air bronchograms, and low lung volume. **B,** Chest radiograph of the same premature infant after surfactant administration, demonstrating improved lung volumes. **C,** Photomicrograph of normal alveoli, demonstrating normal microscopic structure of the lung of a newborn infant. Clear areas are the air-containing expanded alveoli. The colored structures that form a honeycomb lattice are the walls that line the alveolar space. **D,** Microscopic structure of the lung from a premature infant who died of RDS. The normal honeycomb lattice is collapsed (atelectasis), the alveolar walls are adherent to each other, and the lung is almost airless. Those air-containing spaces (clear areas) that do remain are lined by a pink-staining layer of inflammatory protein termed the hyaline membrane. Photos courtesy of Drs. David Kaufman and Robin LeGallo.

Large controlled trials have since established that surfactant preparations greatly reduce mortality in preterm infants. Surfactant replacement for prophylaxis or treatment of RDS has reduced the risk of pneumothorax by 30% to 65% and death by about 40%.[45] Early analysis showed a possible decrease in bronchopulmonary dysplasia, but it is now accepted by experts in the field that surfactants do not reduce the overall incidence of chronic lung disease or bronchopulmonary dysplasia.[2] Surfactant administration is also not associated with significant changes in intraventricular hemorrhage (IVH), patent ductus arteriosus (PDA), or retinopathy of prematurity. However in one study, infants weighing more than 1250 g had a lower incidence of IVH and PDA.[46]

Two clinical strategies are currently used: (1) prophylaxis within 30 minutes of birth in small premature infants and (2) rescue treatment a few hours after birth in infants with RDS. Prophylactic surfactant administration grew out of animal data demonstrating decreased epithelial damage and pulmonary edema when surfactant is given in the first 15 minutes of life.[47]

Prophylaxis

Prophylactic surfactant is administered after a period of stabilization in the first 15 minutes of life, compared with 1.5 to 7.4 hours in the rescue group. The use of prophylactic surfactant compared with rescue treatment has been shown to decrease the risk for mortality, pneumothorax, and pulmonary interstitial emphysema.

Studies also demonstrated decreased neonatal mortality as well as a trend toward decreased IVH.[2] Although the evidence is strong for the use of prophylactic surfactant, the majority of studies enrolled infants with less than 30 weeks of gestation. Therefore, there is some debate as to whether a lower threshold for prophylaxis (e.g., <750 g, <1000 g, or <28 to 29 weeks gestation) would define a higher risk group and avoid unnecessary prophylaxis of more mature infants. In addition, in these studies lower rates of antenatal steroid use were reported and this may have affected the rates of RDS, air leak, IVH, and mortality. The discussion also involves whether immediate stabilization with nasal continuous positive airway pressure (NCPAP) in the delivery room may have similar favorable outcomes in high-risk preterm infants.[48,49] Data, however, demonstrated poorer outcomes (including severe RDS, PDA, IVH, and mortality) with initial NCPAP in infants less than 750 g or with less than 26 weeks gestation, or needing positive pressure ventilation in the delivery room. Therefore, prophylactic surfactant should be strongly considered in these infants.[50] Strategies for surfactant administration are summarized in Table 16-4.

Rescue and Multiple Treatments

In patients to whom prophylactic surfactant is not given or for redosing of surfactant, clinical signs and symptoms of RDS can be used to determine the need for surfactant administration (see Table 16-3). Specific criteria for surfactant administration are still an area of discussion. A few studies have demonstrated some short-term, but not long-term, benefits with retreatment at a low threshold (still intubated, mean airway pressure > 6 cm H_2O, with a fraction of inspired oxygen [FIO_2] > 0.030), versus high threshold (still intubated, mean airway pressure > 7 cm H_2O and FIO_2 > 0.040) or an increase in FIO_2 up to 0.10.[51] Early rescue compared with late rescue strategies have demonstrated decreased mortality and decreased incidence of pneumothorax.[52] In rescue surfactant strategies, infants with signs and symptoms of RDS despite NCPAP support are given surfactant. They then may be extubated immediately to NCPAP or maintained on mechanical ventilation and weaned to extubational settings.

There has been renewed study of the benefits early NCPAP may have in the management of RDS and timing of surfactant delivery. One study evaluated NCPAP success as first-line therapy in very low birth weight infants at risk for RDS. In this study, a late rescue approach was used and surfactant was administered if the FIO_2 was more than 0.60 in order to maintain oxygen saturations at or above 90%.[50] This approach examined the use of NCPAP immediately in the delivery room and was not powered to evaluate the effect on mortality and air leak compared

with prophylactic or early rescue surfactant. There were poorer outcomes (severe RDS, mortality, PDA, and IVH) in infants less than 750 g, less than 26 weeks of gestation, and/or needing positive pressure ventilation in the delivery room. However, this may be an appropriate strategy for more mature and larger infants.

To further investigate this approach of using NCPAP in those extremely preterm infants not requiring intubation at birth, Morley and co-workers randomized infants born at 25 to 28 weeks of gestation, who were not intubated at 5 minutes of life, to either NCPAP or intubation with ventilation.[53] A distending pressure of 8 cm H_2O was used in the NCPAP group, which is higher than in some centers. The authors' rationale was that distending pressure is important for maintaining functional residual capacity and for improving lung compliance and oxygenation, and 8 cm H_2O had been shown to be more effective than a lower pressure.[54] In the NCPAP group 46% required later intubation, with a rate of 55% for infants born at 25 or 26 weeks of gestation and 40% for those born at 27 or 28 weeks of gestation. The total days requiring intubation and ventilation were less in the NCPAP group ($P < 0.001$). The need for surfactant use was 50% less in the NCPAP group (38% vs. 77%; $P < 0.001$). Pneumothorax was more common in the NCPAP group (9.1% vs. 3%; $P < 0.001$), with 98% of those infants needing intubation, but there was no increase in intracranial hemorrhage. There was no difference in oxygen requirement at 36 weeks of gestational age, mortality, or length of hospitalization. This approach is safe and the optimal amount of NCPAP needs further investigation.[55,56]

Natural versus Synthetic Preparations

At present there are several different types of exogenous commercial surfactants[57,58] (Table 16-5): minced bovine lung lipid extracts enriched with synthetic lipids (Survanta [Abbott Nutrition, Columbus, Ohio] and Surfacten [Mitsubishi Tanabe Pharma, Osaka, Japan]), bovine lung lavage lipid extracts (Infasurf [Forest Pharmaceuticals, St. Louis, Mo] and Alveofact [Boehringer Ingelheim, Ingelheim, Germany]), minced porcine lung enriched by chromatography (Curosurf; Chiesi Farmaceutici, Parma, Italy), and a mixture of synthetic lipids (Exosurf [GlaxoSmithKline, London, UK]). The bovine surfactants contain SP-B and SP-C, but not SP-A. Infasurf contains much more SP-B and SP-C than does Survanta. The synthetic surfactants contain no proteins. Compared with older synthetic surfactants, natural surfactants have a more rapid onset of action, allow the fraction of inspired oxygen to be reduced faster, and decrease the incidence of pneumothorax as well as mortality. Clinical trials comparing different natural surfactants have not clearly demonstrated

---

TABLE 16-4

Surfactant Delivery

	Comments	Studies
Timing		
Prophylaxis	Surfactant given in first minutes of life (<15 min), before symptoms appear	↓ PTX and mortality in infants < 31 wk[116]
Treatment	At time of clinical signs and symptoms	↓ PTX and mortality[2]
Subsequent dosing	Required if inactivation or insufficient delivery of surfactant	Surfactant may be redosed in the first 48 h after presentation
		Usually one or two doses is sufficient. Third and fourth doses did not improve outcomes[117]
Administration		
Adapter	ETT with side adapter *or* Y-adapter attached to ETT	Minimizes desaturation due to disconnection from positive pressure ventilation or the ventilator for administration
Delivery	Bolus intratracheal administration	• Bolus administration → homogeneous distribution
		• Slow infusion → nonhomogeneous distribution pattern in animals
		• Aerosolization → not effective; only small amounts of aerosolized surfactant are delivered to the lung[118]
Dose	75-100 mg/kg	• 75-100 mg/kg to overcome destruction by macrophages and inhibition by plasma proteins.
		• 100 and 120 mg/kg produced better results than 50 and 60 mg/kg[119,120]
		• Equal efficacy of 100 and 200 mg/kg of porcine surfactant[121,122]
Surfactant products and dose (phospholipid/dose)	Intratracheal administration	• Calfactant (Infasurf): 3 cc/kg (105 mg) q6h up to four doses
		• Poractant (Curosurf): 2.5 cc/kg (200 mg), then 1.25 cc/kg (100 mg) q12h
		• Beractant (Survanta): 4 cc/kg (100) q6h up to four doses
Aliquots	To enhance delivery distribution in the lung	No difference if dose is divided into two or four aliquots[123]
Positioning	To enhance delivery distribution in the lung	Although recommended, it is not necessary to move the infant into different positions during instillation because exogenous surfactant has remarkable spreading properties
Monitoring		
	Oxygenation	• Side effects include the following: cyanosis, bradycardia, reflux of surfactant into the ETT, and airway obstruction
		• Surfactant delivery should be paused until vital signs recover and ETT clears of visible surfactant. Infant may need to be repositioned prone and positive pressure ventilation increased for lung inflation. Rate of surfactant bolus delivery may need to be slower
	Heart rate	
	Presence of surfactant in the ETT	

ETT, Endotracheal tube; PTX, pneumothorax.

---

one product to be better than another.[2] A new generation of synthetic surfactants incorporating genetically engineered SP-B or SP-C protein equivalent (Pumactant [Zofac; airPharma, Overland Park, Kans] and Surfaxin [lucinactant; Discovery Laboratories, Warrington, Pa], respectively) are currently being studied. In trials, lucinactant appears to offer a level of efficacy similar to that of natural surfactants.[1,59-61]

Nonresponders

Although most infants respond favorably to treatment, about 20% of infants thought to have RDS have little or no response. These infants may have other disease processes such as pneumonia, pulmonary hypoplasia, or congenital heart disease. Full-term infants with RDS, surfactant nonresponders, and infants who cannot be extubated in the first weeks of life because of their respiratory

TABLE 16-5

Types of Surfactant

Surfactant Type: Generic (Trade Name)	COMPOSITION		Advantages	Disadvantages
	% DPPC	Protein		
Synthetic Surfactants				
Colfosceril (Exosurf)	84.5	None	• No risk of disease transmission	• Lower resistance to inactivation
Pumactant (ALEC)	70	None	• Less immunological rejection	• Lacks surface-active apoproteins
			• Inexpensive	• Less rapid improvement in gas exchange
			• Completely defined formulation	
Lucinactant (Surfaxin)	70	Sinapultide (KL-4) = SP-B equivalent		Not yet available
rSP-C (Venticute)	67	rSP-C		
Modified Natural Surfactants				
Bovine			• Contains surfactant apo-protein SP-B and SP-C	• Transmission risk
Surfactant TA (Surfacten)	50	BC	• Higher resistance to inactivation	• Unwanted constituents
Beractant (Survanta)	50	BC		• May contain proinflamma-tory mediators
SF-RI-1 (Alveofact)*		BC		• May be immunogenic
CLSE	53	BC		
CLSE (Infasurf)*	50	BC		
Porcine				
Poractant alfa (Curosurf)	35	BC		

BC, Surfactant proteins B and C; DPPC, dipalmitoyl phosphatidylcholine; rSP-C, recombinant surfactant protein-C; SP, surfactant protein.
* Obtained from lung lavage as opposed to minced lung extracts.

condition should be evaluated for SP-B deficiency, alveo-lar capillary dysplasia, and α_1-antitrypsin deficiency.

Pulmonary Hemorrhage

Blood is a strong inactivator of surfactant, with several of its components (such as hemoglobin, fibrin, fibrin-ogen, red blood cell membrane lipids, immunoglobu-lins, and plasma proteins) contributing to this process. Inactivation can occur as a result of pulmonary hemor-rhage, hemorrhagic edema, or blood aspiration during birth or trauma.

Pulmonary hemorrhage or hemorrhagic edema occurs in 3% to 5% of infants with RDS.[62] The presence of a PDA is a risk factor because of the potential large systemic-to-pulmonary vascular pressure difference between the descending aorta and pulmonary vascula-ture. Pulmonary hemorrhage can occur after subsequent surfactant administration as it decreases pulmonary vascular resistance further and increases the potential for a large pressure gradient if a PDA is present. The effi-cacy of surfactant therapy was reported in 15 neonates with respiratory deterioration due to pulmonary hem-orrhage.[63] Mean oxygen index improved from 24.6, at 0 to 3 hours presurfactant, to 8.6 at 3 to 6 hours postsur-factant ($P < 0.001$). No patient deteriorated after surfac-tant therapy.

Meconium Aspiration Syndrome

Meconium aspiration syndrome (MAS) affects 5% to 10% of all infants born through meconium-stained fluid. The pathophysiology of MAS includes mechani-cal airway obstruction, chemical pneumonitis, and sec-ondary infection. Mounting evidence also points to the role of surfactant inactivation in the development of MAS.[64,65] Mechanisms of surfactant inactivation in MAS include the following[11]:

• Disruption of the surfactant monolayer by fatty acids present in the meconium
• Production of holes in type II cells by phospholipids, causing asymmetry of the surfactant monolayer
• Bile acid–induced Ca^{2+} influx in type II cells
• Influx of neutrophils producing proteases that degrade surfactant 1 to 2 hours after aspiration
• Decreased levels of SP-A and SP-B

These alterations interfere with the ability of surfactant to lower surface tension in children with MAS.

The efficacy of surfactant replacement therapy in MAS has been reported in several uncontrolled, retrospective studies.[66,67] These results were confirmed in random-ized controlled trials. Findlay and co-workers studied 40 term infants receiving mechanical ventilation for MAS and randomized them to either beractant (Survanta) or placebo.[68] They reported that surfactant replacement, started within 6 hours of birth, improves oxygenation, reduces the incidence of air leaks, and reduces the severity of pulmonary morbidity. It also decreased the need for extracorporeal membrane oxygenation (ECMO) from 30% to 5%. Dosing was 6 cc/kg (150 mg) of surfactant, which is slightly higher than used for RDS alone, and surfactant was administered every 6 hours up to four doses.

Lotze and co-workers, in a multicenter, randomized, double-blind, placebo-controlled trial of beractant versus placebo, demonstrated that surfactant significantly decreased the need for ECMO in the treatment of term newborns with respiratory failure.[69] There may also have been benefit for infants in this study with persistent pulmonary hypertension and sepsis. This was not associated with increase in the risk of complications, including no change in the incidence of air leak. Findlay and co-workers demonstrated improved outcomes with earlier administration compared with Lotze and co-workers (6 h vs. 31 h).

Finally, the Chinese Collaborative Study Group for Neonatal Respiratory Diseases published the results of a multicenter, controlled trial of 61 term infants with severe MAS randomized to receive Curosurf (200 mg/kg) versus placebo. There was a significant improvement in oxygenation in the Curosurf-treated group, with no change in the incidence of major complications or difference in survival (no patients received ECMO).[70]

The use of dilute surfactant lavage has also been studied in severe MAS. The principle is that both surfactant delivery and meconium removal can be achieved by lavage, because surfactant facilitates the removal of foreign debris. A few pilot trials were performed with various amounts and methods of lavage. Preliminary trials[71] have been performed in term infants treated with a 48-cc/kg lavage of Surfaxin and saline (for comparison, Findlay and co-workers used 6 cc/kg). Although the authors reported not statistically significant trends toward more rapid extubation and decreased F_{IO_2} requirements for Surfaxin-lavaged infants, the large volume combined with the amount of saline may actually have been injurious to the lung epithelium. In the study, one third of the patients had bloody effluents and more infants in the lavage group (one third) met failure criteria. In addition, surfactant–saline lavage was associated with significant oxygen desaturation during administration, resulting in interruption of the procedure in 20% of the subjects because of hypoxemia or hypotension. Randomized trials are needed to compare surfactant lavage strategies versus standard surfactant administration, as they may have the same efficacy. In addition, future therapies involving surfactant lavage need to demonstrate safer administration. Saline may not be an ideal fluid for lung lavage and perfluorocarbons (used in liquid ventilation

trials) may offer an attractive alternative because they have gas exchange properties.

Pneumonia and Sepsis

Infection and inflammation are associated with inflammatory mediators (transforming growth factor-β, tumor necrosis factor-α, interleukin [IL]-1, IL-5, IL-6, and IL-8) that lead to surfactant alteration, some degree of capillary leak, and pulmonary edema.[72] The combination of edema and leak of plasma proteins into the alveolus leads to surfactant dysfunction. Microorganisms may also directly injure type II cells. Specific microbes may produce substances that downregulate SP-B and SP-C production, catalyze phospholipid hydrolysis (breakdown), and alter fatty acid composition. In animal studies of group B *Streptococcus* pneumonia, surfactant decreased bacterial proliferation, and improved compliance compared with controls.[73,74]

A retrospective study of 118 infants with group B *Streptococcus* infection demonstrated improvement in oxygenation and mean airway pressure.[75] The authors compared the infected surfactant-treated group with infants with RDS and noted that the infected patients had a slower response and were more likely to need repeated doses. In the multicenter placebo-controlled trial in neonates by Lotze and coworkers discussed earlier, 30% of the enrolled infants in both groups had sepsis.[69] Surfactant decreased the need for ECMO and the effect was greatest in the infants with an oxygen index between 15 and 22, suggesting that earlier treatment may improve outcomes.

Congenital Diaphragmatic Hernia

Infants with congenital diaphragmatic hernia (CDH) have immature lung development. In addition, relative surfactant deficiency has been demonstrated in animal models as well as in infants with CDH.[76,77] Exogenous surfactant replacement first demonstrated some efficacy in infants with CDH in a series of small case reports.[78-80] Several large series have reported improved outcomes (survival and no need for ECMO) in infants with CDH. In these studies patients received surfactant as part of a gentle ventilation strategy aimed at limiting barotrauma and volutrauma (with either conventional or high-frequency ventilation), with some patients also receiving nitric oxide.[81-85] The use of surfactant in infants with CDH has been incorporated into the treatment protocols of patients with CDH at many centers. Analysis of data from the CDH registry regarding surfactant use in infants with CDH did not demonstrate any benefit.[86-89] However, the subjects were not randomized, only a subset of the registry was analyzed, and there were no specific guidelines for surfactant use or criteria for ECMO. Therefore, it is possible that the more severely affected infants with CDH received surfactant, skewing the results. Randomized controlled trials in this area are needed to clarify the potential benefits of surfactant replacement therapy in infants with CDH.

Extracorporeal Membrane Oxygenation

Extracorporeal membrane oxygenation (ECMO) and cardiopulmonary bypass are associated with the development of an inflammatory-mediated capillary leak syndrome. This leads to fluid and neutrophil accumulation in the lungs and interstitial tissues, resulting in pulmonary edema and in turn prolonging time receiving ECMO. Inflammatory mediators attract and activate white blood cells possibly contributing to lung injury and edema. Some infants receiving ECMO are unable to wean and may benefit from surfactant administration if surfactant inhibition is contributory to their respiratory failure. A blinded, randomized, controlled study of multiple-dose surfactant therapy demonstrated decreased ECMO duration as well as reduced disease complications.[90] Four doses of modified bovine lung surfactant extract (beractant) were administered to the surfactant group (n = 28), and an equal volume of air was administered to the control group (n = 28). The ECMO treatment period was significantly shorter in the surfactant group ($P = 0.023$). The overall incidence of complications after ECMO was also decreased in the surfactant group (18% vs. 46%; $P = 0.025$).

Infants with CDH requiring ECMO are a challenging patient group to manage. After surgery, failure to wean off of ECMO may be due to:

- Severe pulmonary hypoplasia (as indicated by ECMO requirement for their management)
- Severe pulmonary hypertension
- Pulmonary edema
- Surfactant inactivation
- Complications of surgery

One study examined whether surfactant administration could improve outcomes and decrease the duration of ECMO for infants with CDH.[91] These infants received either four doses of surfactant (beractant, n = 9) or an equal volume of air (control group, n = 8). Tracheal aspirate SP-A concentrations were initially low, and then increased over time in both CDH groups. Lung compliance, time to extubation, time on oxygen, and total number of hospital days were not different between the two groups.

Acute Respiratory Distress Syndrome

Significant impairments of surfactant production and composition have been demonstrated in the lungs of patients with ARDS. Surfactant alterations include reduced phospholipid content and, in particular, reduced DPPC levels as well as decreased levels of surfactant-associated proteins.[29,92,93] These changes result in decreased surface activity resulting in the atelectasis and decreased lung compliance characteristic of ARDS.

Three large trials failed to demonstrate a benefit of surfactant therapy in adult patients with ARDS.[94-96] In children with ARDS, the efficacy of surfactant therapy has been assessed in several pilot studies. Infasurf administration to children with hypoxemic respiratory failure resulted in immediate improvement in oxygenation (Figure 16-8) as well as a 32% reduction in time requiring mechanical ventilation and a 30% reduction in stay in the pediatric intensive care unit.[97]

In a separate study, 20 children with an acute pulmonary disease and severe hypoxemia (13 with systemic or pulmonary disease and 7 with cardiac disease) received Curosurf. There was a moderate improvement in oxygenation among patients with systemic or pulmonary disease but not in children with hypoxemic pulmonary pathology in the postoperative period of cardiovascular surgery. The improvement of the patients who survived was greater than that of those who died.[98]

A multicenter, randomized control trial was published comparing 153 children with respiratory failure from acute lung injury and assigned to 2 doses of Calfactant 12 hours apart versus placebo.[99] Calfactant acutely improved oxygenation with a decrease in the oxygen index from 20 to 13.9. In addition, there was a significant decrease in mortality in the Calfactant group, with an odds ratio of 2.32 (95% confidence interval, 1.15 to 4.85). In this study, no difference in duration of mechanical ventilation, intensive care unit stay, and hospital stay was noted. Adverse effects of the therapy were minimal and in those patients who did not benefit

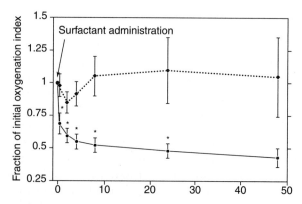

FIGURE 16-8 Changes in oxygenation after surfactant administration. *Circles,* surfactant group; *diamonds,* placebo group.

it did not cause harm. The authors of this study have discussed that although this treatment is still under investigation, patients with direct lung injury such as near drowning, pneumonia, or trauma with severe pulmonary compromise may benefit, whereas patients with diseases involving ongoing capillary leak (e.g., sepsis) do not respond.

Although promising, the results of these studies are confounded by variability in dosing, time of administration, and type of surfactant. In addition, attention to patient population, immune status, and mechanism of lung injury should be integrated into the design of future surfactant trials for ARDS.

Viral Bronchiolitis

Impairment in surfactant function has been reported in patients with viral bronchiolitis,[100] including reduced levels of SP-A, SP-B, and SP-D as well as decreased DPPC.[101,102] In a small randomized control trial of Curosurf in 20 infants with severe RSV bronchiolitis surfactant therapy appeared to improve gas exchange, reduce peak inspiratory pressure, and shorten time on conventional ventilation and duration of intensive care unit stay.[103] In a second randomized trial 19 ventilated infants with RSV bronchiolitis received Survanta or placebo. Again, patients in the surfactant group had improved oxygenation, improved lung compliance, and shortened time on ventilation.[104]

Asthma

Decreased SP-A levels have been reported in sputum from patients with acute asthma.[105] In addition, antigen challenge of patients with asthma results in altered phospholipid properties and increased surface tension.[106] A pilot placebo-controlled trial of surfactant replacement therapy (Surfacten) was conducted in 11 adult patients with acute asthma. Respiratory functions were significantly improved in all patients in the surfactant group, including forced vital capacity, forced expiratory volume in 1 second, and arterial partial pressure of oxygen. No difference was detected in arterial partial pressure of carbon dioxide.[107] However, in 12 children with asthma, there was no significant improvement in airflow obstruction and bronchial responsiveness to histamine after surfactant nebulization (Alveofact).[108]

Cystic Fibrosis

Multiple studies have looked at surfactant in patients with cystic fibrosis (CF), with contrasting results that may be explained in part by the age of the patients. In young patients, no difference in SP-A levels are noted; however, with the development of inflamma-

tion increased levels are observed.[109] In patients with more chronic CF, SP-A levels decrease.[110,111] Griese and co-workers also demonstrated deficient surface tension ability of phospholipids in patients with CF when compared with healthy control subjects.[112] In contrast, Postle and co-workers found no difference in phospholipids.[111] In 2005, the surfactant function of 20 patients with CF was studied longitudinally. The study demonstrated a progressive loss of surfactant function, which correlated with increased inflammation and decreased lung function. In this study, the concentrations of SP-A, SP-C, and SP-D did not change, whereas that of SP-B increased.[113]

No therapeutic trials in children have been published. A pilot study of Alveofact versus placebo in adults with severe CF showed no improvement in lung function or oxygenation.[114]

FUTURE DIRECTIONS

Today, thanks to surfactant replacement therapy, RDS is an uncommon cause of death in the preterm infant. Annual deaths from RDS in the United States have decreased from 10,000 to 15,000/year in the 1950s to less than 1000 in 2002. If surfactant replacement is unequivocally effective in treating surfactant-deficient preterm infants, current evidence suggests that it may prove useful as an adjunctive therapy when surfactant dysfunction is a contributing factor in acute respiratory failure. Thus surfactant replacement offers promise to improve disturbed lung physiology and allow moderation of ventilator support in children with acute respiratory failure.

However, challenges remain in the area of surfactant uses and delivery. Technical aspects including timing of delivery, number of doses, and mode of delivery need to be studied in relation to specific disease type. One exciting development is the potential delivery of surfactant via a laryngeal mask airway, obviating the need for intubation and possibly mechanical ventilation.[115] In addition, synthetic surfactants containing genetically engineered surfactant-associated proteins are now in clinical trials. These synthetic surfactants are potentially more effective because of their constant and known composition, but they also offer less risk to the patient. And because they can be produced in bulk, they are likely to be less expensive and available to more patients worldwide.

Finally, increased understanding of individual genetic polymorphism regarding surfactant-associated proteins may lead to the identification of patients who will or will not benefit from surfactant administration.

CLINICAL SCENARIOS

CASE 1

An 800-g 26-week gestation baby boy is born by spontaneous vaginal delivery due to cervical incompetence. The infant is active with Apgar scores of 5 and 6, and needs positive pressure ventilation to establish regular respirations. Grunting presents immediately and a nasal continuous positive airway pressure (NCPAP) of 5 cm H_2O is applied after positive pressure ventilation at 5 minutes. The chest radiograph demonstrates a homogeneous ground-glass pattern. The infant's first arterial blood gas determination at 30 minutes of life on 70% oxygen produces the following results: pH 7.10; P_{CO_2}, 78 mm Hg; P_{O_2}, 52 mm Hg.

What would you do at this point? (*Note:* More than one answer may be acceptable.)
1. Continue NCPAP
2. Perform endotracheal intubation
3. Perform endotracheal intubation and administer surfactant
4. Increase the F_{IO_2}

CASE 2

A full-term infant is delivered by stat C-section for fetal heart rate decelerations. Thick meconium is noted when membranes are ruptured during the C-section. The obstetrician suctions the infant and then the pediatrician performs endotracheal intubation and suctions the airway. On physical examination, the infant has significant grunting and intercostal retractions. The trachea is reintubated and the infant is placed on high-frequency oscillatory ventilation. He requires an F_{IO_2} of 1.0 and has preductal saturations of 90% and postductal saturations of 85%. The chest radiograph demonstrates bilateral streaky densities throughout the lung fields.

What is this infant at risk for? (*Note:* More than one answer may be acceptable.)
1. Pneumothorax
2. Persistent pulmonary hypertension of the newborn
3. Respiratory distress syndrome
4. Aspiration pneumonia

CLINICAL SCENARIOS—cont'd

ASSESSMENT QUESTIONS

See Evolve Resources for answers.

1. What is/are the most abundant components of surfactant?
    I.   Dipalmitoyl phosphatidylcholine (DPPC)
    II. Surfactant protein (SP)-B
    III. SP-C
    IV. Phosphatidylglycerol
    A. I
    B. II and III
    C. I, II, and III
    D. All of the above
2. Surfactant inactivation and dysfunction have *not* been described in which of the following diseases?
    A. Meconium aspiration syndrome
    B. Asthma
    C. Cystic fibrosis
    D. Congenital heart disease
    E. Sepsis
3. Natural surfactant preparations come from which of the following mammals?
    I.   Pigs
    II. Cows
    III. Calves
    IV. Horses
    V.   Whales
    A. I
    B. I, II, and III
    C. IV and V
    D. I, II, III, and IV
    E. All of the above

Continued

ASSESSMENT QUESTIONS—cont'd

4. Which air sac in the following diagram requires higher pressure to inflate (assuming similar surface tension)?

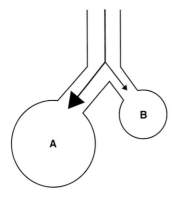

   A. Air sac A
   B. Air sac B

5. Which surfactant-associated protein deficiency is fatal in infancy without lung transplantation?
   A. SP-A deficiency
   B. SP-B deficiency
   C. SP-C deficiency
   D. SP-D deficiency

6. Which surfactant protein(s) is/are important in defense against infection?
     I. SP-A
    II. SP-B
   III. SP-C
   IV. SP-D
   A. I
   B. II and III
   C. I and IV
   D. I, II, and IV
   E. All of the above

7. What are the complications of surfactant administration?
     I. Cyanosis
    II. Airway obstruction
   III. Pulmonary hemorrhage
   IV. Infection
    V. Hypotension
   A. I
   B. II and III
   C. I, II and III
   D. I, II, and IV
   E. All of the above

8. What are the benefits of surfactant replacement therapy in infants with respiratory distress syndrome (RDS)?
     I. Reduction in the severity of RDS

ASSESSMENT QUESTIONS—cont'd

    II. Reduction in the incidence of air leaks (pneumothorax and pulmonary interstitial emphysema)
   III. Reduction in mortality from RDS by 40% to 60%
   IV. Reduction in the incidence of bronchopulmonary dysplasia
    V. Reduction in the incidence of intraventricular hemorrhage
   A. I
   B. II and III
   C. I, II and III
   D. I, II, and IV
   E. All of the above

9. What component(s) of natural surfactant increase(s) efficacy compared with synthetic surfactants?
     I. SP-B
    II. Percentage of DPPC
   III. SP-C
   IV. Cholesterol
   A. I
   B. I and III
   C. I, II and III
   D. I, II, and IV
   E. All of the above

10. What are the radiographic findings typical of a child with RDS?
     I. Large lung volume
    II. Atelectasis
   III. Air bronchograms
   IV. Pulmonary interstitial emphysema
    V. Ground-glass pattern
   A. I
   B. II and III
   C. I, II and III
   D. II, III, and V
   E. All of the above

References

1. Pfister RH, Soll RF: New synthetic surfactants: the next generation? *Biol Neonate* 2005;87:338.
2. Suresh GK, Soll RF: Overview of surfactant replacement trials, *J Perinatol* 2005;25(suppl 2):S40.
3. Obladen M: History of surfactant up to 1980, *Biol Neonate* 2005;87:308.
4. von Neergaard K: Neue Auffassungen uber einen Grundbegriff der Atemmechanik: Die Retraktionskraft der Lunge, abhangig von der Oberflachenspannung in den Alveolen, *Z Gesamte Exp Med* 1929;66:373.
5. Macklin CC: The pulmonary alveolar mucoid film and the pneumonocytes, *Lancet* 1954;266:1099.

6. Mead J, Lindgren I, Gaensler EA: The mechanical properties of the lungs in emphysema, *J Clin Invest* 1955;34:1005; see also Avery ME: Surfactant deficiency in hyaline membrane disease: the story of discovery, *Am J Respir Crit Care Med* 2000;161:1074.

7. Clements J: Surface tension of lung extracts, *Proc Soc Exp Biol Med* 1957;95:170.

8. Pattle RE: Properties, function and origin of the alveolar lining layer, *Nature* 1955;175:1125.

9. Avery ME, Mead J: Surface properties in relation to atelectasis and hyaline membrane disease, *Am J Dis Child* 1959;97:517.

10. Fujiwara T et al: Artificial surfactant therapy in hyaline-membrane disease. Lancet 1980;1(8159):55. As cited in Halliday HL: History of surfactant from 1980, *Biol Neonate* 2005;87:317.

11. Wiswell TE: Expanded uses of surfactant therapy, *Clin Perinatol* 2001;28:695.

12. Poynter SE, LeVine AM: Surfactant biology and clinical application, *Crit Care Clin* 2003;19:459.

13. Finer NN: Surfactant use for neonatal lung injury: beyond respiratory distress syndrome, *Paediatr Respir Rev* 2004;5(suppl A):S289.

14. Jobe AH, Ikegami M: Biology of surfactant, *Clin Perinatol* 2001;28:655.

15. Fujiwara T et al; Surfactant-TA Study Group: Surfactant replacement therapy with a single postventilatory dose of a reconstituted bovine surfactant in preterm neonates with respiratory distress syndrome: final analysis of a multicenter, double-blind, randomized trial and comparison with similar trials, *Pediatrics* 1990;86:753.

16. Williams MC: Uptake of lectins by pulmonary alveolar type II cells: subsequent deposition into lamellar bodies, *Proc Natl Acad Sci USA* 1984;81:6383.

17. Creuwels LA, van Golde LM, Haagsman HP: The pulmonary surfactant system: biochemical and clinical aspects, *Lung* 1997;175:1.

18. Chung J et al: Effect of surfactant-associated protein-A (SP-A) on the activity of lipid extract surfactant, *Biochim Biophys Acta* 1989;1002:348.

19. Curstedt T: Surfactant protein C: basics to bedside, *J Perinatol* 2005;25(suppl 2):S36.

20. Lee MJ et al: Single versus weekly courses of antenatal corticosteroids in preterm premature rupture of membranes, *Obstet Gynecol* 2004;103:274.

21. Banks BA et al: Multiple courses of antenatal corticosteroids are associated with early severe lung disease in preterm neonates, *J Perinatol* 2002;22:101.

22. Zimmermann LJ et al: Surfactant metabolism in the neonate, *Biol Neonate* 2005;87:296.

23. Ballard RA et al; North American Thyrotropin-releasing Hormone Study Group: Antenatal thyrotropin-releasing hormone to prevent lung disease in preterm infants, *N Engl J Med* 1998;338:493.

24. ACTOBAT Study Group: Australian Collaborative Trial of Antenatal Thyrotropin-releasing hormone (ACTOBAT) for prevention of neonatal respiratory disease, *Lancet* 1995;345:877.

25. Geary CA, Whitsett JA: Amniotic fluid markers of fetal lung maturity. In Spitzer AR, editor: Intensive care of the fetus and neonate, Philadelphia: Elsevier Mosby; 2005. pp 122-132.

26. Jobe AH, Ikegami M: Surfactant and acute lung injury, *Proc Assoc Am Physicians* 1998;110:489.

27. Pison U et al: Surfactant abnormalities in patients with respiratory failure after multiple trauma, *Am Rev Respir Dis* 1989;140:1033.

28. Pison U et al: Altered pulmonary surfactant in uncomplicated and septicemia-complicated courses of acute respiratory failure, *J Trauma* 1990;30:19.

29. Gregory TJ et al: Surfactant chemical composition and biophysical activity in acute respiratory distress syndrome, *J Clin Invest* 1991;88:1976.

30. Low RB et al: Bronchoalveolar lavage lipids during development of bleomycin-induced fibrosis in rats: relationship to altered epithelial cell morphology, *Am Rev Respir Dis* 1988;138:709.

31. Young SL et al: Pulmonary surfactant lipid production in oxygen-exposed rat lungs, *Lab Invest* 1982;46:570.

32. Holm BA et al: Pulmonary physiological and surfactant changes during injury and recovery from hyperoxia, *J Appl Physiol* 1985;59:1402.

33. Pison U et al: Phospholipid lung profile in adult respiratory distress syndrome: evidence for surfactant abnormality, *Prog Clin Biol Res* 1987;236A:517.

34. Lewis JF, Jobe AH: Surfactant and the adult respiratory distress syndrome, *Am Rev Respir Dis* 1993;147:218.

35. Veldhuizen RA et al: Pulmonary surfactant subfractions in patients with the acute respiratory distress syndrome, *Am J Respir Crit Care Med* 1995;152:1867.

36. Ueda T, Ikegami M, Jobe A: Surfactant subtypes: in vitro conversion, in vivo function, and effects of serum proteins, *Am J Respir Crit Care Med* 1994;149:1254.

37. Holm BA et al: Type II pneumocyte changes during hyperoxic lung injury and recovery, *J Appl Physiol* 1988;65:2672.

38. Seeger W et al: Alveolar surfactant and adult respiratory distress syndrome: pathogenetic role and therapeutic prospects, *Clin Investig* 1993;71:177.

39. Kobayashi T et al: Inactivation of exogenous surfactant by pulmonary edema fluid, *Pediatr Res* 1991;29:353.

40. Bruni R et al: Inactivation of surfactant in rat lungs, *Pediatr Res* 1996;39:236.

41. Holm BA, Enhorning G, Notter RH: A biophysical mechanism by which plasma proteins inhibit lung surfactant activity, *Chem Phys Lipids* 1988;49:49.

42. Holm BA, Matalon S: Role of pulmonary surfactant in the development and treatment of adult respiratory distress syndrome, *Anesth Analg* 1989;69:805.

43. Hack M et al: Very-low-birth-weight outcomes of the National Institute of Child Health and Human Development Neonatal Network, November 1989 to October 1990, *Am J Obstet Gynecol* 1995;172:457.

44. Fujiwara T et al: Artificial surfactant therapy in hyaline-membrane disease, *Lancet* 1980;1:55.

45. Suresh GK, Soll RF: Current surfactant use in premature infants, *Clin Perinatol* 2001;28:671.

46. Long W et al; American Exosurf Neonatal Study Group I; Canadian Exosurf Neonatal Study Group: A controlled trial of synthetic surfactant in infants weighing 1250 g or more with respiratory distress syndrome, *N Engl J Med* 1991;325:1696.

47. Jobe AH, Mitchell BR, Gunkel JH: Beneficial effects of the combined use of prenatal corticosteroids and postnatal surfactant on preterm infants, *Am J Obstet Gynecol* 1993;168:508.

48. Van Marter LJ et al; Neonatology Committee for the Developmental Network: Do clinical markers of

barotrauma and oxygen toxicity explain interhospital variation in rates of chronic lung disease? *Pediatrics* 2000;105:1194.

49. Thomson MA: Continuous positive airway pressure and surfactant; combined data from animal experiments and clinical trials, *Biol Neonate* 2002;81(suppl 1):16.

50. Ammari A et al: Variables associated with the early failure of nasal CPAP in very low birth weight infants, *J Pediatr* 2005;147:341.

51. Suresh GK, Soll RF: Current surfactant use in premature infants, *Clin Perinatol* 2001;28:671.

52. Yost CC, Soll RF: Early versus delayed selective surfactant treatment for neonatal respiratory distress syndrome, *Cochrane Database Syst Rev* 2000;2:CD001456.

53. Morley CJ et al: Nasal CPAP or intubation at birth for very preterm infants, *N Engl J Med* 2008;358:700.

54. Elgellab A et al: Effects of nasal continuous positive airway pressure (NCPAP) on breathing pattern in spontaneously breathing premature newborn infants, *Intensive Care Med* 2001;27:1782.

55. Morley CJ, Davis PG: Continuous positive airway pressure: scientific and clinical rationale, *Curr Opin Pediatr* 2008;20:119.

56. Morley CJ et al; COIN Trial Investigators: Nasal CPAP or intubation at birth for very preterm infants, *N Engl J Med* 2008;358:700.

57. Lacaze-Masmonteil T: Exogenous surfactant therapy: newer developments, *Semin Neonatol* 2003;8:433.

58. Suresh GK, Soll RF: Current surfactant use in premature infants, *Clin Perinatol* 2001;28:671.

59. Curstedt T, Johansson J: New synthetic surfactants: basic science, *Biol Neonate* 2005;87:332.

60. Moya FR et al: A multicenter, randomized, masked, comparison trial of lucinactant, colfosceril palmitate, and beractant for the prevention of respiratory distress syndrome among very preterm infants, *Pediatrics* 2005;115:1018.

61. Sinha SK et al: A multicenter, randomized, controlled trial of lucinactant versus poractant alfa among very premature infants at high risk for respiratory distress syndrome, *Pediatrics* 2005;115:1030.

62. Lin TW et al: Risk factors of pulmonary hemorrhage in very-low-birth-weight infants: a two-year retrospective study, *Acta Paediatr Taiwan* 2000;41:255.

63. Pandit PB, Dunn MS, Colucci EA: Surfactant therapy in neonates with respiratory deterioration due to pulmonary hemorrhage, *Pediatrics* 1995;95:32.

64. Moses D et al: Inhibition of pulmonary surfactant function by meconium, *Am J Obstet Gynecol* 1991;164:477.

65. Sun B et al: Surfactant improves lung function and morphology in newborn rabbits with meconium aspiration, *Biol Neonate* 1993;63:96.

66. Halliday HL, Speer CP, Robertson B; Collaborative Surfactant Study Group: Treatment of severe meconium aspiration syndrome with porcine surfactant, *Eur J Pediatr* 1996;155:1047.

67. Khammash H et al: Surfactant therapy in full-term neonates with severe respiratory failure, *Pediatrics* 1993;92:135.

68. Findlay RD, Taeusch HW, Walther FJ: Surfactant replacement therapy for meconium aspiration syndrome, *Pediatrics* 1996;97:48.

69. Lotze A et al; Survanta in Term Infants Study Group: Multicenter study of surfactant (beractant) use in the treatment of term infants with severe respiratory failure, *J Pediatr* 1998;132:40.

70. Chinese Collaborative Study Group for Neonatal Respiratory Diseases: Treatment of severe meconium aspiration syndrome with porcine surfactant: a multicentre, randomized, controlled trial, *Acta Paediatr* 2005;94:896.

71. Wiswell TE et al: A multicenter, randomized, controlled trial comparing Surfaxin (Lucinactant) lavage with standard care for treatment of meconium aspiration syndrome, *Pediatrics* 2002;109:1081.

72. Merrill JD, Ballard RA: Pulmonary surfactant for neonatal respiratory disorders, *Curr Opin Pediatr* 2003;15:149.

73. Herting E et al: Surfactant improves lung function and mitigates bacterial growth in immature ventilated rabbits with experimentally induced neonatal group B streptococcal pneumonia, *Arch Dis Child Fetal Neonatal Ed* 1997;76:F3.

74. Herting E et al: Combined treatment with surfactant and specific immunoglobulin reduces bacterial proliferation in experimental neonatal group B streptococcal pneumonia, *Am J Respir Crit Care Med* 1999;159:1862.

75. Herting E et al: Members of the Collaborative European Multicenter Study Group: Surfactant treatment of neonates with respiratory failure and group B streptococcal infection, *Pediatrics* 2000;106:957.

76. Wilcox DT et al: Contributions by individual lungs to the surfactant status in congenital diaphragmatic hernia, *Pediatr Res* 1997;41:686.

77. Moya FR et al: Fetal lung maturation in congenital diaphragmatic hernia, *Am J Obstet Gynecol* 1995;173:1401.

78. Glick PL et al: Pathophysiology of congenital diaphragmatic hernia. III. Exogenous surfactant therapy for the high-risk neonate with CDH, *J Pediatr Surg* 1992;27:866.

79. Bos AP et al: Surfactant replacement therapy in high-risk congenital diaphragmatic hernia, *Lancet* 1991;338:1279.

80. Bae CW et al: Exogenous pulmonary surfactant replacement therapy in a neonate with pulmonary hypoplasia accompanying congenital diaphragmatic hernia: a case report, *J Korean Med Sci* 1996;11:265.

81. Dubois A et al: [Congenital hernia of the diaphragm: a retrospective study of 123 cases recorded in the Neonatal Medicine Department, URHC in Lille between 1985 and 1996]. *Arch Pediatr* 2000;7:132.

82. Somaschini M et al: Impact of new treatments for respiratory failure on outcome of infants with congenital diaphragmatic hernia, *Eur J Pediatr* 1999;158:780.

83. Kays DW et al: Detrimental effects of standard medical therapy in congenital diaphragmatic hernia, *Ann Surg* 1999;230:340.

84. Langham MR Jr et al: Twenty years of progress in congenital diaphragmatic hernia at the University of Florida, *Am Surg* 2003;69:45.

85. Boloker J et al: Congenital diaphragmatic hernia in 120 infants treated consecutively with permissive hypercapnea/spontaneous respiration/elective repair, *J Pediatr Surg* 2002;37:357.

86. Colby CE et al: Surfactant replacement therapy on ECMO does not improve outcome in neonates with congenital diaphragmatic hernia, *J Pediatr Surg* 2004;39:1632.

87. Doyle NM, Lally KP: The CDH Study Group and advances in the clinical care of the patient with congenital diaphragmatic hernia, *Semin Perinatol* 2004;28:174.

88. Lally KP et al: Surfactant does not improve survival rate in preterm infants with congenital diaphragmatic hernia, *J Pediatr Surg* 2004;39:829.

89. Van Meurs K: Is surfactant therapy beneficial in the treatment of the term newborn infant with congenital diaphragmatic hernia? *J Pediatr* 2004;145:312.

90. Lotze A et al: Improved pulmonary outcome after exogenous surfactant therapy for respiratory failure in term infants requiring extracorporeal membrane oxygenation, *J Pediatr* 1993;122:261.

91. Lotze A et al: Surfactant (beractant) therapy for infants with congenital diaphragmatic hernia on ECMO: evidence of persistent surfactant deficiency, *J Pediatr Surg* 1994;29:407.

92. Greene KE et al: Serial changes in surfactant-associated proteins in lung and serum before and after onset of ARDS, *Am J Respir Crit Care Med* 1999;160:1843.

93. Baker CS et al: Damage to surfactant-specific protein in acute respiratory distress syndrome, *Lancet* 1999;353:1232.

94. Anzueto A et al; Exosurf Acute Respiratory Distress Syndrome Sepsis Study Group: Aerosolized surfactant in adults with sepsis-induced acute respiratory distress syndrome, *N Engl J Med* 1996;334:1417.

95. Gregory TJ et al: Bovine surfactant therapy for patients with acute respiratory distress syndrome, *Am J Respir Crit Care Med* 1997;155:1309.

96. Spragg RG et al: Effect of recombinant surfactant protein C–based surfactant on the acute respiratory distress syndrome, *N Engl J Med* 2004;351:884.

97. Willson DF et al; Members of the Mid-Atlantic Pediatric Critical Care Network: Instillation of calf lung surfactant extract (calfactant) is beneficial in pediatric acute hypoxemic respiratory failure, *Crit Care Med* 1999;27:188.

98. Lopez-Herce J et al: Surfactant treatment for acute respiratory distress syndrome, *Arch Dis Child* 1999;80:248.

99. Willson DF et al: Effect of exogenous surfactant (calfactant) in pediatric acute lung injury: a randomized controlled trial, *JAMA* 2005;293:470.

100. Dargaville PA, South M, McDougall PN: Surfactant abnormalities in infants with severe viral bronchiolitis, *Arch Dis Child* 1996;75:133.

101. Skelton R et al: Abnormal surfactant composition and activity in severe bronchiolitis, *Acta Paediatr* 1999;88:942.

102. Kerr MH, Paton JY: Surfactant protein levels in severe respiratory syncytial virus infection, *Am J Respir Crit Care Med* 1999;159:1115.

103. Luchetti M et al: Porcine-derived surfactant treatment of severe bronchiolitis, *Acta Anaesthesiol Scand* 1998;42:805.

104. Tibby SM et al: Exogenous surfactant supplementation in infants with respiratory syncytial virus bronchiolitis, *Am J Respir Crit Care Med* 2000;162:1251.

105. Kurashima K et al: Surface activity of sputum from acute asthmatic patients, *Am J Respir Crit Care Med* 1997;155:1254.

106. Hite RD et al: Surfactant phospholipid changes after antigen challenge: a role for phosphatidylglycerol in dysfunction, *Am J Physiol Lung Cell Mol Physiol* 2005;288:L610.

107. Kurashima K et al: A pilot study of surfactant inhalation in the treatment of asthmatic attack, *Arerugi* 1991;40:160.

108. Oetomo SB et al: Surfactant nebulization does not alter airflow obstruction and bronchial responsiveness to histamine in asthmatic children, *Am J Respir Crit Care Med* 1996;153:1148.

109. Hull J et al: Surfactant composition in infants and young children with cystic fibrosis, *Am J Respir Crit Care Med* 1997;156:161.

110. Griese M, Birrer P, Demirsoy A: Pulmonary surfactant in cystic fibrosis, *Eur Respir J* 1997;10:1983.

111. Postle AD et al: Deficient hydrophilic lung surfactant proteins A and D with normal surfactant phospholipid molecular species in cystic fibrosis, *Am J Respir Cell Mol Biol* 1999;20:90.

112. Griese M et al: Nebulization of a bovine surfactant in cystic fibrosis: a pilot study, *Eur Respir J* 1997;10:1989.

113. Griese M et al: Sequential analysis of surfactant, lung function and inflammation in cystic fibrosis patients, *Respir Res* 2005;6:133.

114. Griese M et al: Nebulization of a bovine surfactant in cystic fibrosis: a pilot study, *Eur Respir J* 1997;10:1989.

115. Trevisanuto D et al: Laryngeal mask airway used as a delivery conduit for the administration of surfactant to preterm infants with respiratory distress syndrome, *Biol Neonate* 2005;87:217.

116. Soll RF, Morley CJ: Prophylactic versus selective use of surfactant in preventing morbidity and mortality in preterm infants, *Cochrane Database Syst Rev* 2001;2:CD000510.

117. OSIRIS Collaborative Group (Open Study of Infants at High Risk of or with Respiratory Insufficiency): Early versus delayed neonatal administration of a synthetic surfactant—the judgment of OSIRIS. 1. The role of surfactant, *Lancet* 1992;340:1363.

118. Berggren E et al: Pilot study of nebulized surfactant therapy for neonatal respiratory distress syndrome, *Acta Paediatr* 2000;89:460.

119. Gortner L et al: High-dose versus low-dose bovine surfactant treatment in very premature infants, *Acta Paediatr* 1994;83:135.

120. Konishi M et al: Surfactant replacement therapy in neonatal respiratory distress syndrome. A multi-centre, randomized clinical trial: comparison of high- versus low-dose of surfactant TA, *Eur J Pediatr* 1988;147:20.

121. Halliday HL et al: Multicentre randomised trial comparing high and low dose surfactant regimens for the treatment of respiratory distress syndrome (the Curosurf 4 trial), *Arch Dis Child* 1993;69:276.

122. Herting E et al: [Effect of 2 different dosages of a porcine surfactant on pulmonary gas exchange of premature infants with severe respiratory distress syndrome], *Monatsschr Kinderheilkd* 1993;141:721.

123. Zola EM et al: Comparison of three dosing procedures for administration of bovine surfactant to neonates with respiratory distress syndrome, *J Pediatr* 1993;122:453.

Chapter 17

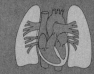

Mechanical Ventilators

KATHERINE FEDOR

LEARNING OBJECTIVES

After reading this chapter the reader will be able to:
- Explain the ventilator classification system
- Appraise the principal modes of operation of commonly used infant and pediatric ventilators

- Identify specific features of commonly used infant and pediatric ventilators

The mechanical ventilators originally used to ventilate infants and older pediatric patients were modifications of adult ventilators.[1] In the early 1970s, however, Kirby and associates[2] described a "new" pediatric ventilator, and the relatively simple continuous-flow time-cycled machine became the predominant design of infant ventilators produced after that time. Although Kirby and colleagues described their machine as a volume ventilator, the practice of pressure limitation became so popular that the terms *infant ventilator* and *pressure ventilator* were often used interchangeably. Older pediatric patients continued to be ventilated with modified adult, or volume, ventilators or with machines with the same design characteristics as adult ventilators.

---

* See Evolve Resources for a detailed description of this ventilator.

More recent advances in ventilator technology, particularly the use of microprocessor control, have greatly increased the sophistication of mechanical ventilators and blurred traditional boundaries between ventilator types and ventilation techniques. It is now common for ventilators to offer a choice of pressure or volume (more accurately, flow) control as well as a variety of inspiratory flow waveforms. In addition, a number of ventilators incorporate the concept of pressure and volume ventilation in a dual mode that is pressure controlled and volume targeted. Microprocessors, and the electromechanical valves that they control, are capable of adjusting flows rapidly and in a wide range, eliminating many of the limitations to flow and tidal volume delivery inherent in the design of earlier ventilators. As a result, it is often possible for a single ventilator to be used to ventilate a wider range of patients. Even the distinction between infant ventilator and adult ventilator is no longer always clear-cut.

In this chapter, a system is presented for classifying mechanical ventilators and for understanding ventilator function. Descriptions of specific, commonly used ventilators are presented, detailing the available features of each. In addition, information about select models of older ventilators can be found at the Evolve website that accompanies this text. Models selected for inclusion at the Evolve site may still be used in some facilities but are no longer widely used, or the manufacturer no longer supports the equipment.

VENTILATOR CLASSIFICATION

Citing the problems with traditional classification schemes, Chatburn proposed a new approach to the understanding and classification of mechanical ventilators.[3-5]

The remainder of this section summarizes Chatburn's classification system, which uses input power, power conversion and transmission, control, and output as a framework for describing mechanical ventilators.

Input Power

Input power refers to the power source (or sources) required by the ventilator to perform the work of ventilation. Input power can be pneumatic or electric. Pneumatic power is usually provided by compressed gas pressurized to about 50 pounds per square inch gauge (psig). Electric power can be either alternating current (AC) or the direct current (DC) of a battery.

Ventilators can be designed to use either one or both input power sources.[6] The original Baby Bird (Bird Products) is an example of a pneumatically powered ventilator. Electrically powered ventilators such as the Puritan Bennett MA-1 (Covidien, Mansfield, Mass) and the Emerson 3-MV (J.H. Emerson) may use a pneumatic

source to increase the oxygen concentration of inspired gas, but interruption of the gas source does not disrupt basic ventilator function. Most ventilators currently in use require both pneumatic and electric power for operation. Typically, pneumatic power provides the ventilator's driving force whereas electricity powers the mechanism or mechanisms controlling the particular manner in which the gas is delivered.

Power Conversion and Transmission

Power conversion and transmission describe the mechanism or mechanisms that the ventilator uses to create and control gas flow to the patient. Together these devices can be referred to as the *drive mechanism* and include the ventilator's compressor and output control valves.

The pressure needed to generate a flow of gas may be initiated by a device outside of the ventilator (an external compressor) or by a device that is part of the ventilator's design (an internal compressor). Pistons and cylinders, diaphragms, bellows, and rotating vanes have been used most often as internal compressors.

A ventilator's compressor is often described in conjunction with the motor used to drive it and the linkage between the motor and compressor. Motor and linkage types can be categorized as electric motor/rotating crank and piston, electric motor/rack and pinion, and direct-drive electric motor. In addition, compressed gas can be considered as the motor that drives a compressor. For example, compressed gas can be used to power a diaphragm or bellows, which, in turn, supplies flow to the patient. Compressed gas may also be used to inflate the lungs directly. The pressure of compressed gas is generally reduced to a "usable" level by a regulator.

The valves used to control the gas flow created by the compressor are called *output control valves*. These devices operate under the influence of the control circuit and include inspiratory flow control valves and exhalation valves. Common types of output control valves are pneumatic diaphragms (frequently used as exhalation valves), pneumatic poppet valves, electromagnetic poppet valves (solenoids), and electromagnetic proportional valves. The latter type of valve regulates flow by varying the size of the valve opening and is often used to "pattern" inspiratory flow.

Control
Control Circuit

The control circuit is the subsystem that performs the logic and decision-making functions of the ventilator and regulates the drive mechanism or output control valves, or both, to produce the desired ventilator output. Ventilators may use one or more types of control circuit, which have been categorized as follows:

- Mechanical control circuits (used in early ventilators) use levers, pulleys, and cams.
- Pneumatic control circuits rely on gas pressure to operate diaphragms, Venturi devices, and pistons.
- Fluidic control circuits use minute gas flows to operate pressure switches and timing mechanisms.
- Electric control circuits use only simple switches. Electronic control circuits use components such as resistors, capacitors, and transistors or combinations of components in integrated circuits. The most sophisticated form of electronic control is provided by a microprocessor.

A ventilator's control scheme can be open loop or closed loop. With both types of control, an input (pressure, volume, or flow setting) is added to a system to obtain a desired output. Control is closed loop when an output variable is measured and compared with a reference (the control settings), and the input is modified as needed to more closely approximate the desired output. Closed loop control is also known as feedback or servo control.

If an input is selected and no information is fed back to modify the input (i.e., close the loop), the system is open loop.

Control Variables and Waveforms

The variables involved in the mechanics of ventilation are pressure, volume, and flow. The relationships among these variables are described by a mathematical model, the equation of motion for the respiratory system. A simplified form of this equation can be found in Figure 17-1. The equation of motion demonstrates that if any single variable is specified, the specified variable is independent of anything else in the equation. Furthermore, the other two variables are dependent on the specified (independent) variable.

Because only one variable can serve as the independent variable at a given time, consequently, only one variable can be controlled by a ventilator at any one time. The variable that a ventilator controls to effect inspiration is the control variable. Pressure, volume,

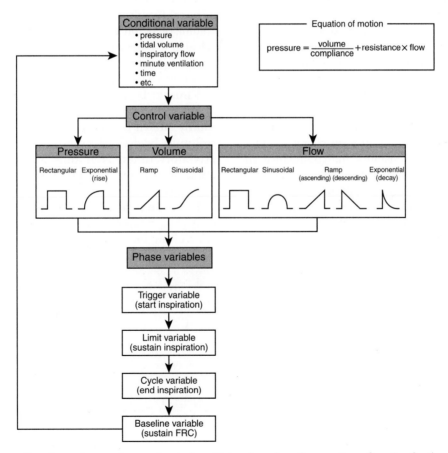

FIGURE 17-1 A paradigm for understanding mechanical ventilators based on the equation of motion for the respiratory system. The model illustrates that during inspiration the ventilator can control only one variable at a time. The diagram shows common waveforms for each control variable. Pressure, volume, flow, and time are also used as phase variables that determine the characteristics of each ventilatory cycle. The diagram is drawn as a flow chart to emphasize that each breath may have a different set of control and phase variables, depending on the mode of ventilation used.

and flow generally serve as control variables, although a ventilator can theoretically control time (the implied variable) as well.

The pattern that a variable produces during inspiration is its inspiratory waveform. A waveform plots the magnitude of a variable (vertical axis) over inspiratory time (horizontal axis). Common inspiratory waveforms for each of the control variables are shown in Figure 17-1. Although these waveforms are idealized, they are representative of waveform types produced by ventilators in current use.

The control variable is characterized by the ability to maintain a constant behavior despite the load, that is, changes in respiratory system resistance and compliance, imposed on the ventilator. Therefore the ability of a particular variable to retain its characteristic waveform in the face of changes in compliance and resistance distinguishes it as the control variable. The criteria for determining the control variable used by a ventilator are set forth in the algorithm in Figure 17-2.

Pressure. If the pressure waveform does not change with changes in patient compliance and resistance, the control variable is pressure. If the ventilator causes airway pressure to rise to greater than body surface pressure to effect inspiratory gas flow, the ventilator is a positive-pressure controller. Infant ventilators are generally used as positive-pressure controllers. If the ventilator causes body surface pressure to drop to less than airway pressure to create the gradient for gas flow, the ventilator is a negative-pressure controller (e.g., the Emerson iron lung; J.H. Emerson).

Volume. If the pressure waveform changes significantly with changes in resistance and compliance, the volume waveform is examined. If the volume waveform remains unchanged, the flow waveform also remains unchanged because volume and flow are functions of each other (i.e., flow is the change of volume over time and volume is flow divided by time).

The factor that distinguishes a volume controller from a flow controller is that a volume controller must measure volume and use the signal to control the volume waveform. Volume can be directly measured as the displacement of a piston or bellows (or similar device). With ventilators that use a piston or bellows compressor drive mechanism, controlling the excursion of the device controls the volume waveform. Examples of this type of volume controller are the Puritan Bennett MA-1 and the Emerson 3-MV. Alternatively, a volume signal can be derived from the integration of a flow signal.

Flow. If the volume (and flow) waveform remains essentially unchanged with changes in patient compliance and resistance, and delivered volume is not directly measured or used as a feedback signal, flow is the variable controlled by the ventilator. The Servo 900C (Maquet, Bridgewater, NJ), Servo 300A (Maquet), SERVO-i (Maquet), Evita 4 (Dräger Medical, Lübeck, Germany), Puritan Bennett 840 (Covidien), AVEA and Vela (Cardinal Health, Dublin, Ohio), Hamilton-G5 (Hamilton Medical, Bonaduz, Switzerland), Engström Carestation (GE Healthcare, Waukesha, WI), and V.I.P. Bird (Bird Products/Cardinal Health) are all flow controllers when delivering volume preset breaths, that is, they all measure flow and calculate volume. An infant ventilator that does not reach its preset pressure limit can be considered a flow controller rather than a pressure controller.

Time. If both pressure and volume outputs (and therefore pressure and volume waveforms) are significantly altered by changes in the imposed load, control must be defined in terms of the inspiratory and expiratory times. Thus time is the control variable. Some high-frequency ventilators can be best classified as time controllers.

Dual Control of the Inspiratory Phase. Dual control is possible if a ventilator has the ability to switch from one control variable to another if a certain

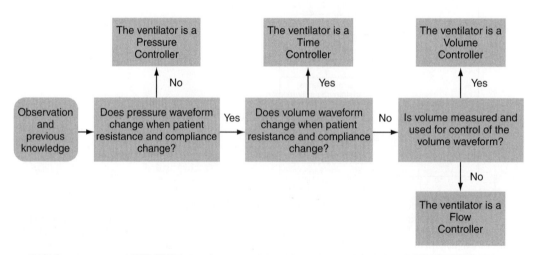

FIGURE 17-2 Criteria for determining the control variable during a ventilator-assisted inspiration.

condition is met, or not met, during the inspiratory phase.[7] Examples of dual control inspiration are volume-assured pressure-support ventilation, volume guarantee (VG), pressure-regulated volume control (PRVC), volume control plus (VC+), adaptive pressure control (APV), and volume support. With volume-assured pressure-support ventilation, inspiration is initially pressure controlled with variable gas flow to meet the patient's inspiratory demand. If a target tidal volume is not delivered during the pressure-controlled portion of the breath, the ventilator switches to flow control with a constant inspiratory flow to meet the tidal volume target.

Phase Variables

Mushin and colleagues[8] divided the ventilatory cycle into four phases:

Phase 1: The change from expiration to inspiration
Phase 2: Inspiration
Phase 3: The change from inspiration to expiration
Phase 4: Expiration

Phase variables (Figure 17-3) are the variables (pressure, volume, flow, and time) that are measured and used by the ventilator to initiate, sustain, or end a ventilatory phase.

Trigger. The variable responsible for initiating inspiration (the changeover from expiration to inspiration) is referred to as the *trigger variable*. Time is the trigger variable if inspiration is initiated by the ventilator at the end of a period determined by the set ventilator rate, whether

or not spontaneous breathing occurs. If the inspiratory phase is initiated by patient effort, one of the remaining variables—pressure, volume, or flow—is used as the trigger variable. Commonly, a ventilator senses patient effort as the drop in baseline pressure to a preset value. Volume and flow can also be used as trigger variables. Frequently, ventilators include a control that permits mandatory breaths to be manually triggered by the operator.

Considerable interest has been generated in the potential benefits of patient synchronization in the infant population. The Babylog 8000 *plus* (Dräger Medical) permits volume triggering of mandatory breaths.

The V.I.P. Bird infant–pediatric ventilator (Bird Products/Cardinal Health); the Servo 300, Servo 300A, and SERVO-i (Maquet); the Puritan Bennett 840 (Covidien); the AVEA (Cardinal Health), and the Evita 4 and EvitaXL (Dräger Medical) all incorporate a flow trigger. With the Star Sync option, the Puritan Bennett Infant Star 500 (Covidien) can be triggered by the change in pressure caused by the movement of the abdomen preceding inspiration.

The degree of patient effort required to trigger inspiration is referred to as the ventilator's *sensitivity*, which is adjusted by changing the set value of the trigger variable.

Limit. A variable that reaches a preset value before the end of inspiration is referred to as a *limit variable*. Pressure, volume, and flow can be limited. Time, however, cannot be a limit variable. If a preset time is reached during inspiration, the inspiration must be terminated.

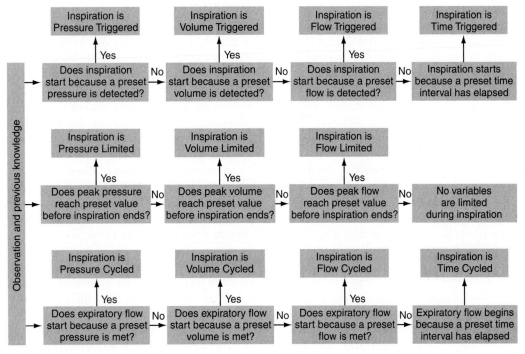

FIGURE 17-3 Criteria for determining the phase variables during a ventilator-assisted breath.

Infant ventilators are generally pressure limited. During inspiration, circuit pressure rises and is maintained at the preset pressure level until inspiration is terminated at the end of the inspiratory time interval. Ventilators used to deliver volume preset breaths often limit flow to a preset peak value. Inspiration is volume limited if an inspiratory pause is added to the inspiratory time of a volume preset breath.

Cycle. The end of inspiration (i.e., the changeover from inspiration to expiration) occurs because a particular measured variable reaches a preset value. The variable responsible for terminating the inspiratory phase is the cycle variable. Pressure, volume, flow, and time can all act as cycle variables.

Many of the newer microprocessor-controlled ventilators require selection of a peak flow and tidal volume, suggesting that inspiration is cycled because a certain volume has been delivered. In fact, these ventilators do not measure volume. Rather, they control flows over an interval of time necessary to deliver the desired tidal volume at the selected flow to produce a predetermined flow waveform. Because the inspiratory phase is cycled at the end of this predetermined inspiratory time interval, the breath is actually time cycled.

Pressure support breaths are typically cycled when inspiratory flow falls to a predetermined flow or percentage of the peak flow needed to reach the set pressure limit. Infant ventilators are generally time cycled. A ventilator may also have a backup or safety cycle variable. For example, inspiration may be pressure cycled if airway pressure reaches the value set on the high airway pressure alarm. Another example of a backup safety cycle variable is time; if inspiration does not meet preset pressure or flow criteria, the ventilator will cycle into exhalation on the basis of a predetermined time interval.

Baseline. With the changeover to expiration, flow, volume, and pressure return to their baseline values. Normally, expiratory flow ceases (and pressure and volume return to baseline) before the end of the expiratory phase. The variable controlled by the ventilator during the expiratory phase is the baseline variable. Although it is theoretically possible to control pressure, volume, or flow during the expiratory phase, the easiest variable to control from a practical standpoint is pressure. Positive end-expiratory pressure (PEEP) or continuous positive airway pressure (CPAP) is baseline pressure that is positive in relation to body surface pressure.

Modes of Ventilation

Figure 17-2 emphasizes that each breath has a specific pattern of control and phase variables and that the pattern may change from one breath to the next. A ventilator may deliver only mandatory breaths, may allow spontaneous breaths between mandatory breaths, or may combine different types of mandatory and spontaneous breaths. The type of breath, or combinations of breath types, permitted by a particular ventilator are dictated by the operational modes available on the ventilator. However, a mode name does not specifically describe the pattern or patterns of ventilation for that given mode. Thus a mode of ventilation can be more precisely described as a specific pattern of control and phase variables for both mandatory and spontaneous breaths.

Conditional Variables

Depending on the mode of ventilation, the ventilator must choose which pattern of control and phase variables to implement for each breath. The ventilator selects a particular pattern when a certain variable reaches a preset threshold value. A variable responsible for causing the ventilator to select a particular pattern of control and phase variables is the conditional variable. If the conditional variable reaches a certain preset value, one pattern is selected; if not, another pattern is selected.

For example, a ventilator may use pressure and time as conditional variables in the synchronized intermittent mandatory ventilation (SIMV) mode. In this example, breaths are either patient (pressure) triggered or machine (time) triggered, depending on whether the SIMV timing window is "open" or "closed" and on whether patient effort is detected.

Spontaneous versus Mandatory Breaths

All breaths may be categorized as either spontaneous or mandatory, depending on the degree of control the patient can exert over the initiation and termination of the breath. A breath is spontaneous if it is initiated by the patient and can be terminated with sufficient activity of the ventilatory muscles or by the effects of respiratory system mechanics. A mandatory breath is a ventilator-assisted breath that is either initiated or terminated by the ventilator.

Spontaneous breaths can be ventilator assisted (e.g., pressure support) or unassisted. Spontaneous breaths from demand flow systems or from continuous flow through the patient circuit are unassisted breaths. To provide demand flow, however, the ventilator responds to patient effort throughout the spontaneous inspiratory phase, so it is appropriate to describe the breath in terms of its phase variables. Because the ventilator provides flow in an attempt to maintain a constant baseline pressure, inspiration is pressure limited. When continuous flow alone is used, the ventilator does not respond to patient effort, and these spontaneous breaths are not controlled.[9]

Output

As a breath is delivered, changes in volume, pressure, and flow occur simultaneously over the course of inspiratory time. The magnitude of the changes in volume, pressure, and flow and the patterns produced by these variables constitute the ventilator's output and are represented by output waveforms.

The ventilator determines the control waveform, which by definition should not be significantly altered by the load imposed on the ventilator. The shapes of the other waveforms are a function of the control waveform and the patient's compliance and resistance. However, waveforms used to represent ventilator output are idealized. Because no ventilator is an ideal controller, even the control waveform will only approximate the ideal. Also, waveforms recorded during ventilation may be deformed by artifact caused by vibration and turbulence in the patient circuit.

The location of the devices used to measure output variables affects the output values and the shape of output waveforms. Pressure, volume, and flow measurements made inside the ventilator are invariably different from measurements made at the patient airway because of the effects of the patient circuit. Pressure measured back inside the ventilator on the inspiratory side is higher than pressure measured at the airway because of both the resistance and compliance of the patient circuit. Circuit compliance also causes volume and flow at the patient airway to be less than that leaving the ventilator. The relative amount of volume "lost" in the patient circuit may be particularly significant with the ventilation of infants and small children. Measurement of exhaled volume made inside the ventilator includes volume compressed in the patient circuit during inspiration and will not reflect the changes in compressed volume that may occur.

Some ventilators incorporate circuit compliance calculations in the preuse set-up, which allows the internal measurements to more accurately reflect actual exhaled volumes. It must be noted that all measurements (regardless of the source) are affected by patient airway leaks, and other variables such as active chest tube vacuum.

Alarm Systems

The purpose of ventilator alarms is to warn of inadvertent changes in ventilator performance and patient status. Thus ventilator alarm systems have been designed to monitor the mechanical and electronic functions of the ventilator and the variables involved in the mechanics of breathing—pressure, volume, flow, and time. Alarms can be categorized according to the same framework used to classify other ventilator functions.

Input Power Alarms

Alarms that signal loss of the power source or sources required for ventilator operation are the input power alarms. Alarms that indicate loss of electric power are activated with the interruption of that power, or they may signal a low battery state if the ventilator is operating on battery power. An alarm that indicates loss of pneumatic power is activated when there is a loss or critical reduction of compressed air or oxygen pressure.

Control Circuit Alarms

Activation of control circuit alarms may signal that a control is set improperly or warn of the incompatibility of a combination of control settings (e.g., an inverse inspiratory to expiratory [I/E] ratio). Control circuit alarms may also signal a fault in the control circuit itself, such as a failure of a microprocessor or related system. Alarms of this type may carry a generic warning such as "ventilator inoperative" or may include specific error codes to facilitate troubleshooting.

Output Alarms

Output alarms are activated when the value of a control variable or other ventilator output (e.g., inspired gas) falls outside an acceptable range. Alarm thresholds may be able to be adjusted by the operator, may automatically be set by the ventilator on the basis of control settings, or may have fixed thresholds set at the factory. Output alarms may signal changes in patient status or changes in ventilator performance.

Pressure alarms include those for high and low peak airway pressure, high and low mean airway pressure, high and low baseline pressure, and failure of airway pressure to return to baseline within a specified period. Alarms for high and low exhaled tidal volume and high and low exhaled minute ventilation warn of unacceptable values for volume and flow output, respectively. Alarms associated with time include those for high and low respiratory rate, an inspiratory time that is too long or too short, and an expiratory time that is too short or too long. Apnea alarms (an expiratory time that is too long) fall into this category. Alarms for inspired gas include those for high and low gas temperature and high and low fraction of inspired oxygen (FIO_2). Expired gas alarms include those for exhaled carbon dioxide tension and exhaled oxygen tension.

NEONATAL/INFANT CRITICAL CARE VENTILATORS

Bear Medical Systems Bear Cub 750vs

See Evolve Resources for information about the Bear Cub 750vs (Bear Medical Systems/Cardinal Health).

Dräger Medical Babylog 8000 *plus*

The Babylog 8000 *plus* (Dräger Medical) (Figure 17-4) is a pneumatically and electrically powered infant ventilator. The Babylog employs an electronic (microprocessor) and pneumatic control circuit to regulate a drive mechanism composed of pressure regulators, a bank of electromagnetic flow control valves, and a pneumatic diaphragm exhalation valve. The ventilator can be used as a pressure or flow controller. Mandatory breaths are volume or time triggered, pressure or flow limited, and time cycled. Continuous flow is available for spontaneous breathing. Alternatively, spontaneous breaths can be volume triggered, pressure limited, and flow cycled.[10]

Power Conversion and Transmission

The Babylog uses compressed air and oxygen in the range of 45 to 90 psig. Air and oxygen regulators reduce and match the source gas pressures and establish the constant pressure necessary for gas blending and flow regulation. The digital blender flow control system is composed of two sets of 10 solenoid valves, one set each for air and oxygen flows. The proportion of open valves for air and oxygen determines the oxygen concentration of inspired

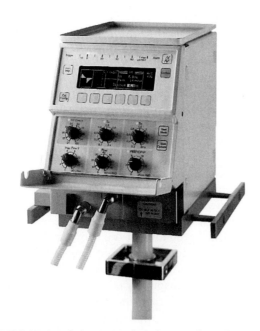

FIGURE 17-4 Babylog 8000 *plus* infant ventilator (Dräger Medical).

gas.[11] Flow from the expiratory limb of the patient circuit is controlled by a pneumatic diaphragm exhalation valve. A solenoid-regulated PEEP–peak inspiratory pressure (PIP) control valve generates the inspiratory and expiratory control pressures applied to the exhalation valve either to direct gas flow to the patient or to maintain baseline pressure. If the pressure in the patient circuit exceeds the pressure on the control side of the diaphragm, excess gas is vented out through the exhalation valve. An injector (Venturi) built into the exhalation valve block produces a negative pressure designed to prevent inadvertent PEEP in the patient circuit. Pressure is measured at the exhalation block by the expiratory pressure sensor.

Control

The Babylog can be operated in the following modes: IMV/continuous mandatory ventilation (CMV), SIMV, assist/control (A/C), and CPAP. A pressure support ventilation (PSV) mode and a volume guarantee (VG) option are also available in the SIMV, A/C, and PS modes.

Pressure-controlled mandatory breaths are pressure limited at the set inspiratory pressure limit (10 to 80 cm H_2O) and time cycled at the end of the set inspiratory time interval. The inspiratory flow is determined by the inspiratory flow setting (1 to 30 L/min). If airway pressure does not reach the set pressure limit, mandatory breaths are flow controlled and flow limited. Inspiration is pressure cycled before the end of set inspiratory time if the high inspiratory pressure alarm is activated.

In the IMV/CMV mode, mandatory breaths are time triggered at the set breath rate. The mandatory breath rate is determined as function of the inspiratory time (0.1 to 2 s) and expiratory time (0.2 to 30 s) settings and has a range of 2 to 150 breaths/minute. In the A/C and SIMV modes, a mandatory breath is volume triggered if the patient's measured inspiratory volume equals the set trigger volume (0.2 to 3 ml). Volume is derived from flow measured by a direction-sensitive hot wire anemometer flow sensor integrated into the Y-connector of the patient circuit. The flow signal is leak compensated so as to decrease the potential for autotriggering. If a spontaneous breath is not detected in the A/C and SIMV modes, a mandatory breath is time triggered at the end of an interval determined by the set breath rate. Mandatory breaths can be triggered manually in all modes.

Spontaneous breathing between mandatory breaths and in the CPAP mode is passively supported by continuous flow. The rate of continuous flow available for spontaneous breathing may be set separately from the inspiratory flow for mandatory inspiration, using the VIVE (variable inspiratory flow–variable expiratory flow) function. If this function is not used, the set inspiratory flow determines the continuous flow available for spontaneous breathing.

In the PSV mode, all breaths are patient triggered, pressure limited to the set inspiratory pressure level, and cycled to expiration when the inspiratory flow drops to 15% of the measured peak inspiratory flow. Alternatively, inspiration is time cycled if inspiratory flow does not fall to the flow-cycling threshold before the end of the set inspiratory time interval. Patient triggering occurs if spontaneous inspiratory volume meets the set volume-triggering criteria. In the absence of spontaneous effort, pressure-limited breaths are time triggered at a "backup" rate dictated by the inspiratory and expiratory time settings; flow cycling remains in effect.

With the volume guarantee (VG) option, a target tidal volume (2 to 100 ml) is set. On the basis of the exhaled tidal volume measurements from previous breaths, the ventilator adjusts the inspiratory pressure limit breath to breath, as needed, to deliver the target tidal volume. Thus VG is volume targeted and pressure controlled. VG can be used in the A/C, SIMV, and PSV modes. VG does not affect the triggering and cycling criteria otherwise applicable in each mode. Cycling criteria may be adjusted up to 30% of the peak inspiratory flow to compensate for leaks.

Baseline pressure is set in a range of 0 to 25 cm H_2O with the PEEP–CPAP control. The inspired oxygen concentration is set between 21% and 100% with the oxygen concentration control. The optional nebulizer uses room air at a flow of 2 L/min, so actual F_{IO_2} will decrease for the duration of the nebulizer treatment.

Table 17-1 summarizes the control and phase variables for mandatory and spontaneous breaths in the operational modes available on the Babylog 8000 *plus*.

Output

Waveforms. If mandatory breaths are pressure controlled, the inspiratory pressure waveform can be nearly rectangular or exponential, depending on specific control settings. The resultant volume and flow waveforms are exponential. Used as a flow controller, the ventilator produces an approximately rectangular inspiratory flow waveform. Pressure and volume waveforms are approximately ramp shaped.

Monitoring. The pressure or flow waveform is displayed in real time on the ventilator's monitoring screen. The sweep speed and scaling of waveforms are automatically adjusted.

Airway pressure is calculated from measurements made by the inspiratory and expiratory pressure sensors. The ventilator displays peak pressure, mean airway pressure, and baseline pressure (PEEP). Airway pressure is also continuously displayed on a bar graph.

Volume measurements include tidal volume, minute volume, and the fraction of minute volume contributed by spontaneous breathing. Endotracheal tube leakage is calculated from the difference between inspiratory and expiratory volumes. Displayed volumes are derived from flow measurements; because the flow sensor is positioned immediately adjacent to the endotracheal tube adapter, the measurements are not affected by continuous gas flow or compressible volume loss within the patient circuit. The measurement range of the flow sensor is 0.2 to 30 L/minute. Breathing frequency and breathing effort are also calculated from the flow signal.

TABLE 17-1

Control and Phase Variables for Mandatory and Spontaneous Breaths in the Operational Modes Available With the Dräger Medical Babylog 8000 *plus* Infant Ventilator

Mode	MANDATORY				SPONTANEOUS			
	Control	Trigger*	Limit	Cycle	Control	Trigger	Limit	Cycle
IMV/CMV	Pressure, flow[†]	Time	Pressure, flow[†]	Time, pressure[‡]	—	—	—	—
A/C[§]	Pressure, flow[†]	Time, volume	Pressure, flow[†]	Time, pressure[‡]	N/A	N/A	N/A	N/A
SIMV[§]	Pressure, flow[†]	Time, volume	Pressure, flow[†]	Time, pressure[‡]	—	—	—	—
CPAP	—	—	—	—	—	—	—	—
PSV[§]	N/A	N/A	N/A	N/A	Pressure	Volume, time	Pressure	Flow, time,[‡] pressure[‡]

Modified from Chatburn RL, Lough MD, Primiano FP Jr: Mechanical ventilation. In Chatburn RL, Lough MD, editors: *Handbook of respiratory care,* ed 2, St. Louis: Mosby; 1990. pp 159-223.
A/C, Assist/control; CMV, continuous mandatory ventilation; CPAP, continuous positive airway pressure; IMV, intermittent mandatory ventilation; N/A, not applicable; PSV, pressure support ventilation; SIMV, synchronized intermittent mandatory ventilation; —, ventilator does not respond.
* Mandatory breaths can be manually triggered in all modes.
[†] Applies if airway pressure does not reach the set pressure limit.
[‡] Secondary or safety cycle variable.
[§] When the volume guarantee (VG) option is active, the ventilator varies the inspiratory pressure limit as needed to deliver a target tidal volume. Thus VG breaths are pressure controlled. VG does not alter the trigger and cycle variables otherwise in effect.

The Babylog 8000 *plus* calculates and displays the lung mechanics parameters of resistance, dynamic compliance, respiratory time constants, C20/C (the ratio of compliance of the last 20% of the curve (C20) to total compliance [C]), and the rate-to-volume ratio. Inspired oxygen concentration is measured by the internal oxygen sensor near the ventilator's main flow outlet. A 24-hour trend of values for F_{IO_2}, as well as minute volume, mean airway pressure, compliance, resistance, and rate-to-volume ratio, is accessible.

The Babylog is equipped with analog and digital output connections.

Alarms

Ventilator alarms and alerts are grouped hierarchically as advisory, caution, and warning messages and are communicated in text on the ventilator's display screen. In addition, each grouping has a distinct audible signal intended to communicate an appropriate level of urgency. Alarm and alert messages are stored in the ventilator's "log," along with time of occurrence.

Input Power Alarms. A low air or low oxygen pressure alarm is activated if the respective gas pressure drops to less than 43.5 psig. The failure of one gas source causes the blender and flow control valves to be supplied with the remaining gas source. An electric power alarm occurs if operating voltages fall outside an acceptable range. If gas supply or electric power fails, ambient air can be drawn into the circuit via the nonreturn valve for spontaneous breathing.

Control Circuit Alarm. Failure of the microprocessor or associated components activates a ventilator malfunction alarm, which is accompanied by a specific error code message. Advisory messages signal faults in the electronic circuitry for individual ventilator controls. Failure of the pressure or flow sensor is also identified. A failure of the flow sensor inactivates patient triggering, flow/volume monitoring and associated alarms, as well as the volume guarantee function.

In addition, the ventilator alerts the operator to incompatible ventilator settings (i.e., mandatory breath rate exceeding 150 breaths/min and inspiratory pressure set at less than 5 cm H_2O above PEEP) or to settings that fall outside of "usual" ranges (i.e., inverse I/E ratio, inspiratory pressure greater than 40 cm H_2O, PEEP greater than 8 cm H_2O).

Output Alarms. Alarm limits for high inspiratory pressure and for low and high baseline pressure are automatically set relative to the specific control settings. If excess pressure builds in the circuit, the ventilator responds by opening the exhalation valve. The safety valve vents pressure if other high-pressure safety mechanisms fail. Airway pressure measurements are also used to trigger alarms that signal circuit obstruction or a leak

in the patient circuit. An alarm that indicates endotracheal tube obstruction is activated if the flow sensor does not detect gas movement during a complete mandatory breath cycle.

A high breath rate alarm limit and high and low thresholds for exhaled minute volume are operator selected. An apnea alarm condition occurs when no ventilation is detected (by the flow sensor) within the set apnea time interval. High and low oxygen concentration alarms are automatically set to ±4% of the selected oxygen concentration.

Puritan Bennett Infant Star 500

See Evolve Resources for information about the Puritan Bennett Infant Star 500 ventilator (Covidien).

Sechrist IV-200 With SAVI System

The Sechrist IV-200 ventilator with SAVI (synchronized assisted ventilation of infants) system (Sechrist Industries, Anaheim, Calif) (Figure 17-5) is a pneumatically and electrically powered ventilator that employs pneumatic, electronic, and fluidic control of a pneumatic diaphragm exhalation valve. The Sechrist IV-200 is a pressure or flow controller. Mandatory breaths are time triggered, pressure or flow limited, and time cycled. Inspiration may also be triggered and cycled by a thoracic impedance signal. Continuous flow is available for spontaneous breathing.[12]

Power Conversion and Transmission

Compressed air and oxygen at 50 psig supply an internal gas blender. The compressed air source also feeds the fluidic

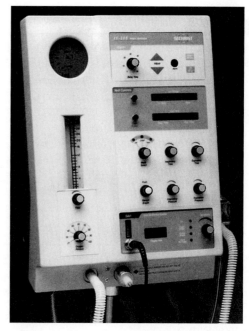

FIGURE 17-5 Sechrist IV-200 infant ventilator (Sechrist Industries).

control circuit. The blender mixes air and oxygen to the desired concentration and a flow control needle valve regulates continuous gas flow to the patient circuit.

All gas flow from the expiratory limb of the patient circuit is controlled by a pneumatic diaphragm exhalation valve. A microprocessor-controlled solenoid valve regulates the backpressure that acts on the fluidic control circuit, determining which of two control pressures (inspiratory or baseline) is transmitted to the exhalation valve diaphragm. During the inspiratory phase, the inspiratory control pressure is applied to the diaphragm, closing the exhalation valve and directing gas flow to the patient. When pressure in the patient circuit reaches the control pressure, the exhalation valve vents excess gas flow to maintain the set pressure limit. With a switch from inspiratory to baseline control pressure, gas from the patient circuit flows out through the exhalation valve and pressure in the patient circuit is maintained at the baseline setting.

An injector jet in the exhalation block creates a slight negative pressure on the patient side of the exhalation valve, eliminating inadvertent PEEP caused by circuit resistance to continuous and expiratory gas flow.

Control

The Sechrist IV-200 can be operated in two modes: vent and CPAP. The vent mode can be used to provide either IMV or assist-control ventilation. Mandatory breaths are pressure or flow controlled.

When the ventilator is used to provide IMV, mandatory breaths are time triggered at a rate determined by the inspiratory time (0.10 to 2.9 s) and expiratory time (0.3 to 60 s) settings. Thus the ventilator has a breath rate range of 1 to 150 breaths/minute. The selected inspiratory and expiratory times, as well as the resulting breath rate and I/E ratio, are displayed digitally.

Mandatory breaths are pressure limited at the set inspiratory pressure (5 to 70 cm H_2O) and time cycled at the end of the selected inspiratory time interval. If set so that pressure in the patient circuit does not reach the set pressure limit, the ventilator functions as a flow controller and inspiration is flow limited. The proximal airway pressure waveform control is a needle valve that varies the response time of the exhalation valve. The waveform control can be set to produce a pressure waveform ranging from nearly rectangular to approximately sinusoidal.

The SAVI system uses the change in electrical impedance caused by chest movement during inspiration and expiration to patient trigger mandatory breaths. With SAVI, IMV becomes A/C ventilation. SAVI processes the impedance signal generated by a neonatal cardiorespiratory monitor. As the chest expands during inspiration, impedance increases. When the impedance value reaches the set sensitivity threshold, SAVI sends a trigger signal to the ventilator's microprocessor to initiate a machine-assisted inspiratory phase as described previously. Sensitivity is set with a nongraduated control with a range of minimum to maximum. Moving the sensitivity setting from minimal toward maximal increases the trigger sensitivity by decreasing the impedance value that SAVI must detect as the trigger value.

When SAVI is employed, the inspiratory phase is cycled to expiration by the impedance signal if the change in thoracic impedance indicates the onset of active expiration before the end of the set inspiratory time interval. If SAVI is switched off, or if the impedance signal is lost, the Sechrist IV-200 reverts to IMV and breaths are time triggered, pressure limited, and time cycled according to the ventilator settings.

The continuous gas flow (0 to 32 L/min) is regulated with the blender flowmeter and determines the flow for mandatory inspiration as well as the continuous flow available for spontaneous breathing in both the vent and CPAP modes. Expiratory pressure (baseline pressure) can be set in an approximate range of –2 to 20 cm H_2O. A slightly negative baseline pressure is possible because of the action of the injector jet at the exhalation valve.

Mandatory breaths can be manually triggered in both operational modes. Inspiration is pressure limited and sustained for as long as the manual breath button is depressed. The manual breath control is independent of ventilator electronics; therefore manual breaths can be given as long as pneumatic power is available.

The oxygen concentration control on the Sechrist air–oxygen mixer is set between 21% and 100%. A spring-loaded safety pressure relief valve can be set in an approximate range of 15 to 85 cm H_2O.

Table 17-2 summarizes the control and phase variables for both mandatory and spontaneous breaths in the Sechrist IV-200 operational modes.

Output

Waveforms. If the waveform control is set to produce a rectangular pressure waveform, the flow waveform exhibits an exponential decay and the volume waveform shows an exponential rise. A sinusoidal pressure waveform dictates that the volume and flow waveforms are also sinusoidal. If the ventilator functions as a flow controller, the inspiratory flow waveform is approximately rectangular and the pressure and volume waveforms are ascending ramp shaped.

Monitoring. An electronic pressure manometer on the ventilator provides a bar graph display of airway pressure that simulates the movement of a mechanical pressure gauge. Mean airway pressure is displayed digitally and is the average of the mean pressure of the last four machine-delivered breaths updated with each breath.

TABLE 17-2

Control and Phase Variables for Mandatory and Spontaneous Breaths in the Operational Modes Available With the Sechrist IV-200 Ventilator With SAVI System

Mode	Mandatory				Spontaneous			
	Control	Trigger*	Limit	Cycle	Control	Trigger	Limit	Cycle
Vent-IMV	Pressure, flow[†]	Time	Pressure, flow[†]	Time	—	—	—	—
Vent-A/C[‡]	Pressure, flow[†]	Time, patient[§]	Pressure, flow[†]	Time, patient[§]	N/A	N/A	N/A	N/A
CPAP	—	—	—	—	—	—	—	—

Modified from Chatburn RL, Lough MD, Primiano FP Jr: Mechanical ventilation. In Chatburn RL, Lough MD, editors: *Handbook of respiratory care*, ed 2, St. Louis: Mosby; 1990. pp 159-223.

A/C, Assist/control; CPAP, continuous positive airway pressure; IMV, intermittent mandatory ventilation; N/A, not applicable; SAVI, synchronized assisted ventilation of infants; —, ventilator does not respond.

* Mandatory breaths can be manually triggered in all modes. Inspiration extends for as long as the manual button is pressed.

[†] Applies if airway pressure does not reach the set limit.

[‡]Available only if the SAVI system is employed.

[§] With SAVI, mandatory breaths are patient triggered, and may be cycled to expiration, by the change in electrical impedance caused by chest movement during inspiration and expiration.

The SAVI unit displays information related to patient triggering. A bar graph provides a visual indicator of the changes in thoracic impedance over the inspiratory/expiratory cycle. A trigger breath indicator flashes with every patient-triggered breath and the patient trigger rate is digitally displayed.

Alarms

Input Power Alarms. No specific ventilator alarms signal the failure of either electric or pneumatic power. However, the Sechrist air–oxygen mixer is equipped with a low inlet pressure alarm. An inlet pressure differential of more than 23 psig triggers an audible pneumatic alarm. This condition also causes a proportioning system bypass so that the gas of the higher pressure supplies the patient circuit.

Control Circuit Alarms. If set inspiratory time exceeds expiratory time, the ventilator's inverse I/E light illuminates. With the SAVI system on, the control breath indicator flashes with every time-triggered (non–patient-triggered) breath. Persistent failure to detect a patient trigger (impedance signal) results in a progression from an alert to an alarm condition. If SAVI cannot detect an impedance signal, the ventilator reverts to IMV.

Output Alarms. High and low airway pressure alarms are incorporated into the electronic pressure manometer. Limits for the pressure alarm are operator adjustable. The low-pressure alarm is activated in response to a number of conditions, including circuit leaks (low airway pressure), circuit disconnection (loss of pressure), microprocessor failure (failure to trigger or cycle a breath), electric or pneumatic power loss, and prolonged inspiration.

The Sechrist model 600 airway pressure monitor is an accessory that can be used with the Sechrist IV-200 to enhance monitoring and alarm capabilities. The monitor can also be equipped with a vent-to-ambient pressure feature that vents patient circuit pressure to near ambient pressure if an overpressure condition is detected. Importantly, the reset button should not be pressed before the cause of an overpressure condition is resolved because resetting the system allows pressure to be generated in the patient circuit.

UNIVERSAL NEONATAL/INFANT/PEDIATRIC/ADULT CRITICAL CARE VENTILATORS

V.I.P. Bird

See Evolve Resources for information about the V.I.P. Bird and V.I.P. Gold ventilator.

Cardinal Health AVEA

The AVEA ventilator (Cardinal Health) (Figure 17-6) is a pneumatically and electrically powered, electronically (microprocessor) and pneumatically controlled ventilator approved for use in neonatal, pediatric, and adult patients. The AVEA is a flow or pressure controller. Mandatory breaths are time or flow triggered; flow, volume, or pressure limited; and time cycled. Spontaneous breaths are flow or pressure triggered, pressure limited, and flow or pressure cycled.[13]

Power Conversion and Transmission

The AVEA software-driven ventilator uses compressed air and oxygen in a range of 20 to 80 psig. An internal battery backup will last for up to 2 hours should electrical power be interrupted.

Control

The AVEA can be operated in the A/C (volume controlled, pressure controlled, PRVC, and time-cycled

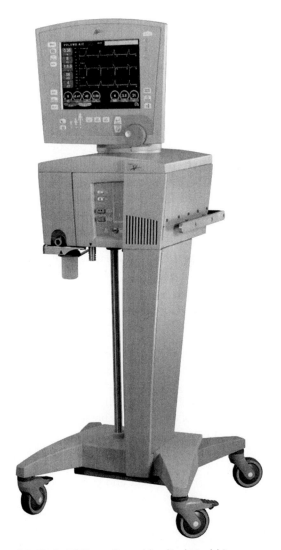

FIGURE 17-6 AVEA ventilator (Cardinal Health).

pressure-limited TCPL), SIMV (volume controlled, pressure controlled, PRVC, and time-cycled pressure-limited TCPL), CPAP/PSV noninvasive, and biphasic (APRV) modes. The PRVC and biphasic options are available for pediatric and adult use, whereas the TCPL option is available only in the neonatal mode.

In volume breath delivery the breaths are flow controlled, volume or pressure limited, and volume or time cycled. Demand flow is available to patients at any point during inspiration to enhance patient comfort. During pressure or TCPL breath delivery breaths are pressure controlled, pressure or time limited, and time or flow cycled. In PRVC breath delivery breaths are pressure or volume controlled, pressure or time limited, and time or pressure cycled. In biphasic modes pressure support breath augmentation can occur during the high-PEEP or low-PEEP phase.

Clinician-controlled parameters are as follows: respiratory rate, 1 to 120 breaths/minute; tidal volume (V_T):

2 to 300 ml (neonatal), 25 to 500 ml (pediatric), and 100 to 2500 ml (adult); PIP, 0 to 80 cm H_2O (neonatal) and 0 to 90 cm H_2O (adult/pediatric); peak flow: 0.4 to 30 L/minute (neonatal), 1 to 75 L/minute (pediatric), and 3 to 150 L/minute (adult); inspiratory time, 0.15 to 3.0 second (neonatal) and 0.2 to 5.0 second (adult/pediatric); PSV, 0 to 80 cm H_2O (neonatal) and 0 to 90 cm H_2O (adult/pediatric); PEEP, 0 to 50 cm H_2O; flow trigger, 0.1 to 20 L/minute; APRV PEEP limits: high, 0 to 90 cm H_2O; and low, 0 to 45 cm H_2O with time limits of 0.20 to 30 seconds (high and low).

Other useful features include the following: suction breaths in which FIO_2 is increased to 100% in the adult/pediatric mode and by 20% above set FIO_2 in the neonatal mode, and apnea ventilation in A/C, SIMV, CPAP/PSV, and APRV modes. The rise feature in pressure-controlled (PC) and pressure-supported (PS) breath delivery allows the clinician to adjust the slope of pressure rise during inspiration (from 1 to 9, with 1 the slowest), and the PSV cycle allows for adjustments in inspiratory flow criteria to terminate PS breaths (5% to 45%). During the ventilator check procedure circuit volume loss is calculated and compensated for in the volume breath delivery and pressure breath delivery V_T calculations.

There are a number of limits on the AVEA that set criteria for volume and time during breath delivery. The Tmax time in PSV sets a time termination for PS breaths ranging from 0.15 to 3.0 seconds (neonatal) and from 0.2 to 5.0 seconds (adult/pediatric). The volume limit sets a maximal inspiratory V_T during pressure-based breaths and provides a visual indication that this has occurred. The machine volume controls the minimal inspiratory V_T delivered during pressure-based breaths by adding flow to meet the minimal V_T. PEEP compensation is also provided by adding flow to the patient circuit when baseline pressure is not maintained. Sigh breaths are available if selected in the adult/pediatric modes.

Output

Waveforms. Decelerating or square waveforms can be selected for volume breath delivery; pressure-based delivery results in decelerating waveforms but will be influenced by the rise setting.

Monitoring. The AVEA has extensive monitoring capabilities, including patient parameters; pressure, flow, and volume waveforms; and flow–volume loops. Esophageal pressure volume loops and tracheal pressure volume loops can be monitored with the optional esophageal balloon and tracheal catheters. The patient monitoring screen can be configured by the operator to include 5 monitored parameters in the main screen and 15 monitored parameters in the monitor screen.

The neonatal mode allows for airway monitoring with an airway sensor placed proximal to the patient.

Alarms

The ventilator incorporates a safety valve whenever a condition exists that results in lack of operation (VENT INOP); this allows the patient to breath room air spontaneously. All alarms are prioritized on the basis of the severity of the alarm condition and are classified as high, medium, or low priority.

Input Power Alarms. A loss of air or oxygen pressure below 18 psig results in a high-priority alarm; if one gas pressure is affected the remaining gas line will provide sufficient gas flow. If both gas sources are lost or if any condition resulting in VENT INOP occurs the safety valve will open and allow for spontaneous breathing.

Control Circuit Alarms. The AVEA incorporates default alarm parameters based on the patient selection; however, the operator may adjust the default alarm parameters to be consistent with set patient parameters. Adjustable alarm settings include the following: low peak airway pressure, high peak airway pressure, low PEEP, low minute volume, high minute volume, high V_T, apnea, and high respiratory rate. Preset alarms exist for high and low F_{IO_2}, I/E ratios, and inspiratory time limit.

Dräger Medical Evita 4 and EvitaXL

The Evita 4 (Dräger Medical) (Figure 17-7) is a pneumatically and electrically powered, electronically (microprocessor) and pneumatically controlled ventilator designed for adult and pediatric use. An option for extending use to the neonatal range is also available with the NeoFlow option. The Evita 4 is a flow or pressure controller. Mandatory breaths are time or flow triggered; flow, volume, or pressure limited; and time cycled. Spontaneous breaths are flow or pressure triggered, pressure limited, and flow or pressure cycled.[14,15]

Power Conversion and Transmission

The Evita 4 uses compressed air and oxygen in a range of 43.5 to 87 psig. The gases are regulated down to a pressure of about 29 psig before entering parallel air/oxygen electromagnetic proportional flow control valves. Each valve is composed of a linear motor and driver that regulates the size of the valve opening. A microprocessor controls the position of the motor and driver of both valves to proportion the gases to the set oxygen concentration and to provide the required inspiratory gas flow. The inspiratory gas flow is calculated by the microprocessor from the gas pressure and the size of the inspiratory valve opening as determined by the position of the valve driver. Blended gas flows past the oxygen sensor and the inspiratory pressure transducer before entering the patient circuit.

Gas from the expiratory limb of the patient circuit is controlled by a pneumatic exhalation valve. The PEEP/PIP solenoid valve generates a control pressure that is applied to the exhalation valve diaphragm. During the inspiratory phase of a mandatory breath, the inspiratory control pressure is applied, closing the exhalation valve. During pressure-controlled ventilation, this "floating" exhalation valve opens and closes as needed to maintain the target pressure limit and to accommodate the patient's spontaneous breathing activity. Excess gas flow is vented through the valve to atmosphere. With the onset of the expiratory phase, control pressure to the exhalation diaphragm switches to the PEEP setting.

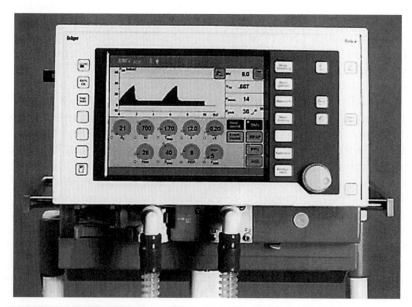

FIGURE 17-7 Evita 4 ventilator (Dräger Medical).

The exhalation valve diaphragm moves away from the valve opening, allowing exhalation to occur, and circuit pressure drops to baseline. The expiratory pressure sensor monitors pressure at the exhalation valve. The expiratory flow sensor measures expiratory gas flow.

Control

The Evita 4 can be operated in the following ventilation modes: CMV, SIMV, mandatory minute ventilation (MMV), pressure-controlled ventilation (PCV), airway pressure release ventilation (APRV), and CPAP. Pressure support can be used to augment spontaneous breaths in the SIMV, PCV, MMV, and CPAP modes. The AutoFlow and pressure-limited ventilation (PLV) extensions can be used to modify mandatory breaths in the CMV, SIMV, and MMV modes. The EvitaXL also offers a noninvasive (NIV) mode with automatic leak compensation up to 30 L/minute. In addition, an apnea ventilation mode is available. Selection of the adult or pediatric patient range determines the range of available tidal volume, set inspiratory flow, and maximal inspiratory flow availability (adult, 180 L/min; pediatric, 60 L/min; neonatal, up to 30 L/min with the NeoFlow option). The ventilator can be configured to choose default ventilation control settings on the basis of the entered ideal patient body weight.

NeoFlow is an available option that extends the patient range of the Evita 4 and EvitaXL to infants and neonates as small as 0.5 kg. NeoFlow uses a hot wire anemometer-type flow sensor located at the patient Y-connector. The flow sensor provides the signal for patient triggering as well as flow and volume monitoring. These flow and volume measurements are compensated for gas leakage around the endotracheal tube. When NeoFlow is used in the CMV, SIMV, and MMV modes, AutoFlow is always active. With NeoFlow, the Evita 4 provides a base gas flow of 6 L/minute through the patient circuit and an inspiratory gas flow of up to 30 L/minute.

The "basic" mandatory breath in the CMV, SIMV, and MMV modes is flow controlled and requires setting tidal volume (adult, 100 to 2000 ml; pediatric, 20 to 300 ml; neonatal, 3 to 100 ml), a breath rate of 0 to 100 breaths/minute (0 to 150 breaths/min with NeoFlow), inspiratory flow (adult, 6 to 120 L/min; pediatric/neonatal, 6 to 30 L/min), and inspiratory time (0.1 to 10 s). During inspiration, gas is delivered at the set flow (flow limit) for the duration of time necessary to deliver the set tidal volume; the inspiratory phase is time cycled at the end of the set inspiratory time interval. If the tidal volume is delivered before the end of the set inspiratory time, inspiratory flow ceases and an inspiratory pause occurs for the remainder of the inspiratory time interval. Depending on the duration of the inspiratory pause, inspiratory pressure may plateau.

If the PLV option is used, a maximal pressure (P_{max}) is set. The mandatory breath is initially delivered at the set flow, as described earlier. However, if peak inspiratory pressure reaches the set P_{max}, the ventilator effectively becomes a pressure controller, limiting inspiratory pressure to the set P_{max}. In this case, the inspiratory gas flow does not remain constant. If the measured inspiratory volume reaches the set tidal volume before the end of the set inspiratory time interval, inspiratory gas flow ceases and volume is held (limited) until the end of the inspiratory phase. If inspiratory gas flow does not reach zero before the end of set inspiratory time, the set tidal volume will not be delivered.

If the AutoFlow function is used, the ventilator acts as a pressure controller. Set tidal volume becomes a target tidal volume. On the basis of the measured tidal volume and inspiratory pressure of previously delivered mandatory breaths, the ventilator incrementally adjusts the pressure limit for subsequent breaths to maintain the target tidal volume. Thus inspiration is pressure limited at the pressure that the ventilator calculates is necessary to deliver the target tidal volume and time cycled at the end of set inspiratory time. Alternatively, the inspiratory phase is volume cycled before the end of the set inspiratory time interval if measured volume reaches the set high inspired tidal volume alarm setting. With AutoFlow, the ventilator coordinates the action of the inspiratory flow control valves and exhalation valve to accommodate spontaneous breathing at any point during both the inspiratory and expiratory phases.

In the CMV mode, all breaths are mandatory. These breaths are either time triggered at an interval determined by the set breath rate or flow triggered if a patient's spontaneous inspiratory flow meets the set flow trigger sensitivity (1 to 15 L/min; 0.3 to 15 L/min with NeoFlow). In SIMV, mandatory breaths are time or flow triggered at the set SIMV breath rate. Spontaneous breaths between mandatory breaths are supported with demand flow. Demand flow is triggered when circuit pressure falls 0.2 cm H_2O below set PEEP and is provided, as needed, to maintain the PEEP setting. In the CPAP mode, all breaths are spontaneous and are supported by demand flow. Spontaneous breaths in the CPAP and SIMV modes may also be pressure supported as described later.

The MMV mode provides mandatory breaths only to the extent that spontaneous minute volume does not meet the preselected minimal minute ventilation. Minimal minute volume is a product of the breath rate and tidal volume settings. If exhaled minute volume drops below minimum, mandatory breaths are time or flow triggered, as needed, to maintain the target minute volume. In MMV, spontaneous breaths may be pressure supported or simply supported with demand flow.

In the pressure-controlled ventilation (PCV) mode, mandatory breaths are time or flow triggered at the set breath rate, pressure limited at the set inspiratory pressure level, and time cycled at the end of the set inspiratory time interval. As with AutoFlow, spontaneous breathing is permitted at any point during either the inspiratory or expiratory phase. Pressure support can be set to augment spontaneous breaths that occur between mandatory breaths.

Pressure support ventilation (PSV) must be patient triggered. With PSV, patient triggering occurs if the spontaneous inspiratory flow reaches the set flow-trigger sensitivity or if inspired volume exceeds 25 ml (12 ml in the pediatric mode; 1 ml with NeoFlow). PSV is pressure limited to the set pressure support level (0 to 80 cm H_2O) and cycled to expiration when inspiratory flow falls to a percentage of peak flow determined by the patient range selection. The flow cycling threshold is 25% of peak inspiratory flow in the adult mode, 6% of peak flow in the pediatric mode, and 15% of peak flow in the neonatal mode. Alternatively, inspiration is time cycled if inspiratory flow does not fall to the flow-cycling threshold within 4 seconds (1.5 s in the pediatric mode; at the end of the set inspiratory time interval with NeoFlow).

Airway pressure release ventilation (APRV) permits spontaneous breathing at two levels of positive airway pressure. The magnitude, as well as the duration, of the high and low levels of positive pressure is set separately. Typically, the patient breathes spontaneously at the higher pressure with only brief periods of release to the lower pressure level.

The pressure rise time setting determines the rate of increase in airway pressure from baseline (at the onset of inspiration) to the set pressure limit for all pressure-controlled breaths. Rise time is set in a range of 0 to 2 seconds and influences the ventilator's initial inspiratory gas flow. With rise time set to zero, the ventilator seeks to reach target pressure almost immediately, requiring a relatively high initial inspiratory flow. Increasing rise time causes peak pressure to be reached later in the inspiratory phase. For example, setting rise time to 0.5 second directs the ventilator to reach the target inspiratory pressure 0.5 second from the onset of inspiration. Increasing rise time effectively reduces the peak inspiratory flow delivered during inspiration. Rise time can be used to modify mandatory breaths in the pressure-controlled ventilation (PCV) mode, AutoFlow mandatory breaths in all modes, and PSV breaths. In addition, rise time determines how quickly the high-pressure level is reached during APRV.

Baseline pressure is set in a range of 0 to 35 cm H_2O, using the PEEP/CPAP control. Activation of the intermittent PEEP function provides increased end-expiratory pressure ("expiratory sighs") for two mandatory breaths every 3 minutes in the CMV mode. Oxygen concentration is set in a range of 21% to 100%. Oxygen concentration can be temporarily increased above what is set by pressing the Suction O_2 key. Activation of the "Neb" control key supplies gas flow to a micronebulizer for up to 30 minutes. Pressing and holding the inspiratory hold button creates an inspiratory pause for up to 15 seconds. Apnea ventilation provides mandatory ventilation at predetermined settings if the ventilator detects apnea.

Table 17-3 summarizes the control and phase variables for mandatory and spontaneous breaths in the operational modes available on the Evita 4 ventilator.

Output

Waveforms. To deliver volume-preset, flow-controlled breaths, the Evita 4 uses a constant inspiratory flow that produces an approximately rectangular inspiratory flow waveform. The resulting pressure and volume waveforms take the shape of an ascending ramp. If set volume is delivered before the end of set inspiratory time, both the pressure and volume waveforms tend to form a plateau from the point at which inspiratory gas flow stops. If circuit pressure reaches the set P_{max} (added using the PLV function), the flow waveform exhibits exponential decay beginning at the point at which the pressure limit is reached. The pressure waveform, which is initially ramp shaped, forms a plateau.

The inspiratory pressure waveform for pressure-controlled mandatory breaths (PCV and AutoFlow) is greatly influenced by the pressure rise time setting. If rise time is set to 0, the pressure waveform is essentially rectangular. The addition of rise time creates a ramp up to the pressure plateau. The ramp becomes less steep as rise time is increased. With pressure control, the resulting inspiratory flow waveform exhibits an exponential decay and the volume waveform shows an exponential rise. As rise time is added, the magnitude of the inspiratory flow waveform decreases (reflecting a decrease in peak flow).

Monitoring. The Evita 4 monitoring screen can be operator configured to display various combinations of numeric and graphic data. Values for peak pressure, mean airway pressure, plateau pressure, and PEEP are displayed numerically on the ventilator's monitoring screen. Exhaled tidal volume and minute ventilation are derived from measurements made by the ventilator's hot wire anemometer-type expiratory flow sensor. However, these measurements are corrected to eliminate the effects of gas compressed in the patient circuit and thus reflect effective volume delivery. When the NeoFlow option is used, monitored flow and volume

TABLE 17-3

Control and Phase Variables for Mandatory and Spontaneous Breaths in the Operational Modes Available on the Dräger Medical Evita 4 Ventilator

Mode	MANDATORY				SPONTANEOUS			
	Control*	Trigger[†]	Limit	Cycle	Control*	Trigger	Limit	Cycle
CMV	Flow, pressure[‡]	Time, flow	Flow, volume, pressure[‡]	Time, volume,[§] pressure[§]	N/A	N/A	N/A	N/A
CMV-AutoFlow	Pressure	Time, flow	Pressure	Time, volume,[§] pressure[§]	N/A	N/A	N/A	N/A
SIMV	Flow, pressure[‡]	Time, flow	Flow, volume, pressure[‡]	Time, volume,[§] pressure[§]	Pressure	Pressure	Pressure	Pressure
SIMV-AutoFlow	Pressure	Time, flow	Pressure	Time, volume,[§] pressure[§]	Pressure	Pressure	Pressure	Pressure
MMV	Flow, pressure[‡]	Time, flow	Flow, volume, pressure[‡]	Time, volume,[§] pressure[§]	Pressure	Pressure	Pressure	Pressure
MMV-AutoFlow	Pressure	Time, flow	Pressure	Time, volume,[§] pressure[§]	Pressure	Pressure	Pressure	Pressure
PCV+	Pressure	Time, flow	Pressure	Time, pressure[§]	Pressure	Pressure	Pressure	Pressure
CPAP	N/A	N/A	N/A	N/A	Pressure	Pressure	Pressure	Pressure
PS[¶]	N/A	N/A	N/A	N/A	Pressure	Flow	Pressure	Flow, time,[§] pressure[§]
APRV	Pressure	Time	Pressure	Time	Pressure	Pressure	Pressure	Pressure

Modified from Chatburn RL, Lough MD, Primiano FP Jr: Mechanical ventilation. In Chatburn RL, Lough MD, editors: *Handbook of respiratory care*, ed 2, St. Louis: Mosby; 1990. pp 159-223.

CMV, Continuous mandatory ventilation; N/A, not applicable; SIMV, synchronized intermittent mandatory ventilation; MMV, mandatory minute ventilation; CPAP, continuous positive airway pressure; PS, pressure support; PCV+, pressure-controlled ventilation; APRV, airway pressure release ventilation.

* The Rise Time setting can be used to modify the shape of the inspiratory pressure waveform for all mandatory pressure-controlled breaths and pressure-supported spontaneous breaths.

[†] Mandatory breaths can be manually triggered.

[‡] Applies if the pressure-limited ventilation (PLV) function is used.

[§] Secondary or safety cycle variable.

[¶] Considered here as a separate mode, but can be used to support spontaneous breaths in the SIMV, MMV, PCV+, and CPAP modes.

values reflect measurements made at the patient airway (Y-connector). Breath rate includes both mandatory and spontaneous breaths.

The Evita 4 has the ability to calculate and display a number of pulmonary mechanics measures, including compliance, resistance, intrinsic (auto) PEEP, the volume of trapped gas, and occlusion pressure ($P = 0.1$ maneuver). The ventilator integrates data from its mainstream end-tidal carbon dioxide and flow sensors to yield volumetric carbon dioxide–related values for carbon dioxide production ($\dot{V}_{CO_2}$), dead space, and dead space-to-tidal volume ratio. Graphics monitoring includes waveforms for pressure, flow, volume, and exhaled carbon dioxide as well as flow–volume and pressure–volume loops. Oxygen concentration is measured by a sensor located near the inspiratory flow control valve. Values for most of the preceding monitored values are stored and may be displayed as trends.

Analog and digital output connections are available.

Alarms

Alarms and alerts on the Evita 4 are prioritized and identified by differing audible and visual signals and text messages to indicate the specific level of urgency.

Input Power Alarms. A low air or oxygen supply pressure alarm is activated if the respective gas pressure falls below 43.5 psig. A high gas supply pressure alarm occurs if either gas pressure exceeds 87 psig. Loss of either supply gas will cause an automatic switchover to the remaining supply gas. A failure-to-cycle alarm activates if no gas flow is delivered by the ventilator.

Control Circuit Alarms. A number of alarm messages signify problems with the ventilator's control components. These include failure of the flow sensor, malfunction of the gas blender, loss of the expiratory pressure measurement, and malfunction of the exhalation valve.

Output Alarms. Output alarms include an operator-adjustable high airway pressure alarm and a low airway pressure alarm that is automatically set 5 cm H_2O above the PEEP setting. A high-PEEP alarm activates owing to a sustained increase in circuit pressure. Alarm limits for high tidal volume, high and low minute volume, apnea, and high spontaneous breath rate are operator adjustable. The low-volume alarm indicates that the delivered inspiratory tidal volume did not reach the set tidal volume. Alarm limits for high and low oxygen concentration are automatically set relative to the selected oxygen concentration. High and low alarm limits for end-tidal carbon dioxide can also be set.

Puritan Bennett 840

The Puritan Bennett 840 (Covidien) (Figure 17-8) is a pneumatically and electrically (AC or internal battery)

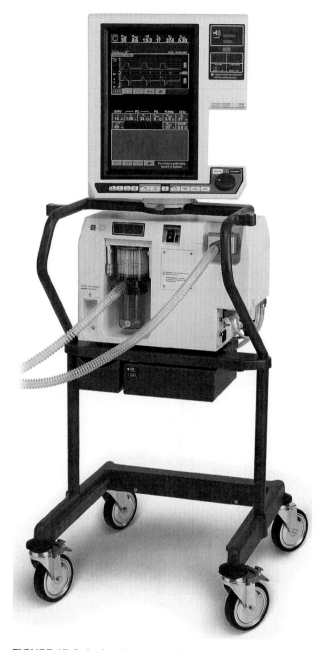

FIGURE 17-8 Puritan Bennett 840 ventilator (Covidien).

powered, electronically (microprocessor) controlled ventilator designed for use with infant, pediatric, and adult patients. Power conversion and transmission are accomplished with pressure regulators, dual proportional solenoid flow control valves, and an electromagnetic exhalation valve. The Puritan Bennett 840 is a flow or pressure controller. Mandatory breaths are time, pressure, or flow triggered; flow, volume, or pressure limited; and time cycled. Spontaneous breaths are flow or pressure triggered, pressure limited, and flow cycled.[16,17]

Power Conversion and Transmission

The Puritan Bennett 840 uses compressed air and oxygen in a range of 35 to 100 psig. Compressed air can be supplied by the optional 806 compressor unit. Air and oxygen gas pressures are reduced and matched to approximately 11 psig for use at separate proportional solenoid flow control valves. A microprocessor regulates the opening size of each solenoid to proportion gases to the set oxygen concentration and to provide the required inspiratory gas flow. The flow for each valve is calculated by the microprocessor as a function of the driving pressure of each gas and the size of the valve opening as determined by the position of the solenoid. Blended gas passes a safety valve and the inspiratory pressure transducer before entering the patient circuit.

Gas from the expiratory limb of the patient circuit is controlled by an electromagnetic exhalation valve. The exhalation valve adjusts rapidly and in small increments (in conjunction with the inspiratory flow control valves) to regulate breath phasing. During the inspiratory phase, the exhalation valve closes so that inspiratory gas flow is directed to the patient. During pressure-controlled ventilation, the exhalation valve opens and closes as needed to maintain the set inspiratory pressure limit. At the end of the inspiratory phase for all breath types, the valve opens to permit exhalation and then adjusts as necessary to maintain the set baseline pressure. Circuit pressure is measured at the exhalation valve by the expiratory pressure transducer, and gas flow through the valve is measured by the expiratory flow sensor.

Control

The Puritan Bennett 840 can be operated in the following modes: A/C, SIMV, spontaneous, and noninvasive. Mandatory breaths in the A/C and SIMV modes can be set as either pressure control or volume control. Pressure support can be used to augment spontaneous breaths in all modes that permit spontaneous breathing. An apnea ventilation mode and a safety ventilation mode are also available. BiLevel, mode VC+, and noninvasive ventilation are available options.

When the volume-controlled mandatory breath type is chosen, tidal volume, peak flow, and flow pattern must be set. The tidal volume range of the ventilator is 5 to 2500 ml dependent on patient category selection criteria. However, the ideal body weight (IBW; range, 0.5 to 150 kg) entered during the patient setup procedure determines the absolute limits for tidal volume and peak flow settings. The peak flow range is 1 to 150 L/minute for adult patient selection, 3 to 60 L/minute for pediatric patient selection, and 1 to 30 L/minute for neonatal patient selection. The inspiratory flow pattern can be set to square (rectangular) or descending ramp shaped. On the basis of the patient circuit compliance calculated by the ventilator, tidal volume is compensated for compressible volume loss, so that the volume actually delivered to the patient more closely approximates set tidal volume.

To deliver a volume-controlled mandatory breath, the ventilator determines the inspiratory time interval necessary to deliver the set tidal volume at the set peak flow to produce the selected flow pattern. The ventilator accomplishes compliance compensation by increasing the actual inspiratory flow above the set level, so that the compensated volume is delivered in the originally determined inspiratory time interval. Because the ventilator regulates inspiratory flow in a fixed pattern until the end of a predetermined inspiratory time interval, volume-controlled mandatory breaths are more specifically flow controlled, flow limited, and time cycled. Alternatively, a volume-controlled breath is cycled to expiration if circuit pressure reaches a high-pressure alarm threshold. Setting a plateau time (0 to 2 s) creates an inspiratory pause and increases total inspiratory time.

When the volume control plus (VC+) mandatory breath type is chosen the target tidal volume range is 5 to 2500 ml. Mandatory breaths will be delivered at the set target tidal volume or 7.5-ml/kg IBW setting (whichever is greater), following a test breath to determine the pressure required to deliver the desired V_T. Changes in target pressures are predetermined, on the basis of the IBW setting, not to exceed 3 cm H_2O in patients weighing less than 15 kg, 6 cm H_2O in patients weighing 15 to 25 kg, and 10 cm H_2O in patients weighing more than 25 kg. Other predetermined parameters also influence breath delivery: actual peak inspiratory pressure must exceed PEEP by 5 cm H_2O and must not exceed the high-pressure limit. Although this mode is a volume mode, the rise time percent and inspiratory time must be set because the actual breath delivery is pressure based.

Pressure-controlled mandatory breaths are pressure limited to the set inspiratory pressure level (5 to 90 cm H_2O above PEEP) and cycled to expiration at the end of the set inspiratory time interval. With changes in the set breath rate, inspiratory time is ultimately determined by the selection of one of the following three parameters as the primary timing parameter: inspiratory time (0.1 to 8 s), expiratory time (minimum, 0.2 second), or I/E ratio (maximum, 4:1). Pressure-controlled breaths are alternately cycled to expiration if circuit pressure reaches a ventilator-determined pressure above the set pressure limit.

When a pressure-controlled breath is triggered, the ventilator delivers gas at the flow necessary to reach and maintain the set pressure limit. Maximal inspiratory flow with pressure control is 200 L/minute for the adult patient category, 80 L/minute for the pediatric patient category, and 30 L/minute for the neonatal patient category. Inspiratory flow is also influenced by the flow acceleration percentage (rise time percent) setting (1% to 100%). The flow acceleration percentage setting dictates how quickly inspiratory pressure rises to the set pressure limit after the initiation of a pressure-controlled breath. Increasing the flow acceleration percentage value directs the ventilator to reach the pressure limit more quickly, resulting in a higher peak inspiratory flow. Setting the flow acceleration percentage too low may result in flow starvation and patient discomfort or dyssynchrony; the default flow acceleration for all patient category selections is 50%.

In A/C, all breaths are mandatory and are either time triggered at the end of a time interval dictated by the ventilator rate setting (1 to 150 breaths/min) or patient triggered by spontaneous breathing effort. In SIMV, mandatory breaths are time or patient triggered at the set ventilator breath rate.

The patient trigger variable can be set as either pressure or flow. Pressure triggering requires spontaneous patient effort to drop the circuit pressure below baseline by an amount equal to the set trigger sensitivity (0.1 to 20 cm H_2O below PEEP). To accomplish flow triggering the ventilator delivers a base gas flow through the patient circuit during the expiratory phase of all breaths. This base flow is equal to the flow set as the trigger sensitivity plus 1.5 L/minute. As the patient breathes from the base flow, the ventilator detects a difference in the inspiratory and expiratory flow measurements. Flow triggering occurs when this flow differential equals the value set as the trigger sensitivity (0.1 to 20 L/min). A backup pressure-triggering threshold of –2 cm H_2O is in effect when flow triggering is selected.

Spontaneous breaths in the SIMV, spontaneous, noninvasive, and BiLevel modes can be pressure supported, volume supported, or supported by the ventilator's demand flow system. Pressure-supported breaths are patient (pressure or flow) triggered, pressure limited to the set pressure support level (0 to 70 cm H_2O set above PEEP), and flow cycled to expiration when the measured inspiratory flow falls to an operator-selected expiratory sensitivity setting. Expiratory sensitivity is set as a percentage (1% to 80%) of the peak inspiratory flow needed to reach the set pressure limit. Peak inspiratory flow is also influenced by the set flow acceleration percentage. Increasing the flow acceleration percentage increases the initial inspiratory flow (and vice versa) as described earlier for pressure-controlled mandatory breaths. As a safety mechanism, pressure support is cycled to expiration if inspiratory flow does not fall to the set flow-cycling threshold at the end of a

ventilator-determined time interval based on the entered ideal body weight. Higher expiratory sensitivity settings might be used in patients with uncuffed endotracheal tubes or in weak patients unable to meet the flow termination requirements to cycle the breath into expiration. Higher expiratory sensitivity settings may also result in premature breath termination and inadequate tidal volume delivery. Pressure support is also pressure cycled if circuit pressure exceeds the set pressure limit by a ventilator-determined increment.

Volume support describes spontaneous breath delivery triggered by pressure or flow. When patient effort is detected, the ventilator delivers a pressure support breath that is volume targeted. The breath is terminated when the target V_T is reached or the patient meets the inspiratory flow criterion. Like pressure support, breath termination in volume support is influenced by the flow acceleration percentage and the expiratory sensitivity. Limitations in target pressure changes are the same as VC+ based on IBW.

Demand flow, like pressure support, is patient (pressure or flow) triggered. When a patient effort is detected, the ventilator regulates the flow control valves to provide the gas flow necessary to reach and maintain set PEEP plus 1.5 cm H_2O (the pressure limit). Demand flow is terminated by the same cycling criteria described for pressure support.

The optional BiLevel mode establishes two levels of positive airway pressure: low PEEP (0 to 45 cm H_2O) and high PEEP (5 to 90 cm H_2O). Spontaneous breathing— with or without pressure support—is permitted on both levels of positive pressure; however, the pressure support level delivered to the patient is calculated on the basis of centimeters of water above the low PEEP setting. The change from one pressure level to the other is determined primarily by operator-selected time intervals. However, the ventilator attempts to synchronize the change in pressure level to the patient's spontaneous breathing activity and uses the set patient triggering criteria to switch from the low-pressure to the high-pressure level. This results in minimal variations in the inspiratory time and I/E ratios. To synchronize the change from the high- to low-pressure level, the ventilator uses the cycling criterion outlined for pressure support and demand flow. When the high and low PEEP time intervals are set to create only a brief drop to the low PEEP level, the mode resembles airway pressure release ventilation (APRV). The high PEEP time interval can be set to a maximum of 30 seconds.

Apnea ventilation provides a backup mode of ventilation if the ventilator detects an apnea condition. Apnea ventilation settings are operator selected and include the choice of pressure-controlled or volume-controlled mandatory breaths. A safety ventilation function institutes default ventilation settings intended to be safe for all patient types (infant to adult) if the ventilator senses circuit connection before the completion of the startup sequence.

The PEEP control sets baseline pressure in a range of 0 to 45 cm H_2O. The $O_2\%$ setting determines the oxygen concentration (21% to 100%). Oxygen breaths are available at 100% for up to 2 minutes and may be canceled at any time during delivery. An inspiratory pause of up to 7 seconds or an expiratory pause of up to 20 seconds can be operator initiated. A mandatory breath can be manually triggered in all modes, using the manual inspiration key. The characteristics of a manually triggered breath are determined by current ventilator settings. Pressing the manual inspiration key when the ventilator is set in the BiLevel mode causes a change from one pressure level to the other.

The Puritan Bennett 840 offers an optional mode of spontaneous breath augmentation: tube compensation, or TC. This choice is available only for size 4.5 endotracheal or tracheal tubes and larger. TC is designed to estimate and compensate for the resistance of the artificial airway. The user chooses the percentage of TC to apply during spontaneous breathing from 40% up to 100%, with higher percentages providing full compensation for the resistance. In the noninvasive mode patient breathing effort can be augmented with CPAP and/or PS, and the ventilator volume alarm parameters can be turned off to compensate for leaks in the system.

Proportional assist ventilation (PAV) is an optional spontaneous adaptive mode of ventilation for patients with a 6.0-mm endotracheal tube or larger. PAV monitors the overall work of breathing and allows the user to select a percentage of support resulting in variable pressure support breath delivery. A color-coded bar graph assists the user in determining the appropriate percentage.

Table 17-4 summarizes the control and phase variables for both mandatory and spontaneous breaths in the Puritan Bennett 840 operational modes.

Output

Waveforms. Flow-controlled (volume control) mandatory breaths can be delivered in either a rectangular or a descending ramp-shaped inspiratory flow pattern. If the rectangular inspiratory flow waveform is selected, the resulting pressure and volume waveforms are ascending ramp shaped. If the descending ramp flow waveform is chosen, the pressure and volume waveforms tend to rise exponentially.

The shape of the inspiratory pressure waveform produced during the delivery of a pressure-controlled mandatory breath is influenced by the flow acceleration

percentage setting. A flow acceleration setting of 100% causes inspiratory pressure to rise rapidly to the set pressure limit. In this case, the inspiratory pressure waveform is approximately rectangular. If the flow acceleration percentage is decreased, inspiratory pressure rises more slowly, causing the initial portion of the pressure waveform to be ramp shaped. The resulting inspiratory flow and volume waveforms exhibit an exponential rise. The magnitude of the inspiratory flow waveform (peak flow) decreases as the flow acceleration percentage setting is decreased.

Monitoring. The Puritan Bennett 840 presents output data both numerically and graphically. Graphics options include pressure time, flow time, volume time, and pressure–volume displays. The breath type display indicates the type (control, assist, or spontaneous) and phase (inspiration or exhalation) of the currently delivered breath.

Airway pressure values are calculated from measurements made by the pressure sensors located in the ventilator's inspiratory and expiratory compartments. These include end-expiratory pressure, end-inspiratory (plateau) pressure, maximal circuit pressure, and mean circuit pressure. Measurements of intrinsic (auto-) PEEP and total PEEP are made during an operator-initiated expiratory pause. In addition, static compliance and resistance are calculated during an inspiratory pause maneuver.

Exhaled tidal volume, spontaneous minute volume, and (total) exhaled minute volume values are derived from the flow measurement made by a hot wire anemometer flow sensor located at the exhalation valve. These volume measurements are circuit compliance compensated. Total (spontaneous and mandatory) respiratory rate and I/E ratio are also displayed. Delivered $O_2\%$ reflects oxygen concentration measured by the internal oxygen sensor. The oxygen sensor can be enabled or disabled by the operator.

The Puritan Bennett 840 is equipped with a digital output connection.

Alarms

The Puritan Bennett 840 classifies alarms as low, medium, and high urgency and uses both visual and audible signals to indicate the appropriate level of urgency. In addition, the ventilator suggests actions to remedy specific alarm conditions. Alarm events are chronologically entered into an alarm log. The log can store up to 50 alarm messages for subsequent review.

Input Power Alarms. If either gas pressure falls below the minimum required for ventilator operation, the no-air supply or no-oxygen supply alarm activates to indicate the specific gas loss and the ventilator continues operation with the remaining available gas. Failure

TABLE 17-4

Control and Phase Variables for Mandatory and Spontaneous Breaths in the Operational Modes Available on the Puritan Bennett 840 Ventilator

| Mode | MANDATORY | | | | SPONTANEOUS | | | |
	Control	Trigger*	Limit	Cycle	Control	Trigger	Limit	Cycle
A/C-volume control	Flow	Time, pressure, flow	Flow, volume	Time, pressure[†]	N/A	N/A	N/A	N/A
A/C-pressure control	Pressure	Time, pressure, flow	Pressure	Time, pressure[†]	N/A	N/A	N/A	N/A
SIMV-volume control	Flow	Time, pressure, flow	Pressure	Time, pressure[†]	Pressure	Pressure, flow	Pressure	Flow, time,[†] pressure[†]
SIMV-pressure control	Pressure	Time, pressure, flow	Pressure	Time, pressure[†]	Pressure	Pressure, flow	Pressure	Flow, time,[†] pressure[†]
BiLevel[‡]	Pressure	Time, pressure, flow	Pressure	Time, flow, pressure	Pressure	Time, flow, pressure	Pressure	Time, pressure, flow
Spontaneous	N/A	N/A	N/A	N/A	Pressure	Pressure, flow	Pressure	Flow, time,[†] pressure[†]
Pressure support	N/A	N/A	N/A	N/A	Pressure, flow	Pressure	Pressure	Flow, time,[†] pressure[†]

Modified from Chatburn RL, Lough MD, Primiano FP Jr: Mechanical ventilation. In Chatburn RL, Lough MD, editors: *Handbook of respiratory care*, ed 2, St. Louis: Mosby; 1990. pp 159-223.
* Mandatory breaths can be manually triggered in all modes.
† Secondary or safety cycle variable.
‡ For the purpose of illustrating ventilator behavior in the BiLevel mode, the high PEEP level is here considered the mandatory breath and the low PEEP level the spontaneous breath. In fact, spontaneous breathing is permitted at both the high and low PEEP levels.
§ Considered here as a separate mode, but can be used to support spontaneous breaths in the SIMV, spontaneous, and BiLevel modes.

of the optional air compressor activates the compressor inoperative alarm.

The low AC power alarm indicates that external electrical power has dropped below a level acceptable for ventilator operation. The AC power loss alarm indicates that AC power is not available and that the internal battery is supporting ventilator function. A fully charged battery generally sustains operation for at least 30 minutes. The inoperative battery alarm indicates that a battery is installed but not functional. The low battery alarm activates when less than 2 minutes of battery power remains. The loss of power alarm signals that both AC and battery power are insufficient for ventilator operation.

Control Circuit Alarms. A device alert is triggered if a system fault is detected during ongoing testing of the ventilator's electronic and pneumatic function. A high-urgency device alert causes a ventilator-inoperable condition and opening of a safety valve to allow the patient to breathe spontaneously from room air. A procedure error alarm activates if the patient is attached to the ventilator before completion of the startup procedure.

Output Alarms. Most of the ventilator's adjustable output alarm limits are initially set on the basis of the entered patient ideal body weight, but they may be subsequently operator adjusted. Operator-set alarms include those for apnea, high circuit pressure, high and low exhaled minute volume, low exhaled spontaneous tidal volume, low exhaled mandatory tidal volume, high exhaled tidal volume (spontaneous and mandatory), high inspiratory spontaneous tidal volume, high (spontaneous and mandatory) are active in the volume ventilation plus mode, and high respiratory rate.

The "inspiration too long" alarm activates if, during the delivery of a spontaneous breath, inspiratory flow does not decrease to the flow-cycling threshold (expiratory sensitivity setting) before the end of the ventilator-determined maximal inspiratory time. The ventilator is also equipped with a circuit disconnect alarm, a high internal pressure alarm, and a circuit occlusion alarm. If a severe circuit occlusion is detected, the ventilator discontinues normal operation, opens its safety valve, and periodically attempts to deliver a pressure-controlled breath (occlusion status cycling) while monitoring for the persistence of the occlusion.

The Puritan Bennett 840 is equipped with a remote alarm connection.

Newport Wave VM200

See Evolve Resources for information about the Newport Wave VM200 infant/pediatric/adult ventilator (Newport Medical Instruments, Costa Mesa, Calif).

Maquet Servo 300A

See Evolve Resources for information about the Servo 300A ventilator (Maquet).

Maquet SERVO-i

The SERVO-i (Maquet) (Figure 17-9) is the newest generation servo ventilator. It is a pneumatically and electrically (AC and battery modules) powered, electronically controlled ventilator designed for neonatal, pediatric, and adult use. Mandatory breaths are time, flow, or pressure triggered; flow, volume, or pressure limited; and time cycled. Spontaneous breaths are flow or pressure triggered, pressure limited, and flow cycled.[18]

Power Conversion and Transmission

The operation of the SERVO-i is patterned after the 300/300A model. The changes are outlined in the following text.

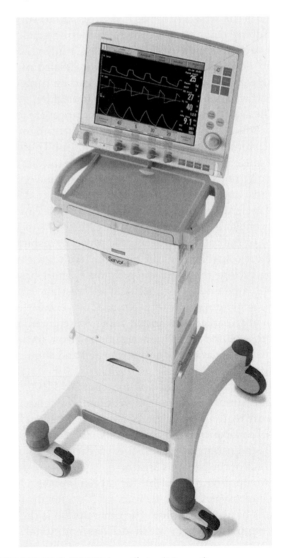

FIGURE 17-9 SERVO-i ventilator (Maquet).

Gas flow from the expiratory limb of the patient circuit enters the expiratory cassette and is measured by ultrasonic transducers while the pressure is measured by the expiratory pressure transducer and PEEP measurements are regulated by the expiratory valve. The exhalation valve is a microprocessor-controlled floating valve that controls PEEP, allowing for changes in expiratory flows.

Control

Additional modes available on the SERVO-i are as follows: SIMV (pressure-regulated volume control), BiVent, and noninvasive ventilation (NIV) with pressure control or pressure support and neurally adjusted ventilation assistance (NAVA). The patient selection mode is reduced to one of two patient ranges: adult or infant.

During the preuse check of the ventilator, oxygen cells are calibrated and circuit compliance is calculated. From this calculation the SERVO-i delivers a V_T that matches the set V_T. At times it is necessary to turn off the tubing compensation when ventilating small premature infants with extremely small V_T ranges secondary to nuisance alarms (especially low exhaled minute volume). The tubing compensation can be turned on and off without repeating the preuse procedure.

The available tidal volume and flow ranges are as follows: Adult flow range is from 0 to 3.3 L/second (or 0 to 180 L/min) with a V_T range of 100 to 2000 ml. The infant flow range is from 0 to 0.55 L/second (or 0 to 33 L/min) with a V_T range of 0 to 350 ml. Inspiratory time is set as seconds, and an inspiratory pause time (0% to 30% of total cycle time) can also be added. Combined inspiratory time and pause times cannot exceed 80% (4:1 I/E ratio) of the total ventilator cycle time. An inspiratory cycle off control allows the operator to alter the exhalation cycling threshold for pressure support breaths, thus compensating for mechanical leaks (an increase in the inspiratory cycle off settings allows exhalation to occur at an earlier point in the peak flow requirements). During volume ventilation additional flow (adaptive ventilation) is available on patient demand should the set flow be inadequate.

In pressure-regulated volume control (PRVC) and volume support modes, the ventilator calculates the pressure required to deliver the preset V_T based on a single volume-controlled breath with an inspiratory pause of 10%; adjustments to subsequent breaths are made on the basis of the previous breath.

Two options are available for oxygen breaths. One is standard oxygen breath delivery at 100% for up to 20 breaths or up to 1 minute. The other option is the suction support feature, which delivers additional supplemental oxygen (as set by the clinician) for up to 2 minutes before suctioning and 60 seconds after the

patient is reconnected to the ventilator. During the use of suction support, select alarms associated with suctioning procedures are inactivated.

The optional open lung tool is designed to assist the clinician in determining the opening and collapsing pressures of the lung, to establish the most effective PEEP levels. When PEEP levels are optimal, PIP–PEEP will be lowest. The clinician will need to determine whether the patient can clinically tolerate the optional PEEP value.

The automode is enhanced in the SERVO-i ventilator to allow the patient to earn additional time to the preset apnea interval by maintaining a spontaneous effort at a rate of 1% of the set apnea time. This earned apnea time assures that the patient does not violate the preset apnea time setting.

NAVA is a new mode of mechanical ventilation that applies pressure in proportion to the electrical activation of the diaphragm (Edi). This electrical activity is obtained with a multiple-array esophageal electrode that doubles as a feeding tube. This new and novel mode of ventilation may offer true synchronization.

The SERVO-i also has an integrated ultrasonic nebulizer, ensuring that additional flow is not added to the circuit during inspiration and therefore ventilator adjustments are not necessary.

Table 17-5 summarizes the control and phase variables for mandatory and spontaneous breaths in the additional modes available on the SERVO-i ventilator.

Output

Waveforms. The SERVO-i has an integrated graphics screen that displays graphic waveforms and monitored ventilator data. There is also a trend screen that allows the user to scroll back up to 24 hours. The trend screen marks each alarm event and user interface, which is displayed on the screen when accessed. In the neonatal mode an airway flow sensor may be added. This appears to clean up some of the graphics and provide more accurate airway measurements in very small infants (< 2 kg) with endotracheal tube leaks.

Monitoring. Patient monitored parameters are vertically displayed on the graphics screen and can be defined by the user; preset oxygen concentration, PEEP, respiratory rate, and V_T or pressure control settings are horizontally displayed at the bottom of the screen, correlating with quick access controls to change settings. Up to three ventilator waveform presentations can be chosen for display.

Alarms

The SERVO-i offers a variety of user-defined alarms in each mode that can be customized to fit the patient ventilatory status. In the noninvasive ventilation modes the audible alarms for minute volume, respiratory rate, and low PEEP can be silenced.

TABLE 17-5

Control and Phase Variables for Mandatory and Spontaneous Breaths in the Additional Available Modes on the Maquet SERVO-i Ventilator

Mode	MANDATORY				SPONTANEOUS			
	Control§	Trigger*	Limit	Cycle	Control§	Trigger*	Limit	Cycle
SIMV PRVC‡	Pressure	Time, flow, pressure	Pressure	Time, pressure†	Pressure	Flow, pressure	Pressure	Flow, pressure,† time†
BiVent	Pressure	Time, flow, pressure	Pressure	Time, pressure†	Pressure	Flow, pressure	Pressure	Flow, pressure,† time†
NIV PC	Pressure	Time, flow, pressure	Pressure	Time, pressure†	N/A	N/A	N/A	N/A
NIV PS	N/A	N/A	N/A	N/A	Pressure	Flow, pressure	Pressure	Flow, pressure,† time†
NIV CPAP	N/A	N/A	N/A	N/A	Pressure	Flow, pressure	Pressure	N/A

CPAP, Continuous positive airway pressure; N/A, not applicable; NIV, noninvasive; PC, pressure controlled; PRVC, pressure-regulated volume control; PS, pressure supported; SIMV, synchronized intermittent mandatory ventilation.
* Mandatory breaths can be manually triggered in all modes. *Note:* Only flow triggering is available in the neonatal mode.
† Secondary or safety cycle variable.
‡ For the purpose of illustrating ventilator behavior in the BiVent mode, the high PEEP level is here considered the mandatory breath and the low PEEP level the spontaneous breath. In fact, spontaneous breathing is permitted at both the high and low PEEP levels.
§ Considered here as a separate mode, but can be used to support spontaneous breaths in the SIMV, spontaneous, and BiVent modes.

Input Power Alarms. If the ventilator loses AC power the machine will automatically switch over to battery power. Each of the battery modules provides 30 minutes of power when fully charged, with the battery time displayed on the graphics screen. If one source gas is lost then gas is diverted from the other gas module to maintain V_T or PC settings. FIO_2 will either be 21% or 100% depending on the functioning module.

Hamilton Medical Hamilton-G5

The Hamilton-G5 ventilator (Hamilton Medical) (Figure 17-10) is the next-generation ventilator based on the GALILEO platform. It is a pneumatically and electrically powered, electronically controlled ventilator designed for neonatal, pediatric, and adult patients. Mandatory breaths are time, flow, or pressure triggered, flow volume or pressure limited, and time cycled. Spontaneous breaths are flow or pressure triggered, pressure limited, and flow cycled.[19]

Power Conversion and Transmission

The Hamilton-G5 has an internal battery with an operational time of approximately 1 hour; optional external extended batteries will provide an additional 1 hour per battery. The ventilator operates on a compressed air and oxygen supply ranging from 29 to 86 psig.

Control

The Hamilton-G5 can be operated in the following modes: APVcmv (adaptive pressure control + CMV), APVsimv (adaptive pressure control + SIMV), P-CMV (pressure-controlled mandatory ventilation), P-SIMV (pressure-controlled synchronized mandatory ventilation), SPONT (pressure-supported ventilation), DuoPAP (dual positive airway pressure-biphasic), APRV (airway pressure release ventilation), (S)CMV (synchronized controlled mandatory ventilation-volume) available for adult and pediatric patients only, SIMV (synchronized mandatory ventilation-volume) available for adult and pediatric patients only, NIV (noninvasive ventilation) available for adult and pediatric patients only, and ASV (adaptive support ventilation-minute volume based) available for adult and pediatric patients only.

The Hamilton-G5 requires the use of an airway sensor and offers two sizes: pediatric/adult and infant. The dead space of the pediatric/adult sensor is 9 ml, whereas that of the infant sensor is 2 ml. The relatively large dead space volume in the infant sensor may prohibit its use with low birth weight babies. The sensors will calibrate automatically or manually and will alert the user to sensor errors or calibration requirements. Tidal volume can be measured down to 2 ml; however, the minimal set tidal volume available in all volume modes of ventilation is 10 ml. The actual tidal volume range is 10 to 2000 ml.

Circuit compliance is determined during the preuse check and is compensated for. Standard features include a peak flow range of 1 to 180 L/minute, flow or pressure triggering capabilities, I/E ratios of up to 4:1, controlled breath rates of 5 to 120 breaths/minute, SIMV breath rates of 1 to 60 breaths/minute, pressure control and pressure support capabilities of up to

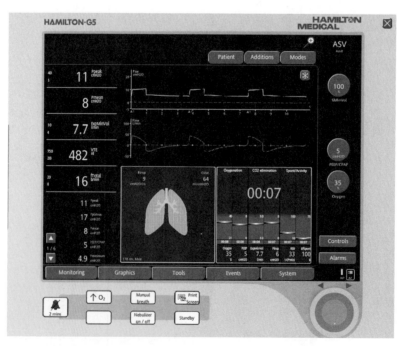

FIGURE 17-10 Hamilton-G5 ventilator (Hamilton Medical).

100 cm H_2O, PEEP at 0 to 50 cm H_2O, and an inspiratory time of 0.1 to 10 seconds. Other standard features include visual indicators of lung function, integrated graphics and trends, a nebulizer unit that nebulizes on inspiration from the inspiratory flow, a manual 100% oxygen breath delivery system, and backup ventilation.

Other patient controls include the expiratory trigger sensitivity ranging from 5% to 70% of inspiratory peak flow to compensate for patient airway leaks; flow pattern selection of sine, square, 100% decelerating, or 50% decelerating; and pressure ramping from 25 to 200 milliseconds.

One feature unique to the Hamilton-G5 is the closed loop ventilation termed ASV (adaptive support ventilation). This mode of ventilation is a version of mandatory minute ventilation in which the ventilator calculates the appropriate respiratory rate and tidal volume on the basis of user-defined percentage of support desired (from 25% to 350%), IDW (ideal body weight) and patient height are vital in the calculation of minute ventilation. This feature can be incorporated in all SIMV and spontaneous breathing modes but is not available for neonatal patients. Continuous monitoring of patient status and adaptation to changing clinical conditions may enhance weaning efforts. Some studies suggest that this mode of ventilation may decrease ventilator days in certain patients.

Optional features include heliox application and volumetric carbon dioxide determinations. Heliox application replaces air administration through the high-pressure air inlet and automatically corrects volume measurements at all F_{IO_2} levels.

Table 17-6 summarizes the control and phase variables for mandatory and spontaneous breaths in the additional modes available on the Hamilton-G5.

Output

Waveforms. The Hamilton-G5 has integrated waveform displays allowing the clinician to view up to four user-selected waveforms or two loops at any time. The pressure–volume curve maneuver displays a lower inflection point to assist in determining the proper PEEP setting and an upper inflection point to identify the maximal safe pressure delivery to avoid overdistention of the lung.

Monitoring. The ventilator stores 37 monitored parameters available for evaluation over a 24-hour period. Real-time lung condition is displayed in picture format and is surrounded by a color-coded outline to provide the user a rapid assessment of lung function and ventilator efficiency. Lung mechanics, ventilator, and patient parameters are also continuously displayed.

Alarms

The Hamilton-G5 has a comprehensive alarm package that allows the user to customize alarm limits to the individual patient. Alarm event logs will store up to the last 1000 events (dated and timed). The audible alarm loudness can be adjusted from 1 to 10.

Input Power Alarms. If the ventilator loses AC power, conversion to battery backup occurs without interruption in ventilation. Low battery and gas supply alarms are also included.

GE Healthcare Engström Carestation

The Engström Carestation ventilator (GE Healthcare) (Figure 17-11) provides many features integrated into the ventilator itself. It is a pneumatically and electrically powered, electronically controlled ventilator designed for neonatal, pediatric, and adult patients. Mandatory breaths are time, flow, or pressure triggered, flow volume or pressure limited, and time cycled. Spontaneous breaths are flow or pressure triggered, pressure limited, and flow cycled. In addition to standard monitoring features the Engström Carestation offers the ability to perform metabolic measurements without the need to bring additional equipment to the bedside. It has a module feature allowing the clinician to integrate ventilation information into the critical care monitoring system.[20]

Power Conversion and Transmission

The Engström Carestation has an internal battery with an operational time of approximately 90 minutes. The ventilator operates on a compressed air and oxygen supply ranging from 35 to 94 psig but will operate with a single gas supply. The oxygen sensor uses a paramagnetic oxygen system that has an unlimited life, eliminating the need for oxygen cell replacements. There is an optional SpiroDynamics pulmonary mechanics monitoring system available for use in pediatric and adult patients, which may allow for more accurate lung mechanics measurements without the use of a separate bedside monitor. The SpiroDynamics system measures intratracheal pressures through a 2-mm O.D. sensor positioned within the airway, approximately 2 cm below the tip of the ETT.

Control

The Engström Carestation can be operated in the following modes: VCV (volume-controlled ventilation, PCV (pressure-controlled ventilation), PCV-VG (pressure-controlled ventilation-volume guaranteed), SIMV-VC (synchronized intermittent mandatory ventilation-volume controlled), SIMV-PC (synchronized

TABLE 17-6

Control and Phase Variables for Mandatory and Spontaneous Breaths in the Additional Available Modes on the Hamilton-G5 Ventilator

Mode	MANDATORY				SPONTANEOUS			
	Control[§]	Trigger*	Limit	Cycle	Control[§]	Trigger*	Limit	Cycle
APVcmv P-CMV	Pressure	Time, flow, pressure	Pressure	Time, pressure[†]	N/A	N/A	N/A	N/A
(S)CMV	Volume	Time, flow, pressure	Volume	Time, volume[†]	N/A	N/A	N/A	NA
APVsimv P-SIMV	Pressure	Time, flow, pressure	Pressure	Time, pressure[†]	Pressure	Flow, pressure	Pressure	Flow, pressure,[†] time[†]
DuoPAP APRV	Pressure	Time, flow, pressure	Pressure	Time, pressure[†]	Pressure	Flow, pressure	Pressure	Flow, pressure,[†] time[†]

APRV, Airway pressure release ventilation; APVcmv, adaptive pressure control + CMV; APVsimv, adaptive pressure control + SIMV; DuoPAP, dual positive airway pressure-biphasic; P-CMV, pressure-controlled mandatory ventilation; P-SIMV, pressure-controlled synchronized mandatory ventilation; N/A, not applicable; (S)CMV, synchronized controlled mandatory ventilation-volume.
* Manual breaths can be triggered in all modes. Note: only flow triggering is available in the infant mode.
[†] Refers to the primary parameter to end the inspiratory cycle.
[§] Refers to the primary control of mandatory breaths.

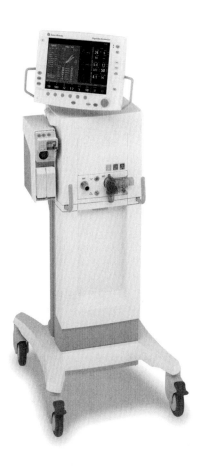

FIGURE 17-11 Engström Carestation ventilator (GE Healthcare).

intermittent mandatory ventilation-pressure controlled), SIMV-PCVG (synchronized intermittent mandatory ventilation-pressure controlled-volume guaranteed), APRV (BiLevel airway pressure ventilation), BiLevel-VG (BiLevel with volume guarantee), NIV (noninvasive ventilation), and CPAP/PSV (continuous positive airway pressure with pressure support ventilation).

Ventilator control settings are variable and the ranges by which they operate and adjusted depend on patient selection (neonate, pediatric, or adult). Standard features include a peak flow range of 1 to 200 L/minute, controlled breath rates of 3 to 120 breaths/minute (up to 150 breaths/min in neonatal mode), SIMV breath rates of 1 to 60 breaths/minute, a tidal volume range of 3 to 2000 ml, pressure control and pressure support capabilities of up to 100 cm H_2O, PEEP at 0 to 60 cm H_2O, an inspiratory time of 0.1 to 15 seconds, flow- or pressure-triggering capabilities, and I/E ratios of up to 4:1. Other available features include an ultrasonic nebulizer and an oxygen breath delivery feature (100%

for pediatric and adult, 25% above set F_{IO_2} for neonatal patients) that is manually adjustable if desired. Other patient-specific controls include circuit leak ranging from 10% to 90% for more accurate delivery of volume-guaranteed breaths and end flow levels ranging from 5% to 50% to terminate pressure-supported breaths to compensate for patient airway leaks, rise time ranges from 0 to 500 milliseconds, airway resistance compensation for airway sizes of 5.0 to 10.0 mm, and end-tidal carbon dioxide determinations.

Table 17-7 summarizes the control and phase variables for mandatory and spontaneous breaths in the additional modes available on the Engström Carestation.

Output

Waveforms. The Engström Carestation ventilator has integrated waveform displays allowing the user to view up to three user-selected waveforms at any time. The optional SpiroDynamics allows for up to two loops to be superimposed on the screen for evaluation when requested (not available for neonatal use). This feature allows for multiple lung mechanics measurements that can be used to optimize mechanical ventilation, including (but not limited to) functional residual capacity measurement, inspiratory and expiratory inflection points for PEEP determination, and others.

Monitoring. The ventilator stores all measured and set ventilator parameters for evaluation over a 14-day period. At a glance, the five most recent alarm conditions are available without accessing trends; a help screen is also available to assist the user in resolving alarm conditions.

Alarms

The Engström Carestation has a comprehensive alarm package that allows the user to customize alarm limits to the individual patient. Alarm event logs will be found in the trends display (dated and timed). The audible alarm is an escalating alarm system that intensifies if a high-priority alarm is unattended; alarm limits are either manually set by the user or automatically set on the basis of measured values.

Input Power Alarms. If the ventilator loses AC power, conversion to battery backup occurs without interruption in ventilation. Low battery and gas supply alarms are also included. A status indicator reflects the ventilation mode, battery level, and clock.

HOME CARE VENTILATORS
Puritan Bennett LP10

See Evolve Resources for information about the Puritan Bennett LP10 ventilator.

TABLE 17-7

Control and Phase Variables for Mandatory and Spontaneous Breaths in the Additional Available Modes on the Engström Carestation Ventilator

Mode	MANDATORY				SPONTANEOUS			
	Control§	Trigger*	Limit	Cycle	Control§	Trigger*	Limit	Cycle
VCV SIMV-VC	Volume	Time, flow, pressure	Volume	Time, volume†	Volume	Time, flow, pressure	Volume	Time, volume†
PCV SIMV-PC	Pressure	Time, flow, pressure	Pressure	Time, pressure†	Pressure	Time, flow, pressure	Pressure	Time, pressure†
SIMV-PCVG PCV-VG‡	Pressure	Time, flow, pressure	Pressure	Time, pressure†	Pressure	Flow, pressure	Pressure	Flow, pressure,† time†
BiVent	Pressure	Time, flow, pressure	Pressure	Time, pressure†	Pressure	Flow, pressure	Pressure	Flow, pressure,† time†
CPAP/PSV	NA	NA	NA	NA	Pressure	Flow, pressure	Pressure	Flow, pressure,† time†

CPAP/PSV, Continuous positive airway pressure with pressure support ventilation; PCV, pressure-controlled ventilation; PCV-VG, pressure-controlled ventilation-volume guaranteed; SIMV-PC, synchronized intermittent mandatory ventilation-pressure controlled; SIMV-PCVG, synchronized intermittent mandatory ventilation-pressure controlled-volume guaranteed; SIMV-VC, synchronized intermittent mandatory ventilation-volume controlled; VCV, volume-controlled ventilation.
* Refers to the type of trigger from the patient to initiate a response from the ventilator to deliver a breath.
† Refers to the primary parameter to end the inspiratory cycle.
§ Refers to the primary control of mandatory breaths.

Puritan Bennett Companion 2801

The Puritan Bennett Companion 2801 ventilator (Covidien) (Figure 17-12) is electrically powered (AC, internal battery, or external 12-V battery) and electronically (microprocessor) and pneumatically controlled. For power conversion and transmission, the ventilator uses an electric motor–driven piston and an external pneumatic exhalation valve. The Companion 2801 is primarily a volume controller that can also function as a pressure controller. Mandatory breaths are time or pressure triggered, flow or pressure limited, and volume cycled. Spontaneous breaths are not actively supported.[21]

Power Conversion and Transmission

Gas flow is created by the movement of a rotating crank and piston driven by an electric gear motor. During the backstroke of the piston (expiratory phase), gas is drawn into the piston chamber through a one-way inlet valve and filter located on the right side panel of the ventilator. The forward stroke of the piston displaces the cylinder volume, directing gas past two pressure-limiting valves and through the one-way outlet valve into the patient circuit.

The exhalation valve solenoid controls a separate gas flow to a mushroom valve in the exhalation manifold of the patient circuit. During the inspiratory phase, this gas flow pressurizes (closes) the valve, directing gas flow to the patient.

Control

The Companion 2801 can be operated in control, A/C, and SIMV modes. A no-ventilation mode setting permits recharging of the internal battery without other ventilator functions.

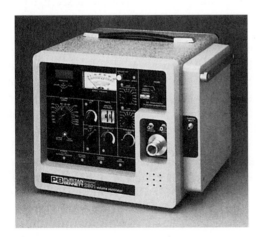

FIGURE 17-12 Puritan Bennett Companion 2801 ventilator (Covidien).

All operational modes require setting tidal volume (50 to 2800 ml), flow (average inspiratory flow, 20 to 120 L/min), and breath rate (1 to 69 breaths/min). To ensure the set tidal volume, the microprocessor determines the position to which the piston moves during its backstroke (refilling). When a mandatory breath is triggered, the microprocessor directs the electric motor to move the piston at the speed needed to deliver the cylinder volume at the set flow (i.e., flow limit). Inspiration cycles to expiration when the cylinder volume is completely displaced by the movement of the piston to its full forward position. Inspiratory time is a function of set tidal volume and flow. Inspiration is prematurely cycled if circuit pressure reaches the high-pressure alarm setting.

Mandatory breaths may be pressure controlled with the pressure limit control, a spring-loaded mechanical valve with a range of 10 to 100 cm H_2O. The pressure limit control is not graduated and must be set while observing circuit pressure on the ventilator's pressure gauge. If inspiratory pressure reaches the pressure limit setting, the pressure-limiting valve vents the remainder of the piston cylinder volume to atmosphere, maintaining the set pressure limit. The set flow and tidal volume influence how quickly pressure reaches the set limit.

In the control and A/C modes, all breaths are mandatory. In the control mode, mandatory breaths are time cycled at the set breath rate. In A/C mode, breaths are either time triggered or patient triggered if inspiratory effort drops circuit pressure to the pressure set with the sensitivity control (–10 to 10 cm H_2O).

In the SIMV mode, mandatory breaths are time or pressure (patient) triggered at the set breath rate. To accomplish spontaneous breathing between mandatory breaths, the patient must draw gas through the piston chamber or through the exhalation valve during the expiratory phase. If the breath rate is set to less than 8 breaths/minute in the SIMV mode and the ventilator fails to detect a patient inspiratory effort within 45 seconds, the ventilator switches to apnea ventilation. In apnea ventilation, mandatory breaths are delivered at a rate of 12 breaths/minute; all other breath variables are determined by the control settings as described earlier.

Sigh breaths can be delivered in all operational modes. When activated, three successive sigh breaths are delivered every 10 minutes at the set sigh volume (50 to 2800 ml). Sigh breaths can also be manually triggered. PEEP can be created by adding a PEEP valve to the external exhalation manifold. Patient trigger sensitivity can be set to as high as approximately 10 cm H_2O to compensate for externally applied PEEP. Supplemental oxygen can be supplied with an optional oxygen accumulator that attaches to the ventilator's right side panel.

Table 17-8 summarizes the control and phase variables for mandatory and spontaneous breaths in the operational modes available on the Puritan Bennett Companion 2801 ventilator.

Output

Waveforms. The motion of the Companion 2801's piston creates a sinusoidal inspiratory flow (and volume) waveform. The resulting inspiratory pressure waveform is also sinusoidal. When the ventilator is set to pressure limit inspiration, the pressure waveform exhibits a plateau and may approximate a rectangular shape depending on the specific control settings.

Monitoring. Proximal airway pressure is displayed throughout the inspiratory and expiratory cycle on an analog pressure gauge. A digital monitoring window with a three-position switch displays electronically measured values for average inspiratory flow, I/E ratio, and the volume of gas displaced by the piston. A sensitivity indicator flashes with each patient breathing effort that drops proximal airway pressure to the set sensitivity threshold. The sigh indicator illuminates when the next mandatory breath is scheduled to be a sigh breath.

Alarms

Input Power Alarms. With the loss of AC electric power, the Companion 2801 automatically switches to battery power and signals the changeover by an audible "chirping." The power indicator shows which of the three power sources is in use. A low-battery alarm indicates that the voltage of the battery in use (internal or external) is below approximately 11.9 V. Complete battery discharge is signaled by continuous long audible pulses.

Control Circuit Alarms. A continuous nonpulsating audio alarm and flashing front panel lamps indicate a microprocessor malfunction. The ventilator also alerts the operator when control settings result in an inverse I/E ratio of 1:0.8 or less, or result in the inability of the ventilator to deliver breaths at the set rate.

Output Alarms. The Companion 2801 is equipped with operator-adjustable high and low circuit pressure alarms. The apnea alarm activates if the ventilator fails to detect a patient inspiratory effort within a 15-second time interval (in SIMV) or if airway pressure remains above the low-pressure alarm setting for 15 seconds or two breath cycles.

The Companion 2801 is equipped with a remote alarm connection.

Respironics LIFECARE PLV-100 and PLV-102

The LIFECARE PLV-100 and PLV-102 (Philips Respironics, Murrysville, Pa) (Figure 17-13) are microprocessor -controlled, electrically powered volume ventilators. Tidal volume is controlled by a rotary motor–driven piston, which determines flow of gas to the patient.[22]

Power Conversion and Transmission

The LIFECARE PLV-100 and PLV-102 use AC power, external battery power, or internal battery power. A separate gas flow supplies the exhalation valve of the patient circuit. During the inspiratory phase, this gas source inflates the exhalation valve balloon, closing the valve and diverting the main gas flow to the patient. In the absence of gas flow to the exhalation valve during the expiratory phase, the balloon depressurizes to allow exhalation. PEEP is maintained with an external spring-loaded expiratory resistance valve.

Control

The LIFECARE PLV-100 and PLV-102 can be operated in one of the following three modes: control, A/C, and SIMV.

Ventilator controls include volume (50 to 3000 ml), breath rate (2 to 40 breaths/min), and peak flow (10 to 120 L/min). On the basis of the set tidal volume, the ventilator's microprocessor controls the stop position of the piston during its backstroke (refilling). During the inspiratory phase of a mandatory breath, the microprocessor regulates piston speed so that the gas volume is delivered at a rate determined by the peak flow setting (the flow limit). Thus inspiratory time is a function of the volume and flow settings. Inspiratory-to-expiratory time ratio is displayed on the front panel as a function of the rate and inspiratory flow settings. Inspiration is volume cycled when the piston reaches its full forward position, completely displacing cylinder volume. Inspiration is pressure cycled before the set volume is delivered if circuit pressure reaches the set high pressure alarm value.

In the control mode, mandatory breaths are time triggered at an interval determined by the set breath rate. In A/C, all breaths are mandatory and are either time triggered or patient triggered if inspiratory effort causes circuit pressure to fall to the set assist sensitivity setting (-6 to 3 cm H_2O in the PLV-100 model, which is displayed as less or more on the control knob and ranging from -6 to +18 cm H_2O in the PLV-102 model). In SIMV, mandatory breaths are either time or pressure (patient) triggered at the set breath rate. Spontaneous breathing is permitted between mandatory breaths in both the SIMV and control modes. The patient must draw in the gas for spontaneous breathing either through the air inlet (located in the back of the machine) or an IMV "H" valve placed within the dry side of the inspiratory circuit. Use of an "H" valve will

TABLE 17-8

Control and Phase Variables for Mandatory and Spontaneous Breaths in the Operational Modes Available on the Puritan Bennett Companion 2801 Ventilator

Mode	MANDATORY				SPONTANEOUS			
	Control	Trigger*	Limit	Cycle	Control	Trigger	Limit	Cycle
Control	Volume, pressure[†]	Time	Flow, pressure[†]	Volume, pressure[‡]	–	–	–	–
A/C	Volume, pressure[†]	Time, pressure	Flow, pressure[†]	Volume, pressure[‡]	N/A	N/A	N/A	N/A
SIMV	Volume, pressure[†]	Time, pressure	Flow, pressure[†]	Volume, pressure[‡]	–	–	–	–

Modified from Chatburn RL, Lough MD, Primiano FP Jr: Mechanical ventilation. In Chatburn RL, Lough MD, editors: *Handbook of respiratory care*, ed 2, St. Louis: Mosby; 1990. pp 159-223.
A/C, Assist/control; N/A, not applicable; SIMV, synchronized intermittent mandatory ventilation; –, ventilator does not respond.
* Refers to the type of trigger from the patient to initiate a response from the ventilator to deliver a breath.
† Secondary or safety cycle.
‡ Applies only if pressure limit control is used to limit inspiratory pressure.
* Sigh breaths can be manually triggered.
†Applies only if pressure limit control is used to limit inspiratory pressure.
‡Secondary or safety cycle variable.

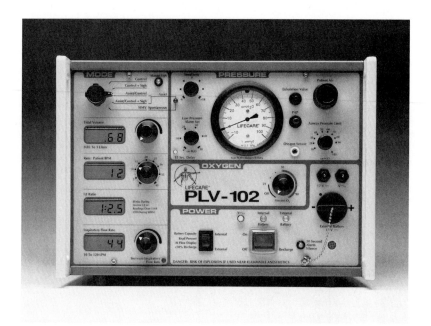

FIGURE 17-13 LIFECARE PLV-102 (Philips Respironics).

alter the sensitivity-sensing capability and must be considered when choosing this option.

When using an external PEEP valve the assist sensitivity can be set up to 18 cm H_2O to compensate for the externally applied PEEP. Supplemental oxygen can be delivered by bleeding in low oxygen flow to the inspiratory circuit on the PLV-100 model or by using the high-pressure gas blender available on the PLV-102.

Output

Waveforms. The motion of the PLV piston produces sinusoidal inspiratory flow and volume waveforms. The resulting inspiratory pressure waveform is also sinusoidal.

Monitoring. Airway pressure, measured in the patient circuit, is displayed throughout the ventilatory cycle on an analog pressure gauge. Tidal volume, peak flow, and I/E ratio are also displayed. During SIMV and A/C the displayed respiratory rate will be the total respiratory rate.

Alarms

Input Power Alarms. The power source change alarm activates when the ventilator switches from a higher to lower priority electric power source (e.g., from AC to external battery). A low internal or external battery alarm indicates that battery power is at less than 9.5 V. Failure of the internal power supply or battery power insufficient to operate the ventilator results in a ventilator-inoperative condition.

Control Circuit Alarms. There are various ventilator-inoperative alarms that activate if the ventilator fails to

cycle, resulting in a "fast beep" alarm sound that cannot be silenced. In all cases the patient can breathe spontaneously through the patient air inlet.

Output Alarms. High- and low-pressure alarms are operator adjustable. The apnea alarm is a function of the low-pressure alarm and is activated if the ventilator fails to detect an inspiratory effort within 15 seconds. The reference point of origin is the low-pressure alarm setting in centimeters of water.

Pulmonetic Systems LTV Series 900/950/1000/1200

The LTV ventilators (Pulmonetic Systems/Cardinal Health) (Figure 17-14) are microprocessor-controlled, electrically powered, pneumatic ventilators. The LTV 900 and 950 versions are most frequently used in the home care setting whereas the LTV 1000 and 1200 versions are often used as transport ventilators. The LTVs are approved for use in patients greater than 5 kg and do require a specific LTV patient-monitoring circuit. The ventilator can be flow or time triggered; volume or pressure limited; and time, pressure, or flow cycled.[23]

Power Conversion and Transmission

The LTVs use AC power, external battery power, or internal battery power. Gas enters through an inlet filter and is routed to the turbine rotary compressor. Patient gas flow then enters the flow valve, which controls patient gas delivery. Flow through the flow valve is ultimately controlled by differential pressure transducers that monitor pressures and flows. A small portion of the gas exiting the flow valve is connected to the

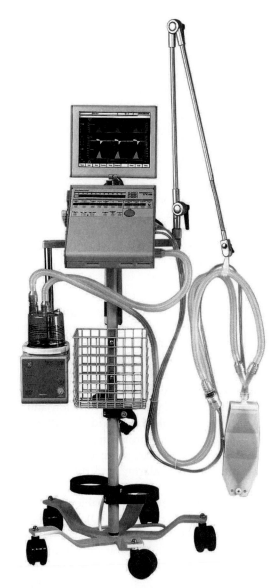

FIGURE 17-14 LTV 1000 (Pulmonetic Systems/Cardinal Health).

external exhalation valve that controls inspiratory flow, expiration, and PEEP.

Control

The LTVs can be operated in one of the following modes: control, A/C, SIMV VC, or PC (models 950, 1000, and 1200 only) with or without PS, CPAP, and NPPV.

The following patient settings are available on the LTV ventilators: breath rate, 0 to 80 breaths/minute; V_T, 50 to 2000 ml; inspiratory time, 0.3 to 9.9 seconds; PS, 0 to 60 cm H_2O; PEEP, 0 to 20 cm H_2O; bias flow, 10 L/minute; trigger sensitivity, 1 to 9 L/minute; and PC, 0 to 99 cm H_2O (available only with LTV models 950, 1000, and 1200). PC and PS settings are referenced to a baseline pressure of "zero" rather than the PEEP

setting, necessitating that the user mathematically calculate the PC and PS levels delivered to the patient. The LTV 1200 model has an internal PEEP valve, changing the way in which the PC and PS parameters are set. Oxygen can be precisely controlled on the LTV 1000 model by connecting to a high-pressure gas source or by bleeding in oxygen to the low-flow inlet, which sends gas to the turbine for mixing before patient breath delivery (all versions). The LTVs offer sensitivity leak compensation for patients with uncuffed tracheostomy tubes. Within the extended menu there are additional settings that allow the clinician to customize various controls to be patient specific; these include adjustments of the rise time, flow termination, time termination, leak compensation for sensitivity control, and PC flow termination. The extended menu also allows the operator to customize various alarm operations for the ventilator.

Output

Waveforms. Volume ventilation produces an aggressive decelerating waveform while PC and PS breaths produce a less aggressive decelerating waveform. Inspiratory times are limited on the basis of V_T volume settings both in VC and PC breath delivery.

Monitoring. A digital display of PIP, mean airway pressure (MAP), PEEP, frequency (f), exhaled tidal volume (Vte), minute ventilation (VE), I/E ratio, and flow calculations (Vcalc) automatically scroll within the display window. Individual displays may also be manually selected by depressing the "select" keypad.

Alarms

Input Power Alarms. The power source change alarm activates when the ventilator switches from the electric power source to internal or external battery power. A low-battery alarm has two thresholds: one when the battery is low (<9.5 V) and one when the battery nears empty (this alarm cannot be silenced). When the battery is fully depleted the ventilator will shut down and become inoperative ("INOP").

Control Circuit Alarms. The ventilator has an "INOP" alarm that shuts down the ventilator while allowing the patient to breathe room air spontaneously; alternative ventilation should be provided whenever this condition exists. A "DISC/SENSE" alarm will activate if the sensing line is pinched, blocked, or occluded, or is disconnected, and remains activated until the alarm condition is no longer present. During the "DISC/SENCE" alarm breath delivery does not occur.

Output Alarms. There are a number of operator-adjustable alarms, including the following: high-pressure alarm, low-pressure alarm, and low minute volume alarm. Within the extended menu the operator can customize the following default alarms: alarm volume

(60 to 85 dBA [A-weighted decibels; an expression of the relative loudness of sounds in air as perceived by the human ear]), apnea interval (10 to 60 s), high-pressure alarm delay (zero-, one-, or two-breath delay), high-frequency (5 to 80/min or off), low peak pressure (LPP; all breaths or VC/PC breaths only), and high-PEEP (3 to 40 cm H_2O or off) alarms.

Newport HT50

The Newport HT50 ventilator (Newport Medical Instruments) (Figure 17-15) is a microprocessor-controlled, electronically powered, pneumatic ventilator and is approved for use in patients who weigh more than 10 kg. It can be pressure or time triggered; volume or pressure limited; and time, pressure, or flow cycled. Newport Medical Instruments recommends specific exhalation valves and circuits for use with the HT50.[24]

Power Conversion and Transmission

The HT50 uses AC power, internal battery power, or external power. A new, fully charged internal battery can last up to 10 hours. A central microprocessor is responsible for electrically activating the internal dual micropiston for gas delivery. A separate proportional solenoid valve controls the internal exhalation valve. A user setup procedure calibrates the exhalation valves and allows for PEEP leak compensation.

Control

The HT50 operates in the CMV, A/C, SIMV, or SPONT modes with volume or pressure breath delivery and PS in the SIMV and SPONT modes.

The following settings are available on the HT50: tidal volume, 100 to 2200 ml; respiratory rate, 1 to 99/

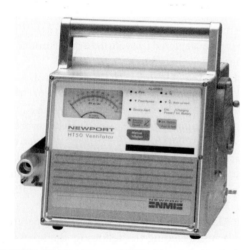

FIGURE 17-15 Newport HT50 (Newport Medical Instruments).

minute; inspiratory time, 0.1 to 3.0 seconds; PEEP, 0 to 30 cm H_2O; PS, 0 to 60 cm H_2O; PC, 5 to 60 cm H_2O; and trigger sensitivity, -9.9 to 0 cm H_2O. Oxygen delivery is accomplished with an optional air–oxygen entrainment mixer to deliver precise FIO_2 levels, or with an oxygen-blending bag kit that produces variable oxygen concentrations depending on minute volume.

Output

Monitoring. The following parameters are monitored continuously on the HT50: peak airway pressure (Paw P), mean airway pressure (Paw M), baseline pressure (Paw B), inspired V_T, inspired minute volume (Vi), and breath rate (f). The peak airway pressure and baseline pressure readings are also displayed on the analog manometer.

Alarms

Input Power Alarms. A power switchover alarm is activated when the ventilator switches from AC to DC power, a low-battery alarm activates when a minimum of 30 minutes of battery life remain, and a "battery empty" alarm indicates a minimum of 15 minutes of battery life.

Control Circuit Alarms. The device alert will activate when there is a ventilator malfunction and alternative ventilation should be provided. Other alarms that terminate effective ventilation are the "occlusion alarm," in which the primary solenoid is malfunctioning, the "system failure alarm," and the "system error alarm."

Output Alarms. Operator-adjustable alarms include high airway pressure (4 to 99 cm H_2O), low airway pressure (3 to 98 cm H_2O), high and low baseline pressure (automatically set), high inspiratory minute volume (1.3 to 50 L/min), low inspiratory minute volume (0.3 to 49 L/min), and apnea (30 s) (automatically set).

Commonly used home care ventilators include the TBird (Bird Products/Cardinal Health) and the Puritan Bennett Achieva (Covidien), both of which provide PS and internal PEEP.

SUMMARY

Understanding the mechanics and features available on ventilators is important to maximize the effectiveness of their use with patients. Most of the ventilators manufactured today possess similar technology marketed under a variety of nomenclatures. When choosing or operating a ventilator for purchase or patient use, the clinician must evaluate the types of patients being helped and the overall needs of those patients. Technology needs and financial constraints will both influence decisions.

ASSESSMENT QUESTIONS

See Evolve Resources for answers.

1. Which of the following power sources are typically required by mechanical ventilators to provide positive pressure ventilation?
   A. Hydraulic
   B. Electric
   C. Pneumatic
   D. Solar
   E. Both B and C

2. The variables involved in the mechanics of ventilation are pressure, volume, and flow. How many of the following variables are controlled by the ventilator during inhalation?
   A. 1
   B. 2
   C. 3
   D. Both a and b

3. Dual control is possible if a ventilator has the ability to switch from one control variable to another if a certain condition is met, or not met, during the inspiratory phase. The following are all examples of dual control modes *except*?
   A. Volume-assured pressure-support ventilation
   B. Volume guarantee (VG)
   C. Pressure-regulated volume control (PRVC)
   D. Volume controlled pressure-support

4. Which of the following safety features allows breath cycling to occur if the predetermined percentage of peak flow cycling criteria cannot be achieved due to an endotracheal tube leak in an infant?
   A. Pressure control
   B. Dual control criteria
   C. Backup inspiratory time
   D. High pressure limit

5. The following are all exclusive neonatal ventilators that are not capable of ventilating adults *except*:
   A. Puritan Bennett Infant Star 500
   B. Sechrist IV-200
   C. Bear Medical Systems
   D. Cardinal Health AVEA
   E. Bear Cub 750vs

6. The Evita ventilator can be operated using all of the following modes *except*:
   A. CMV
   B. SIMV
   C. Machine volume
   D. MMV
   E. CPAP

7. The patient trigger variable(s) on the Puritan Bennett 840 is achieved by the patient based on a change in:
   A. Flow
   B. Pressure

ASSESSMENT QUESTIONS—cont'd

   C. Volume
   D. Both A and B

8. Neurally Adjusted Ventilatory Assist (NAVA) is a mode found on the Servo-I ventilator that may provide improved synchronization between the patient and the ventilator by applying flow and pressure in proportion to the electrical activation of the:
   A. Diaphragm muscle
   B. Medulla oblongata
   C. Pons
   D. Myocardium

References

1. Banner MJ, Blanch P, Desautels DA: Mechanical ventilators. In Kirby RR, Banner MJ, Downs JB, editors: *Clinical applications of ventilatory support*, New York: Churchill Livingstone; 1990. pp 401–503.
2. Kirby RR et al: A new pediatric volume ventilator, *Anesth Analg* 1970;50:533.
3. Chatburn RL: A new system for understanding mechanical ventilators, *Respir Care* 1991;36:1123.
4. Chatburn RL: Classification of mechanical ventilators, *Respir Care* 1992;37:1009.
5. Chatburn RL, Lough MD, Primiano FP Jr: Mechanical ventilation. In Chatburn RL, Lough MD, editors: *Handbook of respiratory care*, ed 2, St. Louis: Mosby; 1990. pp 159–223.
6. Spearman CB, Sanders HG Jr: Physical principles and functional designs of ventilators. In Kirby RR, Banner MJ, Downs JB, editors: *Clinical applications of ventilatory support*, New York: Churchill Livingstone; 1990. pp 63–104.
7. Branson RD, MacIntyre NR: Dual control modes of mechanical ventilation, *Respir Care* 1996;41:294.
8. Mushin M, Rendell-Baker W, Thompson PW: *Automatic ventilation of the lungs*, ed 3, Oxford: Blackwell-Scientific; 1980. pp 62–166.
9. Branson RD, Chatburn RL: Technical description and classification of modes of ventilator operation, *Respir Care* 1992;37:1026.
10. Dräger Medical: *Operating instructions: Babylog 8000 plus infant care ventilator*, software 5.n, ed 1, Telford, Pa: Dräger Medical; 1997.
11. Frembgen S: Extending the power of conventional ventilation, *Neonatal Intensive Care* 1991;4:30.
12. Sechrist Industries: *User's manual: model IV-200 SAVI system*, rev 7, Anaheim, Calif: Sechrist Industries; 1997.
13. Viasys Healthcare: *Operators manual: AVEA ventilating system*, Palm Springs, Calif: Viasys Healthcare, Critical Care Division; 2002.
14. Dräger Medical: *Operating instructions: Evita 4 intensive care ventilator*, Chantilly, Va: Dräger Medical; 1996.

15. Dräger Medical: *NeoFlow neonatal mode: addendum to operating instructions: Evita 4* [as of software 2.n], *Evita 2 dura* [as of software 3.10], Telford, Pa: Dräger Medical; 1999.

16. Nellcor Puritan Bennett: *Operator's and technical reference manual: 840™ ventilator system*, Carlsbad, Calif: Nellcor Puritan Bennett; 1998.

17. Nellcor Puritan Bennett: *BiLevel option/800 series ventilators*, Carlsbad, Calif: Nellcor Puritan Bennett; 1998.

18. Maquet Critical Care: *User's manual: SERVO-i ventilator system* [E313E], Solna, Sweden: Maquet Critical Care; 2002.

19. See www.hamilton-medical.com/New-Hamilton-G5-ventilator.648.0.html. Retrieved September 2008.

20. See http://www.gehealthcare.com/usen/respiratory_care/docs/Engstrom_Brochure_US_2_08.pdf. Retrieved September 2008.

21. Puritan Bennett: *Operating instruction manual—issue B: companion 2801 volume ventilator*, Lenexa, Kans: Puritan Bennett; 1990.

22. Respironics Lifecare: *Operator's manual: PLV volume ventilator*, Lafayette, Colo: Respironics Lifecare; 1991.

23. Pulmonetic Systems: *Operator's manual: LTV series ventilator*, Minneapolis, Minn: Pulmonetic Systems; 2004.

24. Newport Medical Instruments: *Operating manual Newport HT50 ventilator*, Newport Beach, Calif: Newport Medical Instruments; 2001.

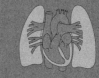

Chapter 18

Continuous Positive Airway Pressure

ROBERT M. DiBLASI ● PETER RICHARDSON

OUTLINE

Indications
Contraindications
Hazards and Complications
Physiologic Effects
Delivery Systems and Patient Interfaces
    Mechanical Ventilator CPAP
    Bubble Nasal CPAP
    Infant Flow Nasal CPAP

Management Strategies
    Application
    Monitoring
    Bedside Care and Airway Management
    Weaning
Advancing Concepts
    Infant Flow SiPAP

LEARNING OBJECTIVES

After reading this chapter the reader will be able to:

- Provide a brief history of the various methods used to generate continuous positive airway pressure (CPAP) in infants
- Describe the indications/contraindications for CPAP
- Describe the various physiologic effects of CPAP
- Identify commonly used delivery systems and nasal interfaces for delivering CPAP
- Discuss potential differences in the operation and patient response between gas delivery systems and CPAP interfaces

- Determine various strategies used to manage patients receiving CPAP and how these may impact outcomes
- Describe monitoring strategies for determining positive and negative responses to CPAP
- Identify common complications and how they can be avoided when using CPAP
- Review bedside care procedures, performed by clinicians, that contribute to the successful use of CPAP in infants
- Describe various weaning strategies that have been used for withdrawing CPAP in infants

Continuous positive airway pressure (CPAP) is a constant gas pressure that is applied to the airway opening of spontaneously breathing infants throughout the entire respiratory cycle. CPAP is used to maintain lung expansion under conditions that cause the alveoli and small airways to collapse or fill with fluid.[1] CPAP has been a standard of care for managing critically ill infants for nearly 4 decades and has had a significant impact on improving patient outcomes,

particularly when considering the morbidity and mortality of low birth weight, premature infants. CPAP use in neonates was first described by Gregory and colleagues in 1971,[2] during an era when efforts to mechanically ventilate infants with respiratory distress often resulted in pulmonary air leaks and death. Their rationale for applying CPAP was to reproduce the physiologic effects of expiratory grunting, exhibited by infants in respiratory distress, to maintain functional residual

305

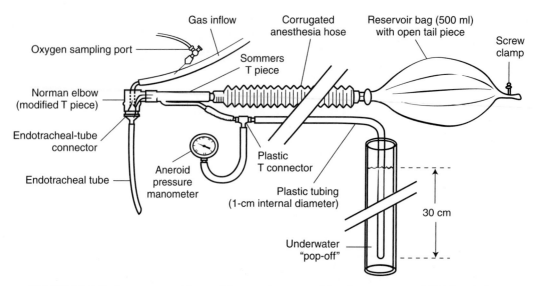

FIGURE 18-1 Early system used for applying continuous positive airway pressure (CPAP) to infants through an endotracheal tube.

capacity. They accomplished this by allowing intubated subjects to breathe spontaneously through a modified T-piece system using a blended, humidified gas source and a flow-inflating resuscitation bag with a screw-clamp at the tail of the bag, which maintained pressure by restricting flow to the atmosphere (Figure 18-1). In another method, nonintubated subjects were placed into a sealed head chamber that was pressurized with fresh gas to produce effects similar to endotracheal tube CPAP but without the potential risks associated with the use of an endotracheal tube.[2]

In early attempts made to provide a noninvasive form of CPAP to the lung, infants were placed in a box with their head out through a loose-fitting cuff around the neck and negative pressure was applied continuously to the infant's chest wall.[3-5] Further efforts to avoid intubation were accomplished with the application of nasal prong CPAP, which was first described by Kattwinkel and colleagues in 1973.[6] Today, nasal prong CPAP is the most common method by which CPAP is delivered to spontaneously breathing infants with respiratory disease.

This discussion focuses primarily on nasal CPAP delivery systems and interfaces that are most commonly used in clinical practice for newborn infants. These systems include ventilator-derived CPAP (V-CPAP), bubble CPAP (B-CPAP), and Infant Flow CPAP (IF-CPAP). Box 18-1 lists terms that are frequently used to describe these modes and methods described in this chapter. Chapter 19 (Mechanical Ventilation of the Neonatal and Pediatric Patient) discusses CPAP delivery through the mechanical ventilator when using an endotracheal or tracheostomy tube. Chapter 21 (Noninvasive Mechanical Ventilation of the Infant and Child) discusses noninvasive forms of support,

Box 18-1	Terms Used to Describe Noninvasive Pressure

CPAP: Continuous positive airway pressure
V-CPAP: Ventilator-derived continuous positive airway pressure
B-CPAP: Bubble continuous positive airway pressure
IF-CPAP: Infant Flow continuous positive airway pressure
IF-SiPAP: Infant Flow "sigh" positive airway pressure

including CPAP, that are commonly used in larger infants and pediatric patients.

INDICATIONS

CPAP is clinically indicated in infants with both obstructive and restrictive lung diseases. Box 18-2 lists the indications and contraindications regarding CPAP use. The use of CPAP can clinically impact lung disease predominantly to improve oxygenation, counter atelectasis,[7-12] and stabilize the chest wall.[13] CPAP is also used to stent open airways and hence lower airway resistance to gas flow in patients with obstructive lung disease and apnea.[14-19] CPAP is frequently used to maintain airway patency in infants with obstructive apnea[17,20-24] and obstructive airway diseases.[16,25-28] Figure 18-2 shows the effect of CPAP on the anatomic structures of the upper airways.

According to American Association for Respiratory Care (AARC, Irving, Tex) clinical practice guidelines,[29] neonates presenting with respiratory rate greater than 30% of normal, and paradoxical chest wall movement[30] with suprasternal and substernal retractions, grunting, nasal flaring, and cyanotic skin color[31,32] should be considered for CPAP administration as long as they are able

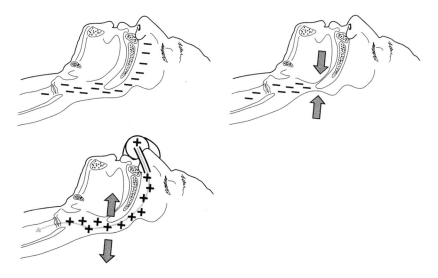

FIGURE 18-2 Top left, Normal patent upper airway. *Top right,* Tongue obstructing upper airway. *Bottom,* CPAP distending structures of oropharynx, preventing obstruction by the tongue and soft palate.

Box 18-2	Indications/Contraindications of Continuous Positive Airway Pressure

INDICATIONS
1. Premature infants
   a. Respiratory distress syndrome
   b. Apnea of prematurity
   c. After extubation and mechanical ventilation
2. Obstructive airway diseases
   a. Obstructive apnea
   b. Laryngeal or tracheal malacia
   c. Bronchopulmonary dysplasia
   d. Viral bronchiolitis
3. Pneumonia
   a. Viral or bacterial
   b. Aspiration
4. Meconium aspiration syndrome
5. Congestive heart failure
6. Pulmonary edema
7. Transient tachypnea of the newborn
8. Postoperative respiratory management
   a. Congenital heart disease
   b. Congenital diaphragmatic hernia
   c. Gastroschisis or omphalocele
9. Used in conjunction with:
   a. Surfactant administration
   b. Nitric oxide administration
   c. Extracorporeal membrane oxygenation
10. Paralysis of a hemidiaphragm

CONTRAINDICATIONS
1. Criteria for CPAP failure requiring mechanical ventilation
   a. $Paco_2$ > 60 mm Hg consistently
   b. pH < 7.25
2. Upper airway abnormalities
   a. Choanal atresia
   b. Cleft palate
   c. Tracheoesophageal fistula
3. Untreated congenital diaphragmatic hernia
4. Neuromuscular disorders
5. CNS depressant medications
6. Central or frequent apnea

CPAP, Continuous positive airway pressure; $Paco_2$, arterial partial pressure of carbon dioxide.

to demonstrate adequate ventilation as defined by an arterial partial pressure of carbon dioxide ($Paco_2$) less than 60 mm Hg and a pH greater than 7.25.[29]

CPAP is an effective option for preventing extubation failure.[33-42] CPAP has been successful in the treatment of pneumonias,[43] transient tachypnea of the newborn, meconium aspiration syndrome,[44,45] and paralysis of the hemidiaphragm. It has been employed for infants with pulmonary edema and patent ductus arteriosus.[46]

CPAP has been shown to improve lung function in postoperative congenital heart disease[47-49] and after surgical repair of abdominal wall defects; however, increased abdominal pressure may adversely affect pulmonary function.[50] CPAP use in infants with diaphragmatic hernia is indicated only after surgical repair. CPAP is used in conjunction with the administration of surfactant,[51-57] nitric oxide,[58] and as a source of high airway pressure in infants receiving extracorporeal membrane oxygenation.[59]

CONTRAINDICATIONS

Infants in respiratory distress with persistent apneic episodes and who are unable to maintain $Paco_2$ less than 60 mm Hg and pH greater than 7.25 should not be given CPAP or, if already receiving CPAP, mechanical ventilation is indicated.[29] Infants with congenital anomalies such as choanal atresia, cleft palate, tracheoesophageal fistula, or preoperative diaphragmatic hernia should not receive CPAP.[60] CPAP is contraindicated in infants with neural muscular disorders, infants receiving CNS depressants, and infants with central apnea or frequent apneic episodes resulting in desaturation and/or bradycardia.[29]

HAZARDS AND COMPLICATIONS

Noninvasive application of CPAP is considered a "gentler" method of support when compared with mechanical ventilation; however, CPAP is still associated with some of the same hazards and complications that are frequently associated with mechanical ventilation. Pneumothorax is a complication that is occasionally reported in infants receiving CPAP.[61] This is a result of inadvertent positive end-expiratory pressure related to gas trapping when infants are tachypneic and do not have a sufficient expiratory time. This may also occur after surfactant replacement therapy, when pulmonary compliance improves and the infant has not been weaned appropriately and, thus, is exposed to excessive airway and hence alveolar pressure. Other forms of air leak caused by inappropriately high CPAP levels may include pulmonary interstitial emphysema, pneumomediastinum, and pneumatocele.[62-66] Although extremely rare, vascular air embolism has been described in infants receiving CPAP.[67] This occurs when a laceration in the lung parenchyma introduces air into the cardiovascular system. Increased intracranial pressures related to lung overdistention may also occur as a result of CPAP.[68] CPAP has been reported as having an adverse impact on renal effects including decreased urine output and glomerular filtration rate.[69] Gastrointestinal blood flow has been cited as a potential complication of endotracheal CPAP and may well manifest similarly in nasal CPAP.[70] Bowel distention is often noted with CPAP.[71] Infants may swallow gas and this can result in bulging flanks, increased abdominal girth, and visibly dilated intestinal loops on X-ray.[72]

A study comparing spontaneously breathing unassisted premature infants with infants receiving CPAP showed that there were no detectable differences in hemodynamic values including stroke volume and cardiac output as measured by echocardiogram.[73] This implies that there is no need to withhold CPAP support to prevent circulatory complications; however, hemodynamic compromise should always be considered as a factor when using any positive pressure device. Complications that have been described regarding problems with equipment include desaturation due to loss of airway pressure caused by inappropriate fit of nasal prongs or leak around a nasal mask. Nasal masks may also result in leaks around the eyes and damage to facial tissue from improper fixation. An open mouth can lead to a loss in airway pressure due to leaks.[74] Obstruction of nasal prongs from mucous plugging or tips pressed against the nasal mucosa can lead to losses in airway pressure unmeasured by low-pressure alarm systems and increase work of breathing.[74] Leaks or obstruction can also lead to a loss in the inspired fraction of oxygen (Fio_2). Fluctuations in baseline pressure and increase in work of breathing can be caused by insufficient gas flow.[75]

Local irritation and trauma[76] to the nasal septum may occur because of misalignment or improper fixation of nasal prongs.[77] Nasal snubbing and circumferential distortion (widening) of the nares can be caused by nasal prongs, especially if CPAP is being used for more than just a few days.[78] Breakdown and erosion low on the septum at the base of the philtrum can occur when using nasal masks.[79,80] Columella necrosis has been reported after only a few days of CPAP use (Figure 18-3). Inadequate humidification can lead to nasal mucosal damage.[81] Skin irritation of the head and neck from improperly secured bonnets or CPAP head harnesses can also occur.[29] Equipment failure and dysfunction should always be considered as a potential source for complicating an infant's condition when providing CPAP.

PHYSIOLOGIC EFFECTS

Applying CPAP to infants with respiratory distress syndrome increases functional residual capacity and arterial

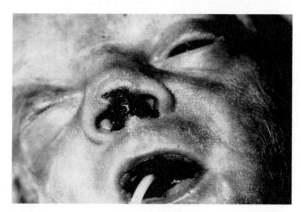

FIGURE 18-3 Columella necrosis resulting from short-term nasal CPAP.

partial pressure of oxygen (Pa_{O_2}),[11] improves lung mechanics,[82,83] reduces thoracoabdominal asynchrony,[24,84] stabilizes the chest wall,[85] improves the ventilation-to-perfusion ratio,[44,86-88] and improves the distribution of ventilation.[11] CPAP in spontaneous breathing infants with respiratory failure improves the breathing strategy as reflected by improved work of breathing, increased tidal volume, and a reduction in "labor breathing index".[84] CPAP decreases the respiratory rate and increases the expiratory time and the time constant of the respiratory system.[88] The characteristic protective expiratory braking observed in premature newborn infants is abolished by CPAP.[88] A decreased respiratory rate is not due to altered ventilatory response to carbon dioxide.[89] Decreases in minute volume are likely due to reductions in alveolar dead space.[2] Box 18-3 shows physiologic effects that are commonly associated with CPAP.

An increasing body of evidence demonstrates that by using CPAP mechanical ventilation can be avoided, resulting in a lower incidence of lung injury and hence chronic lung disease.[53,90] By applying CPAP, the airways can be protected from mechanical injury and colonization related to the endotracheal tube.[91] Infants treated with CPAP have been found to have a lower incidence of complications related to mechanical ventilation, including respiratory-related nosocomial infections, apnea, intraventricular hemorrhage, retinopathy of prematurity, and chronic lung disease, when compared with infants who were intubated and treated with mechanical ventilation.[43] Although a thorough discussion describing the effects of ventilator-induced lung injury in infants is beyond the scope of this chapter, it is important to realize that a major goal of CPAP is to eliminate or reduce the need for prolonged ventilator support.

Postnatal lung development in low birth weight infants, specifically, primary and secondary septation forming saccules and alveoli[91-93] and angiogenesis,[94] may be arrested or altered[95,96] by mechanical ventilation,[97-99] placing the infant at risk for developing chronic lung disease.[93] Considering that CPAP decreases indicators of lung injury,[100,101] the goal of early prophylactic application of CPAP[91,102,103] is to reduce the need for intubation[104,105] and counter the arrest of postnatal lung development in infants, possibly decreasing the incidence of chronic lung disease.[101]

DELIVERY SYSTEMS AND PATIENT INTERFACES

The term *delivery system* describes the mechanism by which fresh gas flow is generated and positive pressure is maintained at the patient's airway. A number of devices are commonly used clinically to deliver CPAP to infants. They are characterized by their ability to provide either a constant or variable flow source. These systems also include a humidifier, circuit, and oxygen analyzer. Gas temperature and humidity are important aspects when maintaining the neutral thermal environment of a newborn infant and thus should be adjusted to provide a temperature between 37° and 39° F and 100% humidity to the patient. The humidifier servoregulates temperature on the basis of measurements acquired at the humidifier probe and thus should not be placed within an incubator or directly beneath a radiant warmer. The circuit should be constructed of flexible and lightweight material to prevent traction and torque on the nasal interface. This helps minimize patient discomfort and nasal injury.[106] The delivery system should include a "pop-off device" placed close to the airway to protect the patient from overpressurization, thereby limiting excessive volume delivery to the respiratory system.[32]

The term *patient interface device* describes the mechanism by which gas flow from the delivery system is delivered to the airway of the infant. Historically, various interface devices have been applied to administer CPAP to infants. These include enclosure of the head in a plastic pressure chamber, a pressurized plastic bag fitted over the infant's head, face chambers, face masks, tight-fitting face masks, devices requiring a neck seal, endotracheal tubes, nasopharyngeal tubes, and long and short binasal pharyngeal prongs.[107]

Today, CPAP is most often administered through short binasal prongs, and this method is considered the most effective interface option for delivering CPAP to infants.[107,108] This is attributed primarily to infants being regarded as obligate nose breathers,[5] resulting in CPAP

Box 18-3	Physiologic Effects of Continuous Positive Airway Pressure

- Increases functional residual capacity
- Increases tidal volume
- Decreases intrapulmonary shunt
- Increases pulmonary compliance
- Decreases airway resistance
- Stabilizes the chest wall
- Improves the distribution of ventilation
- Improves ventilation-to-perfusion ratio
- Improves gas exchange
- Decreases work of breathing
- Reduces alveolar dead space
- Protects the developing lung
- Decreases cellular indicators of lung injury
- Reduces the need for intubation and mechanical ventilation

delivering relatively constant airway pressures. Nasal prongs also facilitate mobilization and oral feeding.[109] Because these other methods are used infrequently in the clinical setting, this chapter focuses primarily on short binasal prongs and nasal masks for interfacing with these systems.

Clinicians have often speculated that differences in the level of imposed resistance and hence imposed work of breathing (WOB_I) between the systems are clinically relevant to infants and may contribute to CPAP failure. Nasal prongs have been reported to have lower resistance to gas flow when compared with other commonly used nasal interfaces.[110] These differences are related to the length and internal diameters of the interfaces but are also associated with the delivery system and how CPAP is maintained by this system. Table 18-1 shows the pressure drop at various flow rates in the devices that have traditionally been used to interface with CPAP delivery systems. The WOB_I is related to the resistance to gas flow when breathing through the various elements imposed by the CPAP system and interface. The WOB_I is superimposed on the physiologic WOB; which in turn increases the total amount of WOB done by the patient.[111] Imposed expiratory resistance can also impact the inspiratory WOB in spontaneously breathing infants.[112] Exhalation is considered active in infants with lung disease and therefore expiratory resistance is an important consideration.[113] This also becomes important because most infants, especially premature infants, do not have adequate energy stores and high caloric requirements often resulting in rapid deterioration of the respiratory status.

Early systems that used flow resistors (screw clamp; see Figure 18-1) for exhalation were associated with higher resistance and hence a higher amount of energy was expended to breathe; currently available systems, on the other hand, use low-resistance threshold-type resistors.[114] In theory, a threshold resistor produces no resistance to exhalation and maintains CPAP by applying an opposing force that is equal to the amount of the desired system pressure.[115] Infant mechanical ventilators have been shown to have higher imposed expiratory resistance compared with an endotracheal tube.[116] However, imposed resistance and hence WOB are likely to be lower when breathing through a ventilator with nasal prongs than with an endotracheal tube.[110] The water seal in

TABLE 18-1

Dimensions of Nasal Continuous Positive Airway Pressure Devices and Pressure Drop at Various Flows

Device	Size	Prong Length* (mm)	Internal Diameter[†] (mm)	Outer Diameter[†] (mm)	Pressure Drop (cm H_2O) at Various Flows				
					4 L/min	5 L/min	6 L/min	7 L/min	8 L/min
Duotube	2.5	40	1.4	2.5	9.7	15	21	29	38
	3.0	40	1.8	3.0	3.0	4.5	6.2	8.3	10.5
	3.5	40	2.5	3.5	1.1	1.7	2.3	3.1	3.9
Single prong[‡]	2.5	50	2.5	3.8	2.2	3.3	4.4	5.9	7.3
	3.0	50	3.0	4.3	1.1	1.5	2.1	2.7	3.3
	3.5	50	3.5	4.9	0.6	0.9	1.2	1.6	1.9
Argyle prong	Extra small	6	1.8	3.1	1.7	2.6	3.6	4.8	6.2
	Small	8	2.3	4.0	0.9	1.4	1.9	2.5	3.2
	Large	10	2.3	4.8	0.7	1.1	1.5	2.1	2.6
Hudson prong	0	11	2.3	3.7	1.4	2.2	3.1	4.2	5.4
	1	11	2.6	3.9	0.8	1.3	1.8	2.5	3.3
	2	11	3.0	4.6	0.3	0.5	0.6	0.9	1.1
	3	12	3.5	4.9	0.2	0.3	0.4	0.5	0.6
	4	15	4.0	5.4	0.1	0.2	0.3	0.5	0.6
Infant Flow driver	Small	6	3.0	3.9	0.2	0.2	0.3	0.4	0.5
	Medium	7	3.5	4.3	-0.1	-0.2	-0.3	-0.4	-0.5
	Large	7	4.0	4.6	-0.2	-0.3	-0.5	-0.7	-0.9

From De Paoli AG et al: In vitro comparison of nasal continuous positive airway pressure devices for neonates, *Arch Dis Child Fetal Neonatal Ed* 2002;87:F42 .

* Does not include the length proximal to the bridge between the prongs.
[†] Internal and outer diameters were measured at the prong tip.
[‡] Refers to Mallinckrodt endotracheal tube cut down to 5 cm in length and attached to a standard endotracheal tube adapter with pressure side port.

B-CPAP functions as a pure threshold-type resistor and has been shown to have low imposed expiratory resistance.[117] The IF-CPAP device has been shown in a lung model to have one quarter of the imposed WOB compared with other forms of CPAP.[118] IF-CPAP has also been shown to significantly reduce inspiratory WOB in preterm infants and to improve compliance better compared with mechanical ventilator CPAP.[119-121] In another study comparing differences in the WOB for infants randomized to B-CPAP or IF-CPAP, resistive WOB was lower for infants treated with IF-CPAP; however, these results did not reflect any clinically significant differences in the total inspiratory WOB done by the patient.[122]

Mechanical Ventilator CPAP

Time-cycled pressure-limited constant-flow infant ventilators were introduced in the mid-1970s and are still a simple and efficient method for nasal CPAP delivery to infants.[86,122,123] V-CPAP, often described as "conventional CPAP," has been accomplished by placing ventilators in the CPAP mode and setting a constant flow rate while interfacing with the system using long binasal prongs, a single nasopharyngeal tube, or an endotracheal tube inserted into the nasopharynx. Time-cycled pressure-limited ventilators use exhalation valves to maintain CPAP. The convenience of a blended gas source, alarm options, and low cost made this a popular choice among clinicians. If intubated patients failed V-CPAP, or if the patient was extubated from conventional ventilation, then the ventilator was available at the bedside without having to set up a separate delivery system.

Today, a number of commercially available microprocessor-controlled infant ventilators allow noninvasive application of V-CPAP. In these systems CPAP is maintained with a variable demand–flow system. Flow rate and airway pressure are regulated by servo-controlling the aperture size of the exhalation valve. These ventilators also include the following:

- Highly responsive demand–flow systems
- Leak compensation
- Airway graphics monitoring
- Apnea backup breaths

The interface that is most commonly used with this delivery system is the Hudson nasal prongs (Hudson RCI/Teleflex, Research Triangle Park, NC) (Figure 18-4). The prongs are adjusted so that there is never contact between the prongs and the nasal septum.[79] The prong size is established on the basis of weight, using a sizing chart provided by the manufacture (Table 18-2). The prongs stay in place by attaching the circuitry to a premade hat, using safety pins and rubber bands. A proximal pressure line or "pop-off" can be attached at a Luer adapter at the nasal interface, or this can also be plugged.

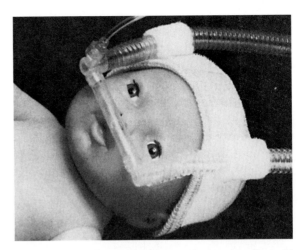

FIGURE 18-4 Hudson RCI infant nasal prong interface with bonnet fixation.

Bubble Nasal CPAP

B-CPAP (also known as the "water seal" or "bubbly bottle" method) is a simple, safe, inexpensive constant flow delivery system that has been used for nearly four decades to deliver CPAP.[124-127] This method was implemented by Jen-Tien Wung in the 1970s at Columbia University Medical Center (New York, NY).[124] It is constructed with readily available equipment and materials that can usually be found in most respiratory care equipment storage areas. A commercially available version of this system (Fisher & Paykel Healthcare, Auckland, New Zealand) is currently being used in Europe and Australia. Materials include the following (see Figure 18-5)[71,106]:

- An infant dual-limb heated wire ventilator circuit
- A humidifier and blended gas source
- A pressure transducer
- A water column filled to 10 cm with either sterile water or a 25% acetic acid solution

A measuring tape is attached to the outside of the water column. The CPAP level is maintained by submerging the distal end of expiratory circuit straight down into

TABLE 18-2

Sizing Chart for Hudson RCI Infant Nasal Prong CPAP

Weight Range (g)	Suggested Cannula Size
Less than 700	0
700 to 1250	1
1250 to 2000	2
2000 to 3000	3
More than 3000	4
1 to 2 years of age	5

Adapted from http://www.hudsonrci.com.

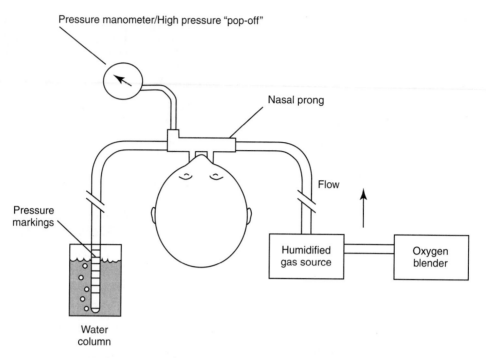

FIGURE 18-5 A simple system for delivering bubble nasal CPAP.

the fluid from the surface of the water line to a measured depth in centimeters, thus creating the amount of CPAP in centimeters of water. If a higher level of CPAP is needed, the tube can be advanced further down into the fluid column. The flow rate of humidified gas (6 to 10 L/min) is set to meet the inspiratory flow rate requirements of the patient, maintain the CPAP level, and rinse the system of exhaled carbon dioxide.[106] The pressure measured at the nasal prong could be slightly higher than the submersion depth of the expiratory tubing below the water surface when higher flow rates are used; therefore, airway pressure should always be monitored at the nasal prong to assure proper CPAP levels. A high-pressure pop-off can be placed as close to the patient as possible should the expiratory limb become occluded.[32] This system has few alarms or monitoring options and therefore it is extremely important to evaluate patients frequently, because vital signs may be the only effective alarm for alerting clinicians to airway disconnects, prong occlusion, and mechanical system failure.

At present, the interface that is most commonly used with this delivery system is Hudson nasal prongs (see Figure 18-4). The prongs are adjusted so that there is never contact between the prongs and the nasal septum.[79] The prong size is established on the basis of weight, using a sizing chart provided by the manufacturer (see Table 18-2). The prongs stay in place by attaching the circuitry to a premade hat, using Velcro or safety pins and rubber bands. A proximal pressure line can be attached at a Luer adapter at the nasal interface, or this can also be plugged.

Various Internet resources provide step-by-step methodologies that are useful when setting up this system.[32]

The use of B-CPAP in infants has been shown to significantly reduce minute volume and respiratory rate with no changes in transcutaneous carbon dioxide or oxygen saturation, compared with mechanical ventilator CPAP.[121] Small pressure fluctuations created by the back pressure of bubbles in the underwater seal are transmitted to the airway, thereby producing a noisy component that may enhance lung recruitment and gas mixing in a fashion similar to mechanisms that are present during high-frequency oscillatory ventilation.[128-131]

Subjective accounts of a visible "thoracic wiggle" from these bubble effects are often reported by clinicians caring for infants supported with B-CPAP. The use of higher flow rates can result in more vigorous bubbling and hence higher pressure fluctuations in the delivery system; however, this does not appear to improve gas exchange.[132] In premature animals, the use of B-CPAP has resulted in improvements in gas exchange, lung mechanics, and lung volume, which suggest enhanced alveolar recruitment when compared to V-CPAP.[129] Additional clinical research needs to be done to confirm similar effects in human infants.

Infant Flow Nasal CPAP

Infant Flow CPAP (IF-CPAP) (Cardinal Health, Dublin, Ohio) is a commercially available variable flow device that is specifically designed to deliver CPAP in newborns. The "flow driver" provides the source gas (Figure 18-6)

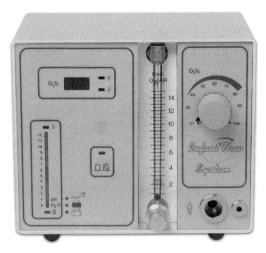

FIGURE 18-6 Infant Flow driver.

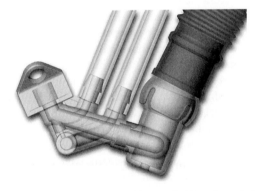

FIGURE 18-7 Infant Flow generator nasal interface device.

and consists of an internalized flow metering system, a blender with an FIO_2 control knob, a digitalized pressure LED, an alarm system, and a pressure relief system.[133] An external auxiliary gas flow meter is used to provide gas source identical to the set FIO_2 for nebulizers and manual resuscitators. Blended gas is humidified and delivered to the nasal interface "flow generator" (Figure 18-7), using a proprietary patient circuit. Despite setting a constant flow on the flow driver, the unique geometric design of the flow generator incorporates unique physical properties that allow control of gas delivery to and from the patient and is thus considered variable. The set flow rate is based on the fluctuation of the baseline pressure measurement, which is made at the flow generator, as indicated by the light-emitting diode bars on the front panel of the flow driver. If the nasal prongs or mask are sized and fitted properly, a flow rate of 8 L/minute should maintain a CPAP level of approximately 5 cm H_2O.[133]

The design of the flow generator uses a fluidic flip valve, which is designed with nonmoving parts and

provides fresh gas to the infant during inhalation and directs flow away from the infant during exhalation. Gas delivery is accomplished on the basis of the Bernoulli effect, whereby gas flow is provided to each nostril through the fresh gas inlet and passes through twin nasal jet injector nozzles at high velocity, which in turn converts the flow into a constant pressure.[72] If the patient requires any additional inspiratory flow, a Venturi-type effect created by the jet injector nozzles entrains more gas to be delivered. When the infant makes a spontaneous expiratory effort, exhaled gas passes freely and unimpeded by the flow of incoming air. This is accomplished by the Coandă effect, which triggers the "fluidic flip" and redirects incoming flow and exhaled gases through the expiratory channel simultaneously. Once the expiratory effort stops and expiratory flow ceases, the flow immediately switches back to the inspiratory position.[72]

The IF-CPAP system has been shown to deliver more consistent pressure, lowers the WOB, is less sensitive to leaks, and is more effective at alveolar recruitment compared with other forms of CPAP.[119,134] IF-CPAP use has also been shown to reduce the need for supplemental oxygenation in extremely low birth weight infants after extubation compared with infants randomized to receive V-CPAP with nasal prongs.[135] The ability of the Infant Flow driver to provide consistent pressure at the airway lowers WOB by applying greater stability to the infant respiratory system mechanics for a given change in intrapleural pressure.[118] The decreased variability of the airway pressure and fast response times of the IF-CPAP may also be due to the fact that the flow regulation mechanism is located at the nasal interface device whereas other CPAP devices (i.e., V-CPAP) regulate flow downstream from the patient (exhalation valve).

IF-CPAP is delivered to infants by using either a proprietary nasal mask or nasal prongs (Figure 18-8). The nasal prongs and masks are made from a soft silicone-based elastomer and are attached directly to the Infant Flow generator, which is then held in place once the interface is fastened by attachment to a soft cap or bonnet (Figure 18-9). The thin, soft material that constructs these nasal devices may provide important mechanical effects when using nasal prongs by flaring out during gas inflow, thus increasing the effective internal diameter and decreasing the leak around the prongs.[120] A mask does not rely on a prong entering the nares and may be more beneficial when trying to secure the nasal device onto an infant with craniofacial abnormalities. Nasal prongs have been shown to result in nasal and septal wall skin breakdown whereas nasal masks have been associated with breakdown low on the septum or at the base of the philtrum.[80] Some clinicians prefer switching back and forth when using nasal masks and prongs to

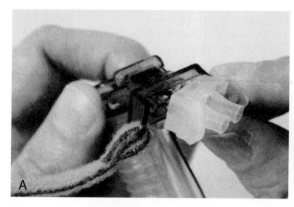
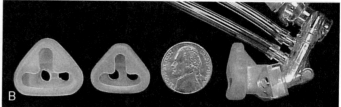

FIGURE 18-8 Silicone nasal prongs **(A)** and masks **(B)** attached to an Infant Flow driver.

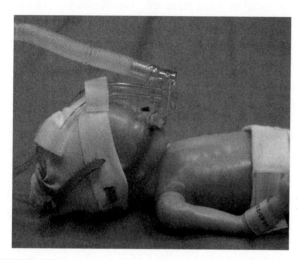

FIGURE 18-9 Proper fixation for the Infant Flow CPAP system.

MANAGEMENT STRATEGIES

CPAP is frequently used in newborn intensive care to avoid endotracheal intubation and mechanical ventilation. Mechanical ventilation in preterm infants is associated with increased risk of sepsis, lung injury, arrested lung development, and chronic lung disease.[136-138] There is no consensus regarding the most effective management strategy or delivery system to administer CPAP in newborn infants.[110] Management is based more on clinical experience than research trials. In one institution, where elective B-CPAP has been the initial form of support for newborn infants for nearly 4 decades, this practice has resulted in less frequent use of mechanical ventilation and surfactant replacement therapy.[126] This practice has been associated with significant reductions in chronic lung disease compared with other centers that use mechanical ventilation as an initial strategy for managing infants. Some institutions support early elective surfactant therapy, brief ventilation, and extubation to nasal CPAP. This practice is also associated with significant reductions in the need for mechanical ventilation,

eliminate these soft tissue injuries. Figure 18-10 shows the proper measurement techniques and Table 18-3 presents the sizing chart used to select the properly sized bonnet and nasal interface for use with the IF-CPAP device.

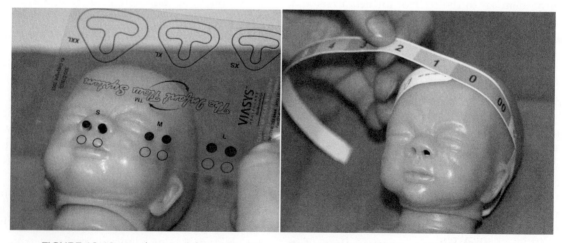

FIGURE 18-10 Nasal prong *(left)* and head circumference *(right)* measurements for the Infant Flow CPAP system.

TABLE 18-3

Cardinal Health Infant Flow Nasal CPAP Bonnet Sizing

Bonnet Size	Bonnet Color	Tape Measurement (cm)*
000	White	18-20
00	Gray	20-22
0	Pink	22-24
1	Light brown	24-26
2	Yellow	26-28
3	Light blue	28-30
4	Gold	30-32
5	Light green	32-34
6	Light burgundy	34-36
7	Orange	36-38
8	Dark green	38-40
9	Navy	40-42

* Tape measurement indicates the measured head circumference.
Courtesy of Cardinal Health (Dublin, Ohio).

fewer air leak syndromes, and lower incidence of chronic lung disease compared with a strategy of selective surfactant administration and continued ventilator support.[55]

A large randomized study conducted by the Vermont Oxford Network[139] will address the clinical benefits when managing infants in the delivery room using the following disparate practices:

- Intubation, prophylactic surfactant administration shortly after delivery, and subsequent stabilization on ventilator support
- Early stabilization on CPAP with selective intubation and surfactant administration for clinical indications
- Intubation, prophylactic surfactant administration shortly after delivery, and rapid extubation to CPAP

This study may help to standardize the respiratory strategy for managing newborn infants.

Application

CPAP is effective at reducing the incidence and duration of severe apneic episodes.[140,141] However, before CPAP can be applied, it is important to emphasize that infants experiencing frequent and sustained apneas and/or severe respiratory failure should not be considered for this form of support. It is essential that infants have a sufficient stimulus to breathe because CPAP is intended only for spontaneously breathing infants. Infants who do not respond to CPAP and continue to have frequent unresponsive apnea have failed this form of support. In most situations, ventilatory failure is indicated when $Paco_2$ exceeds 60 mm Hg and pH is less than 7.25.[29,104,142]

The primary clinical objectives for managing infants with CPAP are to *recruit* collapsed lung units, *stabilize* the lung volume, *maintain* adequate lung expansion, *avoid* hyperinflation and apnea, *improve* gas exchange, and *eliminate* the need for mechanical ventilation. This practice requires a team of clinicians who are properly trained in the technical aspects of the CPAP equipment as well as understand the pathophysiology of the infant pulmonary system. This team usually consists of the respiratory therapist and the nurse caring for the patient. Patients receiving CPAP are often more time-consuming than patients requiring mechanical ventilation.

CPAP of 4 to 6 cm H_2O is a common starting point for initiating CPAP.[103,143-145] Optimal CPAP levels in premature infants with respiratory distress syndrome may be as high as 12 cm H_2O.[86] Infants with obstructive lung disease may initially require higher CPAP levels in order to stent the airways open while allowing adequate ventilation.[26,27] At first, the Fio_2 should be set at the level the patient was receiving before CPAP administration. Higher levels may be used to maintain adequate oxygen saturations or Pao_2. Once CPAP is applied, it may take some time for the patient to adjust to breathing through this system. Often, they resist the initial placement of the equipment but then relax once they have become used to it. If the infant continues to appear anxious, agitated, and inconsolable, then swaddling and/or small amounts of sedation can be given once hypoxia and airway obstruction are ruled out. It is important to adopt "minimal handling" awareness and whenever possible cluster the patient care duties to limit infant stress.[144]

During the *recruitment* stage, it is not uncommon for the patient to remain at a higher Fio_2 until the lung volumes are stabilized. Often, an increase in Fio_2 may have no effect on oxygenation because of intrapulmonary shunting and thus additional pressure is required. A 40% increase in Fio_2 during the first 24 hours of nasal CPAP may represent a useful clinical marker to identify infants at high risk for developing a pneumothorax.[61] Physiologic changes associated with pneumothorax include decreased arterial blood pressure, heart rate, and respiratory rate, narrowed pulse pressure, and decreased Po_2.[62]

Once recruitment occurs, then Fio_2 should be weaned promptly in order to avoid complications caused by hyperoxemia.[146] The CPAP level is generally increased in increments of 1 or 2 cm H_2O; 12 cm H_2O is the maximum pressure attainable when applying CPAP. The pressure and Fio_2 are increased to attain the desired Pao_2. However, it is best to change only one parameter at a time.

The patient is thought to be approaching *stabilization* once an adequate level of CPAP is attained. Oxygenation, ventilation, and chest X-ray appearance begin to improve. Reductions in the work of breathing, respiratory rate, and incidence of apnea are also important findings that indicate that the patient is improving.[147]

Box 18-4	Indications of Stabilization With Continuous Positive Airway Pressure Support

- Reduced respiratory rate
- Reduced grunting, nasal flaring, and retractions
- $Paco_2$ of 50 to 60 mm Hg or less*
- pH > 7.25
- Fi_{O_2} requirement less than 0.60 with Pao_2 greater than 50 mm Hg†
- Improvement in chest X-ray appearance
- Reduction in severity and frequency of apneic episodes

Adapted in part from Czervinske M: AARC clinical practice guideline: application of continuous positive airway pressure to neonates via nasal prongs, nasopharyngeal tube, or nasal mask—2004 Revision and update, *Respir Care* 2004;49:1100.
Fi_{O_2}, fraction of inspired oxygen; $Paco_2$, arterial partial pressure of carbon dioxide; Pao_2, arterial partial pressure of oxygen.
* Higher ranges may apply in infants with chronic carbon dioxide retention.
† Range should be consistent with clinical state and the presence of congenital heart disease and/or persistent pulmonary hypertension of the newborn.

Box 18-5	Recognizing Failure of Continuous Positive Airway Pressure Support

- Increased WOB, nasal flaring, and retractions
- Decreasing pH (<7.25)
- $Paco_2$ greater than 60 mm Hg with intractable metabolic acidosis*
- Fi_{O_2} requirement exceeding 0.6 to 0.7 with Pao_2 less than 50 to 60 mm Hg†
- Nasal CPAP exceeding 12 cm H_2O
- Frequent apnea with cyanosis and bradycardia (not responding to caffeine therapy)

Adapted in part from Chan KM, Chan HM: The use of bubble CPAP in premature infants: local experience, *HK J Paediatr* 2007;12:86.
CPAP, continuous positive airway pressure; Fi_{O_2}, fraction of inspired oxygen; $Paco_2$, arterial partial pressure of carbon dioxide; WOB, work of breathing.
* Higher ranges may apply in infants with chronic carbon dioxide retention.
† Range should be consistent with clinical state and the presence of congenital heart disease and/or persistent pulmonary hypertension of the newborn.

Box 18-4 lists the clinical signs indicating clinical *stabilization* of patients supported with CPAP. More tolerant guidelines for pH and $Paco_2$ or "permissive hypercapnia" have become widely accepted clinical practices when treating critically ill infants.[148] This alone has likely reduced the number of intubations in infants receiving CPAP. However, it is also important to evaluate ventilation frequently by means of capillary blood gas readings or with a calibrated transcutaneous monitor, because extreme hypercapnia increases the risk for developing intraventricular hemorrhage in small infants.[149]

If the patient is not responding to CPAP it is usually because the lungs are not opening with the amount of support the clinician has chosen. If the CPAP level is set below the opening pressure of the terminal respiratory units, then *recruitment* is unlikely to occur.[72] Breathing at low functional residual capacity can also lead to atelectrauma.[150] Proper assessment of tissue perfusion is vital. Increased intrathoracic pressure may result in worsening hemodynamic status. This is common when patients have low intravascular blood volumes or poor cardiac output. Intravenous fluid bolus can help eliminate this problem. If the patient develops apnea that does not require intubation, a loading dose of caffeine citrate (20 mg/kg) followed by a daily maintenance dose of 5 mg/kg (up to 10 mg/kg) can reduce the incidence of apnea.[151]

A rise in $Paco_2$, or fall in Pao_2, after increasing the CPAP pressure may indicate that the optimal CPAP level has been exceeded.[86,152] An increase in mean airway pressure can result in increased alveolar dead space due to mechanical compression of the pulmonary microvasculature.[2] If gas exchange worsens in a patient who appeared to be improving, the pressure can first be reduced; otherwise intubation is indicated.

Criteria used to recognize when a patient has failed CPAP and requires intubation and mechanical ventilation should be established by the medical team before placing a patient on CPAP. There are no definitive recommendations at this time and most institutions rely on anecdotal experience when identifying respiratory failure in infants receiving CPAP support. Box 18-5 lists some clinical signs indicating that CPAP has failed and that intubation and mechanical ventilation are indicated. Extremely low birth weight (<1000 g) infants, born at less than 26 weeks of gestation, are among the patients who most commonly fail nasal CPAP.[103] CPAP is only about 50% effective at eliminating the need for ventilation in infants born at less than 26 weeks of gestation.[153] Recognizing CPAP failure, and the need for intubation and mechanical ventilation, is paramount for the neonatal patient because failure can ensue rapidly as the result of respiratory muscle failure, worsening gas exchange, and apnea.

Monitoring

Monitoring is an essential component in managing patients receiving CPAP. The patient and CPAP system should be assessed frequently and at regular intervals to evaluate the effectiveness of the level of support and plan for subsequent care.[154] The physical assessment can be helpful when identifying early warning signs of respiratory impairment. Frequent assessment and measurements of vital signs and gas exchange can aid in the early diagnosis of air leak (e.g., pneumothorax) and other complications associated with the use of CPAP.

Equipment monitoring should be incorporated into this assessment in order to verify proper function and eliminate equipment failure as a variable, should the patient's condition deteriorate. Physical assessment should include documentation of breath sounds, heart rate, blood pressure, skin color, work of breathing, chest rise, level of activity, condition of the nares and nasal septum, secretions, oxygen saturation, transcutaneous carbon dioxide and periodic arterial blood gas analyses. Brief disconnection from a bubble CPAP device may be indicated in order to properly assess breath sounds. Blood gases should be obtained if there is an acute deterioration in status but only after the patient becomes stabilized. If the $Paco_2$ correlates closely or trends with the transcutaneous carbon dioxide, then blood gas monitoring should be minimized because of the low circulating blood volume in infants and the possibility for contamination with pathogens. Oxygen can be weaned on the basis of measurements obtained with a pulse oximeter.

Equipment monitoring includes assessment of pressure at the patient airway, and verification of the presence of an attached low-pressure or disconnect alarm. However, besides loss of pressure to the patient, back pressure from the resistance across the prongs may prevent the low-pressure or disconnect alarm from sounding. A high-pressure "pop-off" (at least 15 cm H_2O) should be placed in-line with the system and assessed for proper function.[2,33] Other monitors with alarms, such as a pulse oximeter, transcutaneous monitor, or bradycardia alarm, should also be used with a low-pressure, or disconnect, alarm.

When using a B-CPAP device, the frequency of "bubbling" should be evaluated. A continuous bubbling usually indicates adequate gas delivery to the patient. If bubbling ceases during the breath cycle, this may indicate gas loss or a large leak at the patient interface or the patient circuit. Small fluctuations in pressure are common because of the frequency and amplitude of the bubbles; however, if large fluctuations are noted and coincide with the inspiratory phase of the infant, then additional flow should be added to the system. Frequent monitoring of the water level height should be done to prevent changes in system pressure caused by condensation and evaporation. Water should be added or suctioned out to accommodate the desired CPAP level.

In the IF-CPAP and mechanical ventilator CPAP systems, low-pressure alarms usually indicate a leak caused by nasal prongs that are too small or an excessive oropharyngeal leak. The oropharynx acts as a safety valve preventing excessive accumulation of pressure in the airway.[66] Oropharyngeal leaks are more common when using CPAP levels exceeding 8 to 10 cm H_2O.[123] A chin strap, or pacifier, can be helpful at gently sealing the leak and re-establishing the CPAP level.[106] The set flow rate delivered by the CPAP device should not be increased until large leaks have been identified and resolved. The flow rate should then be adjusted to minimize large fluctuations in the system pressure as measured by a pressure manometer placed at the airway.

A functional manual resuscitator with the proper positive end-expiratory pressure setting as well as intubation equipment should be at the bedside, in the event that the patient requires manual ventilation and/or intubation. Transcutaneous carbon dioxide monitors should be calibrated on the basis of manufacturer specifications. Humidification devices should also be documented as being on and set at the proper temperature and humidity levels. Water levels should also be frequently evaluated and maintained when using B-CPAP.

Chest X-rays are a valuable clinical tool for estimating lung expansion during the recruitment phase and for visualizing potential air leaks in the lung parenchyma.[155] Chest X-rays can also be helpful in determining whether the patient has any gastric distention from air entering the abdomen, which is more common when using CPAP levels exceeding 10 to 12 cm H_2O.[123] This can decrease respiratory compliance, limit contraction of the diaphragm, and add significantly to respiratory distress. Gastric distention can be alleviated or prevented by inserting an oral gastric tube or by applying suction via a properly sized suction catheter.

Bedside Care and Airway Management

The proper bedside care of an infant receiving CPAP is, perhaps, the single most important aspect regarding outcomes and successful use of CPAP therapy.[79] It has also been recognized that these improved outcomes correlate well with the level of skill, familiarity, and experience of the clinicians after implementation of a new CPAP strategy in infants.[123,144] This includes caregivers who are adequately trained and are proficient at troubleshooting and selecting the proper-sized hat and nasal prongs or mask. The prongs should fill the entire nares without blanching the external nares.[79] Selecting prongs that are too small can result in increased resistance and WOB, prong displacement, and excessive leaks.[127]

The fixation technique is also an important aspect of airway care in infants receiving CPAP support. The hat should be tight fitting, covering the ears and extending to the base of the neck.[79] Lateral attachment of straps should provide equal and gentle tension to avoid pressure points on the skin while securing the nasal interface to the infant.[106] The lack of stabilization and, hence, excessive movement of the prongs could result in worsening nasal injury, airway displacement, and loss of system pressure.

Another important consideration regarding bedside care that relates to airway management includes proper positioning of the infant. Infants can be positioned prone, supine, or on their side and should be turned every 2 to 4 hours.[106] The use of a small folded towel roll beneath the shoulders or chest can help support the infant and help maintain a patent airway.[106]

On occasion, the nasal prongs should be removed from the infant, and delicate suctioning through the mouth and nasopharynx should be done with a 5-French suction catheter. Nasal resistance is elevated in the neonate compared with the adult and is therefore rapidly elevated by a partial airway obstruction caused by mucous accumulation or swelling.[118] Therefore, infants who are suctioned usually have noticeable changes in WOB afterward. After suctioning, the nose should be evaluated for any signs of skin breakdown or nasal trauma and the prongs should be checked for the presence of kinking or mucus. Table 18-4 shows a nasal breakdown scoring system used for premature infants requiring CPAP.

The safe and effective delivery of aerosolized medications has been accomplished in-line using various delivery methods.[156] These drugs include bronchodilators, corticosteroids, surfactant, and ribavirin. Often, clinicians remove patients from the CPAP system to deliver bronchodilators. This should be done only if the patient tolerates being without CPAP; otherwise the risks of giving the medications outweigh their intended benefit.

Weaning

Attempts at weaning patients from CPAP should be considered when the patient is considered to be stable, has no incidents of apnea, and exhibits acceptable vital signs, blood gas values, and chest radiographic findings. Ideally, the F_{IO_2} should be weaned aggressively. If infants require oxygen chronically (due to pulmonary hypertension) then it is helpful to wean to an oxygen level that can be maintained reasonably with a separate oxygen delivery device. Some institutions wean F_{IO_2} to 0.21 and then pressure is weaned in increments of 1 to 2 cm H_2O to a level between 3 and 5 cm H_2O. Several methods regarding weaning strategies have been described. The most common methods for weaning and withdrawal include (1) decreasing CPAP to a predefined level of airway pressure, and then stopping CPAP completely; (2) removing CPAP for a predetermined number of hours each day (also known as "CPAP holidays"[157]) and gradually increasing the amount of time off CPAP each day until it can be stopped completely; and (3) stopping CPAP and starting high-flow heated humidified air (and oxygen if required) via nasal cannula.[158] Methods using high-flow humidified nasal cannular devices in lieu of CPAP are frequently reported. Although there may be some clinical advantages regarding the use of humidified high-flow nasal cannular devices,[120,159] there are limited data concerning the safety of these devices in humans. The lack of monitoring airway pressures and means for providing a high-pressure "pop-off" mechanism raise legitimate concerns.[120]

ADVANCING CONCEPTS

Infant Flow SiPAP

Infant Flow "sigh" positive airway pressure (IF-SiPAP) (Cardinal Health) is a new device that uses the Infant Flow driver design and a new flow generator (Figure 18-11) to allow the infant to breath spontaneously at two separate CPAP levels. This is accomplished by

TABLE 18-4

Nasal Breakdown Scoring System for Premature Infants Requiring Continuous Positive Airway Pressure

	SCORE				
	0 = Normal	1 = Pale or Pink/Red	2 = Bleeding, Ulcer, Eschar	3 = Skin Tear	Nasal Compression (+ if Present)
Internal nares					
External nares					
Philtrum					
Bridge					
Septum					

Courtesy of Walsh BK, Kaufman D, Zanelli S, Hicks T: University of Virginia Medical Center (Charlottesville, Va).

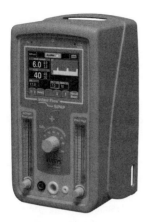

FIGURE 18-11 IF SiPAP flow generator.

complete cycle of the sigh breath. Figure 18-12 shows the sequence of spontaneous breathing of a low birth weight infant during the pressure sigh created by the IF-SiPAP.

This concept is not intended to serve as a noninvasive pressure support mode but, rather, to aid in the recruitment and stabilization of unstable alveoli and thus preserve functional residual capacity. Unlike pressure support, the small delta pressure is held in the lung longer and the patient is not allowed to terminate the breath on the basis of certain criteria; rather, the patient breathes spontaneously throughout the entire respiratory cycle. In theory, these "sigh" breaths should also improve gas exchange and work of breathing, and serve as a stimulant for apneic infants. The application of spontaneous breathing, as compared with the absence of spontaneous breathing, during a sustained pressure-hold has been shown to promote reopening of atelectatic lung regions and improve end-expiratory lung volume.[160] To date, there is only one published report that shows that the use of bilevel nasal CPAP results in significant improvements in gas exchange compared with standard nasal CPAP in preterm infants.[161]

setting the baseline CPAP level, followed by a slow unsynchronized secondary pressure (sigh breath) set at approximately 2 to 3 cm H_2O higher than the baseline pressure. The inspiratory time is set at about 1 to 3 seconds. The respiratory rate controls the frequency of the intermittent "sigh" breaths. The infant is thus allowed to breathe spontaneously throughout the

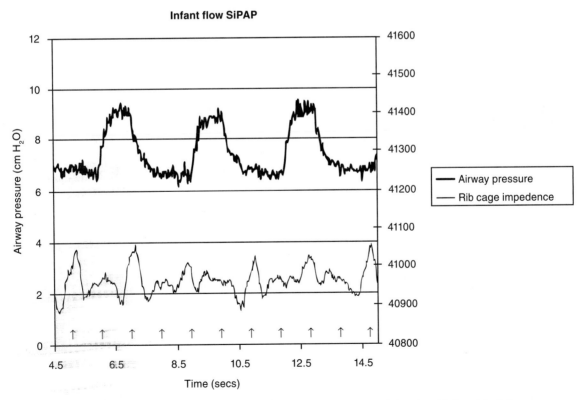

Infant flow SiPAP

FIGURE 18-12 IF SiPAP: spontaneous breathing measurements made in a low birth weight infant. Airway pressure was obtained at the nasal interface and the rib cage impedence (relative volume change) measurements were obtained with respiratory impedance plethysmography bands. The arrows indicate spontaneous breathing efforts made by the patient.

ASSESSMENT QUESTIONS

See Evolve Resources for answers.

1. The most common interface used to deliver CPAP to spontaneously breathing infants is:
   A. Infant hood
   B. Nasal prongs
   C. Nasophayngeal endotracheal tube
2. Physiologic effects of CPAP include all of the following *except:*
   A. Improved respiratory system compliance and resistance
   B. Stabilization of the chest wall
   C. Increased mucous production
   D. Less lung injury than with mechanical ventilators
3. CPAP is contraindicated in infants with which of the following congenital anomalies?
   A. Preoperative congenital diaphragmatic hernia
   B. Postoperative heart surgery
   C. Postoperative congenital diaphragmatic hernia
4. CPAP levels greater than 8 cm H_2O are commonly associated with which of the following conditions?
   A. Gastric distension
   B. Orophayngeal leaks
   C. Acute pulmonary edema
   D. Both A and B
5. Which of the following clinical indicators best describes methods for detecting early pneumothorax while monitoring infants receiving nasal CPAP?
   A. Persistent coughing and nasal flaring
   B. Widened pulse pressure
   C. An increased FiO_2 over the first day of CPAP support
   D. A significant increase in respiratory distress
   E. Diminished bilateral breath sounds
6. The following factors are essential when constructing a B-CPAP system, *except:*
   A. A positive end-expiratory pressure/exhalation valve
   B. Hudson nasal prongs
   C. A blended gas source
7. Early attempts to create systems to provide CPAP to spontaneously breathing infants were aimed at trying to mimic which of the following important physiologic factors that affect gas delivery to the lung?

ASSESSMENT QUESTIONS—cont'd

   A. Nasal flaring
   B. Chest rise
   C. Work of breathing
   D. Grunting
8. The most important aspect of CPAP that can impact the outcome and success of CPAP is
   A. The device being used to generate CPAP
   B. Suctioning and airway clearance techniques
   C. Proper bedside care and level of experience of clinicians using the CPAP device
   D. The physician writing the orders
9. The proper arrangement for any nasal CPAP system includes all of the following *except:*
   A. The hat should be loose fitting, covering the nose and extending to the base of the neck.
   B. Lateral attachment should provide gentle tension on the nasal interface.
   C. The prongs should be properly sized to eliminate migration from the nares.
   D. The hat should be tight fitting, covering the ears and extending to the base of the neck.
10. All of the following devices are considered acceptable for measuring and delivering nasal CPAP safely to infants, *except:*
    A. V-CPAP
    B. B-CPAP
    C. IF-SiPAP
    D. High-flow nasal cannula

References

1. Courtney SE, Barrington KJ: Continuous positive pressure airway pressure and noninvasive ventilation, *Clin Perinatol* 2007;34:73.
2. Gregory GA et al: Treatment of the idiopathic respiratory-distress syndrome with continuous positive airway pressure, *N Engl J Med* 1971;284:1333.
3. Bancalari E, Gerdardt T, Monkus E: Simple device for producing negative pressure in infants with IRDS, *Pediatrics* 1973;52:128.
4. Chernick V, Vidyasager D: Continuous negative chest wall pressure in hyaline membrane disease: one year experience, *Pediatrics* 1972;49:753.
5. Bancalari E, Garcia OL, Jesse MJ: Effects of continuous negative pressure on lung mechanics in idiopathic respiratory distress syndrome, *Pediatrics* 1973;51:485.
6. Kattwinkel J et al: A device for administration of continuous positive airway pressure by the nasal route, *Pediatrics* 1973;52:131.
7. Ho JJ et al: Continuous distending pressure for respiratory distress syndrome in preterm infants, *Cochrane Database Syst Rev* 2000;4:CD002271.

8. Krouskop RW, Brown EG, Sweet AY: The early use of continuous positive airway pressure in the treatment of idiopathic respiratory distress syndrome, *J Pediatr* 1975;87:263.

9. Harris H et al: Nasal continuous positive airway pressure: improvement in arterial oxygenation in hyaline membrane disease, *Biol Neonate* 1976;29:231.

10. Yu VY, Rolfe P: Effect of continuous positive airway pressure breathing on cardiorespiratory function in infants with respiratory distress syndrome, *Acta Paediatr Scand* 1977;66:59.

11. Richardson CP, Jung AL: Effects of continuous positive airway pressure on pulmonary function and blood gases of infants with respiratory distress syndrome, *Pediatr Res* 1978;12:771.

12. Polin RA, Sahni R: Newer experience with CPAP, *Semin Neonatol* 2002;7:379.

13. Heldt GP: Development of stability of the respiratory system in preterm infants, *J Appl Physiol* 1988;65:441.

14. Miller MJ et al: Effects of nasal CPAP on supraglottic and total pulmonary resistance in preterm infants, *J Appl Physiol* 1990;68:141.

15. Gaon P et al: Assessment of effect of nasal continuous positive airway pressure on laryngeal opening using fiber optic laryngoscopy, *Arch Dis Child Fetal Neonatal Ed* 1999;80:F230.

16. Miller RW et al: Effectiveness of continuous positive airway pressure in the treatment of bronchomalacia in infants: a bronchoscopic documentation, *Crit Care Med* 1986;14:125.

17. Miller MJ, Carol WA, Martin RJ: Continuous positive airway pressure selectively reduces obstructive apnea in preterm infants, *J Pediatr* 1985;106:91.

18. Jones RA: Apnea of immaturity. 1. A controlled trial of theophylline and face mask continuous airway pressure, *Arch Dis Child* 1982;57:761.

19. Henderson-Smart DJ, Subramaniam P, Davis PG: Continuous positive airway pressure versus theophylline for apnea in preterm infants, *Cochrane Database Syst Rev* 2001;4:CD001072.

20. Robertson NJ, Hamilton PA: Randomized trial of elective continuous positive airway pressure (CPAP) compared with rescue CPAP after extubation, *Arch Dis Child Fetal Neonatal Ed* 1998;79:F58.

21. Martin RJ, Carlo WA: Role of the upper airway in the pathogenesis of apnea in infants, *Respir Care* 1986;31:615.

22. Kattwinkel J: Neonatal apnea: pathogenesis and therapy, *J Pediatr* 1977;90:342.

23. Kurz H: Influence of nasopharyngeal CPAP on breathing pattern and incidence of apnoeas in preterm infants, *Biol Neonate* 1999;76:129.

24. Locke R et al: Effect of nasal CPAP on thoracoabdominal motion in neonates with respiratory insufficiency, *Pediatr Pulmonol* 1991;11:259.

25. Speidel BD, Dunn PM: Effect of continuous positive airway pressure on breathing pattern of infants with respiratory-distress syndrome, *Lancet* 1975;1:301.

26. Davis S et al: Effect of continuous positive airway pressure on forced expiratory flows in infants with tracheomalacia, *Am J Respir Crit Care Med* 1998;158:148.

27. Panitch HB et al: Effects of CPAP on lung mechanics in infants with acquired tracheobronchomalacia, *Am J Respir Crit Care Med* 1994;150:1341.

28. Weigle CG: Treatment of an infant with tracheobronchomalacia at home with a lightweight, high-humidity, continuous positive airway pressure system, *Crit Care Med* 1990;18:892.

29. Czervinske M: AARC clinical practice guideline: application of continuous positive airway pressure to neonates via nasal prongs, nasopharyngeal tube, or nasal mask—2004 revision and update, *Respir Care* 2004;49:1100.

30. Kiciman NM et al: Thoracoabdominal motion in newborns during ventilation delivered by endotracheal tube or nasal prongs, *Pediatr Pulmonol* 1998;25:175.

31. Jonson B et al: Continuous positive airway pressure: modes of action in relation to clinical applications, *Pediatr Clin North Am* 1980;27:687.

32. Auckland District Health Board: Newborn Services clinical guidelines: continuous positive airway pressure (CPAP). 2004 [Internet]. http://www.adhb.co.nz/newborn/guidelines.htm. Retrieved September 2008.

33. Engelke SC, Roloff DW, Kuhns LR: Postextubation nasal continuous positive airway pressure: a prospective controlled study, *Am J Dis Child* 1982;136:359.

34. Higgins RD, Richter SE, Davis JM: Nasal continuous positive airway pressure facilitates extubation of very low birth weight neonates, *Pediatrics* 1991;88:999.

35. Davis PG, Henderson-Smart DJ: Nasal continuous positive airways pressure immediately after extubation for preventing morbidity in preterm infants, *Cochrane Database Syst Rev* 2000;3:CD000143.

36. Davis PG, Henderson-Smart DJ: Extubation from low-rate intermittent positive airways pressure versus extubation after a trial of endotracheal continuous positive airway pressure in intubated preterm infants, *Cocrane Database Syst Rev* 2001;4:CD001078.

37. Davis P et al: Randomised, controlled trial of nasal continuous positive airway pressure in the extubation of infants weighing 600 to 1250 g, *Arch Dis Child Fetal Neonatal Ed* 1998;79:F54.

38. Chan V, Greenough A: Randomised trial of methods of extubation in acute and chronic respiratory distress, *Arch Dis Child* 1993;68:570.

39. Dimitriou G et al: Elective use of nasal continuous positive airways pressure following extubation of preterm infants, *Eur J Pediatr* 2000;159:434.

40. Annibale DJ et al: RAndomized, controlled trial of nasopharyngeal continuous positive airway pressure in the extubation of very low birth weight infants, *J Pediatr* 1994;124:455.

41. So BH et al: Application of nasal continuous positive airway pressure to early extubation in very low birthweight infants, *Arch Dis Child Fetal Neonatal Ed* 1995;72:F191.

42. Tapia JL et al: Does continuous positive airway pressure (CPAP) during weaning from intermittent mandatory ventilation in very low birth weight infants have risks or benefits? A controlled trial, *Pediatr Pulmonol* 1995;19:269.

43. Jeena P, Pillay P, Adhikari M: Nasal CPAP in newborns with acute respiratory failure, *Ann Trop Paediatr* 2002;22:201.

44. Lin HC et al: System-based strategy for the management of meconium aspiration syndrome: 198 consecutive cases observations, *Acta Paediatr Taiwan* 2005;46:67.

45. Fow WW et al: The therapeutic application of end-expiratory pressure in the meconium aspiration syndrome, *Pediatrics* 1975;56:214.

46. Roberton NRC: Prolonged continuous positive airways pressure for pulmonary oedema due to persistent ductus arteriosus in the newborn, *Arch Dis Child* 1974:49:585.

47. Gregory GA et al: Continuous positive airway pressure and pulmonary and circulatory function after cardiac surgery in infants less than three months of age, *Anesthesiology* 1975;43:426.

48. Cogswell JJ et al: Effects of continuous positive airway pressure on lung mechanics of babies after operation for congenital heart disease, *Arch Dis Child* 1975;50:799.

49. Hatch DJ et al: Continuous positive airway pressure after open-heart operations in infancy, *Lancet* 1973;2:469.

50. Buyukpamukcu N, Hicsonmez A: The effect of CPAP upon pulmonary reserve and cardiac output under increased abdominal pressure, *J Pediatr Surg* 1977;12:49.

51. Verder H et al: Nasal continuous positive airway pressure and early surfactant therapy for respiratory distress syndrome in newborns of less than 30 weeks' gestation, *Pediatrics* 1999;103:E24.

52. Verder H et al: Danish–Swedish Multi-center Study Group: Surfactant therapy and nasal continuous positive airway pressure for newborns with respiratory distress syndrome, *N Engl J Med* 1994;331:1051.

53. Kamper J et al: Early treatment with nasal continuous positive airway pressure in very low-birth-weight infants, *Acta Paediatr* 1993;82:193.

54. Kribs A et al: Early surfactant in spontaneously breathing with nCPAP in ELBW infants—a single center four year experience, *Acta Paediatr* 2008;97:293.

55. Stevens TP, Blennow M, Soll RF: Early surfactant administration with brief ventilation vs selective surfactant and continued mechanical ventilation for preterm infants with or at risk for RDS, *Cochrane Database Syst Rev* 2002;2:CD00.063.

56. Tooley J, Dyke M: Randomized study of nasal continuous positive airway pressure in the preterm infant with respiratory distress syndrome, *Acta Paediatr* 2003;92:1170.

57. Ancora G et al: Efficacy of INSURE approach (intubation-surfactant-extubation) followed by nasal continuous positive airway pressure (nCPAP) in preterm infants with respiratory distress syndrome (RDS) [abstract 2248], *Pediatric Res* 2001;49:392A.

58. Horbar JD et al: Trends in mortality and morbidity for very low birth weight infants, 1991-1999, *Pediatrics* 2002;110:143.

59. Keszler M et al: A prospective, mulitcenter, randomized study of high versus low positive end-expiratory pressure during extracorporeal membrane oxygenation, *J Pediatr* 1992;120:107.

60. Thompson JE, Farrell E, McManus M: Neonatal and pediatric airway emergencies, *Respir Care* 1992;37:582.

61. Migliori C et al: Pneumothorax during nasal-CPAP: a predictable complication? *Pediatr Med Chir* 2003;25:345.

62. Ogata ES et al: Pneumothorax in the respiratory distress syndrome: incidence and effect on vital signs, blood gases, and pH, *Pediatrics* 1976;58:177.

63. Hall RT, Rhodes PG: Pneumothorax and pneumomediastinum in infants with idiopathic respiratory distress syndrome receiving CPAP, *Pediatrics* 1975;55:493.

64. Gessler P et al: Lobar pulmonary interstitial emphysema in a premature infant on continuous positive airway pressure using nasal prongs, *Eur J Pediatr* 2001;160:263.

65. Gurakan B et al: Persistent pulmonary interstitial emphysema in an unventilated neonate, *Pediatr Pulmonol* 2002;34:409.

66. de Bie HM et al: Neonatal pneumatocele as a complication of nasal continuous positive airway pressure, *Arch Dis Child Fetal Neonatal Ed* 2002;86:F202.

67. Wong W et al: Vascular air embolism: a rare complication of nasal CPAP, *J Paediatr Child Health* 1997;33:444.

68. Palmer KS et al: Effects of positive and negative pressure ventilation on cerebral blood volume of newborn infants, *Acta Paediatra* 1995;84:132.

69. Tulassay T et al: Effects of continuous positive airway pressure on renal function in prematures, *Biol Neonate* 1983;43:152.

70. Furzan JA et al: Regional blood flor in newborn lambs during endotracheal continuous negative pressure breathing, *Pediatr Res* 1981;15:84.

71. Jaile JC et al: Benign gaseous distension of the bowel in premature infants treated with nasal continuous airway pressure: a study of contributing factors, *AJR Am J Roentgenol* 1992;152:125.

72. Wiswell TE, Srinivasan P: Continuous positive airway pressure. In Goldsmith JP, Karotkin EH, editors: Assisted ventilation of the neonate, ed 4, Philadelphia: WB Saunders; 2004. pp 127-147.

73. Moritz B et al: Nasal continuous positive airway pressure (n-CPAP) does not change cardiac output in preterm infants, *Am J Perinatol* 2008;25:105.

74. De Paoli AG, Morley C, Davis PG: Nasal CPAP for neonates: what do we know in 2003? *Arch Dis Child Fetal Neonatal Ed* 2003;88:F168.

75. Bonta BW et al: Determination of optimal continuous positive airway pressure for the treatment of IRDS by measurement of esophageal pressure, *J Pediatr* 1977;91:449.

76. Peck DJ et al: A wandering nasal prong: a thing of risks and problems, *Paediatr Anaesth* 1999;9:77.

77. Loftus BC, Ahn J, Haddad J Jr: Neonatal nasal deformities secondary to nasal continuous positive airway pressure, *Laryngoscope* 1994;104:1019.

78. Robertson NJ et al: Nasal deformities resulting from flow driver continuous positive airway pressure, *Arch Dis Child Fetal Neonatal Ed* 1996;75:209.

79. McCoskey L: Nursing care guidelines for prevention of nasal breakdown in neonates receiving nasal CPAP, *Adv Neonatal Care* 2008;8:116.

80. Yong SC, Chen SJ, Boo NY: Incidence of nasal trauma associated with nasal prong versus nasal mask during continuous positive airway pressure treatment in very low birthweight infants: a randomised control study, *Arch Dis Child Fetal Neonatal Ed* 2005;90:F480.

81. Lee SY, Lopez V: Physiological effects of two temperature settings in preterm infants on nasal continuous airway pressure ventilation, *J Clin Nurs* 2002;11:845.

82. Saunders RA, Milner AD, Hopkin IE: The effects of continuous positive airway pressure on lung mechanics and lung volumes in the neonate, *Biol Neonate* 1976;29:178.

83. Greenspan JS, Abbasi S, Bhutani VK: Sequential changes in pulmonary mechanics in the very low birth weight (less than or equal to 1000 grams) infant, *J Pediatr* 1988;113:732.

84. Elgellab A et al: Effects of nasal continuous positive airway pressure (NCPAP) on breathing pattern in spontaneously breathing premature newborn infants, *Intensive Care Med* 2001;27:1782.

85. Heldt GP, McIlroy MB: Distortion of chest wall and work of diaphragm in preterm infants, *J Appl Physiol* 1987;62:164.

86. Landers S et al: Optimal constant positive airway pressure assessed by arterial alveolar difference for CO_2 in hyaline membrane disease, Pediatr Res 1986;20:884.

87. Corbet AJ et al: Effect of positive-pressure breathing on $aADN_2$ in hyaline membrane disease, *J Appl Physiol* 1975;38:33.

88. Magnenant E et al: Dynamic behavior of respiratory system during nasal continuous positive airway pressure in spontaneously breathing premature newborn infants, *Pediatr Pulmonol* 2004;37:485.

89. Durand M, McCann E, Brady JP: Effect of continuous positive airway pressure on the ventilatory response to CO_2 in preterm infants, *Pediatrics* 1983;71:634.

90. De Klerk AM, De Klerk RK: Nasal continuous positive airway pressure and outcomes of preterm infants, *J Paediatr Child Health* 2001;37:161.

91. Narendran V et al: Early bubble CPAP and outcomes in ELBW preterm infants, *J Perinatol* 2003;23:195.

92. Thibeault DW et al: Collagen scaffolding during development and its deformation with chronic lung disease, *Pediatrics* 2003;111:766.

93. Jobe AH, Bancalari E: Bronchopulmonary dysplasia, *Am J Respir Crit Care Med* 2001;163:1723.

94. Parker TA, Abman SH: The pulmonary circulation in bronchopulmonary dysplasia, *Semin Neonatol* 2003;8:51.

95. Abman SH: Bronchopulmonary dysplasia: "a vascular hypothesis," *Am J Respir Crit Care Med* 2001;164:1755.

96. Kinsella JP, Greenough A, Abman SH: Bronchopulmonary dysplasia, *Lancet* 2006;367:1421.

97. Coalson JJ, Winter V, deLemos RA: Decreased alveolarization in baboon survivors with bronchopulmonary dysplasia, *Am J Respir Crit Care Med* 1995;152:640.

98. Coalson JJ et al: Neonatal chronic lung disease in extremely immature baboons, *Am J Respir Crit Care Med* 1999;160:1333.

99. Albertine KH et al: Chronic lung injury in preterm lambs: disordered respiratory tract development, *Am J Respir Crit Care Med* 1999;159:945.

100. Jobe AH et al: Decreased indicators of lung injury with continuous positive expiratory pressure in preterm lambs, *Pediatr Res* 2002;52:387.

101. Thomson MA et al: Treatment of immature baboons for 28 days with early nasal continuous positive airway pressure, *Am J Respir Crit Care Med* 2004;169:1054.

102. Gittermann MK et al: Early nasal continuous positive airway pressure treatment reduces the need for intubation in very low birth weight infants, *Eur J Pediatr* 1997;156:384.

103. Finer NN et al: Delivery room continuous positive airway pressure/positive end-expiratory pressure in extremely low birth weight infants: a feasibility trial, *Pediatrics* 2004;114:651.

104. Morley CJ et al: Nasal CPAP or intubation at birth for very preterm infants, *N Engl J Med* 2008;358:700.

105. Dani C et al: Early extubation and nasal continuous positive airway pressure after surfactant treatment for respiratory distress syndrome among preterm infants <30 weeks' gestation, *Pediatrics* 2004;113:560.

106. Bonner KM, Mainous RO: The nursing care of the infant receiving bubble CPAP therapy, *Adv Neonatal Care* 2008;8:78.

107. De Paoli AG et al: Devices and pressure sources for administration of nasal continuous positive airway pressure (CPAP) in preterm neonates, *Cochrane Database Syst Rev* 2008;1:CD002977.

108. Davis P, Davies M, Faber B: A randomised controlled trial of two methods of delivering nasal continuous positive airway pressure after extubation to infants weighing less than 1000 g: binasal (Hudson) versus single nasal prongs, *Arch Dis Child Fetal Neonatal Ed* 2001;85:82.

109. Sung V et al: Estimating inspired oxygen concentration delivered by nasal prongs in children with bronchiolitis, *J Paediatr Child Health* 2008;44:14.

110. De Paoli AG et al: In vitro comparison of nasal continuous positive airway pressure devices for neonates, *Arch Dis Child Fetal Neonatal Ed* 2002;87:F42.

111. Banner MJ, Kirby RR, Blanch PB: Differentiating the work of breathing into its component parts: essential for appropriate interpretation, *Chest* 1996;109;1141.

112. Moomjian AS et al: The effect of external expiratory resistance on lung and pulmonary function in the neonate, *J Pediatr* 1980;96:908.

113. Emeriaud G et al: Diaphragm electrical activity during expiration in mechanically ventilated infants, *Pediatr Res* 2006;59:705.

114. Pilbeam SP: Introduction to ventilators. In: Cairo JM, Pilbeam SP, editors: Mosby's respiratory care equipment, ed 7, St. Louis, Mo: Mosby; 2004. pp 317-384.

115. Kacmarek RM, Chipman D: Basic principles of ventilator machinery. In: Tobin MJ, editor: Principles and practice of mechanical ventilation, New York: McGraw-Hill; 2006. pp 53-95.

116. DiBlasi RM et al: The impact of imposed expiratory resistance in neonatal mechanical ventilation: a laboratory evaluation, *Respir Care* 2008;7(1): 28.

117. Marini JJ, Culver BH, Krik W: Flow resistance of exhalation valves and positive end-expiratory pressure, *Am Rev Respir Dis* 1985;131:850.

118. Klausner JF, Lee AY, Hutchison AA: Decreased imposed work with a new nasal continuous positive airway pressure device, *Pediatr Pulmonol* 1996;22:188.

119. Pandit PB et al: Work of breathing during constant- and variable-flow nasal continuous positive airway pressure in preterm neonates, *Pediatrics* 2001; 108:682.

120. Courtney SE et al: Lung recruitment and breathing pattern during variable versus continuous flow nasal continuous positive airway pressure in premature infants: an evaluation of three devices, *Pediatrics* 2001;107:304.

121. Lee KS et al: A comparison of underwater bubble continuous positive airway pressure with ventilator-derived continuous positive airway pressure in premature neonates ready for extubation, *Biol Neonate* 1998;73:69.

122. Liptsen E et al: Work of breathing during nasal continuous positive airway pressure in preterm infants: a comparison of bubble vs variable-flow devices, *J Perinatol* 2005;25:453.

123. Chernick V: Continuous distending pressure in hyaline membrane disease: of devices, disadvantages, and a daring study, *Pediatrics* 1973;52:114.

124. Chan KM, Chan HB: The use of bubble CPAP in premature infants: local experience, *HK J Paediatr* 2007;12:86.

125. Kaur C et al: A simple circuit to deliver bubbling CPAP, *Indian Pediatr* 2008;45:312.

126. A very ME et al: Is chronic lung disease in low birth weight infants preventable? A survey of eight centers, *Pediatrics* 1987;79:26.

127. Kahn DJ et al: Unpredictability of delivered bubble nasal continuous positive airway pressure: role of bias flow magnitude and nares-prong air leaks, *Pediatr Res* 2007;62:343.

128. Pillow JJ, Travadi JN: Bubble CPAP: is the noise important? An in vitro study, *Pediatr Res* 2005;57:826.

129. Pillow JJ et al: Bubble continuous positive airway pressure enhances lung volume and gas exchange in preterm lambs, *Am J Respir Crit Care Med* 2007;176:63.

130. Suki B et al: Life-support system benefits from noise, *Nature* 1998;393:127.

131. Morley CJ et al: Nasal continuous positive airway pressure: does bubbling improve gas exchange? *Arch Dis Chil. Fetal Neonatal Ed* 2005;90:343.

132. Watson KF: Infant and pediatric ventilators, In: Cairo JM, Pilbeam SP, editors: Mosby's respiratory care equipment, ed 7, St. Louis, Mo: Mosby; 2004, pp 663-726.

133. Moa G et al: A new device for administration of nasal continuous positive airways pressure in the newborn: an experimental study, *Crit Care Med* 1998;16:1238.

134. Stefanescu BM et al: A randomized, controlled trial comparing two different positive pressure airway systems for the successful extubation of extremely low birth weight infants, *Pediatrics* 2003;112:1031.

135. Stoll BJ et al: Late-onset sepsis in very low birth weight neonates: a report from the national institute of child health and human development neonatal research network, *J Pediatr* 1996;129:63.

136. Thomson MB et al: Delayed extubation to nasal continuous positive airway pressure in the immature baboon model of bronchopulmonary dysplasia: lung clinical and pathological findings, *Pediatrics* 2006;118:2038.

137. Hillman NH et al: Brief, large tidal volume ventilation initiates lung injury and a systemic response in fetal sheep, *Am J Respir Crit Care Med* 2007;176:575.

138. Vermont Oxford Network: Delivery room management trial of premature infants at high risk of respiratory distress syndrome. In: ClinicalTrials.gov [Internet]. Bethesda, Md: National Library of Medicine (US); 2000. Available from: http://clinicaltrials.gov/ct2/show/NCT00244101. Retrieved September 2008.

139. Martin RJ et al: The effect of a low continuous positive airway pressure on the reflex control of respiration in the preterm infant, *J Pediatr* 1977; 90:976.

140. Martin RJ, Abu-Shaeesh JM: Control of breathing and neonatal apnea, *Biol Neonate* 2005;87:288.

141. Chatburn RL: Similiarities and differences in the management of acute lung injury in neonates (IRDS) and in adults (ARDS), *Respir Care* 1988;33:539.

142. Lindner W et al: Delivery room management of extremely low birth weight infants: spontaneous breathing or intubation? *Pediatrics* 1999;103:961.

143. Aly H et al: Does the experience with the use of nasal continuous positive airway pressure improve over time in extremely low birth weight infants? *Pediatrics* 2004;114:697.

144. Thia LP et al: Randomised controlled trial of nasal continuous positive airways pressure (CPAP) in bronchiolitis, *Arch Dis Child* 2008;93:45.

145. Flynn JT et al: A cohort study of transcutaneous oxygen tension and the incidence and severity of retinopathy of prematurity, *N Engl J Med* 1992;326:1050.

146. Kurtz H: Influence of nasopharyngeal CPAP on breathing pattern and apnoeas in preterm infants, *Biol Neonate* 1999;76:129.

147. Miller JD, Carlo WA: Safety and effectiveness of permissive hypercapnia in the preterm infant, *Curr Opin Pediatr* 2007;19:142.

148. Fabres J et al: Both extremes of arterial carbon dioxide pressure and the magnitude of fluctuations in arterial carbon dioxide pressure are associated with severe intraventricular hemorrhage in preterm infants, *Pediatrics* 2007;119:299.

149. Clark RH et al: Lung injury in neonates: causes, strategies for prevention, and long term consequences, *J Pediatr* 2001;139:478.

150. Schmidt B et al: Caffeine for Apnea of Prematurity Trial Group: Long-term effects of caffeine therapy for apnea of prematurity, *N Engl J Med* 2007;357:1893.

151. Andreasson B et al: Measurement of ventilation and respiratory mechanics during continuous positive airway pressure (CPAP) treatment in infants, *Acta Paediatr Scand* 1989;78:194.

152. Ammari A et al: Variables associated with the early failure of nasal CPAP in very low birth weight infants, *J Pediatr* 2005;147:341.

153. Branson RD et al: AARC clinical practice guideline patient–ventilator system checks, *Respir Care* 1992;37:882.

154. Giedion L, Haefliger H, Dangel P: Acute pulmonary radiograph changes in hyaline membrane disease treated with artificial ventilation and positive end expiratory pressure (PEP), *Pediatr Radiol* 1973;1:145.

155. Smedsaas-Löfvenberg A et al: Nebulization of drugs in a nasal CPAP system, *Acta Paediatr* 1999;88:89.

156. Greenough A, Premkumar M, Patel D: Ventilatory strategies for the extremely premature infant, *Pediatr Anes* 2008;18:371.

157. Jardine LA, Inglis GDT, Davies MW: Strategies used for the withdrawal of nasal continuous positive airway pressure (CPAP) in preterm infants: protocol, *Cochrane Database Syst Rev* 2008;1:CD006979.

158. Shoemaker MT et al: High flow nasal cannula versus nasal CPAP for neonatal respiratory disease: a retrospective study, *J Perinatol* 2007;27:85.

159. Wrigge H et al: Spontaneous breathing improves lung aeration in oleic acid–induced lung injury, *Anesthesiology* 2003;99:376-384.

160. Migliori C et al: Nasal bilevel vs. continuous positive airway pressure in preterm infants, *Pediatric Pulmonol* 2005;40:426.

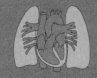

Chapter **19**

Mechanical Ventilation of the Neonate and Pediatric Patient

BRIAN K. WALSH • ROBERT M. DiBLASI

OUTLINE

LEARNING OBJECTIVES

After reading this chapter the reader will be able to:

- Explain when mechanical ventilation is indicated in neonates and pediatrics
- Describe the basic fundamentals for managing patients undergoing mechanical ventilation
- Identify complications associated with mechanical ventilation
- Explain various approaches for minimizing complications with ventilators

- Compare differences in operation between pressure, volume, and dual-control breath types
- Provide reasons why one mode of ventilation would be chosen over another for certain conditions
- Determine initial ventilator settings for various patient sizes
- Recognize factors that could improve interaction between the patient and the mechanical ventilator
- Define and discuss various weaning strategies

Neonatal and pediatric mechanical ventilation presents some of the most clinically challenging situations in respiratory care. The neonatal and pediatric population encompasses a broad range of weights, ages, sizes, and diseases; therefore ventilator practices can vary widely. In this chapter, a *neonate* is defined as any newborn infant younger than 44 weeks of gestation and a *pediatric patient* represents any child older than 1 month of age. Children are not small adults, and infants are not small children.[1] Most of the concepts presented in this chapter are the same for both pediatric and neonatal applications; however, there are other situations that are quite unique to the neonatal or pediatric patient. At present, there is no consensus regarding optimal ventilator strategies for this patient population. A tremendous amount of research still needs to be done to determine best practices for managing neonatal and pediatric patients receiving mechanical ventilation. To manage neonatal and pediatric mechanical ventilation effectively, the clinician must combine the principles described in this chapter with the knowledge of how airway anatomy and pulmonary pathophysiology are impacted by various diseases. It is beyond the scope of this chapter to provide an in-depth review of ventilator equipment or guidelines for disease-specific ventilator management. These aspects are covered in greater detail in Chapter 17 (Mechanical Ventilators) and Chapter 28 (Congenital and Surgical Disorders that Affect Respiratory Care).

OBJECTIVES AND INDICATIONS FOR MECHANICAL VENTILATION

The physiologic objectives for mechanical ventilation in a neonatal or pediatric patient are basically the same as for those in an adult patient:
- To manipulate alveolar ventilation
- To improve oxygenation
- To optimize lung volume
- To reduce the work of breathing
- To minimize risks associated with ventilator-induced lung injury

In general, mechanical ventilation is initiated to increase oxygenation, correct respiratory acidosis, reduce respiratory distress, prevent or reverse atelectasis, reduce respiratory muscle fatigue, manage intracranial pressure, lower oxygen consumption, and stabilize the chest wall for adequate lung expansion. Box 19-1 lists clinical situations in which mechanical ventilation is indicated.[1,2]

TYPES OF MECHANICAL VENTILATION

Mechanical ventilator breath types have traditionally been classified by the type of mechanical ventilator being used but can now be employed in a variety of ways, which are defined mainly by the control variable.[3] The two most common breath types are pressure and volume. Figure 19-1 compares the differences between the flow and pressure waveforms of volume and pressure ventilation. Modern microprocessor ventilators incorporate gas delivery systems that can produce a wide variety of flow and pressure waveforms and are capable of delivering volume and pressure ventilation as well as hybrid modes that combine various aspects of volume and pressure.

Pressure Ventilation

Pressure ventilation uses a pressure setting as the main feature to define inflation. Pressure ventilators are classified as positive pressure or negative pressure.[3] Positive-pressure ventilators use a high external pressure gradient to drive a gas mixture into the lungs and produce inflation.

Negative-pressure ventilation permits gas flow into the lungs by using a vacuum to externally expand the thorax. The chest wall pressure drops, thereby creating a decrease in pleural pressure that is less than the airway opening pressure, and air flows into the lungs. The main advantage of a negative-pressure ventilator is that it may avoid endotracheal intubation or tracheotomy. Because negative-pressure ventilation is provided without an artificial airway, it is sometimes referred to as *noninvasive ventilation*; however, it should be understood that all forms of mechanical ventilation provide ventilation in an "unnatural" form. In addition, both positive and negative pressure ventilation produce positive transpulmonary pressures and may have similar complications as a result.

Time-cycled, pressure-limited ventilation (TCPL) has been the most common form of ventilation used in neonates and infants for nearly 3 decades, mainly because it has been the traditional ventilation for that population. To define the inflation cycle of each breath, TCPL uses a preset (1) constant flow during both inspiration and expiration, (2) inspiratory time, (3) frequency or inspiratory-to-expiratory (I/E) ratio, and (4) pressure setting.[4] Because flow is constant, pressure is variable throughout the inflation cycle.

Microprocessor ventilators are also capable of delivering preset pressure breaths and are useful for neonate and pediatric ventilation. This form of pressure ventila-

Box 19-1	Clinical Indications for (But Not Limited to) Mechanical Ventilation

PULMONARY DISORDERS

RESTRICTIVE PROCESS

- Respiratory distress syndrome
- Acute respiratory distress syndrome
- Pulmonary hemorrhage
- Pulmonary hypoplasia/agenesis
- Congenital pneumonia
- Pneumothorax/air leaks
- Pleural effusion/chylothorax
- Aspiration syndromes (blood, amniotic fluid)
- Flail chest
- Bronchopleural fistula
- Abdominal distention
- Diaphragmatic hernia
- Congenital lung cysts, tumors
- Rib cage anomalies
- Extrinsic masses

OBSTRUCTIVE PROCESS

- Meconium aspiration
- Congenital lobar emphysema
- Asthma
- Bronchiolitis
- Cystic fibrosis
- Bronchopulmonary dysplasia

AIRWAY

- Laryngomalacia
- Tracheomalacia
- Choanal atresia
- Pierre Robin syndrome
- Micrognathia
- Nasopharyngeal tumor
- Subglottic stenosis

EXTRAPULMONARY DISORDERS

NEUROLOGIC/MUSCULAR

- Myasthenia gravis
- Muscular dystrophy

- Guillain-Barré syndrome
- Cerebral edema
- Cerebral hemorrhage
- Spinal cord injury/disease
- Phrenic nerve damage

HYPOVENTILATION

- Sleep apnea - *from obesity*
- Overdose/poisoning
- Postoperative recovery

INCREASED INTRACRANIAL PRESSURE

- Infection
- Head trauma
- Near-drowning
- Reye's syndrome - *aspirin*

CARDIOVASCULAR DYSFUNCTION

- Cardiac shunting
- Cyanotic heart disease
- Circulatory collapse
- Hypovolemia
- Anemia
- Polycythemia
- Congestive heart failure
- Postoperative cardiac surgery
- Persistent pulmonary hypertension

METABOLIC

- Acidosis
- Hypoglycemia
- Hypothermia
- Hyperthermia

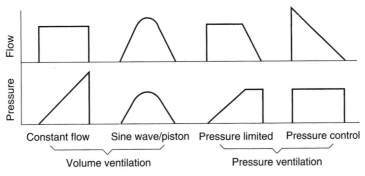

FIGURE 19-1 Flow and pressure waveforms of four types of ventilation.

tion is called *pressure-controlled ventilation* (PCV). Usually a preset pressure level, inspiratory time, and frequency are chosen by the operator. Flow, however, is variable and is a function of driving pressure and peaks almost instantly to attain the defined pressure level. Pressure is maintained constant throughout the inspiratory time, and flow decelerates rapidly.[5,6] However, the total flow delivered to the respiratory system is regulated by the ventilator to assure that pressure is maintained throughout the entire inspiratory time. The majority of the tidal volume is delivered early in the inflation stage, while pressure is held constant. Compared with other types of ventilation, the resulting distribution of alveolar pressures sustained by tidal volume may lead to a lower dead space–to–tidal volume (V_D/V_T) ratio, improved ventilation, and improved oxygenation.[7,8] PCV can offer lower work of breathing and improved comfort for patients with increased and variable respiratory demand.[9] Although the peak pressure level is constant or nearly constant, PCV results in a higher mean airway pressure ($\overline{Paw}$) than do other types of ventilation. The disadvantages or advantages of a higher $\overline{Paw}$ should be considered when instituting PCV. Another disadvantage is that when using any type of pressure ventilation, tidal volume will vary with changes in lung compliance and constant alveolar minute ventilation may be difficult to obtain.

Volume Ventilation

Volume control ventilation (VCV) is most often used in adult patients and is chosen when ventilating a pediatric patient. Adult volume-cycled ventilators were used initially in newborn intensive care in the early 1970s and fell from favor with the invention of pressure-controlled ventilators that were designed specifically for use in neonates. Because of improved sensor and ventilator technology, it is now possible to use volume ventilation in all patients.[10] A constant tidal volume and flow rate characterize volume ventilation, and the resulting peak inspiratory pressure varies with changes in respiratory system compliance and resistance. When a flow-controlling valve is used, tidal volume is calculated by measuring the flow delivered over a preset inflation time.[11]

VCV with a constant flow has the advantage of a lower $\overline{Paw}$ compared with pressure ventilation. This is often a critical factor after cardiac surgery in infants and children. Many currently available ventilators offer the option of delivering this constant flow with either a traditional square-wave flow pattern or a 50% decelerating flow pattern in VCV. In theory, tidal volume does not vary with changing lung compliance or airway resistance during volume ventilation. As lung impedance increases, however, tidal volume may

decrease if the ventilator cannot correct for volume losses resulting from gas compression in the patient circuit. Delivered tidal volume may also be affected by leaks from cuffless endotracheal tubes, which are commonly used during neonatal mechanical ventilation. When ventilating a larger patient, the volume loss may be negligible; however, in a small child or infant it may be a significant portion of the delivered tidal volume. Failure to consider this volume loss may result in hypoventilation and hypercapnia of the patient. The compressed volume can also affect the calculations of respiratory compliance, oxygen consumption, carbon dioxide production, and dead space volume.[12] To account for this loss, an effective tidal volume should be calculated (Box 19-2).[13] A piston-driven volume ventilator also delivers a constant volume with a variable peak pressure. Because of the piston action, flow peaks in the middle of the inflation when stroke speed is the greatest. Although piston ventilators are seldom used in the pediatric critical care setting, they become an inexpensive and practical choice for the nonacute care or home setting.

Many home ventilators also allow the use of pressure limitation by setting a desired maximal pressure level. Using this feature decreases tidal volume from the volume set on the ventilator, but exactly how it affects volume depends on the specific ventilator and inflation time settings. A piston-generated pressure preset mode is not appropriate for the pediatric or

---

Box 19-2 Calculation of Effective Tidal Volume

$$V_{Teff} = V_{Tset} - [(\text{Pstatic*} - \text{PEEP}) \times \text{Circuit}]$$

DETERMINATION OF COMPLIANCE FACTOR OF CIRCUIT
1. With the circuit assembled and connected to the ventilator, the patient connection to the circuit is occluded.
2. A known volume of gas is delivered into the circuit through the ventilator, and the resulting peak inspiratory pressure is noted.
3. The resulting pressure is divided by the delivered volume to obtain the compliance factor of the circuit. This is generally 1 ml/cm H_2O for infant circuits and 2 to 3 ml/cm H_2O for larger circuits.

V_{Teff}, Effective tidal volume; V_{Tset}, tidal volume set on ventilator; Pstatic, static (plateau) pressure measured during inflation; PEEP, positive end-expiratory pressure set on ventilator; Circuit, compliance or compression factor of circuit.
*If static or plateau pressure measurement cannot be obtained because of airway leaks, the peak inspiratory pressure may be used as an approximation.

infant home setting. Using a microprocessor-based turbine-driven portable ventilator is a better home care choice in such a situation.

Dual-control Ventilation

Advances in ventilator sensors, response times, and microprocessor technologies have introduced new features into mechanical ventilators. "Dual control" or "volume-targeted" refers to a ventilation mode that allows the clinician to set a volume target while the ventilator delivers pressure-controlled breaths.[14] Although it is impossible to control two variables simultaneously (volume and pressure), this form of ventilation can be thought of simply as a pressure controller that servo-controls the pressure levels automatically in response to measurements of volume or compliance. These modes are commonly used in the neonatal and pediatric populations. These "hybrid modes" allow the comfort of pressure control with the maintenance of a tidal volume target by servo-controlling pressure on the basis of feedback obtained at the ventilator pneumotachometer or proximal flow sensor. As lung compliance and airway resistance improves or worsens, the microprocessor will measure these changes and increase or decrease the pressure level on the basis of a breath-to-breath analysis, a multiple-breath average, or within-breath measurement. Some of these modes use more than one flow control signal at the flow valve and may switch from PCV to VCV within a single breath to establish a minimal tidal volume goal. These modes can provide the patient with some of the best features of PCV and VCV. Dual-control modes can be effective at maintaining a more consistent tidal volume and hence alveolar minute ventilation in patients who are prone to abrupt changes in pulmonary compliance.

Limited data exist concerning whether these modes are superior to traditional approaches to mechanical ventilation of humans. On the basis of these limited data, the future of these modes looks promising. A meta-analysis of trials comparing PCV with various volume-targeted modes in premature infants resulted in trends favoring volume targeting for reduction in duration of ventilation, rates of pneumothorax, severe intraventricular hemorrhage, and (to a lesser degree) incidence of bronchopulmonary dysplasia.[15] These modes have also been shown to be effective in avoiding hypo/hypercapneic episodes in premature infants, in whom cerebral blood flow is impacted by small changes in carbon dioxide.[16] Future randomized controlled clinical trials are necessary to determine clinical significance in improving survival without complications in

premature infants when using dual-control modes over other modes of ventilation.

Pressure-regulated volume control (PRVC) attempts to maintain a minimal target tidal volume with a constant pressure by manipulating the flow waveform. The ventilator initially performs a test breath sequence, which measures dynamic or static system compliance. Subsequent adjustments in pressure or tidal volume are made on the basis of the previous breath or a historical average of breaths. Some ventilators initiate a "test breath" sequence during PRVC by implementing a brief inspiratory pause during a volume-controlled breath. The static pressure measured during the pause will be the pressure control level for the next breath. The following breaths will increase or decrease the pressure control level by a maximal value of 3 cm H_2O to try to achieve the set tidal volume with the lowest possible pressure. Within a few sequential breaths, the tidal volume goal may be reached. Certain conditions can restart the test breath sequence for optimal accuracy, including high-pressure limitation, V_T in excess of 150% of the set V_T, and after-setting settings changes. Other modes that implement similar volume strategies as PRVC are volume support ventilation (VSV), Vsynch, VC plus, and Auto-flow. Most new microprocessor ventilators can provide these modes within Assist-control and synchronized intermittent mandatory ventilation (SIMV).

Volume-assured pressure support (VAPS) uses pressure support ventilation while maintaining a minimal tidal volume with each breath. If the patient does not receive the minimal tidal volume during a breath, the flow rate is held constant and the pressure is increased until the volume is received.[17] This mode is useful in patients who have good respiratory effort but may rely on the ventilator to ensure a steady volume goal when pulmonary compliance and resistance are variable.

Another form of dual-controlled ventilation in neonatal and pediatric mechanical ventilation is machine volume (MV), which uses an intrabreath pressure adjustment to target volume. This mode is further classified as Auto-set-point control. Auto-set-point control is a more advanced version of a dual-control mode. The breath can start out as pressure controlled and automatically switch to volume controlled within the same breath.[18] The ventilator flow control valve measures compliance every 2 milliseconds within the breath and can increase or decrease the pressure adjustment within this time by manipulating the flow rate if the delivered volume is not being met or if the patient requires more flow. The ventilator calculates a target flow rate on the basis of the minimal volume set at the ventilator and the inspiratory time. The breath begins as a PCV breath with a variable-decelerating flow signal and once the minimal tidal volume has been met, the breath is terminated at the preset inspiratory time and ends as a PCV breath. If the minimal tidal volume goal has not been delivered, then the ventilator transitions from a decelerating flow to a continuous flow signal to reach the tidal volume goal within the preset inspiratory time. The high-pressure limit must be set appropriately to protect against high pressure. The operator can set a volume limit feature, which will terminate the breath once this preset volume is exceeded either at the proximal flow sensor or at the ventilator flow control valve. This mode is similar to VAPS and pressure augmentation but different in that the inspiratory time will not by increased in order to deliver the set tidal volume. The clinician must set an uncorrected minimal tidal volume when using this mode in neonates. This includes the volume of gas delivered to the patient as well as the volume of gas delivered to the ventilator circuit.

Volume guarantee (VG) is another form of dual-control ventilation that is used in one type of neonatal ventilator. The operator sets a tidal volume, inspiratory time, and flow rate. This mode can also be applied to pressure support ventilation. The ventilator incorporates a proximal flow sensor at the patient airway. The microprocessor assesses an eight-breath historical average of expired tidal volume and will increase pressure on the basis of these measurements up to the pressure limit to deliver the target volume. If compliance or resistance improves dramatically then the ventilator will terminate breath delivery if the delivered tidal volume exceeds 130% of the set tidal volume. Pressure will also wean as the result of improving compliance, based on the breath average. Because the ventilator makes manipulations on the basis of expiratory tidal volume, this mode can correct for compressible volume loss of inspired gases and small endotracheal tube leaks and is useful in the neonatal population. The practitioner should be careful when using this mode with excessive endotracheal tube leaks. "In the presence of a substantial leak around the endotracheal tube, there are concerns that this system will falsely underestimate the actual tidal volume delivered to the lung and overcompensate the subsequent breaths with excessive tidal volumes."[19]

Many clinicians maintain that constant pressure ventilation is superior to other types of ventilation in neonates or pediatric patients who have leaks around a cuffless endotracheal tube. However, a leak around an endotracheal tube reduces ventilation during constant pressure ventilation just as it does with other types of ventilation.[20]

FLOW AND PRESSURE WAVEFORM PATTERNS

To fully understand mechanical ventilation, the clinician should relate each change in a ventilator setting with the effect it will have on respiratory variables. Using this approach helps the clinician to understand the relationship of each ventilator setting to the respiratory system, rather than memorizing a long list of cause-and-effect relationships.[3] The concepts of flow and pressure as they relate to time are helpful in relating ventilator settings to the goals of mechanical ventilation. The pressure and flow waveforms are altered each time a ventilator setting is changed. These waveforms can be viewed as two-dimensional pictures of the changes that occur in the lungs as the ventilator settings are adjusted. Tidal volume and $P\overline{aw}$ as they relate to flow and pressure waveforms is shown in Figure 19-2. Assuming constant lung conditions and inflation time, an increase in the inspired volume per unit time results in an increase in peak pressure and an increase in both tidal volume and $P\overline{aw}$. Similarly, if the tidal volume control on a ventilator increases, flow, peak pressure, and $P\overline{aw}$ also increase. Note that once a change occurs in one variable it results in changes in other variables. Two-dimensional images such as this help to illustrate

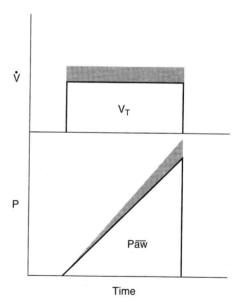

FIGURE 19-2 Flow ($\dot{V}$) and pressure (P) waveforms during constant flow–volume ventilation. The *unshaded area* below each waveform represents tidal volume (V_T) and mean airway pressure ($P\overline{aw}$). The *shaded area* represents the increase in V_T and $P\overline{aw}$ when flow is increased.

concepts as they relate to ventilator management or other ventilator functions.

TIME CONSTANTS

The concept of a time constant in the lung represents how fast pressure equilibrates between the circuit and the alveoli. Conversely, it represents the maximal rate at which exhalation occurs. The time constant is a mathematic and physiologic concept that is not consistently applied clinically. Previously, accurately obtaining the values necessary for calculating a time constant was technically difficult. Advances in pulmonary function measurement techniques have made these data more available.

A time constant is the product of multiplying compliance and resistance. The time constant relates to both inspiratory filling and expiratory emptying of the lungs. Mouth pressure or proximal airway pressure equilibrates with alveolar pressure in three to five time constants.[21] In a healthy newborn this is 0.33 second. In severely premature infants with respiratory distress syndrome with decreased lung compliance, one time constant can be as short as 0.05 second.[22] This means that pressure equilibration will occur in 0.15 to 0.25 second, which is the minimal inspiratory time required to ensure complete delivery of the tidal volume. When airway resistance is high, such as in meconium aspiration syndrome, the time constant is longer. This would indicate using longer inspiratory times, lower inspiratory flows, and longer exhalation times to ventilate these infants.

Monitoring respiratory system mechanics to derive time constants assists in properly adjusting adequate inspiratory time and expiratory time during ventilation. The time component is important when using rapid rates to allow adequate exhalation without developing breath stacking and automatic positive end-expiratory pressure

(auto-PEEP) and to minimize iatrogenic lung damage. Using serial measurements of resistance and compliance directs the setting of ventilator parameters to match the changing pathophysiology of the patient.[23]

TRIGGERING

Patient triggering is one of the most important links to the ventilator. Proper triggering can reduce work of breathing, allows a patient to be more comfortable, reduces oxygen consumption, and can result in a shorter duration of ventilation.[24] There are four types of sensing: flow, pressure, motion, and neurally adjusted ventilatory assist (Table 19-1). Many ventilators can do one if not two of the types of sensing. When types of triggering are considered, the placement of the triggering device and its effects on the patient are evaluated. Flow triggering is the most frequently used in the neonatal patient population.

Flow Sensing

Many ventilators now offer flow triggering as the primary mechanism by which a breath is initiated by a patient from the ventilator. A pneumotachometer between the circuit and the patient senses effort by measuring inspiratory flow or volume. Two types of pneumotachometer can be used to sense flow: the heated-wire anemometer and the variable-orifice pneumotachometer. These units have fast response times, usually in the 30- to 70-millisecond range, and provide reliable synchronization at all rates.[25,26] However, flow sensors add dead space to the airway, and the potential increase in tidal volume associated with SIMV may be negated by an increase in carbon dioxide retention. Flow sensors may also be affected by secretions and require frequent cleaning. Flow sensing and triggering can also be done with the internal ventilator pneumotachometer and can be sensitive enough for most patients. With these

---

TABLE 19-1

Synchronizing Systems for Mechanical Ventilators

Type	Source	Advantages/Disadvantages
Flow sensor	Pneumotachometer (heated wire, variable orifice, differential pressure)	Fast response; provides volume measurement; adds dead space; affected by secretions
Pressure sensor	Proximal airway, ventilator demand valve	No dead space; requires good patient effort; low transit time
Motion sensor	Abdominal sensor (impedance electrode)	Requires correct placement; false-positive measurements; no volume measurement
Neurally adjusted ventilatory assist	Nasogastric tube (EAdi)	No dead space; unaffected by secretions, auto-PEEP, and leaks; requires catheter (invasive); no volume measurement

EAdi, Electrical activity of the diaphragm; *PEEP,* positive end-expiratory pressure.

improvements in making the ventilator more receptive to patient effort, problems associated with secretions, condensation, system/patient leaks, and active cardiac pulsation could lead to erroneous triggering of the ventilator (auto-cycling).

Pressure Sensing

Some ventilators use a drop in the pressure signal sensed at the airway to trigger the ventilator with the patient's breath. For the pressure in the circuit to drop to less than the trigger level, or sensitivity setting, approximately 2 ml of volume must be displaced. This often accounts for a large portion of the neonatal tidal volume and thus is not well tolerated. A low birth weight infant may not consistently produce the level of effort necessary to trigger the ventilator. During pressure sensing, the response time tends to be slow because of delay from the progression of the pressure drop through the ventilator tubing. Because of this, synchronization is difficult to achieve at ventilator rates greater than 35 to 40 breaths/minute.

Motion Sensing

Two types of motion-sensing devices are used to detect patient effort and synchronize the ventilator. The first device incorporates a Graseby capsule taped to the infant's abdomen. Abdominal movement occurs 100 milliseconds before air flow is initiated.[27] This movement compresses the capsule and sends a signal to the processing unit, which, in turn, triggers the ventilator. This system demonstrated slightly shorter response times than did flow sensors.[28] Another type of motion sensor uses impedance monitoring and receives the signal from the bedside cardiac and respiration monitor. The respiration signal is sent to a microprocessor in the ventilator, which triggers a mechanical breath. This system appears to have response times comparable to those of other systems and is successfully used in very low birth weight infants.[29]

Each of these systems accomplishes synchronization in different ways. Proper setting of the sensitivity and placement of the sensor is required to make the sensor work properly. Frequently, an infant may have abdominal movement not associated with a respiratory effort, which causes a false trigger. Impedance-monitoring technology is prone to problems in the event of airway obstruction.

Neurally Adjusted Ventilatory Assist

Neurally adjusted ventilatory assist allows the patient full neurological control of the triggering, magnitude, and timing of the mechanical support provided, regardless of changes in respiratory drive, mechanics, and muscle function.[30] Neurally adjusted ventilatory assist uses a nasogastric tube with specialized sensors that obtain signals from the electrical activity of the diaphragm to control the timing and pressure of the ventilation delivered.[31] In theory, this form of triggering and support is particularly useful for patients with gas trapping and auto-PEEP who have high work of breathing due to triggering. This form of triggering is not affected by leaks and secretions; therefore auto-cycling and hypocapnia in newborns can be eliminated. However, this modality is invasive and placement of the nasogastric tube could be uncomfortable to the patient.

MODES OF VENTILATION

The mode of ventilation is defined by how a ventilator is going to interface with the patient's breathing efforts. These modes can use pressure, flow, or other signals to trigger. The main control variables may be volume, pressure, or flow and may use either positive or negative pressure as the driving force. Most ventilators are capable of providing multiple modes, and some even combine modes to enhance the patient–ventilator interface. Figure 19-3 illustrates various modes of ventilation and how they interface with spontaneous breathing.

Control Mode

The control mode is used when the clinician needs to maintain complete control over a patient's ventilation variables. To attain complete control, the patient-triggering mechanism is made inactive and all breaths are delivered at a preset volume or pressure, frequency, and inspiratory flow rate.[17] The patient should be sedated and paralyzed to avoid asynchrony between ventilator inflations and patient breathing efforts. Control ventilation may be desirable when extreme ventilation variables are required, and asynchrony may result in complications such as pneumothorax. Such situations may occur during mechanical ventilation of the patient with severe acute respiratory distress syndrome (ARDS) or asthma.

Assist/Control Mode

Like the control mode, the assist/control (A/C) mode allows the clinician control over most of the patient's ventilation variables except for rate. The volume or pressure, frequency, and inspiratory flow rate are preset, and the ventilator supports every breath. However, the patient is allowed to use his or her own ventilatory drive to trigger the ventilator and receive a breath at the preset volume or pressure. If the patient fails to take a breath during a specific period, the ventilator delivers the defined breath at a preset rate. Control and A/C are then defined as patient-triggered and machine-triggered continuous mandatory ventilation.[32] Some ventilators

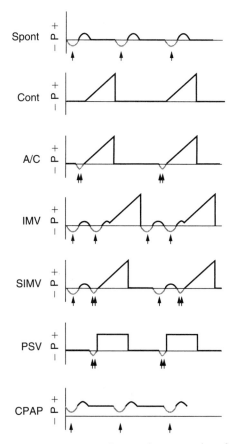

FIGURE 19-3 Pressure waveforms of seven modes of ventilation. *Single arrows* denote spontaneous inspiratory efforts. *Double arrows* denote ventilator breaths triggered by inspiratory efforts. Spont, spontaneous breathing; Cont, controlled ventilation; A/C, assist/control ventilation; IMV, intermittent mandatory ventilation; SIMV, synchronized intermittent mandatory ventilation; PSV, pressure support ventilation; CPAP, continuous positive airway pressure.

have control and A/C as the same mode, with the sensitivity setting being the only difference. The sensitivity of the triggering mechanism is set sufficiently low to be activated by any attempted breath. The sensitivity must also be set sufficiently high to prevent activation (autocycling), by artifacts such as cardiac activity, airway leaks, or patient care procedures. The A/C mode may be useful for older children or adolescents. It is being used more frequently in neonates and small children who are more susceptible to lung injury, especially when using volume and dual-control modes. The advantage of the A/C mode is that every breath delivered to the patient, whether patient or machine triggered, has a guaranteed volume or pressure. There are several disadvantages to this mode. In neonates, infants, or small children with high respiratory rates, hyperventilation, hyperinflation and respiratory alkalosis may occur. The work of breathing may be increased, especially for patients who

are not breathing in synchrony with the machine or who are "fighting the ventilator." Sedating the patient may alleviate this. If the sensitivity of the triggering mechanism is not set adequately, the patient's inspiratory effort may be increased and result in an increase in oxygen consumption.[2]

Synchronized Intermittent Mandatory Ventilation

Early models of mechanical ventilators used primarily intermittent mandatory ventilation (IMV). With IMV the ventilator was incapable of sensing patient effort and would deliver mandatory breaths on top of spontaneous breaths. To avoid patient–ventilator asynchrony, a sensing mechanism is built into most modern ventilators. The ventilator presets a rate for the delivery of mandatory breaths (of preset volume or pressure and flow rate) and attempts to synchronize the breaths with the patient's spontaneous effort. If no patient effort is sensed within a specific window of time, a mandatory breath is given. Airway pressure or flow is the usual triggering mechanism for SIMV; however, a few designs incorporate abdominal motion and, more recently, a sensor that triggers inhalation and exhalation on the basis of an electric signal generated by the diaphragm. Small volumes and rapid rates characterize an infant's spontaneous breathing effort, which makes synchronizing ventilator inflation difficult. With the latest advances in sensor technology, SIMV is now a feasible option in neonates and infants.[24,33,34] Advantages of this mode are that it allows the patient to perform part of the ventilatory work while maintaining a backup of mandatory ventilation and that it is useful in weaning the patient from mechanical ventilation (Box 19-3). Hyperventilation and respiratory alkalosis are risks just

Box 19-3	Benefits of Synchronized Intermittent Mandatory Ventilation

- Better distribution of ventilation by coordinating air flow with respiratory muscle effort
- Improved oxygenation by reducing ventilation-perfusion mismatch
- Better tidal volume at the same positive inspiratory pressure
- Improved minute ventilation through the minimization of ineffective breaths
- Reduced incidence of pneumothorax
- Reduced incidence of intraventricular hemorrhage due to less variation in cerebral blood flow
- Decreased use of sedation and paralysis
- Reduced length of ventilation

as with the A/C mode, but they are less likely to occur. Another risk associated with SIMV is increased work of breathing during spontaneous ventilation. This may be the result of inadequate inspiratory flow, ventilator response to the patient's inspiratory effort, ventilator circuitry, or endotracheal tube resistance.[2]

Continuous Positive Airway Pressure

During continuous positive airway pressure (CPAP), also termed *constant airway pressure,* a constant, above-ambient pressure is applied to the airways and maintained through the entire respiratory cycle.[35] Respiratory efforts are spontaneous and not supported by mandatory ventilator inflations.[17] However, many ventilators provide a "back-up" mode of ventilation that provides full support in the event that the patient becomes apneic. In the pediatric setting, CPAP is applied to improve oxygenation by increasing the functional residual capacity, as in aspiration pneumonitis, or to stent floppy anatomic structures, as in tracheomalacia or disorders associated with sleep apnea.[25,36] CPAP should be considered as a primary mode to improve lung compliance and oxygenation in spontaneously breathing patients when the potential adverse effects of high peak airway pressures and volutrauma must be avoided.[25-28] It is frequently in intubated and tracheotomized patients when weaning from mechanical ventilation. High levels of CPAP may overdistend the lungs, increase the work of breathing, and reduce compliance (Chapter 18 [Continuous Positive Airway Pressure] for a discussion of CPAP for the neonate).

Airway Pressure Release Ventilation

Airway pressure release ventilation (APRV) is another form of CPAP, in which a CPAP level and a pressure release level are set along with the frequency and time of the pressure release. This mode of ventilation is usually indicated when a patient has intrapulmonary shunting from RDS or ARDS that is not responding to traditional approaches with a conventional mechanical ventilator. A high level (CPAP) is held in the lung for up to 2 seconds for infants and 4 seconds for pediatrics, and the patient is able to breathe spontaneously during this pressure hold. The ventilator will continue to provide inspiratory flow to the patient during spontaneous breathing in order to maintain the high CPAP level. This is accomplished because the expiratory valve is active throughout inhalation and exhalation and the patient is allowed to exhale during inspiration as long as the inflation pressure is still being held in the ventilator system. Spontaneous breathing at a higher pressure not only aids in alveolar recruitment but through the

application of pleural pressure change, improvements in the distribution of lung volume to diseased lung units may improve functional residual capacity (FRC) and pulmonary compliance.[37] The short intermittent decreases in the CPAP level allow alveolar emptying of gases. Unlike conventional CPAP, however, the intermittent release of pressure augments ventilation and allows elimination of carbon dioxide.[38,39] APRV has been used in neonatal, pediatric, and adult forms of respiratory failure.[37] APRV has been referred to as *bilevel positive airway pressure* (BiPAP) but is inherently different in that it is usually implemented in an intubated patient who is failing conventional mechanical ventilation because of refractory hypoxemia. Noninvasive BiPAP does not require that a patient be tracheally intubated. In this mode, the pressure level changes between inspiration and expiration. Although its use in preventing sleep apnea is similar to that of conventional CPAP, it may be helpful in overcoming ventilation difficulties and avoiding tracheotomy in individuals afflicted with neuromuscular diseases, such as spinal muscular atrophy.[40]

Pressure Support Ventilation

Pressure support ventilation (PSV) is a spontaneous ventilation mode in which each breath must be triggered by the patient. It incorporates a constant pressure inflation that is triggered by the patient and terminated when inspiratory flow decays to a certain threshold (usually a percentage of peak flow). PSV improves the efficiency of inspiratory work of breathing, decreases the respiratory rate, reduces the oxygen cost of breathing, and is associated with faster weaning times.[41,42] It may be associated with an improved sense of breathing comfort by the patient.[43,44] PSV is popularly used to augment breaths in conjunction with SIMV or as a mode for weaning patients from mechanical ventilation.[45] Combining PSV with SIMV may help reduce some of the work associated with demand valves and small endotracheal tubes, but it may also increase $\overline{Paw}$. The PSV level that is chosen to deliver a full tidal volume breath is referred to as PSV_{max}, and PSV used solely to overcome the imposed work of breathing is referred to as the PSV_{min}. Caution should be used in clinical situations in which increased $\overline{Paw}$ may be harmful. PSV is useful as a stand-alone mode or for weaning patients receiving short- and long-term mechanical ventilation. If the patient develops an endotracheal tube leak, the flow termination criteria may not be met, thereby creating a "breath hold." Ventilators have been introduced that allow adjustment of the flow termination criteria, which may help alleviate this problem. Current ventilators have incorporated a preset or adjustable backup time termination setting that will cycle the breath into exhalation should a leak occur and the flow cycling criteria are not met.

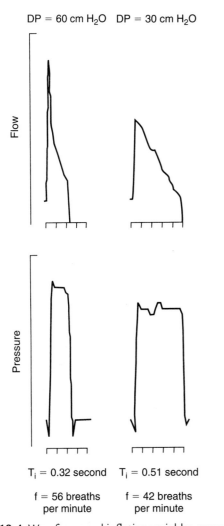

DP = 60 cm H_2O DP = 30 cm H_2O

Flow

Pressure

T_i = 0.32 second T_i = 0.51 second

f = 56 breaths
per minute

f = 42 breaths
per minute

FIGURE 19-4 Waveforms and inflation variables comparing a high driving pressure (DP) (60 cm H_2O) and a low DP (30 cm H_2O) to generate flow during pressure support ventilation of an infant. f, Frequency (breaths/min); T_i, inspiratory time.

Effective PSV can result in adequate tidal volume and minute ventilation at a lower respiratory rate.[46] Figure 19-4 compares inflation variables when high and low driving pressures are used to generate flow during PSV

in an infant. Other modes that adapt PSV to meet tidal volume or minute volume criteria are also available. Such modes provide true pressure support inflation but then alter an inflation to meet a minimal tidal volume if not met during the PSV inflation.[17]

Inverse Ratio Ventilation

Inverse ratio ventilation (IRV) is a nonconventional mode of ventilation in which an I/E ratio greater than 1:1 is used during controlled ventilation. The patient is usually deeply sedated or paralyzed, or both, to avoid dyssynchrony with the ventilator. It is most often used in patients with ARDS. The major goals of IRV are to improve oxygenation by increasing the $\overline{Paw}$ and to allow recruitment of pulmonary units by increasing inspiratory time. Complications associated with IRV are pulmonary volutrauma and compromised cardiac output. Patients may also require substantial amounts of sedation and neuromuscular blocking agents to be comfortable when using this approach. There are currently few data demonstrating the advantage of IRV over other, more conventional modes of ventilation.[2]

MANAGING VENTILATOR SETTINGS

Proper management of ventilator settings requires monitoring of arterial blood gases, chest X-rays, ventilator waveforms, and physical assessment of the patient. Table 19-2 shows commonly used initial ventilator settings suggested for different patient sizes; however, certain conditions or severity of disease may require a different initial approach.

Manipulating Arterial Carbon Dioxide Tension

One of the main goals of mechanical ventilation is to manipulate the arterial carbon dioxide tension ($Paco_2$), which is affected by changing the minute ventilation. The minute ventilation is directly related to ventilation frequency and tidal volume and is inversely related to the $Paco_2$.

TABLE 19-2						
Initial Mechanical Ventilator Settings						
	Premature Infant	**Infant**	**Toddler**	**Small Child**	**Child**	**Adolescent**
Respiratory rate (breaths/min)	40-60	25-40	20-35	20-30	18-25	12-20
V_T (ml/kg)	4-6	5-8	5-8	6-9	7-10	7-10
Inspiratory time (s)	0.25-0.4	0.3-0.5	0.6-0.7	0.7-0.8	0.8-1	1-1.2
PEEP (cm H_2O)	3-5	5	5	5	5	5
Fio_2	*	*	*	*	*	*

Fio_2, Fraction of inspired oxygen; PEEP, peak end-expiratory pressure; V_T, tidal volume.
*Start 10% higher than preintubation Fio_2 or 100%.

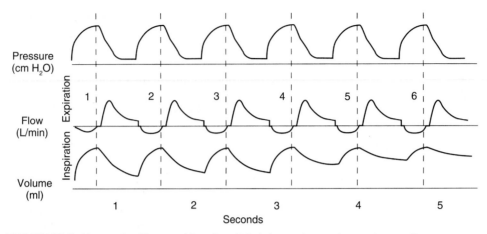

FIGURE 19-5 Air trapping illustrated in a flow (L/min) over time scalar. Expiratory flow never returns to baseline before the ventilator cycles again.

Frequency

Frequency or rate is generally the first method used to increase minute ventilation. At low rates and conventional I/E ratios or during weaning, adjusting frequency is the most desirable option. Two disadvantages exist when manipulating frequency at higher rates or inverse I/E ratios. The first is that as frequency increases, air trapping is likely to occur.[47,48] Figure 19-5 illustrates this in a flow/time scalar graphic. Notice that flow does not come back to baseline. The second is that when the I/E ratio is kept constant, minute ventilation does not change.

Tidal Volume

An alternative to adjusting frequency is to change any variable that affects tidal volume and hence affects minute ventilation and $Paco_2$. The goal is to select a variable that will increase the area under the flow waveform. This is accomplished by increasing flow or inspiratory time. The tidal volume control on a microprocessor ventilator adjusts flow or times to derive an increase in tidal volume. Another variable that is available on some ventilators is the I/E ratio. Adjusting it to provide a longer inspiratory time may also improve elimination of carbon dioxide. Altering tidal volume variables is useful in situations such as severe asthma, in which the goal is to minimize the rate and air trapping while maximizing exhalation time and ventilation. Figure 19-6 illustrates the three ways in which the flow waveform can change to increase tidal volume and minute ventilation.

Research has shown that the largest contribution to ventilator-induced lung injury results from lung overdistention caused by excessive tidal volume (volutrauma); followed by the repetitive opening and closing of the terminal lung units (atelectrauma).[49] Therefore, more

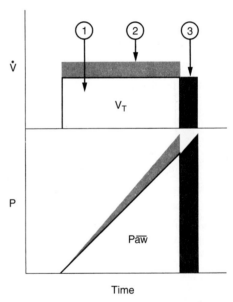

FIGURE 19-6 Control variables that affect minute ventilation by increasing the area under the flow (V̇) waveform to increase tidal volume (V_T). *1*, Increase V_T or rate; *2*, increase inspiratory flow; *3*, increase inspiratory time. Also shown is the associated change in mean airway pressure (Pa̅w̅). P, pressure.

emphasis is being placed on setting lower tidal volumes, improvements in tidal volume monitoring, and setting adequate PEEP levels. The tidal volume setting in neonates varies from 4 to 6 ml/kg in low birth weight premature infants, to 5 to 8 ml/kg in term infants, and to 7 to 10 ml/kg in pediatric and adolescent patients.[19,49] Lower volumes have been shown to be effective for patients with restrictive lung disease such as RDS and ARDS.[50,51] Tidal volume should be corrected for compressible volume loss or a proximal flow sensor should be used.

Careful monitoring of breath sounds, chest expansion, arterial blood gas values, and chest radiographs is essential in determining adequate tidal volume.

During pressure ventilation, increasing the pressure limit may also increase tidal volume. When the pressure limit is reached, flow decelerates. The increase in tidal volume is the result of the delay in flow deceleration and widening of the area under the flow waveform. An increase in the pressure limit during PCV and PSV causes the initial flow to increase. The result is a larger decelerating flow waveform and larger tidal volume. Figure 19-7 illustrates the way a change in the pressure limit affects both forms of pressure ventilation.

Manipulating Arterial Oxygen Tension
Fraction of Inspired Oxygen

The most obvious way to improve oxygen delivery is to increase the alveolar oxygen tension by increasing the fraction of inspired oxygen (FIO_2). A simple method to determine the FIO_2 needed for a desired arterial oxygen tension (PaO_2) is derived from the arterial-to-alveolar oxygen tension ratio. Assuming constant barometric pressure, $PaCO_2$, and stable lung conditions, the equation simplifies to:

$$FIO_2 \text{ desired} = PaO_2 \text{ desired} \times FIO_2 \text{ known}/PaO_2 \text{ known}$$

Because prolonged exposure to high levels of oxygen may be toxic, the lowest acceptable FIO_2 should be used.[52]

However, high levels of oxygen may be necessary to correct hypoxemia when treating severe lung disease or persistent pulmonary hypertension of the newborn. To avoid these complications, other variables that relate to improving oxygenation must also be considered, such as $P\overline{aw}$, nitric oxide, and positive end-expiratory pressure (PEEP).

Mean Airway Pressure

Improvement in PaO_2 is directly related to an increase in $P\overline{aw}$. (It may have an inverse relationship in right-to-left cardiac shunts or in pulmonary volutrauma.[53,54]) This improvement is believed to be caused by recruitment of collapsed alveoli or the redistribution of lung fluid, or both.[12] $P\overline{aw}$ is the area under the pressure waveform from the beginning of inflation to the beginning of the next inflation divided by the total cycle time. A simple equation for estimating $P\overline{aw}$ is as follows:

$$P\overline{aw} = 1/2 \times \text{peak pressure} \times (\text{inspiratory/time/inspiratory} + \text{expiratory times})$$

Several control variables affect $P\overline{aw}$, including inspiratory time, peak pressure, frequency, flow, and PEEP. The denominator of the equation for $P\overline{aw}$ is cycle time or frequency. As frequency increases, cycle time decreases so that the result is an increase in the value of $P\overline{aw}$. Figure 19-8 demonstrates how the pressure waveform can be altered by these variables to increase $P\overline{aw}$. The desired $P\overline{aw}$ is one in which both oxygenation and

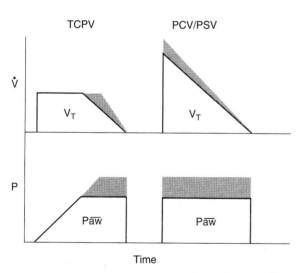

FIGURE 19-7 Waveforms comparing the mechanism of increasing tidal volume (V_T) by adjusting pressure limit during time-cycled pressure-limited ventilation (TCPV) to pressure-control or pressure-support ventilation (PCV/PSV). Flow changes during PCV/PSV, but only the length of time changes before flow decelerates during TCPV. $P\overline{aw}$, mean airway pressure; $\dot{V}$, flow.

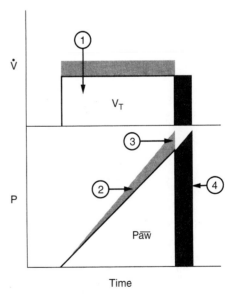

FIGURE 19-8 Control variables that alter mean airway pressure ($P\overline{aw}$) by increasing the area under the pressure waveform. *1,* Increase tidal volume (V_T) or rate; *2,* increase inspiratory flow; *3,* increase peak pressure; *4,* increase inspiratory time. Also shown is the associated change in V_T. P, pressure; $\dot{V}$, flow.

ventilation are optimized, and the risks of pulmonary volutrauma, impaired hemodynamics, and fluid retention are minimized.

Flow Rate

The flow rate will directly affect P$\overline{aw}$. Ideally, inspiratory flow should be set to match the patient's peak inspiratory demands and depends largely on the following:

- The patient's spontaneous effort
- The work of breathing
- Patient–ventilator synchrony

Too much or not enough flow can increase the work of breathing or cause dyssynchrony.[55,56] Figure 19-9 presents a flow–volume loop illustrating when there is inadequate flow. Flow and pressure waveforms vary among ventilators. The flow required for spontaneous breathing is provided by means of continuous flow or a demand valve that is triggered by the patient's inspiratory effort.[2]

Inspiratory Time and I/E Ratio

The inspiratory time and I/E ratio also directly affect P$\overline{aw}$. Although there are few specific data regarding guidelines for inspiratory time and I/E ratio, it is suggested that the appropriate inspiratory time and I/E ratio depend on the patient's ventilation and oxygenation status as well as on the level of spontaneous breathing. Ventilators are often set at an inspiratory time of 0.25 to 0.5 second for neonates, 0.6 to 0.9 second for toddlers and children, and 1 to 1.2 seconds for adolescents, with an I/E ratio of 1:2 to 1:3. Increasing the inspiratory time or I/E ratio is performed in an effort to increase P$\overline{aw}$ and improve oxygenation. When this is carried out,

however, the impact on patient comfort, the need for sedation, and the development of auto-PEEP, hemodynamic compromise, and breath stacking must be considered[57] (see previous discussion of IRV mode). Figure 19-10 presents what is seen on the ventilator graphics if the inspiratory time is excessive.

Positive End-expiratory Pressure

The most significant variable affecting P$\overline{aw}$ is PEEP. Figure 19-11 shows the relationship of PEEP to the pressure waveform and P$\overline{aw}$. PEEP affects pressure throughout the entire respiratory cycle and alters the simple formula given previously for P$\overline{aw}$ to

P$\overline{aw}$ = 1/2 × (Peak pressure − PEEP) × (Inspiratory time/Inspiratory time + Expiratory time) + PEEP

PEEP improves gas exchange by improving PaO_2, recruiting collapsed alveoli, increasing functional lung volume, decreasing intrapulmonary shunting, and improving lung compliance.[58-60]

An adequate PEEP level is the amount of PEEP necessary to attain an acceptable PaO_2 at the lowest FIO_2,

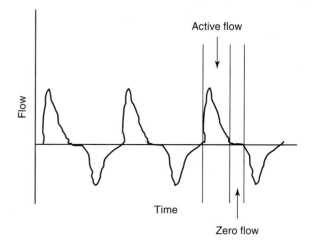

FIGURE 19-10 Excessive inspiratory time on flow/time scalar. Flow returns to baseline before the ventilator cycles into expiration.

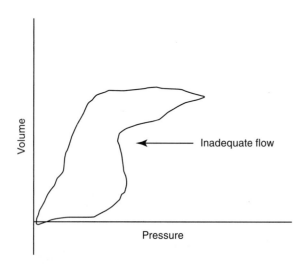

FIGURE 19-9 Inadequate flow support on flow–volume loop. A normal loop should look like a football at a 45-degree angle. The inspiratory phase of this loop is concave, owing to inadequate flow.

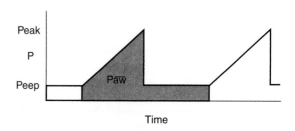

FIGURE 19-11 The relationship of positive end-expiratory pressure (PEEP) to the pressure waveform. Note that mean airway pressure (P$\overline{aw}$) is the area under the waveform during the entire respiratory cycle. P, pressure.

although avoidance of high PEEP levels is desirable.[61] It is determined by many physiologic factors, which may or may not be monitored in any given clinical situation. A conservative but acceptable Pao_2 is 45 to 65 mm Hg for neonates younger than 33 weeks of gestation and 60 to 80 mm Hg for pediatric patients at an Fio_2 of 0.4 to 0.5. PEEP usually begins at 3 to 5 cm H_2O, with increases made in increments of 2 cm H_2O.[62,63] A method of judging adequate PEEP levels is to monitor static lung compliance or to calculate it by dividing the effective tidal volume formula by the end-inspiratory pause pressure minus PEEP. When the functional residual capacity is low, static compliance increases as PEEP increases because of shifting of the ventilating volume to the optimal point on the compliance curve. When optimal distention is reached, lung compliance is maximal. If PEEP is increased further, overdistention, reduced compliance, and decreased oxygen transport may result.[58] A static compliance measurement can be difficult to obtain in patients with cuffless endotracheal tubes that have a leak.

Monitoring the $Paco_2$ to end-tidal carbon dioxide gradient may also be useful in judging PEEP levels (Chapter 10, Invasive Blood Gas Analysis and Cardiovascular Monitoring). Overdistention and reduced cardiac output resulting from excessive PEEP cause the gradient to widen. Caution must be exercised with this method because other abnormalities causing a low cardiac output may also increase this gradient.[8,64] Because excessive levels of PEEP affect cardiac function, monitoring mean blood pressure, central venous pressure, mean pulmonary artery pressure, and other hemodynamic variables is also important while monitoring PEEP levels. When pulmonary artery catheters are used, cardiac output and the pulmonary shunt fraction are useful measures. A reduction of the shunt fraction, normally to less than 15%, is the goal when applying PEEP in patients with ARDS.[59] When using this variable to adjust PEEP and the shunt fraction is reduced to less than 15%, levels of PEEP in excess of 25 cm H_2O are usually required.[60] This aspect of using PEEP in the pediatric population is generally prohibited in patients with a cuffless endotracheal tube because of the leakage around the tube.

Not only can PEEP be applied as a ventilating variable, but it also can be present in the form of auto-PEEP (intrinsic, occult, or inadvertent PEEP).[65,66] Auto-PEEP is the difference between alveolar pressure and external airway pressure at end expiration.[6] Causes include impedance to exhalation related to airway resistance, expiratory muscle activity, imposed resistance caused by endotracheal tubes and exhalation valves, water obstructing the exhalation circuit, rapid breathing frequency, and inverse I/E ratio.[2] Auto-PEEP has the same clinical effects as therapeutically applied PEEP. The two possible goals to manage auto-PEEP are either (1) to minimize it or (2) to use it as a ventilation variable in manipulating $\overline{Paw}$. In either case, recognizing and monitoring auto-PEEP are clinically important. The use of PEEP in obstructive lung disease, such as asthma, is controversial, with some investigators reporting improved gas exchange and decreased airway resistance whereas others found increased air trapping and hemodynamic compromise.[67,68] More recent research has shown that higher set PEEP levels can be helpful in decreasing the work of breathing in mechanically ventilated, spontaneously breathing pediatric patients with obstructive airway disease.[69] In theory, external PEEP holds the airways open and allows better exhalation, thus reducing the auto-PEEP and making it easier for patients to trigger ventilator breaths. Multiple variables affect ventilation and oxygenation. It must be understood that manipulating a ventilator setting with the objective of improving one condition may result in undesirable effects on another.[2] Balancing these variables allows the clinician to meet the goals of mechanical ventilation, as well as to optimize oxygen delivery, recruit lung volume, improve gas distribution, and alter minute ventilation.

PATIENT–VENTILATOR INTERFACE

Understanding the ventilator circuit is an integral aspect of ventilator management. The *circuit* is the interface between the ventilator and the patient system.[70] There are five major factors to consider when assessing the impact of the circuit on ventilation:

- Compressible volume
- Air leak
- Dead space
- Resistance
- Humidification

Compressible Volume

The influence of compressible volume on effective tidal volume during volume ventilation was discussed earlier (see Dual-control Ventilation). Ventilator circuit compression influences tidal volume during pressure ventilation as well.[20] When the ventilator delivers a breath, pressure inside the circuit increases and compresses the gas volume delivered. This compressed volume never reaches the patient, and the inspired volume is less than the set volume. During expiration, however, the compressed volume passes through the exhalation valve and is measured as part of the patient's exhaled volume. This results in the patient's actual inflation volumes being less than that recorded as exhaled volume. If the actual volume delivered to the lungs of critically ill infants and young children is not accurately known, the patient may be at risk for atelectasis, hypoxia, and hypercapnia.[71] A circuit compliance or compression factor can be calculated, as illustrated in Box 19-2. Thus some clinicians describe this as volume "lost" in the tubing. The compressible volume of disposable tubing is generally greater than that of reusable tubing.[72] The humidifier also represents a source for gas compression and is included in calculating compressible volume. Using a constant-level self-feeding humidifier is necessary to minimize variations in compressible volume in all pediatric ventilation situations.[73] When tidal volumes are measured with a proximal flow sensor placed at the endotracheal tube, ventilator circuit compliance and the confounding circuit variables are no longer pertinent factors.[71]

Air Leak

In the pediatric clinical setting, it is important not to confuse compressible volume losses with air leaks. Air leaks are most notable around a cuffless endotracheal or tracheostomy tube. Accurately monitoring tidal volume is difficult in the presence of an air leak. An excessive air leak compromises tidal volume delivery, reduces lung-distending pressures, and may adversely affect the ventilator triggering mechanism. In general, air leaks are monitored by the difference between the tidal volume delivered by the ventilator and the patient's exhaled tidal volume.[20] Another way to identify an air leak is via flow graphics. Figure 19-12 illustrates an air leak on a volume–time scale. In most clinical situations, an air leak greater than 15% of the delivered tidal volume makes volume ventilation difficult. Even though the leak still occurs during constant pressure ventilation, switching to a higher flow rate and pressure setting may deliver a satisfactory tidal volume. Usually reintubation is necessary to maintain consistent volume ventilation and adequate triggering of the ventilator.

Dead Space and Resistance

Dead space is the portion of the circuit distal to the main bias flow or circuit where gas can be rebreathed. This includes the volume of the circuit Y-connector, elbow, any monitoring device attached to the endotracheal tube connector, the endotracheal tube, and the conducting airways. The conducting airways are known as *anatomic dead space* and are not influenced by the circuit. However, the dead space added to the circuit is *mechanical dead space*. With smaller pediatric volumes, mechanical dead space may result in undesired rebreathing of carbon dioxide. Specially designed pediatric or infant monitoring devices and circuits help minimize this. Overzealous application of low dead space monitoring devices may result in increased resistance at the airway if the proper size is not used. Another component to evaluate as a choke point for gas flow is the adaptor connecting the tubing to the elbow or the endotracheal tube. A rule of thumb is that the endotracheal tube should be the point of highest circuit resistance. If a circuit component is smaller in cross-sectional area than the endotracheal tube, another circuit or component should be used.[74]

Humidification

The humidification system is an integral part of the patient–ventilator system. When the normal heating and humidification systems of the body are bypassed or are inadequate, it is necessary to artificially heat and humidify the inhaled gases. Optimal humidity and temperature are dependent on the clinical situation. Usually a temperature of 37 °C and a water content of 44 mg/L are adequate.[75] Servo-controlled, heated humidifiers that possess a small compressible volume are used most often in pediatric patients who require mechanical ventilation. Complications associated with these humidifiers include overheating and nosocomial infection. Water condensation in the ventilator circuit may also lead to nosocomial infection as well as to the accidental drainage of water into the patient's lungs. With the use of a servo-controlled heated wire circuit, complications are not as frequent in the pediatric population as they once were. However, awareness of the operational characteristics of the humidifier and its controlling mechanisms is important in the ventilator management of the pediatric patient.

COMPLICATIONS OF MECHANICAL VENTILATION

Each of the physiologic effects of mechanical ventilation has an associated risk. Box 19-4 lists the complications associated with mechanical ventilation.[2]

Overdistention

Alveolar overdistention is a primary cause of complications encountered during mechanical ventilation and is

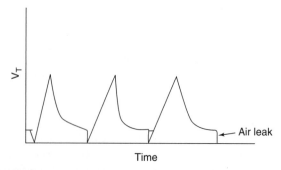

FIGURE 19-12 Air leak shown on a volume/time scalar. Volume never returns to baseline before ventilator cycles again. V_T, tidal volume.

Box 19-4	Complications of Mechanical Ventilation

- Barotrauma
- Volutrauma
- Atelectrauma
- Biotrauma
- Pulmonary interstitial emphysema
- Subcutaneous emphysema
- Pneumothorax
- Pneumomediastinum
- Pneumopericardium
- Pneumoperitoneum
- Bronchopulmonary dysplasia
- Nosocomial infection
  - Acute respiratory distress syndrome
  - Pneumonia
- Patient–ventilator asynchrony
  - Auto-PEEP
  - Hyperventilation
  - Respiratory alkalosis
  - Increased work of breathing
- Noncardiopulmonary complications
  - Psychologic distress
  - Renal dysfunction
    - Fluid retention
  - Gastrointestinal dysfunction
    - Vomiting
    - Ulceration and bleeding

- Increased intracranial pressure
- Interventricular hemorrhage
- Periventricular leukomalacia
- Airway complications
  - Sinusitis
  - Vocal cord injury
  - Inadvertent extubation
  - Retention of secretions
  - Glottic injury
    - Glottic edema
    - Glottic stenosis
    - Glottic erosion
  - Tracheal injury
    - Tracheal erosion
    - Tracheomalacia
    - Tracheal dilation
    - Tracheal–innominate artery fistula
  - Airway obstruction
    - Main stem intubation
    - Kinking of endotracheal tube
    - Plugging of endotracheal tracheostomy tube
- Cardiovascular compromise
  - Decreased venous return
  - Decreased cardiac output
- Oxygen toxicity
- Retinopathy of prematurity

PEEP, Positive end-expiratory pressure.

a result of high ventilating pressures (barotrauma), large tidal volumes (volutrauma), and repetitive opening and closing of the terminal lung units at low lung volumes (atelectrauma). Extrapulmonary air leaks, in the form of pneumothorax, pneumomediastinum, pneumoperitoneum, and subcutaneous emphysema, are the most notable complications and are the result of overdistention of alveolar and peribronchial tissues.[76] Treatment consists of detecting the leak, decreasing tidal volume, and decreasing the PEEP, relieving the leak with a chest tube if necessary. Permissive hypercapnia could also be a useful tool in the treatment of an air leak.[77] Nonconventional rescue modes such as high-frequency jet ventilation, high-frequency oscillatory ventilation, and extracorporeal membrane oxygenation are implemented for excessive air leakage that is not responding during conventional ventilation.

Overdistention also causes a decrease in static compliance, an increase in the work of breathing, an increase in anatomic dead space, an increase in the air leak around the endotracheal tube, and possible difficulties in weaning. As compliance diminishes, the Pa_{CO_2} may rise or fail to improve. To counter this, ventilation is increased, which may lead to further distention.

Because volumes are smaller in the neonatal and pediatric patient than in the adult, avoiding and detecting overdistention is a critical aspect of ventilator management. Alarms that may help detect this are indirect and can be activated by other problems. These alarms include high $\overline{Paw}$; exhaled minute ventilation, which is useful during SIMV and other spontaneous modes; high peak pressure; high PEEP; high respiratory frequency; and inverse I/E ratio. Measures such as using an end-expiratory pause to look for incomplete exhalation and an increase in PEEP or to detect auto-PEEP, measuring optimal static compliance, inspecting pressure-volume loops to determine overdistention or exhaled resistance, monitoring changes in $\overline{Paw}$, and obtaining a chest radiograph all help to detect overdistention.

The formation of a bronchopleural fistula presents an especially challenging clinical situation. Because the volume of gas delivered by the ventilator will follow the path of least resistance, a substantial part of the tidal volume will move into the pleural space during inspiration and escape through the chest tube. This volume is seen as the air bubbles through the water seal chamber of the chest tube drainage system, and the amount may be determined by noting the difference between the inspiratory and expiratory volumes. Although most bronchopleural fistulas are insignificant, if the leak is large enough it may result in inadequate ventilation and lead to ventilation–perfusion mismatch and further hypoxemia. Conventional treatment consisting of low pressures and volumes allowing permissive hypercapnia and allowing the patient to breathe spontaneously as much as possible may aid in decreasing flow through the fistula and facilitate its closure. When this is not possible in patients with severe ventilation problems, nonconventional modes of treatment may be needed. Independent lung ventilation or high-frequency ventilation may be considered, as may the use of valves to occlude the chest tube during inspiration.[78,79]

Cardiovascular Complications

Reduced cardiac output from cardiac septal deviation, increased pulmonary vascular resistance, reduced venous return, and reduced myocardial blood flow is a complication of mechanical ventilation. In most cases, it is a result of increased intrathoracic pressures. In the neonatal and pediatric patient it can usually be prevented by increasing the circulating fluid volume.[60,80] Vasopressor drugs may also be used to maintain cardiac output during ventilation regimens that include high distending volumes.[53] An increase in intrathoracic pressure may be applied in some clinical situations to reduce left-to-right shunting, raise pulmonary vascular resistance, and impede pulmonary blood flow. However, other means such as carbon dioxide or nitrogen–oxygen gas mixtures with less than 21% oxygen may also accomplish this without risk of increasing intrathoracic pressures and reducing blood flow to other organ systems.

Oxygen Toxicity

Oxygen toxicity is another concern during mechanical ventilation. High F_{IO_2} levels that have been applied for an extended period may result in tissue injury that alters lung function and gas distribution.[52] High F_{IO_2} levels have also been associated with an increase in chronic lung disease and retinopathy of prematurity among low birth weight infants.[81] Incorporating a high F_{IO_2} alarm and minimizing the F_{IO_2} to the level necessary to attain adequate tissue oxygenation, as well as using pulse oximetry and blood gas monitoring, are essential in attempting to prevent tissue damage.

Hypoventilation/Hyperventilation

The primary cause of hypoventilation during mechanical ventilation is disconnection from the ventilator and accidental extubation.[82,83] Care must be used when moving the patient connected to a ventilator, especially during transport and patient care procedures such as chest physiotherapy. A low-pressure or disconnect alarm is essential to alert the clinician when this occurs. Hypoventilation may also result from high impedance to inflation, which can be due to high resistance (resulting from anatomic, pathologic, or circuit design) or loss of pulmonary compliance.[84] A low-volume monitor will not detect these changes unless it is located at the airway connection. Underventilation can be avoided by calculating effective tidal volume or airway monitoring of ventilation variables, routinely monitoring or calculating compliance and resistance, monitoring pressure-volume and flow–volume loops, and using sufficient driving or working pressures to minimize attenuation of the inflating flow waveform. A chest radiograph also may be helpful in detecting underaeration.

Hypoventilation may also be related to "operator error" in establishing ventilation. Hypoventilation caused by minute ventilation, frequency, volume, or flow rate that is insufficient to meet inspiratory demand results in increased work of breathing and muscle fatigue. These conditions may also be present when weaning from the ventilator and may cause weaning failure. The alert patient may communicate feelings of respiratory distress. Retractions, use of accessory muscles, head bobbing, and a 10% to 20% increase in heart rate and spontaneous respiratory frequency are clinical signs of insufficient ventilation. In a sedated, paralyzed, or critically ill patient, however, this problem may not be as evident. Using pressure–volume and flow–volume loops, monitoring carbon dioxide production and oxygen consumption, and obtaining other measurements such as a diaphragm electromyogram may help detect this problem. Ensuring that the initial inspiratory flow rate meets the patient's inspiratory demand is usually the best method of avoidance.[85,86] An example of a pressure–volume loop demonstrating insufficient flow caused by insufficient driving pressure during PSV is shown in Figure 19-13. Figure 19-14 shows the effect of a faulty flow transducer on a diaphragm electromyogram tracing during PSV, leading to increased work of breathing.

Hyperventilation can also be a problem if the patient's lung compliance improves (i.e., through surfactant administration or prone/supine positioning) in a pressure control or pressure support mode. Autocycling of the ventilator due to endotracheal tube leak, secretions in the circuit or flow sensor, and inappropriate sensitivity setting can lead to hyperventilation. Hyperventilation and low carbon dioxide in low birth weight infants can result in cerebral vasoconstriction, which can cause a cystic brain lesion called periventricular leukomalacia.[87] Close monitoring of transcutaneous carbon dioxide levels, sensitivity, tidal volume, and minute ventilation with alarms has proved to be useful in reducing this problem.

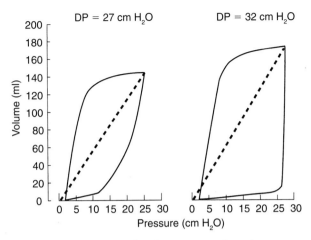

FIGURE 19-13 An example of a pressure–volume loop demonstrating insufficient flow caused by setting the driving pressure (DP) too low during pressure-support ventilation of a child. With DP set at 27 cm H_2O, the peak pressure *(top right-hand corner of the loop)* is reached at the end of inflation. With the DP set at 32 cm H_2O, the peak pressure is reached early during inflation *(lower right-hand corner of the loop)*. Note the perpendicular right side of the loop.

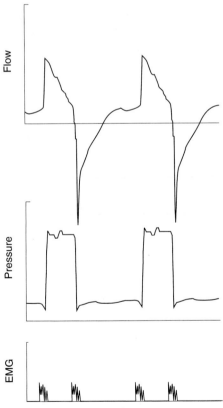

FIGURE 19-14 A recording of the electromyographic (EMG) signal shows muscle activity to initiate inflation during pressure-support ventilation. The flow transducer on this ventilator is defective, and the electromyogram shows abnormal muscle activity, not seen by clinical observation, at the end of inflation to stop the breath. Transdiaphragmatic pressure measurements would also help detect this situation.

MONITORING DURING MECHANICAL VENTILATION

Monitoring effective ventilation is accomplished by using the techniques discussed previously. Box 19-5 lists monitoring applications as they apply to pediatric mechanical ventilation. Most ventilators monitor airway pressures, flow, ventilatory frequency, tidal volume, and minute volume. Essential aspects of monitoring include the following:

- Calculation of effective tidal volume
- Close observation of the patient for clinical signs of adequate ventilation as well as respiratory distress, such as chest expansion and retractions
- Noninvasive methods of determining oxygenation and ventilation status, such as pulse oximetry, transcutaneous monitoring, and end-tidal carbon dioxide monitoring
- Direct measurement of blood gas values

Box 19-5	Monitoring Applications in Pediatric Mechanical Ventilation

MEASURED VENTILATOR VARIABLES
- Effective tidal volume
- Minute ventilation
- Mean airway pressure ($\overline{Paw}$)
- Low–high positive end-expiratory pressure (PEEP)
- High peak pressure
- Fraction of inspired oxygen (FIO_2)
- Pause pressure
- Inspiratory-to-expiratory ratio
- Pressure waveform
- Flow waveform
- Static compliance
- Respiratory time fraction
- Dynamic compliance
- Airway resistance
- Respiratory time constant
- Maximal inspiratory occlusion pressure
- Maximal expiratory occlusion pressure
- Maximal minute ventilation
- Vital capacity

SUPPLEMENTAL MONITORS
- Pulse oximetry
- End-tidal carbon dioxide
- End-tidal carbon dioxide to $PaCO_2$ gradient
- Pressure–volume loop
- Esophageal pressure
- Transpulmonary pressure
- Dead space-to-tidal volume ratio
- Ineffective-to-effective tidal volume ratio
- Work of breathing
- Pressure–time product
- Pressure–time index

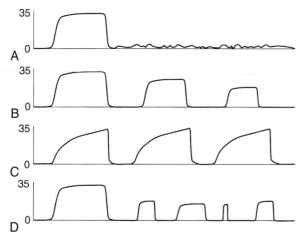

FIGURE 19-15 End-tidal carbon dioxide recordings. **A,** Abrupt disconnection from the ventilator. **B,** Falling partial pressure of end-tidal carbon dioxide (PET_{CO2}), possibly from an increase in tidal volume or, if $PaCO_2$ is unchanged, a reduction in pulmonary blood flow from overdistention or low cardiac output. **C,** Dampened waveform from severe air flow obstruction or side stream sampling tube obstruction. **D,** System leak or secretions in the sampling chamber.

Figure 19-15 demonstrates possible problems detected with an end-tidal carbon dioxide monitor.[66,88]

Esophageal Pressure Monitoring

Some ventilators have the ability to monitor esophageal pressure. Esophageal pressure monitoring uses an air-filled, balloon-tipped catheter placed in the midsection of the esophagus, where pleural pressure measurements can be closely estimated. Esophageal pressure measurements can be extremely helpful in understanding the physiology of the respiratory system during mechanical ventilation.[89] It is essential that proper placement of the balloon catheter be confirmed in order to accurately measure esophageal pressure. These pressure measurements can be displayed graphically or incorporated into a number of pulmonary mechanics calculations. Calculations that require esophageal pressure include chest wall compliance, lung compliance, transpulmonary pressure, work of breathing, change in esophageal pressure, and auto-PEEP.

Evaluation of the esophageal pressure waveform can be compared graphically with other ventilator graphics and provides important clinical information regarding interactions between the patient and the ventilator. Esophageal balloon technology can also guide the clinician during difficult weaning from mechanical ventilation without increased patient intolerance.[90]

Estimating Lung Volumes

At present, the ability to determine whether ventilator breaths are delivered at, below, or above their ideal functional residual capacity is deduced from surrogate measurements, including lung appearance on the chest radiograph, vital sign trends (particularly oxygenation), and dynamic pressure–volume (P–V) curves generated by modern ventilators.

Automated Slow Flow Rate Pressure–Volume Curves

Pressure–volume curves can provide important information about the compliance of the respiratory system when supporting mechanically ventilated patients with restrictive lung diseases. Ventilators have incorporated automated slow-flow or "quasi-static" P–V curves that use a slow inspiratory flow rate delivered during a single breath. This method reduces the pressure increase due to the resistive elements (endotracheal tube, high flow rates) and more closely approximates the alveolar pressure.

The slope of the line is measured to determine compliance of the respiratory system (line C, Figure 19-16). These technologies also provide algorithms that measure the upper and lower inflection points of a nonlinear respiratory system compliance curve. These points represent areas on the P–V loop during lung inflation and deflation, where there is a substantial decrease in compliance. Figure 19-16 shows three lines that comprise the inflation limb (lower curve) of a static P–V curve. Line B represents an area of low compliance related to the opening of atelectatic lung units early during inflation of the lung. The point at which the slope of the line changes (where line A intersects line B) reflects an area where there is an acute improvement in compliance; this is known as the *lower inflection point*. Mechanical ventilator practices that adopt an "open lung approach" set PEEP to a pressure just above the lower inflection point. In theory, as long as the PEEP is set above the lower inflection point on the inflation or deflation limb, then oxygenation improves by resolving atelectasis and increasing the functional residual capacity. Lung injury can also be reduced because the patient is ventilated above the closing pressure of the lung and thus repetitive cycling of the lung at low volumes decreases atelectrauma. Figure 19-16 also distinguishes a second point where compliance decreases (where line A intersects line C); this is known as the *upper inflection point*. This point represents overdistention of the respiratory system. Ventilator pressures and/or tidal volume settings can be set below this point to avoid lung overdistention or volutrauma.

Nitrogen Multiple Breath Washout Technique

Nitrogen multiple breath washout technique has been used in a number of clinical studies, and is considered

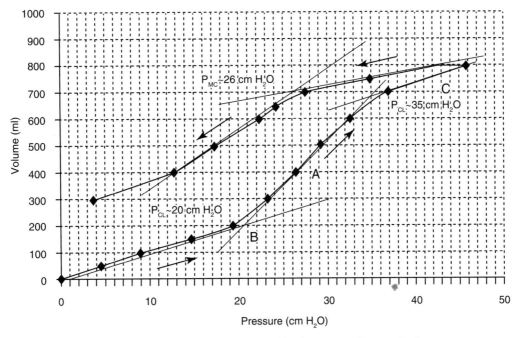

FIGURE 19-16 Pressure–volume curve as determined by the super-syringe method.

to be the "gold standard" in the measurement of lung volume.[91-94] At present, the most accurate way to measure the volume of the lung is through dilution of a known amount of a gas with low solubility by rebreathing in a closed system. The changes in concentration with sequential breaths allow calculation of the volume of distribution of the gas. One gas that has been used for this purpose is nitrogen,[95] appealing because of its ubiquitous presence in the environment. Measurement of nitrogen gas concentrations, however, is available only by gas chromatography or mass spectrometry, neither of which is clinically practical. A technique has been validated by which the partial pressure of nitrogen is calculated as the residual of partial pressures of oxygen gas, carbon dioxide gas, and nitrogen gas, which together comprise the only three important gases in a ventilator circuit. The former two gases are readily measured in a ventilator circuit in real time, but of course vary widely with the metabolic state of the patient. Olegård and coworkers have developed the nitrogen multiple breath washout technique to calculate FRC on the basis of changes in exhaled oxygen and carbon dioxide, manipulating inspired oxygen concentration to alter fraction of inspired nitrogen.[96] Measurement of FRC by this methodology in a lung model of known oxygen consumption and lung volumes[96] revealed excellent precision (mean FRC, 103% ± 5%) even when using incremental changes in FiO_2 from 0.9 to 1.0. Measurement in adult patients with respiratory insufficiency also revealed excellent precision. However, it

has not been well validated in patients with tidal volumes less than approximately 200 ml.

WEANING FROM MECHANICAL VENTILATION

Initiation

Weaning is the gradual process by which mechanical ventilation is discontinued and the patient resumes spontaneous breathing. The process may be rapid or slow, depending on the individual clinical situation. It is difficult to define at exactly what point during mechanical ventilation the weaning process should begin; however, most would agree that ideally it is after significant resolution or reversal of the pathologic condition for which it was initiated. Before weaning begins, the patient's condition should be stable and the patient should be receiving adequate nourishment and be able to breathe spontaneously and maintain a clinically acceptable $Paco_2$. The ventilator should be on acceptable settings: usually PEEP less than 8 cm H_2O; peak pressure less than 30 cm H_2O; ventilator rate less than 20 breaths/minute for a neonate, 15 breaths/minute for an infant/toddler, and 10 breaths/minute for a child or adolescent; and FiO_2 less than 0.4 to 0.5.[6,84,88,97,98]

Various methods exist for measuring respiratory muscle endurance and predicting successful weaning. Simple observations such as accessory or paradoxical muscle activity, respiratory rate, tidal volume, and minute ventilation are the first indicators of weaning readiness.[99,100] An increase in respiratory frequency of 15% to 20% or a reduction in tidal volume is associated with impending fatigue. Maintaining normal or clinically acceptable Pa_{CO_2} with normal minute ventilation (0.5 to 1 L/min for an infant to 4 to 9 L/min for an adult) would indicate that the patient might tolerate weaning. Normal carbon dioxide production in an infant is 6 ml/kg/minute, and it is 3 ml/kg/minute in an adult.[101] Excessive carbon dioxide production indicates a hypermetabolic state and may be corrected by adjusting nutritional elements to lower the respiratory quotient. Another helpful determinant of the ability to wean is the $V_D:V_T$ ratio. The normal value is 0.3; however, intubation and mechanical ventilation may alter this. A value of less than 0.6 to 0.7 may predict successful weaning. Another clinically measurable variable that roughly approximates the $V_D:V_T$ ratio is the ineffective-to-effective tidal volume ratio. Abnormal values may indicate continued pulmonary or cardiac dysfunction. Measurement of the end-tidal carbon dioxide to Pa_{CO_2} gradient may also help detect continued pulmonary or cardiac dysfunction. In this case, cautious weaning may be indicated, although resolution of the clinical condition is most likely indicated.[97]

Other predicting factors may also be considered. A flow–volume loop may help discover impedance to inspiratory or expiratory flow that will precipitate fatigue. A pressure–volume loop may help determine work of breathing and evaluate various weaning modes. Measurements of dynamic and static compliance, resistance, transpulmonary pressure tracing, work of breathing, respiratory time fraction, the pressure time product (PTP), and the pressure time index (PTI) are useful variables in monitoring the course of weaning. The PTP reflects the metabolic work of the respiratory system and is an electronically integrated value derived from tidal volume, compliance, esophageal pressure, and duration of the breath.[102] The PTI combines the PTP and the respiratory time fraction and correlates directly with muscle fatigue and oxygen consumption.[103] Spontaneous maximal inspiratory and expiratory occlusion pressures may also be of value. These measurements are routine weaning values in many adult units, along with maximal spontaneous minute ventilation and vital capacity measurements. Unlike these measurements, however, occlusion pressure measurements do not require that a patient understand the breathing techniques necessary to effectively determine the values.

Techniques of Weaning

The basic weaning techniques used in neonates and pediatric patients include CPAP, SIMV, and PSV. Using CPAP during weaning is common among pediatric patients. The positive airway pressure is used to provide the physiologic PEEP, which is bypassed when the patient is intubated.[29] Two techniques for using CPAP are practiced. The first is applied when there is sufficient respiratory drive and endurance but the physiologic effects of PEEP are still required. In this case, the CPAP is gradually reduced during the weaning process. The second technique is a postoperative weaning technique. The usefulness of this technique in pediatrics may be limited, however, because of the high resistance of the small-diameter airways. It may occasionally be employed to build respiratory muscle endurance by using a bias flow during short-duration exercises alternating with long periods of complete rest. The exercise periods are slowly increased as the resting periods are decreased. The process continues until the patient can breathe without support for a specified time. This technique is typically used only when the goal is to wean the patient to intermittent periods off the ventilator, such as with certain neuromuscular diseases or quadriplegia or in preparation for phrenic nerve pacing.

SIMV involves a gradual decrease in the ventilator frequency, usually in increments of 2 to 5 breaths/minute. As the ventilator rate is reduced, the patient is required to contribute more spontaneous efforts to the overall ventilation frequency. How quickly the SIMV rate is decreased depends on assessment of the patient's clinical status and blood gas values. The more slowly the process is performed, the more time the patient has to acclimate to less ventilator support. Factors such as ventilator system resistance, a sluggish demand valve, an inappropriately sized endotracheal tube, or insufficient inspiratory flow may affect the success of weaning with SIMV. Weaning with SIMV is generally uncomplicated and is usually successful in older patients with endotracheal tube sizes large enough to minimize excessive inspiratory resistance. When weaning patients with smaller tube sizes, the goal is to wean to a rate of 20 breaths/minute for an endotracheal tube less than 3.5 mm (internal diameter), 15 breaths/minute for endotracheal tube sizes of 4.0 to 5.0 mm, and 10 breaths/minute for anything greater than a 5.0-mm tube, and then extubate. When using continuous flow, a common practice is to set a standard flow rate on all ventilators in the neonatal patient population. Figure 19-17 shows the relationship of continuous flow to resistance. The smaller the diameter of the endotracheal tube, the more likely that changes in flow rate influence exhaled resistance. Using a rate less than those just stated is thought to contribute to fatigue and unsuccessful weaning because of endotracheal resistance.

Weaning with PSV provides sufficient positive pressure to minimize the metabolic requirements for ventilation during weaning.[6,42,97,100] In addition, PSV allows the patient to initiate the breath, preventing atrophy of the inspiratory muscles. Figure 19-18 illustrates a pressure–volume loop and other respiratory variables used to evaluate the effect of PSV and CPAP on an infant who is proving difficult to wean. Once weaning is indicated and PSV is selected, the pressure support level should be adjusted to deliver a tidal volume of 3 to 4 ml/kg. Frequency should be monitored and the driving pressure adjusted to attain an appropriate flow rate. Once satisfactory volume, flow, and frequency are set, the pressure support level can be reduced in increments of 2 to 5 cm H_2O. While at a higher pressure level, the patient contributes only the muscle work required to trigger the inflation. As the pressure is reduced, the patient progressively shares more of the work of breathing.[77] The pressure support should be weaned at a rate that is reasonable for each clinical situation. Endotracheal or tracheostomy tube leaks can hinder this progress. The patient who has been mechanically ventilated for only a short time, such as the stable postoperative patient, can be weaned at a rapid pace. The patient who has been undergoing long-term mechanical ventilation requires patience and persistence in reducing the support level by only 1 or 2 cm H_2O over a longer period, such as a day or even a week. In these patients, weaning can be slowed by clinical events such as a viral illness or fluid and electrolyte imbalance. Once these clinical conditions are resolved, usually weaning can be continued with a successful outcome.[6]

ADVANCING CONCEPTS

Advances and improvements in technologies and practices such as high-frequency ventilation, nitric oxide, corticosteroids, prone positioning, permissive hypercapnia, extracorporeal membrane oxygenation, and surfactant replacement all influence future design and approaches to conventionally ventilating the neonate and pediatric patient.

Automated regulation of the inspired oxygen (closed-loop F_{IO_2}) is a novel concept that is awaiting U.S. Food and Drug Administration approval for use in one mechanical ventilator. This feature requires the clinician to set a patient saturation range (i.e., 85% to 92%) on the ventilator. A pulse oximeter is attached to the patient and signal extraction software within the ventilator obtains these measurements from the oximeter probe. If the saturation measurement increases above or below the target range, then the ventilator will adjust the F_{IO_2} in order to keep oxygen saturations within the prescribed range. This can potentially reduce the frequency of hypo/hyperoxic episodes in very low birth weight infants receiving mechanical ventilation. It has been speculated that long-term closed-loop F_{IO_2} control may reduce clinician time spent to maintain adequate oxygenation and reduce the risks of morbidity (retinopathy of prematurity and bronchopulmonary dysplasia) associated with supplemental oxygen and frequent episodes of hypoxemia and hyperoxemia.[104]

Ventilators are increasingly becoming "partial support" in that they must work dynamically with the patient. Proportional assist ventilation is an innovative new mode of ventilation that is currently being investigated for neonatal and pediatric mechanical ventilation. This mode uses an algorithm that varies pressure support or pressure control levels on the basis of patient effort and changes in patient elastic and resistive loads during inhalation and exhalation. Preliminary work suggests that this mode may result in improvements in patient synchrony, oxygenation index, and overall cardiovascular stability.[19] New-generation ventilator companies are incorporating many modes, triggers, and graphics to help the clinician pick and choose

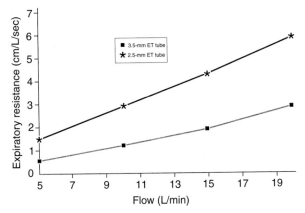

FIGURE 19-17 Exhaled resistance using 2.5- and 3.5-mm-diameter endotracheal (ET) tubes at various continuous flow rates through the ventilator circuit.

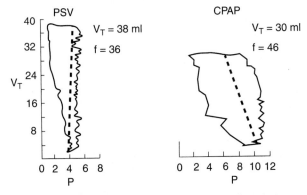

FIGURE 19-18 Pressure–volume loops of an infant during weaning, demonstrating the effectiveness of using 5 cm H_2O of PEEP and 1 cm H_2O of pressure-support ventilation instead of using 10 cm H_2O of continuous positive airway pressure (CPAP). f, frequency (breaths/min); P, pressure; PSV, pressure-support ventilation; V_T, tidal volume.

what is best for an individual patient's needs. This fosters a dynamic relationship between the ventilator and patient. Negative-pressure ventilation is also finding its way back into the critical care setting. Cardiopulmonary interactions are being investigated in children after simple cardiac surgery.[105]

Electrical impedance tomography (EIT) capitalizes on changes in impedence in air-filled versus tissue-filled spaces to characterize and quantify regional distribution of lung volumes at the bedside. Significant work has been done to validate this technology in animals[106] and in humans.[106,107] This monitoring system uses a series of 16 electrodes placed across the patient's chest (Figure 19-19). Through complex algorithms, the impedance signal is extracted and integrated to show a two-dimensional image (Figure 19-20). This has been shown to correlate with clinical and radiographic changes in patients.[108] In 10 mechanically ventilated adults with ARDS, end-expiratory lung volume as determined by nitrogen washout correlated well with end-expiratory lung impedance.[109] The ability to estimate lung volume noninvasively and in real time may aid in mechanical ventilator techniques designed to improve outcomes in patients with lung injury.

There is a growing body of evidence regarding exhaled breath condensate changes in airway lining fluid (ALF) pH in acute and chronic respiratory diseases that are characterized, at least in part, by inflammation. It has been demonstrated that the pH of ALF is low (acidic) in multiple pulmonary inflammatory diseases including asthma,[110] cystic fibrosis,[111] pneumonia, and ARDS.[112,113] This pH measurement can be detected continuously, safely, and noninvasively in exhaled breath condensate (EBC).[113] The pH of EBC may be a safe, noninvasive screening tool for progression of ARDS, and of lung recruitment. It has been shown to predict respiratory failure and impending respiratory infection.[113] Figure 19-21 shows that the EBC pH is a marker exhibiting rapid

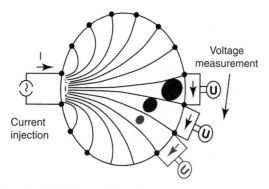

FIGURE 19-19 Electrical impedance tomographic images are created with a series of electrodes placed across the chest, each of which sends and receives electrical impulses from one another.

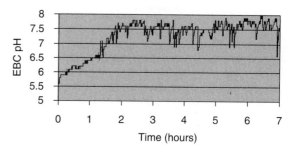

FIGURE 19-21 Sample tracing of exhaled breath condensate (EBC) pH over time in an intubated 14-year-old child with asthma. Note the responsiveness of EBC pH to the patient's improving condition.

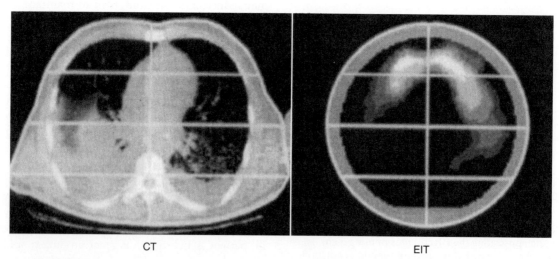

CT   EIT

FIGURE 19-20 Computed tomography (CT) and electrical impedance tomographic (EIT) images in a patient with acute lung injury. Note that the EIT image provides functional and anatomic information regarding the presence of ventilated lung fields.

turnover and thus may be valuable for real-time monitoring of lung pathology. A continuous exhaled breath condensate pH collection and assay system (ALFA monitor; Respiratory Research, Austin, Tex) consists of a condenser attached to the expiratory limb of the ventilator. Exhaled breath condensate is collected continuously from the expiratory port and condensed in a cooling chamber, and carbon dioxide is removed and collected in an inferior chamber where pH is continuously read. This yields a continuous, responsive measure from ventilated patients, which (1) takes samples from an exhaust port on the outside of the ventilator circuit, and (2) adds no measurable resistance to the ventilator circuit. The measurement of EBC in patients with lung injury may serve as an early marker of lung health.

ASSESSMENT QUESTIONS

See Evolve Resources for answers.

1. Which of the following issues would most likely explain why a newborn infant's measured respiratory rate would rise from 40 to 100 breaths/minute on a ventilator after the patient was turned and an audible endotracheal tube leak was heard?
   A. Pneumothorax
   B. Auto-cycling
   C. Secretions
   D. Bradypnea

2. A 10-year-old child is intubated and receiving mechanical ventilation. The tidal volume is set at 280 ml, the peak airway pressure is 38 cm H_2O, the plateau pressure is 20 cm H_2O, and the PEEP is 5 cm H_2O. The tubing compliance factor is 1.5 ml/cm H_2O. What is the delivered V_T to this patient?
   A. 255 ml
   B. 157 ml
   C. 230 ml
   D. 330 ml

3. A term infant is being ventilated with a microprocessor ventilator and the physician would like to wean the infant from the ventilator. The clinician has tried turning the patient's set rate on SIMV down to 10 breaths/minute, but the infant immediately becomes tachypneic and desaturates to 85%. Which of the following should be done at this time?
   A. Increase the PEEP
   B. Initiate pressure support ventilation
   C. Increase the inspiratory time
   D. Place on nasal CPAP

ASSESSMENT QUESTIONS—cont'd

4. A 600-g neonate is being mechanically ventilated in pressure control ventilation with the following ventilator settings: peak inspiratory pressure (PIP), 24 cm H_2O; PEEP, 4 cm H_2O; FIO_2, 0.45; respiratory rate, 40 breaths/minute. Which inspiratory time should the clinician recommend?
   A. 0.6 second
   B. 0.3 second
   C. 0.8 second
   D. 1.0 second

5. The physician would like to begin dual-control ventilation of a 500-g infant. What would be the initial corrected volume target?
   A. 5 ml/kg
   B. 10 ml/kg
   C. 3 ml/kg
   D. 8 ml/kg

6. While observing a ventilator flow graphic for a 12-year-old patient with asthma, the clinician notices that expiratory flow does not return to baseline and the patient's auto-PEEP level is 6 cm H_2O. Which ventilator manipulation might help this patient the most?
   A. Increase the respiratory rate by 8 breaths/minute
   B. Decrease the inspiratory time
   C. Decrease the peak inspiratory flow
   D. Increase the PEEP

7. A neonatal patient with respiratory syncytial virus (RSV) is receiving mechanical ventilation in the pressure control mode with the following current settings: PIP, 14 cm H_2O; PEEP, 5 cm H_2O; FIO_2, 0.50; respiratory rate, 28 breaths/minute. The patient has poor chest rise bilaterally, and breath sounds are underaerated with faint wheezes bilaterally. You notice that the measured tidal volume is 3 ml/kg and the respiratory rate is 80 breaths/minute. The patient has nasal flaring, retractions, and head bobbing. What should be suggested at this time?
   A. Placing the patient on a high-frequency oscillator
   B. Suctioning and then increasing the PIP
   C. Decreasing the respiratory rate
   D. Using a neuromuscular blocking agent

8. TCPL is fundamentally different from PCV in that a(n) _____ must be set:
   A. Constant flow rate
   B. External PEEP resistor
   C. High pressure limit alarm
   D. Apnea alarm

Continued

ASSESSMENT QUESTIONS—cont'd

9. Which nonconventional ventilator approach would be good for a 10-year-old boy with severe ARDS who is spontaneously breathing while undergoing ventilation?
   A. TCPL
   B. APRV
   C. CPAP
   D. IRV
10. Which of the following factors does not affect mean airway pressure?
    A. PEEP
    B. I-time
    C. Time constant
    D. PIP

References

1. Mellins R et al: *Respiratory care in infants and children*, New York: American Lung Association; 1971. p 3.
2. American College of Chest Physicians: Consensus conference: mechanical ventilation, *Chest* 1993;104:1835.
3. Chatburn R: A new system for understanding mechanical ventilators, *Respir Care* 1991;36:1123.
4. Reynolds EO: Effect of alterations in mechanical ventilator settings on pulmonary gas exchange in hyaline membrane disease, *Arch Dis Child* 1971;46:152.
5. Branson RD et al: Altering flow rate during maximum pressure support ventilation: effects on cardiorespiratory function, *Respir Care* 1990;35:1056.
6. Czervinske MP et al: Effects of working pressure on respiratory pattern and airway pressure during pressure support ventilation in infants with chronic lung disease, *Respir Care* 1988;33:930.
7. Bergman NA: Effect of varying respiratory waveforms on distribution of inspired gas during artificial ventilation, *Am Rev Respir Dis* 1969;100:518.
8. Czervinske MP, Jiao JH, Teague WG: Improved effective to ineffective tidal volume ratio during pressure control ventilation of infant pigs, *Respir Care* 1989;34:1067.
9. Campbell RS, Davis BR: Pressure-control versus volume-controlled ventilation: does it matter? *Respir Care* 2002;47:416.
10. Singh J et al: Mechanical ventilation of very low birth weight infants: is volume or pressure a better target variable? *J Pediatr* 2006;149:308.
11. Hakanson DO: Positive pressure ventilation: volume-cycled ventilators. In Goldsmith JP, Karrotkin EH, editors: *Assisted ventilation of the neonate*, Philadelphia: WB Saunders; 1981. pp 161-179.
12. Tobin MJ: Monitoring of pressure, flow, and volume during mechanical ventilation, *Respir Care* 1992;37:1081.
13. Demers RR, Pratter MR, Irwin RS: Use of the concept of ventilator compliance in the determination of static total compliance, *Respir Care* 1981;26:644.
14. Branson RD, Johannigman JA: What is the evidence base for the newer ventilation modes? *Respir Care* 2004;49:743.
15. McCallion N, Davis P, Morley CJ: Volume-targeted versus pressure-limited ventilation in the neonate, *Cochrane Database System Rev* 2005;3:CD003666.
16. Dawson C, Davies MW: Volume-targeted ventilation and arterial carbon dioxide in neonates, *J Paediatr Child Health* 2005;41:518.
17. Branson RD, Chatburn RL: Technical description and classification of modes of ventilator operation, *Respir Care* 1992;37:1026.
18. Chatburn RL: Computer control of mechanical ventilation, *Respir Care* 2004;49:507.
19. Sinah SK, Donn SM: Volume controlled ventilation. In Goldsmith JP, Karotkin EH, editors: *Assisted ventilation of the neonate*, Philadelphia: WB Saunders; 2003. pp 171-182.
20. Perez-Fontan JJ, Heldt GP, Gregory GG: The effect of a gas leak around the endotracheal tube on the mean tracheal pressure during mechanical ventilation, *Am Rev Respir Dis* 1985;132:339.
21. Boros SJ et al: The effect of independent variations in inspiratory–expiratory ratio and end expiratory pressure during mechanical ventilation in hyaline membrane disease: the significance of mean airway pressure, *J Pediatr* 1977;91:794.
22. Carlo WA, Martin RJ: Principles of assisted ventilation, *Pediatr Clin North Am* 1986;33:221.
23. Reynolds EOR: Pressure waveform and ventilator settings for mechanical ventilation in severe hyaline membrane disease, *Int Anesthesiol Clin* 1974;12:259.
24. Greenough A et al: Synchronized mechanical ventilation for respiratory support in newborn infants, *Cochrane Database Syst Rev* 2008;1:CD000456.
25. Abbey NC et al: Measurement of pharyngeal volume by digitized magnetic resonance imaging: effect of nasal continuous positive airway pressure, *Am Rev Respir Dis* 1989;140:717.
26. Katz JA, Marks JD: Inspiratory work with and without continuous positive airway pressure in patients with acute respiratory failure, *Anesthesiology* 1985;63:598.
27. Chatburn RL: Similarities and differences in the management of acute lung injury in neonates (IRDS) and in adults (ARDS), *Respir Care* 1988;33:539.
28. Smith RA et al: Morphometric changes in a dog model of the adult respiratory distress syndrome after early therapy with continuous positive airway pressure, *Respir Care* 1987;32:525.
29. Berman LS et al: Optimum levels of CPAP for tracheal extubation of newborn infants, *J Pediatr* 1976;89:109.
30. Kelly J: New method permits neural control of mechanical ventilation. *Pulmonary Rev* 2000;5. Accessed from http://www.pulmonaryreviews.com/may00/pr_may00_neuralcontrol.html. Retrieved October 2008.
31. Sinderby C et al: Inspiratory muscle unloading by neurally adjusted ventilatory assist during maximal inspiratory efforts in healthy subjects, *Chest* 2007;131:711.
32. Greenough A, Greenall F: Patient triggered ventilation in premature neonates, *Arch Dis Child* 1988;63:77.
33. MacDonald K et al: Effect of patient flow-triggered ventilation pulmonary mechanics in neonates, *Respir Care* 1991;36:1315.
34. Sassoon CSH: Mechanical ventilator design and function: the trigger variable, *Respir Care* 1992;37:1056.
35. American College of Chest Physicians-American Thoracic Society Joint Committee on Pulmonary Nomenclature: Pulmonary terms and symbols, *Chest* 1975;67:583.

36. Waldhorn RE et al: Long-term compliance with nasal continuous positive airway pressure therapy of obstructive sleep apnea, *Chest* 1990;97:33.

37. Habashi NM: Other approaches to open lung ventilation: airway pressure release ventilation, *Crit Care Med* 2005;3:229.

38. Stock MC, Downs JB: Airway pressure release ventilation: a new approach to ventilatory support during acute lung injury, *Respir Care* 1987;32:517.

39. Stock MC, Downs JB, Frolicher DA: Airway pressure release ventilation, *Crit Care Med* 1987;15:426.

40. Bach JR, Alba AS: Management of chronic alveolar hypoventilation by nasal ventilation, *Chest* 1990;97:52.

41. Kacmarek RM: The role of pressure support ventilation in reducing work of breathing, *Respir Care* 1988;33:99.

42. MacIntyre NR: Weaning from mechanical ventilatory support: volume-assisting intermittent breaths versus pressure-assisting every breath, *Respir Care* 1988;33:121.

43. MacIntyre NR: Pressure support ventilation, *Respir Care* 1986;31:189.

44. Brochard L et al: Inspiratory pressure support prevents diaphragmatic fatigue during weaning from mechanical ventilation, *Am Rev Respir Dis* 1989;139:513.

45. Brochard L et al: Inspiratory pressure support compensates for the additional work of breathing caused by the endotracheal tube, *Anesthesiology* 1991;75:739.

46. Forrette TL et al: Changes in pediatric ventilatory dynamics during mechanical ventilation with PSV, *Respir Care* 1990;35:1128.

47. Ramsden CA, Reynolds EOR: Ventilator settings for newborn infants, *Arch Dis Child* 1987;62:529.

48. Boros SJ et al: Using conventional ventilators at unconventional rates, *Pediatrics* 1984;74:487.

49. Kezler M: Volume-targeted ventilation, *Neoreviews* 2006;7:5:250.

50. Clark RH, Slutsky AS, Gerstmann DR: Lung protective strategies of ventilation in the neonate: what are they? *Pediatrics* 2000;105:112.

51. Eisner MD et al; Acute Respiratory Distress Syndrome Network: Efficacy of low tidal volume ventilation in patients with different clinical risk factors for acute lung injury and the acute respiratory distress syndrome, *Am J Respir Crit Care Med* 2001;164:231.

52. Jenkinson SG: Oxygen toxicity in acute respiratory failure, *Respir Care* 1983;28:614.

53. Ciszek TA et al: Mean airway pressure: significance during mechanical ventilation in neonates, *J Pediatr* 1981;99:121.

54. Gallagher TJ, Banner MJ: Mean airway pressure as a determinant of oxygenation, *Crit Care Med* 1980;8:244.

55. Kirby R: Improving ventilator patient interaction: reduction of flow dyssynchrony, *Crit Care Med* 1997;25:10.

56. Amal J: Inspiratory flow rate: more may not be better, *Crit Care Med* 1999;27:4.

57. Kacmarek RM: Essential gas delivery features of mechanical ventilators, *Respir Care* 1992;37:1045.

58. Suter PM, Fairley HB, Isenberg MD: Optimum end-expiratory pressure in patients with acute pulmonary failure, *N Engl J Med* 1975;292:284.

59. Kirby RR et al: High level positive end-expiratory pressure in acute respiratory insufficiency, *Chest* 1977;71:18.

60. Kirby RR: Best PEEP: issues and choices in the selection and monitoring of PEEP levels, *Respir Care* 1988;33:569.

61. Witte MK et al: Optimal positive end-expiratory pressure therapy in infants and children with acute respiratory failure, *Pediatr Res* 1988;24:217.

62. Carroll CG et al: Minimal positive end-expiratory pressure (PEEP) may be "best PEEP," *Chest* 1988;93:1020.

63. Nelson LD, Civetta JM, Hudson-Civetta J: Titrating positive end-expiratory pressure therapy in patients with early moderate arterial hypoxemia, *Crit Care Med* 1987;15:14.

64. Bilen Z, Colhen IL: Auto-PEEP characterization and consequences, *Anesthesiol Rep* 1990;3:255.

65. Benson MS, Pierson MD: Auto-PEEP during mechanical ventilation of adults, *Respir Care* 1988;33:557.

66. Murray JP et al: Titration of PEEP by the arterial minus end tidal carbon dioxide gradient, *Chest* 1984;85:100.

67. Marini JJ: Should PEEP be used in airflow obstruction? *Am Rev Respir Dis* 1989;140:1.

68. Smith PG, El-Khatib MF, Carlo WA: PEEP does not improve pulmonary mechanics in infants with bronchiolitis, *Am Rev Respir Dis* 1993;147:1295.

69. Graham AS et al: Positive end-expiratory pressure and pressure support in peripheral airways obstruction: work of breathing in intubated children, *Intensive Care Med* 2007;33:120.

70. Czervinske MP: Mechanical ventilator: a life support system [letter], *Crit Care Q* 1984;7:1.

71. Hamel DS, Cheifetz IR: Measuring pediatric tidal volumes, *RT for Decision Makers in Respiratory Therapy* 2002:June/July. Available at http://www.rtmagazine.com/issues/articles/2002–06_05.asp. Retrieved October 2008.

72. Hess D, McCurdy S, Simmons M: Compression volume in adult ventilator circuits: a comparison of five disposable circuits and nondisposable circuits, *Respir Care* 1991;36:1113.

73. Haddad C, Richards CC: Mechanical ventilation of infants: significance and elimination of ventilator compression volume, *Anesthesiology* 1968;29:365.

74. Rasanen J, Leijala M: Breathing circuit respiratory work in infants recovering from respiratory failure, *Crit Care Med* 1991;19:31.

75. Irlbeck D: Normal mechanisms of heat and moisture exchange in the respiratory tract, *Respir Care Clin North Am* 1998;4:2.

76. Dreyfuss D et al: High inflation pressure pulmonary edema: respective effects of high airway pressure, high tidal volume, and positive end expiratory pressure, *Am Rev Respir Dis* 1988;137:1159.

77. MacIntyre NR: Pressure support ventilation: effects on ventilatory reflexes and ventilatory muscle workloads, *Respir Care* 1987;32:447.

78. Gallagher TJ et al: Intermittent inspiratory chest tube occlusion to limit bronchopleural cutaneous airleaks, *Crit Care Med* 1976;4:328.

79. Bevelaqua FA, Kay S: A modified technique for the management of bronchopleural fistula in ventilator-dependent patients: a report of two cases, *Respir Care* 1986;31:904.

80. Walkinshaw M, Shoemaker WC: Use of volume loading to obtain preferred levels of PEEP, *Crit Care Med* 1980;8:81.

81. STOP-ROP Multicenter Study Group: Supplemental Therapeutic Oxygen for Prethreshold Retinopathy Of Prematurity (STOP-ROP), a randomized, controlled trial. I. Primary outcomes, *Pediatrics* 2000;105:295.

82. Dellinger PR: Complications of mechanical ventilation, *Pulmonol Crit Care Update* 1989;5:2.
83. Strieter RM, Lynch JP: Complications in the ventilated patient, *Clin Chest Med* 1988;9:127.
84. Mathewson HS, Linn RC, Gish GB: Pediatric mechanical ventilators, *J Kansas Med Soc* 1983;84:255.
85. Marini JJ, Capps JS, Culver BH: The inspiratory work of breathing during assisted mechanical ventilation, *Chest* 1985;87:612.
86. Shannon DC: Rational monitoring of respiratory function during mechanical ventilation of infants and children, *Intensive Care Med* 1989;15:S13.
87. Fabres J et al: Both extremes of arterial carbon dioxide pressure and the magnitude of fluctuations in arterial carbon dioxide pressure are associated with severe intraventricular hemorrhage in preterm infants, *Pediatrics* 2007;119:299.
88. Harris K: Noninvasive monitoring of gas exchange, *Respir Care* 1987;32:544.
89. Benditt JO: Esophageal and gastric pressure measurements, *Respir Care* 2005;50:68.
90. Gluck EH, Barkoviak JM: Medical effectiveness of esophageal balloon pressure manometry in weaning patients from mechanical ventilation, *Crit Care Med* 1995;23:504.
91. Heinze H et al: The accuracy of the oxygen washout technique for functional residual capacity assessment during spontaneous breathing, *Anesth Analg* 2007;104:598.
92. Newth CJ, Enright P, Johnson RL: Multiple-breath nitrogen washout techniques: including measurements with patients on ventilators, *Eur Respir J* 1997;10:2174.
93. Whiteley JP, Gavaghan DJ, Hahn CE: A mathematical evaluation of the multiple breath nitrogen washout (MBNW) technique and the multiple inert gas elimination technique (MIGET), *J Theor Biol* 1998;194:517.
94. Zinserling J et al: Measurement of functional residual capacity by nitrogen washout during partial ventilatory support, *Intensive Care Med* 2003;29:720.
95. Wrigge H et al: Determination of functional residual capacity (FRC) by multibreath nitrogen washout in a lung model and in mechanically ventilated patients: accuracy depends on continuous dynamic compensation for changes of gas sampling delay time, *Intensive Care Med* 1998;24:487.
96. Olegård C et al: Estimation of functional residual capacity at the bedside using standard monitoring equipment: a modified nitrogen washout/washin technique requiring a small change of the inspired oxygen fraction, *Anesth Analg* 2005;101:206.
97. Pierson DJ: Weaning from mechanical ventilation in acute respiratory failure: concepts, indications, and techniques, *Respir Care* 1983;28:646.
98. Venkataraman ST: Validation of predictors of extubation success and failure in mechanically ventilated infants and children, *Crit Care Med* 2000;28:2991.
99. Manczur TI: Comparison of predictors of extubation from mechanical ventilated in children, *Pediatric Crit Care Med* 2000;1:28.
100. Doershuk CF, Orenstein DM: Pulmonary function and exercise testing. In Lough MD, Doershuk CF, Stern RC, editors: *Pediatric respiratory therapy*, Chicago: Year Book Medical; 1979. p 250.
101. Sassoon CSH et al: Pressure–time product during continuous positive airway pressure, pressure support ventilation, and T-piece during weaning from mechanical ventilation, *Am Rev Respir Dis* 1991;143:469.
102. Grassino A, Macklem P: Respiratory muscle fatigue and ventilator failure, *Annu Rev Med* 1984;35:625.
103. Bancalari E et al: Closed-loop controlled inspired oxygen concentration for mechanically ventilated very low birth weight infants with frequent episodes of hypoxemia, *Pediatrics* 2001;107:1120.
104. Shekerdemian LS: Cardiopulmonary interactions in healthy children and children after simple cardiac surgery: the effects of positive and negative pressure ventilation, *Heart* 1997;78:587.
105. Frerichs I et al: Reproducibility of regional lung ventilation distribution determined by electrical impedance tomography during mechanical ventilation, *Physiol Meas* 2007;28:S261.
106. Hinz J et al: End-expiratory lung impedance change enables bedside monitoring of end-expiratory lung volume change, *Intensive Care Med* 2003;29:37.
107. Wolf GK et al: Regional lung volume changes in children with acute respiratory distress syndrome during a derecruitment maneuver, *Crit Care Med* 2007;35:1972.
108. Hunt JF et al: Endogenous airway acidification: implications for asthma pathophysiology, *Am J Respir Crit Care Med* 2000;161:694.
109. Tate S et al: Airways in cystic fibrosis are acidified: detection by exhaled breath condensate, *Thorax* 2002;57:926.
110. Kostikas K et al: pH in expired breath condensate of patients with inflammatory airway diseases, *Am J Respir Crit Care Med* 2002;165:1364.
111. Effros RM: Exhaled breath condensate acidification in acute lung injury, *Respir Med* 2004;98:682, author reply 3.
112. Gessner C et al: Exhaled breath condensate acidification in acute lung injury, *Respir Med* 2003;97:1188.
113. Walsh BK et al: Exhaled-breath condensate pH can be safely and continuously monitored in mechanically ventilated patients, *Respir Care* 2006;51:1125.

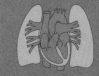

Chapter 20

Neonatal and Pediatric High-frequency Ventilation

KEITH S. MEREDITH ● MARK ROGERS

OUTLINE

LEARNING OBJECTIVES

After reading this chapter the reader will be able to:
- Define high-frequency ventilation
- Describe how gas is delivered and exhaled during high-frequency jet ventilation
- Describe how gas is delivered and exhaled during high-frequency oscillatory ventilation
- Describe the relative role frequency and tidal volume play during high-frequency ventilation
- Explain the relationship between lung volume and oxygenation during high-frequency ventilation
- Identify lung volume strategies for a given pathophysiology

We have witnessed the development and implementation of several exciting modalities for the respiratory care of newborns and pediatric patients. These new tools range from enhancements in the pharmacologic management of distinct cardiopulmonary disorders to tremendous strides in mechanical ventilation. Critical to the successful application of these new treatments is the development of disease-specific strategies, which also include ways in which some therapies may positively interact with others. High-frequency ventilation (HFV) continues to play an important role in this growth.[1-4]

The link between mechanical ventilation, oxygen, and subsequent acute and chronic lung disease was made in both pediatric and adult patients shortly after the introduction of conventional ventilation (CV) into clinical practice.[5,6] More recent trials indicate that ventilating patients with acute respiratory distress syndrome with higher tidal volumes contributes to further lung damage.[7,8] The various techniques of HFV emerged later from efforts to develop methods of managing respiratory failure that would minimize the negative pulmonary consequences of ventilatory support. At that time, our understanding of the mechanisms of these injuries was limited to the observed interactions between oxygen, pressure, and time.[9] Ironically, some of our early insights into the undesired interactions between the surfactant-deficient lung and mechanical ventilation occurred during experiments designed to determine whether HFV would be beneficial at all.[10] This gap in the fundamental understanding of concepts of ventilator-induced lung injury explains both the early controversies regarding HFV strategies and the conflicting clinical reports.[11,12] The finding, at least in animal models, that a lung-protective ventilator strategy is possible helped spawn a growing body of data describing lung injury mechanisms and, therefore, prevention techniques.[10] These remain the focus of ongoing research and commentary.[13,14] Whereas initial clinical uses of HFV were in rescue situations, the primary focus of HFV research was to protect the lung from injury. This lung protection focus

continues and should not be confused with rescue attempts to treat the already injured lung.

This chapter reviews (1) basic concepts of HFV, (2) current understanding of mechanisms of gas exchange during HFV, (3) basic approaches to the use of approved devices, (4) disease-specific HFV strategies, and (5) special patient care considerations. This chapter also introduces the emerging understanding of the interaction between new pharmacologic therapies and HFV.

DEFINITIONS

High-frequency ventilation is defined as mechanical ventilation using tidal volumes less than or equal to the dead space volume and delivered at supraphysiologic rates. Tidal volume, dead space volume, and breathing rate magnitude vary with patient age and size (tidal and dead space volumes vary inversely with increasing age, whereas breathing rate varies directly). The U.S. Food and Drug Administration (FDA) has chosen to define HFV devices as those that provide breathing rates exceeding 150 breaths/minute. This discussion is limited to those devices currently approved by the FDA for use in neonates and/or pediatric patients. These ventilators operate at breathing rates of 4 to 10 Hz (1 Hz = 60 breaths/min or 1 cycle/s) and deliver the requisite small tidal volumes. Several types of HFV device have been tested and reported in the literature. They differ functionally by the way each breath is generated, their relationship to conventional ventilator settings (if any), the range of breathing rates, and the nature of the expiratory portion of the respiratory cycle (Table 20-1).

High-frequency Conventional and Positive-pressure Ventilation

High-frequency CV is a modification of conventional pressure-limited infant ventilators that provides breathing rates up to 150 breaths/minute (2.5 Hz).[15] The limitations of this approach include larger delivered tidal volumes than with traditional HFV and the potential for intrapulmonary gas trapping. High-frequency positive-pressure ventilation (HFPPV) was

TABLE 20-1

Functional High-frequency Device Characteristics

Device Characteristic	HFFI	HFJV	HFOV
Breath generation	Interrupted variable flow	Pulsed high flow	Bias flow piston agitation
Relationship to conventional ventilator	In tandem or independent	In tandem (independent use on protocol)	Independent only
Operational frequencies	2-28 Hz	4-11 Hz	3-15 Hz
Expiratory flow	Passive or Venturi assisted	Passive	Active

HFFI, High-frequency flow interruption; HFJV, high-frequency jet ventilation; HFOV, high-frequency oscillatory ventilation.

first described in the anesthesia literature as a tool for managing patients during bronchoscopic or laryngeal surgery.[16] HFPPV subsequently received brief exposure as a management tool for more chronic conditions in adults and underwent brief trials in a small series of infants with respiratory distress.[17,18] These definitions are included here for completeness only because the use of FDA-approved HFV devices has generally replaced the routine use of these techniques in infants.

High-frequency Flow Interruption

High-frequency flow interrupters (HFFIs) deliver pressure-regulated, short-duration, low tidal volume breaths, frequently in conjunction with CV breaths. Each HFV breath is inserted proximal to the endotracheal tube (ETT), allowing the ETT to filter proximal pressures and minimize intratracheal and intrapulmonary pressure amplitudes. Exhalation of inspired gases takes place by passive chest recoil or by negative pressure assist at the exhalation valve. Continuous flow from a CV provides the baseline pressure. This nomenclature may seem unnecessarily confusing because these devices are essentially hybrids of jet (passive exhalation) or oscillatory (assisted exhalation) ventilators.

High-frequency Jet Ventilation

High-frequency jet ventilation (HFJV) devices deliver short pulsed jets distal to the proximal end of the ETT. Functional tidal volumes are a combination of the jet breath and entrainment volumes that are "dragged" along with each jet. Techniques using a modified triple-lumen ETT and those employing catheters placed in a standard ETT have been described.[19,20] These devices combine CV breaths with jet breaths and, like HFFI, rely on passive chest recoil for gas egress. Baseline pressures are provided by continuous flow from the CV. Initial difficulties with necrotizing tracheobronchitis have been overcome by unique design modifications that improved humidification of the jet breaths.[21] Tandem use with a CV is usually required.

High-frequency Oscillatory Ventilation

Of all HFV techniques, high-frequency oscillatory ventilation (HFOV) devices may be the most variable. Initial techniques included loudspeakers whose output was attached to the ETT and a host of piston pump devices with various performance characteristics.[22-25] Common to all of these devices is the provision of extremely small tidal volumes and very high rates of 8 to 30 Hz, as well as the presence of a continuous distending pressure (CDP) or mean airway pressure ($\overline{\text{Paw}}$). The outward flow of expiratory gases is enhanced by the active exhalation phase of the piston cycle. This last feature distinguishes HFOV from all other HFV methods. All current devices use a standard ETT, allow precise control over $\overline{\text{Paw}}$ and pressure amplitude, and in general are not used in tandem with conventional ventilators. The ability to accurately adjust continuous (or mean) and phasic pressures and the inspiratory-to-expiratory (I/E) ratio varies among devices. Ventilator output is delivered to the proximal ETT (at the ETT circuit connection). Because the ETT behaves as a low-pass filter at these rapid breathing rates, pulmonary structures "see" markedly dampened phasic pressures.

MECHANISMS OF GAS EXCHANGE

The HFV techniques previously described represent different locations on the mechanical ventilation spectrum. On this spectrum, CV occupies one extreme with relatively large tidal volumes and low breathing rates and HFOV resides at the other extreme with very small tidal volumes and high breathing rates. The techniques of HFCV, HFPPV, HFFI, and HFJV lie in between. As one traverses this ventilatory spectrum, the classic roles of convection to deliver bulk gas to small airways and diffusion to distribute the gas among the gas-exchanging surfaces become blurred. Most of the research attempting to refine our understanding of gas transport and exchange during HFV has been accomplished in adult animal models with normal or injured lungs. At best, the injured states mimic secondary (not natural) surfactant deficiency, and adult pulmonary time constants and airway rigidity differ significantly from those of the neonatal lung.

Enhanced diffusion is found in large and medium airways in which alterations in gas flow velocity profiles occur. This is thought to be responsible for delivery of gas farther into the lung than can be explained by pure convection.[26] There is significant interdependence between adjacent alveolar units because the walls of any alveolar unit are shared with juxtaposed alveoli, each providing stability to the other. Once inflated, these units, which may have different time constants, can equilibrate gases by swinging ventilation between them. This phenomenon, called *pendelluft*, tends to equilibrate gas concentrations in conducting airways and serves to improve gas exchange from distal pulmonary units. In addition, the impact of enhanced diffusion, the product of tidal volume and rate, and the relationship between pulmonary units may all vary depending on the HFV technique used, the settings chosen, the patient's lung size, and pathologic conditions.[27] Obviously, our understanding of this complex set of gas exchange dynamics remains incomplete.

Ventilation

Classic physiology teaches that elimination of carbon dioxide is directly related to the product of breathing rate and tidal volume (minute ventilation, where $\dot{V}CO_2 = f \times V_T$); however, the volume that effectively removes carbon dioxide is alveolar volume, that is, the difference between tidal and dead space volumes. On the basis of this, if tidal volume is less than dead space, this difference, zero, and its product with breathing rate does not yield a meaningful number. Because all of the HFV methods described are effective means of ventilation, even with tidal volumes less than dead space, a new explanation is needed. Fredberg and coworkers[23] provided insight into this apparent paradox by describing elimination of carbon dioxide as follows:

$$(\dot{V}CO_2) = (f)^x \times (V_T)^y$$

where x is 0.5 to 1 and y is 1.5 to 2.2 (depending on the device). From this relationship we see that tidal volume is more critical to ventilation than rate is during HFV, and HFV appears to reduce the impact of dead space volume on ventilation.

Unlike oxygenation, in which the relationship of $\overline{Paw}$ to mean lung volume (MLV) and subsequent optimization of gas exchange is similar between CV and HFV, the elimination of carbon dioxide by CV and HFV is drastically different. This difference lies not only in the alterations to the minute ventilation equation just described but also in the nature of HFV devices themselves. In this regard, Fredberg and colleagues[23] made several interesting observations during an evaluation of multiple neonatal HFV devices. They noted that not only is carbon dioxide elimination during HFV more sensitive to changes in tidal volume than in rate but also the tidal volume output of HFV devices is sensitive to changes in ETT diameter and lung compliance. As ETT dimensions and compliance decreased so did tidal volume output from the HFV tested. This occurred in the presence of stable ventilator settings. Therefore any clinical change causing a decrease in ETT diameter, such as reintubation with a different-sized ETT or partial ETT obstruction with tracheal secretions, alters the delivered tidal volume. Furthermore, improvements in lung compliance (e.g., volume recruitment) and decrements in lung compliance (e.g., patent ductus arteriosus or alveolar derecruitment) have a direct effect on tidal volume.

In addition, the relationship between ventilator frequency and carbon dioxide elimination is nonintuitive. Changes in ventilator rate at a given pressure amplitude cause an inverse change in tidal volume. Thus, when ventilation must be improved, a reduction in breathing frequency improves ventilation because the increased volume output per stroke has a greater impact on ventilation than does the decrease in stroke frequency. The converse is also true. When less ventilation is needed and pressure amplitude is already minimized, increasing breathing frequency will further decrease tidal volume and allow weaning from ventilation. Figure 20-1 depicts data collected during volume measurement experiments with a SensorMedics 3100A high-frequency oscillator (Cardinal Health, Dublin, Ohio). Observe that although varying $\overline{Paw}$ (10 and 20 cm H_2O) had no impact on tidal volume output at any given oscillatory amplitude, there was a substantial difference in tidal volume with

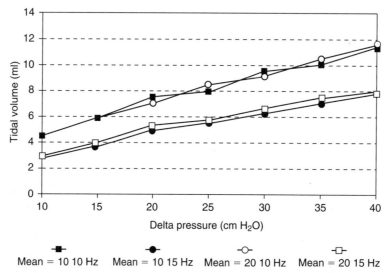

FIGURE 20-1 Tidal volume output measured during high-frequency oscillatory ventilation (HFOV) with a SensorMedics 3100A at a mean airway pressure ($\overline{Paw}$) equal to 10 and 20 cm H_2O and a frequency equal to 10 and 15 Hz. There is a nearly linear relationship between oscillatory amplitude and tidal volume. At each oscillatory amplitude tested, tidal volume at 10 Hz is higher than at 15 Hz. $\overline{Paw}$ has no effect.

differing frequencies. Volumes at 10 Hz are much higher than those at 15 Hz for each oscillatory amplitude tested.

Oxygenation

Although from a mechanistic perspective gas exchange remains complex, the clinical management of oxygenation is more straightforward. Excluding adjustments of fraction of inspired oxygen (Fio_2), oxygenation is improved during CV and HFV by recruiting or maintaining lung volume. In fact, there is a direct and linear relationship between lung volume and oxygenation (Figure 20-2). The exception to this occurs when the lung is either under or over inflated. In each circumstance the relationship between ventilation and perfusion is disturbed and oxygenation is impaired. Achieving an optimal MLV, then, optimizes ventilation–perfusion matching while avoiding impaired cardiac output. Adjusting several CV settings, such as tidal volume, peak pressure, inspiratory time, and end-expiratory pressure, accomplishes this. The resulting Paw is an indirect expression of the pressure effort required to achieve and sustain the desired MLV. Phasic pressures delivered with CV during attempts to recruit lung volumes can damage the fragile, yet noncompliant, infant airways and lung parenchyma. Thus conventional tidal volume breathing applied to lungs with nonuniform compliances, as in the premature surfactant-deficient lung, results in nonhomogeneous gas distribution, with overinflation of compliant areas and underinflation of noncompliant regions. During spontaneous or conventional mechanical breathing, the lung swings past the MLV and mean Paw during the cycles of inspiration and expiration, residing at the MLV (and Paw) for only brief periods. With normal lung mechanics, a stable functional residual capacity is maintained and oxygenation is not impaired. In the lung prone to atelectasis, however, residual lung volumes are dynamic. Although volume may seem adequate at peak inflation, stable lung volumes may not exist and oxygenation will be significantly impaired (even in the presence of positive end-expiratory pressures).[28,29]

The methods used to create and maintain Paw (or CDP during HFOV) therefore have a profound effect on the consequences of reaching the MLV. Conventional methods require the use of relatively high peak pressures to recruit collapsed noncompliant pulmonary units. The potential negative impact has already been described. The approach taken during HFV strategies, in contrast, is the application of a CDP without the use of high phasic pressures. In fact, direct control over CDP (Paw) is possible, with ventilation occurring around a relatively fixed intrapulmonary pressure and, therefore, relatively stable MLV. The danger of this technique, as mentioned earlier, is lung overdistention and resultant decreases in venous return and cardiac output. This can occur without changes in ventilation pressures during CV and HFOV when lung volume is silently recruited as compliance improves.

The optimal MLV, during high-volume strategies (see the later section, Ventilator Management), is reached when distending pressure exceeds alveolar opening pressures, and, as a result, the arterial-to-alveolar oxygen tension ratio [P(a–A)O_2] is maximized. This measure of oxygenation is useful because it normalizes measured arterial partial pressure of oxygen (PaO_2) for delivered Fio_2.[30] Perfect oxygenation, unobtainable in nature, yields a ratio of 1:1. The safe application of pressures adequate to achieve a stable MLV during management of the uninjured, atelectasis-prone lung is the goal of mechanical ventilation. Data from both animal and human infant studies suggest that improved oxygenation, with acceptable ventilation, does occur safely with HFV techniques while using distending pressures that are initially higher than in CV controls.[12,31,32] Attempts to achieve improved oxygenation using mean pressures lower than those used in CV, although attractive in theory, have not proved fruitful except in short-term studies and in patients with pulmonary interstitial emphysema (PIE) in whom low-volume strategies are desired and intentional (see the later section, Ventilator Management). Experiments performed by McCulloch and coworkers,[33] using the surfactant-deficient rabbit model, elegantly demonstrated the relationship between lung inflation strategy and resultant lung volume and gas exchange. In this work, animals with similar pressure–volume relationships after lavage were managed for a 7-hour study period with conventional mechanical ventilation, HFOV with a low lung volume strategy, or HFOV with a high lung volume strategy. Figure 20-3 graphically demonstrates the impact of these approaches on lung volumes. Note the significantly higher volumes obtained in the animals receiving HFOV and a high

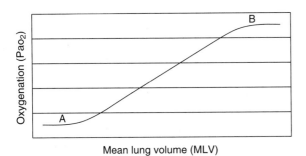

FIGURE 20-2 Relationship between mean lung volume and oxygenation (by inference, between Paw or CDP and MLV). **A,** Unopened lung. **B,** Overinflated lung.

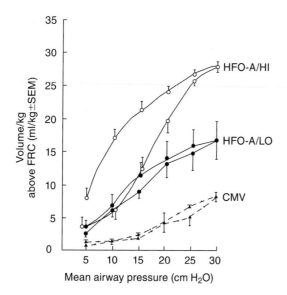

FIGURE 20-3 Respiratory system pressure–volume curves obtained after 7 hours of ventilation in surfactant-depleted rabbits. Note the intergroup differences in total respiratory system compliance and lung volumes. The differences in hysteresis (inflation–deflation limb separation) are also significant between groups. CMV, Conventional mechanical ventilation; FRC, functional residual capacity; HFO-A, high-frequency oscillatory ventilation with an active expiratory phase; HFO-A/HI, HFO-A at a high lung volume; HFO-A/LO, HFO-A at a low lung volume.

lung volume at an equivalent $\overline{Paw}$. As anticipated, this group also had a fivefold higher Pao_2 and less evidence of significant bronchiolar epithelial injury.[33]

Figure 20-3 also illustrates that an equivalent $\overline{Paw}$ does not imply equivalent lung volumes. As patient compliance changes, so does the $\overline{Paw}$ required to maintain optimal MLV. Obviously, a direct measure of MLV or compliance during HFV would be extremely useful; however, neither is currently available for routine bedside use. Clinical measures to properly wean patients and avoid inadvertent overdistention are discussed later in this chapter.

INDICATIONS

Neonatal Patients

The bulk of clinical data regarding appropriate application of HFV devices has been acquired from neonatal animals and humans. From these studies, two clear indications for HFV use during either routine or rescue circumstances have evolved. They include diffuse, homogeneous lung disease (or the atelectasis-prone lung), in which CV management is failing or may lead to increased risk of pulmonary morbidity, and existing pulmonary air leak syndromes (e.g., pneumothorax and PIE). Diffuse homogeneous lung disease includes natural surfactant deficiency (respiratory distress syndrome), shock

lung in the newborn, and diffuse pneumonia. Other diagnoses, including congenital pulmonary hypoplasia (both the congenital diffuse variety and that associated with congenital diaphragmatic hernia), may be additional indications. The efficacy of HFV for pulmonary hypoplasia is promising but not yet clearly established.[34]

Each of the lung diseases just mentioned has been successfully managed with extracorporeal membrane oxygenation (ECMO).[35] The role of pre-ECMO HFV has been the subject of wide debate, with at least one published report describing a 50% reduction in the need for ECMO among infants referred to an ECMO center and who met ECMO criteria and began HFOV on admission.[36] However, there are also data that imply an increased risk of pulmonary morbidity among infants avoiding ECMO with HFV. The timing of HFV intervention, the parameters determining HFV failure, and the decision for discontinuing HFV and initiating ECMO are currently empirical.[37]

There is no question that exogenous surfactant replacement is changing the course of respiratory distress syndrome (RDS) in affected infants. As a consequence, the role of HFV in patients treated with surfactant may differ from that in the presurfactant era. Proponents of early HFV for patients with RDS argue that tidal volume ventilation is damaging to immature lung structures after only a few minutes. In fact, there is no consensus regarding the timing of HFV initiation or surfactant administration in those treated with high-volume HFV. Encouraging, but not yet irrefutable, data are available regarding the early use of HFV in surfactant-treated infants.[38,39] Findings do show strong trends toward the need for fewer surfactant doses, less chronic lung disease and more pulmonary reserve at discharge, and decreased cost of hospitalization.

HFV continues to be indicated for infants in whom air leak syndromes develop, but, gratefully, the incidence of intractable air leak has decreased. This is probably the result of surfactant use, improved ventilatory techniques and devices, and better patient monitoring. Other conditions common to the neonate but not clearly benefited by HFV include particulate meconium aspiration, congenital lobar emphysema, bronchopulmonary dysplasia, and viral pneumonia. Further data from controlled trials with defined patient populations and treatment strategies are needed to offer clearer recommendations about HFV use in these conditions.

Pediatric Patients

Controlled trials in pediatric patients have been fairly limited.[40] However, as would be anticipated, proper strategic HFV use has had positive results in children with acute RDS and pulmonary air leak. In general, HFOV (now approved for pediatric patients) is applied as a rescue therapy in those failing CV. (A more powerful HFOV device, the SensorMedics 3100B, is being evaluated for use in larger pediatric patients.) An additional interesting HFV application is HFJV use during and after cardiac surgery, especially for children undergoing right ventricular outflow tract diversion or repair. At least two groups of investigators have reported improved hemodynamic measurements in children managed with the Life Pulse HFJV (Bunnell, Salt Lake City, Utah) in both intraoperative and postoperative environments.[41,42] The ability to provide adequate ventilation with low mean and peak pressures in children with otherwise normal lungs offers a substantial advantage of HFJV over HFOV and CV. Furthermore, this feature makes HFJV a more efficacious method of treating traumatic or acquired bronchopleural fistulas than other forms of respiratory support.

VENTILATOR SETTINGS

Frequency

Breathing frequency ranges between 2 and 28 Hz, depending on the device. Rates lower than 4 Hz and greater than 15 Hz are rarely used. The impact of the breathing rate on ventilation during HFV is less than the impact of tidal volume. Frequency is therefore not usually changed, and management of ventilation occurs with changes in delivered volume. Changes in frequency are made when operating at machine limits of tidal volume (both low and high limits). Choices of breathing frequency depend on understanding optimal functional characteristics of each device and the nature of the patient and the disease treated. For example, with a similar disease, such as acute RDS, neonatal and pediatric patients are managed with different frequencies during HFOV. The smaller child requires a lower tidal volume and therefore a higher frequency. Preliminary data in mature animals suggest that, at an equivalent arterial partial pressure of carbon dioxide ($Paco_2$), higher frequencies during HFOV are less damaging to airways than lower frequencies.[43]

Oscillatory Amplitude or Peak Pressure

Each of the ventilators available in the United States is pressure limited. Changes in delivered pressure amplitude have a direct influence on tidal volume delivery. The purpose of measuring peak inspiratory pressure is to offer both patient safety and ease of adjustment of delivered tidal volume. Although HFJV provides separate control and display of distal ETT peak pressure, HFFI and HFOV do not. The latter two devices display oscillatory amplitude (the peak-to-trough pressure difference). Measurement of pressures (whether peak or peak-to-trough) distal to the insertion point of HFV breaths in the patient circuit is important to avoid underestimation of pressures seen by pulmonary structures. Transducers, amplifiers, and measuring circuit fidelity must be adequate and unfiltered to properly measure peak-to-peak pressures at these breathing frequencies.

During HFOV and HFFI, peak and trough pressures are measured, although they are not usually displayed. Because of the impact of the ETT on transmitted pressure, these values have only relative significance. Of more importance is the difference between peak and trough pressures, known as *oscillatory amplitude* or simply the *delta P*. Delivered volume is directly proportional to this peak–trough difference, and adjustments result in changes in tidal volume (see Figure 20-1). During both HFOV and HFFI, the relationship between oscillatory amplitude and tidal volume actually delivered to the lung is subject to the same constraints as peak-to–end-expiratory pressure differences during pressure-limited CV. Changes in downstream compliance and impingement on the ETT lumen cause tidal volumes to vary without changes in displayed pressure amplitudes. Control over tidal volume during HFJV occurs by modifications in distally measured peak pressures. Although this measurement is less vulnerable to variations in the ETT lumen, total volume delivery during HFJV is a combination of jet pulse and gas entrained with each breath from the proximal ETT connection. This entrainment volume is vulnerable to reductions in the ETT lumen.

Positive End-expiratory Pressure

Like peak pressure, the attempt to apply a conventional setting to an HFV technique can lead to confusion. One can easily measure trough pressures during HFV, but the meaning and value are unclear. With CV, we relate oxygenation to levels of end-expiratory pressure because this setting contributes so significantly to $\overline{Paw}$. With HFJV and HFFI this remains true because end-expiratory pressure is set by adding it from the CV. During HFOV, however, it is set directly, and true end-expiratory pressure (or trough pressure) is meaningless. In fact, to avoid confusion some authors suggest that CDP (rather than $\overline{Paw}$) be used to describe the constant pressure delivered during HFOV.

Fraction of Inspired Oxygen

The principles for management of Fio_2 with CV also apply to HFV and are pulmonary disease dependent. There are no additional considerations for this setting during HFV.

Mean Airway Pressure or Continual Distending Pressure

Mean airway pressure or CDP controls MLV. During CV, this setting is the consequence of a combination of ventilator settings, and although it is a true mathematical average of pulmonary pressures, the lung maintains this pressure (and hence volume) for only brief periods. During HFV, especially HFOV, this pressure is directly controlled by the combination of bias flow and expiratory valve aperture. In this circumstance, the HFV static pressure (or CDP) truly creates a static lung volume, the magnitude of which depends on lung compliance. All the devices described provide a display of $\overline{Paw}$. During HFJV and HFFI, control over this parameter is achieved by changing the settings of the tandem CV. It cannot be overstated that as lung volume increases, so does compliance. In fact, at the very lung volume where oxygenation is optimized, compliance is as well. The importance of this concept is that ventilation is influenced if lung volume is too high, or too low, during HFV. Thus $\overline{Paw}$ facilitates oxygenation *and* permits optimal ventilation (see Figure 20-2). Therefore using $\overline{Paw}$ to maintain the correct lung volume is doubly critical.

Flow

The use of flow to control ventilator settings is variable among the devices described. During HFJV, jet pulses are delivered by means of a timing circuit with minimal control of flow. Pressures, and therefore volumes, are determined by variations of jet on-time and frequency. HFFI incorporates multiple solenoid technology to determine rate of pressure rise and end-expiratory pressures during CV, which has little impact on HFV functions. HFOV CDP is determined by the combination of circuit bias flow and the back-pressure created by the expiratory valve opening. Even though desired CDP may be achieved with complete valve closure, care should be taken to avoid this because rapid rebreathing followed by circuit (and patient) overpressurization will occur.

Inspiratory Time

Inspiratory time adjustments result in alterations in ventilator rate, I/E ratio, and tidal volume, all of which are significant, to differing degrees, for each type of HFV. Inspiratory time during HFJV is adjusted by changing jet on-time. Depending on ventilator frequency, this alters the I/E ratio and influences tidal volume output. Jet on-times of 20 to 34 milliseconds are common. With HFOV, inspiratory time varies with ventilator rate but the I/E ratio is singularly meaningful. The recommendation is a 33% inspiratory time for the HFOV devices approved in the United States. The result is that for each completed respiratory cycle, one third is inspiratory and two thirds is expiratory. The importance of this lies in the enhancement of gas egress during exhalation because the 1:2 ratio favors

the expiratory phase, thereby reducing inadvertent air trapping or breath stacking. This becomes a more significant factor as ventilator frequencies increase. Increases in inspiratory time at any given rate will increase tidal volume, but there is an obligatory reduction in I/E ratio that may offset any desirable effects. The inspiratory time during HFFI is fixed at 18 milliseconds. Changes in ventilator rate are made with changes in expiratory time, and the I/E ratio varies with frequency. In comparison with the other ventilators, adjustments in tidal volume cannot be made by increasing inspiratory time, and I/E ratios will vary with frequency.

HIGH-FREQUENCY VENTILATORS ON THE U.S. MARKET

Bunnell Life Pulse Jet Ventilator

The Life Pulse jet ventilator (Bunnell) (Figure 20-4) is the jet device approved by the FDA for use in infants. It was released in 1989 for rescue of air leak syndromes and respiratory failure after CV. Not intended as a stand-alone device, it is recommended for use with a conventional ventilator. Operational frequencies range from 4 to 11 Hz. Patients can be managed with a Hi–Lo jet ETT (see Figure 20-5), with jet pulses delivered to the airways through a separate side lumen (the ETT is available in standard neonatal sizes) or through an ETT adapter (LifePort; Bunnell) (Figure 20-4). This latter feature mitigates the need for reintubation and facilitates a smooth transition to HFJV. The proximal lumen of the ETT is connected to the CV circuit, and a third (distal) lumen permits servo control of jet peak pressure. Inspiratory times are controllable from 20 to 34 milliseconds, creating I/E ratios in excess of 1:6. This

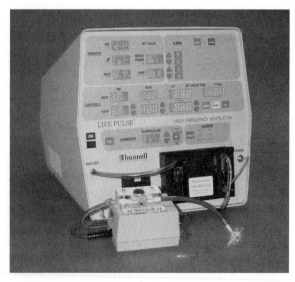

FIGURE 20-4 Bunnell Life Pulse high-frequency jet ventilator.

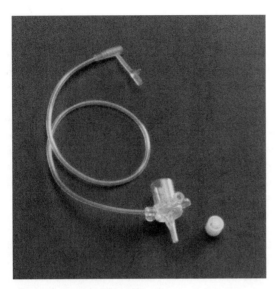

FIGURE 20-5 LifePort ETT adapter. Jet pulses are delivered through the side lumen of the ETT, and servo control over jet pressures is maintained by feedback from pressures sampled at the distal ETT lumen. Connection to a conventional ventilator is provided at the proximal ETT opening. This ETT adapter made specifically for this device now makes reintubation optional. (Courtesy Bunnell Inc., Salt Lake City, Utah.)

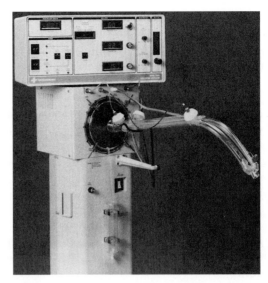

FIGURE 20-6 SensorMedics 3100A high-frequency oscillatory ventilator.

minimizes the possibility of intrapulmonary gas trapping. $\overline{Paw}$ is the consequence of both HFJV and CV settings. During a multicenter controlled trial comparing HFJV and CV in premature infants with PIE, significant improvements with greater survival and fewer treatment failures were seen in HFJV-treated patients.[44] Furthermore, a multicenter trial evaluating the use of HFJV compared with simple CV in uncomplicated RDS among preterm infants implied a clear benefit for HFV-managed patients, with less chronic lung disease and fewer patients requiring home oxygen at discharge.[45,46]

SensorMedics 3100A and 3100B High-frequency Oscillatory Ventilators

The SensorMedics 3100A (Cardinal Health) (Figure 20-6) is the HFOV device approved by the FDA for general use in infants with respiratory failure and for pulmonary rescue. This device permits operator control over frequency, CDP (or $\overline{Paw}$), inspiratory time, and pressure amplitude. Frequencies range from 5 to 15 Hz, and inspiratory time ranges from 30% to 75% of the total cycle time. (The total cycle time is defined as one complete machine breath from the beginning of inspiration to end expiration.) Pressure amplitude is adjusted by increasing electric power to the piston diaphragm (7 to 100 cm H_2O); peak and trough pressures are consequential. Varying the bias flow and expiratory valve aperture controls CDP (or $\overline{Paw}$). Data from two presurfactant studies of infants with RDS treated with

this device and compared with control patients treated with simple CV have shown reductions in both acute and chronic lung injury in HFOV-treated infants.[12,31] Subsequent publications that repeated these experiments in surfactant-treated patients showed benefit in residual lung disease and the cost of care for HFOV-treated patients.[38,47] Unfortunately, other authors have found mixed results.[11] Some, but not all, of these variations in findings can be attributed to differences between studies in devices used (data from institutions outside the United States may have been obtained with ventilators not available in the United States), nature of the patient population (gestational age or birth weight), and duration of CV before surfactant administration and initiation of HFOV. An attempt to resolve this confusing data set was undertaken by performing a meta-analysis of HFOV clinical trials. The authors concluded that studies using HFOV strategies designed to optimize lung volume (high-volume strategy) have consistently shown improvement in short-term indices of chronic lung disease without increases in morbidity.[39,48]

The SensorMedics 3100B was approved by the FDA in 2001 for the treatment of acute respiratory failure in adults and large children weighing more than 35 kg. On the basis of the established technology of the model 3100A HFOV ventilator, the 3100B increases the performance capabilities required for ventilation in larger patients. It has the ability to deliver high-frequency oscillations with a larger volume piston and to use higher distending pressure levels. Yet it maintains the ability to provide a protective low-stretch lung ventilation strategy. One randomized controlled trial comparing HFOV and conventional ventilation in an adult patient population with severe acute respiratory distress syndrome demonstrated that HFOV in adults is both safe and effective and resulted in a 29% relative reduction in mortality.[49] Neonatal and adult trials indicate earlier use of HFOV is associated with improved outcomes.[50-54]

Circuit Considerations

To achieve adequate gas exchange for both oxygenation and ventilation, high-frequency ventilators have unique design requirements. With the exception of HFCV, all HFV devices have special patient circuit considerations. Each of them must

- Use very low circuit compliance to reduce compressible volume and increase precision of control over the small volumes delivered
- Have intrinsic timing mechanisms to allow breathing frequencies between 4 and 28 Hz (varying by device)
- Provide control over inspiratory times and circuit design to allow sufficient time for gas egress during exhalation
- Adequately humidify gases
- Include alarms and fail-safe devices for patient safety

As a consequence of these considerations, circuit configurations cannot be altered without careful investigation because function and safety are extremely sensitive to small changes in engineering.

A unique device-specific option is the use of the high-low jet ETT (see Figure 20-5) with the Bunnell Life Pulse HFJV. This ETT was initially an integral feature of this device. Jet pulses are delivered through the side lumen of the ETT, and servo control over jet pressures is maintained by feedback from pressures sampled at the distal ETT lumen. Connection to a conventional ventilator is provided at the proximal ETT opening. An ETT adapter made specifically for this device now makes reintubation optional.

The SensorMedics 3100A originally operated with a nonstandard, semirigid circuit that required creative efforts on the part of caregivers to optimize patient positioning. Now a redesigned flexible circuit is available and frees the infant from many of the position constraints of the older circuit design.

A thorough understanding of the limits of breathing frequency, tidal volume, P̄aw control, circuit design, ETT requirements, and specifics of ventilator design is critical to the safe and optimal use of each high-frequency ventilator.

VENTILATOR MANAGEMENT

Each HFV device was initially developed for specific lung disease states. Because of ethical, scientific, and legal constraints, use in human infants was at first confined to rescue patients in whom conventional methods were failing. With increasing anecdotal success noted by several groups, it became apparent that strategies applied to these infants were unique to each device. Subsequently, refinements in patient management led to tailoring device design, with a resultant narrowing of the spectrum of lung diseases to which they could be applied. For example, HFJV was directed toward air leak syndromes and HFOV toward diffuse alveolar disease. Studies have now shown that P̄aw recruitment of the atelectasis-prone lung can be accomplished with different HFV types with similar successes in gas exchange, histologic evidence of uniform gas distribution, and decreased hyaline membrane formation.[55,56] Conversely, Clark and associates[57] reported successful HFOV treatment of a series of infants with PIE and supported the value of HFOV use in patients with air leaks. In another study of infants with PIE, Keszler and coworkers[44] reported a clear superiority of HFJV over CV in a carefully controlled multicenter trial. Keszler and coworkers[45] have subsequently had success in managing infants with RDS with HFJV. These findings imply that successful management of infants with significant pulmonary disorders is best accomplished by device-specific strategies directed toward specific lung pathophysiologic processes rather than by specific HFV types.

Initial Settings

Clinical protocols guiding decisions to implement HFV techniques should be in place in each institution before these devices are used. Personnel involved in patient management must demonstrate proficiency in the use of the device and clinical expertise to ensure patient safety. Active training programs within each institution should be mandatory and include a demonstration by personnel that they understand ventilator controls and circuit design, basic troubleshooting, and management strategies. Before the initiation of HFV, each device and circuit should be inspected to ensure proper calibration and function. Specific care should be taken to ensure that (1) proper gas temperature and humidity are present, (2) ventilator and circuit position is such that a smooth transition can occur, and (3) initial settings are lower than anticipated requirements to allow a slow increase toward desired levels and prevention of inadvertent injury. Finally, other appropriate primary therapies (e.g., surfactant replacement for surfactant deficiency and vasopressor support for impaired myocardial function) are not replaced by HFV and should be optimized along with ventilatory management.

Until more recently, HFV use was limited to patients in whom CV was failing. The literature and experience with neonates are changing this impression, so that

HFV is increasingly being used before rescue situations develop. These developments are changing current protocols for changing patients from CV to HFV. Because of this, it is necessary to focus on the concepts that need to be considered when applying HFV to patients, rather than describing specific ventilator settings. The evolving literature and device-specific manufacturer's recommendations should be consulted for more details.

CLINICAL MANAGEMENT STRATEGIES

Successful application of any HFV device requires accurate comprehension of individual patient pulmonary pathophysiology and selection of an appropriate ventilatory strategy. At present, there are two fundamentally differing strategies that are designed to approach contrasting pulmonary pathophysiologic processes.

High-volume Strategy

For the patient with an atelectasis-prone lung (e.g., natural or acquired surfactant deficiency), the primary therapeutic goal is to optimize lung inflation so that ventilation–perfusion mismatching is minimized while reducing inflation–deflation breathing patterns that initiate a cascade of events leading to lung tissue injury.[10,33] This has been termed the *high-volume strategy*. Two separate means of achieving this goal have evolved.

One method is to increase the distending pressures (Paw or CDP) in small increments (1 to 2 cm H_2O) while watching for improvement in oxygenation (arterial blood gas determinations, transcutaneous oxygen measurements, or pulse oximetry saturations) and MLV (chest radiograph). Mean airway pressure is increased until oxygenation improves significantly or until MLV reaches desired levels, or both, which may be determined by the presence of a well-inflated lung on a radiograph (Figure 20-7). While using this method, care must be taken to anticipate silent lung recruitment and to reduce Paw as appropriate to avoid serious impairment to venous return and reduction in cardiac output. Silent lung recruitment is gradual lung inflation taking place with static Paw settings (Figure 20-8). Clinical clues heralding this include rapid improvements with subsequent unexplained decrements in oxygenation, decreasing $PaCO_2$ without changes in oscillatory amplitude (improving compliance), and, finally, clinical changes in perfusion. These problems often can be avoided with diligence and anticipation. Silent recruitment, although more common during initial HFV management, can occur any time attempts are made to optimize MLV. Data confirm the pulmonary, central nervous system, and cardiovascular safety and efficacy of this technique.[12,31,32,58,59]

The other approach to recruiting the collapsed lung is the use of sustained inflations (SIs), that is, applying plateau pressures at levels in excess of expected alveolar opening pressures for periods of 5 to 30 seconds. This technique should result in incremental improvement in oxygenation if pressure levels are adequate. Furthermore, because of lung hysteresis, the inter-SI Paw can frequently be reduced to levels slightly less than can be achieved with the other lung inflation method. SIs are usually repeated until no change in oxygenation is noted or until oxygenation decreases. Both imply that the lung is at the upper limits of lung capacity. The need for repeat SI maneuvers is determined by the level of inter-SI Paw used and the amount of subsequent alveolar derecruitment. The SI method may achieve optimal MLV more rapidly and, because of the lower inter-SI Paw, avoid silent recruitment. However, potential disadvantages include the risk of using too little pressure (minimal recruitment) or too much pressure (airway injury, air leak, and reductions in cardiac output). Data from excised baboon lungs suggest that lung recruitment responses to SI maneuvers are dependent on lung pathophysiology. Thus there is a difference in the response of surfactant-sufficient collapsed lungs and uninjured surfactant-deficient lungs.[3] This method has been used successfully in infants with minimal complications.[2,58] Definite superiority of one technique over the other has not been demonstrated.

Note the contrast between CV and HFV. With CV, lung recruitment is achieved by increasing inspiratory time, end-expiratory pressure, and the resultant mean airway pressure, whereas HFV uses Paw alone to achieve lung recruitment. Supplying adequate oscillatory amplitude around the baseline Paw provides ventilation during HFFI and HFOV. With HFJV, ventilation is determined by changes in jet-pulse tidal volume delivery and by the amount of background CV used. It is critical to avoid the temptation to use HFV phasic pressure to recruit underinflated lung units. Table 20-2 suggests an algorithm for implementation of the high-volume strategy.

Low-volume Strategy

In contrast to the lung inflation strategies described, management of infants with PIE, pneumothorax, or air trapping requires the employment of alternative strategies because attempts to achieve optimal MLV in these patients will exaggerate existing lung overinflation or serve to further damage injured lung. Here the primary objective should be to offer a ventilatory strategy that allows the lung to slowly deflate, or one that minimizes ongoing air leakage while providing tolerable ventilation while accepting higher FiO_2. This

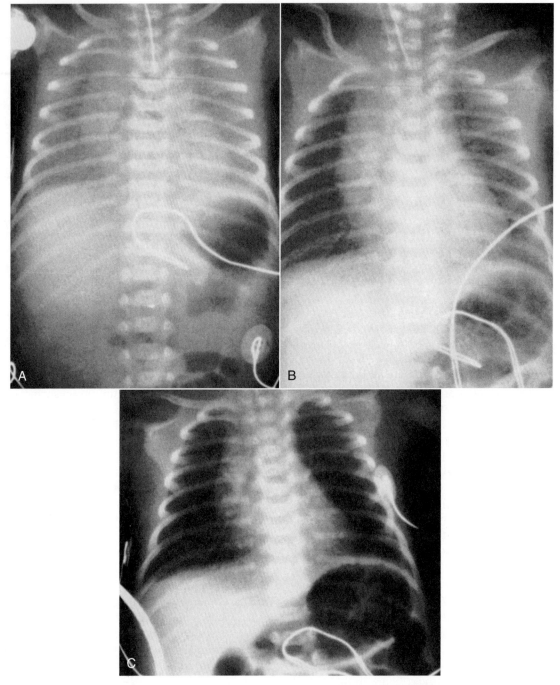

FIGURE 20-7 Radiographs during the first day of life for a 30-week premature infant with respiratory distress syndrome (RDS) managed with HFOV to achieve optimal mean lung volume (MLV). **A,** Initial $\overline{Paw}$ equal to 10 cm H_2O, fraction of inspired oxygen (FIO_2) equal to 1. **B,** At 12 hours of age, with $\overline{Paw}$ equal to 15 cm H_2O and FIO_2 equal to 0.45. **C,** At 24 hours of age with $\overline{Paw}$ equal to 12 cm H_2O and FIO_2 equal to 0.28.

is accomplished with all HFV systems by using a lower $\overline{Paw}$ than that creating the problem. (These patients are usually undergoing CV before being switched to HFV.) This allows the lung to derecruit and isolates damaged areas from inflation pressures. The consequence of this, however, is the frequent requirement for a higher FIO_2.

In addition, tidal volume delivery must be decreased to further reduce tidal volume exposure while using I/E ratios and ventilatory frequencies that maximize gas egress. A $Paco_2$ between 50 and 60 mm Hg is frequently tolerated in these patients as long as the arterial pH exceeds 7.25 (these parameter limits will likely

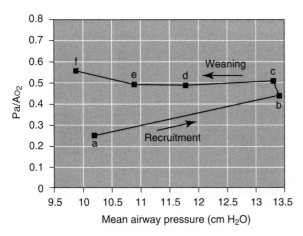

FIGURE 20-8 Mean arterial-to-alveolar oxygen tension ratio [P(a–A)O$_2$] and P$\overline{aw}$ of 21 premature infants managed with HFOV immediately after surfactant replacement. Note that increasing P$\overline{aw}$ initially results in increased P(a–A)O$_2$ (alveolar recruitment); subsequent P$\overline{aw}$ weaning does not reduce oxygenation but is associated with gradual improvement in P(a–A)O$_2$. The line between points *b* and *c* represents silent lung recruitment as assessed by improving P(a–A)O$_2$ with essentially stable P$\overline{aw}$. (*a*) Surfactant replacement; (*b*) 12 hours later; (*c*) 12 to 24 hours later; (*d*) 24 to 48 hours later; (*e*) 48 to 72 hours later; and (*f*) 72 to 96 hours later.

TABLE 20-2			
Generic Oxygenation and Ventilation Strategies for Use During High-frequency Ventilation in Patients With Diffuse Lung Disease			
Oxygenation Strategies			
Pao$_2$	Increased	Normal	Decreased
Lung inflation	Normal	Normal	Normal
Primary response	Decrease FIO$_2$	None	Increase FIO$_2$
Secondary response	None	None	None
Pao$_2$	Increased	Normal	Decreased
Lung inflation	Decreased	Decreased	Decreased
Primary response	Increase P$\overline{aw}$	Increase P$\overline{aw}$	Increase P$\overline{aw}$
Secondary response	Decrease FIO$_2$	None	Increase FIO$_2$
Pao$_2$	Increased	Normal	Decreased
Lung inflation	Increased	Increased	Increased
Primary response	Decrease P$\overline{aw}$	Decrease P$\overline{aw}$	Decrease P$\overline{aw}$
Secondary response	Decrease FIO$_2$	None	Increase FIO$_2$
Ventilation Strategies			
Paco$_2$	Increased	Normal	Decreased
Primary response	Increase OA	None	Decrease OA
Secondary response	Decrease frequency	None	Increase frequency

FIO$_2$, Fraction of inspired oxygen; OA, oscillatory amplitude; Paco$_2$, arterial partial pressure of carbon dioxide; Pao$_2$, arterial partial pressure of oxygen; P$\overline{aw}$, mean airway pressure.

vary between institutions). Once there is radiographic evidence that the lung has adequately deflated and air leaks have resolved (for at least 12 to 24 h), the lung is reinflated by one of the preceding lung inflation strategies. Air leak rarely recurs with this approach. This method is successful in at least 66% of infants with PIE. Those with PIE under tension and myocardial compromise are more difficult to manage and have poorer outcomes (Figure 20-9).[12,57] This approach has been dubbed the *low-volume strategy*.

The choice of strategy is lung disease specific. Although simplistic, it is reasonable to try to inflate an underinflated lung and deflate an overinflated or air-trapped one.

WEANING

At this stage of HFV development, weaning remains a challenge. Weaning ventilation is for the most part simple. Minute ventilation can be weaned by reducing oscillatory amplitude during HFFI and HFOV and by decreasing peak pressure and on-time with HFJV. Changes in ventilation rarely have an impact on oxygenation because lung volume is preserved. Conversely, weaning P$\overline{aw}$ with improving compliance and increasing lung inflation is less straightforward. Radiographic assessment of lung volume and FIO$_2$ may provide empirical information guiding

management sufficiency. The well-inflated lung requires a reduction in mean pressure to avoid the negative consequences of excessive lung volumes. However, too rapid a reduction in distending pressures can cause alveolar derecruitment in the unstable lung, and reinflation will be necessary. In general, P$\overline{aw}$ should be reduced slowly (0.5 to 1 cm H$_2$O) every 2 to 3 hours as long as there are no signs of overdistention (suggesting much more rapid decreases are necessary) or alveolar derecruitment (decrements in oxygenation). By taking advantage of lung hysteresis, gradual reductions in mean pressure generally do not cause significant changes in oxygenation or, by inference, lung volume (see Figure 20-8). Simple and reproducible bedside measures of lung volume are on the horizon. The application of these techniques to weaning may be useful in the future.[60]

Radiographic assessment of lung volume takes considerable practice. The novice is cautioned that although,

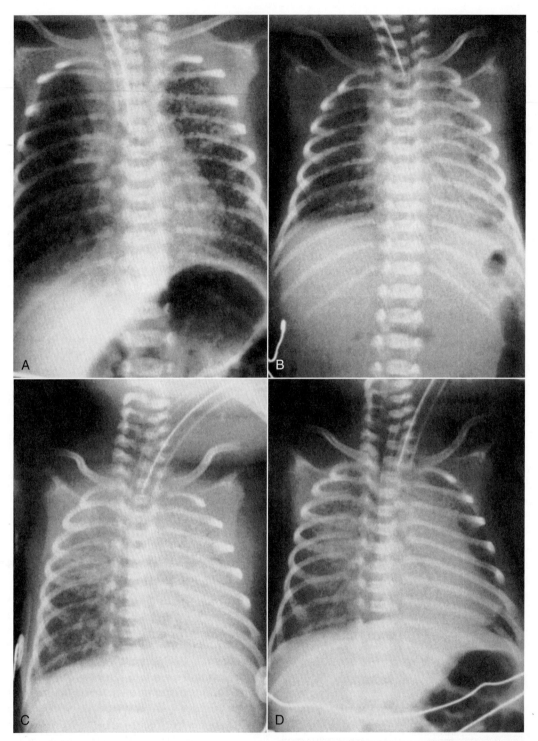

FIGURE 20-9 Radiographs of a 2-day-old preterm infant with pulmonary interstitial emphysema (PIE). **A,** $\overline{Paw}$ equal to 16 cm H_2O and Fio_2 equal to 0.65. **B,** Six hours later, $\overline{Paw}$ equal to 8 cm H_2O and Fio_2 equal to 1. **C,** Twelve hours later, settings were unchanged, PIE was resolved, and lung was nearly totally deflated. **D,** Thirty-six hours later, reinflation was beginning, $\overline{Paw}$ was equal to 12 cm H_2O, and Fio_2 was equal to 0.45.

in general, lung volume can be assessed by counting the number of posterior ribs seen above the diaphragm, radiographs of neonates are usually anterior-to-posterior views and counting ribs requires the juxtaposition of an anterior structure (the diaphragm) against a posterior structure (the rib interfacing with the diaphragm). This method assesses a three-dimensional object (the lung) with a two-dimensional picture (the radiograph) and is vulnerable to technician-selected focus angles. It is possible, then, to underestimate or overestimate inflation.

The present inability to routinely measure lung volume or compliance at the bedside and the ease with which acceptable oxygenation is achieved with relatively high $\overline{Paw}$ can confuse the clinician about the speed with which weaning should occur. Experience seems to be the best teacher in this situation. The consequences of failing to wean the patient quickly enough are significant pulmonary overdistention and impairment of cardiac output. In neonates, this complication can increase the risk of intracranial hemorrhage because venous return from vessels draining the head is impeded and venous hypertension and vessel rupture can ensue. Conversely, rapid weaning of $\overline{Paw}$ can result in alveolar derecruitment requiring reinitiation of lung recruitment procedures. Efforts are currently underway to develop a simple, reproducible, safe, and inexpensive method to frequently estimate lung volumes at the bedside.[60]

CARE OF THE PATIENT

Positioning

As mentioned earlier, patient positioning is constrained with the use of the older SensorMedics HFOV circuits. The unique nature of the patient circuit challenges caregivers to ensure ETT stability. Positioning the patient appropriately by rotating among supine, prone, and left and right lateral decubitus positions remains as important during HFV as during CV. Protocols describing approaches to positioning have been described.[61]

Endotracheal Tube

Initially, the HFJV Bunnell Life Pulse required the use of a triple-lumen high-low ETT (see Figure 20-5). This was necessary for placement of jet breaths through a separate lumen located in the mid-portion of the ETT, sampling of pressure at the distal ETT, and proximal ETT connection to the tandem CV. With the introduction of the Bunnell LifePort ETT adapter, the use of a special ETT is no longer required. The SensorMedics does require a specific ETT. Care must be taken to ensure that the ETT bevel is not against the tracheal wall. This will decrease the functional opening of the ETT and impair volume transmission. The application of HFV techniques to the tracheotomized patient has not been extensively explored.

Suctioning

Suctioning techniques vary among institutions. One technique consists of quickly disconnecting the patient from the HFV circuit, performing suctioning, and reapplying HFV without bagging between disconnections. Because suctioning can reduce lung volume by the sudden drop in airway pressure at disconnection and by the negative pressures applied during the procedure, lung derecruitment can occur. For some patients, this requires a temporary increase in $\overline{Paw}$ to regain baseline oxygenation. Closed tracheal suction systems with connections appropriate for the ventilator circuit used may be used.

Monitoring

As during CV, the frequency of blood gas sampling is related to the patient's clinical status. Blood gas measurements should be obtained frequently during the early course of ventilatory management and in patients in extremis (e.g., every 1 to 4 h). Intervals between samples should be increased as clinical conditions improve. For trending purposes, pulse oximetry and transcutaneous Po_2 and Pco_2 monitoring should be used. Because of rapid changes in $Paco_2$ noted especially during initial HFV management, transcutaneous monitoring is strongly recommended. There is no alteration in performance of these noninvasive gas exchange methods for patients receiving HFV.[62]

CIRCUITS AND HUMIDIFICATION

The SensorMedics circuit is constructed of smooth-walled semirigid tubing, unlike more flexible CV circuits. A larger diameter tube provides the inspiratory gas flow, whereas a narrower length of tubing is used for exhalation. The circuit is constructed to minimize compressible volume losses and is specific to the ventilator (i.e., the ventilator cannot be used with conventional neonatal ventilator circuits). A standard mushroom valve controls pressures that develop in the circuit, whereas two additional valves provide a selectable upper $\overline{Paw}$ limit (usually 2 to 3 cm H_2O greater than the actual $\overline{Paw}$) and a preset high mean pressure limit (50 cm H_2O). Proximal airway pressure is monitored at the patient airway. An input distal to the ventilator and proximal to the patient conducts humidified bias flow with the selected F_{IO_2} into the inspiratory limb of the circuit. Airway temperature is monitored to control temperature and humidity. Each circuit is calibrated for each ventilator before use. The Bunnell Life Pulse uses regular pressure ventilator circuits, with the jet tubing attached to the patient via the middle port of the Hi-Lo jet ETT or the LifePort ETT adapter.

Humidification is provided via an integral metered system, and bias flow for volume entrainment is provided by the continuous flow of the tandem neonatal CV. Current departmental policies for conventional mechanical ventilator circuit changes may be followed when using HFV devices; these policies vary among institutions.

Early HFV rescue experiences noted the presence of necrotizing tracheobronchitis, and at least one group believed that poor humidification was in part responsible for this airway complication.[63] Manufacturers of all FDA-approved HFV devices have addressed this problem with specific instructions for the provision of gas humidification.

TROUBLESHOOTING

The approach to troubleshooting HFV devices should not be different from that during CV. Either deterioration of the patient's vital signs or a ventilator alarm may alert the clinician. In either circumstance, it is necessary to ensure that the patient is in no further jeopardy before proceeding with a detailed troubleshooting procedure. High-frequency ventilators are dependent on patient airway caliber for adequate volume delivery. A change in airway diameter (e.g., by accumulation of secretions or by migration of the tip of the ETT against the tracheal wall) may significantly reduce delivered volumes. The first step should be a quick assessment of chest wall movement to ensure unchanged ventilation. If chest wall motion is substantially decreased, a return to or increase in CV or hand bagging may dramatically improve the situation. Steps should be taken to correct any problems with the ETT lumen or position (i.e., suctioning, chest radiograph).

Like CV, there are conditions in which HFV techniques are not uniformly successful. HFV seems especially vulnerable to the state of myocardial performance. In patients with poor cardiac output (e.g., decreased intravascular volume or reduced contractility), lung inflation with high Paw can result in abrupt and serious cardiac output impairment. Ensuring the adequacy of cardiac output before initiating HFV can mitigate this. Low-volume strategies will have less impact on cardiac output. For this reason, HFJV is successful during cardiac surgery and in circumstances in which lung compliance is normal and cardiac output is reduced.[41,42]

Because a relatively high MLV is necessary for both HFFI and HFOV (when no SI or intermittent CV breaths are used), these two techniques are not optimal for use in normal lungs. Furthermore, in conditions in which airway resistance is increased, such as fresh particulate meconium aspiration, bronchopulmonary dysplasia, and reactive airway disease, HFOV and HFFI may not be optimal. Because of the tremendous impedance to flow created by reductions in airway lumen with these disorders (thus increasing pulmonary time constants), decreases in delivered tidal volume or gas trapping, or both, cause derangement in gas exchange. In contrast, HFJV using larger tidal volumes and lower breathing frequencies may be more efficacious in conditions in which airway time constants are pathologically prolonged. These impressions are based on theoretical considerations and anecdotal experiences. Extensive controlled data supporting these contentions are not currently available.

Each ventilator manufacturer has developed detailed approaches to troubleshooting the mechanical problems of its own device, and these recommendations should be followed, tempered by actual clinical experience. A regular preventive maintenance program will help reduce mechanical failures.

EMERGING CLINICAL APPLICATIONS

The learning curve for these techniques continues to progress. Clinicians using HFV early in patients with respiratory distress syndrome believe that hospital courses are reduced and significant pulmonary morbidity is decreased.[12,31,47] The impact of HFJV on patients with PIE has been clearly demonstrated.[44] The precise role of HFV with respect to long-term outcome and cost of care continues to be defined. The availability of exogenous surfactant replacement, newer modes of CV for primary management, and ECMO and inhalational nitric oxide for patients with intractable respiratory failure continue to impact HFV use.[35,64-67] Ongoing investigations into the field of liquid ventilation, particularly partial liquid ventilation, are likely to stimulate new applications and enhance patient outcomes.

Surfactant Replacement

There remains little doubt that surfactant replacement therapy for immature infants with RDS is valuable. Issues that still confront surfactant replacement include the nature of the surfactant used, the timing of surfactant replacement (especially with HFV), and the method of delivery during HFV. As newer surfactants become available, the determination of the best product to use becomes complex (see Chapter 16, Surfactant Replacement). Furthermore, the use of surfactants during HFV, which may permit uninterrupted and progressive lung recruitment, presents alternatives for timing and method of drug delivery. Many investigators, especially in European countries, prefer surfactant replacement once optimal lung volume is achieved, whereas others consider more traditional prophylactic treatment.[48] No data exist that confirm the value of one method over the other. However, bolus surfactant delivery, even during HFV, seems more effective in ensuring uniform drug distribution.

Inhaled Nitric Oxide

The discovery that endothelial relaxing factor is nitric oxide has supplied medicine with a natural therapy for unwanted pulmonary vasoconstriction. Neonatal persistent pulmonary hypertension remains a problematic condition in critically ill near-term infants. Although it appears that inhaled nitric oxide is valuable in many circumstances, the delivery of this agent to the gas-exchanging surface is critical to its success. The uniform nature of gas delivery that occurs during HFV makes this method of ventilation an excellent delivery vehicle. Studies evaluating HFOV and CV with inhaled nitric oxide have convincingly supported the value of HFV for this indication.[67,68] This having been said, clear indications for inhaled nitric oxide therapy (with or without HFV) remain to be defined.

Liquid Ventilation

Liquid ventilation relies on the concept that liquid perfluorocarbons carry much more oxygen than gases and can move carbon dioxide with ease (see Chapter 22, Administration of Gas Mixtures).[69,70] Using liquid instead of gas to inflate the collapsed lung increases the uniformity of inflation with less injury. The addition of HFV to a liquid-filled lung permits ease of ventilation and may reduce lung injury.[71,72] This novel approach to RDS management has been the subject of ongoing evaluation with little new movement toward clinical introduction.

ASSESSMENT QUESTIONS

See Evolve Resources for answers.

1. High-frequency ventilation is defined by the U.S. FDA as delivering more than:
   - A. 150 breaths/minute
   - B. 12 breaths/second
   - C. 120 breaths/minute
   - D. 150 breaths/second
2. High-frequency jet ventilation delivers gas by:
   - A. Intermittently occluding a high flow of gas with a rotating vane
   - B. Pulsing gas down the endotracheal tube at a high velocity
   - C. Passing gas past the endotracheal tube and agitating it with a piston
   - D. The same method as conventional ventilation, just at a higher frequency.
3. High-frequency oscillatory ventilation delivers gas by:
   - A. The same method as conventional ventilation, just at a higher frequency
   - B. Pulsing gas down the endotracheal tube at a high velocity
   - C. Alternating gas in and out via a rotating vane
   - D. Passing gas past the endotracheal tube and agitating it with a piston.
4. The exhalation phase of HFOV differs from other forms of high-frequency ventilation because:
   - A. Exhaled gas is actively pulled out via the patient as the piston moves back.
   - B. Exhalation is passive, whereas on the HFJV gas is pulled out via a Venturi effect.
   - C. Exhalation is active during HFOV due to a separate vacuum assist device.
   - D. Exhaled gases passively exit the patient due to passive chest recoil.
5. Which of the following most accurately describe(s) the relationship of lung volume and P̄aw:
   - I. Increasing P̄aw increases lung volume and improves ventilation–perfusion matching.
   - II. Increasing P̄aw increases the pressure gradient, allowing more oxygen to cross the alveolar capillary membrane.
   - III. Increasing P̄aw improves the efficiency of the jet or piston.
   - IV. At very high and very low lung volumes ventilation–perfusion matching is impaired.
   - A. I
   - B. II
   - C. I, III, IV
   - D. I and IV

Continued

ASSESSMENT QUESTIONS—cont'd

6. The goal in treating atelectatic prone lung is
   A. High lung volume to recruit alveolar lung units
   B. Low lung volumes to reduce the chance of barotrauma
   C. High tidal volumes during convention ventilation to assist in carbon dioxide removal
   D. High lung volume to recruit the lung and large tidal volumes to aid ventilation

7. The goal in treating infants with pulmonary interstitial emphysema or active air leak is
   A. High lung volume to recruit alveolar lung units
   B. Low lung volume to reduce the chance of creating or worsening an air leak
   C. High lung volume to recruit the lung and large tidal volumes to aid ventilation
   D. Low tidal volumes combined with high lung volumes

8. A neonate is progressing satisfactorily on HFOV, with a mean airway pressure of 15 cm H_2O. The physician consults the respiratory clinician to determine in what increments the Paw should be weaned. What should the respiratory therapist recommend?
   A. 4–6 cm H_2O
   B. 3–4 cm H_2O
   C. 1–2 cm H_2O
   D. No increment; simply extubate

9. A clinician prepares to suction a patient undergoing HFV. What is the most likely consequence of suctioning?
   A. Hypoxia, requiring a temporary increase in Paw to resolve
   B. Pulmonary hemorrhage, requiring ETT epinephrine
   C. Negative-pressure pulmonary edema, requiring a temporary increase in Paw to resolve
   D. None of the above

10. An infant has just been placed on HFJV. What trending monitor(s) should be recommended?
    A. In-line blood gas analyzer
    B. Pulse oximetry
    C. Transcutaneous monitoring
    D. B and C

References

1. Bancalari E, Goldberg RN: High-frequency ventilation in the neonate, *Clin Perinatol* 1987;14:581.
2. Froese AB, Bryan AC: High frequency ventilation, *Am Rev Respir Dis* 1987;135:1363.
3. Gerstmann DR, deLemos RA: High-frequency ventilation: issues of strategy, *Clin Perinatol* 1991;18:563.
4. Clark RH, Gerstmann DR: Controversies in high-frequency ventilation, *Clin Perinatol* 1998;25:113.
5. Nash G, Blennerhassett JB, Pontoppidan H: Pulmonary lesions associated with oxygen therapy and artificial ventilation, *N Engl J Med* 1967;276:368.
6. Northway WH, Rosan RC, Porter DY: Pulmonary disease following respirator therapy of hyaline membrane, *N Engl J Med* 1967;276:357.
7. American Thoracic Society, European Society of Intensive Care Medicine, Société de Réanimation de Langue Française: International Consensus Conferences in Intensive Care Medicine: ventilator-associated lung injury in ARDS, *Am J Respir Crit Care Med* 1999;160:2118.
8. Acute Respiratory Distress Syndrome Network: Ventilation with lower tidal volumes as compared with traditional tidal volumes for acute lung injury and the acute respiratory distress syndrome, *N Engl J Med* 2000;342:1301.
9. Taghizadeh A, Reynolds EOR: Pathogenesis of bronchopulmonary dysplasia following hyaline membrane disease, *Am J Pathol* 1976;82:241.
10. Meredith KS et al: Role of lung injury in the pathogenesis of hyaline membrane disease in premature baboons, *J Appl Physiol* 1989;66:2150.
11. HiFi Study Group: High-frequency oscillatory ventilation compared with conventional mechanical ventilation in the treatment of respiratory failure in preterm infants, *N Engl J Med* 1989;320:88.
12. Clark RH et al: Prospective randomized comparison of high-frequency oscillatory and conventional ventilation in respiratory distress syndrome, *Pediatrics* 1992;89:5.
13. Jobe AH: Too many unvalidated new therapies to prevent chronic lung disease in preterm infants, *J Pediatr* 1998;132:200.
14. Clark RH, Slutsky AS, Gertsmann DR: Lung protective strategies of ventilation in the neonate: what are they? *Pediatrics* 2000;105:112.
15. Bland RD et al: High frequency mechanical ventilation in severe hyaline membrane disease, *Crit Care Med* 1980;8:275.
16. Borg U, Eriksson I, Sjostrand U: High-frequency positive pressure ventilation (HFPPV): a review based upon its use during bronchoscopy and for laryngoscopic and microlaryngeal surgery under general anesthesia, *Anesth Analg* 1980;59:594.
17. Sjostrand U: High-frequency positive pressure ventilation (HFPPV): a review, *Crit Care Med* 1980;8:345.
18. Heijman L, Sjostrand U: Treatment of the respiratory distress syndrome: preliminary report, *Opusc Med* 1974;19:235.
19. Boros SJ et al: Neonatal high-frequency jet ventilation: four years' experience, *Pediatrics* 1985;75:657.
20. Carlo WA et al: Decrease in airway pressure during high-frequency jet ventilation in infants with respiratory distress syndrome, *J Pediatr* 1984;104:101.
21. Chatburn RL, McClellan LD: A heat and humidification system for high-frequency jet ventilation, *Respir Care* 1982;27:1386.
22. Lunkenheimer PP et al: Intrapulmonaler Gasweschsel unter simulierter Apnoe durch transtrachealen, periodischen intrathorakalen Druckwechsel, *Anaesthesist* 1973;22:232.
23. Fredberg JJ et al: Factors influencing mechanical performance of neonatal high-frequency ventilators, *J Appl Physiol* 1987;62:2485.

24. Jouvet P et al: Assessment of high-frequency neonatal ventilator performances, *Intensive Care Med* 1997;23:208.

25. Hatcher D et al: Mechanical performances of clinically available, neonatal, high-frequency, oscillatory-type ventilators, *Crit Care Med* 1998;26:1081.

26. Fredberg JJ: Augmented diffusion in the airways can support pulmonary gas exchange, *J Appl Physiol* 1980;49:232.

27. Fredberg JJ et al: Alveolar pressure non-homogeneity during small amplitude high-frequency oscillation, *J Appl Physiol* 1984;57:788.

28. Chang HK: Mechanisms of gas transport during ventilation by high-frequency oscillation, *J Appl Physiol* 1984;56:553.

29. Robertson B: Pathology of neonatal surfactant deficiency, *Perspect Pediatr Pathol* 1987;11:6.

30. Gilbert R, Keighley JF: The arterial/alveolar oxygen tension ratio: an index of gas exchange applicable to varying oxygen concentrations, *Am Rev Respir Dis* 1974;109:142.

31. HiFO Study Group: Randomized study of high-frequency oscillatory ventilation in infants with severe respiratory distress syndrome, *J Pediatr* 1993;122:609.

32. Kinsella JP et al: High-frequency ventilation versus intermittent mandatory ventilation: early hemodynamic effects in the premature baboon with hyaline membrane disease, *Pediatr Res* 1991;29:160.

33. McCulloch PR, Forkert PG, Froese AB: Lung volume maintenance prevents lung injury during high-frequency oscillatory ventilation in surfactant deficient rabbits, *Am Rev Respir Dis* 1988;137:1185.

34. Gerstmann DR et al: Treatment of congenital diaphragmatic hernia with high-frequency oscillatory ventilation. Presented at the Eleventh Conference on High-Frequency Ventilation of Infants, Snowbird, Utah, April 1994.

35. Bartlett RH et al: Extracorporeal circulatory support in neonatal respiratory failure: a prospective randomized study, *Pediatrics* 1985;76:479.

36. Carter JM et al: High-frequency oscillatory ventilation and extracorporeal membrane oxygenation for the treatment of acute neonatal respiratory failure, *Pediatrics* 1990;85:159.

37. Paranka MS et al: Predictors of failure of high-frequency ventilation in term infants with severe respiratory failure, *Pediatrics* 1995;95:400.

38. Gerstmann DR et al: The Provo Multicenter Early High-frequency Oscillatory Ventilation Trial: improved pulmonary and clinical outcome in respiratory distress syndrome, *Pediatrics* 1996;98:1196.

39. Henderson-Smart DJ et al: Elective high frequency oscillatory ventilation versus conventional ventilation for acute pulmonary dysfunction in preterm infants, *Cochrane Database Syst Rev* 2000;2:CD000104.

40. Duval EL et al: High-frequency ventilation in pediatric patients, *Neth J Med* 2000;56:177.

41. Dekeon MK et al: High-frequency jet ventilation in post-operative Fontan patients. Presented at the Seventh Conference on High-frequency Ventilation of Infants, Snowbird, Utah, April 1990.

42. Davis D et al: High-frequency jet ventilation: intraoperative application during neonatal cardiac surgery. Presented at the Ninth Conference of High-frequency Ventilation of Infants, Snowbird, Utah, April 1992.

43. Choong K: Low frequency oscillation is potentially more injurious than high frequency oscillatory ventilation. Presented at the Seventeenth Conference on High-frequency Ventilation of Infants, Snowbird, Utah, April 2000.

44. Keszler M et al: Multicenter controlled trial comparing high-frequency jet ventilation and conventional mechanical ventilation in newborns with pulmonary interstitial emphysema, *J Pediatr* 1991;119:85.

45. Keszler M et al: Multicenter controlled trial of high-frequency jet ventilation in preterm infants with uncomplicated respiratory distress syndrome, *Pediatrics* 1997;100:593.

46. Bhuta T, Henderson-Smart DJ: Elective high frequency jet ventilation versus conventional ventilation for respiratory distress syndrome in preterm infants, *Cochrane Database Syst Rev* 2000;2:CD000104.

47. Plavka R et al: A prospective randomized comparison of conventional mechanical ventilation and very early high frequency ventilation in extremely premature newborns with respiratory distress syndrome, *Intensive Care Med* 1999;25:68.

48. Cools F, Offringa M: Meta-analysis of elective high frequency ventilation in preterm infants with respiratory distress syndrome, *Arch Dis Child Fetal Neonatal Ed* 1999;80:F15.

49. Derdak S et al: High frequency oscillatory ventilation for acute respiratory distress syndrome in adults: a randomized, controlled trial, *Am J Respir Crit Care Med* 2002;166:801.

50. Courtney SE et al: High-frequency oscillatory ventilation versus conventional mechanical ventilation for very-low-birth-weight infants, *N Engl J Med* 2002;347:643.

51. Fort P et al: High frequency oscillatory ventilation for adult respiratory distress syndrome: a pilot study, *Crit Care Med* 1997;25:937.

52. Mehta S et al: Prospective trial of high-frequency oscillation in adults with acute respiratory distress syndrome, *Crit Care Med* 2001;29:1360.

53. David M et al: High frequency oscillatory ventilation in adult acute respiratory distress syndrome, *Intensive Care Med* 2003;29:1656.

54. Mehta S et al: High-frequency oscillatory ventilation in adults: the Toronto experience, *Chest* 2004;126:518.

55. Froese AB: High-frequency ventilation: strategy and device differences. Presented at the Seventh Conference on High-frequency Ventilation of Infants, Snowbird, Utah, April 1990.

56. Hamm CR et al: High frequency jet ventilation preceded by lung volume recruitment decreases hyaline membrane formation in surfactant deficient lungs, *Pediatr Res* 1990;27:305A.

57. Clark RH et al: Pulmonary interstitial emphysema treated by high-frequency oscillatory ventilation, *Crit Care Med* 1986;14:926.

58. Ogawa Y et al: A multicenter randomized trial of high-frequency oscillatory ventilation as compared with conventional ventilation in preterm infants with respiratory failure, *Early Hum Dev* 1993;32:1.

59. Clark RH et al: Intraventricular hemorrhage and high-frequency ventilation: a meta-analysis of prospective clinical trials, *Pediatrics* 1996;98:1058.

60. Palmer C: Personal communication, August 2000.

61. Avila K et al: High-frequency oscillatory ventilation: a nursing approach to bedside care, *Neonatal Network* 1994;13:23.

62. Meredith KS: Clinical evaluation of non-invasive blood gas monitoring. Presented at the Eighth Conference on High-frequency Ventilation of Infants, Snowbird, Utah, April 1991.

63. Ophoven JP et al: Tracheobronchial histopathology associated with high-frequency jet ventilation, *Crit Care Med* 1984;12:829.

64. Randel RC, Manning FL: One lung high-frequency ventilation in the management of an acquired neonatal pulmonary cyst, *J Perinatol* 1989;9:66.

65. Bloom BT et al: Respiratory distress syndrome and tracheoesophageal fistula: management with high-frequency ventilation, *Crit Care Med* 1990;18:447.

66. Fujiwara T et al: Artificial surfactant therapy in hyaline membrane disease, *Lancet* 1980;1:55.

67. Kinsella JP et al: Randomized, multicenter trial of inhaled nitric oxide and high-frequency oscillatory ventilation in severe, persistent pulmonary hypertension of the newborn, *J Pediatr* 1997;131:55.

68. Kinsella JP, Abman SH; Nitric Oxide Study Group: High-frequency oscillatory ventilation augments the response to inhaled nitric oxide in persistent pulmonary hypertension of the newborn, *Crit Care Med* 1998;26:993.

69. Leach CL et al; LiquiVent Study Group: Partial liquid ventilation with perflubron in premature infants with severe respiratory distress syndrome, *N Engl J Med* 1996;335:761.

70. Weis CM, Wolsfson MR, Shaffer TH: Liquid-assisted ventilation: physiology and clinical application, *Ann Med* 1997;29:509.

71. Sukumar M et al: High-frequency partial liquid ventilation in respiratory distress syndrome: hemodynamics and gas exchange, *J Appl Physiol* 1998;84:327.

72. Kinsella JP et al: Independent and combined effects of inhaled nitric oxide, liquid perfluorochemical, and high-frequency oscillatory ventilation in premature lambs with respiratory distress syndrome, *Am J Respir Crit Care Med* 1999;159:1220.

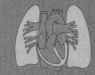

Chapter 21

Noninvasive Mechanical Ventilation of the Infant and Child

PRADIP KAMAT ● W. GERALD TEAGUE

OUTLINE

LEARNING OBJECTIVES

After reading this chapter the reader will be able to:

- Describe the effects of noninvasive positive-pressure ventilation on respiratory function
- Differentiate the effects on respiratory function of noninvasive positive-pressure ventilation and continuous positive airway pressure
- Identify the respiratory disorders most amenable to a trial of noninvasive ventilation
- Explain the inspiratory pressure support feature of commercial bilevel pressure ventilators

- Discuss how adjustments in inspiratory and expiratory positive airway pressures affect respiratory function
- Recall the principles of interface selection so as to optimize the effectiveness and comfort of noninvasive positive-pressure ventilation
- Discuss common complications and contraindications to noninvasive positive-pressure ventilation

Methods of respiratory assistance that do not require an indwelling artificial airway are termed *noninvasive*. Noninvasive positive-pressure ventilation (NPPV) systems include an external mask interface and positive-pressure mechanical venti- lator. Negative-pressure–assisted ventilation, a second method of noninvasive ventilation, involves the inter- mittent application of subatmospheric pressure exter- nal to the rib cage by means of a tank or chest mold. Continuous positive airway pressure (CPAP) therapy is a third method of noninvasive ventilation. CPAP is administered through an external mask interface with a simple constant flow source or through a pressure-targeted bilevel ventilator in the CPAP mode. This chapter addresses noninvasive ventilation in children in general, but the focus is primarily on NPPV.

Starting in the early 1990s, NPPV has rapidly grown as a method of assisted ventilation in pediatric-age patients. The growing popularity in the use of NPPV is explained in part by the high complication rate associated with mechanical ventilation via an indwelling (invasive) airway in children. For example, positive-pressure–assisted ventilation by means of tracheotomy (TPPV) is considered standard therapy for the long-term management of complicated pediatric respiratory disorders. Although highly effective, TPPV can result in significant medical complications, loss of mobility, and social isolation.[1] As a result, clinicians dissatisfied with TPPV look to NPPV as a less invasive alternative. A second factor promoting the use of NPPV is the improved survival of children with catastrophic lung injury who are left with significant chronic lung disease. Noninvasive modes of respiratory assistance are increasingly attempted in these children to facilitate early extubation and for long-term care. Finally, commercial availability of compact NPPV systems and improved external interfaces have expanded the use of NPPV from highly specialized units dedicated to pediatric respiratory care to other sites including the emergency room and postoperative recovery area.

Clinicians who attempt NPPV in pediatric-age patients should know that modern bilevel pressure ventilators were designed to treat adult and not pediatric patients. Common shortfalls in the implementation of NPPV in pediatric patients include poor mask fit, incorrect adjustment of the inspiratory and expiratory pressures, and failure of small infants to trigger the ventilator in the spontaneous mode. These issues must be resolved for NPPV to be effectively used in very small patients.

The respiratory clinician must carefully evaluate a number of variables before attempting NPPV. Foremost, the clinician should assess the age and pattern of respiratory dysfunction in the child to decide whether a trial of NPPV is even warranted. Then the appropriate equipment and settings should be considered. After initiation of NPPV, the child must be assessed immediately to be certain that the work of breathing has decreased and that there is sufficient improvement in respiratory gas exchange. An approach to these and other problems is addressed in this chapter.

OBJECTIVES OF NONINVASIVE VENTILATION

Noninvasive Positive-pressure Ventilation

The objective(s) of noninvasive ventilation are identical to those of invasive mechanical ventilation (see Chapter 19, Mechanical Ventilation of the Neonate and Pediatric Patient). The primary objectives are to decrease the work of breathing, restore adequate carbon dioxide elimination, improve oxygenation, maintain upper airway stability, and restore lung volume (Box 21-1). There are a number of methods to determine the effectiveness of noninvasive ventilation in meeting these goals in the clinical setting, each with advantages and disadvantages. Whatever the method(s) used, each member of the respiratory team must carefully document in the medical record the patient's response to treatment. This requires that the therapist carefully evaluate the patient both before and after initiation of noninvasive ventilation to document that the goals of treatment have been achieved. As important, a rescue plan that includes notification of the physician must be evident to assist children who fail a trial of noninvasive ventilation.

In the acute setting, the primary goal of noninvasive ventilation is to decrease the patient's work of breathing. Children with acute respiratory distress typically breathe rapidly and shallowly, visibly recruit the accessory muscles of respiration, and have prolonged

---

Box 21-1 | Objectives of Noninvasive Ventilation in Pediatric Patients With Respiratory Disorders

DECREASE THE WORK OF BREATHING
- Assist the respiratory muscles
- Decrease the respiratory rate
- Decrease retractions (thoracoabdominal asynchrony)
- Decrease energy use associated with breathing
- Decrease auto-PEEP

INCREASE ALVEOLAR VENTILATION
- Increase tidal volume
- Decrease arterial and end-tidal Pa_{CO_2}

INCREASE FUNCTIONAL RESIDUAL CAPACITY
- Decrease the alveolar–arterial oxygen tension difference
- Prevent atelectasis

MAINTAIN UPPER AIRWAY PATENCY
- Decrease the number and length of occlusive apneas and hypopneas

Pa_{CO_2}, Arterial partial pressure of carbon dioxide; PEEP, positive end-expiratory pressure.

periods of paradoxical rib cage/abdominal motion, referred to as *retractions*. These symptoms manifest a high level of respiratory muscle work maintained by neural activation. However, children with neuromuscular disorders often do not demonstrate the classic signs and symptoms of respiratory distress despite severe derangement in respiratory gas exchange. In such patients and in young infants, arterial blood gas analysis is necessary to assess the degree of respiratory dysfunction and to determine the effectiveness of noninvasive ventilation.

In the chronic setting, the goals of noninvasive ventilation are often different than in the acute setting. In children with chronic disorders complicated by alveolar hypoventilation, intermittent NPPV at night can be offered as a clinical benefit as a means to improve the quality of sleep and to reduce the severity of daytime symptoms associated with hypercarbia—headache and fatigue.[2] Although the ultimate goal of NPPV in this setting is to increase carbon dioxide elimination, this goal may not be reached for a number of days to weeks while the patient may report significant subjective improvement.

The daytime $PaCO_2$ (arterial partial pressure of carbon dioxide) should decrease 1 to 2 weeks after initiation of intermittent NPPV treatment at night in patients with restrictive disorders and chronic hypercarbia.[3] The mechanism for this improvement is uncertain, but it is likely caused by restoration of the central ventilatory responsiveness to changes in pH as a result of increased nocturnal carbon dioxide elimination. We have found that intermittent NPPV treatment in pediatric patients with chronic hypoventilation disorders effectively improves daytime carbon dioxide elimination for at least a period of 1 year and that this improvement is associated with a decrease in total serum levels of bicarbonate.[4,5] Other improvements in respiratory function that might result from long-term NPPV treatment include prevention of atelectasis and maintenance of functional residual capacity, increased lung compliance, and increased endurance of the respiratory muscles as a result of periods of rest. However, none of these potential benefits has been conclusively found in clinical studies.

Continuous Positive Airway Pressure

The primary goal of CPAP therapy is to increase end-expiratory lung volume, thereby improving oxygenation. CPAP therapy may or may not improve tidal volume and alveolar ventilation. In children and especially neonates with restrictive respiratory dysfunction and decreased lung compliance, CPAP therapy can raise tidal volume. However, in children with lung overexpansion and increased compliance, CPAP therapy may actually decrease tidal volume. In clinical practice, the results of arterial or capillary blood gas analysis in combination with the pattern of respiratory dysfunction and cardiovascular stability determine the mode of treatment. CPAP is likely as good a choice as NPPV in situations in which the predominant respiratory derangement is hypoxemia from ventilation–perfusion inequality with preserved alveolar ventilation. In addition, there is a mode of CPAP that alternates the level of CPAP in a low-frequency unsynchronized fashion that mimics lung recruitment maneuvers specifically in neonates.[6-10] Although not conclusive, it appears to be an alternative to full NPPV or intubation and may reduce the respiratory distress in this select patient population. NPPV is preferred when hypoventilation is present and the child has sufficient inspiratory effort to trigger the inspiratory pressure support function of the NPPV device.

EXPERIENCE WITH NPPV IN PEDIATRIC PATIENTS

Acute Respiratory Distress

Until recently NPPV therapy in children with acute respiratory distress has been described only in case reports and uncontrolled studies.[11,12] This is particularly true in the setting of acute hypoxemic respiratory failure, in which the experience with NPPV in children, although promising, has not been subjected to carefully controlled trials. This situation is in marked contrast to a growing body of evidence in support of NPPV as superior to standard care in preventing intubation of adult patients with acute hypercarbic exacerbations of chronic obstructive lung disease.[13] However, a few small prospectively controlled trials have shown great promise. In 1998 Padman and colleagues[14] prospectively studied 34 patients admitted to the pediatric intensive care unit with various diagnoses (pneumonia, postextubation stridor, asthma, acute chest syndrome, obstructive sleep apnea, and postoperative hypoventilation with atelectasis) and who required airway or oxygenation/ventilation support. They found that initiation of NPPV caused a decrease in respiratory rate, heart rate, and dyspnea score and an improvement in oxygenation in more than 90% of the patients studied, with only 8% of patients needing intubation.

Thill and colleagues[15] prospectively studied 20 pediatric-age patients admitted to the pediatric intensive care unit with lower airway obstruction. Compared with standard therapy NPPV treatment decreased the overall work of breathing as manifested by decreased respiratory rate, decreased accessory muscle use, and decreased dyspnea. Whereas no randomized controlled trials have been conducted in children with acute respiratory distress, it is not known whether NPPV can reduce the incidence of intubation altogether or simply delay intubation. Nonetheless, NPPV is widely used in this setting and has been found in published case reports to be generally safe when used appropriately. Therefore despite the absence of high-level clinical evidence, pediatric patients with acute hypoxemic and/or hypercarbic respiratory failure (Box 21-2) could be offered a trial of NPPV in the appropriate setting. This recommendation assumes careful selection of patients to exclude those with known contraindications (hemodynamic instability, altered mental status, and inability to handle airway secretions).

Chronic Respiratory Dysfunction

In contrast to the acute setting, there is a better-defined role for NPPV in children with chronic disorders of the respiratory system complicated by alveolar hypoventilation (Box 21-3). Children with even moderately severe chronic respiratory failure can compensate reasonably well for months to years as a result of the renal adaptation to hypercarbia. In the presence of lower respiratory tract infection or the stress of general anesthesia, the kidneys cannot compensate sufficiently, resulting in acute respiratory acidosis. In this setting, NPPV can be applied in the intensive care unit or postoperative recovery area as a means to avoid endotracheal intubation. NPPV appears to work best when there is significant atelectasis and less so when the patient is agitated or the derangement in lung mechanical function is severe (see earlier). NPPV also shows promise as a weaning adjunct from invasive mechanical ventilation. In this role, NPPV has been used effectively in children with acute decompensation after adenotonsillar removal and to stabilize airway function after laryngotracheoplasty.[16,17]

Chronic Neuromuscular Disease

Intermittent (nocturnal) NPPV has the potential to evolve as preferred therapy in pediatric patients with

---

Box 21-2	Causes of Acute Respiratory Failure in Pediatric Patients Amenable to a Trial of NPPV Treatment*

- ARDS (early phase only)
- Acute chest syndrome
- Pneumonia
- Pulmonary edema
- Postoperative upper airway obstruction
- Atelectasis
- Hypercarbic exacerbations of cystic fibrosis lung disease
- Status asthmaticus complicated by severe hypoxemia
- Acute decompensation of neuromuscular diseases (SMA, Duchenne's muscular dystrophy, spinal cord injury)
- Postextubation respiratory distress
- Acute pulmonary hemorrhage (only if hemoptysis not present)
- Respiratory distress with cerebral palsy and other "overlap syndromes"
- Acute intrapulmonary aspiration
- Near drowning

ARDS, Acute respiratory distress syndrome; SMA, spinal muscular atrophy.
* In each disorder the recommendation is based on careful observation of the patient with implementation in a setting appropriate for a child with respiratory distress and documentation of the effectiveness of NPPV in each application.

Box 21-3	Role of NPPV in Children with Chronic Dysfunction of the Respiratory System

NEUROMUSCULAR DISORDERS
- Duchenne's muscular dystrophy
- Spinal muscular atrophy (type II)
- Nemaline myopathy

RIB CAGE AND CHEST WALL ANOMALIES
- Progressive idiopathic and juvenile scoliosis
- Mild forms of asphyxiating thoracic dystrophy
- Advanced cystic fibrosis complicated by hypercarbia

OBESITY HYPOVENTILATION DISORDERS
- Prader-Willi syndrome
- Morbid obesity with obstructive sleep apnea

OVERLAP SYNDROMES (UPPER AIRWAY OBSTRUCTION AND RESTRICTIVE LUNG DYSFUNCTION)
- Spina bifida (pulmonary complications: Arnold-Chiari malformation, restrictive lung dysfunction, upper airway obstruction)
- Cerebral palsy (laryngeal obstruction and restrictive lung dysfunction)

CHRONIC UPPER AIRWAY OBSTRUCTION
- Obstructive apnea syndrome complicated by hypercarbia
- Down's syndrome (maxillary hypoplasia, large tongue)
- Craniofacial syndromes with midfacial or mandibular hypoplasia

CHRONIC OBSTRUCTIVE AIRWAY DISEASES
- Advanced cystic fibrosis

NPPV LESS WELL ESTABLISHED IN TREATMENT BUT SHOWING PROMISE
- Laryngotracheomalacia
- Disorders with central alveolar hypoventilation

stable but chronic hypoventilation disorders caused by neuromuscular weakness. The pattern of respiratory dysfunction in these children is often complex, and includes both upper airway obstruction and reduced forced vital capacity. Children with advanced neuromuscular disorders may go through an early stage of sleep disruption characterized by recurrent arousals and brief episodes of obstructive apnea/hypopnea with transient desaturation.[18,19] Rapid eye movement sleep in particular may be a relatively dangerous time for these patients because the upper airway muscle tone decreases, resulting in episodes of complete or partial airway occlusion. We have found that a long-term trial of NPPV administered at night in children with restrictive, obstructive hypoventilation and overlap (restrictive dysfunction with upper airway obstruction) disorders acutely improves sleep quality and reduces the number of occlusive events.[20] In a 1-year follow-up period, patient and family adherence to NPPV was better than expected and few patients required tracheotomy died as a result of respiratory complications.[4]

Advanced Cystic Fibrosis Lung Disease

Advanced cystic fibrosis lung disease is characterized by persistent hypoxemia and hypoventilation, especially in patients with pancreatic insufficiency and malnutrition. In previous reports, NPPV ameliorated nocturnal hypoventilation with supplemental oxygen therapy.[21] In long-term use NPPV was an effective "bridge" treatment to help survival before lung transplantation.[22] Although NPPV therapy in cystic fibrosis does not appear to improve lung function or clearance of secretions, it does appear to improve respiratory gas exchange.[23]

NONINVASIVE VENTILATION WITH POSITIVE-PRESSURE DEVICES

Bilevel Pressure-targeted Ventilators

In daily practice a bilevel pressure-targeted ventilator is most often used for NPPV in pediatric patients. Bilevel devices set in the spontaneous mode respond to a step change in inspiratory flow rate by delivering a preset level of positive pressure, which is similar to the pressure-support function of contemporary ventilators designed for invasive mechanical ventilation. The result is an increase in tidal volume that is dependent on the compliance and resistance of the respiratory system and the gradient between the inspiratory and expiratory pressure adjustments.[24] Most bilevel ventilators

available for commercial use are remarkably adept at delivering sufficient flow to reach the targeted level of inspiratory pressure.[25] These devices have a flow compensation feature so that small leaks around the interface or through the mouth do not seriously impair performance. However, the capacity of NPPV devices to compensate for severe leaks is limited. This can significantly impair the effectiveness of NPPV administered by a nasal mask interface in children with nasal pharyngeal obstruction, who commonly adapt by breathing via the oral route.

Other features standard on bilevel pressure-targeted ventilators include an expiratory positive airway pressure adjustment (EPAP), back-up ventilatory rate, and mode selection. Most do not have an independent oxygen blend feature.

The advantages of pressure-targeted ventilators designed for NPPV include ease of adjustment, portability, and relatively low cost. Newer devices (such as the BiPAP Vision ventilator support system; Philips Respironics, Murrysville, Pa) are equipped with built-in oxygen blender, alarm systems, graphics, and an internal battery pack. The BiPAP Pro 2 with Bi-Flex (Philips Respironics) has a memory chip for recording events, useful in the management of patients with obstructive sleep apnea. Furthermore, there is no U.S. Food and Drug Administration (FDA) approval for the first generation of bilevel ventilators for use as an invasive mode of mechanical ventilation in children. Although this has not been an issue for inpatient application, it is a major impediment for outpatient use. Most home care companies require that physicians sign an indemnification agreement releasing them from liability should the device fail.

Volume-regulated Ventilators

NPPV can be accomplished through portable ventilators designed to cycle in the volume mode. The features of these ventilators are reviewed in Chapter 46 (Home Care). Most portable volume-regulated ventilators used in the home do not have a pressure support feature and must be adjusted carefully to ensure patient comfort. The potential advantages of volume-regulated devices for NPPV include superior performance when used in the synchronized intermittent mandatory ventilation mode for patients who, with significant neuromuscular weakness or central hypoventilation, may not trigger bilevel ventilators. Furthermore, they can provide assisted ventilation in patients with poor compliance; use three to eight times less electricity for the same battery capacity, permitting longer periods of mobility; are quieter; do not require expiratory positive airway pressure (to prevent rebreathing); can result in lower mean thoracic pressures; and can be used to operate abdominal exsufflation belts.[26] Major drawbacks of portable volume-regulated ventilators for NPPV in pediatric patients include their relative size, limited portability, and, most importantly, limited attainment of high levels of inspiratory flow to support spontaneous respiratory efforts. Newer generations of portable ventilators are smaller and provide flow rates that support spontaneous breathing, including pressure support.

To appropriately adjust a volume-regulated ventilator for NPPV, the delivered tidal volume should be approximately twice that of the child's physiologic tidal volume to accommodate the dead space of the nasopharynx and conducting airways. Setting the tidal volume above the physiologic range and adjusting the peak inspiratory pressure until the required tidal volume is achieved can accomplish this. This method, often referred to as *pressure plateau ventilation,* is commonly used for invasive long-term mechanical ventilation in pediatric patients.[27]

NONINVASIVE VENTILATION WITH NEGATIVE-PRESSURE DEVICES

Negative-pressure ventilation is a form of respiratory assistance in which subatmospheric pressure is applied intermittently through a cuirass or tank device external to the chest wall. Expiration occurs as the pressure around the chest wall is allowed to return to atmospheric levels. This method of assisted ventilation is effective in pediatric patients with hypoventilation associated with acquired neurologic injury from trauma or infection and chronic restrictive lung disorders.[28] More recently it has also shown some promise in patients with congenital hypoventilation syndromes and bronchiolitis-related apnea.[29,30] An advantage of negative-pressure ventilation is that it can improve carbon dioxide elimination without a tracheostomy. However, both the cuirass and tank devices require a fairly complete seal around the chest margins to be effective, and the tank device is large and difficult to move. Another important drawback of negative-pressure ventilation is significant disruption of sleep in patients with neuromuscular disorders and poor control of the muscle group supporting the upper airway. In these patients, treatment with negative-pressure ventilation can be complicated by recurrent episodes of obstructive apnea/hypopnea culminating in transient hypoxemia. Whereas NPPV is effective in preventing such episodes in children with unstable upper airway function, it is increasingly being used in lieu of a trial of negative-pressure ventilation for pediatric patients with chronic hypoventilation disorders.

NPPV MODES

Most bilevel pressure-targeted ventilators suitable for NPPV feature CPAP, spontaneous, timed, and spontaneous/timed (assist-control) operating modes. In the CPAP mode, these devices provide constant flow to maintain a target level of continuous positive airway pressure. Inspiratory pressure support is not provided. In the spontaneous mode, the ventilator responds to a threshold level of inspiratory flow or to a change in volume that is initiated by the patient's spontaneous respiratory effort. At the inspiratory flow threshold, the ventilator delivers additional gas flow to reach the preset inspiratory positive airway pressure (IPAP). Exhalation occurs after the inspiratory flow peaks and then decreases to a threshold level. In the timed mode, the ventilator does not flow trigger but delivers intermittent pulses of positive airway pressure at a set rate. In the spontaneous/timed mode, the flow-trigger feature is activated. The ventilator cycles in the timed mode only in the event of prolonged apnea.

Pediatric patients are typically managed with NPPV in the spontaneous/timed mode. The chief advantage of this mode is patient comfort. This results when the child's inspiratory efforts are assisted with the inspiratory pressure support feature. A significant barrier to effective NPPV in young or very small patients is their inability to achieve sufficient inspiratory flow to trigger the inspiratory pressure support feature.[31] This problem may be solved by replacing the connector circuit between the mask interface and ventilator from standard tubing supplied by the manufacturer to shorter, less compliant tubing. However, this is clearly a departure from standard procedure that is not recommended by the manufacturer and should be attempted only in centers with experience in pediatric NPPV.

Another common problem with NPPV in the spontaneous mode in pediatric patients is the effects of significant gas leaks around the mask or through the mouth. In the presence of a significant leak, the inspiratory pressure target is never reached, resulting in a long inflation time as the unit delivers massive amounts of inspiratory flow in an attempt to attain the preset inspiratory pressure. Some modern bilevel ventilators (VPAP III ST, ResMed, Poway, Calif; BiPAP Vision, Philips Respironics) designed for NPPV feature an adjustable inflation time that can be set to prevent this problem. There is little published experience with pediatric patients treated with NPPV exclusively in the timed mode. In this mode the ventilator essentially functions as a time-cycled, pressure-limited device.

MONITORING THE PATIENT AND VENTILATOR CIRCUIT

Selection of patient and ventilator monitors with NPPV is based primarily on the clinical setting and the acuity of the patient. In critically ill children with acute respiratory failure, NPPV is frequently attempted to prevent intubation. Under these conditions NPPV serves a life support function. The optimal location for patients receiving NPPV depends on the capacity for adequate monitoring, staff skill, experience with and knowledge of the equipment used, and awareness of potential complications. The patient should thus be monitored with arterial oxygen saturation (Sao_2), arterial blood gases, work of breathing, development of hemodynamic instability or altered mental status, and failure to tolerate the device (see Case Report).[32,33] Each monitor device should have alarm limits set by an experienced respiratory therapist and nurse.

Frequently, NPPV is used for stable patients with respiratory dysfunction as a clinical benefit. A hospital ward, sleep laboratory, or step-down unit is an appropriate setting for NPPV in this capacity. A pulse oximeter alone may be sufficient monitoring provided the child is clinically stable and not likely to decompensate in the event of equipment failure or removal of the interface. Intermittent NPPV can be accomplished safely at home without any patient or ventilator monitors. However, children with limited capacity to spontaneously increase minute ventilation, such as an advanced neuromuscular disorder or congenital central hypoventilation syndrome, do require both a cardiorespiratory impedance monitor and pulse oximeter for NPPV in the outpatient setting. End-tidal carbon dioxide should also be monitored in children with congenital central hypoventilation syndrome. This is often a challenge with NPPV because of dilution of exhaled carbon dioxide by the continuous flow present between the nasal opening and mask interface.

PRESSURE TITRATION IN NONINVASIVE VENTILATION

With modern bilevel pressure ventilators, the IPAP adjustment determines the target distending airway pressure attained during flow-triggered or timed ventilator inflations. The IPAP should be set above the EPAP to raise the child's tidal volume, "unload" the respiratory muscles, and decrease respiratory distress. The differential between the IPAP and EPAP adjustment determines the tidal volume. Although second-generation bilevel devices are capable of achieving IPAP levels of 30 cm H_2O, children typically do not tolerate pressures higher than 20 cm H_2O without some type of sedation. There may be a delay

of several hours before a step increase in IPAP achieves a reduction in $Paco_2$. In this event, other factors can be used to determine the effectiveness in NPPV (Table 21-1). In day-to-day clinical practice an IPAP setting of between 8 and 12 cm H_2O is typically sufficient to achieve the goals of NPPV in pediatric-age patients.

The EPAP adjustment with NPPV primarily determines the end-expiratory lung volume and maintains the stability of the upper airway. In a typical pediatric application of NPPV, EPAP levels of 6 to 8 cm H_2O are effective in improving oxygenation and preventing obstructive

TABLE 21-1

Methods to Determine the Clinical Effectiveness of Noninvasive Ventilation

Outcome Expected	Method and Limitations
Decrease in work of breathing	*Physical examination:* Acute decrease in respiratory rate, retractions, and use of accessory muscles. Not reliable in patients with neuromuscular and central disorders
Improvement in respiratory gas exchange	*Pulse oximetry:* Acute improvement in Sao_2. Not reliable in the assessment of hypoventilation. Interpretation obscured by concurrent O_2 treatment
	Blood gas sampling: Increase in pH, decrease in $Paco_2$, increase in Pao_2; invasive—$Paco_2$ may not decrease for hours if at all in some disorders
	End-tidal CO_2 monitoring: Acute reduction in end-tidal CO_2. High background flow in NPPV circuit can wash out expired CO_2
	Transcutaneous CO_2 monitoring: Subacute reduction in transcutaneous CO_2 monitoring; accuracy dependent on careful electrode placement, changes lag minutes behind change in actual $Paco_2$
Increase in functional residual capacity	*Routine chest radiography:* Increased lung expansion, decreased atelectasis; difficult to accomplish during therapy; changes can lag days behind
Maintenance of upper airway patency	*Sleep polysomnography:* Subacute reductions in the number of airway-occlusive episodes decrease with the degree of thoracoabdominal asynchrony. Not amenable to acute clinical setting

$Paco_2$, Arterial partial pressure of carbon dioxide; Pao_2, arterial partial pressure of oxygen; Sao_2, arterial oxygen saturation.

apnea. Most children, regardless of the setting or indication, poorly tolerate EPAP levels above 10 cm H$_2$O.

Overtitration of airway pressures is a common mistake when NPPV is attempted in pediatric patients. In children with normal lung compliance, typically those with neuromuscular lung diseases, optimal results are seen at relatively low distending pressures. Raising the pressure to compensate for leaks around the nasal mask or through the mouth often is poorly tolerated in children and can lead to central hypoventilation. The mechanism behind this is uncertain, but it is also seen in adult patients with obesity hypoventilation syndrome treated with nasal CPAP.[34]

In negative-pressure-assisted ventilation the applied subatmospheric pressure is decreased incrementally to raise the tidal volume. A significant hazard in exposing patients with neuromuscular disorders to intermittent external subatmospheric pressures while leaving the head and neck exposed to ambient atmospheric pressure is episodic obstructive apnea and hypopnea. In clinical practice this can be minimized by concomitant nasal CPAP therapy with negative-pressure-assisted ventilation.

INTERFACE SELECTION AND FIT

Interface devices appropriate for NPPV include nasal masks, nasal-oral masks, and nasal plugs or pillows. Studies promote the use of helmet devices in adults with acute respiratory distress. Experience with these is limited in children, and would likely be difficult because of the child's natural apprehension. One study in adults compared different interfaces and showed that although nasal masks are more acceptable to patients, facial masks and nasal plugs delivered higher minute ventilation with better carbon dioxide elimination than nasal masks.[35] In most clinical scenarios the nasal mask is the preferred interface in pediatric-age patients. Newer generation nasal masks have a soft gel cushion (e.g., the Phantom nasal mask: SleepNet, Manchester, NH) that conforms to the contour of the face and forehead and are thus more comfortable. These models also minimize air leaks and facial trauma.

However, in critically ill patients even small oral air leaks are undesirable. Nasal-oral masks should be considered when absolute avoidance of an oral air leak is necessary. However, nasal-oral masks may pose a significant risk of aspiration of gastric contents in the event of emesis, and also may increase anxiety in young children. Under these conditions, sedation is often necessary, and the child should not be fed.

Nasal plugs or pillows can be substituted for nasal masks in children who complain of discomfort with the nasal mask. Nasal plugs or pillows are not used as often because most children eventually adapt to the nasal mask very well. They may have some role in teenagers as they place no pressure on the face and do not interfere with vision.

Nasal masks are commercially available in a wide range of sizes and shapes to fit children and adolescents. Unfortunately, soft nasal masks are not widely available for small infants. Masks may be custom-molded to fit individual patients in specific circumstances, such as in children with midfacial syndromes associated with maxillary hypoplasia. The nasal mask should fit snugly around the nasal margins. When the mask is too large, significant tension on the head straps is necessary to prevent mask leaks, thereby promoting dermal ulceration at the nasal bridge. Long-term intermittent NPPV by means of a nasal mask may impair maxillary bone growth. This concern, although not clearly supported by available evidence, is considered significant by caregivers of children treated with NPPV.

COMPLICATIONS AND CONTRAINDICATIONS TO NPPV

Pediatric-age patients are at relatively higher risk for complications to NPPV as a result of unique physiologic differences from adults (Table 21-2). However, in clinical experience, major complications with NPPV are unusual, while approximately 50% of children experience one or more minor complications. The most common minor complications reported include skin irritation due to the nasal mask, nasal dryness or discomfort, epistaxis, and eye irritation. One study found that prolonged use of maintenance steroids was an additional risk factor for development of skin ulcers during NPPV.[36] Epistaxis can be prevented by humidification,

TABLE 21-2

Factors Unique to Pediatric Patients That Promote Complications of NPPV

Complication	Factor Unique to Children
Aspiration	Immaturity of airway reflexes
Reflux	Impaired gastroesophageal sphincter function during infancy
Upper airway obstruction	Anatomic factors, difficulty clearing secretions
Large oral leak	Tendency to mouth breathe
Agitation	Anxiety, incomplete understanding, developmental disorders

whereas conjunctival irritation may be prevented by selection of appropriate-sized nasal mask. Despite these complaints, preliminary reports of adherence to intermittent NPPV in children with chronic hypoventilation disorders are surprisingly good and better than those reported for adult patients treated with nasal CPAP.[4]

The only absolute contraindication to a trial of NPPV in pediatric-age patients with acute respiratory distress is cardiovascular instability. Relative contraindications include nasopharyngeal obstruction, inability to handle oral secretions, and extreme agitation or anxiety.

FUTURE OF NONINVASIVE VENTILATION

A major impediment to the future of NPPV in infants and children is the reluctance of companies that manufacture bilevel ventilators to seek FDA approval of their devices for pediatric-age patients. This is primarily because of the cost of FDA approval and the relatively low volume of units expected to be sold in the pediatric market. The result is that clinicians who care for children with chronic hypoventilation disorders and who are attracted to NPPV as an alternative to TPPV become involved in funding disputes and legal conflicts with companies that dispense durable medical equipment.

Despite these constraints, the future for NPPV in pediatric-age patients is promising. Smaller interfaces and flow-triggered, pressure-targeted units suitable for small children are appearing for home use. Second-generation bilevel units already can achieve target inspiratory pressures of 30 cm H_2O and are equipped with independent oxygen adjustment settings. These units also come with a maximal inspiratory time setting so as to prevent prolonged inflations in the presence of uncompensated leaks. Proportion assist ventilation, a method of assisted ventilation that is responsive to the resistive and elastic properties of the respiratory system, can be administered by means of a nasal mask. This method of assisted ventilation is well beyond preliminary trials in adults and may have significant advantages over NPPV with current bilevel devices. At present NPPV treatment should be restricted to carefully selected children, and only in centers equipped with the appropriate equipment and experienced personnel. Randomized trials comparing early NPPV versus standard treatment in well-characterized patient populations are needed to clearly define the role of NPPV in children.

1. A patient is being masked and ventilated. What is the term for a method of respiratory assistance that does not require an indwelling artificial airway?
   A. Noninvasive
   B. Invasive
   C. Positive pressure
   D. Negative pressure
2. What complications(s) of NPPV can be specifically found in children?
   A. Aspiration and/or reflux
   B. Upper airway obstruction or large oral leak
   C. Agitation
   D. All of the above
3. What pitfall(s) is/are associated with NPPV in the pediatric patient?
   A. Poor fit
   B. Incorrect adjustments for inspiratory and expiratory pressures
   C. Insufficient sensitivity for infants
   D. All of the above
4. A 6-year-old patient has just been placed on NPPV. What is *not* the objective?
   A. To decrease the work of breathing
   B. To avoid intubation at all cost
   C. To increase alveolar ventilation
   D. To increase functional residual capacity
5. Why is NPPV not attempted more often?
   A. Lack of patient interfaces for the majority of the population
   B. It is easier to sedate and mechanically ventilate patients via an endotracheal tube
   C. Lack of conclusive evidence showing benefit when compared with invasive mechanical ventilation
   D. A and C
6. Name an advantage(s) of negative-pressure ventilation.
   A. Carbon dioxide may be removed without the need for a tracheostomy.
   B. It is more physiologic than positive-pressure ventilation.
   C. It is easily transportable.
   D. A and B
7. What is a relative contraindication to negative-pressure ventilation?
   A. Hypoventilation
   B. Thoracic trauma requiring an open wound or chest tubes
   C. Airway obstruction
   D. Chronic respiratory disease

Continued

ASSESSMENT QUESTIONS—cont'd

8. A patient is receiving ventilation at an IPAP setting of 10. What is IPAP?
   A. Inspiratory positive airway pressure
   B. Inspiratory position airway posture
   C. Peak positive airway pressure
   D. None of the above

9. How should the IPAP be set?
   A. To 5 cm H_2O above EPAP
   B. Above EPAP to increase tidal volume and "unload" the respiratory muscles, reducing the work of breathing
   C. Until an audible leak around the mask is heard, determining lung filling
   D. To 2 cm H_2O for every year of age, until the age of 10

10. A patient in the pediatric intensive care unit undergoes respiratory failure and has just been placed on NPPV. How should this device be monitored?
    A. As a piece of life support equipment
    B. It does not require monitoring
    C. Alarms are not required
    D. PRN spot checks

References

1. Make BJ et al: Management of pediatric patients requiring long-term ventilation, *Chest* 1998;113:289S-344S.
2. Marcus CL: Sleep disordered breathing in children, *Am J Respir Crit Care Med* 2001;164:16.
3. Hill NS et al: Efficacy of nocturnal nasal ventilation in patients with restrictive thoracic disease, *Am Rev Respir Dis* 1992;145:365.
4. Teague WG: Long term mechanical ventilation in infants and children. In Hill NS, editor: *Long-term mechanical ventilation*, New York. Marcel Dekker; 2001. pp 177-213.
5. Teague WG, Harsch A, Lesnick B: Non-invasive positive pressure ventilation as a long-term treatment for pediatric patients with chronic hypoventilation disorders [abstract], *Am J Respir Crit Care Med* 1999;159:297a.
6. Lin CH et al: Efficacy of nasal intermittent positive pressure ventilation in treating apnea of prematurity, *Pediatr Pulmonol* 1998;26:349.
7. Lemyre B, Davis PG, De Paoli AG: Nasal intermittent positive pressure ventilation (NIPPV) versus nasal continuous positive airway pressure (NCPAP) for apnea of prematurity, *Cochrane Database Syst Rev* 2000;3:CD002272.
8. Barrington KJ, Bull D, Finer NN: Randomized trial of nasal synchronized IMV compared with CPAP after extubation of VLBW infants, *Pediatrics* 2001;107:638.
9. Nabeel Khalaf M et al: A prospective randomized, controlled trial comparing synchronized nasal intermittent positive pressure ventilation versus nasal continuous positive airway pressure as modes of extubation, *Pediatrics* 2001;108:13.
10. Moretti C et al: Comparing the effects of nasal synchronized intermittent positive pressure ventilation (nSIPPV) and nasal continuous positive airway pressure (nCPAP) after extubation in very low birth weight infants, *Early Hum Dev* 1999;56:167.
11. Teague WG: Noninvasive ventilation in the pediatric intensive care unit for children with acute respiratory failure, *Pediatr Pulmonol* 2003;35:418.
12. Teague WG et al: Non-invasive positive pressure ventilation (NPPV) in critically ill children with status asthmaticus [abstract], *Am J Respir Crit Care Med* 1998;157:542a.
13. Keenan SP et al: Which patients with acute exacerbation of chronic obstructive pulmonary disease benefit from noninvasive positive-pressure ventilation? *Ann Intern Med* 2003;138:861.
14. Padman R, Lawless S, Kettrick RG: Noninvasive ventilation via bi-level positive airway pressure support in pediatric practice, *Crit Care Med* 1998;26:169.
15. Thill PJ et al: Noninvasive positive pressure ventilation in children with lower airway obstruction, *Pediatr Crit Care Med* 2004;5:337.
16. Rosen GM et al: Postoperative respiratory compromise in children with obstructive sleep apnea syndrome: can it be anticipated? *Pediatrics* 1994;93:784.
17. Hertzog JH et al: Noninvasive positive pressure ventilation facilitates tracheal extubation after laryngotracheal reconstruction in children, *Chest* 1999;116:260.
18. Khan Y, Heckmatt JZ: Obstructive apnoeas in Duchenne muscular dystrophy, *Thorax* 1994;49:157.
19. Labonowski M, Schmidt-Nowara W, Guilleminault C: Sleep and neuromuscular disease: frequency of sleep disordered breathing in a neuromuscular disease clinic population, *Neurology* 1996;47:1173.
20. Teague WG et al: Nasal bi-level positive airway pressure acutely improves ventilation and oxygen saturation in children with upper airway obstruction [abstract], *Am Rev Respir Dis* 1991;143:505a.
21. Gozal D: Nocturnal ventilatory support in patients with cystic fibrosis: comparison with supplemental oxygen, *Eur Respir J* 1997;10:1999.
22. Padman R et al: Noninvasive positive pressure ventilation in end-stage cystic fibrosis: a report of seven cases, *Respir Care* 1994;39:736.
23. Moran F et al: Noninvasive ventilation for cystic fibrosis, *Cochrane Database Syst Rev* 2007;3:CD002769.
24. Strumpf DA et al: An evaluation of the Respironics BiPAP bi-level CPAP device for delivery of assisted ventilation, *Respir Care* 1990;35:415.
25. Kacmarek RM: Characteristics of pressure-targeted ventilators used for noninvasive positive pressure ventilation, *Respir Care* 1997;42:380.
26. Bach JR: Prevention of morbidity and mortality with the use of physical medicine aids. In: Bach JR, editor: *Pulmonary rehabilitation: the obstructive and paralytic conditions*, Philadelphia: Hanley and Belfus; 1996. pp 303-329.
27. Keens TG, Jansen MT, DeWitt PK: Home care for children with chronic respiratory failure, *Semin Respir Med* 1990;11:269.
28. Samuels MP, Southall DP: Negative extrathoracic pressure in the treatment of respiratory failure in infants and young children, *BMJ* 1989;299:1253.

29. Hartmann H et al: Negative extrathoracic pressure ventilation in central hypoventilation syndrome, *Arch Dis Child* 1994;70:418.

30. Al-balkhi A et al: Review of treatment of bronchiolitis related apnea in two centres, *Arch Dis Child* 2005;90:224.

31. Fauroux B et al: Chronic stridor caused by laryngomalacia in children: work of breathing and effects of noninvasive ventilatory assistance, *Am J Respir Crit Care Med* 2001;164:1874.

32. Antonelli M et al: Risk factors for failure of non-invasive ventilation in acute hypoxemic respiratory failure: a multicenter study, *Intensive Care Med* 1999;25:S56.

33. American Thoracic Society, European Respiratory Society, European Society of Intensive Care Medicine, Société de Réanimation de Langue Française: International consensus conferences in intensive care medicine: noninvasive positive pressure ventilation in acute respiratory failure, *Am J Respir Crit Care Med* 2001;163:283.

34. Piper AJ, Sullivan CE: Effects of short-term NIPPV in the treatment of patients with severe obstructive sleep apnea and hypercapnia, *Chest* 1994;105:434.

35. Navales P et al: physiologic evaluation of noninvasive mechanical ventilation delivered with three types of mask in patients with chronic hypercapnic respiratory failure, *Crit Care Med* 2000;28:1785.

36. Meecham Jones DJ, Braid GM, Wedzicha JA: Nasal masks for domiciliary positive pressure ventilation: patient usage and complications, *Thorax* 1994;49:811.

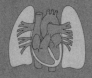

Chapter 22

Administration of Gas Mixtures

MARK ROGERS

OUTLINE

Nitric Oxide
  Physiological Basis of Action
  Application
Helium–Oxygen Mixtures
  Physiologic Basis of Action
  Application

Hypoxic and Hypercarbic Gas Mixtures
  Physiologic Basis of Action
  Application
Anesthetic Mixtures
  Physiologic Basis of Action
  Application

LEARNING OBJECTIVES

After reading this chapter the reader will be able to:
- Identify the basic chemical properties of nitric oxide
- Describe the process of smooth muscle contraction and relaxation
- Differentiate between intravenous vasodilators (such as nitroprusside or prostaglandin E) and inhaled nitric oxide regarding ventilation–perfusion matching and shunt
- Identify the potential side effects of inhaled nitric oxide
- Describe the beneficial properties of helium when used medically
- Describe how heliox affects nebulizers, flowmeters, and mechanical ventilators

- Describe what effects hypoxic and hypercarbic gas mixtures have on pulmonary circulation, and what types of patients would benefit from its use
- List safeguards that must be used to ensure patient safety when using hypoxic or hypercarbic gas mixtures
- List the inhaled anesthetic agents that are commonly used to treat status asthmaticus
- Identify which inhaled anesthetic agents are best tolerated by mask
- List the physiologic effects of inhaled anesthetic agents

One of the primary goals of critical care is to optimize oxygen delivery to the tissues. Frequently this entails the delivery of supplemental oxygen. However, other gases may be used to improve oxygen delivery, based on the patient's clinical diagnosis. The gases discussed in this chapter dilate the pulmonary vasculature, constrict the pulmonary vasculature, reduce airway resistance, and relax bronchial smooth muscle tone.

NITRIC OXIDE

Nitric oxide (NO) is a colorless, sweet-smelling, non-flammable toxic gas. Nitric oxide, not to be confused with *nitrous* oxide (N_2O, an anesthetic), is also an unstable, highly reactive, lipophilic, diatomic free radical. Because of its high reactivity, NO is often combined with nitrogen in various concentrations and stored in aluminum alloy cylinders. The most common concentration available commercially is 800 ppm, although higher and lower concentrations are available as well.

Physiologic Basis of Action

Nitric oxide is a ubiquitous substance produced by nearly every cell and organ in the human body (Box 22-1). Directly or indirectly, NO performs numerous functions, including vasodilation, platelet inhibition, immune regulation, enzyme regulation, and neurotransmission.[1] This chapter, however, focuses on smooth muscle relaxation of the pulmonary vascular bed.

Pulmonary Smooth Muscle Relaxation and Contraction

An understanding of the mechanism of smooth muscle relaxation in the pulmonary vascular bed is based on the regulation of smooth muscle tone. In general, smooth muscle tone is regulated by chemical, hormonal, nervous, and physical interactions.[2] Current understanding suggests that vascular smooth muscle is largely dependent on intracellular calcium ion (Ca^{2+}) concentration. Smooth muscle tissue comprises bundles of myofibrils, threadlike contractile fibers encased by the sarcoplasmic reticulum, a network of tubes or channels that store Ca^{2+}. Muscle contraction begins with the release of Ca^{2+} from the sarcoplasmic reticulum. Calcium ion binds with the protein calmodulin. The calcium-calmodulin complex activates the enzyme myosin light-chain kinase, enabling phosphorylation of the myosin,

resulting in contraction of the cell. Contraction continues until Ca^{2+} is reabsorbed into the sarcoplasmic reticulum. Therefore, any process that inhibits the release of Ca^{2+} will interrupt smooth muscle contraction.

In the body, the process of smooth muscle relaxation uses cyclic guanosine monophosphate (cGMP) to reduce Ca^{2+} levels. In smooth muscle cells, cGMP activates cGMP-dependent kinase, preventing the release of Ca^{2+} from the sarcoplasmic reticulum, resulting in smooth muscle relaxation. In the early 1980s, researchers reported a potent smooth muscle–relaxing agent, endothelium-derived relaxing factor (EDRF),[3] now understood to be endogenous nitric oxide. Formation of EDRF results in increased levels of cGMP in smooth muscle cells. EDRF and cGMP are conceivably the two most important substances in regulating smooth muscle tone.[2,4]

Nitric Oxide Synthase and Endogenous Nitric Oxide Production

In the body, NO is produced by the combination of nitric oxide synthase (NOS) enzymes with the amino acid L-arginine and molecular oxygen. This combination results in the formation of the amino acid L-citrulline and NO (Figure 22-1). The two types of NOS enzymes are constitutive and inducible. The *constitutive* NOS (cNOS) enzymes are normally expressed in tissues and consist of two isoforms: eNOS (endothelial in origin) and nNOS (neuronal in origin).[1] The one *inducible*

Box 22-1	Organs and Cells Involved in the Endogenous Production of Nitric Oxide

- Brain
- Peripheral nerves
- Skeletal muscle
- Liver
- Myocytes
- Epithelium
- Platelets
- Adrenals
- Macrophages
- Lungs

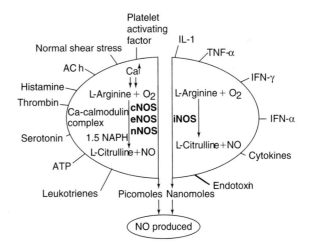

FIGURE 22-1 Endogenous nitric oxide (NO) production. Under normal conditions, picomoles of NO are produced. When inducible nitric acid synthase is activated in conditions of sepsis or inflammation, nanomoles of NO are produced. ACh, Acetylcholine; ATP, adenosine triphosphate; cNOS, constitutive nitric oxide synthase; eNOS, endogenous nitric oxide synthase; IFN, interferon; IL, interleukin; iNOS, induced nitric oxide synthase; nNOS, neuronal nitric oxide synthase; TNF, tumor necrosis factor.

NOS enzyme, iNOS, results from enzyme induction.[5] The cNOS enzymes, which are calmodulin dependent, produce relatively small amounts of NO (picomoles). The iNOS enzyme functions independently of calmodulin and produces relatively large amounts of NO (nanomoles). NO resulting from iNOS is most often produced in sepsis and is probably responsible for the pathologic decrease in systemic vascular resistance observed in septic shock.

Once NO is formed and bound to hemoglobin, guanylyl cyclase is activated, which converts cyclic guanidine triphosphate to cGMP. This increased cGMP results in reduced Ca^{2+} and smooth muscle relaxation.

Inhaled Nitric Oxide

The underlying principle of inhaled nitric oxide (iNO) is its selectivity as a pulmonary vasodilator.[6] Inhaled NO will relax only pulmonary smooth muscle adjacent to functioning alveoli. Atelectatic or fluid-filled lung units will not participate in iNO uptake. Therefore, if the pulmonary vasculature is constricted in atelectatic regions of the lung, pulmonary blood flow will remain minimal in these regions, reducing intrapulmonary shunt (Figure 22-2). This is in contrast to intravenous vasodilators such as nitroprusside or prostacyclin. These drugs will relax pulmonary vasculature globally, reducing pulmonary vascular resistance, but also increasing blood flow past nonfunctioning alveoli and intrapulmonary right-to-left shunt.

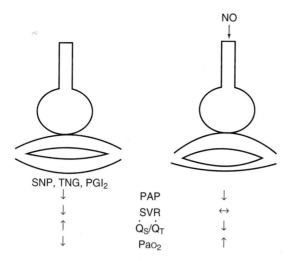

FIGURE 22-2 Comparison of the vasodilator effects from systemic drugs and NO. Both reduce pulmonary artery pressure, but the systemic vasodilators also dilate the blood vessels not participating in gas exchange, thereby increasing the intrapulmonary shunt. Pa_{O_2}, Arterial partial pressure of oxygen; PAP, pulmonary artery pressure; PGI_2, prostacyclin; $\dot{Q}_S/\dot{Q}_T$, intrapulmonary shunt; SNP, sodium nitroprusside; SVR, systemic vascular resistance; TNG, nitroglycerin.

Newborn Hypoxic Respiratory Failure. The concept of treating pulmonary hypertension of term or near-term infants with iNO has been advocated in many early reports and randomized controlled trials. These studies confirmed that iNO improved oxygenation and reduced the need for extracorporeal membrane oxygenation. In 2000 the first U.S. Food and Drug Administration (FDA) approval of iNO as a noninvestigative drug was for the treatment of primary pulmonary hypertension of the term or near-term (>34 weeks gestational age) neonate with hypoxic respiratory failure associated with evidence of pulmonary hypertension. Hypoxic respiratory failure may be primary or a secondary effect of another disorder (meconium aspiration, congenital diaphragmatic hernia, pneumonia, etc.).

Dosing strategies should be focused on physiologic end points.[7] This involves titrating the delivered NO in increments until a positive response is achieved. Several studies[8-13] have used an increase in oxygen saturation of 20% over baseline as an indication that the infant is responsive. These studies and others[14,15] have suggested that optimal dosing is usually in the 20- to 30-ppm range. Some infants will not respond positively. The Neonatal Inhaled Nitric Oxide Study (NINOS) trial[16] indicated that only 6% of nonresponders will demonstrate a positive response when given NO at 80 ppm. Typically, a response would be seen almost immediately; however, it is recommended[7] that determining an infant's response last no longer than 4 hours to limit the exposure to NO. Endogenous NO is downregulated when the patient receives iNO. This may result in a worsening of pulmonary hypertension and hypoxemia.[17,18]

Although there is strong evidence for the use of iNO in term or near-term infants, its efficacy in premature babies is less clear. Nitric oxide has been shown to improve oxygenation and outcomes in a few studies. However, larger randomized controlled trials[19-22] and a systematic review[23] have demonstrated similar improvements in oxygenation, but survival outcomes were unchanged. The preterm population is at increased risk for intraventricular hemorrhage and chronic lung disease. These larger, more recent trials did not show any increase in these comorbidities. Therefore, although its usefulness is still in question, NO does appear to be safe in the premature infant population.

Acute Respiratory Distress Syndrome. Current research is investigating the use of NO in acute respiratory distress syndrome (ARDS) and acute lung injury. ARDS is a complex syndrome characterized by noncardiogenic pulmonary edema, diminished lung compliance, and pulmonary hypertension. Current therapy for ARDS is primarily supportive, allowing time for the lung to heal. Although no definitive studies show improved outcomes, iNO has been suggested to improve oxygenation and ventilation–perfusion ($\dot{V}/\dot{Q}$) matching, consequently lowering airway pressure and oxygen concentration. However, studies investigating the use of iNO for the treatment of ARDS or acute lung injury have failed to demonstrate improved outcomes. NO will reach more capillary endothelium by opening collapsed alveoli. In turn, a greater degree of vasorelaxation should occur. Studies have shown that responsiveness to iNO may be enhanced by the application of positive end-expiratory pressure, and perhaps turn nonresponders into responders (to iNO therapy).[24-26] In the pediatric population, Kinsella and colleagues[27] reported improved outcomes when using high-frequency oscillatory ventilation (HFOV) combined with iNO compared with HFOV or iNO alone. Mehta and colleagues[28] also studied the combined effects of iNO and HFOV; the rationale being that if lung volume were optimized they could further enhance the effects of iNO. They demonstrated that the use of HFOV did improve oxygenation response to iNO.[37] Further studies are warranted to determine whether this combination is clinically useful.

Application

Multiple methods have been advocated for the delivery of iNO.[29,30] Early systems were custom-built in-house and comprised two basic subsystems: delivery and monitoring. In these systems, NO is bled into the breathing circuit through a flowmeter or blender. NO and NO_2 levels are monitored with an NO/NO_2 analyzer (Figure 22-3). These systems were cumbersome and were often difficult to assemble. Now that the use of iNO has increased, a few vendors have developed systems incorporating NO delivery with NO and NO_2 monitoring. These devices come in a variety of designs. Some are larger and designed for in-hospital use (Figure 22-4). Others are small battery-operated devices and may be used for interfacility transport (Figure 22-5).

In general, NO is bled into the breathing circuit before the humidifier. To analyze *inspired* NO and NO_2 concentrations, gas is sampled before the patient–circuit interface. These devices provide alarms to monitor these values, as well as oxygen. The Datex-Ohmeda INOVent (GE Healthcare, Waukesha, Wis) and ViaNOx-ds (PulmoNOx Medical, Tofield, Alberta, Canada) measure ventilator circuit gas flow. These flow measurements allow the device to modulate NO output to provide a stable concentration throughout the breath.

Nitrogen Dioxide

As discussed earlier, when combined with oxygen, NO produces NO_2, a toxic gas. Although rare, the patient as well as health care providers can be adversely affected. Factors influencing NO_2 production are oxygen concentration, NO concentration, and time of contact between NO and oxygen. Therefore the patients most at risk of NO_2 delivery include those receiving high oxygen concentrations and low ventilator flow rates.

Decreasing the NO or oxygen concentration is usually not an option; therefore, to reduce NO_2 delivery to the patient, reduce the duration of contact between NO and oxygen. Two methods accomplish this: (1) increase the inspiratory flow or (2) add the NO as close to the patient as possible. Each of these methods has practical limitations. Increasing the ventilator flow will reduce the time of contact between NO and oxygen before

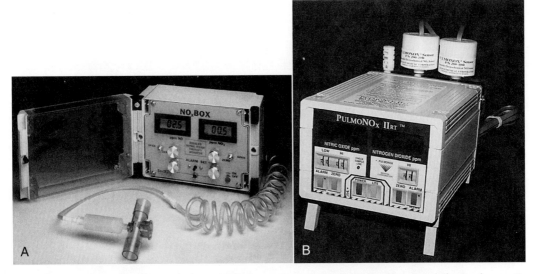

FIGURE 22-3 Small, battery-operated, stand-alone NO/NO_2 monitors: **A,** No$_x$BOX (Bedfont Scientific, Rochester, Kent, UK); **B,** PulmoNO$_x$ IIRT (PulmoNOx Medical, Tofield, Alberta, Canada).

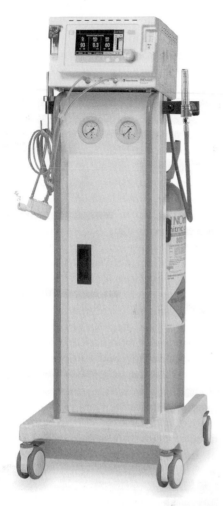

FIGURE 22-4 Datex-Ohmeda INOVent (GE Healthcare, Waukesha, Wis), a stand-alone NO delivery and monitoring device. Versions are available for use in the operating room and for transport.

reaching the patient, but it may also affect inspiratory time, tidal volume, mean airway pressure, and so on. Adding NO into the inspiratory limb of the ventilator circuit close to the patient will reduce contact time, but it also creates monitoring difficulties. The practitioner must allow an adequate distance for proper mixing to ensure accurate NO measurement.

In addition, the local atmosphere could become contaminated with NO and NO_2. Although this is rare, early systems included means for the scavenging of expiratory and wasted gases. Usually this was accomplished by the collection of gases into a gas evacuation system similar in design to those used in anesthesia. Gas was collected in a large reservoir and removed continuously through the hospital's vacuum system. At first, scavenging was advocated to reduce the possible harmful inhalation of nitrogen dioxide by other personnel in the vicinity. Studies have shown this to be unnecessary because of the relatively small amounts of NO_2 present at the bedside. Modern hospitals have adequate room air exchange rates, and the chance of NO or NO_2 accumulation is remote. A possible caveat involves interfacility transport. Pressurized aircraft may not allow an adequate cabin air exchange rate to ensure safety. The aircraft crew must be made aware of this so that proper measures are taken to reduce this risk.

Methemoglobin

The half-life of iNO is extremely short, about five seconds. Once NO crosses the vascular endothelium, it is rapidly bound by hemoglobin, forming nitrosyl hemoglobin (methemoglobin). Methemoglobin production results from the oxidation of the iron in the hemoglobin.[31] The quantity of methemoglobin depends on iNO

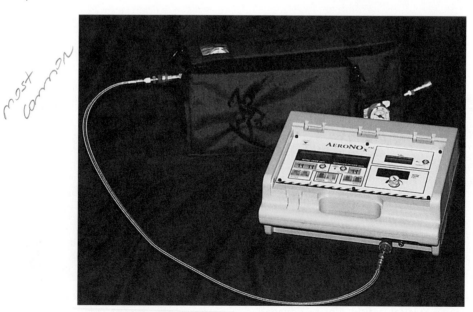

FIGURE 22-5 AeroNO$_x$ (International Biomedical, Austin, Tex), a small stand-alone delivery and monitoring device designed for transport.

concentration and concurrent nitrate-based drug therapy (e.g., nitroprusside, nitroglycerin). If the methemoglobin level is excessive, a reduction in iNO or other nitro-based vasodilators is warranted. Ultimately, NO metabolites are excreted, primarily by the kidneys, as nitrates and nitrites.[32]

HELIUM–OXYGEN MIXTURES

Helium (He) was discovered in 1895 by Sir William Ramsay and independently by Langley and Cleve. Helium is one of the lightest elements, second only to hydrogen. It is a colorless, odorless, tasteless, and physiologically inert noble gas. Helium is present in dry air at a concentration of 0.0005%. At present, the majority of helium comes from natural gas mines in the United States. The supply is limited, and until the Helium Privatization Act of 1996, production was under the control of the U.S. government.

Helium is remarkable for its low density and high viscosity (Table 22-1). Pure helium gas has a density of 0.179 g/L, one-seventh the density of air. A common misconception is that because of its low density, helium has low viscosity. Actually, helium is slightly more viscous than air. However, its kinematic viscosity (the ratio of absolute viscosity to density) is almost seven times greater than that of air. Therefore, from the standpoint of fluid dynamics, helium is much more viscous than air.[33]

Physiologic Basis of Action

The use of helium-oxygen mixtures in treating airway obstruction was first described in 1934 by Barach.[34-37] Barach's studies reported a decrease in work of breathing in patients with both upper and lower airway obstruction. Helium is an inert gas, has no pharmacologic properties of its own, and does not participate in or interfere with any biochemical activity in the body. Its sole purpose is to lower the total density of any gas mixture.

It is important to note that helium is not used to treat the underlying cause of increased airway resistance, but rather to decrease the work of breathing until more definitive therapies are effective. When helium is combined with oxygen, the resulting gas mixture density is one third that of air. Poiseuille's law states: if the diameter of a tube is reduced by half, the pressure gradient to achieve the same flow increases 16 times. Graham's law states that the flow of gas through an orifice is inversely proportional to the square root of its density.[38] In other words: if the driving pressure remains constant, a gas with lower density will have higher flow than a gas with higher density. Alternatively, less pressure is required to maintain a given flow through a fixed orifice. This physical property of helium may be useful in overcoming airway resistance and obstruction.

In normal human anatomy, inspired gas is turbulent between the glottis and the tenth-generation airways, primarily because of the high gas flow and larger radii of the airways. Physics dictates that greater pressure is required to move gas through a tube (or airway) under turbulent conditions compared with the same volume of gas during laminar flow. A quick review of Reynold's equation shows that decreasing density and increasing viscosity will reduce turbulent flow, decreasing the pressure and work required to move the gas (Box 22-2). Likewise, gas flow through a large, partially obstructed airway will create the same turbulent flow. Decreasing turbulent flow reduces the amount of pressure required to move the gas through the airways, decreasing the work required to breathe.

Application

Helium must be combined with oxygen when used clinically, thus the term *heliox*. Several concentrations of medical-grade helium are available commercially: 80% helium–20% oxygen heliox mixture (80:20), 70% helium–30% oxygen (70:30), and 100% helium–0% oxygen (100%). The 80:20 mixture has essentially the same concentration of oxygen as air; the nitrogen and trace gases are replaced with helium. The 70:30 mixture is useful for patients with airway obstruction who require increased oxygen concentration. The 100% helium concentration is unique; it must be used with oxygen to be compatible with life. Extreme caution and close monitoring must be employed when using this concentration as it is possible to deliver a hypoxic gas mixture to the patient, possibly resulting in asphyxiation and death.

For the purposes of this chapter, only the use of nonhypoxic gas mixtures is discussed. Heliox cylinders containing at least 20% oxygen are brown and white (or brown and green) and use a CGA-280 fitting.

TABLE 22-1

Comparison of Inhaled Gas Densities and Viscosities

	Density (g/L)	Viscosity (μP)
Helium	0.179	188.7
Nitrogen	1.25	167.4
Air	1.29	170.8
Oxygen	1.42	192.6

Box 22-2 — Reynold's Equation for Turbulent Flow

$$\text{Reynold's Number} = \frac{\text{Flow} \times \text{Diameter} \times \text{Density}}{\text{Viscosity}}$$

Laminar ≤ 2000 ≥ Turbulent

Aerosol Delivery

Multiple studies have investigated the use of helium–oxygen mixtures and the deposition of aerosolized particles.[39-42] Anderson and colleagues[39] studied patients with stable asthma. Ten patients inhaled radiolabeled particles of Teflon suspended in air or a helium–oxygen mixture. The study concluded there was more aerosol deposition in the lung and less deposition in the upper airways when breathing helium–oxygen mixtures. In a similar study, 42 patients were randomly assigned to receive β-agonists with helium–oxygen mixtures or air.[43] Patients who used the helium–oxygen mixtures showed more improvement in expiratory peak flows than the group using air. These studies support the concept that aerosol has deeper and prolonged deposition in the lung when it is delivered with heliox as the carrier gas.

Heliox mixtures will cause pneumatic nebulizers to perform differently than if air or oxygen is used. When driving a pneumatic nebulizer with helium, the nebulizer will produce smaller particles, nebulize more slowly, and have reduced output compared with similar devices driven with air. When using a conventional pneumatic nebulizer driven with heliox, it is advisable it increase gas flow.[44] This will increase drug output by producing denser aerosol and larger particles.

Flowmeters

Helium is less dense, and therefore more diffusible than oxygen. As a consequence, standard oxygen flowmeters will indicate an incorrect flow when used with helium-containing mixtures. This error will cause the indicated flow to be erroneously low. An 80:20 heliox mixture is 1.8 times more diffusible than oxygen. To correct for the difference in gas density, the indicated flow on the flowmeter is multiplied by 1.8. A 70:30 heliox mixture is 1.6 times more diffusible than oxygen. To obtain the accurate flow rate for this mixture, the indicated flow is multiplied by 1.6. This error will be present in most gas-measuring devices (see later discussion in this section).

Spontaneously Breathing Patients

Spontaneously breathing patients with upper or lower airway obstruction can be given heliox via mask. Because the goal of heliox therapy is to reduce the density of the inspired gas, it is important to deliver the greatest concentration of helium. Therefore, the patient must be able to tolerate the lowest possible fractional concentration of inspired oxygen (FIO_2), and room air entrainment must be minimized, resulting in a higher fractional concentration of inspired helium (FI_{He}). Nasal cannulas and simple masks allow far too much room air entrainment, thereby diluting the helium concentration. Therefore, a close-fitting nonrebreathing mask should be used. This limitation makes the treatment of young patients difficult. Children in distress may not tolerate the tightly fitting mask required to minimize air entrainment. Stillwell and colleagues[45] investigated the use of heliox mixtures delivered through an infant hood. Not surprisingly, they found a greater concentration of helium at the top of the hood (due to its lower gas density), away from the infant's nose and mouth. This resulted in a lower FI_{He} and therefore a denser gas being delivered to the infant.

Mechanically Ventilated Patients

Unfortunately, many patients with airway obstruction must be mechanically ventilated to manage respiratory failure and to reduce their work of breathing. This presents the practitioner with a new set of challenges. Patients with severe lower airway obstruction (as seen in status asthmaticus) have reduced expiratory flows. The resulting increased expiratory times could lead to air trapping, barotrauma, and hemodynamic compromise. The use of heliox mixtures has been advocated to minimize air trapping and to reduce peak inspiratory pressures when mechanically ventilating a patient with severe lower airway obstruction.

The primary obstacle to heliox delivery via a mechanical ventilator is error in volume and flow measurement. Many mechanical ventilators rely on gas density to measure flows and volumes. Most errors result from underestimation of flow due to the low-density characteristics of helium. Volume is typically a mathematical integration of flow and time; therefore volumes will be equally affected. In one study the Servo 900C (Maquet, Bridgewater, NJ) demonstrated a statistically significant (approximately 10%) underestimation in volume measurement at a helium concentration of 50%, increasing to a 20% error at a helium concentration of 80%.[46] This error in flow and volume is also seen in external monitors as well. In the same study the VenTrak pulmonary monitor (Novametrix/Philips Respironics, Murrysville, Pa) underestimated volume by 20% at a helium concentration of 20%, increasing to a 40% error at a helium concentration of 80%.

The most popular method to deliver helium–oxygen mixtures via mechanical ventilation is to connect the heliox mixture to the air inlet of the mechanical ventilator. The practitioner then uses the ventilator's oxygen concentration control to adjust helium and oxygen to the desired mixture. This allows the practitioner to deliver a helium concentration up to the concentration of the heliox cylinder. It is important to note that some ventilators may not function properly with helium as a source gas. For example, the Puritan Bennett 7200 or 840 (Covidien, Mansfield, Mass) will not function properly if helium is connected to the air inlet. This anomaly appears to be related to the heated-wire flow anemometer on the gas inlets. The high thermal conductivity of helium rapidly cools the wires, simulating a high-flow condition. The microprocessor responds by closing the gas inlet valve to such a degree that the ventilator will not function. As always, it is important to monitor oxygen concentration when using heliox.

Four devices in the United States have been cleared by the U.S. FDA for use with helium mixtures: the AVEA (Cardinal Health, Dublin, Ohio), the Servo-*i* (Maquet, Bridgewater, NJ), Hamilton G5 (Hamilton Medical, Reno NV), and the Datex-Ohmeda Aptaér (GE Healthcare, Madison, WI).

HYPOXIC AND HYPERCARBIC GAS MIXTURES

The primary goal of the practitioner is to maximize oxygen delivery to the tissues. To achieve this goal, hypoxic (less than 21% oxygen) or hypercarbic gas mixtures may be used. Oxygen is a potent pulmonary vasodilator, and conversely, carbon dioxide is an equally potent pulmonary vasoconstrictor. Knowing these effects allows the practitioner to alter pulmonary and systemic blood flow by manipulating pulmonary vascular resistance (PVR) in infants with congenital cardiac lesions.

Physiologic Basis of Action

Hypoxic or hypercarbic gas therapy may be beneficial in infants with certain lesions when pulmonary blood flow may be excessive through the ductus arteriosus, as in hypoplastic left-sided heart syndrome (HLHS) and single-ventricle syndromes. Cardiac lesions are addressed in Chapter 30 (Congenital Cardiac Defects); this section focuses on HLHS as a representative physiology.

Infants with HLHS present with a constellation of cardiac disorders, including small or absent left ventricle, aortic and mitral stenosis, and hypoplasia of the ascending aorta. Because little or no blood is ejected from the left ventricle, pulmonary as well as systemic blood flow originates from the right ventricle. Blood returning from the lungs is shunted from the left atrium to the right atrium via an atrial septal defect. Systemic blood flow is supplied entirely from right-to-left flow through a patent ductus arteriosus (PDA). Preoperative survival of the patient depends on a PDA and an elevated PVR. Preoperatively, the PDA is maintained with prostaglandin E_1 and judicious use of oxygen.

In these patients a delicate balance exists between pulmonary blood flow ($\dot{Q}p$) and systemic blood flow ($\dot{Q}s$). Changes in PVR and systemic vascular resistance affect $\dot{Q}p$ and $\dot{Q}s$ directly. This relationship can be expressed as the ratio between $\dot{Q}p$ and $\dot{Q}s$. A $\dot{Q}p/\dot{Q}s$ ratio greatly exceeding 1.0 will result in systemic hypoperfusion, circulatory shock, decreased renal blood flow, and metabolic acidosis. A $\dot{Q}p/\dot{Q}s$ ratio much less than 1.0 results in pulmonary hypoperfusion leading to systemic oxygen debt.[47,48] In general, $\dot{Q}p$ should be approximately one third to one half of $\dot{Q}s$.[49]

Supportive therapy before palliative or corrective surgery may require the use of hypoxic gas mixtures to increase PVR, thereby promoting systemic blood flow. Because PVR and systemic vascular resistance are not typically measured in infants, other means are needed to gauge the $\dot{Q}p/\dot{Q}s$ ratio. Typically, these patients are managed on an F_{IO_2} of 0.18 to 0.21, achieving an arterial oxygen saturation of 75% to 85%. Clinically, extremity temperature, color, and blood pressure are usually sufficient to assess systemic blood flow. If the patient has cool extremities but is pink, $\dot{Q}p/\dot{Q}s$ is probably too high. Conversely, if the patient has warm extremities but is cyanotic, $\dot{Q}p/\dot{Q}s$ is probably too low. Ongoing clinical examinations are required to assess the appropriateness of hypoxic gas mixture therapy.

At times the PVR cannot be increased without decreasing F_{IO_2} to precipitous levels (<18%). Increasing the infant's partial pressure of arterial carbon dioxide (Pa_{CO_2}) would be clinically advantageous. Although it is possible to allow the infant's Pa_{CO_2} to increase secondary to alveolar hypoventilation, this technique may lead to atelectasis. The use of hypercarbic gas therapy has been advocated to increase PVR further while maintaining a safe F_{IO_2} and alveolar ventilation. These patients are typically managed on a fractional concentration of inspired carbon dioxide ($F_{I_{CO_2}}$) of 0.02 to 0.05.

Extracorporeal Membrane Oxygenation

Some patients require extracorporeal membrane oxygenation to achieve adequate gas exchange (see Chapter 23, Extracorporeal Life Support). As gas from a blender passes through the oxygenator cartridge, gas exchange occurs. The oxygen in this gas oxygenates the blood. Carbon dioxide diffuses from the blood into the sweep gas. The membrane oxygenator in the extracorporeal membrane oxygenation circuit is efficient, and sometimes too efficient, in exchanging gases with the blood. When the sweep gas (gas flow through the membrane lung; usually 100% oxygen) through the oxygenator removes too much CO_2 from the blood, carbogen may be substituted as the sweep gas to inhibit excessive CO_2 removal. Carbogen is a mixture of 95% oxygen and 5% carbon dioxide.

Application

In principle the application of hypoxic gas therapy is straightforward. The gas delivery device (oxygen hood or mechanical ventilator) is set to deliver 21% oxygen. Nitrogen is then added to the gas flow before humidification (Figure 22-6). Whenever hypoxic gas mixtures

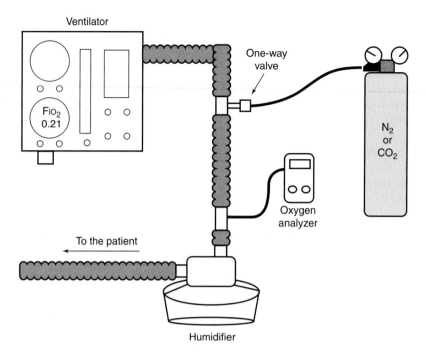

FIGURE 22-6 Subambient oxygen therapy is achieved by introducing a flow of nitrogen (N_2) into the inspired gas stream of a ventilator circuit before it reaches the humidification system.

are used, extreme care must be used to monitor the gas delivered to reduce the chance of suffocation. The oxygen analyzer must be capable of measuring the lowest oxygen concentration to be used (17% to 18%). In addition, low-oxygen alarms must be set at that low oxygen concentration. Many commercially available oxygen analyzers limit the low-oxygen alarm, and therefore the practitioner must ensure that the analyzer used is capable of monitoring (with alarms) at an oxygen concentration of 17% to 18%.

In general, the delivery of hypercarbic gas mixtures follows the same procedure as for hypoxic gas mixtures. Carbon dioxide is added to the main gas flow of the device (oxygen hood or mechanical ventilator) before any humidification. The resulting mixture is analyzed near the patient for oxygen and carbon dioxide. Hypoxic gas and hypercarbic gas may be combined for increased effect.

ANESTHETIC MIXTURES

Patients in status asthmaticus (SA) can be placed on helium–oxygen therapy as a temporizing measure to reduce the work of breathing until other therapy (β-agonists, methylxanthines, and corticosteroids) is effective. However, these patients frequently have bronchospasm that is refractory to conventional therapy. Certain volatile inhaled anesthetics are known for their bronchodilatory properties. Although no clinical trials have investigated the use of inhaled anesthetics (IAs) in the routine treatment of SA, several case reports exist.[50-55]

Of the several IAs used clinically for anesthesia, only a few (halothane, isoflurane, enflurane, and sevoflurane) have been widely reported as potential treatments for SA. *Halothane* is an alkane derivative and has been the volatile anesthetic of choice in reducing bronchospasm in asthmatic patients. Sevoflurane, a methyl ethyl ether, has been shown to be as effective as halothane in reducing lung resistance; however, safety studies for its use in children with asthma are needed.[51,56,57] Isoflurane and enflurane are also methyl ethyl ethers and are often used in the acute treatment of SA. Each has advantages and disadvantages in treating bronchospasm (Table 22-2).

Physiologic Basis of Action

Volatile IAs reduce bronchospasm through a number of pathways: β-adrenergic receptor stimulation, direct smooth muscle relaxation, antagonism of acetylcholine and histamine, and inhibition of hypocapneic bronchoconstriction.[58] In essence, they reduce central afferent parasympathetic activity.[59] Therefore a patient receiving standard bronchodilators may see an additional response with the addition of an IA.[60]

Application

The setup and delivery of IAs must be performed by qualified individuals, usually anesthesiologists. Most states expressly prohibit respiratory care practitioners from delivering anesthetic agents; some, however, will allow their use for nonanesthetic purposes (e.g., for bronchodilation).

TABLE 22-2

Comparison of Inhaled Anesthetic Agents

	Halothane	Isoflurane	Enflurane	Sevoflurane
Mean arterial pressure	↓	↓↓↓	↓↓	↓
Pulmonary vascular resistance	—	↓↓	↓	↓
Heart rate	↓	↑	↑↑	↑
Cardiac output	↓↓	—	↓↓↓	—
Airway irritant	—	↑↑	↑↑	—
Respiratory depression	↑	↑	↑↑	↑
Myocardial sensitization to catecholamines	↑↑↑↑	—	—	—
Risk of explosion	—	—	—	—

In general, the anesthesiologist performs the initial setup and troubleshooting. Adjustments are usually done by the intensive care physician or anesthesiologist. The bedside caregiver handles routine monitoring procedures. All caregivers must understand the pharmacology of the IA being delivered and its side effect profile.

The two ways to deliver IAs are by face mask for the spontaneously breathing patient and through a mechanical ventilator. In either system the setup is similar to that used in the operating room. Both methods require similar equipment: vaporizers for the volatile anesthetic, scavenging devices, anesthetic gas analyzers, and vital sign monitoring.

Inhaled Anesthetics via Face Mask

To avoid intubation and mechanical ventilation, treating the spontaneously breathing patient with an IA could be advantageous. The systems used for spontaneous breathing of IAs are complicated, but are similar to full-face noninvasive continuous positive airway pressure circuits. The expiratory gases pass through a carbon dioxide absorber and then return to the inspiratory limb, creating a circle. A fresh gas supply (including the IA) is introduced after the carbon dioxide absorber. This design is called a *rebreathing circuit.*

The face mask must be tight fitting to prevent the leakage of the IA into the room and to ensure that the patient receives the IA. Because patients may be somewhat awake, they must be cooperative enough not to remove the mask. The IA must also be compatible with face mask administration. Enflurane and isoflurane are irritants to the upper airway and are unpleasant to breathe while conscious, especially for the pediatric patient. These vapors may produce laryngospasm and fighting. Isoflurane and enflurane are more suited for use with an intubated and mechanically ventilated patient. Conversely, halothane and sevoflurane are neutral-smelling vapors and may be accepted more readily via mask.

Typically, halothane is the IA of choice when delivering to a conscious, spontaneously breathing patient. The dose range for halothane is approximately 0.25% to 0.5%. The patient usually is sufficiently awake to communicate in short sentences. Bronchodilation is usually rapid (15 to 20 min). The patient benefits by the reduced resistance as well as the sedative effect.

Inhaled Anesthetics via Mechanical Ventilation

Almost universally, the Servo 900C is used to deliver IAs to mechanically ventilated patients. Although not the most modern pediatric ventilator, the 900C is designed for inhalation anesthesia. Using a conversion kit, the 900C can easily be converted to a device with anesthesia capability. The ventilator itself is set up in the usual way; the outlet of the anesthesia vaporizer is then connected to the low-pressure inlet of the 900C.

Waste anesthetic agent may pose a risk for staff and visitors. Therefore, exhaled and waste gases need to be scavenged from the circuit. These waste gases are typically collected in a 2- to 3-L anesthesia bag device connected to the hospital vacuum system. As the bag fills, the suction system is activated, and the bag contents are emptied.

ASSESSMENT QUESTIONS

See Evolve Resources for answers.

1. Which of the following is/are chemical properties of nitric oxide?
   A. Lipophilic
   B. Highly reactive
   C. Unstable free radical
   D. All of the above

ASSESSMENT QUESTIONS—cont'd

2. Which chemical is most associated with smooth muscle contractility?
   A. Iron
   B. Calcium
   C. Citric acid
   D. l-Arginine
3. Inhaled nitric oxide reduces shunt by:
   A. Vasodilating only pulmonary capillaries adjacent to atelectatic lung units
   B. Decreasing pulmonary vascular resistance
   C. Increasing systemic oxygenation
   D. Vasodilating only pulmonary capillaries adjacent to functioning lung units
4. Which of the following are potential side effects of iNO administration?
   A. Nitrous oxide formation in the ventilator circuit
   B. Fetal hemoglobin formation
   C. Decrease in guanylyl cyclase in the sarcoplasmic reticulum
   D. Methemoglobin formation
5. Which of the following are useful properties of helium when used to treat patients in status asthmaticus?
   I. Lower density
   II. Lower viscosity
   III. Higher viscosity
   IV. Low thermal conductivity
   A. I and II
   B. I and III
   C. I, II, and IV
   D. I, III, and IV
6. All of the following are effects of heliox on mechanical ventilation except:
   A. Measured flow is falsely low when using a differential pneumotachometer.
   B. Nebulizer output is decreased.
   C. Actual flow from the flowmeter is lower than indicated.
   D. Measured flow is falsely high when using a hot-wire anemometer.
7. Hypoxic and hypercarbic gas mixtures
   A. Increase pulmonary blood flow
   B. Are useful in patients with pulmonary hypertension
   C. Decrease pulmonary blood flow
   D. Increase systemic blood flow
8. Which of the following is not an inhaled anesthetic agent used to treat status asthmaticus?
   A. Halothane
   B. Sevoflurane
   C. Enflurane
   D. Nitrous oxide

ASSESSMENT QUESTIONS—cont'd

9. Which of the following inhaled anesthetic agents are best tolerated by the patient when breathing spontaneously from a mask?
   A. Isoflurane and enflurane
   B. Halothane and sevoflurane
   C. Enflurane and sevoflurane
   D. Isoflurane, halothane, and sevoflurane
10. What IA should not be used in patients receiving catecholamines?
    A. Enflurane
    B. Isoflurane
    C. Sevoflurane
    D. Halothane

References

1. Hurford WE: The biological basis of inhaled nitric oxide, *Respir Care Clin North Am* 1997;3:357.
2. Dagby RM, Corey-Kreyling MD: Structural aspects of the contractile machinery of smooth muscle: is the organization of contractile elements compatible with a sliding filament mechanism? In Stephens NL, editor: *Smooth muscle contraction*, New York: Marcel Dekker; 1984. pp 47-74.
3. Furchgott RF, Zawadzki JV: The obligatory role of endothelial cells in the relaxation of arterial smooth muscle by acetylcholine, *Nature* 1980;288:373.
4. Miller CC, Miller J: Pulmonary vascular smooth muscle regulation: the role of inhaled nitric oxide gas, *Respir Care* 1992;37:1175.
5. Aranda A, Pearl RG: The biology of nitric oxide, *Respir Care* 1999;44:156.
6. Bigatello LM, Hurford WE, Hess D: Use of inhaled nitric oxide for ARDS, *Respir Care Clin North Am* 1997;3:437.
7. Macrae DJ et al: Inhaled nitric oxide therapy in neonates and children: reaching a European consensus, *Intensive Care Med* 2004;30:372.
8. Barefield ES et al: Inhaled nitric oxide in term infants with hypoxemic respiratory failure, *J Pediatr* 1996;129:279.
9. Clark RH et al; Clinical Inhaled Nitric Oxide Research Group: Low-dose nitric oxide therapy for persistent pulmonary hypertension of the newborn, *N Engl J Med* 2000;342:469.
10. Davidson D et al: Inhaled nitric oxide for the early treatment of persistent pulmonary hypertension of the newborn: a randomized, doublemasked, placebo-controlled, dose-response, multicenter study, *Pediatrics* 1998;101:325.
11. Day RW et al: Acute response to inhaled nitric oxide in newborns with respiratory failure and pulmonary hypertension, *Pediatrics* 1996;98:698.
12. Neonatal Inhaled Nitric Oxide Study Group (NINOS): Inhaled nitric oxide in full-term and nearly fullterm infants with hypoxic respiratory failure, *N Engl J Med* 1997;336:597.

13. Roberts JD Jr et al; Inhaled Nitric Oxide Study Group: Inhaled nitric oxide and persistent pulmonary hypertension of the newborn, *N Engl J Med* 1997;336:605.
14. Finer NN et al: Inhaled nitric oxide in infants referred for extracorporeal membrane oxygenation: dose response, *J Pediatr* 1994;124:302.
15. Demirakça S et al: Inhaled nitric oxide in neonatal and pediatric acute respiratory distress syndrome: dose response, prolonged inhalation and weaning, *Crit Care Med* 1996;24:1913.
16. Neonatal Inhaled Nitric Oxide Study Group (NINOS): Inhaled nitric oxide in full-term and nearly fullterm infants with hypoxic respiratory failure, *N Engl J Med* 1997;336:597.
17. Dötsch J et al: Recovery from withdrawal of inhaled nitric oxide and kinetics of nitric oxide–induced inhibition of nitric oxide synthase activity *in vitro*, *Intensive Care Med* 2000;26:330.
18. Black SM et al: Inhaled nitric oxide inhibits NOS activity in lambs: potential mechanism for rebound pulmonary hypertension, *Am J Physiol* 1999;277:H1849.
19. Kinsella JP et al: Inhaled nitric oxide in premature neonates with severe hypoxemic respiratory failure: a randomised controlled trial, *Lancet* 1999;354:1061.
20. Franco-Belgium Collaborative NO Trial Group: Early compared with delayed inhaled nitric oxide in moderately hypoxemic neonates with respiratory failure: a randomised controlled trial, *Lancet* 1999;354:1066.
21. Van Meurs KP et al; Preemie Inhaled Nitric Oxide Study: Inhaled nitric oxide for premature infants with severe respiratory failure, *N Engl J Med* 2005;353:13.
22. Field D et al; INNOVO Trial Collaborating Group: Neonatal ventilation with inhaled nitric oxide versus ventilatory support without inhaled nitric oxide for preterm infants with severe respiratory failure: the INNOVO Multicentre Randomised Controlled Trial (ISRCTN 17821339), *Pediatrics* 2005;115:926.
23. Barrington KJ, Finer NN: Inhaled nitric oxide for respiratory failure in preterm infants, *Cochrane Database Syst Rev* 2006;1:CD000509.
24. Puybasset L et al: Factors influencing cardiopulmonary effects of inhaled nitric oxide in acute respiratory failure, *Am J Respir Crit Care Med* 1995;152:318.
25. Okamoto K et al: Combined effects of inhaled nitric oxide and positive end-expiratory pressure during mechanical ventilation in acute respiratory distress syndrome, *Artif Organs* 2000;24:390.
26. Johannigman JA et al: Positive end-expiratory pressure and response to inhaled nitric oxide: changing nonresponders to responders, *Surgery* 2000;127:390.
27. Kinsella JP et al: Randomized, multicenter trial of inhaled nitric oxide and high-frequency oscillatory ventilation in severe, persistent pulmonary hypertension of the newborn, *J Pediatr* 1997;131:55.
28. Mehta S et al: Acute oxygenation response to inhaled nitric oxide when combined with high-frequency oscillatory ventilation in adults with acute respiratory distress syndrome, *Crit Care Med* 2003;31:383.
29. Hess D, Ritz R, Branson RD: Delivery systems for inhaled nitric oxide, *Respir Care Clin North Am* 1997;3:371.
30. Branson RD et al: Inhaled nitric oxide systems and monitoring, *Respir Care* 1999;44:281.
31. Curry S: Methemoglobinemia, *Ann Emerg Med* 1982;11:214.
32. Jacob TD et al: Hemodynamic effects and metabolic fate of inhaled nitric oxide in hypoxic piglets, *J Appl Physiol* 1994;76:1794.
33. Papamoschou D: Theoretical validation of the respiratory benefits of helium–oxygen mixtures, *Respir Physiol* 1995;99:183.
34. Barach AL: Use of helium as a new therapeutic gas, *Proc Soc Exp Biol Med* 1934;32:462.
35. Barach AL: The therapeutic use of helium, *JAMA* 1936;107:1273.
36. Barach AL: The use of helium in the treatment of asthma and obstructive lesions of the larynx and trachea, *Ann Intern Med* 1935;9:739.
37. Barach AL: The use of helium as a new therapeutic gas, *Anesth Analg* 1935;14:210.
38. Nunn JF: Diffusion and alveolar/capillary permeability. In: *Applied respiratory physiology*, London: Butterworth; 1987. pp 184-206.
39. Anderson M et al: Deposition in asthmatics of particles inhaled in air or helium–oxygen, *Am Rev Respir Dis* 1993;147:524.
40. Svartengren M et al: Human lung deposition of particles suspended in air or in helium/oxygen mixture, *Exp Lung Res* 1989;15:575.
41. Bandi V et al: Deposition pattern of heliox-driven bronchodilator aerosol in the airways of stable asthmatics, *J Asthma* 2005;42:583.
42. Corcoran TE et al: Aerosol drug delivery using heliox and nebulizer reservoirs: results from an MRI-based pediatric model, *J Aerosol Med* 2003;16:263.
43. Melmed A et al: The use of heliox as a vehicle for β-agonist nebulization in patients with severe asthma [abstract], *Am J Respir Crit Care Med* 1995;151:A269.
44. Hess DR et al: The effect of heliox on nebulizer function using a β-agonist bronchodilator, *Chest* 1999;115:184.
45. Stillwell PC et al: Effectiveness of open-circuit Oxyhood delivery of helium–oxygen, *Chest* 1989;95:1222.
46. Rogers MS et al: Volume accuracy of the Siemens Servo 900C and Novametrix Ventrak when delivering helium oxygen mixtures [abstract], *Respir Care* 1995;40:1206.
47. El-Lessy HN: Pulmonary vascular control in hypoplastic left-heart syndrome: hypoxic- and hypercarbic-gas therapy, *Respir Care* 1995;40:737.
48. Jobes DR et al: Carbon dioxide prevents pulmonary overcirculation in hypoplastic left heart syndrome, *Ann Thorac Surg* 1992;54:150.
49. Mayer JE: Initial management of the single ventricle patient, *Semin Thorac Cardiovasc Surg* 1994;6:2.
50. Wheeler DS et al: Isoflurane therapy for status asthmaticus in children: a case series and protocol, *Pediatr Crit Care Med* 2000;1:55.
51. Restrepo RD, Pettignano R, DeMeuse P: Halothane, an effective infrequently used drug, in the treatment of pediatric status asthmaticus: a case report, *J Asthma* 2005;42:649.
52. Bishop MJ, Rooke GA: Sevoflurane for patients with asthma [letter], *Anesth Analg* 2000;91:245.
53. Habre W et al: Respiratory mechanics during sevoflurane anesthesia in children with and without asthma, *Anesth Analg* 1999;89:1177.
54. Padkin AJ, Baigel G, Morgan GA: Halothane treatment of severe asthma to avoid mechanical ventilation, *Anesthesia* 1997;52:994.

55. Miyagi T et al: Prolonged isoflurane anesthesia in a case of catastrophic asthma, *Acta Paediatr Jpn* 1997;39:375.

56. Rooke GA, Choi JH, Bishop MJ: The effect of isoflurane, halothane, sevoflurane, and thiopental/nitrous oxide on respiratory system resistance after trachea intubation, *Anesthesiology* 1997;86:1294.

57. Habre W, Wildhaber JH, Sly PD: Prevention of methacholine induced changes in respiratory mechanics in piglets with sevoflurane and halothane, *Anesthesiology* 1997;87:585.

58. Hirschman CA et al: Mechanism of action of inhalational anesthesia on airways, *Anesthesiology* 1982; 56:107.

59. Stoelting R: *Pharmacology and physiology in anesthetic practice*, Philadelphia: J.B. Lippincott; 1987. p 45.

60. Johnson RG et al: Isoflurane therapy for status asthmaticus in children and adults, *Chest* 1990;97:698.

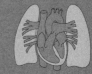

Chapter 23

Extracorporeal Life Support

DOUGLAS R. HANSELL

LEARNING OBJECTIVES

After reading this chapter the reader will be able to:
- Provide a brief history of the development of extracorporeal life support techniques
- Describe the rationale for the use of extracorporeal membrane oxygenation support for neonatal and pediatric respiratory failure

- Compare extracorporeal and human circulatory physiology
- Compare and contrast venoarterial and venovenous extracorporeal membrane oxygenation support
- Describe the basic components of extracorporeal membrane oxygenation circuitry

Extracorporeal circulation is the technique of supporting the function of the heart or lungs, or both, with external artificial organs. This support was originally developed for use in the operating room during cardiac surgery and was limited to several hours' duration. In more recent years, extracorporeal support has been applied in the intensive care unit in critically ill patients with pulmonary problems for days and even weeks. In this setting, extracorporeal circulation enables the practitioner to minimize the ventilator's support, thereby avoiding iatrogenic damage to the lungs and the problems associated with high mean airway pressures while allowing the disease process to run its natural course. This form of support is known as extracorporeal membrane oxygenation (ECMO), or extracorporeal life support (ECLS).

HISTORY

Hooke, writing of allowing "blood to circulate through a vessel, so as it may be openly exposed to air," recorded one of the earliest references to extracorporeal oxygenation in 1667.[1] His speculation, well ahead of its time, had no impact on medicine. In reality, the technique of ECLS evolved directly from the cardiopulmonary bypass procedure developed for cardiac surgery. Gibbon, the inventor of the mechanical oxygenator, is considered the "father" of extracorporeal circulation.[2] In 1937, he reported the use of cardiopulmonary bypass during pulmonary artery occlusion in animals.[3] It was not until 1953, however, that Gibbon first successfully performed extracorporeal circulation in a human. His invention substituted a roller pump for the heart. To achieve gas exchange, blood was distributed in a film along stainless steel screens vertically suspended in a plastic chamber. The thinness of the advancing blood film allowed uptake of oxygen and release of carbon dioxide by diffusion.

During the 1950s, studies in extracorporeal gas exchange involving cross-circulation in animals were performed with biological lungs for gas exchange. Lillehei and associates[4] were the first to perform cross-circulation in humans. In 1955, they reported a series of eight pediatric patients in whom cardiac surgery was performed, using the parent as the oxygenator. All patients and donors survived, and no long-lasting donor morbidity was noted. Subsequently, a bubble oxygenator was designed and successfully used in seven patients.[5] With bubble oxygenators, however, the duration of bypass was limited to a few hours because the direct blood–gas interface resulted in hemolysis, denatured plasma proteins, and thrombus formation. Investigation continued for an extracorporeal circuit that was more biocompatible and capable of extended use.

The observation that blue venous blood entering a hemodialysis membrane turned red when the blood exited the membrane spurred interest in developing a membrane oxygenator.[6] In 1956, Clowes[7] reported the first clinical use of a membrane for gas exchange. The membrane oxygenator was constructed of polyethylene and Teflon and for the first time eliminated the direct blood–gas interface. Because gas exchange was inefficient, however, the membrane had to be large, thus limiting its clinical application. Subsequently, silicone

rubber was found to have gas transfer characteristics far superior to polyethylene, and in 1963 a silicone membrane similar to the one used today was developed.[8] With this device the first extended bypass procedure was performed in animals, which demonstrated minimal hematologic effect for up to 1 week.[9] This development paved the way for the successful application of long-term extracorporeal support.

In 1969, Dorson and colleagues[10] attempted to perfuse a 1.16-kg premature neonate with respiratory distress syndrome. The infant was supported with ECMO for 21 hours before death from intraventricular hemorrhage (IVH). Subsequently, 10 days of extracorporeal support in a 28-week premature neonate was reported.[11] Although this infant also died of IVH, the findings demonstrated that prolonged extracorporeal support was possible. The first successful use of ECMO was reported in 1972 in a 24-year-old man with multiple trauma and respiratory failure.[12] He was maintained on extracorporeal support for 75 hours, during which time his lung injury resolved.

Other trials in adults followed, with anecdotal reports of success. This prompted the National Institutes of Health (NIH, Bethesda, Md) to sponsor a multicenter, randomized prospective study of ECMO in adults with acute respiratory failure, and a collaborative study was published in 1979.[13] Nine institutions randomized 90 adults with adult respiratory distress syndrome (ARDS) to either conventional mechanical ventilation (CMV) or ECMO. The results were dismal, with only eight survivors: four in the CMV group and four in the ECMO group. The authors were forced to conclude that although ECMO could support gas exchange, it could not improve survival of patients with ARDS. Critics of the study have suggested that the results may be misleading.[14] Some of the centers involved had no experience with ECMO before the study. In addition, because of the stringent entry criteria, a significant proportion of the patient population had irreversible lung injury that was subsequently noted at autopsy. Perhaps most important, although the purpose of ECMO was to allow resting of the lungs, most patients were still subjected to high ventilator settings and fractional concentration of inspired oxygen (FIO_2) while receiving ECMO. Bleeding complications were also significant, with an average blood loss of 2 L/day. Regardless of the shortcomings of the study, adult ECMO in the United States was virtually abandoned.

Despite these disappointing results, the search continued to identify a population with reversible lung disease that could potentially benefit from ECMO. In 1976, Bartlett and Harken[15] at the University of California–Irvine (Irvine, Calif) pioneered neonatal ECMO, developed the standard circuit, and successfully used ECMO in a neonate with meconium aspiration syndrome (MAS). Their success continued, and in 1982, Bartlett and colleagues[16] reported 55% survival in a series of 45 neonates treated with ECMO. By the mid-1980s, two prospective randomized trials comparing ECMO to CMV were published. The study by Bartlett and colleagues reported 100% survival of the 11 patients receiving ECMO and 0% survival in the control group.[17] This study was met with skepticism because only one patient constituted the control group. O'Rourke and colleagues[18] subsequently reported 100% survival for nine ECMO patients compared with 33% for six CMV-treated newborns, but they too encountered criticism for the study design.

Meanwhile in Europe, interest in adult ECLS continued, and with the addition of several innovations, results improved. Gattinoni and colleagues[19] believed that high airway pressures could cause progressive lung injury and that extracorporeal support could be employed to eliminate the need for high-pressure ventilator support. With an emphasis on carbon dioxide removal, using a large membrane surface area and a venovenous route, they treated 43 adults selected on the basis of the same selection criteria used in the NIH adult ECMO study. They referred to this technique as "extracorporeal carbon dioxide removal" ($ECCO_2R$) and in 1986 reported an astounding 49% survival in adults.

In the United Kingdom, a randomized controlled clinical trial was conducted to determine the role of ECMO in the adult population. This trial, known as CESAR (Conventional Ventilation or ECMO for Severe Adult Respiratory Failure), compared conventional ventilation methods with extracorporeal membrane oxygenation for the treatment of severe acute respiratory failure in adults. Trials concluded in 2006 and results have become available. Details regarding the trial are available at http://www.cesar-trial.org/. Lead clinical investigator Giles J. Peek, MD, FRCS, from the University of Leicester, Glenfield, United Kingdom, reported the findings of the trial at the Society of Critical Care Medicine 37th Critical Care Congress, February, 2008. A total of 180 patients from 68 centers were randomly assigned to receive conventional ventilation (n = 90) or ECMO (n = 90). Of the 90 patients assigned to receive ECMO, 22 did not receive ECMO, most often because they improved without it. Patient characteristics were well matched between groups.

Of the patients randomly assigned to receive ECMO, 57 of 90 met the primary endpoint of survival or absence of severe disability at 6 months compared with 41 of 87 evaluable patients in the conventional ventilation group. This translated to a relative risk in favor of the ECMO group of 0.69 (95% confidence interval, 0.05 − 0.97; P = 0.03). Extracorporeal membrane oxygenation

(ECMO) increased survival among adult patients with severe but potentially reversible respiratory failure compared with conventional ventilatory support, and resulted in 1 extra survivor for every 6 patients treated.

Since Bartlett's first reported success with ECMO in neonates, the number of ECLS centers has continued to grow, with 114 active ECLS centers reported in 2002. In 1989 the ECLS centers formed a national organization known as the Extracorporeal Life Support Organization (ELSO, Ann Arbor, Mich). ELSO's purpose is to coordinate clinical research on extracorporeal support, develop ECLS guidelines, and maintain ECMO National Registry data. This registry is a databank of all reported ECLS cases from the active ELSO centers and contains information about more than 31,000 neonatal, pediatric, and adult cases to date.[20]

NEONATAL TREATMENT

The majority of the reported ECLS cases (76%) are neonates. In the 1990s, ECLS in this population became a standard mode of therapy for acute respiratory failure unresponsive to maximal medical therapy. This acceptance occurred despite the lack of a randomized controlled clinical trial proving the efficacy of ECMO in the treatment of ARDS. Finally, in 1996 the UK Collaborative ECMO Trial Group[21] reported the results of a trial to assess whether a policy of referral for ECMO has a beneficial effect on survival to 1 year without severe disability in comparison with conventional management. Recruitment to the trial was stopped early (November 1995) because the data accumulated showed a clear advantage with ECMO. Of 185 infants in two groups, 81 (44%) died before leaving the hospital, and 2 died after discharge. Death rates differed between the two groups; 30 of 93 infants in the ECMO group died compared with 54 of 92 in the conventional care group. The results, reported in 1996, leave little doubt that ECMO is an effective lifesaving treatment for neonates with severe respiratory failure.

Persistent Pulmonary Hypertension of Newborn

Persistent pulmonary hypertension of the newborn (PPHN), the abnormal continuance of fetal circulation after birth, continues to be the major pathophysiologic condition treated with ECLS.[22]

There are two distinctive intracardiac structures in the fetus. The ductus arteriosus is a large vessel between the pulmonary artery and the aorta. The foramen ovale is a hole with a tissue flap, situated in the atrial septum. In utero, pulmonary vascular resistance (PVR) is greater than systemic vascular resistance, resulting in higher pressures in the right atrium than in the left atrium.

Consequently, blood is diverted through the foramen ovale to the left atrium and through the ductus arteriosus to the aorta, thereby bypassing the pulmonary circulation. With the first breath, PVR is immediately reduced because of the effects of mechanical lung expansion and the increase in oxygenation. This reduction leads to an increase in pulmonary blood flow and a reversal of atrial pressures, resulting in functional closure of the foramen ovale. Concurrently, increased oxygen partial pressure (Po_2) causes constriction and functional closure of the ductus arteriosus, completing the transition to the postnatal circulatory pattern. A hypoxic state after birth can increase PVR, which in turn promotes the reinstitution of right-to-left shunting at both the atrial and ductal levels, sustaining or reestablishing the fetal circulation.

PPHN can result from any underlying neonatal condition leading to hypoxia.[23] Most often it is associated with MAS, perinatal asphyxia, congenital diaphragmatic hernia (CDH), sepsis, and respiratory distress syndrome. The presentation and clinical course depend on the primary disease.[24] Immediate presentation of PPHN is the norm in perinatal asphyxia and CDH. Presentation at 4 to 12 hours of age is seen in the infant with MAS. Late presentation may be seen at 24 hours or more in the septic population. The majority of these neonates can be managed with pharmacologic and ventilatory support.[25,26] A small percentage are unresponsive to conventional therapy, however, and before ECLS, they would have died. Institution of ECLS interrupts the cycle of pulmonary hypertension, minimizes the need for escalating mechanical ventilation, and avoids barotrauma while the underlying condition resolves. Table 23-1 summarizes the survival of neonates treated with ECMO.[20]

Meconium Aspiration Syndrome

The introduction of ECLS in neonates with MAS has resulted in the highest survival rate of all the neonatal diseases commonly treated. Meconium is a sterile, dark green substance that is normally present in the fetal colon. Meconium staining of amniotic fluid is common in 10% of all deliveries but is rare in neonates born at less than 37 weeks of gestation.[27] Premature passage of the meconium into the amniotic fluid may occur under several conditions, most notably fetal hypoxia.[27] Therefore the presence of meconium-stained fluid may indicate fetal distress.

The diagnosis of MAS is made if the infant has a history of meconium-stained fluid, the presence of meconium in the trachea at birth, and a variable radiographic pattern of patchy infiltrates with hyperinflation to consolidation.[28] The neonate's degree of respiratory distress may be mild to severe. The resulting hypoxia and acidosis can increase PVR, leading to right-to-left shunting and further hypoxia.

Sepsis

The most common organism to cause sepsis in the neonate is group B *Streptococcus*. The organism is found primarily in the intestinal tract, with colonization occurring in the mother's vagina.[29] Although sepsis is more often associated with early rupture of membranes, the fetus can still become infected with the membranes intact. This bacterial infection can be serious in the immediate newborn period, with mortality approaching 45%.[30] It can present as either pneumonia or overwhelming vascular collapse, referred to as *septic shock*. Other organisms such as *Escherichia coli* and *Listeria* can follow the same clinical course as group B *Streptococcus*. The overall survival in this group is lower than in the group with MAS because cardiovascular instability and difficulties in coagulation management lead to a more complicated and prolonged course of ECLS.

Congenital Diaphragmatic Hernia

CDH occurs in approximately 1 in 2200 births.[31] It is characterized by the incomplete formation of the fetal diaphragm and usually occurs on the left side. The most common herniation is the posterolateral type known

TABLE 23-1

Neonatal Extracorporeal Membrane Oxygenation Cases by Diagnosis

Diagnosis	No. of Patients	No. of Survivors	Percentage Surviving
Meconium aspiration syndrome	6805	6388	94
Congenital diaphragmatic hernia	3816	2063	54
Sepsis/pneumonia	2699	1987	74
Persistent pulmonary hypertension of newborn	3077	2405	78
Respiratory distress syndrome	1398	1174	84
Air leak syndrome	100	71	71
Other	1336	849	64

Data from ELSO National Registry Report. Ann Arbor, Mich: University of Michigan; 2005.

as Bochdalek's hernia. This defect allows herniation of the abdominal contents into the thoracic cavity, affecting fetal lung development. It compresses the lung on the affected side but also shifts the mediastinum to the opposite side and compresses the contralateral lung, resulting in various degrees of bilateral pulmonary hypoplasia. Infants who are symptomatic within the first 6 hours of life have the highest mortality.[32] The distressed newborn has a scaphoid abdomen and diminished or no breath sounds on one side and has a chest radiograph that demonstrates gastrointestinal structures in the thorax.

CDH continues to have the lowest cure rate of all common neonatal diseases treated with ECLS. Identifying the characteristics of infants who have pulmonary hypoplasia incompatible with survival has long been an elusive goal.[33] Since the introduction of ECLS, many predictors of mortality have been proposed; however, because of differences in clinical management, none has been reproducible from institution to institution.[34] Kays and colleagues[35] found that infants who are maintained with "gentle ventilation" methods, including permissive hypercapnia, moderate hypoxemia, minimal use of sedatives, and minimal stimulation, are less likely to require ECMO and have significantly improved survival.

Patient Selection Criteria

The success of neonatal ECLS depends on the disease process. Most neonatal respiratory failure results in PPHN, which is completely reversible. However, the escalating ventilator pressures and F_{IO_2} used to treat PPHN can lead to secondary lung injury. Knowing the correct time to cease exposing the neonate's lungs to these iatrogenic complications becomes a concern for ensuring long-term survival and limiting morbidity.

In the early years of neonatal ECLS, deciding when to employ ECLS was purely subjective. Subsequently, several methods were proposed to standardize ECLS criteria. Bartlett and colleagues[36] developed the "neonatal pulmonary insufficiency index," which plotted pH and F_{IO_2} over time to a point at which the risk of mortality exceeded 80%. However, the index became unsuitable for patients who had induced iatrogenic alkalosis as a treatment for PPHN.

Krummel and colleagues[37] reported that an alveolar–arterial oxygen gradient [P_{AO_2}–P_{aO_2}; also $(A-a)D_{O_2}$] greater than 620 mm Hg for 6 to 12 hours was indicative of an 80% risk of mortality. However, this criterion was not useful in the neonate who failed rapidly. Ortega and colleagues[38] proposed the oxygenation index (OI), a calculation based on mean airway pressure ($\overline{Paw}$), F_{IO_2}, and arterial oxygenation (P_{aO_2}), as follows:

$$OI = \overline{Paw} \times (F_{IO_2}/P_{aO_2}) \times 100$$

The authors found that when the OI exceeded 40, risk of mortality exceeded 80%. Their results have been reproduced by other institutions, and the OI is currently the most widely accepted predictor of mortality in neonates with respiratory failure on conventional ventilators. As experience with neonatal resuscitation improves, however, and as more institutions employ high-frequency ventilation as rescue therapy before ECLS, the value of the OI and other guidelines will require constant reassessment.

In addition to statistical indicators for employing ECLS, other criteria need to be considered for the candidate for ECLS. In early ECLS studies, IVH was a common complication among infants born at less than 35 weeks of gestation. They recommended that neonates born at less than 35 weeks of gestation and those with preexisting IVH should be excluded from ECLS until anticoagulation management techniques used during ECLS are improved. At present, several centers are reporting reduced extension of grade 1, 2, or 3 IVH with the use of antifibrinolytic therapy.[39] However, all candidates should have an ultrasound before initiation of ECLS. A "subependymal" or grade 1 bleed is currently considered only a relative contraindication. Because bleeding is the major complication of ECLS, active bleeding or uncorrectable coagulopathies are also considered relative contraindications.

Ultimately, the patient's pulmonary disease should be reversible; therefore prior mechanical ventilation for more than 14 days is considered a contraindication for ECLS because of the potential iatrogenic lung injury. Preexisting major cardiac defects should be ruled out before considering ECLS; this is done by performing an echocardiogram. If a major defect is detected, surgical intervention should be the first option. If lung disease prevents surgical correction, the surgical team may consider stabilizing the patient with ECLS until resolution of the pulmonary disease. Other congenital and medical conditions associated with poor prognosis may be contraindications for ECLS. Box 23-1 summarizes current patient selection criteria.

Box 23-1	Neonatal Extracorporeal Life Support Selection Criteria

- Oxygen index > 40
- No major cardiac defect
- Reversible lung disease
- Gestational age > 33 weeks
- Mechanical ventilation < 14 days
- No major intraventricular hemorrhage
- No significant coagulopathy or bleeding complications (relative contraindication)

PEDIATRIC TREATMENT

Beyond infancy, there is no pulmonary condition as completely reversible as PPHN. In older children, most conditions leading to respiratory failure involve pulmonary parenchymal injury, including posttraumatic respiratory failure; viral or bacterial pneumonia; and blood, gastric acid, and foreign substance aspiration. These conditions all present a picture more closely related to ARDS than to PPHN. In the mid-1970s, risk of mortality from ARDS in children was 80%.[40] It continued to remain equally high in the late 1980s despite changes in ventilator strategies.[41]

Although interest in ECLS for the older patient population was virtually abandoned after the NIH study in the 1970s, the successful European ECLS experience in older patients, along with refinements in technology and coagulation control, has revitalized interest in using this technique in the pediatric population. Several small studies reported survival of nearly 50% with long ECLS runs and many complications.[42-44] Of particular note, one child cannulated via the right common carotid artery experienced left hemiparesis and seizures, suggesting an increased risk when using the carotid artery for cannulation in older patients.[44]

O'Rourke and colleagues[45] reviewed pediatric ECMO reports in the ELSO Registry, which contained 285 cases in which ECLS was used for pediatric respiratory failure. Although 56 centers contributed at least one case, 50% of all the cases were contributed by only 7 centers, indicating that most neonatal centers had limited experience with pediatric ECLS. Despite concerns about carotid artery ligation in the older child, venoarterial ECLS via the right internal jugular vein and the right common carotid artery was employed in most cases. Traditional predictors of severity, such as those for neonatal ECLS, were not routinely used. The principal indication for ECLS in pediatric patients was based on the probability that the patient's condition was potentially reversible and that death was otherwise certain. Table 23-2 lists the principal diagnoses for which ECLS was employed, along with survival.

The report from O'Rourke and colleagues further noted that survivors were younger and had higher arterial pH values and lower peak and mean airway pressures before ECLS than did the nonsurvivors. The duration of pre-ECLS ventilatory support (0 to 129 d) and the mean duration of ECLS (10 d) were not significantly different between the neonatal and pediatric patients, although a higher incidence of complications was reported in the pediatric group. This may have been due to either longer ECLS runs that stressed the limits of the technology or the severity of illness in these patients. Finally, it was noted that death in this series occurred secondary to either progressive pulmonary failure or multisystem organ failure. The investigators suggested that selection criteria include reversibility indicators of both pulmonary and other organ dysfunction.[45] This recommendation was supported by Weber and colleagues,[46] who reported their ECLS experience in 32 pediatric patients. Overall survival was 41%, but 75% of the patients with isolated pulmonary disease survived, in contrast to only 8% of those with failure of even one other organ system.

More recently, Swaniker and colleagues[47] from the University of Michigan (Ann Arbor, Mich) evaluated data from 128 pediatric patients with acute respiratory failure and found that overall survival to discharge was 71%.

Although it is impossible to provide specific recommendations for the institution of ECLS in postneonatal patients, some guidelines have been suggested. The University of Michigan has proposed a set of guidelines for patient selection (Box 23-2). Until a prospective randomized trial of ECLS in pediatric pulmonary failure can be undertaken, these guidelines are a reasonable attempt to bring some standardization to this area.[48]

EXTRACORPOREAL PHYSIOLOGY

Venoarterial System

Oxygen delivery in ECLS is provided by a combination of blood flow from the ECLS circuit and blood flow from the patient's own cardiopulmonary system.[48] The delivery of oxygen is a function of both the oxygen

TABLE 23-2

Pediatric Extracorporeal Membrane Oxygenation Cases by Diagnosis

Diagnosis	No. of Patients	No. of Survivors	Percentage Surviving
Viral pneumonia	793	499	63
Acute respiratory distress syndrome	374	203	54
Aspiration	172	114	66
Bacterial pneumonia	334	184	55
ARF, non-ARDS	625	297	48
Pneumocystis carinii infection	24	11	44
Other	796	423	53

ARDS, Acute respiratory distress syndrome; ARF, acute renal failure.
Data from ELSO National Registry Report. Ann Arbor, Mich: University of Michigan; 2005.

Box 23-2	University of Michigan Pediatric and Adult Extracorporeal Membrane Oxygenation Criteria

INDICATIONS

- Poor gas exchange despite "optimal" ventilator and pharmacologic therapy
- Age < 60 years
- Ventilator support < 6 days
- Neurologic status responsive
- Oxygenation decreased: shunt > 30%
- Pao_2/Fio_2 100

and/or

- Carbon dioxide clearance decreased: $Paco_2$ > 45 mm Hg despite minute ventilation > 0.2 L/kg

CONTRAINDICATIONS

RELATIVE

- Ventilator support > 6 to 10 days
- Immunosuppression
- Systemic sepsis
- Active bleeding

ABSOLUTE

- Septic shock
- Cardiac arrest
- Brain injury
- Terminal disease
- Metabolic acidosis (base deficit > 5 mEq/L for 12 h)

Fio_2, Fractional inspired oxygen concentration; $Paco_2$, arterial carbon dioxide tension; Pao_2, arterial oxygen tension.
From Bartlett RH: *Extracorporeal life support manual for adult and pediatric patients,* Ann Arbor, Mich: University of Michigan Medical Center; 1993.

content of the blood and the cardiac output. Both variables (oxygenation and cardiac function) can be controlled by the venoarterial ECLS route. In this format a venous cannula, inserted via the right internal jugular vein, drains blood from the right atrium. An arterial cannula, inserted into the right common carotid artery, reinfuses the oxygenated blood into the aortic arch (Figure 23-1).

By increasing the flow rate, blood is preferentially diverted into the circuit. At maximal performance, approximately 80% of the cardiac output can be replaced by the circuit, which is often reflected by a dampened pulse pressure. The oxygenated blood returning from the ECLS circuit combines in the aortic arch with the desaturated blood from the patient's native circulation. The oxygen content of the patient's blood therefore depends on the relative contributions of each system. For example, as more blood is diverted into the ECLS circuit, less blood is contributed by the native lungs, and Pao_2 increases. Because of this parallel circulation, an increase in systemic Pao_2 during ECLS may reflect either improving lung function (increased Pao_2 in the native circulation) or decreasing native cardiac output (less flow from the patient's circulation). Changes in tissue oxygen consumption and hemoglobin concentration will also alter oxygen content.

In ECLS the arterial carbon dioxide partial pressure ($Paco_2$) also reflects the combination of the perfusate blood mixing with the native cardiac output. Once adjusted, however, the $Paco_2$ remains relatively stable on ECLS, responding only slightly to large changes in pulmonary blood flow and carbon dioxide production.

Although different vessels have been cannulated for venoarterial ECLS, the right internal jugular vein and right common carotid artery are the preferred vessels, especially in the neonate, in whom they are disproportionately large. This cannula orientation provides both pulmonary and cardiac support, a major advantage of this route.

The major disadvantage of the venoarterial approach is the need to ligate the right common carotid artery. In adults, acute disruption of the carotid artery results in strokes. In neonates, however, the risks remain unknown, although some suggest an increase in right-sided brain lesions.[49] Some patients have had the carotid artery reconstructed after ECLS, but the efficacy of this procedure is also unknown.[50]

Additional disadvantages, however, can also arise from the efficiency of venoarterial ECLS at diverting native flow. The ECLS circuit is nonpulsatile. Diverting blood away from the native cardiopulmonary system results in less pulsatile flow to the organs and disruption of the normal blood flow pattern.[51] The combination of

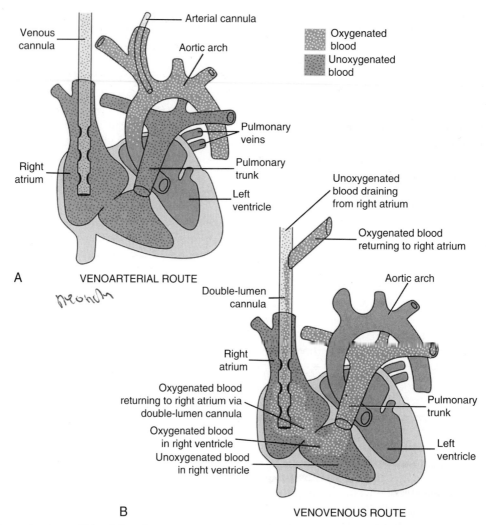

FIGURE 23-1 Mechanisms of blood flow during extracorporeal membrane oxygenation (ECMO). **A,** In the venoarterial route, blood is removed from the right atrium via a cannula inserted in the right internal jugular vein. Oxygenated blood is returned to the aortic arch via a cannula in the right common carotid artery. The shaded area indicates unoxygenated blood. **B,** In the venovenous route, blood is also removed from the right atrium via a cannula inserted in the right internal jugular vein, but the oxygenated blood is returned to the venous circulation. The shaded area indicates unoxygenated blood. Blood in the pulmonary trunk has been oxygenated via the cardiopulmonary bypass machine.

the orientation of the reinfusion cannula (distant aortic arch) and poorly oxygenated blood leaving the left ventricle may potentiate lower oxygen delivery to the coronary arteries.[52] Another potential disadvantage to venoarterial support is that any particle or bubble in the circuit may be directly infused into the arterial circulation, leading to embolus formation.

Venovenous System

In venovenous support, blood is both drained and reinfused back into the venous circulation at the same rate, thereby providing only pulmonary support. The oxygenated perfusate mixes with the venous blood in the right atrium, raising the oxygen content and lowering

the carbon dioxide content. Because both the drainage and reinfusion cannulas are in the venous system, some of the perfusate blood returns to the circuit. This phenomenon, known as *recirculation*, decreases the efficiency of gas transfer between circuit and patient. At present, the degree of recirculation is monitored by comparing the oxygen saturation of the venous drainage ($S\bar{v}o_2$) with the patient's arterial oxygen saturation (Sao_2).[53] If $S\bar{v}o_2$ is greater than Sao_2, the recirculation is excessive, and either the blood flow rate or cannula placement requires adjustment.

Because venovenous ECLS is less efficient than venoarterial ECLS, the maximal Sao_2 achievable can be as low as 80% to 85%. As lung function improves, Sao_2

increases. Because venovenous ECLS is essentially operating in series with the native circulation, alterations in cardiac output will not have a significant effect on oxygenation. The volume of blood removed is equal to the volume reinfused, so there is also no effect on the patient's hemodynamics.

The advantages of venovenous support are that the carotid artery is spared, full pulsatile flow is maintained, and potential emboli from the circuit are trapped in the pulmonary vascular bed.[48] The major disadvantage is lack of cardiovascular support. The presence of mild to moderate myocardial dysfunction, however, should not discourage one from using the venovenous approach. The improved oxygenation and lower airway pressures achieved with implementation of ECLS often improve cardiac output substantially. If myocardial dysfunction worsens during ECLS, however, or if oxygen delivery is insufficient, the conversion to venoarterial support should be instituted by inserting an arterial cannula. Box 23-3 summarizes additional advantages and disadvantages of venoarterial and venovenous ECLS.

Venovenous ECLS can be performed by three different techniques:

- The two-cannula system
- The tidal flow system
- The double-lumen cannula

Two-cannula System

The two-cannula system was the first design to be used. The circuit is identical to that used for venoarterial support. Blood is drained from the right atrium and is reinfused into the femoral vein. Klein and colleagues[54] compared their neonatal experience with this method and venoarterial support between 1981 and 1984. Venovenous support required a longer cannulation time and higher bypass flow rates to achieve a lower Pao_2. Complications included leg edema, frequent wound infections, and alterations in leg growth. Concerns about these issues have tempered enthusiasm for this route in the newborn. The two-cannula method is now most frequently used in pediatric and adult populations because no suitable equipment exists to provide other methods of venovenous support in these patients.

Tidal Flow System

The single-lumen tidal flow system, developed by Kolobow and colleagues,[55] is a method currently

---

Box 23-3   **Advantages and Disadvantages of Venovenous and Venoarterial Extracorporeal Life Support**

VENOVENOUS EXTRACORPOREAL LIFE SUPPORT

ADVANTAGES

- Sparing of carotid artery
- Preservation of pulsatile flow
- Normal pulmonary blood flow
- Perfusion of lungs with oxygenated blood
- Perfusion of coronaries with oxygenated blood
- Avoidance of infusion of possible emboli directly into arterial circulation
- Central venous pressure accurate
- Selective limb perfusion does not occur

DISADVANTAGES

- No cardiac support
- Lower systemic Pao_2
- Recirculation issues

VENOARTERIAL EXTRACORPOREAL LIFE SUPPORT

ADVANTAGES

- Provides cardiac support
- Excellent gas exchange
- Rapid stabilization

DISADVANTAGES

- Carotid artery ligation
- Nonpulsatile flow
- Reduced pulmonary blood flow
- Lower myocardial oxygen delivery
- Direct infusion of possible emboli into arterial circulation
- Central venous pressure inaccurate

Pao_2, Arterial partial pressure of oxygen.

available only in France. A single cannula is placed in the right internal jugular vein. Inflow and outflow are controlled by time-cycled valves that allow alternating drainage and infusion within the same cannula. The time-cycled valves have helped to minimize potential recirculation.[56] Despite reports of success, the introduction of the tidal flow system in the United States has been delayed by lack of U.S. Food and Drug Administration (FDA) approval.[57]

Double-lumen Cannula

The newest and most popular approach in the neonate is the double-lumen cannula. A single cannula is inserted into the right internal jugular vein, and blood is simultaneously drained and reinfused through the two lumens.[58] The larger lumen is used for drainage, and the smaller lumen is the reinfusion port. Although recirculation is also a problem with this method, it can be minimized by proper positioning of the cannula to direct the perfusate blood through the tricuspid valve into the right ventricle (see Figure 23-1). At present, four sizes are commercially available: the 12F, 15F, and 18F OriGen (OriGen Biomedical, Austin, Tex) and the 14F Kendall (Covidien, Mansfield, Mass). Therefore application of this technique is limited to patients weighing 2 to 11 kg.

EXTRACORPOREAL LIFE SUPPORT CIRCUIT

The ECLS circuit is composed of several disposable and nondisposable components. The disposable components consist of the tubing and various connectors, bladder, membrane, heat exchanger, and cannulas. Preassembled sterile tubing packs simplify the setup. At present the circuit is not standardized, leading most ECLS centers to customize their preassembled packs.

The ideal design should promote laminar flow patterns, require minimal blood volume, be constructed for longevity, and be mobile for intrahospital transport. The nondisposable components include the pump, venous servo-regulation system, water bath, coagulating timer, oxygen and carbon dioxide flowmeters, and portable ECLS cart.

With blood flow through a typical venoarterial circuit, blood is drained by gravity from the venous cannula to the bladder (Figure 23-2). From there the blood is pumped through the membrane and the heat exchanger before it is reinfused via the arterial cannula. The bridge is located near the cannula section of the circuit. It allows the patient to be isolated from the circuit while a blood flow rate is maintained to prevent stagnation. The venovenous circuit follows the same pattern except that the reinfusion cannula is inserted into a vein.

Cannulas

The ECLS circuit begins and ends with the cannulas. The cannulas chosen dictate the maximal flow rate that the system can achieve. The ideal cannula should be thin walled to achieve the largest internal diameter possible, stiff enough for insertion, kink resistant, and radiopaque. Wire-reinforced cannulas have many of these characteristics. A standardized rating system, the M number, has been developed to score various devices on their pressure-to-blood flow characteristic.[59] A device with a low M number indicates that a higher blood flow rate is possible at a lower pressure.

The arterial cannula is the source of highest resistance in the circuit because of its small diameter. Because hemolysis can occur at system pressures exceeding 350 mm Hg, it is important to select an arterial cannula large enough to handle the anticipated flow rates

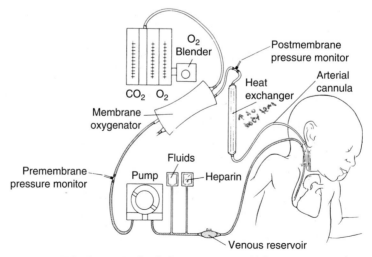

FIGURE 23-2 Circuit for extracorporeal life support.

for a given patient.[60] The major differences between the venous and arterial cannulas are that the lower portion of the venous cannula has multiple side ports for optimal drainage, whereas the arterial cannula is shorter to reduce resistance. In addition to the diameter of the venous cannula, drainage depends on cannula position, right atrial pressure, and the height of the patient above the bladder. Subtle manipulations of these variables may be necessary to optimize flow. The most common causes of a decrease in venous return include malpositioning of the venous cannula, kinking of the cannula, shifting of the mediastinum, or a hypovolemic state.

Pumps

Pumps are classified as either kinetic or positive displacement, depending on the way they exert energy to transport or compress fluid. The two pump systems employed with ECLS are the roller and centrifugal pumps.

Roller Pump

The roller pump, a positive displacement type, is most often used during ECLS. It functions on the principle of compression and displacement and is reliable and easy to operate. Flow is produced by compressing a segment of tubing between two roller heads, spaced 180° apart, and a back plate. Volume is displaced as the rollers travel the length of the "raceway" (tubing contained within the pump's housing), delivering a forward force. The second roller begins compressing the tubing as the first roller is reaching the end. The output depends on the size of the tubing, the rotations per minute, and proper occlusion. *Occlusion* refers to the amount of pressure the roller heads exert on the tubing to prevent fluid from slipping backward. Most roller pumps require manual adjustment of the occlusion before each use.

One drawback to this device is that it is not pressure dependent and will pump to deliver the specified flow rate. Therefore, even if excessive pressure builds up within the system, the pump will continue to operate until the problem is recognized or rupture occurs. For safe operation, a roller pump requires the incorporation of a venous servo-regulation system, either a bladder box or a pressure-monitoring system.

Bladder Box System. The bladder is a small reservoir composed of thin, pliable silicone. Situated between the patient and the ECLS pump, the bladder allows the pump to pull from this reservoir instead of from the right atrium. If there is an acute decrease in venous drainage, the bladder will collapse on itself, preventing excessive negative pressure from being transmitted to the heart. The bladder section of the circuit is the site that is used most often for infusing fluids because of its ability to trap small amounts of air inadvertently administered with medications. Two vents for purging the inadvertent air and for continuous infusions are built into the top. The major complication associated with the bladder is the development of clots caused by the stagnant blood flow pattern near the bottom of the bladder. New streamlined designs, however, are reducing the occurrence of clots.

The bladder box assembly is the safety mechanism for the circuit. It is composed of two brackets to support the silicone bladder and a microswitch or plunger that rests on the bladder surface. When the bladder collapses, the microswitch is released and interrupts the electrical signal, stopping the pump and alerting the clinician with an audible alarm. When corrected, the bladder reexpands and depresses the microswitch, restoring the pump's electric current. The purpose of this bladder box assembly is to prevent the pump's flow rate from exceeding the rate of venous drainage.

Pressure Monitoring System. An alternative to the microswitch-operated bladder box is a servo-regulated pressure monitoring system. A pressure transducer is connected between the patient and the bladder. When flow diminishes, the pressure in the venous line decreases until a predetermined level is reached. At this point the pump is disengaged until adequate drainage is reestablished. This technology allows regulation thresholds as well as absolute limits, so the pump will actually slow down and speed up as the bladder pressure changes.

Centrifugal Pump

The centrifugal pump, a kinetic type, is also used by some centers. Energy is transferred to the blood by a rapidly rotating cone. Blood passes through a vortex created by the spinning motion of the cone and is forced out through the outlet. It automatically responds to the resistance against which it is pumping, resulting in changes in the delivered flow. As line pressure increases, flow decreases. This pressure-limited feature prevents pumping against a high-pressure head and ultimately eliminates potential system ruptures. Another advantage of this system is the elimination of the venous servo-regulating system and the raceway. If venous drainage is inadequate, however, significant negative pressure can be generated, which may cause hemolysis. This risk is why the centrifugal pump is still not universally accepted in the ECLS community, although there is growing use of this pump because of the advent of servo-regulated pump systems.[54]

Gas Exchange Devices
Silicone Rubber Membrane

Most of the experience in ECLS has been with the Medtronic silicone rubber membrane (Medtronic,

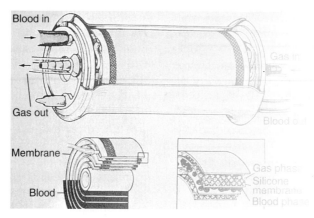

FIGURE 23-3 Diagram of membrane oxygenator *(top)* and the membrane unwound *(bottom)* to demonstrate the large surface area used for gas exchange.

Minneapolis, Minn), originally designed by Kolobow and Bowman.[8] It is a flat silicone membrane envelope wound in a spiral coil around a polycarbonate spool (Figure 23-3). The two compartments in this membrane, for blood and for gas, are separated by the semipermeable silicone membrane. While the blood is pumped through its compartment in the membrane, a ventilating gas, the *sweep gas,* is flushed through the air compartment. Because this sweep gas is providing a constant fresh source of oxygen and is constantly flushing out diffused carbon dioxide, a gradient is established that optimizes transport of oxygen and carbon dioxide across the membrane.

Microporous Membrane

Microporous hollow-fiber devices have also been used in ECLS. The hollow-fiber device is made of woven capillaries of microporous plastic. Gas passes through the capillaries while blood flows around them. The microporous membrane has excellent gas exchange capabilities and low resistance and is easy to prime. Over extended periods, however, condensation, wettability, and plasma leakage make it less desirable for long-term use. This type of membrane was used in the early clinical trials involving heparin-bonded circuits.[61] The introduction of a solid membrane hollow-fiber device (MEDOS Medizintechnik, Stolberg, Germany) combines the best features of both the silicone membrane and hollow-fiber gas exchange devices. These fibers are most often made of polymethylpentene. As of this writing, polymethylpentene devices are not available in the United States although several manufacturers have plans to introduce models for the U.S. FDA approval process in the near future.

Physiologic Basis

Membrane oxygenators are designed to eliminate direct contact between the blood and gas phases. This design avoids unnecessary trauma to the blood and makes membrane oxygenators more suitable than bubble oxygenators for long-term extracorporeal support. Gas transfer across the membrane depends on the nature of the gas, the thickness of the membrane, the surface area, and the difference in the partial pressure of the gases on each side of the membrane. This partial-pressure difference is referred to as the *driving pressure* or the *transmembrane pressure.* The characteristics of a membrane oxygenator that influence gas exchange can be simplified by describing the effect of the transfer rate and the blood film thickness.[48]

Transfer Rate. The transfer rate is equal to the driving pressure times the permeability of the membrane. The driving pressure reflects the tendency of gases to diffuse from an area of high pressure to an area of low pressure. The greater this differential, the greater is the rate of exchange. The more permeable the membrane is for a particular gas, the greater the exchange of that gas.[62]

The driving pressure is different for each gas. If the sweep gas on the membrane is 100% oxygen, the gas-side Po_2 will be 760 mm Hg, and the venous Po_2 will be approximately 40 mm Hg. This difference results in an oxygen driving pressure of 720 mm Hg, moving oxygen into the blood. The driving pressure of carbon dioxide is significantly less: zero on the gas side and 45 mm Hg in the blood. This results in only a 45–mm Hg force moving carbon dioxide into the gas compartment (Figure 23-4). Despite this small driving pressure, however, carbon dioxide exchange is efficient because silicone rubber is six times more permeable to carbon dioxide than to oxygen. To enhance this gradient further, blood and gas flow in a countercurrent direction. This allows a consistently larger and extended gradient as the blood travels through the membrane.

Blood Film Thickness. The transfer rate of oxygen is limited by the thickness of the blood film between the membrane layers. As the blood film becomes thicker, the oxygenating efficiency decreases. In the human

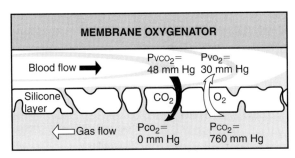

FIGURE 23-4 Schematic drawing of the membrane oxygenator, illustrating separation of blood and gas compartments, with transfer of gases across the silicone membrane because of a pressure gradient. Pco_2, Carbon dioxide partial pressure; Po_2, oxygen partial pressure; $Pvco_2$, mixed venous carbon dioxide pressure; Pvo_2, mixed venous oxygen pressure.

lung, this thickness is only one red cell, compared with a 20-cell to 60-cell layer in membrane oxygenators. The red cells closest to the membrane become saturated with oxygen first; with time, oxygen diffuses deeper into the blood, finally reaching the red cells in the innermost layer. The blood must remain in contact with the membrane long enough for complete saturation to occur. If the blood moves too fast, this will not occur, and the blood leaving the membrane will be less than fully saturated. This limitation, the rated flow, is the flow rate at which venous blood leaves the oxygenator at 95% saturation.[63] Therefore oxygen transfer will continue to increase only until the rated flow is reached. If higher blood flow rates are required, a larger membrane with a larger surface area is needed.

Carbon Dioxide Transfer. Because of the high permeability of silicone to carbon dioxide, the transfer of this gas is not dependent on the blood film thickness or blood flow rate. In practice, transfer depends more on the gas flow rate, the surface area of the membrane, and the driving pressure. Any situation that decreases the surface area (e.g., thrombus) will decrease carbon dioxide transfer. Increasing the sweep gas flow rate will lower the patient's $Paco_2$, principally because it maintains a full driving pressure throughout the gas phase.

Carbon dioxide clearance decreases as water accumulates in the gas compartment of the membrane, because of the temperature difference between the two sides of the membrane. The warm blood and the cooler gas allow condensation to occur. A minimal fresh gas flow is required for continuous flushing of these water droplets. Unfortunately, the minimal flow rate required to remove condensation usually results in excessive elimination of carbon dioxide as well. To compensate for this, sweep gas is often blended to contain carbogen, which reduces the driving pressure across the membrane and maintains normocarbia.

Monitoring the difference between the premembrane Pco_2 and postmembrane Pco_2 is important because carbon dioxide transfer is more selectively sensitive than oxygen transfer. Changes in carbon dioxide can be an early indication of membrane malfunction. Box 23-4 summarizes the relationship between the artificial membrane and its effect on gas exchange.

Pressure Drop. Each membrane oxygenator also has a rated pressure drop across the membrane. If this is exceeded, the membrane may rupture. Pressure drop is the resistance to blood flow produced by the membrane, obtained by subtracting the outlet pressure (postmembrane pressure) from the inlet pressure (premembrane pressure). The normal resistance within the membrane is usually fixed. This pressure difference can increase with internal clotting, higher flow rates, and an increase in blood viscosity. Monitoring of the premembrane and postmembrane pressures allows continuous assessment of the membrane's internal resistance.

Heat Exchanger

As blood travels through the ECLS circuit, heat is continually lost from the exposed surface of the tubing and through the oxygenator because of the cooling effects of the sweep gas and water evaporation. Therefore a disposable heat exchanger, which warms the blood and maintains the body temperature, is placed as the last component in the circuit before reinfusion into the patient. The heat exchanger is designed as a countercurrent system in which blood travels down stainless steel tubes in the center of the exchanger while warm water is pumped up the surrounding cylinders outside the tubes. In this manner the circulating water never has direct contact with the blood. The water itself is heated and pumped through a separate water pump and thermal regulator. To provide additional safety, the heat

---

Box 23-4	Gas Exchange Characteristics of Membrane Oxygenators

CARBON DIOXIDE EXCHANGE
- Independent of blood flow rate
- Dependent on driving pressure
- Dependent on sweep gas flow rate
- Increase sweep gas, decrease $Paco_2$
- Dependent on membrane surface area

OXYGEN EXCHANGE
- Dependent on blood flow rate
- Dependent on blood path thickness
- Independent of sweep gas flow rate
- Increase blood flow rate, increase Pao_2
- Dependent on membrane surface area

$Paco_2$, Arterial partial pressure of carbon dioxide; Pao_2, arterial partial pressure of oxygen.

exchanger also acts as a bubble trap when mounted vertically so that blood enters the top and exits the bottom. In this design a small amount of air can be trapped at the top of the heat exchanger.

Tubing

The tubing used in the ECLS circuit is usually composed of ¼-, ⅜-, or ½-inch diameter polyvinyl chloride. The total length of tubing in the circuit varies from institution to institution. Most of the tubing is subjected to low stress, and component failure is rare. However, the section of tubing housed between the pump heads and the back plate, the raceway, is under continuous strain from the roller heads throughout the run. This has often resulted in rupture of the raceway tubing, which can be a catastrophic event. Therefore many techniques are employed to prevent undue stress on this tubing. The first method, "walking the raceway," involves advancing the tubing to a new section at predetermined intervals, thereby having each section of tubing in the raceway for a limited time only. Another approach is to use larger diameter tubing. Because larger tubing has a greater volume per unit length, the revolutions per minute necessary to generate a given flow rate are reduced. Finally, a new stronger polymer, known as "super Tygon tubing" (S-65-HL), has become available. It is ideally suited for the pump's raceway. Although its qualities would make it ideal for the entire ECLS circuit, because of its high cost it typically is used only for the raceway section.

The ECLS circuit also contains a variety of polycarbonate connectors in various configurations, allowing volume administration and blood sample withdrawing. An attempt is made to minimize the number of connectors because each connector can promote turbulent flow and thrombus formation and each is a potential source of disconnection and leak.

Priming

Before initiating ECLS, the circuit must be prepared by the process of priming, which is divided into four stages[62]:

Stage 1: Carbon dioxide flush
Stage 2: Vacuum
Stage 3: Crystalloid prime
Stage 4: Blood prime

Carbon dioxide is flushed through the circuit for a minimum of 2 minutes. This flushes out the air in the circuit and replaces it with carbon dioxide, which is highly soluble in blood, decreasing the risk of microbubbles.

A line vacuum is applied to the gas ports of the membrane for at least 5 minutes. The reservoirs will gradually collapse, removing the carbon dioxide from the blood

partition of the membrane. This step opens the membrane, allowing more of its surface to be in full contact with the blood. The negative pressure also facilitates the subsequent filling of the circuit with fluid.

A crystalloid solution is added, and the circuit is filled systematically, expelling air as each section of the circuit is primed with fluid. Once completely filled, the vacuum is disconnected and the pump turned on to circulate the fluid. All air must be removed from the circuit. Special attention should be directed to the membrane and heat exchanger to ensure that they are free of bubbles. These components require aggressive shaking and slight tapping. Albumin is then added to the normal saline and circulated. Albumin coats and "pacifies" the internal surface of the circuit to minimize the blood–foreign surface interaction.

The crystalloid–albumin solution is then slowly drained from the priming bag and replaced with packed red blood cells. The blood is treated with heparin for anticoagulation, tromethamine (THAM) or sodium bicarbonate to adjust the pH, and calcium gluconate to reverse the citrate effect of stored blood. The blood is pumped into the circuit as the crystalloid is "chased out," draining into a waste bag. Once the blood is circulating, gas flow is connected to the membrane, and a blood gas determination, activated clotting time, and ionized calcium level are obtained from the circuit. The water bath is also attached to the heat exchanger, and the circulating blood is warmed to 37 °C before initiation of ECLS.

CANNULATION

Once ECLS criteria are met, parental consent is obtained, and blood products are ordered, it is critical that the team move quickly, because candidates for ECLS are by definition critically ill. The patient is positioned with the head at the foot of an elevated bed in the intensive care unit or ECMO unit. The patient's head is then rotated to the left, and the right side of the neck and the chest are prepared in a sterile manner and draped. A small incision is made at the base of the neck, and the right common carotid artery and internal jugular vein are mobilized. The patient is then given heparin at 30 to 100 units/kg; when this has been circulating for several minutes, cannulation is begun.

Concurrently, the ECLS team assembles and primes the circuit at the bedside. While the surgeon is cannulating, it is the responsibility of the nursing team and associated physicians to monitor the patient's vital signs. With the vessels exposed, the artery and vein are distally ligated with absorbable sutures and controlled proximally by vascular clamps. The appropriate cannulas are selected for the patient size and anticipated flow rates. The venous cannula is introduced through the jugular vein into the right atrium. The arterial cannula is introduced into the distal aortic arch via the right carotid artery. Both cannulas are secured to vessels and to the patient's skin to avoid accidental decannulation. At this point the cannulas are connected to the ECLS circuit, avoiding any air bubbles in the system. Once connected, the circuit is turned on, and the flow is slowly increased while the ventilator settings are concomitantly decreased. This usually results in immediate stabilization of the patient's vital signs.

With venovenous ECMO via the double-lumen cannula, only the internal jugular vein is cannulated. This approach is often performed by a "semipercutaneous" technique that obviates the need to ligate the vessel.

MANAGEMENT AND MONITORING

Cardiovascular System

The main goal of ECLS is to provide adequate oxygen delivery. This is assessed by monitoring the $S\overline{v}o_2$, using a fiberoptic catheter inserted into the circuit. An $S\overline{v}o_2$ of 75% is considered acceptable. On venovenous support, the $S\overline{v}o_2$ also reflects the recirculation and consequently cannot be used to assess oxygen delivery. Pulse oximetry provides continuous assessment of the patient's Sao_2, with 90% or greater being acceptable. On full venoarterial support, however, the pulse pressure is narrow and the oximeter may be inaccurate. Because of selective limb perfusion with venoarterial ECLS, the ideal sites for arterial blood gas monitoring are the lower extremities or the umbilical artery.

Once the cannulas are connected to the circuit, the pump's flow rate is slowly increased while the arterial pressure waveform is observed. With venoarterial support the arterial waveform decreases as flow is increased. The flow is increased to a goal of 100 to 120 ml/kg/minute or until the $S\overline{v}o_2$ is 75%. This approximates 70% to 80% of total cardiac output and is usually sufficient to support gas exchange. In a hypermetabolic state, however, the flow requirement may exceed 150 ml/kg/minute. When an adequate flow and $S\overline{v}o_2$ are established, ventilator settings are lowered, and subsequent adjustments in the Pao_2 are made by varying the Fio_2 of the sweep gas. Changes in $Paco_2$ are accomplished by altering the flow rate of the sweep gas, including the carbogen flow rate.

The mean blood pressure range for neonates on ECLS is 40 to 65 mm Hg. If inotropic support was required during cannulation, it can often be rapidly weaned or discontinued, whereas in venovenous ECLS, inotropes are gradually decreased. On occasion, hypertension will occur, requiring antihypertensive administration to maintain a mean blood pressure of less than 65 mm Hg. This is an essential precaution taken to reduce the incidence of IVH.

Anticoagulation

Clotting will occur within the ECLS circuit unless the blood is anticoagulated. When blood is exposed to a foreign surface, several changes take place. A layer of protein adheres to the foreign surface instantly. Some of these proteins "pacify" the surface, whereas others activate platelets and the clotting and complement cascades, resulting in clot formation.

Preventing a thrombus during extracorporeal support requires the administration of an anticoagulant, such as heparin. The effect of heparin is immediate, and it produces no side effects. Heparin has no direct anticoagulant effect on the blood by itself but combines with a cofactor, antithrombin III, to prevent thrombi from forming. This stops the conversion of fibrinogen to fibrin and ultimately prevents blood from clotting. A deficiency in antithrombin III can cause heparin to be ineffective, resulting in use of excessive amounts of heparin. If excessive clotting in the circuit is noted, a deficiency in antithrombin III should be considered.

Activated clotting time is monitored to assess heparin administration. It is a simple whole-blood test performed at the bedside. A small quantity of blood is injected into a test tube containing a catalyst. The test tube is inserted into a spinning well. When a clot is detected, a timer stops. In general, a continuous infusion of 20 to 60 units/kg/hour is required to sustain the activated clotting time at 180 to 200 seconds (normal, 90 to 120 s). Once stable, the activated clotting times are measured at least hourly.

The amount of heparin required can be influenced by several factors. Because heparin binds to platelets, higher doses of heparin are required with platelet transfusions. Conversely, a lower level of heparin is needed when thrombocytopenia exists. Heparin is also excreted in the urine, so a higher dose may be required during significant diuresis.

Hematologic System

Of all the blood components, platelets are most affected by extracorporeal support. Platelets are continuously consumed on ECLS and are generally administered on a daily basis in concentrated form.[64,65] Platelets attach to areas in which fibrinogen is present, become activated, and attract more platelets. These platelet aggregates are continuously formed while the patient receives ECLS. Because platelets adhere to the silicone membrane, they are administered directly to the patient or into the circuit after the membrane. Other blood products also adhere to the circuit, but with less effect.[66]

Although protocols vary among institutions, platelets are generally administered when the count is less than 100,000/mm³, accompanied by additional heparin. The hematocrit, prothrombin time, and fibrinogen are also monitored. Box 23-5 provides an example of protocol guidelines.

If fluid administration is required and the hematocrit is acceptable, 5% albumin should be administered. Fresh frozen plasma or cryoprecipitate is to be considered if a bleeding complication occurs or if factor replacements are necessary.

The effect of ECLS on the red blood cell is usually negligible if the roller pump is adjusted for proper occlusion. If dark plasma or hematuria occurs, however, hemolysis should be suspected. A plasma-free hemoglobin sample should be obtained and a search instituted for either a mechanical or a physiologic cause.

Neurologic System

Paralysis during ECLS is usually avoided except during cannulation and decannulation procedures. The patients are sedated while on ECLS to prevent accidental decannulation or hypertension secondary to agitation and to provide comfort. Fentanyl, midazolam, and lorazepam are typically used. Studies have shown that fentanyl continues to bind to the membrane during ECLS, and increasing amounts are usually required.[67] Narcotic withdrawal can delay recovery after ECLS.[68]

Head ultrasounds are performed to rule out IVH. If IVH does occur, the mean blood pressure is decreased, the range of activated clotting times is lowered, coagulation values are optimized, and an antifibrinolytic drug may be given to avoid extension of the bleed. As with any complication, the risk versus benefit of continuing ECLS should be carefully considered.

Because of the ligation of the internal jugular vein and the right common carotid artery, the head is maintained in the midline position to ensure adequate cerebral drainage and perfusion. Some institutions also insert an additional cannula into the cephalad segment of the right jugular vein to avoid venous obstruction and to enhance drainage.[69]

Box 23-5	Hematologic Guidelines for Extracorporeal Life Support

- Hematocrit > 35 ml/dl
- Platelets > 150,000/mm³
- Fibrinogen > 150 g/dl
- Prothrombin time < 17 seconds
- Activated clotting time = 180 to 220 seconds

Courtesy Wake Forest University Baptist Medical Center (Winston-Salem, NC).

Pulmonary System

After the initiation of venoarterial ECLS, the ventilator is generally reduced to an F_{IO_2} of 0.21 to 0.4, a peak inspiratory pressure of 20 to 25 cm H_2O, a positive end-expiratory pressure of 4 to 10 cm H_2O, and a respiratory rate of 5 to 10 breaths/minute. These resting ventilator settings presumably allow the lung to heal. Pulmonary care should include chest vibrations, manual ventilation with an inspiratory hold, saline instillation, and suctioning. Chest radiographs are taken daily and often exhibit a generalized opacification within the first 24 hours.[70] This phenomenon has been attributed to an abrupt decrease in airway pressure and to the release of vasoactive substances from the blood–circuit interface.

Patients who continue to have persistent pulmonary air leaks while receiving ECLS may require low levels of continuous positive airway pressure for the lungs to heal. Keszler and colleagues[71] have shown accelerated lung recovery by employing positive end-expiratory pressure levels of 12 to 14 cm H_2O. They found less opacification on chest X-ray films and a shorter duration of ECLS. In general, lung recovery usually occurs over 3 to 4 days, and it can be quantified by improvements in the chest radiograph, lung compliance, and gas exchange.[72]

Fluid Balance

Most patients receiving ECLS are edematous because of fluid resuscitation before ECLS. This edematous state can further compromise the lungs and impede lung recovery. Once capillary leak ceases, the goal of fluid management is to promote diuresis while maintaining adequate perfusion. Accordingly, fluid intake and output should be monitored for the duration of ECLS. Insensible water loss from the patient and the membrane cannot be measured but should not be forgotten. Although renal function is usually normal on ECLS, a decrease in urine output may be seen early in the run, especially if the patient sustained a prolonged period of hypoxia or hypotension before cannulation.

If oliguria or anuria occurs, ultrafiltration can be added to enhance output and manage fluid overload.[73] This is accomplished by connecting a hemofilter to the ECLS circuit, which allows a fraction of plasma water and dissolved solutes to pass through the filter's pores, while maintaining the cellular components and proteins. Nutrition is usually started on the third day of life; hyperalimentation and an infusion of a fat emulsion are usually initiated. However, transpyloric feeding can also be considered. In addition, most patients require calcium and potassium replacement while receiving ECLS.

WEANING

The amount of time a patient requires ECLS varies with the diagnosis. The average duration for a neonate is 4 to 6 days. Two approaches are used to wean patients from venoarterial ECLS. In the first approach, as lung function improves, ECLS is withdrawn slowly as ventilator support slowly increases. This is usually carried out over several days. Once the flow rate is decreased to 20 ml/kg/minute, the patient is usually ready for decannulation.

In the second approach the patient is maintained on full flows of 100 ml/kg/minute and minimal ventilator settings. At various intervals the patient is weaned from the ECLS circuit over a few minutes while the ventilator settings are increased. The patient circuit is then clamped off, and blood gases are obtained to assess pulmonary function. The rationale for the second approach is that the longer period of low ventilator support maximizes the (resting) time for the lungs to heal. Both methods are used widely, and neither has been clearly shown to have any advantage over the other.

Weaning from venovenous ECLS is slightly different from weaning from venoarterial ECLS. After increasing the ventilator parameters, both the membrane's gas ports are isolated from the ambient air. Eventually the blood entering and exiting the membrane is in equilibrium and reflects typical venous values. This eliminates any issues associated with clamping of the cannulas, particularly thrombus formation, which allows a longer trial without any pulmonary support.

DECANNULATION

When the patient is ready to be removed from ECLS, the decannulation is performed at the bedside. Sedative and paralytic agents are administered, and all infusions are switched to a peripheral site. Heparin is discontinued; however, its anticoagulating effect is not pharmacologically reversed. In a mirror-image reversal of the original cannulation procedure, the cannulas are removed and the vessels either reconstructed or ligated. Again, when the "semipercutaneous" method of cannulation is used, the cannula is simply pulled out and direct pressure held against the site until the bleeding stops. After the patient recovers from the paralysis, weaning from the ventilator can proceed. Before the patient is discharged from the hospital, it is essential that he or she be referred to a follow-up program within the hospital for further and future evaluations.

COMPLICATIONS

Complications of ECLS can be divided into patient and technical issues. All patient complications may be caused by two physiologic alterations: alterations in the blood-surface interaction and changes in the blood flow pattern. Both these variables can have adverse effects on all the organ systems. As already stated, when blood comes into contact with a foreign surface, a chain of events results in thrombus formation and platelet consumption. This necessitates the use of heparin and consequently contributes to the bleeding complications of ECLS.

Systemic heparinization makes IVH the primary risk of ECLS. The central nervous system, therefore, becomes the major area of concern. The risk of IVH is compounded by blood flow changes from the ligation of both the right internal jugular vein and the right common carotid artery. The effect of this perfusion and drainage interruption to the right side of the brain has been documented by Schumacher and colleagues,[49] who reported several occurrences of right-sided brain lesions after ECMO. Stolar and colleagues,[74] in reviewing the experience of the Neonatal ECMO Registry, reported that neurologic complications were predominant, with a 24% occurrence. The incidence of IVH in the neonate receiving ECLS is approximately 14%. In early ECLS studies, Cilley and colleagues[75] reported a series of eight infants born at less than 35 weeks of gestation and who all experienced IVH while receiving ECLS. This finding has led to the recommendation that ECLS should not be offered to infants born at less than 36 weeks of gestation or until anticoagulation is minimized or eliminated.

Wilson and colleagues[76] reported a different approach to this issue. They successfully employed an antifibrinolytic drug, *aminocaproic acid*, in infants considered at high risk for IVH and other types of hemorrhage. They reported a decrease in IVH from 18% to 0% with the use of this drug, along with a decrease in all postoperative bleeding. Circuit thrombotic complications, however, appeared to be greater with the use of aminocaproic acid.

Venoarterial ECLS alters the blood flow pattern throughout the body, especially the cerebral and pulmonary perfusion. Diverting blood flow through a nonpulsatile pump contributes to diminished pulse pressure. *Cardiac stun*, a term used to describe a dramatic decrease in the cardiac function of a patient receiving ECLS, is characterized by a minimal pulse pressure (<5 mm Hg).[77] This minimal pulse pressure infers nearly absent ventricular contribution, resulting in a Pao_2 almost equalizing the postmembrane Po_2. Cardiac stun occurs infrequently and lasts only transiently. Its exact mechanism is unknown, but cardiac stun is associated with increased mortality.

The ELSO registry contains information from more than 17,000 cases and includes every reported occurrence of both physiologic and mechanical complications (Tables 23-3 and 23-4).

TABLE 23-3

Neonatal Respiratory Failure: Patient Complications*

Complication	Percentage
Dialysis-hemofiltration	16
Hemolysis	11.8
Hypertension	12.7
Seizures	12
Abnormal creatinine value	9.9
Hyperbilirubinemia	8.1
Infection	6.4
Surgical site bleeding	6.1
Pneumothorax	6.1
Myocardial stun	5.5
Cannula site bleeding	6.3
Intraventricular hemorrhage	5.9
Cardiac dysrhythmias	4.0

* Total cases, 19,939.
Data from ELSO National Registry Report. Ann Arbor, Mich: University of Michigan; 2005.

TABLE 23-4

Neonatal Respiratory Failure: Mechanical Complications*

Complication	Percentage
Clots in circuit	18.6
Cannula problems	11.2
Oxygenator failure	5.7
Air in circuit	5.2
Pump malfunction	1.8
Heat exchanger malfunction	0.9
Tubing rupture	0.7

* Total cases, 19,939.
Data from ELSO National Registry Report. Ann Arbor, Mich: University of Michigan; 2005.

ASSESSMENT QUESTIONS

See Evolve Resources for answers.

1. In the ECMO system, the pump functions as the ___ of the circuit.
   A. Heart
   B. Lung
   C. Brain
   D. Monitor
2. In the ECMO system, the gas exchange device functions as the ___ of the circuit.
   A. Heart
   B. Lung
   C. Brain
   D. Monitor

ASSESSMENT QUESTIONS—cont'd

3. In VA ECMO the arterial cannula is inserted into the:
   A. Right atrium
   B. Femoral vein
   C. Right common carotid artery
   D. Superior vena cava
4. In venovenous ECMO the arterial cannula is inserted into the:
   A. Right atrium
   B. Femoral vein
   C. Right common carotid artery
   D. Superior vena cava
5. Which of the following is necessary for venoarterial ECMO to be effective?
   A. Adequate native cardiac output
   B. A well-established FRC
   C. Urine output > 3 ml/kg/hour
   D. None of the above
6. Which of the following is necessary for venovenous ECMO to be effective?
   A. Adequate native cardiac output
   B. A well-established FRC
   C. Urine output > 3 ml/kg/hour
   D. None of the above
7. The two components of oxygen delivery are:
   I. Arterial oxygen concentration
   II. Cardiac output
   III. Pao2
   IV. End-tidal carbon dioxide
   A. I and II
   B. II and III
   C. III and IV
   D. I and IV
8. In general, the criteria for extracorporeal membrane oxygenation is an estimated risk of mortality greater than
   A. 50%
   B. 65%
   C. 80%
   D. 95%
9. The main goal of ECLS is to:
   A. Support cardiac function
   B. Support lung function
   C. Provide adequate tissue oxygen delivery
   D. Remove carbon dioxide
10. The predominant complication reported in the Neonatal ECMO Registry is
   A. Neurologic
   B. Infectious
   C. Pump failure
   D. Thrombolysis

References

1. Comroe JH Jr: *Retrospectroscope insights into medical discoveries*, Menlo Park, Calif: Von Gehr; 1983.

2. Gibbon JH: Application of a mechanical heart lung apparatus to cardiac surgery, *Minn Med* 1954;37:171.

3. Gibbon JH: Artificial maintenance of circulation during experimental occlusion of pulmonary artery, *Arch Surg* 1937;34:1105.

4. Lillehei CW et al: The results of direct vision closure of ventricular septal defects in 8 patients by means of controlled cross-circulation, *Surg Gynecol Obstet* 1955;101:447.

5. Lillehei CW et al: Direct vision intracardiac surgery in man using a simple, disposable artificial oxygenator, *Dis Chest* 1956;29:1.

6. Kolff WJ, Berk HT Jr: Artificial kidney: a dialyzer with a great area, *Acta Med Scand* 1944;117:121.

7. Clowes GH: An artificial lung dependent upon diffusion of oxygen and carbon dioxide through plastic membranes, *J Thorac Surg* 1956;32:630.

8. Kolobow T, Bowman RL: Construction and elimination of an alveolar membrane artificial heart–lung, *Trans Am Soc Artif Intern Organs* 1963;9:238.

9. Kolobow T, Zapol WM, Pierce J: High survival and minimal blood damage in lambs exposed to long term venovenous pumping with a polyurethane chamber roller pump with and without a membrane oxygenator, *Trans Am Soc Artif Intern Organs* 1969;15:172.

10. Dorson WJ et al: A perfusion system for infants, *Trans Am Soc Artif Intern Organs* 1969;15:155.

11. White JJ et al: Prolonged respiratory support in newborn infants with a membrane oxygenator, *Surgery* 1971;70:288.

12. Hill JD: Prolonged extracorporeal oxygenation for acute post-traumatic respiratory failure: use of the Bramson membrane lung, *N Engl J Med* 1972;286:629.

13. Zapol WM et al: Extracorporeal membrane oxygenation in severe respiratory failure: a randomized prospective study, *JAMA* 1979;242:2193.

14. Hirschl RB, Bartlett RH: Extracorporeal membrane oxygenation (ECMO) support in cardio-respiratory failure. In Tompkins R, editor: *Advances in surgery*, Chicago: Year Book Medical; 1987. p 189.

15. Bartlett RH, Harken DE: Instrumentation for cardiopulmonary bypass: past, present, and future, *Med Instrum* 1976;10:119.

16. Bartlett RH et al: Extracorporeal membrane oxygenation for newborn respiratory failure: 45 cases, *Surgery* 1982;92:425.

17. Bartlett RH et al: Extracorporeal circulation in neonatal respiratory failure: a prospective randomized study, *Pediatrics* 1985;76:479.

18. O'Rourke PP et al: Extracorporeal membrane oxygenation and conventional medical therapy in neonates with persistent pulmonary hypertension of the newborn: a prospective randomized study, *Pediatrics* 1989;84:957.

19. Gattinoni L et al: Low frequency positive pressure ventilation with extracorporeal CO_2 removal in severe acute respiratory failure, *JAMA* 1986;256:881.

20. ECMO National Registry, Ann Arbor, Mich: University of Michigan; 2005. http://www.elso.med.umich.edu/)?

21. UK Collaborative ECMO Trial Group: The report of the UK collaborative randomised trial of neonatal extracorporeal membrane oxygenation, *Lancet* 1996;348:75.

22. Fox W, Duara S: Persistent pulmonary hypertension in the neonate: diagnosis and management, *J Pediatr* 1983;103:505.

23. Duara S, Fox W: Persistent pulmonary hypertension of the newborn. In Thibeault DW, Gregory GA, editors: *Neonatal pulmonary care*, ed 2, Menlo Park, Calif: Addison-Wesley; 1986.

24. Vacanti JP et al: The pulmonary hemodynamic response to perioperative anesthesia in the treatment of high risk infants with congenital diaphragmatic hernia, *J Pediatr Surg* 1984;19:672.

25. Wung JT et al: Management of infants with severe respiratory failure and persistence of the fetal circulation without hyperventilation, *Pediatrics* 1985;76:488.

26. Stahlman M: Acute respiratory disorders in the newborn. In Avery GB, editor: *Neonatology*, Philadelphia: Lippincott; 1981. p 390.

27. Miller FC et al: Significance of meconium during labor, *Am J Obstet Gynecol* 1975;122:573.

28. Yeh TF et al: Roentgenographic findings in infants with meconium aspiration syndrome, *JAMA* 1979;242:60.

29. Dillon HC Jr et al: Anorectal and vaginal carriage of group B streptococci in pregnant women, *J Infect Dis* 1984;145:794.

30. Anthony BF, Okada DM: The emergence of group B streptococci in infections of the newborn infant, *Annu Rev Med* 1977;28:355.

31. Puri P: Epidemiology of congenital diaphragmatic hernia. In Puri P, editor: *Modern problems in paediatrics*, New York: Karger; 1989.

32. Harrison MR, deLorimier AA: Congenital diaphragmatic hernia, *Surg Clin North Am* 1981;61:1023.

33. Dibbins AW, Wiener ES: Mortality from diaphragmatic hernia, *J Pediatr Surg* 1974;9:653.

34. Wilson JM et al: Congenital diaphragmatic hernia: predictors of severity in the ECMO era, *J Pediatr Surg* 1991;26:1028.

35. Kays DW et al: Detrimental effects of standard medical therapy in congenital diaphragmatic hernia, *Ann Surg* 1999;230:340.

36. Bartlett RH et al: Extracorporeal circulation (ECMO) in neonatal respiratory failure, *J Thorac Cardiovasc Surg* 1977;74:826.

37. Krummel TM et al: Alveolar–arterial oxygen gradients versus the neonatal pulmonary insufficiency index for prediction of mortality in ECMO candidates, *J Pediatr Surg* 1984;19:380.

38. Ortega M et al: Oxygenation index can predict outcome in neonates who are candidates for extracorporeal membrane oxygenation, *Pediatr Res* 1987;22:462A.

39. Muntean W: Coagulation and anticoagulation in extracorporeal membrane oxygenation, *Artif Organs* 1999;23:979.

40. Murray JF: Conference report: mechanisms of acute respiratory failure, *Am Rev Respir Dis* 1977;115:1071.

41. Bartlett RH et al: A prospective study of acute hypoxic respiratory failure, *Chest* 1986;89:684.

42. Steinhorn RH, Green TP: Use of extracorporeal membrane oxygenation in the treatment of respiratory syncytial virus bronchiolitis: the national experience, 1983 to 1988, *J Pediatr* 1990;116:338.

43. Adolph V et al: Extracorporeal membrane oxygenation for nonneonatal respiratory failure, *J Pediatr Surg* 1991;26:326.

44. Scalzo AJ et al: Extracorporeal membrane oxygenation for hydrocarbon aspiration, *Am J Dis Child* 1990;144:867.

45. O'Rourke PP et al: Extracorporeal membrane oxygenation: support for overwhelming pulmonary failure in the pediatric population: experience from the Extracorporeal Life Support Organization, *J Pediatr Surg* 1993;28:523.

46. Weber TR et al: Prolonged extracorporeal support for non-neonatal respiratory failure, *J Pediatr Surg* 1992;27:1100.

47. Swaniker F et al: Extracorporeal life support outcome for 128 pediatric patients with respiratory failure, *J Pediatr Surg* 2000;35:197.

48. Bartlett RH: Extracorporeal life support for cardiopulmonary failure, *Curr Probl Surg* 1990;27:261.

49. Schumacher RE et al: Rightsided brain lesions in infants following extracorporeal membrane oxygenation, *Pediatrics* 1988;82:155.

50. Moulton SL et al: Carotid artery reconstruction following neonatal extracorporeal membrane oxygenation, *J Pediatr Surg* 1991;26:794.

51. Hickey PR, Buckley MJ, Philbin DM: Pulsatile and nonpulsatile cardiopulmonary bypass: review of a counterproductive controversy, *Ann Thorac Surg* 1983;36:720.

52. Gerstmann DR et al: Left carotid artery and coronary arterial flow partitioning during neonatal ECMO, *Pediatr Res* 1989;25:37A.

53. Otsu T et al: Laboratory evaluation of a double lumen catheter for venovenous neonatal ECMO, *Trans Am Soc Artif Intern Organs* 1989;35:647.

54. Klein MD et al: Venovenous perfusion in ECMO for newborn respiratory insufficiency: a clinical comparison with venoarterial perfusion, *Ann Surg* 1985;201:520.

55. Kolobow T et al: Single catheter venovenous membrane lung bypass in the treatment of experimental ARDS, *Trans Am Soc Artif Intern Organs* 1988;34:35.

56. Zwischenberger JB et al: Total respiratory support with single cannula venovenous ECMO: double lumen continuous flow vs. single lumen tidal flow, *Trans Am Soc Artif Intern Organs* 1985;31:610.

57. Anderson HL et al: Venovenous extracorporeal life support in neonates using a double lumen catheter, *Trans Am Soc Artif Intern Organs* 1989;35:650.

58. Montogia JP, Merz SI, Bartlett RH: A standardized system for describing flow/pressure relationships in vascular access devices, *Trans Am Soc Artif Intern Organs* 1991;34:4.

59. Van Meurs KP et al: Maximum blood flow rates for arterial cannulae used in neonatal ECMO, *Trans Am Soc Artif Intern Organs* 1990;36:679.

60. Toomasian JM et al: Evaluation of Duraflo II heparin coating in prolonged extracorporeal membrane oxygenation, *Trans Am Soc Artif Intern Organs* 1988;34:410.

61. Bartlett RH: *Extracorporeal membrane oxygenation technical specialist manual*, ed 9. Ann Arbor, Mich: University of Michigan; 1988.

62. Galletti PM, Richardson PD, Snider MT: A standardized method for defining the overall gas transfer performance of artificial lungs, *Trans Am Soc Artif Intern Organs* 1972;18:359.

63. Anderson HL et al: Thrombocytopenia in neonates after extracorporeal membrane oxygenation, *Trans Am Soc Artif Intern Organs* 1986;32:534.

64. Moroff G et al: Reduction of the volume of stored platelet concentrations for neonatal use, *Transfusion* 1982;22:125.

65. Zach TL et al: Leukopenia associated with extracorporeal membrane oxygenation in the newborn, *J Pediatr* 1990;116:440.

66. Arnold JH et al: Tolerance and dependence in neonates sedated with fentanyl during extracorporeal membrane oxygenation, *Anesthesiology* 1990;73:1136.

67. Caron E, Maguie DP: Current management of pain, sedation, and narcotic physical dependency of the infant on ECMO, *J Perinatol Neonatal Nurs* 1990;4:63.

68. Vogt JF et al: Cannulation of cephalad segment of internal jugular vein during extracorporeal membrane oxygenation in the neonate. Presented at Children's National Medical Center, Snowmass, Colo, 1989.

69. Taylor GA et al: Diffuse pulmonary opacification in infants undergoing extracorporeal membrane oxygenation: clinical and pathologic correlation, *Radiology* 1986;161:347.

70. Keszler M et al: A prospective multicenter randomized study of high to low positive end-expiratory pressure during extracorporeal membrane oxygenation, *J Pediatr* 1992;120:107.

71. Lotze A, Short BL, Taylor GA: The use of lung compliance as a parameter for improvement in lung function in newborns with respiratory failure requiring extracorporeal membrane oxygenation, *Crit Care Med* 1987;15:226.

72. Heiss KF et al: Renal insufficiency and volume overload in neonatal ECMO managed by continuous ultrafiltration, *Trans Am Soc Artif Intern Organs* 1987;33:557.

73. Stolar CJ, Snedecor SM, Bartlett RH: Extracorporeal membrane oxygenation and neonatal respiratory failure: experience from the Extracorporeal Life Support Organization, *J Pediatr Surg* 1991;26:563.

74. Cilley RE et al: Intracranial hemorrhage during extracorporeal membrane oxygenation in neonates, *Pediatrics* 1986;78:699.

75. Wilson JM et al: AMICAR decreases the incidence of intracranial hemorrhage and other hemorrhagic complications of ECMO, *J Pediatr Surg* 1993;28:536.

76. Martin GR et al: Cardiac stun in infants undergoing extracorporeal membrane oxygenation, *J Thorac Cardiovasc Surg* 1991;101:607.

Pharmacology

ROBERT G. AUCOIN

OUTLINE

LEARNING OBJECTIVES

After reading this chapter the reader will be able to:

- Discuss common pharmacologic agents used in the treatment of pediatric respiratory disease
- Describe routes of administration for each drug
- Discuss each drug's mechanism of action
- Identify potential side effects of respiratory drugs
- Calculate dosage ranges of respiratory drugs
- Discuss the place in therapy of each agent or each family of agents

- Explain special handling and administration issues of selected drugs
- Select disease-specific drug regimens
- Differentiate drug absorption, distribution, and metabolism between neonatal and pediatric patients
- Describe disease-specific pathogens that are susceptible to certain drugs

The purpose of this chapter is to introduce a number of pharmacologic agents used in the treatment of pediatric airway disease. The mechanism of action, side effect profile, dose ranges, and place in therapy are covered. Several of the drugs reviewed require special handling and storage as well as specific administration techniques. These techniques are covered where appropriate.

Although most marketed drugs are used in pediatrics, only about one fourth of the drugs approved by the U.S. Food and Drug Administration (FDA) have a specific indication for use in neonatal and pediatric patients. Many differences exist among neonatal, pediatric, and adult patients regarding a drug's pharmacokinetics, pharmacodynamics, efficacy, and pediatric dosage regimens should not be simply extrapolated from adult data.[1]

Drug absorption, distribution, and metabolism vary greatly in neonatal and pediatric patients. Both physiochemical and physiologic factors affect drug distribution. Effects depend on the drug's specific pharmacologic properties. Clinically, this can lead to increased or decreased requirements for loading doses, dosing interval, metabolic rate, and time to excretion. Drug metabolism is slower in infants than in older children and adults, and even slower in premature infants. Between ages 1 and 9 years, metabolic rate increases to exceed that of the premature infant and the adult. Disease states may also alter drug dosing, metabolism, and elimination.[1]

Great progress has been made in pediatric pharmacokinetics. The FDA Modernization Act of 1997, the 1998 Pediatric Final Rule, and the Children's Health Act of 2000 were designed to help increase pediatric studies of drugs. In 2002, the Best Pharmaceuticals for Children Act was added to promote drug research in pediatrics.[2] Together; these steps provide increased support for pediatric clinical research and require pharmaceutical companies to conduct pediatric drug studies by allowing additional time for market exclusivity to designated drugs.[3]

Between 2007 and Spring 2008 there have been additional legislative actions targeting children and the need for further research and development of drugs.[4]

β-ADRENERGIC AGONISTS

Mechanism of Action

Norepinephrine is the parent compound of all the β_2-agonists. Over the years there have been structural changes and additions to the parent structure of norepinephrine that bestowed the resulting compounds with selectivity for α- or β-receptors, and prolonged duration of action. This alteration is easy to understand when one remembers that norepinephrine differs from

epinephrine only in the terminal amine group. This one difference gives norepinephrine its selective β activity.[5] In like fashion, addition and substitution of molecular entities cause significantly different actions in the resulting compounds.

Activation of β-adrenergic receptor sites on airway smooth muscle results in activation of adenyl cyclase, which increases the production of cyclic adenosine monophosphate (cAMP). This increase results in bronchial smooth muscle relaxation and skeletal muscle stimulation. β-Agonists have additional effects that inhibit the release of inflammatory mediators through stabilization of the mast cell membrane[6] (Figure 24-1). This in turn slows progression of the inflammatory cascade.

Place in Therapy

β_2-Adrenergic agonists are the treatment of choice for managing acute exacerbations of asthma as well as acute episodes of bronchospasm.[7] It has been found that β_2-agonist administration via metered-dose inhaler with a spacer is as effective as nebulized therapy.[8] Oral or intravenous β_2-agonist administration has no place in the treatment of acute asthma.[9]

Adverse Events

Aerosol administration results in effective activation of bronchial β_2-receptors with minimal systemic adverse effects. Adverse effects occur through excessive activation of β-adrenergic receptors and are more common with the use of nonselective β-adrenergic agonists than with the selective β_2-adrenergic agonists given parenterally or orally.[10]

Stimulation of the β_2-receptors in skeletal muscle results in *tremor*, the most common adverse effect observed with the use of selective agents. Tolerance to the tremor generally develops over time. Vasodilation is observed when β_2-receptors in the peripheral vasculature are stimulated. Tachycardia is observed most often as a result of stimulation of the β_1-receptors of the heart. Direct stimulation of cardiac β_2-receptors and reflex mechanisms from the peripheral vasodilation also increase heart rate. Headache, nervousness, dizziness, palpitations, cough, nausea, vomiting, and throat irritation may also occur.[11] All these adverse effects are much less likely with inhalation therapy than with parenteral or oral therapy.[12-14]

Tolerance to the effects of β-adrenergic agonists has been extensively studied both in vitro and in vivo. Although long-term use of systemic β-agonists can lead to some tolerance, tolerance to the pulmonary effects of these drugs is in all likelihood not a major clinical problem for most patients with asthma. This is especially true for those patients who do not exceed recommended

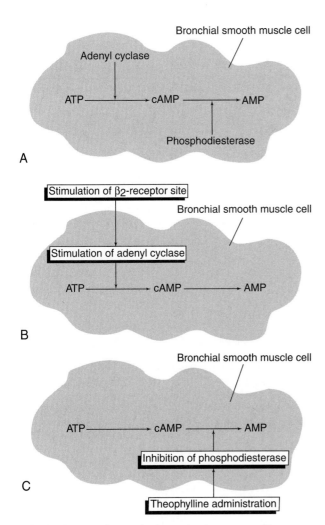

A

B

C

FIGURE 24-1 **A,** Sympathetic mechanisms controlling bronchial muscle tone. The enzyme adenyl cyclase is the catalyst for the conversion of adenosine triphosphate (ATP) to cyclic adenosine monophosphate (cAMP). The enzyme phosphodiesterase breaks down cAMP into adenosine monophosphate (AMP). Increased levels of cAMP result in relaxation of bronchial smooth muscle. Decreased levels of cAMP lead to spasm of susceptible bronchial smooth muscle. **B,** Bronchial muscle receptors are called β_2-receptor sites. Stimulation of these sites results in stimulation of the enzyme adenyl cyclase, which produces an increased level of cAMP, resulting in bronchodilation. **C,** Administration of the methylxanthine theophylline inhibits the enzyme phosphodiesterase, which inhibits the breakdown of cAMP and results in increased levels of cAMP and bronchodilation.

dosages over a long period. Systemic tolerance occurs as a result of chronic administration, which decreases the number of β_2-receptors and decreases the binding affinity of the receptors.[6,11] A *subsensitivity* to allergen and methacholine in patients who regularly use β_2-agonists has been reported.[12] The subsensitivity was not overcome by high-dose albuterol.[15] More studies are needed to determine the clinical importance of this phenomenon.

Overuse of inhaled β_2-agonists has been associated with increased risk of mortality from asthma. This increased risk of sudden death was greater among patients using more than one canister of rescue inhaler each month. The cardiotoxic potential of β_2-agonists may increase the risk of mortality, as may overreliance on medication and the patient's comfort level with β_2-agonist use. Control of symptoms may cause the patient to postpone obtaining adequate medical care in the presence of worsening asthma. With the use of a powerful bronchodilator the perceived need for corticosteroid therapy may not be realized.[16] Salpeter and colleagues[17] published a meta-analysis in 2004 documenting the negative cardiac effects of β-agonists. The increased risk of cardiac ischemia, congestive heart failure, arrhythmias, and sudden death was ascribed to increased heart rate, and reduction in potassium levels. It should be noted that the meta-analysis included patients with both chronic obstructive pulmonary disease and asthma.

Concerns about overuse have led to the recommendation that β-agonists be used only on an "as needed" basis in the treatment of acute episodes.[7,18,19]

Selective Agents

Selective agents have a more specific effect on β_2-receptors, with minimal effect on β_1-receptors; so that less stimulation of the heart rate is observed.[20] Several β-adrenergic agonists are available for the management of airway obstruction. These agents differ in β_2-selectivity, potency, elimination half-life, and availability of dosage formulations.

Albuterol is the official generic name for this agent in the United States, although the name suggested by the World Health Organization (Geneva, Switzerland) is *salbutamol.* Albuterol is indicated for the treatment and prevention of bronchospasm and is available in a variety of dosage forms. The recommended pediatric dosage for the metered-dose inhaler (MDI) in the treatment of acute exacerbations is 4 to 8 inhalations every 20 minutes for 3 doses, and then every 1 to 4 hours. For maintenance therapy in children more than 4 years of age the MDI dose is 1 or 2 inhalations every 4 to 6 hours with a maximum of 12 inhalations per day.[3] Neonatal nebulization consists of 0.05 to 0.15 mg/kg per dose mixed with 1 to 2 ml of normal saline (NS) every 4 to 6 hours as needed. Pediatric nebulization doses range from 0.1 to 0.5 ml in 2 to 3 ml of NS every 2 to 6 hours as needed. Nebulization treatments may be given as often as every 1 hour. In severe cases of status asthmaticus, continuous nebulization may be given. The normal oral dose in children less than 6 years of age is 0.1 mg/kg per dose every 8 hours (three times daily), with a maximal dose of 12 mg/day. Dosages may be increased during acute exacerbation of the disease.[3,21] Table 24-1 lists the bronchodilators available in inhalation form that are commonly used with infant and pediatric patients.

TABLE 24-1

Inhaled Bronchodilators

Agent	Availability	Dose	Adverse Events
Albuterol (Proventil, Ventolin)	MDI: 90 µg/inh HFA: 90 µg/inh Soln for neb: 0.042% (3 ml), 0.083% (3 ml), and 0.5% (20 ml)	Acute: 4 to 8 puffs q 20 min for 3 doses, then q 1 to 4 h; or 1 or 2 puffs q 4-6 h (max, 12 puffs/d) Children: 0.15 mg/kg (min, 2.5 mg) every 20 min for 3 doses, then 0.15-0.3 mg/kg (max, 10 mg) every 1 to 4 h prn	Tachycardia, tremor, nervousness, headache, palpitations, dizziness, nausea, vomiting, hypokalemia (at high doses)
Levalbuterol (Xopenex)	HFA: 45 µg/actuation Soln for neb: 0.31 mg/3 ml, 0.63 mg/3 ml, 1.25 mg/3 ml Conc: 1.25 mg/0.5 ml	Children 2-11 yr: 0.16-1.25 mg Children 6-11 yr: 0.31 mg q 6 to 8 h (max, 3 times daily) Children > 12 yr: 0.63-1.25 mg 3 times daily	Nervousness, tremor, dizziness, headache, tachycardia
Pirbuterol (Maxair)	MDI: 200 µg/puff	Children: 4-8 puffs every 20 min for 3 doses, then every 1-4 h Children > 12 yr: 4-8 puffs every 20 min for up to 4 h, then every 1-4 h Maintenance dose: 2 puffs q 4-6 hours	Tachycardia, tremor, dizziness, nausea, vomiting, headache, nervousness, palpitations
Salmeterol (Serevent)	Pwd for inh: 50 µg/puff	Maintenance: 1 puff every 12 h Prevention of EIA: 1 puff 30 min before exercise. Next dose in 12 h	Prolonged QT interval, tachycardia, palpitations, dizziness, nausea, and vomiting
Formoterol (Foradil)	Pwd for oral inh (capsules): 12 µg/25 mg lactose as carrier	1 inh q 12 h (max, 2 doses daily)	Tachycardia, tremor, nervousness, nausea, vomiting, headache, hypertension, dizziness, viral chest infection, fatigue, tonsillitis
Metaproterenol (Alupent, Metaprel)	MDI: 65 mg/puff Soln for neb: 0.4% and 0.6% in 2.5 ml	Inhalation: Children > 12 yr: 2 or 3 puffs q 3-4 h up to 12 puffs/d Nebulization: Infants/children: 0.5-1 mg/kg (max, 15 mg) q 4-6 h	Tachycardia, tremor, nervousness, nausea, vomiting, headache, hypertension, dizziness
Racemic epinephrine	Neb soln: 2.25%	0.05 mg/kg (max, 0.5 ml) in 2 ml of saline	Tachycardia, tremor, dizziness, nausea, vomiting, headache, nervousness, palpitations
Ipratropium bromide (Atrovent)	HFA: 17 µg/puff Neb soln: 0.2% (2.5 ml) Intranasal: 0.03% and 0.06%	Neonates: Neb: 25 µg/kg/dose, 3 times daily Infants: Neb: 125-250 µg, 3 times daily Acute: Children: 250 µg neb q 20 min for 3 doses, then q 2-4 h Children > 12 yr: 500 µg q 30 min for 3 doses, then q 2-4 h MDI: 4-8 puffs prn Maintenance Tx: 250-500 µg q 6 h or MDI 1-2 inh q 6 h (max, 12 inh/d)	Dry mouth, headache, dizziness, cough, blurred vision, drying of secretions
Terbutaline (Brethine, Brethaire)	Aqueous soln as sulfate: 1 mg/ml	Nebulization: 0.01-0.03 ml/kg (min, 0.1 ml; max, 2.5 ml) every 4-6 h Subcutaneous: 0.01 mg/kg (max, 0.4 mg) q 15-20 min times 3 doses	Tachycardia, tremor, dizziness, nausea, vomiting, headache, nervousness, palpitations

Conc, Concentration; EIA, exercise-induced asthma; HFA, hydrofluoroalkane; inh, inhaled; max, maximum; MDI, metered-dose inhaler; neb, nebulization; prn, as needed; pwd, powder; q, every; soln, solution; Tx, treatment.

Adverse reactions to albuterol are similar to those of other β_2-agonists. One of the documented side effects of albuterol therapy is *hypokalemia,* which may explain the increased mortality of patients using large doses of albuterol. Hypokalemia is caused by a transient activation of the Na^+/K^+ pump and the transport of K^+ intracellularly.[21a] Hypokalemia may predispose the heart to toxic effects by leading to arrhythmias.[17]

Levalbuterol (Xopenex)

Albuterol is composed of both (R)- and (S)-albuterol. The (S)-isomers are not clinically beneficial and may worsen airway reactivity.[22,23] Levalbuterol is the modified name for (R)-albuterol hydrochloride and is the active component of albuterol. Most drugs are available in both dextro (d)- and levo (l)-isomers. The maker of levalbuterol has tested both isomers and found that the l-isomer is the most active compound. It also possesses a longer duration of action and is postulated to have a slightly better side effect profile.

Levalbuterol is indicated for the treatment or prevention of bronchospasm in adults and children 2 years of age and older. In studies of asthma treatment in the pediatric patient, levalbuterol was compared with both racemic albuterol and placebo.[24] In doses of 0.31 and 0.63 mg, levalbuterol produced an equipotent degree of bronchodilation, as measured by percent change from predose forced expiratory volume at 1 second (FEV_1), as comparable doses of 1.25 and 2.5 mg of racemic albuterol. The study found that 0.63 mg of levalbuterol was equipotent to 1.25 mg of racemic albuterol, and 1.25 mg of levalbuterol was equipotent to 2.5 mg of racemic albuterol.[3,20,25]

Levalbuterol is supplied in 3.0–ml unit-dose vials and requires no dilution before administration by nebulization. Each unit-dose vial contains either 0.63 or 1.25 mg of levalbuterol. The suggested nebulization dosage for children more than 12 years of age is a 0.63–mg unit dose administered every 6 to 8 hours. Patients who do not respond adequately to a dose of 0.63 mg may benefit from a dosage of 1.25 mg administered every 6 to 8 hours. The solution is stored in a protective foil pouch and discarded if it is not colorless.[3,20]

Adverse events reported in patients receiving levalbuterol are similar to those observed with racemic albuterol. However, the incidence of tremor and nervousness is reported to be slightly less when using 0.63 mg of levalbuterol.

Metaproterenol (Alupent, Metaprel)

Metaproterenol is classified as a selective β_2-agonist, although it is less selective than albuterol. With the introduction of albuterol and other more specific agents, metaproterenol has fallen into disuse. It is indicated for the treatment of bronchospasm and is available as an oral syrup and tablet, MDI, and solution for nebulization.[6] The recommended dosing regimen for the MDI is 1 to 3 inhalations every 3 to 4 hours, up to a maximal dose of 12 inhalations per day. The recommended pediatric dosage for the 5% nebulized solution is 0.01 to 0.03 ml/kg in 1 to 2 ml of NS every 4 to 6 hours. The nebulized solution may be administered as frequently as every hour for severe bronchospasm. The medication may be administered orally at doses of 0.4 mg/kg per dose every 6 to 8 hours. In the infant population the dosing interval may be expanded to 8 to 12 hours.[3,6]

Terbutaline (Brethine, Brethaire)

Terbutaline is the only selective β_2-agonist available in parenteral form for the emergency treatment of status asthmaticus. It is available as an oral tablet and a sterile aqueous solution for subcutaneous and intravenous administration. The maximal pediatric oral dose recommended is 0.15 mg/kg per dose three times per day, not to exceed 5 mg/day. The aqueous solution is supplied in a 2–ml clear glass ampoule containing 1 mg of terbutaline per 1 ml of solution. Dosage for nebulization is 0.01 to 0.03 ml/kg mixed in 1 to 2 ml of NS every 4 to 6 hours. The minimal dose is 0.1 ml and the maximal dose is 2.5 ml every 4 to 6 hours. Two MDI inhalations every 4 to 6 hours is recommended. The subcutaneous dosage recommended for children is 0.01 mg/kg (maximum, 0.4 mg) every 15 to 20 minutes times three doses.[3,20]

Terbutaline may be administered intravenously as a continuous infusion to pediatric patients refractory to more common inhalation therapy. In most institutions, terbutaline is reserved for the management of acute episodes of severe asthma. Recommended dosing for continuous infusion begins at 2 to 10 µg/kg as a loading dose followed by 0.08 to 0.4 µg/kg per minute, increased as needed to as high as 10 µg/kg per minute. Tachycardia, often a dose-limiting adverse effect, is more frequently observed when using doses in the upper range and is the main dose-limiting side effect.[3,20]

Pirbuterol (Maxair)

Pirbuterol has a relatively fast onset of action, at 5 minutes or less, and a short duration of action at 5 hours. It is indicated for the prevention and reversal of bronchospasm in adults and children more than 12 years old.[3,20] In many respects the adverse reaction profile of pirbuterol is better than for albuterol, with fewer incidences of tachycardia, palpitations, and tremor. Pirbuterol is available as an MDI and in a "Maxair Autohaler (Graceway Pharmaceuticals, Bristol, Tenn)" inhaler formulation. The normal dose for adults and children more than 12 years of age is 2 inhalations (0.4 mg) every 4 to 6 hours. One inhalation (0.2 mg) may be sufficient for some patients.[3,20]

Salmeterol (Serevent)

Salmeterol is a long-acting β_2-agonist indicated for long-term maintenance treatment of asthma and prevention of bronchospasm in patients 4 years of age and older. It is also indicated for the prevention of exercise-induced bronchospasm (EIB). Salmeterol has much the same profile for safety and adverse effects as albuterol. Long-acting β_2-agonists can be beneficial to patients when added to inhaled corticosteroid therapy, especially to control nighttime asthma symptoms.[7] They also attenuate EIB for longer time periods than do short-acting β_2-agonists. Studies suggest that for patients with inadequate symptom control who are receiving low-to-medium doses of inhaled corticosteroids, it may be more beneficial to add salmeterol than to increase the dose of inhaled corticosteroid.[10,20,26,27]

Salmeterol is no longer available in the United States as an MDI. It is available as the Serevent Diskus (GlaxoSmithKline, Research Triangle Park, NC), which delivers 50 µg per inhalation. The normal dose for prevention of asthma symptoms is 50 µg (1 inhalation) of the Diskus twice daily. For the prevention of EIB, 100 µg (2 inhalations) can be given 30 minutes before exercise. Patients using salmeterol twice per day for maintenance therapy do not take an additional dose before exercise.[3,20]

The most common form of salmeterol used today is in combination with fluticasone (Advair). The combination is available in a variety of strengths. See the individual monographs for drug information.

Salmeterol is not used to treat acute asthma symptoms. The onset of action is not immediate and occurs approximately 30 minutes after intake.[28] Instead, a short-acting β_2-agonist is used to relieve acute symptoms. When beginning treatment with salmeterol, instruct patients to discontinue any regular use of the short-acting β_2-agonist and to use the shorter acting agent for symptomatic, quick relief during acute episodes only.

Adverse reactions to salmeterol are similar to those seen with other selective β_2-agonists, including tachycardia, palpitations, tremor, and nervousness. Although uncommon after administration at recommended doses, salmeterol can produce a clinically significant cardiovascular effect in some patients. Changes in the electrocardiogram include flattening of the T wave, prolongation of the QT interval, and ST-segment depression. Fatalities have been reported in association with excessive use. Large doses (12 to 20 times the recommended dose) have been associated with ventricular arrhythmias. Therefore salmeterol is not given more frequently than twice daily at the recommended dose.[3,11,20]

Formoterol (Foradil)

Formoterol is a long-acting, highly β_2-selective bronchodilator. It is indicated for long-term, twice-daily (morning and evening) administration in the maintenance treatment of asthma and prevention of bronchospasm in adults and children 5 years of age and older.[3,10,20] Formoterol is also indicated for the acute prevention of EIB in adults and adolescents 12 years of age and older. It is inherently different from the short-acting inhaled β_2-agonists; formoterol is not used to treat acute symptoms and is not considered a substitute for inhaled or oral corticosteroids. When beginning treatment with formoterol, instruct patients to discontinue any regular use of short-acting β_2-agonists and to use a shorter-acting agent for symptomatic, quick relief during acute episodes only.

Formoterol is available in a hard, gelatin capsule dosage form containing a dry powder blend of 12 µg of formoterol and 25 mg of lactose as a carrier. It is intended for oral inhalation only with the Foradil Aerolizer inhaler (Schering, Kenilworth, NJ); the capsules are not swallowed. The usual dosage is the inhalation of the contents of one 12–µg capsule every 12 hours, with a total daily dose not to exceed one capsule twice daily (total daily dose, 24 µg). If symptoms arise between doses, an inhaled short-acting β_2-agonist is taken for immediate relief. For the prevention of EIB, the usual dosage is the inhalation of the contents of one 12–µg capsule at least 15 minutes before exercise. Regular, twice-daily dosing in preventing EIB has not been studied. Patients who are receiving formoterol twice daily for maintenance treatment of their asthma do not use additional doses for prevention of EIB.[3,20]

Adverse reactions to formoterol include tremor, tachycardia, arrhythmias, palpitation, nervousness, agitation, headache, muscle cramps, dizziness, fatigue, insomnia, dry mouth, nausea, hypokalemia, hyperglycemia, and metabolic acidosis. Adverse events occurring more frequently in children (ages 5 to 12 yr) in need of daily bronchodilator and antiinflammatory treatment include viral infection, rhinitis, tonsillitis, gastroenteritis, abdominal pain, nausea, and dyspepsia. Clinical trials show no evidence of drug dependence with the use of formoterol.[3,20]

Nonselective Agents
Isoproterenol (Isuprel)

The use of isoproterenol in the treatment of asthma has dramatically decreased with the introduction of more selective agents. Administration of isoproterenol results in relaxation of bronchial smooth muscle, cardiac stimulation, and peripheral vasodilation. It may be used intravenously in emergency situations to stimulate the heart rate in patients with bradycardia. Common adverse effects include palpitations, tachycardia, headache, nervousness, dizziness, nausea, vomiting, tremor, and cutaneous flushing.[3,6,20]

Isoproterenol is available as an injectable solution. Intravenous dosages range from 0.05 to 2 µg/kg per minute and should be initiated at 0.05 µg/kg per minute, with incremental increases until the desired effect is achieved.[3,20]

Ephedrine (Neo-Synephrine)

Ephedrine is used primarily as a systemic decongestant. Its therapeutic index is low, with hypertension resulting from doses exceeding two to three times the normal dose. Ephedrine has a therapeutic half-life of 3 to 6 hours. Most excretion occurs through the kidney, with unchanged drug excreted in the urine. The most common adverse effect associated with ephedrine is hypertension. Tachycardia is another common side effect. Children with underlying vascular or cardiac problems should avoid the use of ephedrine if possible. The common pediatric dose for ephedrine in children ages 2 to 6 years is 2 to 3 mg/kg per day divided every 4 to 6 hours, with a maximal dose of 25 mg every 4 hours. Dosing for children ages 7 to 11 years is 6.25 to 12.5 mg every 4 hours with a maximum of 75 mg/day. The nasal spray dose for children age 6 to 12 years is 1 or 2 sprays in each nostril, not more than every 4 hours. Do not exceed more than 3 days of therapy.[3,20]

Epinephrine (Vaponefrin)

Racemic epinephrine inhalant solution is a sympathomimetic that acts on both α-receptors and β-receptors of the respiratory tract. The α-adrenergic effects are thought to result from inhibition of the enzyme adenyl cyclase. Stimulation of the α-receptors results in vasoconstriction and a reduction of mucosal and submucosal congestion and edema. The β-adrenergic effects result from stimulation of adenyl cyclase and increased cAMP production, which results in reduction of airway smooth muscle spasm (see Figure 24-1). Both actions work in concert to reduce airway swelling. In children, racemic epinephrine is used most often to treat postextubation edema and laryngotracheobronchitis.

The solution of racemic epinephrine, 2.25%, is an equal mixture of the *d*- and *l*-isomers of epinephrine. A plastic or glass dropper should be used to prepare the dose because the solution reacts on contact with metals. Do not use the solution if the color is pinkish or darker than slightly yellow, or if it contains a precipitate. Refrigerate the solution once the bottle is opened. The recommended dose for laryngotracheobronchitis is 0.05 ml/kg (maximum, 0.5 ml) in 3 ml of NS nebulized every 1 to 4 hours as needed. Common adverse effects include tachycardia, palpitations, nervousness, tremor, insomnia, headache, loss of appetite, and nausea.[3,6,20]

ANTICHOLINERGICS

Mechanism of Action

The parasympathetic nervous system plays a major role in regulating airway homeostasis and bronchomotor tone. Various noxious stimuli have been demonstrated to increase parasympathetic activity with resultant bronchoconstriction. Vagal nerve fibers that end on muscarinic receptors innervate the larger airway smooth muscles. Cholinergic irritant receptors are also located in the junction between airway mucosal cells. Anticholinergic agents are competitive inhibitors of acetylcholine at the muscarinic receptors and are effective in relieving cholinergic-mediated bronchoconstriction (Figure 24-2). Increasing levels of acetylcholine can overcome this smooth muscle receptor blockade.[11,29]

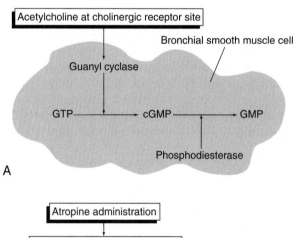

A

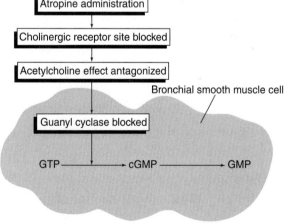

B

FIGURE 24-2 **A,** Parasympathetic mechanisms controlling bronchial smooth muscle tone. Stimulation of the parasympathetic system causes the release of acetylcholine at the cholinergic receptor site. Acetylcholine stimulates the enzyme guanyl cyclase to convert guanosine triphosphate (GTP) to cyclic guanosine monophosphate (cGMP). Phosphodiesterase then breaks down cGMP to guanosine monophosphate (GMP). High cGMP levels result in bronchoconstriction. **B,** Administration of an anticholinergic (atropine) antagonizes the acetylcholinergic effect and prevents cGMP from forming. This relieves the bronchoconstriction.

Place in Therapy

Ipratropium is part of routine therapy in infants, children, and adults with asthma, chronic obstructive pulmonary disease, or both.[9-11] In 2002, Rodrigo and Rodrigo found in their review that multiple doses of ipratropium along with a β-agonist, administered to children with severe asthma exacerbations, reduced the number of hospitalizations and improved lung function.[30] Werner,[31] in a review of the treatment of status asthmaticus, strongly recommended the incorporation of ipratropium in the emergency department treatment plan. Craven and colleagues, in 2001, found no significant difference between treatment groups when randomized to treatment with albuterol plus ipratropium versus albuterol alone.[32] The addition of anticholinergics, specifically ipratropium, to β_2-agonist in the treatment of severe asthma exacerbations shows benefit without significantly increasing risk.[7]

Ipratropium Bromide (Atrovent)

Ipratropium bromide is an anticholinergic agent used in the treatment of bronchospasm associated with chronic obstructive pulmonary disease, chronic bronchitis, and asthma.[9,11] It is a quaternary ammonium derivative of atropine. Ipratropium has little effect on mucociliary clearance and ciliary functions compared with atropine; use of ipratropium avoids accumulation of lower airway secretions. Quaternary compounds are poorly absorbed across mucosal membranes and the blood–brain barrier. Inhalation of ipratropium therefore results in local airway effects with minimal systemic effects.[29,33] Ipratropium inhalation is not sufficiently effective to be used as a single agent in the treatment of acute bronchospasm, but with albuterol is often more effective than either agent alone. This is often the case if the patient has no previous history of β-agonist use.[34,35]

Dosage and Administration

Ipratropium bromide is available as a nasal spray, an MDI, and a nebulization solution. Concentrations of the nasal spray are 0.03% and 0.06%. The dose for the nasal spray is 2 sprays in each nostril two or three times daily.[3,9,10,20] The nasal spray is used only for symptomatic relief of rhinorrhea associated with allergic and nonallergic perennial rhinitis; it does not relieve nasal congestion, sneezing, or postnasal drip.[36]

The inhalation solution is available in unit-dose vials containing 500 µg of ipratropium in 2.5 ml of NS.[3] The vials are packaged in a foil pouch and must be protected from light. The inhalation solution can be mixed in the nebulizer with albuterol or metaproterenol if used within 1 hour. The stability and safety of ipratropium when mixed with other drugs in a nebulizer have not been established. The usual dose for neonates by nebulization is 25 µg/kg per dose three times daily. For infants and children less than 12 years of age the nebulization dose is 125 to 250 µg three times daily. For adults and children more than 12 years of age, with an acute exacerbation, the nebulization dose is 500 µg every 30 minutes for 3 doses and then every 2 to 4 hours as needed. For maintenance therapy the dose is 2 or 3 inhalations every 6 hours, not to exceed 12 inhalations per day.[3]

The MDI dose for children 3 to 12 years old is 1 or 2 inhalations every 4 to 6 hours as needed, with a maximum of 6 inhalations in a 24-hour period. The MDI dose for adults and children over 12 years of age is 2 inhalations every 4 to 6 hours, with a maximum of 12 inhalations in 24 hours. The most common adverse reactions are dry mouth, cough, headache, nausea, dizziness, blurred vision, and drying of secretions. Ipratropium is also available mixed with albuterol (Combivent, DuoNeb), supplied as an MDI and in solution for nebulization. Dosage recommendations for this mixture follow those for ipratropium bromide alone.[3,8,20]

Glycopyrrolate (Robinul)

Glycopyrrolate is a quaternary anticholinergic compound. It is a member of a class of drugs also known as *antimuscarinic* agents. These drugs are used to inhibit the muscarinic actions of acetylcholine at multiple sites. Glycopyrrolate is used specifically to inhibit salivation and excessive secretions of the respiratory tract. It is also used to counter the muscarinic effects of neostigmine and pyridostigmine during reversal of neuromuscular blockade.[29,37] Glycopyrrolate is contraindicated in patients with tachycardia, paralytic ileus, or myasthenia gravis. Use with extreme caution in infants and children. Neonates are at risk for "gasping syndrome" (the quick inhalation and exhalation of breaths—much like gulping for air), secondary to benzyl alcohol content in the injectable form.[3]

The dosage for control of secretions in children is 40 to 100 µg/kg three or four times daily. The intramuscular and intravenous dosage is 4 to 10 µg/kg every 3 to 4 hours. Adverse reactions include tachycardia, ventricular fibrillation, and palpitations. Central effects include drowsiness, headache, and ataxia.[3,37]

INHALED CORTICOSTEROIDS

Mechanism of Action

Corticosteroids are potent anti-inflammatory agents used in the management of asthma. While the term "corticosteroids" is used for most steroids, it is the general term that includes both glucocorticoids and mineralocorticoids. The mechanisms of action include the following:

- Inhibition of the production of leukotrienes and prostaglandins through interference with arachidonic acid metabolism
- Reduction of migration and inhibition of the activity of inflammatory cells
- Increase in the number of β-receptors
- Enhancement of the responsiveness of β-receptors in airway smooth muscle

Glucocorticoids act on mast cells by slowing the synthesis of histamines. This slowing of synthesis does not affect the rate of release of histamines.[10,11,20] The benefits of inhaled corticosteroids include a reduction in airway inflammation and hyperresponsiveness, as well as a decrease in mucous secretion and airway edema.

Place in Therapy

The Expert Panel Report 3 (EPR-3) on asthma[7] states that inhaled corticosteroids are the most effective long-term therapy available for mild, moderate, or severe persistent asthma and that in general they are well tolerated and safe at the recommended dosages. Over the past 5 years the debate concerning long-term use of corticosteroids has subsided. The EPR-3 deems that the risk of adverse effects is far outweighed by the benefit. When used at recommended dosages, corticosteroids are safe and have few untoward effects.[40] There are several points made by the EPR-3 in the discussion of inhaled corticosteroids. The points include the following:

- Potential risks of inhaled corticosteroids are well balanced by their benefits.
- Poorly controlled asthma may delay growth and growth rates are highly variable in children.
- Inhalation therapy allows the topical administration of potent antiinflammatory agents directly at the site of action in the airways.
- Administration directly to the site of action helps decrease the adverse effects observed with systemic corticosteroid therapy.

The five formulations for inhalation therapy currently available in the United States are as follows:

1. Beclomethasone dipropionate (Beclovent, QVAR, Vanceril)
2. Budesonide (Pulmicort)
3. Flunisolide (AeroBid)
4. Fluticasone propionate (Flovent)
5. Triamcinolone acetonide (Azmacort)

All five agents are available as dry powder and/or MDI formulations. Budesonide is also available in suspension for nebulization (Pulmicort Respules; AstraZeneca, London, UK).[10,20] All inhaled products are not created equal. There are significant differences in their efficacy and safety profiles. These differences result from differences in chemical structure. A thorough discussion of these differences is beyond the scope of this chapter.

Dosage and Administration

Table 24-2 lists the antiinflammatory agents that are available for inhalation therapy in children and the recommended dosages. These dosages are often increased depending on the age of the patient and the response to therapy. Once asthma is under control, the initial dose is adjusted to the lowest effective dose to reduce the possibility of side effects. Maximal benefit may not be achieved for 1 to 2 weeks or longer after starting treatment.

Adverse Events

The likelihood of systemic side effects increases when inhaled corticosteroids are used at higher doses and for long periods. Inhaled corticosteroids produce a dose-dependent suppression of adrenal axis steroid production. Use of these agents may also impair growth and decrease bone formation.[38-40] The effects on linear growth are discussed extensively in the literature. Treatment with inhaled corticosteroids was associated with prepubertal growth impairment in one study using beclomethasone as the study drug. The suppression was limited to 1.5 cm/year in children treated with beclomethasone at 400 μg/day. Subsequent studies have shown that inhaled corticosteroid therapy does not clinically affect final adult height.[38,40] Many studies to determine the effects on growth have significant design limitations. Because delayed or impaired growth may be a result of the disease itself, the question remains as to whether the treatment or the underlying disease is the true determinant of linear growth reduction. Further studies have proved that even with this initial reduction in linear growth, the long-term effects do not last. In long-term follow-up, patients with a history of inhaled corticosteroid use achieved height that fell within the expectation based on hereditary models.[41]

The American College of Chest Physicians (Northbrook, Ill), along with three other national organizations, published a review of the current literature with respect to potential complications of inhaled corticosteroid use in asthma.[38] They state that the evidence concludes that the clinical effectiveness of inhaled corticosteroid therapy far outweighs the risk. The National Heart, Lung, and Blood Institute (Bethesda, Md) recommends using the lowest effective dose of

TABLE 24-2

Inhaled Antiinflammatory Agents

Agent	Availability	Dose	Adverse Events/Considerations

Cromolyn sodium (Intal)	MDI: 800 µg/puff
	Soln for neb: 20 mg/2 ml
	Soln, intranasal (spray): 40 mg/ml
		2 puffs 4 times daily
		  Nebulizer: 20 mg (1 vial)
		  4 times daily
			Foul taste, nausea, cough, throat irritation

Nedocromil sodium (Tilade)	MDI: 1.75 mg/puff	2 puffs 4 times daily	Foul taste, nausea, headache
Beclomethasone dipropionate (various)	HFA MDI (QVAR): 40 µg/puff; other brands use CFC as propellant	Low dose: 80-160 µg/d Medium dose: 160-320 µg/d	Hoarseness, dry throat, dysphonia, cough, oropharyngeal candidiasis (thrush)
Budesonide (various)	DPI: 200 µg/inh Flexhaler DPI: 90 µg/puff and 180 µg/puff Intranasal susp: 32 µg/inh Susp for nebulization: 0.25 mg/2 ml and 0.5 mg/2 ml	Intranasal: 32 µg in each nostril once daily Nebulization: 12 mo to 8 yr: 0.25 mg twice daily or 0.5 mg once daily (max dose, 1 mg/daily) MDI: 200 µg twice daily (max dose, 400 µg twice daily)	Facial edema, nervousness, migraine, insomnia, rash, pruritus, HPA axis suppression, hypokalemia, nasal irritation, burning or ulceration, pharyngitis
Flunisolide	MDI: 250 µg/puff CFC free: 80 µg/puff Intranasal soln: 29 µg/actuation	Intranasal: 1 spray in each nostril 3 times daily or 2 sprays in each nostril twice daily MDI: 2 inh twice daily (max, 4 inh twice daily) Non-CFC: 1 inh twice daily (max, 4 inh/d)	Palpitations, hypertension, chest pain, dizziness, rash, HPA axis suppression, oral candidiasis, nausea, vomiting, nasal burning
Fluticasone	MDI: HFA: 44 µg/puff, 110 µg/puff, 220 µg/puff Fluticasone/salmeterol: 100 µg/50 µg, 250 µg/50 µg, 500 µg/50 µg	1–2 puffs q 12 h 1 inhalation q 12 h	Palpitations, hypertension, chest pain, dizziness, rash, HPA axis suppression, oral candidiasis, nausea, vomiting, nasal burning
Triamcinolone acetonide	MDI: 100 µg/puff Intranasal susp: 55 µg/inh	Intranasal: 2 sprays in each nostril twice daily MDI: 1–2 puffs 3–4 times daily (max dose, 12 puffs daily)	Edema, CHF, fatigue, dizziness, malaise, insomnia, HPA axis suppression, oral candidiasis, dry throat, wheezing, cough, hoarseness

CFC, Chlorofluorocarbon; CHF, congestive heart failure; DPI, dry powder inhaler; HFA, hydrofluoroalkane; HPA, hypothalamic–pituitary–adrenal; inh, inhaled; max, maximum; MDI, metered-dose inhaler; neb, nebulization; soln, solution.

these drugs and routine monitoring of patients' growth rates. At the time of this writing there is ongoing controversy regarding the long term effects of inhaled corticosteroids in younger children. As stated in 2006 by Drs Irwin and Richardson, there is continued concern regarding growth retardation and Osteoporosis There is need for further study in this area. Until definitive studies are completed the use of the lowest effective dose of inhaled corticosteroids in children should always be used.[39,40,42–47]

Dose-related local adverse effects include oropharyngeal candidiasis, dysphonia, cough, and dry throat. The dysphonia appears to be the result of a direct effect of the steroid on the musculature that controls the vocal cords. Proper inhalation technique, use of spacer or holding chamber devices, rinsing the mouth and gargling with water, and expectorating after inhalation all may help decrease these local adverse effects. These techniques decrease drug deposition in the mouth.

Increased wheezing has been reported infrequently.[6,12,48] Patients who have undergone long-term steroid therapy may experience hypertension when treatment levels are reduced.[49] Chickenpox and measles may lead to serious or even fatal complications in children taking immunosuppressant drugs. Therefore considerable care must be taken to avoid exposure; if a child is exposed, immunoglobulin therapy may be indicated.[50] Development of cataracts and glaucoma caused by systemic absorption is associated with oral steroids, but no clear association exists with high doses of inhaled corticosteroids.[51] It is useful to keep in mind that the great majority of these side effects are not seen in inhalation therapy.

SYSTEMIC CORTICOSTEROIDS

Systemic corticosteroids are of great value in the treatment of acute exacerbations of asthma.[7] In the emergency department, intravenous and oral corticosteroids are first-line therapy.[7] There is no advantage to using intravenous dosing if the patient is able to tolerate oral dosing.[41,52] The most commonly used intravenous member of this family is methylprednisolone. The oral forms of dexamethasone, prednisone, and prednisolone are also used. There is no evidence of long-term adverse effects if the systemic agents are used for short periods of time (4 to 5 d).[10] Dosages for the systemic agents are listed in Table 24-2.

The mechanism of actions and side effect profiles of the parenteral agents are the same as those of their inhaled counterparts.[3,20]

Methylprednisolone (Solu-Medrol)

Of note is that methylprednisolone sodium succinate injection contains benzyl alcohol, which may cause allergic reactions in susceptible patients. Benzyl alcohol

in large doses (>99 mg/kg/d) has been linked to fatal toxicities (gasping syndrome) in neonates.[3]

Dexamethasone (Decadron)

Dexamethasone is used in the treatment of exacerbations of asthma and related bronchospasm events. It is also used to treat airway edema before extubation. Its use before extubation is dependent on clinical factors, including duration of intubation, and the presence of an air leak.

LEUKOTRIENE MODIFIERS

Leukotrienes were initially known as "slow-reacting substance of anaphylaxis" (SRS-A). They are derived from the metabolism of *arachidonic acid,* a fatty acid found in cell membranes.[40,51] When sensitized mast cells are exposed to allergen triggers, there is synthesis and release of molecules, including histamine and leukotrienes. The leukotrienes work to constrict airway smooth muscle, increase vascular permeability that leads to airway edema, increase mucous production, and both attract and activate inflammatory cells in the airways of patients with asthma.[53]

Leukotriene modifiers are the first new class of asthma medications to be introduced in the United States in more than 20 years. Table 24-3 lists the leukotriene-modifying agents currently available.

TABLE 24-3

Leukotriene-Modifying Agents

Agent	Availability	Dosage	Population	Adverse Events
Synthetic inhibitor				
Zileuton (Zyflo)	600–mg tablet	Children over 12 yr: 600 mg 4 times daily	Approved only for patients more than 12 yr old	Liver function evaluation before beginning medication and monthly times 3, then every 3 mo for 1 yr, then periodically. Abdominal pain, upset stomach, nausea, elevated liver enzymes; Multiple drug interactions
Receptor antagonists				
Zafirlukast (Accolate)	10-mg chewable tablet and 20-mg tablet	Children, 5-11 yr: 10 mg twice daily Children, > 12 yr: 20 mg twice daily	Children 5 yr and over	Headache, dizziness, pain, fever, nausea, diarrhea, abdominal pain, elevated liver enzymes, hepatitis. *Note:* Rare cases of eosinophilic vasculitis (Churg-Strauss) have been reported in patients receiving zafirlukast. No casual relationship has been established
Montelukast (Singulair)	4-mg chewable tablet; 5-mg chewable tablet; 10-mg tablet; granules, 4 mg	6 months-5 yr: 4 mg/d 6-14 yr: 4 mg/d >14 yr: 10 mg/d	Ages 6 mo and over	Headache (most common), heartburn, abdominal pain. rash, fatigue, dizziness, gastroenteritis, fever

Mechanism of Action

Two approaches are available to prevent the action of leukotrienes:

1. Antagonize or block leukotriene binding to its cellular receptor *(receptor antagonists)*
2. Inhibit the production of leukotrienes *(synthesis inhibitors)*

The U.S. FDA has currently approved three oral leukotriene-modifying drugs for use in the United States: *Zafirlukast* (Accolate) and *montelukast* (Singulair) are selective leukotriene receptor antagonists. *Zileuton* (Zyflo) is the only agent that inhibits 5-lipoxygenase, the enzyme responsible for converting arachidonic acid to the leukotrienes.[48,49]

Place in Therapy

The leukotriene modifiers are approved for prophylaxis and chronic treatment of asthma.[50,52] They are not an alternative to using β-adrenergic agonists during an acute asthma attack. However, they are continued during acute exacerbations of asthma.[7] Treatment with leukotriene modifiers is associated with improved asthma symptoms and pulmonary function, including FEV_1 values. They are effective in preventing bronchospasm caused by exercise, cold air, aspirin ingestion, and allergens. The leukotriene inhibitor montelukast was compared with inhaled corticosteroids. Although the inhaled corticosteroid provided better control, montelukast was a viable alternative secondary to its ease of use and better adherence.[9] Leukotriene modifiers also reduce the severity of asthma and allow for a reduction in the dose of inhaled corticosteroids and the need for β-agonist therapy.[54] Potential candidates include patients with poor inhaler technique and those who are noncompliant in taking inhaled corticosteroids.

Montelukast (Singulair)

Montelukast is the most widely used leukotriene modifier. It is an orally administered, selective cysteinyl leukotriene receptor antagonist.[51] The initial response after a single dose of montelukast occurs in 3 to 4 hours. The duration of action approaches 24 hours. In clinical studies, montelukast yielded significant improvement in parameters of asthma control, including improved FEV_1, daytime and nighttime symptoms, and a reduction in both as-needed β-agonist use and inhaled corticosteroid dose.[55] Montelukast also provides significant protection against EIB. It is not a bronchodilator, however, and is not indicated for use in the reversal of bronchospasm in acute asthma attacks. Montelukast has also been shown to improve symptoms when used in combination with loratadine for the treatment of seasonal allergic rhinitis.[56]

Dosage and Administration

Montelukast is available as both a 4-mg and 5-mg chewable, cherry-flavored tablet, as well as a 10-mg film-coated tablet.[3,11,20] The dose for children 2 to 5 years old is one 4-mg tablet daily. The dose for children 6 to 14 years old is one 5-mg tablet daily. The dose for adolescents (15 yr and older) and adults is one 10-mg tablet daily. The safety and efficacy of montelukast were demonstrated in clinical trials, in which it was administered in the evening without regard to the time of food ingestion. No clinical trials have evaluated the relative efficacy of morning versus evening dosing. Therefore it is recommended that the tablets be taken in the evening, with or without food.

Adverse Events

The most common side effect of montelukast is headache. Other side effects are usually mild and include fatigue, fever, abdominal pain, gastroenteritis, heartburn, dizziness, and rash. In rare cases, patients may present with clinical features of vasculitis consistent with *Churg-Strauss syndrome*.[56] These events typically have occurred in patients undergoing a reduction in oral corticosteroid medication.[3,11,20]

Zafirlukast (Accolate)

Zafirlukast is a leukotriene receptor antagonist of leukotrienes D_4 and E_4, components of SRS-A. These leukotrienes are associated with airway edema, smooth muscle constriction, and altered cellular activity associated with the inflammatory process. Zafirlukast is rapidly absorbed after oral administration, with response 3 hours after dosing. The duration of action is approximately 10 hours. Clinical trials demonstrated that zafirlukast improved daytime asthma symptoms, nighttime awakenings, rescue β-agonist use, FEV_1, and morning peak expiratory flow rate.[20] Zafirlukast is not a bronchodilator and is not used to treat acute episodes of asthma.[53]

Dosage and Administration

Zafirlukast is available in a 10-mg chewable tablet and a 20-mg coated tablet.[57] The recommended dose for children 5 to 11 years of age is 10 mg twice daily. The dose for adults and children 12 years and older is 20 mg twice daily. Because food reduces its bioavailability, zafirlukast should be taken at least 1 hour before or 2 hours after meals.[3] Zafirlukast has been reported to inhibit the metabolism of warfarin, resulting in an increased prothrombin time. Patients receiving oral warfarin anticoagulant therapy and zafirlukast should have their prothrombin time closely monitored and anticoagulant dose adjusted accordingly.[3,20]

Adverse Events

Initially it was believed that zafirlukast was relatively free of adverse events. With increasing use, however, side effects have become evident. Headache, nausea, diarrhea, abdominal pain, dizziness, fever, back pain, and vomiting have been reported.[3,20] Elevation of liver enzymes, progressing to hepatitis and hepatic failure, has occurred in patients using zafirlukast. Although most incidents occurred while using doses four times higher than the recommend dose, cases have occurred in patients receiving the recommended daily dose. In most patients the clinical symptoms abated and the enzyme levels returned to normal after discontinuing zafirlukast.

In rare cases, patients had increased theophylline levels, with or without clinical symptoms of theophylline toxicity, after zafirlukast had been added to the existing theophylline regimen.[20] The mechanism of the interaction between zafirlukast and theophylline in these patients is currently unknown.

At least eight patients given zafirlukast presented with systemic eosinophilia, pulmonary infiltrates, cardiomyopathy, and clinical features of vasculitis similar to Churg-Strauss syndrome.[55-57] The patients had severe asthma and were reducing or discontinuing oral corticosteroids after beginning zafirlukast therapy, during which time the reactions occurred. The symptoms reversed when zafirlukast was discontinued and corticosteroid therapy resumed. Although further studies are needed to determine the extent of the association, many believe that the syndrome was unmasked after corticosteroid withdrawal and was not a direct effect of zafirlukast. In 2003 Keogh and Specks published a study from the Mayo Clinic in which they found no correlation between leukotriene use and vasculitis (Churg-Strauss syndrome).[58]

Zileuton (Zyflo)

Zileuton inhibits 5-lipoxygenase, the enzyme that catalyzes the formation of leukotrienes from arachidonic acid, and thus inhibits leukotriene formation.[3,20] It is the only member of the leukotriene synthesis inhibitors currently approved for use. Zileuton has been shown to be effective in the treatment of cold air–induced, aspirin-intolerant, exercise-induced, and nocturnal asthma.[50] Zileuton reduces asthma symptoms and the supplemental use of β-agonists improves FEV_1 values, and may have an additive effect with inhaled steroids.[59,60] It is not indicated for use in the reversal of bronchospasm in acute asthma attacks, although its use can be continued during an acute exacerbation.

Zileuton is a cytochrome *P*-450 enzyme substrate and as such will affect the plasma concentration of other such substrates. Caution should be used when dosing zileuton with theophylline, propranolol, warfarin, and terfenadine.[3,20]

Dosage and Administration

Zileuton is available as a 600-mg tablet. The recommended dosage in adults and children 12 years and older is one 600-mg tablet four times per day for a total daily dose of 2400 mg.[3,20] It can be taken with or without food, although for ease of administration, zileuton should be taken with meals and at bedtime.

Adverse Events

The most common side effects are abdominal pain, upset stomach, and nausea. Zileuton is associated with threefold or greater elevations of liver enzymes (serum aminotransferase) in 2% to 4% of patients. The elevations usually occur during the first 3 months of treatment and return to normal when zileuton is discontinued. Therefore liver function should be evaluated before starting zileuton, monthly for the first 3 months of treatment, and then every 3 months of the first year, and periodically thereafter.[53] The inconvenient, four-times-daily dosing; incidence of elevated liver transaminases; and need for frequent liver function studies have limited the use of zileuton.

METHYLXANTHINES

Methylxanthines relax smooth muscle, stimulate the central nervous system and cardiac muscle, increase mucociliary transport and diaphragmatic contractility, and act on the kidneys to promote diuresis. Their usefulness in promoting relaxation of bronchial smooth muscle is of benefit in the management of asthma.[6]

Theophylline

Although no longer as widely used for the treatment of acute severe asthma, the methylxanthine theophylline is still considered as additive therapy when response to β-agonists is suboptimal. Wheeler and colleagues[61] published a study in 2005 comparing theophylline alone, terbutaline alone, and terbutaline with theophylline in patients with status asthmaticus. These patients were also receiving intravenous corticosteroids and continuous nebulized albuterol. In this patient population it was found that theophylline was superior to either of the terbutaline groups and was much less expensive. When patients present in status asthmaticus and they are resistant to conventional therapy, theophylline should be considered at part of the treatment package.

Mechanism of Action

The mechanism of action of theophylline is not completely understood. Theophylline is known to competitively inhibit phosphodiesterase, the enzyme that degrades cAMP. Increased concentrations of cAMP may mediate the observed bronchodilation (see Figure 24-1).[10,11,20] Other proposed mechanisms of action include inhibition of the release of intracellular calcium and competitive antagonism of the bronchoconstrictor adenosine.[6]

Dosage and Administration

Aerosol administration of theophylline is ineffective; it must be administered systemically. Theophylline is available in a multitude of dosage formulations and strengths, with great variation in the recommended dosing guidelines based on patient age. Sustained-release preparations generally provide more consistent drug levels and allow dosing once, twice, or three times daily, favoring patient compliance. However, the rate of absorption is variable between patients and is influenced by numerous medical interventions and conditions. Multiple factors increase the clearance rate of theophylline and result in higher dose requirements, including smoking, hyperthyroidism, and concurrent use of medications such as phenobarbital and rifampin. Factors that can decrease clearance and lead to toxicity include hypothyroidism, congestive heart failure, liver failure, and the use of oral contraceptives and various antibiotics, including ciprofloxacin and erythromycin.[20]

Initial oral dosing for pediatric patient who have not received theophylline within the past 24 hours is 5 mg/kg. If the patient has received theophylline within the past 24 hours then the dose is 2.5 mg/kg.[3] Maintenance dosing is based on age and weight of the patient. Theophylline has complex pharmacokinetic properties and standard dosing is virtually impossible. In our institution the maintenance dose is based on serum levels. The *Pediatric Dosage Handbook* is an excellent resource for dosing theophylline.[3] The therapeutic serum range for theophylline is 10 to 20 μg/ml. Blood levels are routinely monitored to avoid toxic levels, especially in patients requiring multiple medications. Many patients will respond to lower serum concentrations; 5 to15 μg/ml is accepted as a safe and effective range.[6,20]

Adverse Events

The adverse gastrointestinal effects of theophylline include nausea, vomiting, abdominal pain, cramping, and diarrhea. Adverse CNS effects include insomnia, headache, dizziness, nervousness, and seizures, which are often more severe in children. Seizures may occur as the initial sign of theophylline toxicity without other preceding signs and symptoms of toxicity.[20] Increased tremor in the patient's dominant hand has been reported.[46] Cardiovascular and pulmonary adverse effects include tachycardia, arrhythmias, and tachypnea. Theophylline worsens gastroesophageal reflux disease, potentially resulting in an exacerbation of asthma.

Because of these toxicities, theophylline is often used as a fourth-line asthma medication.

MAGNESIUM SULFATE

Mechanism of Action and Place in Therapy

Magnesium is a cofactor in more than 300 enzymatic reactions in the body. In heart muscle, magnesium acts as a calcium channel blocker. In smooth muscle, it acts as a muscle relaxant. When given intravenously, magnesium promotes bronchodilation.[62] The use of magnesium sulfate ($MgSO_4$) in the treatment of moderate to severe exacerbations of asthma dates back more than 60 years.[63] Current evidence suggests that patients with severe asthma may benefit most from its use.[64-67]

Dosage and Administration

The dose of $MgSO_4$ for bronchodilation is 25 mg/kg; doses as high as 75 mg/kg have been used to treat pediatric status asthmaticus. The literature presents studies of $MgSO_4$ using single as well as multidose schedules.[3] The standard dosage is 25 mg/kg every 4 hours, for a total of 4 doses. Monitor magnesium serum levels during administration. The normal serum value for magnesium is 1.5 to 2.5 mEq/L.[3]

Side effects include severe fatigue, somnolence, and pseudocoma.[68] Deep tendon reflexes are blunted with $MgSO_4$ injection. As the magnesium serum level diminishes, deep tendon reflexes will return in reverse order of attenuation. This agent may be of benefit to patients who are prone to hypomagnesemia secondary to prolonged β-agonist use. $MgSO_4$ should be considered for patients refractory to standard therapy.

NONSTEROIDAL ANTIINFLAMMATORY DRUGS

Cromolyn Sodium (Intal)
Mechanism of Action

Cromolyn has been referred to as a mast cell stabilizer. Although the complete mechanism of action is unknown, it inhibits sensitized mast cell degranulation occurring after exposure to specific antigens. The drug also blocks the release of histamine and slow-reacting substance of anaphylaxis (SRS-A, i.e., leukotrienes) from the mast cell. These actions serve to inhibit the early asthmatic response through stabilization of the mast cell membrane. Cromolyn also inhibits the late asthmatic response. In some patients, cromolyn attenuates bronchospasm caused by exercise, aspirin, and cold air. Cromolyn has no intrinsic bronchodilator, antihistaminic, anticholinergic, or vasoconstrictor activity.[3,10,11]

Place in Therapy

The EPR-3 on asthma reports cromolyn sodium as a component of therapy in the treatment of mild and moderate persistent asthma.[7] Because it has no known long-term systemic effects, cromolyn is often used as first-line antiinflammatory therapy in children with mild or moderate persistent asthma. However, the new guidelines relegate cromolyn to a lower tier in the treatment plan for asthma. It is of little benefit during an acute exacerbation of asthma or in children with severe asthma.[10]

Dosage and Administration

Cromolyn sodium is available as a nebulized solution and as an MDI. The recommended dosage of the solution for nebulization in children older than 2 years is 20 mg (one 2-ml ampoule) four times daily. Protect the ampoule from light by storing it in a foil package, and do not use it if it contains a precipitate or becomes discolored. The recommended dosage of the MDI is 2 inhalations four times daily. For the prevention of bronchospasm after exercise or exposure to cold air, cromolyn is administered 10 to 15 minutes, but not more than 60 minutes, before exposure.[3,11] Long-term prophylaxis of 6 to 12 weeks is necessary to prevent the increased airway hyperactivity associated with specific allergen exposure. Improvement in symptoms usually occurs within the first 4 weeks of administration. Cromolyn is extremely safe and is one of the most nontoxic drugs used in the management of asthma. However, the need for four-times-daily administration tends to decrease patient compliance.[69]

Nedocromil Sodium (Tilade)
Place in Therapy

As with cromolyn sodium, nedocromil sodium is a nonsteroidal anti-inflammatory drug indicated primarily for the prevention of mild persistent to moderate persistent asthma. Although the exact mechanism of action has yet to be elucidated, clinical studies have reported that nedocromil inhibits the bronchoconstrictor response to several challenges, including various antigens, exercise, cold air, and fog. This inhibition is of both early- and late-phase bronchoconstriction. Nedocromil has no intrinsic bronchodilator, antihistamine, or corticosteroid action. Nedocromil has no place in the treatment of acute bronchospasm, particularly during status asthmaticus.[3,7]

Dosage and Administration

Nedocromil is available as an MDI. The recommended dosage for children 6 years of age and older is 2 inhalations four times daily.[3,7] Twice-daily dosing may be effective in some patients. Some reports show nedocromil to have a modest effect in lowering the required dose of corticosteroids. The most common adverse effect is a transient, mild, unpleasant taste. Nausea and headache have also been reported.[3,20,69]

MUCOLYTIC AGENTS

N-Acetylcysteine (Mucomyst)
Mechanism of Action

The viscosity of mucous secretions in the lungs depends on the concentrations of mucoprotein and the presence of disulfide bonds between these macromolecules and DNA. N-Acetylcysteine acts to split the sulfide bonds in the macromolecules, thereby decreasing viscosity, allowing for their removal by normal chest physiotherapy. The action of N-acetylcysteine is pH dependent, with mucolytic action significant at pH ranges of 7.0 to 9.0.[69]

Place in Therapy

N-Acetylcysteine is an aerosolized mucolytic agent often used as adjunctive therapy for pulmonary complications of cystic fibrosis (CF) in combination with vigorous chest physiotherapy.[70] N-Acetylcysteine is also used as an antidote in acetaminophen overdose to prevent or lessen hepatic injury.

Dosage and Administration

The recommended dose of N-acetylcysteine in children is 3 to 5 ml of the 20% solution diluted with an equal volume of water or saline (or 6 to 10 ml of a 10% solution) administered by nebulization three or four times per day.[3,20]

Adverse Events

Adverse effects reported with N-acetylcysteine include stomatitis, vomiting, hemoptysis, and severe rhinorrhea. It has an unpleasant, pungent odor that may lead to an increased incidence of nausea. Bronchospasm has also been reported with N-acetylcysteine therapy.[20]

Recombinant Human DNase (Pulmozyme)

An additional factor that contributes to viscous mucus in patients with CF is extracellular DNA. Bacterial cell death and subsequent cell lysis release DNA into the extracellular environment. This high extracellular DNA content works to thicken airway secretions further.[71] DNase is a highly purified solution of recombinant human deoxyribonuclease I (rhDNase), an enzyme that selectively cleaves DNA.[20] rhDNase has been demonstrated to reduce the viscosity of sputum in patients with CF by hydrolyzing the extracellular DNA. Studies have shown that daily administration of rhDNase results in a definite improvement in the outcome of pulmonary function, as assessed by improved FEV_1 above baseline. Using rhDNase also resulted in a significant reduction in the number of patients experiencing respiratory tract infections requiring parenteral antibiotics.[72,73]

Dosage and Administration

Recombinant human DNase was approved by the FDA in 1993 and currently is indicated in the management of patients with CF to improve pulmonary function and to decrease the frequency of respiratory infections. The recommended dose for most patients with CF is 2.5 mg by nebulization once daily. Some patients may benefit from twice-daily treatments. Safety and efficacy have not been demonstrated in children less than 5 years of age.[3,20]

Adverse Events

Adverse effects are minimal and include voice alteration, pharyngitis, laryngitis, rash, and chest pain. To date there have been no case reports of anaphylaxis. rhDNase should be kept refrigerated and not exposed to room temperature for a total time exceeding 24 hours. Discolored and cloudy solutions of rhDNase should be discarded.[3,20]

Sodium Chloride 3%: Adjunctive Therapy

Hypertonic sodium chloride has been studied for use in the treatment of traumatic brain injury and viral bronchiolitis.[74] Our discussion focuses on aerosolized 3% sodium chloride and its use in viral bronchiolitis. It has been shown that hypertonic sodium chloride will increase mucociliary clearance in patients with cystic fibrosis, patients with asthma, and in healthy subjects.[75-77] It is postulated that the mechanism of action is via absorbing water from the submucosa and the reversal of submucosal and adventitial edema. This decreases the viscosity and dryness of mucous plaques, allowing for easier removal by mucociliary action.

Hypertonic saline may be used in place of normal saline for the administration of albuterol, terbutaline, or epinephrine. The usual dose is 3 to 4 ml of sterile 3% sodium chloride either as the carrier or alone every 2 to 4 hours. The most commonly reported side effect is cough. The 3% sodium chloride is often used in conjunction with inspiratory positive ventilation.[75] In the CF population 7% hypertonic saline solution has been used for nebulization. It is not mixed with any of the standard bronchodilators or adjunctive agents.

KETAMINE

Ketamine is an anesthetic agent that produces anesthesia, sedation, and amnesia without significant respiratory depression. Because of its bronchodilating effects, ketamine has been used as part of rapid-sequence intubation in the pediatric patient with status asthmaticus. It has also been used as a combined bronchodilator and sedative in patients with asthma requiring mechanical ventilation.

Mechanism of Action

The mechanism of action of ketamine appears to be a selective interruption of the association pathways of the brain. The resulting bronchodilation may be of sympathetic origin. There is also a parasympathetic limb of action whereby ketamine diminishes acetylcholine activity on bronchial smooth muscle, resulting in bronchodilation.[78-80]

In July 2005, Allen and Macias[81] published a study of 68 patients with asthma randomized to receive continuous ketamine via the intravenous route or placebo. The study was performed in an emergency room setting with patients who presented with acute asthma exacerbation. They concluded that ketamine given at a dose of 0.2 mg/kg followed by a infusion of 0.5 mg/kg per hour for 2 hours provided no incremental benefit to standard therapy. In the setting of quickly deteriorating asthma, ketamine may be one of several last-resort medications to prevent placing the patient on mechanical ventilation. Its use should be viewed as third- or fourth-line therapy.

Dosage and Administration

Ketamine is given through a central venous catheter as a continuous infusion. The normal sedation dose is listed as 5 to 20 µg/kg per minute. For bronchodilation, the starting dose may be as small as 2 µg/kg per minute and titrated to effect.[82,83] For sedation or minor procedures, the dose is 0.5 to 1 mg/kg. Duration of action of a single dose is 10 to 20 minutes.[3,20,84] State laws vary as to who is allowed to administer and titrate ketamine.

Adverse Effects

Adverse effects seen with ketamine include increased sympathomimetic activity, seizures, delirium, increased laryngeal secretions, and respiratory depression. During the recovery phase, unusual dreams and hallucinations have been reported. Premedication with midazolam (less than 0.1 mg/kg) can attenuate this effect. Intubation equipment must be readily available before administering ketamine, because the sedative effects may result in respiratory failure and the need for emergency intubation. Epinephrine should also be available for possible bradycardia.[3,20]

AEROSOLIZED ANTIBIOTICS

Aminoglycosides, β-Lactams, and Colistin

Direct aerosol delivery of antibiotics reduces systemic adverse effects and is often used for targeted drug delivery. Aminoglycosides (e.g., tobramycin), β-lactams (e.g., ceftazidime), and colistin have all been used with various degrees of success.[68] Preliminary analysis of a study evaluating inhalation of 600 mg of tobramycin every 8 hours has reported a positive response, as demonstrated by favorable improvement in pulmonary status and reduction in *Pseudomonas* sputum density. The mechanism of administration dictates the amount of drug delivered and the dispersion of the drug. Geller and colleagues[85] showed that a new-generation aerosol delivery system (Aerodose 5.5 RP inhaler; Aerogen, Mountain View, Calif) could increase the amount of tobramycin delivered (approximately threefold greater efficiency in less than half the time) compared with an older aerosol delivery model.

Doses currently used for nebulization of colistin (Coly-Mycin) are 150 mg/day divided every 6 to 12 hours. The colistin dose is based on ideal body weight and calculated in colistin units.[3] The recommended dose for tobramycin is 40 to 80 mg two or three times daily. The high-dose regimen for adults and children older than 6 years of age is 300 mg every 12 hours. Colistin is administered in repeated cycles of 28 days "on" the drug followed by 28 days "off" the drug.[3,86]

Pentamidine (NebuPent)

Pneumocystis carinii, along with *Streptococcus pneumoniae* and *Haemophilus influenzae*, are the most common opportunistic infections among patients with acquired immunodeficiency syndrome (AIDS). The risk of mortality from untreated *P. carinii* pneumonia (PCP) approaches 100%. Treatment with agents effective against *P. carinii* (parenteral pentamidine) is associated with a 60% response rate.[87] In severe cases of PCP, for adult patients requiring mechanical ventilation, mortality approaches 50%. PCP is associated with even higher mortality among children. Effective PCP prophylaxis improved the quality of life and reduced mortality among patients with AIDS.[87,88] Prophylaxis does not, however, remove the threat of PCP. There are still treatment failures among persons who are not aware of their disease, or who lack compliance with prophylactic treatment.

The Centers for Disease Control and Prevention (CDC, Atlanta, Ga) recommend aerosolized pentamidine as an effective agent for PCP prophylaxis. Although the mechanism of action is not completely understood, pentamidine inhibits protein and nucleic acid synthesis. The role of aerosolized pentamidine for PCP prophylaxis in children has not been completely evaluated. However, pentamidine may be an effective option in children who are old enough to comply with aerosol administration.

Dosage and Administration

The recommended dose is 300 mg of pentamidine given by nebulization every 4 weeks. This has been shown to be more effective than a dosing regimen of 30 mg given every 2 weeks or 150 mg given every 2 weeks. Pentamidine in doses of 300 mg every 28 days has been shown to prevent first episodes of PCP in 60% to 70% of patients.[3,20] The nebulizer used to administer pentamidine should include a one-way valve assembly.

Adverse Events

Aerosol administration of pentamidine is associated with fewer systemic adverse effects than is oral administration of prophylactic agents. Common side effects include cough, rash, dizziness, nausea, and gagging. Reversible bronchospasm is also a frequent adverse effect. A common practice is to pretreat patients with an inhaled β-agonist to reduce the occurrence of bronchospasm.[3,20]

ANTIVIRAL AGENTS

Respiratory Syncytial Virus Infections

Respiratory syncytial virus (RSV) is a frequent cause of lower respiratory tract infection in infants and young children. More than 50% of infants experience RSV infections during their first year of life, with virtually all children experiencing an RSV infection during the first 3 years of life. Outbreaks are seasonal and most common during the fall and winter months.[89] In the northern hemisphere, RSV season is usually designated as October through March or April. Approximately 0.5% to 2% of infants with severe lower respiratory tract disease require hospitalization and medical intervention, with most of these infants being less than 6 months of age.[90]

Children most susceptible to serious or even fatal disease include those with a history of congenital heart disease, bronchopulmonary dysplasia, pulmonary hypertension, premature birth (gestational age, less than 34 weeks), and immunodeficiency. Patients with severe illness are typically younger than 3 months of age and present with an oxygen saturation less than 95%, respiratory rates greater than 70 breaths/minute, and atelectasis. These patients often require intensive respiratory support that includes mechanical ventilation.[90]

Ribavirin (Virazole)

Ribavirin is a synthetic nucleoside with broad-spectrum antiviral activity. It appears to disrupt viral protein synthesis through inhibition of messenger ribonucleic acid (mRNA) expression.[91] Ribavirin is approved for the treatment of hospitalized children with severe, lower respiratory tract disease caused by RSV. The American Academy of Pediatrics (Elk Grove, Ill) guidelines for ribavirin therapy are stringent because of concerns about cost, benefit, safety, and variable clinical efficacy.[89] Ribavirin is viewed as "possibly effective" in the treatment of RSV and thus has a limited role in routine use.[92]

Dosage and Administration

Ribavirin is recommended for continuous aerosol administration through an oxygen hood, tent, or face mask for 12 to 20 hours daily for a mean of 4 days.[91] Aerosolized ribavirin should be administered only with the aerosol-generating device recommended by the maker of the drug. A 20-mg/ml ribavirin solution is the recommended treatment regimen. Special precautions are essential with mechanically ventilated patients to prevent complications and to reduce the risk of crystalline precipitation in the circuit, with subsequent ventilator dysfunction.[93]

Adverse Events

Adverse events attributed to ribavirin are infrequent but include sudden deterioration adverse cardiovascular effects. The most common adverse effects reported by health care personnel exposed to aerosolized ribavirin include eye irritation (especially in those wearing contact lenses) and headache. Because ribavirin can precipitate on contact lenses, protective goggles or glasses are recommended. Ribavirin has a black box warning pertaining to teratogenic and/or embryocidal effects. These effects have been demonstrated in all animal models tested.[94]

Respiratory Syncytial Virus Immune Globulin Intravenous (RespiGam)

Respiratory syncytial virus immune globulin IV (RSV-IGIV) is sterile, liquid immunoglobulin G (IgG) containing neutralizing antibody to RSV. It is used for RSV prophylaxis. Released in January of 1996, RespiGam was the first antiviral agent approved for the prevention of RSV disease. RespiGam contains IgG antibodies representative of the large number of normal, healthy persons who contributed to the plasma pools from which the product was derived. The immune globulin contains a high concentration of neutralizing and protective antibodies directed against RSV.[95] According to the American Academy of Pediatrics, RespiGam is considered an *immunoprophylactic* agent. When first introduced, RespiGam held much promise for the prevention of RSV infections. The drug was subsequently largely replaced by palivizumab.

Dosage and Administration

RespiGam is approved for use in children less than 24 months of age. It is administered once per month for 4 or 5 months, at the height of the RSV season. In general, 4 monthly doses (for a total of 5 doses) are sufficient to provide protection during the entire RSV season. The dose of RSV-IGIV is 15 ml/kg (750 mg/kg) administered intravenously.[89]

Adverse Events

The most common adverse effects of RespiGam include fever, fluid overload, and decreased oxygen saturation. The decision to initiate RSV-IGIV prophylaxis should be patient specific. Considerations include underlying disease, chance of therapy completion, cost of administration, and socioeconomic environment.[96]

Palivizumab (Synagis)

In 1998, the FDA approved palivizumab (Synagis), the latest drug produced by MedImmune (Gaithersburg, Md) in its quest for an RSV vaccine or prophylactic agent.[95] Palivizumab is a humanized monoclonal antibody for the prevention of disease caused by RSV. In phase III trials, 1502 high-risk infants were treated with palivizumab. The hospitalization rate was 55% less in the palivizumab group than in the placebo-controlled group. Unlike its predecessor RespiGam, which must be administered as an intravenous infusion, palivizumab is an intramuscular formulation. It still must be given for the 5 months of RSV season. Studies have found palivizumab to be safe and well tolerated in the high-risk pediatric population targeted for this product.[93,96-98] This group includes infants born prematurely (less than 35 weeks of gestation), those less than 6 months of age, and infants with bronchopulmonary dysplasia who are less than 24 months of age. Doses of 15 mg/kg given once monthly maintain serum concentrations of greater than 40 µg/ml for most patients.

There are specific guidelines put forth by the American Academy of Pediatrics concerning palivizumab and RSV IGIV.[89] These should be strictly adhered to in order to avoid costly and unnecessary therapy.[83]

MONOCLONAL ANTI-IgE ANTIBODY THERAPY

Omalizumab

Many of the childhood respiratory diseases are associated with an inflammatory process. Asthma has been found to be principally an inflammatory process. Many of the first-line therapies are directed toward reducing inflammation or countering the inflammatory cascade. Corticosteroids, leukotriene modifiers, and non-steroidal agents all target the inflammatory process whereas β_2-agonists counteract the results of the allergen/inflammatory response.

Mechanism of Action

Specific targeting of the IgE antibody was a logical step in the search for new agents in the treatment of asthma. Omalizumab is a recombinant humanized monoclonal anti-IgE antibody. This agent binds to the same region of the IgE molecule that interacts with IgE receptors, that is, the Cε3 domain, thereby inhibiting the allergic cascade by markedly reducing the serum concentration of free IgE.[20,98,99]

Place in Therapy

Omalizumab should be considered for those patients 12 years and older who have moderate to severe persistent asthma and who have had a positive skin test response or in vitro reactivity to a perennial aeroallergen, the symptoms of which are inadequately controlled with inhaled corticosteroids. There is clinical evidence that omalizumab may be of use in patients who have a peanut allergy. It may diminish peanut-induced allergic reactions. Omalizumab is not considered first-line therapy and should be prescribed only by a specialist in pulmonology and immunology.[7,20,99]

Adverse Events

There are many warnings and precautions associated with omalizumab. Omalizumab is not indicated for acute asthma exacerbations. Anaphylactic reactions have occurred after the first and subsequent doses in patients who presented no identifiable triggers. Patients should be monitored and medications for treatment of severe allergic reactions should be available.[3] The practitioner should refer to the package insert for a complete list of warnings and precautions.

Adverse reactions include headache, dizziness, and fatigue; local injection reactions are not uncommon. Respiratory infections, anaphylaxis, hypersensitivity reactions, and viral infections are also possible.

Dosage and Administration

Dosage and frequency are based on the serum total IgE level and body weight. Total IgE levels are elevated with initiation of omalizumab therapy and remain elevated for up to 1 year after discontinuation. Dosage should not be based on serial IgE levels. Administration is via subcutaneous injection. Preparation of the injection should be by qualified personnel.[11,20] Refer to the package insert or other noted text for more information and a schedule of dosing.

ASSESSMENT QUESTIONS

See Evolve Resources for answers.

1. Approximately what percentage of all drugs used for neonatal and pediatric patients is approved by the U.S. Food and Drug Administration?
   A. 100%
   B. 75%
   C. 50%
   D. 25%
2. Overuse of inhaled β_2-agonists has been associated with increased mortality from asthma. It is currently recommended that β_2-agonists be used only on a _____ basis in the treatment of acute episodes.
   A. q 4 hours and prn
   B. q 2 hours and prn
   C. q 2 hours
   D. prn
3. Levalbuterol (Xopenex) differs from albuterol (Ventolin) in that it lacks the _____; this allows longer duration of action and slightly fewer side effects.
   A. *l*-Isomer
   B. (*R*)-Isomer
   C. (*S*)-Isomer
   D. Both A and B
4. Inhaled corticosteroids are potent antiinflammatory agents used in the management of asthma. The mechanisms of action include all of the following, *except:*
   A. Inhibition of the production of leukotrienes and prostaglandins
   B. Increased mucus and lung edema
   C. Inhibition of the activity of inflammatory cells
   D. Increase in the number of β-receptors
   E. Enhancement of the responsiveness of β-receptors in airway smooth muscle
5. J.D. is a 5-year-old patient with chronic asthma. Which of the following drug regimens would he take on a daily basis?
   A. Mucomyst, albuterol, corticosteroid
   B. Albuterol, corticosteroid, leukotriene modifier
   C. Methylxanthine, albuterol, hypertonic saline
6. Which of the following is commonly used to increase mucociliary clearance in patients with bronchiolitis and cystic fibrosis by absorbing water from the submucosa of the airway wall lining, which allows thick mucus to be expectorated more easily?
   A. Pulmozyme
   B. Albuterol
   C. 3% hypertonic sodium chloride
   D. Pentamidine

Continued

ASSESSMENT QUESTIONS—cont'd

7. Racemic epinephrine is a useful decongestant when used in a child who develops moderate respiratory distress and stridor after extubation. Which of the following choices *best* describes the targeting mechanisms of this drug, which reduces airway inflammation by vasoconstriction?
   A. β-Receptors
   B. α-Receptors
   C. Muscarinic receptors
   D. All of the above

8. Palivizumab (Synagis) is a monoclonal antibody indicated for the prevention of the following respiratory virus:
   A. Herpes zoster
   B. Respiratory syncytial virus
   C. Metapneumovirus
   D. Rotavirus

9. A 15-year-old patient with status asthmaticus is admitted to the emergency room. The doctor would like the respiratory therapist to initiate bilevel positive airway pressure (BiPAP) via nasal mask to this patient. The patient is extremely uncomfortable with BiPAP. Which sedative would be most appropriate at this time?
   A. Vecuronium
   B. Propofol
   C. Ketamine
   D. Bronkosol

10. Which of the following drugs would a respiratory therapist suggest for a patient with cerebral palsy with excessive oral secretions and chronic aspiration, and who doesn't show signs of a current pneumonia or thick secretions?
    A. Glycopyrrolate
    B. Albuterol
    C. Intravenous lactated Ringer's
    D. Mucomyst

References

1. Nahata MC, Taketomo C: Pediatrics. In DiPiro JT, Talbert RL, Yee GC, Matzke GR, Wells BG, Posey LM, editors: *Pharmacotherapy: a pathophysiologic approach*, ed 5, New York: McGraw-Hill; 2002. pp 69-78.

2. U.S. Food and Drug Administration Center for Drug Evaluation and Research: *Pediatric drug development*. Available at http://www.fda.gov/cder/pediatric. Retrieved October 2008.

3. Taketomo CK, Hodding JH, Kraus DM, editors: *Pediatric dosage handbook*, ed 14, Cleveland, Ohio: Lexi-Comp; 2007-2008.

4. U.S. Food and Drug Administration Center for Drug Evaluation and Research: *Pediatric drug development*. U.S. Food and Drug Administration Center for Drug Evaluation and Research web site. *Look for: "Lists of*

Determinations including Written Request (UPDATED 10/1/2008) Available at: http://www.fda.gov/cder/pediatric/#bpca. Retrieved October 2008.

5. Barnes PJ: Airway pharmacology. In Mason RJ, Broaddus VC, Murray JF, Nadel JA, editors: *Murray and Nadel's textbook of respiratory medicine*, ed 4, Philadelphia: WB Saunders; 2005. pp

6. Hoffman BB: Catecholamines, sympathomimetic drugs, and adrenergic receptor antagonists. In Hardman JG, Limbird LE, editors: *Goodman and Gilman's the pharmacological basis of therapeutics*, ed 10, New York: McGraw-Hill; 2001. pp 215-268.

7. National Asthma Education and Prevention Program: *Expert Panel Report 3 (EPR-3): guidelines for the diagnosis and management of asthma—summary report 2007*. Available at http://www.nhlbi.nih.gov/guidelines/asthma/asth-summ.htm. Retrieved October 2008.

8. Leversha AM: Costs and effectiveness of spacer versus nebulizer in young children with moderate and severe acute asthma, *J Pediatr* 2000;136:497.

9. Courtney AU et al: Childhood asthma: treatment update, *Am Fam Physician* 2005; 71:1959.

10. Undem BJ, Lichtenstein LM: Drugs used in the treatment of asthma. In Hardman JG, Limbird LE, editors: *Goodman and Gilman's the pharmacological basis of therapeutics*, ed 10, New York: McGraw-Hill; 2001. pp 733-754.

11. Kelly HW, Sorkness CA: Asthma. In DiPiro JT, Talbert RL, Yee GC, Matzke GR, Wells BG, Posey LM, editors: *Pharmacotherapy: a pathophysiologic approach*, ed 6, New York: McGraw-Hill; 2005. pp 503-536.

12. Cockcroft DW: Inhaled β2-agonist and airway responses to allergen, *J Allergy Clin Immunol* 1998;102:S96.

13. Everard ML, LeSouef PN: Aerosol therapy and delivery systems. In Taussig LM, Landau LI, editors: *Pediatric respiratory medicine*, St. Louis: Mosby; 1999. pp 286-299.

14. Dolovich M: Aerosol delivery to children: what to use, how to choose, *Pediatr Pulmonol Suppl* 1999;18:79.

15. Lipworth BJ, Aziz I: A high dose of albuterol does not overcome bronchoprotective subsensitivity in asthmatic subjects receiving regular salmeterol or formoterol, *J Allergy Clin Immunol* 1999;103:88.

16. Spitzer WO et al: The use of β agonists and the risk of death and near death from asthma, *N Engl J Med* 1992;326:501.

17. Salpeter SR et al: Cardiovascular effects of β-agonists in patients with asthma and COPD: a meta-analysis [special report], *Chest* 2004;125:2309.

18. Smith L: Childhood asthma: diagnosis and treatment, *Curr Probl Pediatr* 1993;23:271.

19. Kornecki A, Shemie SD: Bronchodilators and RSV-induced respiratory failure: agonizing about β2-agonists, *Pediatr Pulmonol* 1998;26:4.

20. Kastrup EK et al, editors: Respiratory drugs [update]. In *Drug facts and comparisons*, St. Louis: Facts and Comparisons; 2004. pp 859-874.

21. http://www.mdconsult.com/das/pharm/body/108703481-11/765486630/full/11 Direct link to Indications and Dosages. (Accessed 10/27/2008)

21a. Leinin JB et al: Hypokalemia after pediatric albuterol overdose: a case series, *Am J Emerg Med* 1994;12:64.

22. Handley D: The asthma-like pharmacology and toxicology of (S)-isomers of β-agonists, *J Allergy Clin Immunol* 1999;104(suppl):S69.

23. Spagnolo SV: Status asthmaticus and hospital management of asthma, *Immun Allergy Clin North Am* 2001;21:503.

24. Gawchik SM et al: The safety and efficacy of nebulized levalbuterol compared with racemic albuterol and placebo in the treatment of asthma in pediatric patients, *J Allergy Clin Immunol* 1999;103:615.

25. Qureshi F. Clinical efficacy of racemic albuterol versus levalbuterol for the treatment of acute pediatric asthma, *Ann Emerg Med* 2005;46:29.

26. Condemi JJ et al; Salmeterol Study Group: The addition of salmeterol to fluticasone propionate versus increasing the dose of fluticasone propionate in patients with persistent asthma, *Ann Allergy Asthma Immunol* 1999;82:383.

27. Murray JJ et al: Concurrent use of salmeterol with inhaled corticosteroids is more effective than inhaled corticosteroid dose increases, *Allergy Asthma Proc* 1999;20:173.

28. Pearlman DS et al: A comparison of salmeterol with albuterol in the treatment of mild-to-moderate asthma, *N Engl J Med* 1992;327:1420.

29. Brown JH, Taylor P: Muscarinic receptor agonists and antagonists. In Hardman JG, Limbird LE, editors: *Goodman and Gilman's the pharmacological basis of therapeutics*, ed 10, New York: McGraw-Hill; 2001. pp 155-173.

30. Rodrigo GJ, Rodrigo C: The role of anticholinergics in acute asthma treatment: an evidence-based evaluation, *Chest* 2002;121:1977.

31. Werner HA: Status asthmaticus in children: a review, *Chest* 2001;119:1913.

32. Craven C et al: Ipratropium bromide plus nebulized albuterol for the treatment of hospitalized children with acute asthma, *J Pediatr* 2001;138:51.

33. Garrett JE et al: Nebulized salbutamol with and without ipratropium bromide in the treatment of acute asthma, *J Allergy Clin Immunol* 1997;100:165.

34. Qureshi F et al: Effect of nebulized ipratropium on the hospitalization rates of children with asthma, *N Engl J Med* 1998;339:1030.

35. Schuh S et al: Efficacy of frequent nebulized ipratropium bromide added to frequent high-dose albuterol therapy in severe childhood asthma, *J Pediatr* 1995;126:639.

36. May JR, Smith PH Allergic Rhinitis. In DiPiro JT, Talbert RL, Posey LM, editors: *Pharmacotherapy: a pathophysiologic approach*. ed 6 Norwalk, Conn: McGraw-Hill/Appleton & Lange; 2005. pp 1729-1740.

37. Kastrup EK et al, editors: Gastrointestinal anticholinergics/antispasmodics. In *Drug facts and comparisons*, St. Louis: Facts and Comparisons; 2004. pp 1327-1332.

38. Allen DB et al: Inhaled corticosteroids: past lessons and future issues, *J Allergy Clin Immunol* 2003;112(3 suppl):S1.

39. Irwin RS, Richardson ND: Side Effects With Inhaled Corticosteroids The Physician's Persception *Chest* 2006; 130(1 Suppl): 41S-53S.

40. Wenzel SE: New approaches to anti-inflammatory therapy for asthma, *Am J Med* 1998;104:287.

41. Becker JM et al: Oral versus intravenous corticosteroids in children hospitalized with asthma, *J Allergy Clin Immunol* 1999;103:586.

42. Tinkelman DG et al: Aerosol beclomethasone dipropionate compared with theophylline as primary treatment of chronic, mild to moderately severe asthma in children, *Pediatrics* 1993;92:64.

43. Leone FT: Systematic review of the evidence regarding potential complications of inhaled corticosteroid use in asthma: collaboration of American College of Chest Physicians, American Academy of Allergy, Asthma, and Immunology, and American College of Allergy, Asthma, and Immunology, *Chest* 2003;124:2329.

44. Gregson RK et al: Effect of inhaled corticosteroids on bone mineral density in childhood asthma: comparison of fluticasone propionate with beclomethasone dipropionate, *Osteoporos Int* 1998;8:418.

45. Sanders P et al: Hypertension during reduction of long-term steroid therapy in young subjects with asthma, *J Allergy Clin Immunol* 1992;89:816.

46. Hanania NA, Chapman KR, Kesten S: Adverse effects of inhaled corticosteroids, *Am J Med* 1995;98:196.

47. Agertoft L: Effect of long-term treatment with inhaled budesonide on adult height in children with asthma, *N Engl J Med* 2000;343:1064.

48. Bernstein PR: Chemistry and structure–activity relationships of leukotriene receptor antagonists, *Am J Respir Crit Care Med* 1998;157:S220.

49. Aharony D: Pharmacology of leukotriene receptor antagonists, *Am J Respir Crit Care Med* 1998;157:S214.

50. Chung KF: Leukotriene receptor antagonists and biosynthesis inhibitors: potential breakthrough in asthma therapy, *Eur Respir J* 1995;8:1203.

51. Leff JA et al: Montelukast, a leukotriene-receptor antagonist, for the treatment of mild asthma and exercise-induced bronchoconstriction, *N Engl J Med* 1998;339:147.

52. Knorr B et al: Montelukast for chronic asthma in 6- to 14–year-old children, *JAMA* 1998;279:1181.

53. Drazen J: Clinical pharmacology of leukotriene receptor antagonists and 5-antagonists, *Am J Respir Crit Care Med* 1998;157:S233.

54. Horwitz RJ, McGill KA, Busse WW: The role of leukotriene modifiers in the treatment of asthma, *Am J Respir Crit Care Med* 1998;157:1363.

55. Wechsler ME et al: Pulmonary infiltrates, eosinophilia, and cardiomyopathy following corticosteroid withdrawal in patients with asthma receiving zafirlukast, *JAMA* 1998;279:455.

56. Holloway J et al: Churg-Strauss syndrome associated with zafirlukast, *J Am Osteopath Assoc* 1998;98:275.

57. Knoell DL et al: Churg-Strauss syndrome associated with zafirlukast, *Chest* 1998;114:332.

58. Keogh KA, Specks U: Churg-Strauss syndrome: clinical presentation, antineutrophil cytoplasmic antibodies, and leukotriene receptor antagonists, *Am J Med* 2003;115:284.

59. Isreal E et al: The effect of inhibition of 5-lipoxygenase by zileuton in mild-to-moderate asthma, *Ann Intern Med* 1993;119:1059.

60. Liu MC et al: Acute and chronic effects of a 5-lipoxygenase inhibitor in asthma: a 6-month randomized multicenter trial, *J Allergy Clin Immunol* 1996;98:859.

61. Wheeler DS et al: Theophylline versus terbutaline in treating critically ill children with status asthmaticus: a prospective, randomized, controlled trial, *Pediatr Crit Care Med* 2005;6:142.

62. Skobeloff EM et al: Effect of magnesium chloride on rabbit bronchial smooth muscle, *Ann Emerg Med* 1990;19:1107.

63. Haury VG: Blood serum magnesium in bronchial asthma and its treatment by administration of magnesium sulfate, *J Lab Clin Med* 1940;26:340.

64. McNamera RM et al: Intravenous magnesium sulfate in the management of acute respiratory failure complicating asthma, *Ann Emerg Med* 1989;18:197.

65. Noppen M et al: Bronchodilating effect of intravenous magnesium sulfate in acute severe bronchial asthma, *Chest* 1990;97:373.

66. Okayama H et al: Treatment of status asthmaticus with intravenous magnesium sulfate, *J Asthma* 1991;28:11.

67. Ciarallo L, Sauer AH, Shannon MW: Intravenous magnesium therapy for moderate to severe pediatric asthma: results of a randomized placebo-controlled trial, *J Pediatr* 1996;129:809.

68. *Mosby's Drug Consult,* St. Louis: Mosby; 2005 [magnesium sulfate].

69. Kastrup EK et al, editors: Respiratory inhalant products. In *Drug Facts and Comparisons,* St. Louis: Facts and Comparisons; 2004. pp 788-810.

70. Prescott WA, Johnson CE: Antiinflammatory therapies for cystic fibrosis: past, present, and future, *Pharmacotherapy* 2005;25:555.

71. McEvoy GK: Mucolytic agents. In McEvoy GK, editor: *American hospital formulary service drug information,* Bethesda, Md: American Society of Hospital Pharmacists; 1993. pp 1680-1682.

72. Duplantier D, McWaters DS: Cystic fibrosis: progress against a childhood killer, *US Pharm* 1992;17:34.

73. Ranasinha C et al: Efficacy and safety of short-term administration of aerosolized recombinant human DNase I in adults with stable stage cystic fibrosis, *Lancet* 1993;342:199.

74. Mazzola CA, Adelson PD: Critical care management of head trauma in children, *Crit Care Med* 2002;30(11 Suppl):S393.

75. Eng PA et al: Short-term efficacy of ultrasonically nebulized hypertonic saline in cystic fibrosis, *Pediatr Pulmonol* 1996;21:77.

76. Daviskas E et al: Inhalation of hypertonic saline aerosol enhances mucociliary clearance in asthmatic and healthy subjects, *Eur Respir J* 1996;9:725.

77. Mandelberg A et al: Nebulized 3% hypertonic saline solution treatment in hospitalized infants with viral bronchiolitis, *Chest* 2003;123:481.

78. Kastrup EK et al, editors: General anesthetics. In *Drug facts and comparisons,* St. Louis: Facts and Comparisons; 2004. pp 1129-1143.

79. Strube PJ, Hallam PL: Ketamine by continuous infusion in status asthmaticus, *Anesthesia* 1986;41:1017.

80. Sarma VJ: Use of ketamine in acute severe asthma, *Acta Anaesthesiol Scand* 1992;36:106.

81. Allen JY, Macias CG: The efficacy of ketamine in pediatric emergency department patients who present with acute severe asthma, *Ann Emerg Med* 2005;46:43.

82. Howton JC et al: Randomized, double-blind, placebo-controlled trial of intravenous ketamine in acute asthma, *Ann Emerg Med* 1996;27:170.

83. Hemming A, MacKenzie I, Finfer S: Response to ketamine in status asthmaticus resistant to maximal medical treatment, *Thorax* 1994;49:90.

84. Nehama J et al: Continuous ketamine infusion for the treatment of refractory asthma in a mechanically ventilated infant: case report and review of the pediatric literature, *Pediatr Emerg Care* 1996;12:294.

85. Geller DE et al: Efficiency of pulmonary administration of tobramycin solution for inhalation in cystic fibrosis using an improved drug delivery system, *Chest* 2003;123:28.

86. Milavetz G, Smith JJ: Cystic fibrosis. In DiPiro JT, Talbert RL, Yee GC, Matzke GR, Wells BG, Posey LM, editors: *Pharmacotherapy: a pathophysiologic approach,* ed 6 New York: McGraw-Hill; 2005. pp 591-604.

87. Fletcher CV et al., editors: Human Immunodeficiency Virus Infection. In DiPiro JT, Talbert RL, Yee GC, Matzke GR, Wells BG, Posey LM, editors: *Pharmacotherapy: a pathophysiologic approach,* ed 6 New York: McGraw-Hill; 2005. pp 2255-2278.

88. Cohen DE, Mayer KH. Primary Care Issues for HIV-Infected Patients. *Infectious Disease Clinics of North America* - Volume 21, Issue 1 (March 2007) p 49-70, 89.

89. Pickering LK et al: *Red Book 2003: Report of the Committee on Infectious Diseases,* ed 26, Elk Grove, Ill: American Academy of Pediatrics; 2003. pp 523-528.

90. Meissner HC: Reducing the impact of viral respiratory infections in children, *Pediatr Clin North Am* 2005;52:695.

91. Committee on Infectious Diseases: Use of ribavirin in the treatment of respiratory syncytial virus infection, *Pediatrics* 1993;92:501.

92. Steiner RW: Treating acute bronchiolitis associated with RSV, *Am Fam Physician* 2004;69:325.

93. Welliver RC: Respiratory syncytial virus immunoglobulin and monoclonal antibodies in the prevention and treatment of respiratory syncytial virus infections, *Semin Perinatol* 1998;22:87.

94. Kastrup ED et al, editors: Antiviral drugs. In *Drug Facts and Comparison,* St. Louis: Facts and Comparisons; 2004. pp 1623-1661.

95. Kastrup ED et al, editors: Immune globulins. In *Drug Facts and Comparison,* St. Louis: Facts and Comparisons; 2004. pp 1753-1768.

96. Sandritter TL, Kraus DM: Respiratory syncytial virus–immunoglobulin intravenous (RSV-IGIV) for respiratory syncytial viral infections: part II, *J Pediatr Health Care* 1998;12:85.

97. Subramanian KN et al: Safety, tolerance and pharmacokinetics of a humanized monoclonal antibody to respiratory syncytial virus in premature infants and infants with bronchopulmonary dysplasia, *Pediatr Infect Dis J* 1998;17:110.

98. Bousquet J et al: Predicting response to omalizumab, an anti-IgE antibody, in patients with allergic asthma, *Chest* 2004;125:1378.

99. Poole JA et al: Targeting the IgE molecule in allergic and asthmatic disease: review of the IgE molecule and clinical efficacy, *J Allergy Clin Immunol* 2005;115:S376.

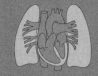

Chapter 25

Thoracic Organ Transplantation

GEORGE B. MALLORY, JR. • OKAN ELIDEMIR • MARC G. SCHECTER

OUTLINE

Heart Transplantation
Heart–Lung Transplantation
Lung Transplantation
Immunosuppressive Regimens
Complications
   Respiratory Problems
   Organ Rejection

Infection
Bronchiolitis Obliterans
Drug Toxicity
Other Complications
Role of the Respiratory Therapist

LEARNING OBJECTIVES

After reading this chapter the reader will be able to:
- Recognize the basic indications for heart and lung transplantation in childhood
- Describe the important respiratory complications after heart and lung transplantation

- Explain the reasons why children can have more complications than adults after thoracic transplantation
- Identify the reasons why lung transplant recipients have increased susceptibility to respiratory infections and their complications

The first heart and lung transplants date back to the 1960s in Cape Town, South Africa, and Jackson, Mississippi, respectively. In each case, the recipients survived for only a few weeks. Despite the continuing development of surgical techniques for thoracic organ transplantation, it was not until effective immunosuppressive regimens became available in the early 1980s that there was a significant increase in the number of successful thoracic organ transplantations (Figure 25-1).[1,2]

In 1982 and 1983, less than a dozen pediatric heart transplants were performed worldwide each year; by 1990, the number had increased to 325 and since then, the worldwide total has ranged from 325 to 390 with no substantive increase since the late 1990s.[1] In contrast, fewer than 10 pediatric lung transplants were performed

in 1986 through 1989.[1] Since 1991, the number of pediatric lung transplants worldwide has ranged from 43 to 84 without a sustained increase in numbers more recently.[1,3] In the mid-1980s, heart–lung transplantation was employed for end-stage pulmonary disease because of the relative easy availability of heart–lung blocks and concerns about surgical challenges intrinsic to isolated lung transplantation. In fact, the peak year for heart–lung transplantation was 1989, when 240 heart–lung transplants were performed.[1]

With the advances in surgical technique in selected adults pioneered by Cooper in Toronto in the 1980s, lung transplantation became the procedure of choice for end-stage lung disease. It is now rare to consider heart–lung transplantation for isolated pulmonary disease.[4]

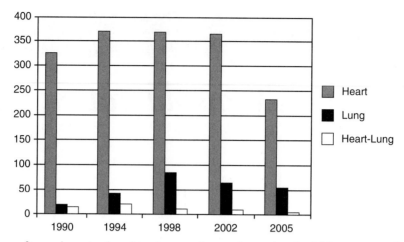

FIGURE 25-1 Frequency of transplantation by selected year and type of transplant in children younger than 18 years of age. The number of pediatric heart and lung transplants remained stable until about 2005, whereas the number of pediatric heart–lung transplants has steadily declined.

TABLE 25-1		
Pediatric Thoracic Organ Transplantation: Primary Indications		
Transplant Type	**Clinical Indication**	
Heart	Cardiomyopathy	
	Congenital heart disease	
Single lung*	Certain forms of interstitial lung disease	
	Bronchopulmonary dysplasia	
	Pulmonary hypertension†	
Bilateral lung	Cystic fibrosis	
	Pulmonary hypertension	
	Bronchiectasis	
Lung with heart repair	Congenital heart disease with pulmonary hypertension but preserved left ventricular function	
Heart–lung	End-stage lung disease with left ventricular failure	
	Irreparable congenital heart disease with pulmonary hypertension	

*Most pediatric programs prefer bilateral lung transplantation because of the growth potential in children and possible skeletal complications from a single lung.

†Although single-lung transplantation was performed successfully in the 1990s for pulmonary hypertension, most programs now use the bilateral lung transplant approach, even with severe right ventricular dysfunction.

In the twenty-first century, heart transplantation is indicated for inoperable congenital heart defects or end-stage myocardial failure and single or bilateral lung transplantation is employed for end-stage pulmonary and pulmonary vascular disease. Heart–lung transplantation is reserved for the infrequent circumstance of combined left ventricular heart failure with pulmonary disease or combined congenital defects of both the heart and lung (Table 25-1).[1-4] In 2004, only 74 heart–lung

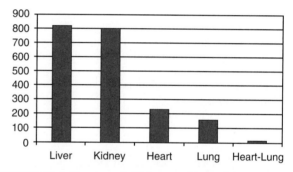

FIGURE 25-2 Number of children awaiting solid organ transplantation by organ type as of November 30, 2005. There are a relatively large number of children awaiting kidney or liver transplantation compared with those waiting for heart, lung, or heart–lung transplantation.

transplants were performed worldwide compared with 1815 lung and 2948 heart transplants in all ages.[4] Of the 74 heart–lung transplants performed around the world in 2004, only 7 were performed in individuals under the age of 18 years.[3,5]

There have been and are significantly fewer children waiting for thoracic organ transplantation compared with those waiting for kidney or liver transplantation (Figure 25-2). Since the late 1990s, there has been a steady increase in the number of pediatric candidates for solid organ transplantation but, until recently, there has been no increase in the number of donors.

In 2003, the Organ Donation Breakthrough Collaborative was formed under public auspices in the United States to enhance organ donation.[6] The average conversion rate, that is, the rate at which families of brain dead individuals consent to organ donation, was 46% at that time. Examination of best practices suggested that 75% conversion rate was achievable and this goal was formally set in the final report of the

Collaborative in September 2003. Since that time, there has been a significant increase in donors for the first time in a decade.

In 2005, the Organ Transplantation Breakthrough Collaborative was formed to increase the number of organs harvested from each donor. In the majority of donors, the liver and kidneys are deemed suitable for transplant but only approximately 25% of the hearts and 10% to 15% of the lungs are deemed intact enough to be transplanted. Lungs are frequently infected and/or atelectatic or injured during prolonged intubation and ventilation, or unsuitable because of pulmonary edema, trauma, or aspiration.[7] By the application of best practices, aggressive donor management can increase both heart and lung donation, although it may take longer to manage the donor until the time of harvest.[8] However, the number of both abdominal and thoracic organs can also be increased by this approach.

It is the goal of the Collaboratives to extend the use of aggressive donor management protocols around the country to increase the yield of transplanted organs. One of the mandates of the Organ Transplantation Collaborative is to treat every donor as a thoracic organ donor with early emphasis on evaluating and resuscitating the lungs and heart. Although there have been great hopes for xenotransplantation (use of animal donors in human solid organ transplantation), ongoing research has discovered vexing hurdles, which pushed the realization of this hope into the distant future.[9] Another innovative approach to the donor shortage is the use of living donor lobar donation for lung transplantation (using a lower lobe from two taller individuals, commonly but not always a parent or relative).[10]

For most children who undergo thoracic organ transplantation, quality of life usually returns to normal.[11,12] Within weeks after the operation, depending on their pretransplant nutritional and physical state, most patients are able to resume age-appropriate activities with improving exercise tolerance. Cardiac function is generally normal in heart transplant patients.[13] Gas exchange and pulmonary function rapidly return to near normal in the first months after lung transplantation.[11,12] Minor childhood illnesses appear to be well tolerated, although it is frequently difficult to ascertain in its initial stage whether a febrile illness represents a minor infection, graft rejection, or a life-threatening infection in the immunocompromised host. Growth delay can be a problem, at least in part resulting from the administration of prednisone, which is continued lifelong in almost all lung and a subset of heart recipients. However, subsequent growth of the patient as well as of the allograft is possible, and it is unlikely that the subject will outgrow the transplanted organ.[14]

HEART TRANSPLANTATION

In the 1980s, the primary indication for heart transplantation was cardiomyopathy. However, in more recent years the proportion of transplantations for congenital heart defects has been increasing (Table 25-2).[1] Congenital lesions are the predominant problem leading to heart transplantation in children younger than 1 year of age, whereas cardiomyopathy predominates in older children.[15] The operative approach in heart transplantation involves a sternotomy with surgical anastomoses to the venae cavae and aorta. Early postoperative mortality arises from graft failure and, less commonly, cardiac rhythm disorders. The newly denervated implanted heart often has an initial intrinsic rhythm too slow to produce an adequate cardiac output. Thus, a temporary external pacemaker is attached at the end of each heart transplant operation. Infectious complications, graft rejection, and central nervous system hemorrhage or embolism occur with lower incidence. The early posttransplant mortality rate after transplantation is higher in younger children, as evidenced by the 25% mortality rate in recipients less than 1 year of age compared with 10% for the 11- to 18-year age group.[15] Late deaths are caused primarily by coronary vasculopathy (chronic rejection). A small number of deaths in the early and late groups have been related to central nervous system complications such as stroke. The death rate from malignancy (primarily lymphoproliferative disease) increases over time and represents 10% of deaths after 5 years.[15] Other morbidities from heart

---

TABLE 25-2

Indications for Heart Transplantation by Percent Frequency in Each Age Group

	1 Year	1–10 Years	11–17 Years
Cardiomyopathy	19.7	52.4	65.4
Congenital heart defects	76.5	37.3	25
Other	2.6	5.0	6.3
Retransplantation	1.2	5.3	3.4

Modified from Hosenpud JD et al: The Registry of the International Society for Heart and Lung Transplantation: eighteenth official report—2001, *J Heart Lung Transplant* 2001;20:805.

transplantation include hypertension in approximately 40% of individuals, renal insufficiency in 20%, and seizures in 25%.[16-18]

A troublesome and life-limiting problem in long-term heart transplant survivors, regardless of age, is the development of premature coronary artery disease or coronary vasculopathy, also known as *graft atherosclerosis*.[15,16,18] This condition may be asymptomatic and may be discovered only at the time of surveillance coronary angiography. In some patients, the disease can be significant enough to cause myocardial ischemia and may contribute to dysrhythmias or sudden death. There is general consensus that premature coronary artery disease is immunologically mediated as a manifestation of chronic graft rejection and therefore may decrease in prevalence with improvements in immunosuppressive regimens.

Neonatal heart transplantation has been successful at some centers. This has been used almost exclusively for hypoplastic left-heart syndrome, which is uniformly fatal if surgical correction or transplantation is not offered. The current experience with either surgical correction or transplantation does not clearly indicate which is more appropriate to optimize survival.[17] Although once considered promising, anencephalic infants have not proven to be suitable donors for other neonates.[19] Young infants are less sophisticated hosts by virtue of their relatively immature immune response and therefore might tolerate the immunologic challenge of transplantation more readily than older subjects. In fact, many pediatric candidates under 18 months of age can receive hearts across the ABO group barriers with long-term success. The survival rate and duration of survival with good cardiac function appear to be the same for children as for adult heart transplant recipients.[15,18]

HEART–LUNG TRANSPLANTATION

Before the surgical technique for successful lung transplantation was developed, heart–lung transplantation was offered for end-stage pulmonary disease. Heart–lung transplantation involves a sternotomy and surgical anastomoses of the trachea, superior and inferior venae cavae, and the aorta and is generally acknowledged to be a technically less challenging operation compared with lung transplantation. With the ability to successfully transplant a single lung or two lungs, the use of heart–lung transplantation for pulmonary disease has decreased.[1,3] There are multiple reasons for this, including the following:

- The limited availability of satisfactory coupled heart–lung donations from a single donor (governed in part by the distribution algorithm unique to each country)

- The practical advantage of using the heart–lung block for three separate donations (one heart and two single lungs)
- The decreased risk of cardiac rejection if isolated lung transplantation is performed
- The decreased risk of premature coronary artery disease

Despite concerns about the impact of right ventricular dysfunction commonly associated with chronic pulmonary disease or severe pulmonary hypertension in the immediate postoperative period, there has generally been an excellent improvement in right ventricular function with single- or double-lung transplantation, and therefore severe right-sided cardiac dysfunction is rarely an indication for heart–lung transplantation, especially in children.[3,11] For patients with congenital heart defects such as atrial septal defect, ventricular septal defect, or patent ductus arteriosus, as well as pulmonary hypertension from Eisenmenger's syndrome, the currently preferred surgery is lung transplantation (single or double) with repair of the congenital heart defect.[20]

The volume of heart–lung transplantation has decreased by more than half since the late 1990s, from a peak of 240 transplants per year in 1989 to 78 per year in 2004.[1,3] The decrease in use of heart–lung transplantation is most dramatic in the United States compared with other countries, notably the United Kingdom.

LUNG TRANSPLANTATION

A common and severe complication of lung transplantation before 1983 was tracheal and bronchial anastomosis failure. When Cooper demonstrated techniques that overcame these problems in the late 1980s, single- and double-lung transplantation became the preferred option for adult patients with chronic pulmonary disease. Table 25-1 lists the diseases appropriate for single- or double-lung transplantation. Figure 25-3 shows the most common chronic lung diseases that, in children, lead to transplantation. Cystic fibrosis is the most common indication for bilateral lung transplantation, almost exclusively in children more than 6 years of age.[1,3]

Enthusiasm for lung transplantation has been tempered by the low survival rate; the initial 1-year survival rate was only slightly more than 50% at 1 year. This compares with early survival rates after heart–lung or double-lung transplants in patients with cystic fibrosis of 60% to 70% at 1 year in the 1990s.[21,22] As overall experience has increased, survival after lung transplantation has improved; the most recent actuarial survival at 1 year after transplant is 84%,[23] with some individual centers reporting even better survival.[18] Longer term survival rates remain disappointing, however, with a 5-year survival of just below 50%.[3,5,23] Post-lung transplant

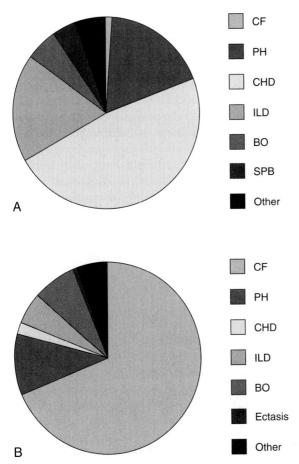

A

CF

PH

CHD

ILD

BO

SPB

Other

B

CF

PH

CHD

ILD

BO

Ectasis

Other

FIGURE 25-3 Frequency of primary diseases leading to lung transplantation in children. **A,** Diagnoses from birth through age 5 years. **B,** Diagnoses from birth through age 6 to 18 years. BO, Bronchiolitis obliterans; CF, cystic fibrosis; CHD, congenital heart disease; Ectasis, bronchiectasis; ILD, interstitial lung disease; PH, pulmonary hypertension; SPB, surfactant protein B deficiency. The category "other" is made up primarily of bronchopulmonary dysplasia or congenital lung defects.

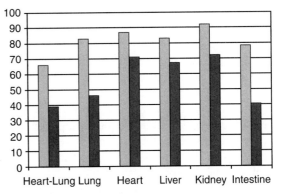

FIGURE 25-4 Overall 1-year *(lighter columns)* and 5-year *(darker columns)* survival rates for solid organ transplant recipients as reported by the United Network for Organ Sharing (Richmond, Va). Although 1-year survival has improved from early experience, lung, intestine, and heart–lung transplantations are not yet as successful in terms of longer term survival as other solid organ transplantations. Note that after graft failure, renal recipients usually survive on dialysis.

survival rates have a long way to go to be comparable with the successes of kidney, heart, pancreas, and liver transplantation (Figure 25-4).[23]

Deaths within the first 90 days after lung transplantation (early deaths) result most commonly from graft failure due to ischemia–reperfusion injury. Less common are surgical problems such as airway anastomotic dehiscence or massive hemorrhage. Even less common are overwhelming infection, either systemic or pulmonary; multiple organ failure; or acute graft rejection. Late deaths are generally related to infection or bronchiolitis obliterans, usually a manifestation of chronic rejection.[6,7]

A particular concern in pediatric lung transplantation is the problem of donor–recipient size matching. In addition to the problems of donor availability among all transplantation candidates, the thoracic dimensions of infants and small children add another obstacle, so that size-appropriate donors are even less frequently available than for adolescents or adults.[24]

A potential solution to this problem is reduced-size transplantation, often from a living donor (e.g., transplanting an adult lower lobe to a pediatric patient to replace the recipient's entire lung[25]). Although initial attempts at living-related donation were disappointing, more recent experience suggests that living donor lobar transplantation can be successful with a 1-year survival of 60% to 80% with only minimal risk to the donor.[26] Therefore living donor lobar transplantation may help overcome the obstacles of donor waiting time, size limitation, and organ availability for the urgently ill transplant candidate. The lung allocation score system, which took effect in the United States in 2005, now lists patients according to a computed score of urgency, reducing the need for living donor lung transplantation.[27]

IMMUNOSUPPRESSIVE REGIMENS

Although children frequently resume normal activity within weeks of transplantation, the medical regimen after thoracic transplantation is extensive, especially in the first year. In addition to an intense new pharmacologic program, there are frequent office visits, multiple blood tests, repeated radiographs, and, in most centers, surveillance biopsies. Even a minor illness can lead to hospitalization to rule out graft rejection or serious infection. With increasing time after transplantation and successful graft function, there are fewer impositions on the lives of the child and family.

When children are referred to centers distant from their home communities, their families usually have to spend months before and often 3 months after transplant in the transplant center community. There are considerable financial and psychosocial costs to this dislocation of children and parents from their homes. As has been said many times, the transplant patient trades one set of problems (the burdens of living with a terminal disease) for another (the long-term immunosuppression and lifelong risk of potential life-threatening complications).

Most immunosuppressive regimens for organ transplantations (thoracic and other solid organs) include the combined use of cyclosporine or tacrolimus, azathioprine or mycophenolate mofetil, and prednisone.[3,15] The administration of cyclosporine or tacrolimus and azathioprine or mycophenolate mofetil is generally needed for the life of the transplant recipient. There has been an increasing trend to embrace a corticosteroid-free immunosuppressant program in pediatric heart transplant centers. Many heart centers wean or attempt to discontinue prednisone within weeks to months after the transplantation. Because lung allografts are more susceptible to both acute and chronic rejection, immunosuppressant dosing is generally higher and more prolonged compared with that in heart transplant recipients. Few lung transplant centers attempt to wean patients from prednisone; at most, some patients can be weaned to alternate-day dosing.

Immunosuppressive drugs are usually given intravenously in the immediate period after transplantation and then are changed to the oral route as patients recover from surgery. We have used tacrolimus via the sublingual route as opposed to the parenteral route with success. There are serious potential side effects from these medications (Table 25-3) as well as a multitude of drug interactions, of which all prescribing physicians need to be aware. Episodes of acute rejection are treated with augmented immunosuppression, generally with 3 days of high-dose intravenous steroid pulse therapy. The clinical response is usually favorable and prompt. On occasion, with repeated episodes of acute rejection or the appearance of chronic rejection, additional immunosuppressive agents may be required, such as anti-lymphocyte globulin, anti-thymocyte globulin, or monoclonal antibodies such as muromonab-CD3 (Orthoclone OKT3).[3] Although chronic rejection is also treated with augmented immunosuppression, the response is less often favorable than with acute rejection.[28,29] Oral agents such as methotrexate and sirolimus are also used in selected patients.

COMPLICATIONS

The complications of thoracic organ transplantation can be grouped into the following categories[3]:
- Respiratory failure and related problems
- Acute rejection
- Infection
- Chronic rejection or bronchiolitis obliterans
- Drug toxicity
- Other complications

Respiratory Problems

All thoracic transplantation patients arrive in the intensive care unit after transplantation and receive mechanical ventilatory support via an endotracheal tube. Most well-conditioned heart transplant patients with good myocardial contractility in the immediate postoperative period can be weaned from mechanical ventilation within the first hours. The surgical incision and thoracostomy tube will result in reduced thoracic

---

TABLE 25-3

Common Side Effects of Immunosuppressive Drugs

	Cyclosporine	Tacrolimus	Azathioprine	Mycophenolate Mofetil	Prednisone
Headache	++	++			
Seizures	++	++			
Hyperglycemia	+	++			++
Hypertension	+++	+++			++
Hyperlipidemia	++	+			+
Renal injury	++	++			
Growth impairment					++
Hirsutism	++				
GI intolerance			+	++	+
Leukopenia			+	++	
Anemia			+/−	+	

GI, Gastrointestinal.

compliance, and both deep inspiration and cough will likely be compromised. With the judicious use of intravenous analgesics, chest physiotherapy, and occasionally regional nerve block or epidural anesthesia, most heart transplant patients, like their counterparts who undergo other cardiac surgical procedures, do well. With the increasing frequency of left ventricular assist devices, there are a growing number of severely deconditioned pediatric cardiac transplant recipients who may require longer periods of ventilator support. A subset of recipients experience severe myocardial failure postoperatively. Extracorporeal membrane oxygenation or a ventricular assist device may be required with or without mechanical ventilatory support for several days. With myocardial failure, some degree of pulmonary edema with reduced lung compliance occurs. These and other patients require aggressive intravenous cardiotonic and diuretic medications. Oxygen supplementation is almost always needed in these patients. Under some circumstances, a relatively large heart graft that is placed in a smaller child may compress the intrathoracic airways, the left mainstem bronchus being particularly vulnerable to such compression. With compression, consolidation with absent breath sounds over the left lower lobe or low-pitched expiratory wheezing with a variable degree of dyspnea may result. Bronchodilators, vigorous chest physiotherapy and noninvasive positive-pressure ventilation may be needed to maintain maximal airway patency, minimize atelectasis, and mobilize retained secretions.

Heart–lung and lung transplant patients are more vulnerable to respiratory complications than are heart transplant patients. The thoracic incision is usually more extensive when lungs are transplanted. Allograft dysfunction after lung transplantation is common but highly variable. The delicate pulmonary capillary bed appears to be more susceptible to ischemic injury than is the myocardium, liver, or kidney in the context of transplantation. So-called ischemia–reperfusion injury in the lung is manifested as pulmonary capillary leak.

This reperfusion injury, which occurs in 10% to 20% of lung transplants, mimics the acute respiratory distress syndrome clinically and radiographically. On chest radiography, pulmonary edema, either immediately after transplantation or within the first 72 hours, is usually a sign of ischemic injury or reperfusion injury (Figure 25-5).[30,31] Interruption of the pulmonary lymphatics, which are cut during the surgery, also contribute to pleural, alveolar and interstitial fluid accumulation. Severe reperfusion injury, now called primary graft dysfunction, affects approximately 25% of adult and pediatric lung transplant recipients with varying severity.[32] Another complication occurring in a small subset of patients in the first week after lung transplantation is

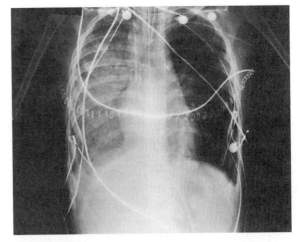

FIGURE 25-5 This chest radiograph demonstrates reperfusion injury to the right lung immediately after double-lung transplantation in an 11-year-old girl with cystic fibrosis. There is a ground-glass haziness with air bronchograms over the right lung field. The staples across the chest are external and used for surgical skin closure. There are surgical clips in each hilar region where the vascular anastomoses were performed. There is also an endotracheal tube, a nasogastric tube, a left subclavian vein catheter, a right internal jugular vein catheter, bilateral chest tubes, and surface electrodes.

the overproduction of mucus (bronchorrhea). Signs and symptoms of abundant lower airway secretions without fever or leukocytosis will often lead to emergent bronchoscopy in which abundant thick mucus is found. With isolated bronchorrhea, cultures are sterile and Gram stains demonstrate mucus, polymorphonuclear leukocytes, and no bacterial organisms.

Vigorous chest physiotherapy and the addition of aerosolized atropine can be helpful. Bronchorrhea slowly subsides over several days to weeks. The cause is unknown, although it may be the result of autonomic imbalance related to vagotomy from the transplantation surgery.

Subacute respiratory failure requiring ventilatory support for 1 to 2 weeks without severe parenchymal disease is seen in some patients who had significant preoperative hypercapnia. Respiratory control mechanisms may require many days to reset after lung or heart–lung transplantation.[33] The keys to management are to avoid oversedation and to provide adequate nutrition and ventilatory support until weaning can be achieved. Noninvasive ventilatory support with bilevel positive airway pressure may help make the transition from the pretransplant hypercarbic state to the posttransplant normocarbic state.

Significant bronchial obstruction may develop after lung or heart–lung transplantation because of stricture or dehiscence at the site of the bronchial anastomosis. Most airway complications will present within

3 months of transplantation, and although a few can be fatal if severe and early, most are treatable with bronchoscopic dilation, laser resection of granulation tissue, or the placement of airway stents.[34,35]

Organ Rejection

The clinical signs and symptoms of organ rejection may be minimal or subtle. Acute rejection of the transplanted heart, if clinically apparent, results in decreased cardiac contractility with signs and symptoms of congestive heart failure. Tachycardia, tachypnea, and malaise may be noted. Echocardiography is the noninvasive diagnostic mode of choice to ascertain the physiologic signs of cardiac rejection. In the lung transplant patient, tachypnea, bibasilar inspiratory crackles on auscultation, increased interstitial infiltrates on chest radiography, and oxygen desaturation are often associated with acute rejection (Figure 25-6). For older patients who can perform spirometry, a drop in pulmonary function, either restrictive or obstructive, is often the most sensitive indicator of acute rejection.

Many transplant centers perform routine surveillance biopsies of the transplanted tissue in an effort to identify and treat early rejection before permanent organ damage occurs.[18,36] When clinically suspected, the diagnosis of rejection is also usually confirmed by biopsy.[4,18] Endomyocardial biopsy by means of biopsy forceps passed through a vascular-accessed catheter is the method of choice in heart transplant patients. Flexible bronchoscopy with transbronchial biopsy in

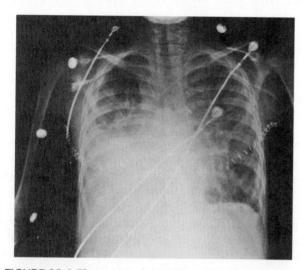

FIGURE 25-6 The same patient in Figure 25–5, seen 3 weeks later during an episode of acute lung rejection. A large right pleural effusion obscures the right hemidiaphragm and the border of the right side of the heart. There is an extensive increase in peribronchial markings in both lungs and a blunted left costophrenic angle. All chest tubes and the endotracheal tube have been removed. A right subclavian vein catheter has been added.

children and adolescents is used to obtain multiple pieces of tissue for histopathologic examination in lung transplant patients. For infants and young children, rigid bronchoscopy or open-lung biopsy may be required, although tiny biopsy forceps may allow biopsy through the flexible bronchoscope even in very small children. Most transplantation physicians are uncomfortable augmenting immunosuppression without tissue confirmation of graft rejection.

Infection

It can be difficult to separate rejection from infection, especially on a clinical diagnostic basis, and in some cases they may coexist.[31] Although pulmonary infections are common because of the immunosuppression required with any solid organ transplant, the pulmonary infection rate for lung transplantation appears to be particularly high.[36] This may be partially explained by the fact that the lung is the only solid organ that after transplantation is regularly in direct contact with the external environment and multiple potential pathogens. Many pulmonary bacterial infections are readily identified and easily treated with antibiotics. Pulmonary viral infections are less frequent but more often fatal, especially if cytomegalovirus is involved.[36] Fungal infections are particularly troublesome in terms of both identification and treatment. Because the transplant patient with cystic fibrosis retains the native trachea and sinuses, there is a potential increase in infections from chronic colonization of the respiratory epithelia in the trachea and from frank infection within the paranasal sinuses.[37] This can be particularly serious if the colonizing organisms have multiple antibiotic resistances.[37,38] In fact, some centers consider infection with *Pseudomonas* species that have no antibiotic sensitivity a contraindication to transplantation.[4] The highly antibiotic-resistant *Burkholderia cepacia* complex organisms have been associated with significant morbidity and mortality in patients with cystic fibrosis.[39] These resistant organisms are found most often in the older patient with advanced lung disease, and this is the patient with cystic fibrosis who most likely needs transplantation. Of concern is the report that *B. cepacia* is particularly lethal to transplant patients with cystic fibrosis who acquire it after transplantation.[40] The role of antibiotic prophylaxis in patients with cystic fibrosis who undergo lung transplantation remains to be clarified. A common and potentially effective prophylaxis for transplant patients with cystic fibrosis involves inhaled antibiotics, usually an aminoglycoside such as tobramycin.

Bronchiolitis Obliterans

Bronchiolitis obliterans is unfortunately a common late complication in both heart–lung and lung transplant recipients.[4,5,28] The exact cause is unknown, but it most likely represents the common pathway for different insults such as chronic rejection, infection, and aspiration. Bronchiolitis obliterans can be initially identified by a decrease in flow rates at low lung volumes during surveillance pulmonary function testing and can be confirmed by transbronchial biopsy or open-lung biopsy (Figure 25-7). Because of the high frequency of false-negative transbronchial biopsies, most clinicians use the clinical definition of "bronchiolitis obliterans syndrome" for both diagnosis and treatment decisions.[41] In the majority of patients, bronchiolitis obliterans is a progressive disease manifested by increasing dyspnea, increased coughing with sputum production, colonization or infection with *Pseudomonas* species, and eventual respiratory failure and death. A small minority of patients responds favorably to augmented immunosuppression, with reversal or stabilization of their airway dysfunction.[29] Bronchiolitis obliterans remains a major obstacle to the success of lung and heart–lung transplantation.

Drug Toxicity

All immunosuppressive regimens place the patient at risk for infection. In addition, each arm of the regimen may cause other complications from side effects or drug toxicity. Cyclosporine and tacrolimus can have multiple side effects (see Table 25-3). Hypertension and nephrotoxicity are most common, but, fortunately, are usually manageable. Experienced transplant physicians expect the incidence of renal failure to increase with increasing survivors and prolonged exposure to immunosuppressive agents. The major complication from both azathioprine and mycophenolate mofetil is a decreased white blood cell count caused by bone marrow suppression, which usually improves with temporary discontinuation of the medicine or a decrease in dose. There may be more symptoms of gastrointestinal disturbance with mycophenolate mofetil compared with azathioprine. Complications of prednisone are quite common in the immediate posttransplantation period when high doses are used, but complications lessen with decreasing doses after several months. Some children and adolescents will experience little or no skeletal growth until the prednisone can be decreased to low daily doses (0.1 to 0.15 mg/kg/d) or to an alternate-day dosage schedule. It is common for patients to assume a cushingoid appearance in the early months after transplantation. Many become glucose intolerant, particularly patients with cystic fibrosis who may have partial glucose intolerance because of intrinsic pancreatic involvement by the disease and the diabetogenic effects of tacrolimus and cyclosporine.

Other Complications

A broad spectrum of other complications occur less frequently after transplantation. For patients receiving heart or heart–lung transplants, accelerated coronary artery disease is a potentially serious problem.[15,16,18] Like bronchiolitis obliterans, it is a form of chronic graft rejection and is usually progressive. Other potential complications include obstructive sleep apnea, cerebrovascular accidents, and aspiration of gastric contents. Epstein-Barr virus–related lymphoproliferative disease is a neoplastic disorder that occurs in relation to the intensity and duration of immunosuppression. The incidence in pediatric thoracic transplantation varies from 1% to 10%.[13,42] It may regress with decreased levels of immunosuppression or progress to fatal malignancy. Other fairly common medical complications include generalized seizures, aggravated acne, and mild suppression of maximal exercise performance. Up to 25% of lung transplant recipients may experience unilateral vocal cord or hemidiaphragm paralysis, which may recover 3 to 6 months after transplant. Equally important are the psychosocial adjustments to the emotional "roller coaster" of thoracic organ transplantation.[43] Although almost all patients can benefit from extensive psychosocial support, occasionally some will require pharmacologic assistance to deal with either anxiety or

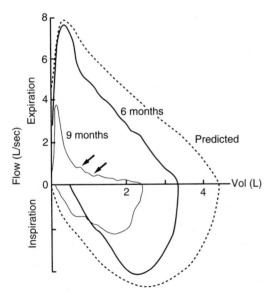

FIGURE 25-7 These curves represent serial flow–volume pulmonary function test data produced by a patient with cystic fibrosis after sequential double-lung transplantation. Flow is presented on the vertical axis, with volume on the horizontal axis. The *dashed line* represents the predicted value for the patient's age, sex, and height. Six months after transplantation, the patient's pulmonary function is nearly normal, with no suggestion of significant airflow limitation. The *curve* at 9 months demonstrates the changes associated with the development of bronchiolitis obliterans; the *arrows* demonstrate the marked flow limitation at mid- and low lung volumes characteristic of this condition.

depression.[43,44] These psychologic or psychiatric complications are quite common, and they are potentially serious. Nonadherence to the medical regimen is often fatal. The entire transplantation team must be alert for any psychologic or psychiatric complications in the hope of either their prevention or their early detection and treatment.

ROLE OF THE RESPIRATORY THERAPIST

There are multiple areas of interaction between the respiratory therapist (RT) and the transplant patient. Care of the patient who undergoes thoracic transplantation always involves teamwork from a variety of health care professionals. The child who receives a lung or heart–lung transplant is especially likely to require an RT on the team. Familiarity with the diseases leading to transplantation, as well as the transplantation process, will help the practitioner provide more comprehensive care to the patient as well as improve interaction with the health care team. Many RTs will already be familiar with the transplant candidate because of their role in providing routine care for the primary disease process, particularly for chronic pulmonary diseases such as cystic fibrosis. The RT may become the true contact with the transplantation candidate in the initial evaluation process or during pulmonary function testing. After the patient has been accepted to the transplantation list, the RT may be involved in providing an exercise evaluation or a rehabilitation program, or both, in an effort to optimize the patient's condition while he or she is awaiting transplantation. Immediately after the transplantation procedure, the RT will be involved with the patient in the intensive care unit, primarily providing mechanical ventilatory support. Because of the temporary interruption of ciliary function, the RT may be asked to provide aerosolized bronchodilators, mechanical aids to assist full inflation and cough, and bronchopulmonary hygiene. For most patients, this therapy is not required on a long-term basis. Shortly after the patient is taken off mechanical ventilation, the RT may be involved in reinstituting the exercise and rehabilitation program that had been initiated before the procedure.

Over the intermediate and long term, patients and families often forget the importance of bronchial denervation in masking symptoms of significant lower respiratory tract disease. Lung transplant recipients can develop airway obstruction related to purulent bronchitis with surprisingly little cough. We have emphasized the importance of monitoring lung function at home as the single most sensitive indicator of lung health. We usually teach our lung transplant recipients how to use the Flutter® device (Cardinal Health, Dublin, Ohio,

USA) as a tool to aid in cough with mucus clearance. Refresher sessions are important during the extended period of follow-up. Last, the RT may be involved in the transplant patient's care by assisting with follow-up pulmonary function tests, instructing the patient in the use of home spirometry, and assisting with bronchoscopies.

ASSESSMENT QUESTIONS

See Evolve Resources for the answers.

1. What is the frequency of transplantations performed in the pediatric-age group, in order from most to least?
   A. Lung > heart–lung > heart
   B. Heart > heart–lung > lung
   C. Lung > heart > heart–lung
   D. Heart > lung > heart–lung
2. What is the major reason why fewer lungs are transplanted per donor compared with heart transplants in childhood?
   A. There are fewer lung transplant candidates than heart transplant candidates in childhood.
   B. There are fewer lung transplant programs than heart transplant programs.
   C. The lungs are more likely to be injured or infected in the brain-dead individual than the heart.
   D. The size of lungs is less adaptable to children of different ages than is the size of the heart.
3. What is the major medical problem in the immediate posttransplantation period for pediatric heart transplant patients?
   A. Graft failure
   B. Weaning patients from mechanical ventilatory support
   C. Cardiac arrhythmias
   D. Graft rejection
4. What is the major medical problem in the immediate posttransplantation period for pediatric lung transplant recipients?
   A. Graft failure
   B. Weaning patients from ventilator support
   C. Pneumonia from the donor
   D. Graft rejection
5. For what condition is heart–lung transplant surgery most commonly performed in pediatric patients?
   A. Cystic fibrosis
   B. Pulmonary hypertension
   C. Infants with lung disease due to the technical difficulties in isolated lung transplantation
   D. Pulmonary hypertension with congenital heart disease

Continued

ASSESSMENT QUESTIONS—cont'd

6. Living donor transplantation has been performed for:
   A. Heart transplantation
   B. Heart–lung transplantation
   C. Lung transplantation
   D. All of the above
   E. None of the above

7. How long is immunosuppression used in lung, heart, and heart–lung transplantation?
   A. Only during the critical 6 months after transplantation; the patient is then weaned.
   B. Lifelong
   C. Lifelong only in lung and heart–lung transplantation because of the higher incidence of graft rejection
   D. Lifelong only in heart and heart–lung transplantation because lung infections become a greater risk to survival after the first year because of immunosuppression

8. Among the most important risks for pulmonary complications after lung transplantation in children are all of the following *except:*
   A. Dangers of childhood vaccines
   B. Absence of cough reflex due to interruption of the nerve supply to the transplanted lungs
   C. Immunosuppression
   D. Frequency of inevitable exposure to community respiratory viruses and other pathogens

9. Organ rejection is
   A. A problem only in lung and heart–lung transplantation
   B. A problem only in the critical first 6 months after thoracic transplants
   C. The most common cause of late death in heart and lung transplantation
   D. Receding as a common problem because of advances in early detection and better immunosuppression

10. What is the role of the respiratory therapist in transplantation?
    A. Unimportant after isolated heart transplantation because the native lungs are, by definition, healthy
    B. Important only in the postoperative period in heart, heart–lung, and lung transplantation, during the variable period of weaning from mechanical ventilatory support
    C. Needed with many intercurrent respiratory infections after lung or heart–lung transplantation because of the blunting of the cough reflex
    D. Critical in evaluating oxygen saturation trends for cardiologists who are unfamiliar with this technology

References

1. Hosenpud JD et al: The Registry of the International Society for Heart and Lung Transplantation: eighteenth official report—2001, *J Heart Lung Transplant* 2001;20:805.
2. Cooper JD: The evolution of techniques and indications for lung transplantation, *Ann Surg* 1990;212:249.
3. Waltz DA et al: Registry of the International Society for Heart and Lung Transplantation: ninth official pediatric lung and heart–lung transplantation report – 2006, *J Heart Lung Transplant* 2006;25:904.
4. Trulock EP: Lung transplantation, *Am J Respir Crit Care Med* 1997;155:789.
5. Trulock EP et al: Registry of the International Society for Heart and Lung Transplantation: twenty third official adult lung and heart–lung transplantation report—2006, *J Heart Lung Transplant* 2006;25:880.
6. Marks WH et al: Organ donation and utilization, 1995-2004: entering the collaborative era, *Am J Transplant* 2006;6:1101.
7. de Perrot M et al: Strategies to optimize the use of current available lung donors, *J Heart Lung Transplant* 2004;23:1127.
8. Kutsogiannis DJ et al: Medical management to optimize donor organ potential: review of the literature, *Can J Anesth* 2006;53:820.
9. Cooper DK et al: Report of the Xenotransplantation Advisory Committee of the International Society for Heart And Lung Transplantation: potential role in the treatment of end-stage cardiac and pulmonary diseases, *J Heart Lung Transplant* 2000;19:1125.
10. Starnes VA et al: Living-donor lobar lung transplantation experience: immediate results, *J Thorac Cardiovasc Surg* 1996;112:1284.
11. Sweet SC et al: Pediatric lung transplantation at St Louis Children's Hospital, 1990-1995, *Am J Respir Crit Care Med* 1997;155:1027.
12. Noyes BE, Kurland G, Orenstein DM: Lung and heart-lung transplantation in children, *Pediatr Pulmonol* 1997;23:39.
13. Baum D et al: Pediatric heart transplantation at Stanford: results of a 15 year experience, *Pediatrics* 1991;88:203.
14. Cohen AH et al: Growth of lungs after transplantation in infants and in children younger than age, *Am J Respir Crit Care Med* 1999;159:1747.
15. Boucek MM et al: The Registry of the International Society of Heart and Lung Transplantation: ninth official pediatric heart transplantation report—2006, *J Heart Lung Transplant* 2006;25:893.
16. Pahl E et al: Coronary arteriosclerosis in pediatric heart transplant survivors: limitation of long-term survival, *J Pediatr* 1990;116:177.
17. Boucek MM et al: Cardiac transplantation in infancy: donors and recipients, *J Pediatr* 1990;116:171.
18. Ross M et al: Ten- and 20-year survivors of pediatric orthotopic heart transplantation, *J Heart Lung Transplant* 2006;25:261.
19. Shewmon DA et al: The use of anencephalic infants as organ sources: a critique, *JAMA* 1989;261:1173.
20. Spray TL et al: Pediatric lung transplantation for pulmonary hypertension and congenital heart disease, *Ann Thorac Surg* 1992;54:216.
21. Ramirez JC et al: Bilateral lung transplantation for cystic fibrosis, *J Thorac Cardiovasc Surg* 1991;103:287.

22. Mendeloff EM et al: Pediatric and adult lung transplantation for cystic fibrosis, *J Thorac Cardiovasc Surg* 1998;115:404.

23. U.S. Organ Procurement and Transplantation Network and the Scientific Registry of Transplant Recipients website: www.optn.org. Retrieved October 2008.

24. Noirclerc M et al: Size matching in lung transplantation, *J Heart Lung Transplant* 1992;11:S203.

25. Starnes VA et al: Current trends in lung transplantation: lobar transplantation and expanded use of single lungs, *J Thorac Cardiovasc Surg* 1992;104:1060.

26. Starnes VA et al: Comparison of outcomes between living donor and cadaveric lung transplant children, *Ann Thorac Surg* 1999;68:2279.

27. Egan T et al: Development of the new lung allocation system in the United States, *Am J Transplant* 2006;6:1212.

28. Boehler A et al: Bronchiolitis obliterans after lung transplantation: a review, *Chest* 1998;114:1411.

29. Date H et al: The impact of cytolytic therapy on bronchiolitis obliterans syndrome, *J Heart Lung Transplant* 1998;17:869.

30. Jurmann MJ et al: Pulmonary reperfusion injury: evidence for oxygen-derived free radical mediated damage and effects of different free radical scavengers, *Eur J Cardiothorac Surg* 1990;4:665.

31. Paradis IL et al: Distinguishing between infection, rejection, and the adult respiratory distress syndrome after human lung transplantation, *J Heart Lung Transplant* 1992;11:S232.

32. Meyers BF et al: Primary graft dysfunction and other selected complications of lung transplantation: a single center experience, *J Thorac Cardiovasc Surg* 2005;129:1421.

33. Trachiotis GD et al: Carbon dioxide response in lung transplant recipients [abstract], *Am Rev Respir Dis* 1992;145:A702.

34. Patterson GA et al: Airway complications after double lung transplantation, *J Thorac Cardiovasc Surg* 1990;99:14.

35. Kaditis AG et al: Airway complications following pediatric lung and heart–lung transplantation, *Am J Respir Crit Care Med* 2000;162:301.

36. Trulock EP et al: The role of trans-bronchial lung biopsy in the treatment of lung transplant recipients: an analysis of 200 consecutive procedures, *Chest* 1992;102:1049.

37. Mauer JR et al: Infectious complications following isolated lung transplantation, *Chest* 1992;101:1056.

38. Nunley DR et al: Allograft colonization and infections with *Pseudomonas* in cystic fibrosis lung transplant recipients, *Chest* 1998;113:1235.

39. Chaparro C et al: Infection with *Burkholderia cepacia* in cystic fibrosis: outcome following lung transplantation, *Am J Respir Crit Care Med* 2001;163:43.

40. Snell GI et al: *Pseudomonas cepacia* in lung transplant recipients with cystic fibrosis, *Chest* 1993;103:466.

41. Cooper JD et al: A working formulation for the standardization of nomenclature and for clinical staging of chronic dysfunction in lung allografts: International Society for Heart and Lung Transplantation, *J Heart Lung Transplant* 1993;12:713.

42. Cohen AH et al: High incidence of posttransplant lymphoproliferative disease in pediatric patients with cystic fibrosis, *Am J Respir Crit Care Med* 2000;161:1252.

43. Kurland G, Orenstein DM: Lung transplantation and cystic fibrosis: the psychosocial toll, *Pediatrics* 2001;107:1419.

44. Craven JL, Bright J, Dear CL: Psychiatric, psychosocial and rehabilitative aspects of lung transplantation, *Clin Chest Med* 1990;11:247.

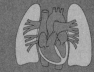

Chapter 26

Pediatric Advanced Life Support

PATRICE JOHNSON • KIM STEVENSON

OUTLINE

LEARNING OBJECTIVES

After reading this chapter you will be able to:
- Define respiratory distress, respiratory failure and respiratory arrest.
- Define shock and its correlation with respiratory failure.
- Identify the clinical findings consistent with respiratory compromise.
- List and describe the components of rapid cardio-pulmonary assessment.
- Describe the techniques utilized in the treatment of a patient in respiratory distress and respiratory failure.

This chapter emphasizes the recognition, based on clinical evaluation, of children at risk for respiratory failure. When a child presents with clinical signs of respiratory distress or failure and does not improve after initial life support interventions, more aggressive therapy should be considered. Respiratory distress and subsequent respiratory failure are the leading causes of arrest in children. The following recommendations are based on the American Heart Association and American Academy of Pediatrics—Pediatric Advanced Life Support Manual; 2006.

RESPIRATORY DISTRESS, RESPIRATORY FAILURE, AND RESPIRATORY ARREST

Pediatric cardiac arrests commonly involve progressive shock or respiratory failure rather than sudden collapse from an arrhythmia. The causes of cardiac arrest vary with the underlying health of the child, the age of the child, and where the event took place. Trauma, submersion, poisoning, choking, seizures, sudden infant death syndrome (SIDS), and pneumonia are a few out-of-hospital events.

In-hospital causes include respiratory failure, drug toxicity, sepsis, arrhythmias, and metabolic disorders.

Many conditions may cause respiratory distress. Typical characteristics of respiratory distress include: altered level of consciousness, tachypnea, hyperpnea, retractions, accessory muscle usage, central cyanosis, diaphoresis, nasal flaring, head bobbing, grunting, stridor, and periodic apnea. Tachycardia is a common response to many types of stress. Monitoring the changes in heart rate in response to therapy or an intervention is helpful. Recognizing respiratory distress and initiating supportive care based on clinical presentation are crucial to preventing further deterioration.

A clinical state of inadequate oxygenation, ventilation, or both is respiratory failure. Due to an increased metabolic rate, infants and children have higher oxygen demands than adults. Factors that may contribute to the progression of respiratory failure include neuromuscular disease, pulmonary disease, and an assortment of airway diseases or complications. Respiratory failure can also occur when there are no signs of respiratory distress (e.g., when a person is under sedation or anesthesia, or has suffered a closed head injury).

Respiratory failure requires immediate intervention for patient survival. Blood gas analysis is not required to identify potential respiratory failure, but may be used to confirm the clinical impression or to evaluate the child's response to therapy.

Respiratory arrest is the absence of breathing. Agonal respirations or gasping respirations should be treated as respiratory arrest.

Box 26-1	**Clinical Fndings Consistent With Respiratory Compromise**

Infants and children may exhibit one or more signs and symptoms leading to respiratory arrest. When any of the following is observed, rapid assessment is required to determine appropriate intervention.
- Nasal flaring
- Cyanosis
- Inspiratory retractions
- Diminished breath sounds
- Increased respiratory rate
- Decreased level of consciousness
- Increased depth of breathing
- Poor skeletal muscle tone
- Head-bobbing
- Inadequate respiratory rate, effort, or chest excursion
- Seesaw respirations
- Tachycardia
- Stridor
- Grunting

SHOCK AND THE RELATIONSHIP WITH RESPIRATORY FAILURE

Shock is characterized by inadequate tissue perfusion resulting in poor delivery of oxygen and metabolic substrates to the tissues. Infants and children have airway compromise more often than circulation compromise, and shock can occur with or without signs of cardiac distress. Oxygenation and ventilation are vital when attempting to restore perfusion in these patients.

The severity of shock is characterized as compensated or decompensated. Infants and children will attempt to maintain blood pressure by increasing heart rate, cardiac contractility, and peripheral vascular tone (compensated shock) until no longer physiologically possible (decompensated shock). Decompensated shock due to hemorrhage may not occur until a significant amount of blood volume is lost. Observing subtle changes in clinical signs is critical (Box 26-1). The combined effect of respiratory failure and shock will invariably lead to a state of cardiopulmonary failure preceding cardiac arrest.

RAPID CARDIOPULMONARY ASSESSMENT

Rapid cardiopulmonary assessment begins the minute you see the patient at the initial assessment. To avoid creating anxiety, the clinician can evaluate the patient from a short distance and without touching. Anxiety and agitation, which can increase with even the simplest physical examination, can alter the patient's baseline status and make treatment difficult or unsuccessful. The general appearance reflects the adequacy of oxygenation, ventilation, brain perfusion, and central nervous system function. The continual re-assessment will actually assess and treat the findings of your initial assessment. The initial assessment should take no longer than 60 seconds. If any of the abnormal findings listed in Table 26-1 are exhibited by the patient,

TABLE 26-1	
Normal and Abnormal Findings in Assessment of General Appearance	
Normal	**Abnormal**
Normal muscle tone	Agitation, irritability, inconsistent responsiveness, or rigid muscle tone
Patient responds to his/her own name	Patient does not recognize caregiver, family, or siblings
All extremities move equally	Limp or rigid extremities
Eyes are open	Hard to arouse, lethargic
Normal speech or cry	Inconsolable crying, hoarse cry or voice

immediate intervention may be required. The steps to rapid cardiopulmonary assessment are outlined in Table 26-2.

INITIAL ASSESSMENT OF APPEARANCE

During the initial assessment, the clinician should pause a short distance from the patient and using the senses of sight and hearing to determine if a life-threatening problem exists that requires immediate intervention. No equipment should be used (e.g., stethoscope, ECG monitor, pulse oximetry, blood pressure cuffs). The goal

is to determine quickly whether the child looks "sick" or "not sick." Remember that the patient's condition can change at any time.

These clinical assessment questions should be asked:
- Is the child moving, or is he or she limp, listless, or flaccid?
- Is the child alert and attentive to his or her surroundings, or uninterested?
- Can the child be comforted by the caregiver or health care professional?
- Does the child follow your movements or just stare?
- Can the child speak or cry? Is the cry strong or weak? Is the voice hoarse or weak?

TABLE 26-2

Steps to Rapid Cardiopulmonary Assessment

GENERAL APPEARANCE

Color	Level of Consciousness	Activity

Patient color is:
  Pale
  Pink
  Blue
  Gray
	Does the patient:
	  Respond to voice?
	  Respond to pain?
	  Appear responsive?
	  Recognize their parents?
		Does the patient:
		  Move all extremities?
		  Have normal muscle tone?

EXAMINATION OF AIRWAY, BREATHING, CIRCULATION

Airway	Breathing	Circulation

Is the airway:
 	
  Clear?
  Able to be maintained without assistance?
  Not able to be maintained without assistance?
	What is the respiratory rate?
	
	  Faster than normal for age
	  Slower than normal for age
	
	What is the patient's respiratory effort and mechanics?
	  Grunting
	  Nasal Flaring
	  Head bobbing
	  Stridor
	  Retractions
	  Abdominal breathing
	What is the air entry/tidal volume?
	
	  Adequate chest expansion
	  Symmetrical chest rise
	  Decreased chest expansion
	What are the breath sounds?
	  Equal
	  Normal
	  Rales
	  Rhonchi
	  Wheezes
	  Silent with no aeration
		Does the patient have a pulse? What is the pulse rate? Is the pulse rate:
		  Normal?
		  Decreased?
		  Increased?
		
		Is the pulse:
		
		  Strong?
		  Weak?
		
		Check the capillary refill. Is capillary refill:
		  < 2 seconds?
		  > 2 seconds?
		
		Are extremities cool to touch?
		  Yes, indicating deterioration in perfusion
		  No
		
		What is the blood pressure? Is it:
		  Low for patient age?
		  Normal for patient age?
		  Elevated for patient age?

INITIAL ASSESSMENT OF AIRWAY/BREATHING

You still have not touched the patient; your continued evaluation of the airway focuses on respiratory rate, breathing effort, audible airway sounds, body position, and visible movement of the chest and abdomen.

Tachypnea

Tachypnea is a rapid rate of breathing. A patient attempts to maintain a normal pH by increasing minute ventilation. Examples of nonpulmonary causes of tachypnea include metabolic acidosis associated with shock, diabetic ketoacidosis, some congenital cardiac abnormalities, metabolic abnormalities, salicylate poisoning, chronic diarrhea, or chronic renal insufficiency. A careful and complete history can be very useful when evaluating tachypnea. Normal breathing rates for infants 1 to 12 months of age range from 30 to 60 breaths per minute (bpm). Toddlers to preschool aged children breathe 20 to 40 bpm normally. School-aged to adolescent children breathe 12 to 30 bpm normally.

A slow or irregular respiratory rate (bradypnea) in an acutely ill infant or child can be threatening sign. Decreased respiratory rate or an irregular respiratory rhythm may indicate deterioration rather than improvement in the patient's clinical condition. The signs of increased breathing effort are described in Table 26-3. Abnormal audible airway sounds are listed in Table 26-4.

Body Position

Body position is a key indicator of respiratory distress. Abnormal body positions include sniffing position, tripod position, and infants with "head bobbing." In the sniffing position the child can sit upright, but will lean forward with the chin raised slightly. Children in the tripod position can sit upright but will want to lean forward usually supported by a bedside table or stack of pillows. Infants who "head bob" are in respiratory

TABLE 26-4

Audible Airway Sounds That Are Abnormal

Gasping	Inhaling and exhaling with quick, difficult breaths
Grunting	Short, low-pitched sound heard at the end of exhalation that represents an attempt to generate positive end expiratory pressure (PEEP) by exhaling against a closed glottis. A compensatory mechanism to help maintain patency of small airways and prevent atelectasis
Snoring	Noisy breathing through the mouth and nose during sleep
Stridor	Harsh, high-pitched sound heard on inspiration associated with upper airway obstruction; frequently described as a high-pitched sound or a cough that sounds like a seal-bark
Wheezing	High-pitched musical sounds produced by air moving through narrowed airway passages

From Aehlert B: PALS Pediatric Advanced Life Support study guide—revised, ed 2, St. Louis, 2007, Mosby.

distress and have an increased work of breathing. The head falls forward with each exhalation and comes up with inhalation.

Patients who present with any of the above body positions will usually have other signs of respiratory distress and increased work of breathing.

Visible Movement

Observing visible movement of the patient's chest and abdomen is important in evaluating the breathing effort. Increased breathing effort results from conditions that increase resistance to airflow or decrease lung compliance. Increased work of breathing often produces nasal flaring and intercostal, subcostal, and suprasternal inspiratory retractions. As work of breathing increases, cardiac output must increase to deliver blood to the respiratory muscles, which increases oxygen demand and produces more carbon dioxide that must be exhaled.

INITIAL ASSESSMENT OF CIRCULATION

The patient still has not been touched as the clinician continues to assess the patient's circulation. Assessment includes evaluation of cardiac output and perfusion of vital organs by evaluating the skin color. Skin color should appear normal for the patient's ethnic group. Skin that appears to be mottled, pallid, or cyanotic are abnormal findings.

TABLE 26-3

Normal and Abnormal Findings in Assessment of the Airway (Breathing Effort)

Normal	Abnormal
Quiet, non-labored respiration	Abnormal body position, sniffing, tripod, head bob, retractions, nasal, flaring, stridor, grunting, gasping, wheezing
Equal chest rise and fall	Accessory muscle tone
Normal respiratory rate	Respiratory rate outside of normal range

Box 26-2	"Hands On" Patient Assessment

Evaluate your patient's airway (should take less than 10 seconds)
- Patent airway?
- Can the patient handle his or her own secretions?
- Can the patient speak or make appropriate sounds for age?

Evaluate your patient's breathing and ventilation (should take less than 10 seconds)
- Awake, alert?
- Pulse oximetry greater than 95%?
- Skin color and temperature normal?
- Respirations spontaneous, unlabored, normal rate for age?
- Chest expansion bilaterally?
- Breath sounds present, clear, and equal bilaterally?

Evaluate your patient's cardiovascular function and tissue perfusion
- Awake and alert?
- Central and peripheral pulses strong and regular?
- Heart rate and blood pressure within normal ranges?
- Skin color normal? Warm and dry?
- Capillary refill less than 2 seconds?
- Any evidence of bleeding? History of trauma?

Completion of the initial assessment should take less then 60 seconds. In the "hands on" phase (Box 26-2), the clinician assesses the patient and treats problems when they are discovered.

Pulse Oximetry

Pulse oximetry should be used to monitor hemoglobin oxygen saturation if a patient is as risk for developing hypoxemia. Arterial blood gases should be analyzed if respiratory impairment (hypercarbia or acidosis) is suspected.

Capillary Refill

Capillary refill time must be evaluated. The ambient temperature should be considered when the patient's skin color and temperature are being evaluated. If the patient has good oxygenation and perfusion and is in a warm environment, skin color and temperature should be consistent over the trunk and extremities. Mucous membranes, nail beds, and the palms of the hands and soles of the feet will be pink if cardiorespiratory function is normal. As perfusion deteriorates, the hands and feet are typically affected first, becoming cool, pale, or dusky. As perfusion worsens, skin over the trunk or extremities may become mottled and cool to the touch. Central cyanosis may be apparent in a patient with hypoxemia, but this clinical sign is affected by several factors (e.g., anemia, polycythemia). Central cyanosis is most likely to occur when low arterial oxygen saturation is combined with low cardiac output.

Assessing the chest and abdomen for respiratory movement includes observing the depth and symmetry of movement with each breath. Determine the respiratory rate by counting the respirations for 30 to 60 seconds. Patients with breathing difficulty often have a respiratory rate outside the normal limits for their age.

Air Entry

Air entry assessment includes the evaluation of tidal volume (chest expansion) and auscultation of breath sounds. Chest expansion should be symmetric; this is true for a patient breathing spontaneously as well as for a patient who requires bag-valve-mask ventilation. Decreased chest expansion may result from inadequate effort and hypoventilation, airway obstruction, atelectasis, pneumothorax, hemothorax, pleural effusion, mucous plug, or foreign-body aspiration.

Listen for air movement not only over the chest but also over the nose and mouth. Stridor, wheezing, snoring, and grunting can be heard throughout the lungs and sometimes over the nose and mouth. Breath sounds should be heard bilaterally. Because the chest of a child is small and the chest wall is thin, breath sounds are easily transmitted from one side to the other. This means that pneumothorax, hemothorax, or atelectasis may not be heard even though it may exist.

Listen over the anterior, posterior, and lateral chest wall. Take a moment and listen to the heart as well.

Perform interventions as needed. These may include oxygen delivery, suctioning the upper airway, placing airway adjuncts, or providing positive pressure ventilation with a resuscitation bag and mask.

Systemic Perfusion

Systemic perfusion is best evaluated by noting the presence and volume of peripheral pulses and assessing end-organ perfusion and function.

Brain

After 2 months of age an infant should normally focus on the faces of his or her parents. Failure to recognize or make eye contact with parents may be an early, ominous sign of cortical hypoperfusion or cerebral dysfunction. Failure to respond to painful stimulus is also an ominous sign in a previously normal child. Parents may be the first to recognize these signs, but may be unable to describe them other than to say something is wrong.

Pulses

Carotid, axillary, brachial, radial, femoral, dorsalis pedis, and posterior tibial pulses should be readily palpable in healthy infants and children, although it may be difficult in obese infants or when the ambient temperature is low. The strength of the pulse is normally related to the stroke volume and pulse pressure (the difference between systolic and diastolic pressures). When cardiac output is low, systemic vascular resistance increases, and narrowing pulse pressure is the result.

Heart Rate

Normal heart rate values for infants and children are listed in Table 26-5. Tachycardia is a common response to many types of stress (e.g., pain, anxiety, hypoxia, fever, hypercapnia, hypovolemia, or cardiac impairment). The development of sinus tachycardia mandates evaluation to determine if it is a sign of shock.

Monitoring the change in heart rate in response to therapy or interventions may also be helpful. Improved detection of dehydration in patients can be obtained by evaluating multiple potential signs of poor perfusion and level of hydration (e.g., delayed capillary refill, dry mucous membranes, and ill general appearance in patients with dehydration).

A very rapid heart rate in infants and children may be caused by an underlying cardiac condition that produces supraventricular tachycardia, atrial flutter, or ventricular tachycardia. Regardless of the reason, a very rapid heart rate increases myocardial oxygen demand while simultaneously impairing myocardial oxygen delivery because the left ventricle is perfused during diastole and diastole is shortened with severe tachycardia. A very rapid rate may also impair diastolic filling of the atria and ventricles, leading to low stroke volume. These factors may lead to cardiogenic shock.

Blood Pressure

Blood pressure normal values for infants and children are listed in Table 26-6. Cardiac output and systemic vascular resistance determine mean blood pressure. When cardiac output falls, normal blood pressure can be maintained only if compensatory vasoconstriction

TABLE 26-6

Normal Blood Pressure in Children

Age	Systolic (mm Hg)	Diastolic (mm Hg)
Birth (12h, <1000g)	39–59	16–36
Birth (12 h, 3 kg)	50–70	25–45
Neonate (96h)	60–90	20–60
Infant (6 mos)	87–105	53–66
Toddler (2Yr)	95–105	53–66
School age (7y)	97–112	57–71
Adolescent (15y)	112–128	66–80

Data compiled from Versmold H, et al: Aortic blood pressure during the first 12 hours of life in infants with birth weight 610 to 4220g, *Pediatrics.*, 1981;67:107.; Horan MJ.: Task force on blood pressure control in children: report of the second task force on blood pressure in children., *Pediatrics* 1987;79:1. From the; Hazinski MF., Children are different. In: Hazinski MF, ed *Nursing care of the critically ill child*, ed 2, St Louis, 1992, Mosby Year Book.

occurs. Hypotension is a late and often sudden sign of cardiovascular decompensation. Even mild hypotension must be treated quickly and vigorously because it signals decompensation.

Skin

When the child is well perfused and the ambient temperature is warm, the hands and feet should be warm and dry and the palms pink to the distal phalanx. With decreases in cardiac output, the skin begins to cool in the fingers and toes and extends toward the trunk. Mottling, pallor, delayed capillary refill, and peripheral cyanosis often indicate poor skin perfusion. Acrocyanosis, on the other hand, may be normal in the newborn or polycythemic patient. Severe vasoconstriction produces a gray or ashen color in newborns and pallor in older children.

Kidneys

Urine output is directly proportional to renal blood flow and glomerular filtration rate. Normal urine output averages 1 to 2 ml/kg per hour in children. Urine output is a good indicator of renal function, but it may not be a good indicator of renal perfusion. An indwelling urinary catheter will facilitate accurate and continuous determination of urine flow.

Assessment and management of the seriously ill or injured child begins with rapid cardiopulmonary assessment. This assessment, which is the foundation of pediatric advanced life support, enables the caregiver to quickly identify potential or actual respiratory failure and shock and provide the appropriate interventions.

Priorities in management after rapid cardiopulmonary assessment not only include initial but continued reassessment. Laboratory studies such as pulse oximetry, arterial blood gas analysis, and chest x-ray may be

TABLE 26-5

Normal Heart Rates (Beats per Minute [bpm]) in Children

Age	Awake Rate	Mean	Sleeping Rate
Newborn to 3 mo	85–205	140	80–160
3 mo to 2 yr	100–190	130	75–160
2 yr to 10 yr	60–140	80	60–90
> 10 yr	60–100	75	50–90

From Gillette PC, Garson AJr, Porter CJ, et al.: Dysrhythmias. In: Adams FG, Emmanouilides GC, Reimenschenider TA, eds., *Moss' heart disease in infants, children and adolescents*, 4th ed. Baltimore, Md: Williams and Wilkins; 1989:l 725–741.

useful. Administering supplemental oxygen, in a non-threatening manner whenever possible, should be an initial consideration for treatment of respiratory distress or shock.

When treating respiratory distress, the caregiver should support of the airway in the neutral position for infants and allow the older patient to assume a position of maximal comfort to minimize work of breathing and airway patency. Maintaining the patient's normal ambient and body temperature and withholding any oral intake is recommended if there is any concern that the patient's condition may deteriorate and invasive interventions be needed.

If signs of respiratory failure are present, establish a patient airway and ensure adequate ventilation with maximum supplemental oxygen. When signs of shock are present, establish vascular access rapidly and provide volume expansion and medications as needed. When cardiopulmonary failure is detected, give initial priority to ventilation and oxygenation (Figure 26-1).

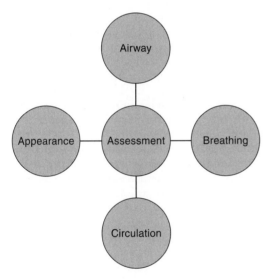

FIGURE 26–1 Rapid cardiopulmonary assessment includes evaluation of patient appearance, airway, breathing, and circulation.

CLINICAL SCENARIOS

Case 1

An anxious seven-year-old girl was well until a few days ago, when she developed fever, cough, and mild shortness of breath. She is wheezing and having difficulty breathing. She is sitting upright, working moderately to breathe, with frequent episodes of tight, nonproductive-sounding cough. Her color is pale with a slight bluish tone to lips and nail beds.

As you begin your rapid assessment, remember to start with what you observe as you walk through the door.
1. What is this patient's general appearance?
2. What are you able to assess about this patient's level of responsiveness?

You note she has moderate suprasternal and intercostal retractions, with a prolonged expiratory phase. Her respiratory rate is 54 bpm. Her breath sounds are symmetric with fair distal air entry and faint scattered expiratory wheezes. She is able to speak only 2 to 3 words at a time. Placement of a pulse oximeter reveals a room air saturation of 88%.
3. What specific characteristics of respiratory distress are identified?
4. At this point what actions would you take in the care of this patient?

During the delivery of inhaled beta-agonist with oxygen at 8 liters per minute the patient's pulse oximetry reading increases to 92%. You note that her radial pulse disappears and reappears in a somewhat rhythmic manner every few heart beats. Her heart rate is 150 beat per minute, her skin is cool when touched, capillary refill 4 seconds. Her blood pressure is not obtainable with a blood pressure monitor, but the RN is able to palpate a systolic blood pressure of 100 mmHg.
5. What specific characteristics are beneficial in assessing this patient's cardiovascular system?
6. Are these characteristics normal or abnormal?

Following the delivery of an inhaled beta-agonist a reassessment of the patient airway and breathing reveal no improvement, a 100% non-rebreather mask is placed and the pulse oximeter reads 88%. She has increased suprasternal and intercostal retractions, and her expiratory phase remains prolonged. Her respiratory rate is 60 bpm. She is very sleepy and hard to arouse. Her heart rate has increased on the monitor to 170 beats per minute.
7. Based on the clinical signs and symptoms, could this patient be categorized as being in respiratory distress or respiratory failure? What are the clinical signs and symptoms to support your decision?
8. If respiratory failure is evident, what preparation is needed for increased support of this patient?

The patient is positioned with an open airway and bag valve mask is implemented to assist the patient, who is now breathing at a rate of 25 bpm. There is extreme difficulty in assisting ventilation of this patient. The patient is unresponsive with agonal (breathing effort with no air movement) respirations. The stomach of the patient is noted to be overdistended.
9. What changes in airway support could be considered that may cause less abdominal distention and offer better air exchange?

Cricoid pressure is maintained during two-person bag-mask ventilation. Breath sounds are equal bilaterally,

Continued

Case 1—cont'd

with symmetrical chest rise and fall. The patient remains unresponsive, and vascular access is obtained. The equipment is obtained for intubation and placement of a 5.5 mm ID uncuffed endotracheal tube is completed.

10. What primary assessments should be made to determine correct endotracheal tube placement?

The tube is secured, and the oxygen saturation increases to 96% of 10-cm H_2O of PEEP. Her heart rate has improved and now is 130 beats per minute. A chest radiograph is obtained to confirm tube placement. After the x-ray plate is removed, the oxygen saturation alarm sounds and reads 80%; the heart monitor shows a heart rate of 80 beats per minute.

11. Your immediate assessment of the patient would include?
12. What could be the cause of this decompensation?

The tube was noted to have been pushed in too far. The tube is adjusted and resecured and heart rate and pulse oximetry return to 130 beats per minute and 96%. Breath sounds are equal bilaterally, with symmetrical chest rise. The patient continues to have bilaterally expiratory wheezes and will receive intermittent pharmacologic beta-agonist administration.

Case 2

A 6 month old presents with a history of fever and cough for the past 3 days. The baby is asleep; respirations are shallow and rapid. Intercostals and subcostal retractions with grunting respirations are present. Color is pale, with circumoral cyanosis. Patient is resting in parents' arms, but arouses with intervention.

1. What is your observation of this patient's general appearance?
2. What are you able to assess about this patient's level of responsiveness and activity?

The patient is placed on a cardiorespiratory monitor. Heart rate is 136 bpm, and respiratory rate is 45bpm. A pulse oximeter is placed and the room air saturation is 82%. The nurse has obtained a blood pressure of 110/60 and a temperature of 103.3° F.

3. At this point what actions would you take in the care of this patient?

The patient becomes agitated with the placement of oxygen. The pulse oximeter reads 90% on a simple face mask running at 10 Lpm. The breath sounds are diminished bilaterally, with crackles over the right posterior lung field. Retractions increase and the baby has pronounced grunting. Over the next few minutes the baby becomes less responsive and the pulse oximeter reads 85%. With a heart rate of 165 bpm and respiratory rate 60 breaths/min.

4. What clinical signs and symptoms indicate this patient is decompensating?

5. What preparation is needed for increased support of this patient?
6. Describe what equipment will be necessary for intubation

The patient has now been receiving manual ventilation using a resuscitator bag and mask for 10 minutes. The baby is unconscious, allowing you to breathe for him/her. The infant is without any sign of respiration. The cardiorespiratory monitor reads a heart rate of 150 and breathing at 25 bpm. You note the chest rises and falls symmetrically, and on auscultation the breath sounds are still diminished with crackles over the right. Due to the level of consciousness and decrease in respiratory drive, intubation will be necessary. Cricoid pressure is maintained during bag-mask ventilation. Vascular access is obtained. The physician prepares the equipment for intubation and selects a 4.5 mm cuffed endotracheal tube.

7. What signs and symptoms would indicate that intubation of this patient is necessary?
8. Would this endotracheal tube be the appropriate size for this patient?

The physician attempts to place a 4.0 mm endotracheal tube after 30 seconds the heart monitor alarms when the heart rate reaches 60 bpm. The saturation monitor is alarming at 75%. The physician continues to attempt visualization.

9. Describe what is causing the intolerance of this intubation procedure and what should be done to stabilize this patient.

The patient is ventilated with 100% oxygen until a heart rate of 120 bpm is obtained. The physician places a 3.5 mm endotracheal tube without complications.

10. What primary assessments should be made to determine correct endotracheal tube placement?

The patient is bagged and an end tidal carbon dioxide detector is placed. The detector display shows a tan color and a "snoring" sound is produced when the resuscitation bag is squeezed. Chest expansion with ventilation is minimal. Oxygen saturation is 92%.

11. What troubleshooting is necessary to improve the ventilation and oxygenation of this patient?

With the pop-off valve engaged, the oxygen saturation is now 96%, chest rise is adequate, but a "snoring" upper airway noise continues to be heard with every inflation. Chest rise is symmetrical with equal breath sounds bilaterally. Chest radiograph indicates good endotracheal tube placement. There is also a consolidation in the right middle and right lower lobe. The "snoring" sounds heard from the upper airway are from a tracheal tube that is too small, producing an air leak.

ASSESSMENT QUESTIONS

See Evolve Resources for answers.

1. Which of the following is more likely to occur in the pediatric population?
   A. Cardiac arrest
   B. Respiratory arrest
   C. Cor pulmonale
   D. Pulmonary thromboembolism
2. Respiratory distress is characterized by which of the following?
   A. Retractions
   B. Tachypnea
   C. Accessory muscle use
   D. All of the above
3. Which of the following best defines respiratory failure?
   A. Inadequate tissue perfusion
   B. Tachypnea and hypertension
   C. Inadequate oxygenation or ventilation or both
   D. The absence of breathing
4. Which of the following is one of the first assessments during the initial assessment of an infant or child?
   A. Determine heart rate and blood pressure to see if they are in compensated or decompensated shock.
   B. Determine the strength of peripheral pulses to see if shock of any kind is present.
   C. Evaluate arterial blood gases to determine the need for intubation.
   D. From a distance assess the airway and breathing by counting respiratory rate, evaluating breathing effort, and noting the color of the skin.
5. Which of the following is the most appropriate initial intervention for a child in mild respiratory distress?
   A. Immediate tracheal intubation
   B. Evaluation of oxyhemoglobin saturation with pulse oximetry and analysis of an arterial blood gas
   C. Administration of humidified supplemental oxygen and continued evaluation
   D. Chest radiograph
6. An intubated patient is transferred to a hospital bed from a stretcher. You note a loud noise coming from the upper airway when the resuscitator bag is squeezed. The pulse oximeter alarm has sounded and it is noted to read 75%. Which of the following is the most likely cause of this deterioration?
   A. Displaced tube
   B. Obstructed tube
   C. Pneumothorax
   D. Disconnection from oxygen

ASSESSMENT QUESTIONS—cont'd

7. Which of the following is an early sign of impending respiratory difficulty?
   A. Increased heart rate
   B. A decrease in blood pressure
   C. An increase in respiratory rate
   D. A decrease in capillary refill
8. Which of the below assessments would be found in the evaluation of the appearance of an infant or child?
   A. Skin color and tone
   B. Audible airway sounds
   C. Shallow respirations
   D. Awake, but limp
9. Select the incorrect statement regarding the correct findings of a correctly placed endotracheal tube.
   A. Gurgling sounds during auscultation
   B. Symmetrical chest rise and fall
   C. Equal bilateral breath sounds
   D. Absent breath sounds over the abdomen
10. A cause of deterioration of the intubated patient includes which of the following:
    A. Correct-sized endotracheal tube with no airway leak
    B. Breath sounds heard over the right chest but not the left
    C. Bag-valve mask ventilation with 100% oxygen
    D. Chest radiograph confirming endotracheal tube adequate placement.

Bibliography

American Heart Association: A reappraisal of mouth-to-mouth ventilation during bystander-initiated cardiopulmonary resuscitation. A statement for healthcare professionals from the Ventilation Working Group of the Basic Life Support and Pediatric Life Support Subcommittees, American Heart Association. *Circulation* 1997; 96(6):2102-2112.

Babbs CF et al: CPR with simultaneous compression and ventilation at high airway pressure in 4 animal models. *Crit Care Med* 1982; 10:501-504.

Berg RA et al: A randomized, blinded trial of high-dose epinephrine versus standard-dose epinephrine in a swine model of pediatric asphyxial cardiac arrest. *Crit Care Med* 1996; 24(10):1695-1700.

Cavallaro DL, Melker RJ: Comparison of two techniques for detecting cardiac activity in infants. *Crit Care Med* 1983; 11:189-190.

Centers for Disease Control, Division of Injury Control, Center for Environmental Health and Injury Control: Childhood injuries in the United States. *Am J Dis Child* 1990; 144:627-646.

Centers for Disease Control: Guidelines for prevention of transmission of human immunodeficiency virus and hepatitis B virus to health care and public safety workers. *MMWR* 1989; 38(6, suppl):1-37.

Eisenberg M, Bergner L, Hallstrom A: Epidemiology of cardiac arrest and resuscitation in children. *Ann Emerg Med* 1983; 12:672-674.

Eisenberg M, Bergner L, Hallstrom A: Epidemiology of cardiac arrest and resuscitation in children. *Ann Emerg Med* 1983; 12:672-674.

Finer NN et al: Limitations of self-inflating resuscitators. *Pediatrics* 1986; 77:417-420.

Flesche CW et al: The ability of health professionals to check the carotid pulse. *Circulation* 1994 (abstract); 90(suppl):1-288.

Frei FJ et al: Respiratory and circulatory arrest in pediatric patients. *Acta Anaesth Scand Suppl* 1997; 111:200-201.

Frishman WH, Vahdat S, Bhatta S: Innovative pharmacologic approaches to cardiopulmonary resuscitation. *J Clin Pharmacol* 1998; 38:765-772.

Gelband H, Rosen M: Pharmacologic basis for treatment of cardiac arrhythmias. *Pediatrics* 1975; 55:59-67.

Gillis J et al: Results of inpatient pediatric resuscitation. *Crit Care Med* 1986; 14:469-471.

Goetting MG, Paradis NA: High-dose epinephrine improves outcome from pediatric cardiac arrest. *Ann Emerg Med* 1991; 20:22-26.

Gutgesell HP et al: Energy dose for ventricular defibrillation of children. *Pediatrics* 1976; 58:898-901.

Hazinski MF: Basic life support: controversial and unresolved issues. *J Cardiovasc Nurs* 1996; 10(4):1-14.

Horowitz BZ, Matheny L: Health care professionals' willingness to do mouth-to-mouth resuscitation. *West J Med* 1997; 167:392-397.

International Consensus on Science: Guidelines 2000 for cardiopulmonary resuscitation and emergency cardiovascular care. *Circulation* 2000; 102(suppl I):1-384.

Lee CJ, Bullock LJ: Determining pulse for infant CPR: time for a change? *Milit Med* 1991; 156:190-191.

Lewis JK et al: Outcome of pediatric resuscitation. *Ann Emerg Med* 1983; 12:297-299.

Losek JD et al: Prehospital countershock treatment of pediatric asystole. *Am J Emerg Med* 1989; 7:571-575.

Ochoa FJ et al: The effect of rescuer fatigue on the quality of chest compressions. *Resuscitation* 1998; 37:149-152.

O'Rourke PP: Outcome of children who are apneic and pulseless in the emergency room. *Crit Care Med* 1986; 14:466-468.

Otto CW, Yakaitis RW, Blitt CS: Mechanism of action of epinephrine in resuscitation from asphyxial arrest. *Crit Care Med* 1981; 9:321-324.

Overholt ED et al: Usefulness of adenosine for arrhythmias in infants and children. *Am J Cardiol* 1988; 61:336-340.

Ronco R et al: Outcome and cost at a children's hospital following resuscitation for out-of-hospital cardiopulmonary arrest. *Arch Pediatr Adolesc Med* 1995; 149(2):210-214.

Sande MA: Transmissions of AIDS: the case against causal contagion. *N Engl J Med* 1986; 314:380-382.

Sanders A, Ewy G, Taft T: Prognostic and therapeutic importance of the aortic diastolic pressure in resuscitation from cardiac arrest. *Crit Care Med* 1984; 12:871-878.

Stokke DB et al: Acid-base interactions with noradrenaline-induced contractile response of the rabbit isolated aorta. *Anesthesia* 1984; 60:400-404.

Thrush DN, Downs JB, Smith RA: Is epinephrine contraindicated during cardiopulmonary resuscitation? *Circulation* 1997; 96(8):2709-2714.

Till J et al: Efficacy and safety of adenosine in the treatment of supraventricular tachycardia in infants and children. *Br Heart J* 1989; 62:204-211.

Torphy DE, Minter MG, Thompson BM: Cardiorespiratory arrest and resuscitation of children. *Am J Dis Child* 1984; 138:1099-1102.

Torres A et al: Long-term functional outcome of inpatient pediatric cardiopulmonary resuscitation. *Pediatr Emerg Care* 1997; 13(6):369-373.

Ushay HM, Notterman DA: Pharmacology of pediatric resuscitation. *Pediatr Clin North Am* 1997; 44(1):207-233.

Walsh CK, Krongrad E: Terminal cardiac electrical activity in pediatric patients. *Am J Cardiol* 1983; 51:557-561.

Weisfeldt ML: Recent advances in cardiopulmonary resuscitation. *Jpn Circ J* 1985; 49:13-24.

Wenzel V et al: Influence of tidal volume on the distribution of gas between the lungs and stomach in the nonintubated patient receiving positive-pressure ventilation. *Crit Care Med* 1998; 26(2):364-368.

Zaritsky A et al: CPR in children. *Ann Emerg Med* 1987; 16:1107-1111.

Zaritsky A, Chernow B: Use of catecholamines in pediatrics. *J Pediatr* 1984; 105:341-350.

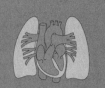

Chapter **27**

Neonatal Pulmonary Disorders

THOMAS L. MILLER • THOMAS H. SHAFFER • JAY S. GREENSPAN

OUTLINE

LEARNING OBJECTIVES

After reading this chapter the reader will be able to:
• Identify common pulmonary disorders in infants
• Describe the pathophysiology underlying common
  infant pulmonary complications

• Recognize and differentiate the causes of neonatal
  respiratory distress
• Choose treatment options for various forms of
  neonatal pulmonary disorders

Most infants are admitted to a neonatal intensive care unit because of respiratory distress.[1] The more premature the neonate is, the more likely that respiratory complications will exist at presentation. However, term and post-term infants can also experience respiratory difficulty resulting from pulmonary as well as nonpulmonary conditions (Table 27-1). Whatever the cause, disorders that result in respiratory distress remain a major reason for morbidity and mortality in the neonate. The more common neonatal pulmonary disorders are addressed in this chapter.

RESPIRATORY DISTRESS SYNDROME

First described in 1903, respiratory distress syndrome (RDS) usually affects premature infants with inadequate lung development. RDS is diagnosed in 60% of infants born at less than 28 weeks' gestation, and occurs in 10% of all preterm infants.[2] According to the most recent data from the American Lung Association, approximately 24,000 infants are born with RDS each year.[2] Despite advances in neonatal care, the mortality rate for infants with RDS is still between 5% to 10%, making RDS the fifth-leading cause of death for infants under 1 year of age.[2,3] There is a higher incidence of RDS, with a greater clinical impact, in infants with very low birth weights. It is most often associated with infants born at less than 37 weeks' gestation, in infants of diabetic mothers, in multiple births, when cesarean section is performed before the onset of labor, in asphyxia, in cold stress, and in infants of mothers who have previously had infants with RDS.[4-7]

TABLE 27-1

Clues to Diagnosis of Types of Respiratory Distress

Information From Maternal History	Most Probable Condition in Infant
Peripartum fever	Pneumonia
Foul-smelling amniotic fluid	Pneumonia
Excessive obstetric manipulation at delivery	Pneumonia
Infection	Pneumonia
Premature rupture of membranes	Pneumonia
Prolonged labor	Pneumonia
Prematurity	Hyaline membrane disease (RDS)
Diabetes	Hyaline membrane disease
Hemorrhage in days before delivery	Hyaline membrane disease
Meconium-stained amniotic fluid	Meconium aspiration syndrome
Hydramnios	Tracheoesophageal fistula
Excessive medications	Central nervous system depression
Reserpine	Stuffy nose
Traumatic or breech delivery	Central nervous system hemorrhage; phrenic nerve paralysis
Fetal tachycardia or bradycardia	Asphyxia
Prolapsed cord or entanglements	Asphyxia
Postmaturity	Asphyxia
Amniotic fluid loss	Hypoplastic lungs

Signs in the Infant	Most Probable Condition
Single umbilical artery	Congenital anomalies
Other congenital anomalies	Associated cardiopulmonary anomalies
Situs inversus	Kartagener's syndrome
Scaphoid abdomen	Diaphragmatic hernia
Erb's palsy	Phrenic nerve palsy
Cannot breathe with mouth closed	Choanal atresia; stuffy nose
Gasping with little air exchange	Upper airway obstruction
Overdistention of lungs	Aspiration, lobar emphysema, or pneumothorax
Shift of apical pulse	Pneumothorax, chylothorax, hypoplastic lung
Fever or rise in temperature in a constant-temperature environment	Pneumonia
Shrill cry, hypertonia, or flaccidity	Central nervous system disorder
Atonia	Trauma, myasthenia, poliomyelitis, amyotonia
Frothy blood from larynx	Pulmonary hemorrhage
Head extended in the absence of neurologic findings	Tracheoesophageal fistula or pharyngeal incoordination
Plethora	Transient tachypnea

From Avery ME, Fletcher BD, Williams RG: *The lung and its disorders in the newborn infant,* Philadelphia, 1981, WB Saunders.

Etiology and Pathophysiology

In 1959, Avery and Mead reported that RDS was associated with a deficiency of pulmonary surfactant and abnormal lung surface tension properties.[8] Since that time, it has been widely accepted that the pathophysiology of RDS is the result of an insufficient amount of surfactant as well as immature cell and vascular development of the lungs.[9,10]

At approximately 16 weeks of gestation, the alveolar type II cells synthesize and store surfactant. Increasing amounts are produced as the fetus approaches term. Between the 28th and 38th weeks of gestation, surfactant is secreted into the alveoli and eventually migrates into the amniotic fluid through the trachea. With its release into the alveoli, surfactant reduces the surface tension and helps to maintain alveolar stability when the lung transitions to a gas filled organ at birth[11-13] (see Chapters 1 and 16). Primitive alveoli form between the 27th and 35th weeks of gestation, with true alveoli forming between the 30th and 36th weeks of gestation.[14,15] Infants born before 28 weeks' gestation have structural underdevelopment of the terminal air spaces with little or no surfactant, leading to a susceptibility to RDS.

Deficient surfactant production or deficient release of surfactant into the immature respiratory alveoli results in an increase in surface forces and lung elastic recoil. Coupled with the extremely compliant chest wall of the preterm infant, this leads to reduced alveolar recruitment (known as atelectasis). This condition is characterized by decreased functional residual capacity (FRC), decreased pulmonary compliance, increased pulmonary resistance, and ventilation-perfusion mismatch.[16] The resulting hypoxia, hypercarbia, and respiratory acidosis constrict the pulmonary arteries and reduce pulmonary blood flow. This results in damage to the cells lining the alveoli.[17] The pulmonary hypertension can lead to increased right-to-left shunting through a patent ductus arteriosus (PDA) and the foramen ovale (extrapulmonary), as well as within the lung itself (intrapulmonary).[18] The shunting of blood results in greater hypoxemia and possibly metabolic acidosis, which increases the pulmonary vascular resistance (PVR) even more. This vicious cycle continues and may even lead to further suppression of surfactant synthesis.

Other pathophysiologic processes contribute to the clinical picture. They include poor gas exchange secondary to inadequate surface area, a compliant chest wall that reduces effectiveness of ventilation, a thickened alveolar-capillary membrane and insufficient vascularization, and poor clearance of lung fluid that can result in pulmonary edema.[19]

Within 2 days of birth immature lungs progress with alveolarization, where true alveoli and an increased number of capillaries continue to develop. If lung damage does not occur, the signs and symptoms of respiratory distress should subside. However, often the therapies needed to treat RDS, such as mechanical ventilation, prolong the symptoms and ultimately alter lung development.[20-22]

Chronic stress seems to protect infants at risk for the development of RDS. Conditions associated with chronic stress include maternal heroin addiction, which is thought to induce surfactant synthesis, and maternal toxemia. Premature rupture of membranes (PROM) for a duration of more than 24 hours preceding birth may also reduce the incidence of RDS.[4]

Disease Progression

In milder cases, the signs and symptoms reach a peak within 72 hours, followed by gradual improvement. Spontaneous diuresis and an increased ability to oxygenate the infant are the first signs of improvement. Severely affected infants may die, usually between days 2 and 7, with death most often associated with pulmonary interstitial emphysema, pneumothorax, or intraventricular hemorrhage (IVH). Surfactant and early use of nasal continuous positive airway pressure (NCPAP) have altered the classic presentation of the progression of RDS. Rapid weaning of ventilator settings and stabilization with low F_{IO_2} can be observed in a matter of hours. Extremely premature infants (23 to 25 weeks' gestation) may have an initial "honeymoon" period in which the patient has stable ventilator settings but will exhibit increased oxygen and ventilator demands as time progresses. These extremely low–birth-weight infants not only have immature lungs but their extreme prematurity also presents challenges because metabolic and cardiac functions are affected.

Larger Infants With Respiratory Distress Syndrome

One group of patients commonly overlooked are the term or near-term infants in whom RDS develops. These infants are typically 34 to 37 weeks' gestational age and are born to diabetic mothers or to mothers with a history of late-gestational infants with RDS. Because of their strength and pulmonary reserve, they may be able to cope with RDS for a longer period; however, they will demonstrate increasing oxygen demands requiring an F_{IO_2} greater than 0.6. These infants often have borderline hypovolemia, low blood pressure, poor oxygenation, and persistent metabolic acidosis. If the condition remains unrecognized, they often experience a sudden, and at times catastrophic, deterioration requiring maximum support before stabilization occurs. It often takes more than 12 hours of mechanical ventilation with high F_{IO_2} levels before ABG values begin to improve.[23]

Complications

The clinical outcome in preterm infants surviving RDS is often associated with chronic lung disease in the form of bronchopulmonary dysplasia (BPD), reactive airway disease, and an increase in and vulnerability to respiratory disorders.[24] Frequently pulmonary function testing demonstrates increased pulmonary resistance and work of breathing as well as decreased lung compliance and a tendency toward oxygen desaturation.[25,26] Other complications encountered include IVH, retinopathy of prematurity, infection, air leaks, and necrotizing enterocolitis (NEC). Current research is focusing on the inflammatory mediators and tissue modeling pathways that link RDS and the management of RDS to the chronic pathologies in an ongoing effort to improve the outcome of these patients.[20,21,27]

Clinical Presentation

The clinical features of RDS include a manifestation of the surfactant deficiency and a highly compliant chest wall. Infants with RDS are usually preterm and exhibit tachypnea or labored breathing, or both, beginning at or immediately after birth. A decrease in the respiratory rate may indicate impending respiratory failure. A characteristic grunt during expiration (which is an attempt to maintain the FRC) and nasal flaring are also present.[28] Intercostal and subcostal retractions are apparent and occur when the negative intrathoracic inspiratory pressures distort the chest wall instead of inflating the stiff lungs.[16] The retractions may have a "seesaw" appearance, with the abdomen protruding as the chest pulls in. Infants frequently look distressed, and the very premature infant may be hypotonic and unresponsive. Chest auscultation reveals diminished air in the alveoli in spite of the increased work of breathing.

Without stabilization of the alveoli, infants with RDS have increasing cyanosis that is relatively unresponsive to oxygen therapy. Larger infants may need minimal oxygen initially but require more as atelectasis becomes progressively worse. Some may have decreased oxygen requirements as acidosis and hypothermia (a result of delivery) are corrected but then have an increased need after 3 to 6 hours of life.

Arterial blood gas (ABG) analysis reveals moderate to severe hypoxemia, varying degrees of hypercarbia, and mixed acidosis (owing to respiratory failure and lactic acid accumulation). The $PaCO_2$ may initially be normal or low, but as the work of breathing increases and the infant begins to fail, there is resulting hypercarbia.

The chest radiograph typically reveals diffuse, fine, granular (reticulogranular) densities, which give a ground-glass appearance. The heart may be slightly enlarged, and the thymus is nearly always present radiographically. The appearance of the chest radiograph in RDS can be described as stages representing increasing severity of the disease. Stage I is described as a fine, diffuse reticulogranular pattern over the lung fields. Stage II reveals a denser lung, with the presence of air bronchograms within the heart border. Stage III shows increased density and the presence of air bronchograms beyond the heart border. Stage IV, termed "white out," describes the radiograph of the infant with severe disease complicated by pulmonary edema.[29] The view of the heart border and edge of the diaphragm may be obliterated in this stage. The disease may progress from one stage to the next, but the severity of the disease is initially described as the stage of RDS on the first chest film.[30]

Diagnosis and Treatment

Diagnosis is based on the history, clinical assessment, chest radiograph, and laboratory evaluation. Acute respiratory distress in the newborn is fairly common and may be caused by a multitude of pathophysiologic conditions. Box 27-1 lists some of the more common neonatal problems that may present as respiratory distress.

Box 27-1   Neonatal Disorders That May Present as Respiratory Distress

AIRWAY DISORDERS
- Pneumonia
- Pulmonary hypoplasia
- Air leaks
- Pulmonary edema
- Pulmonary hemorrhage
- Pleural effusion
- Vascular ring
- Choanal atresia
- Macroglossia
- Micrognathia
- Cysts and tumors
- Laryngomalacia-atresia
- Tracheomalacia-atresia
- Tracheoesophageal fistula
- Wilson-Mikity syndrome
- Respiratory distress syndrome
- Meconium aspiration syndrome
- Transient tachypnea of the newborn

THORACIC DISORDERS
- Thoracic dystrophy
- Osteogenesis imperfecta
- Cysts and tumors

DIAPHRAGM DISORDERS
- Diaphragmatic hernia
- Phrenic nerve paralysis
- Eventration

CARDIOVASCULAR DISORDERS
- Persistent pulmonary hypertension
- Congenital heart disease

Infants at risk for RDS may be identified by several laboratory tests that have been developed to estimate lung maturity. Lung maturity may be determined by assessing the amniotic fluid lecithin-to-sphingomyelin (L:S) ratio. Lecithin, also known as dipalmitoyl phosphatidylcholine, is the most abundant phospholipid found in surfactant. When the lung is mature, there is twice as much lecithin as sphingomyelin. Thus an L:S ratio of more than 2:1 is considered evidence of lung maturity. Nearly 100% of the infants with an L:S ratio less than 1:1 tend to acquire RDS, whereas those with a ratio greater than 2:1 do not. The L:S ratio is unreliable in pregnancies characterized by diabetes and Rh isoimmunization.[30,31] Levels of phosphatidylglycerol (PG), the second-most abundant phospholipid in surfactant, increase toward term. The presence of PG in amniotic fluid indicates a low risk for RDS. A patient with an L:S ratio less than 2:1 and a lack of PG has more than an 80% risk for the development of RDS. However, with the presence of PG and an L:S ratio greater than 2:1, the risk drops to nearly 0%.[4,32] In the foam stability test, amniotic fluid is mixed with different volumes of 95% ethanol. When this mixture is shaken with air, a foam develops that can be seen for several hours at room temperature. If no surfactant is present, the foam will not appear or will appear only briefly, indicating the strong possibility of immature lungs. The shake test is not as specific as a low L:S ratio.[33]

Prevention

Because RDS is associated with incomplete development of the lung at birth, the first line of treatment is prevention. If predictive tests indicate that the infant is at high risk for the development of RDS, elective cesarean section should not be performed. Premature delivery should be delayed, when possible, and glucocorticoids given for at least 2 days before delivery.[34] Antenatal corticosteroid therapy may accelerate lung development and promote pulmonary surfactant secretion.

Surfactant Replacement

Prophylactic and therapeutic surfactant replacement therapy has been shown to reduce morbidity and mortality in infants with RDS (see Chapter 16). Although studies have not found that it decreases the incidence of BPD in RDS survivors, it does seem to reduce the severity of the chronic condition.[35,36] Combining therapy with administering antenatal corticosteroids and surfactant has been shown to reduce the time of mechanical ventilation. This improves survival and neurodevelopment outcome in those preterm infants who require mechanical ventilation.[37]

Oxygen Therapy

Treatment of the infant with RDS entails providing adequate oxygenation, preventing atelectasis, and reducing the risk of complications. Oxygen therapy begins with delivery of oxygen via an oxygen hood in an attempt to maintain the PaO_2 between 50 and 80 mm Hg. The FIO_2 may be increased in increments of 0.10 and oxygenation assessed by means of either ABG analysis or pulse oximetry until the appropriate oxygen level is obtained. Use of the oxygen hood as an initial therapy for mild respiratory distress symptoms should be reserved for those larger infants who require above ambient FIO_2. When applying oxygen therapy, care should be taken to minimize the FIO_2 to no more than necessary. Recent evidence has reinforced the potential for oxygen to contribute to lung damage and lead to BPD.[38]

Continuous Positive Airway Pressure

If oxygenation fails to improve with the oxygen hood, continuous positive airway pressure via nasal prongs may be instituted (NCPAP; see Chapter 20). A CPAP of 4 to 6 cm H_2O is the usual starting point in these infants. In infants weighing more than 1500 g, CPAP levels of 7 to 8 cm H_2O may be needed. As CPAP levels are increased, or when pulmonary compliance improves, alveoli may become overdistended, with impairment of ventilation and pulmonary circulation. Continuous pulse oximetry is imperative to wean oxygen and CPAP to minimally acceptable levels. Frequent ABG analysis should be provided for early detection of respiratory failure.

Early NCPAP in the moderately preterm newborn of 28 to 32 weeks' gestation can reduce the need for intubation.[39,40] Stabilization of the alveoli in this gestational age may allow surfactant production to occur without further intervention. During this time, if the infant requires an FIO_2 of more than 0.40 on NCPAP, it is an indication for intubation and exogenous surfactant treatment. Early intubation and prophylactic administration of surfactant with subsequent extubation within 10 minutes of administration of NCPAP may be effective in reducing the need for prolonged intubation and mechanical ventilation.[41,42] Treatment of the very low–birth-weight infant is often more assertive. In many patient care protocols, management of the newborn younger than 28 weeks' gestation can begin with intubation and prophylactic use of surfactant. Moderately aggressive treatment with these smaller infants can improve clinical outcome in the form of lower risk of pneumothorax, pulmonary interstitial emphysema, and mortality[43] (see Chapter 16).

Mechanical Ventilation

Classic indications for endotracheal intubation and mechanical ventilation occur if the infant requires greater than 80% oxygen with a CPAP of 8 cm H_2O, if there is increasing hypercarbia with respiratory acidosis, or if apneic episodes become prolonged. Some patient care protocols are less tolerant, with intubation, surfactant, and subsequent ventilation occurring at a much lower threshold. In the very low–birth-weight infant (<1000 g), intubation and positive-pressure ventilation may be necessary immediately after birth while the infant is still in the delivery room. Intubation may also be indicated in larger infants with severe respiratory distress or asphyxia. Generally, once the infant is stabilized and in the intensive care unit, a pressure-limited ventilator utilizing a sinusoidal flow pattern is used. Peak inspiratory pressures (PIPs) generally begin at 15 to 25 cm H_2O, depending on the size of the infant and the severity of the disease, to establish a tidal volume between 3 and 5 ml/kg. Positive end-expiratory pressure (PEEP) levels of 3 to 6 cm H_2O are used to prevent further alveolar collapse, and rates of 20 to 50 breaths per minute are used to treat hypercapnia. Inspiratory times should be initiated at 0.3 to 0.4 second. If a longer inspiratory time is required before surfactant administration, it should be lowered to 0.3 second after surfactant is administered.

Most ventilators today utilize pressure and flow measurements to produce real-time pulmonary function data. These numeric data and graphical displays can be used to correct tidal volumes and optimize ventilation parameters to optimize pulmonary mechanical parameters.[44] Ventilator modes such as synchronous intermittent mandatory ventilation or assist-control modes can reduce work of breathing and blood pressure fluctuations if sensitivities are set properly.[45] Modes that maintain a consistent tidal volume reduce the risk of volutrauma, particularly after the administration of surfactant (see Chapter 19). High-frequency ventilation (HFV) may be indicated in infants who cannot be ventilated with the usually effective F_{IO_2} levels, ventilator pressures, and rates (see Chapter 21).

Monitoring

When RDS is characterized by both high surface tension and high-permeability pulmonary edema, fluid input and output should be closely monitored. Excess fluids may contribute to more difficult ventilatory management and to the development of a PDA. Although diuresis has been tried clinically, the results are inconclusive.[4,5,46] Umbilical or peripheral arterial lines should be used initially for ABG measurements. Transcutaneous oxygen and CO_2 monitors, end-tidal CO_2, pulse oximetry, cardiopulmonary monitors, and Doppler flow studies can be used to monitor the infant's progress. Routine daily chest radiographs may be useful in managing the very low–birth-weight infant who is mechanically

ventilated. Abnormalities ranging from malposition of the endotracheal tube to pulmonary interstitial emphysema can occur from one day to the next.[47]

TRANSIENT TACHYPNEA OF THE NEWBORN

First described by Avery and colleagues in 1966, transient tachypnea of the newborn (TTN) is a relatively benign, typically self-correcting disease.[48] Also known as RDS type II and wet lung syndrome, it occurs in approximately 11 of every 1000 live births. It is more common in boys and in infants with perinatal asphyxia.[49] The incidence after elective cesarean section delivery without labor is as high as 23%. Although TTN does appear in infants born prematurely, it occurs more frequently in term infants. Box 27-2 lists factors that are associated with the occurrence of TTN.[50]

Etiology and Pathophysiology

Although the precise cause is unknown, TTN is believed to be due to delayed resorption of fetal lung fluid and may be caused by any condition that elevates central venous pressure and delays the clearance of pulmonary liquid by the lymphatics. This delay in pulmonary fluid absorption by the lymphatics and pulmonary capillaries results in a decrease in pulmonary compliance, a decreased tidal volume, and an increase in dead space.[51] TTN usually does not require intervention and is generally resolved by 72 hours after birth with no reports of permanent pulmonary damage.[52]

Clinical Presentation

The infant with TTN may be mildly depressed at birth with fairly good Apgar scores. Tachypnea (60 to 150 breaths per minute), cyanosis, grunting, retractions, and nasal flaring begin within a few hours. ABG analysis reveals mild to moderate hypoxemia, hypercapnia, and

Box 27-2	Factors Associated With Transient Tachypnea of the Newborn

- Cesarean section delivery
- Term or preterm infant/near
- Maternal analgesia during labor
- Maternal anesthesia during labor
- Maternal fluid administration
- Maternal asthma
- Maternal diabetes
- Maternal bleeding
- Perinatal asphyxia
- Prolapsed umbilical cord

respiratory acidosis. These symptoms are nearly identical to RDS, hence the term RDS type II. Some have referred to TTN as "persistent postnatal pulmonary edema" because tachypnea is not a consistent finding (it is often masked by drugs given to the mother during labor) and also because some of the fluid may enter the lungs postnatally from the pulmonary circulation.

The chest radiograph shows pulmonary vascular congestion, prominent perihilar streaking, fluid in the interlobular fissures, hyperexpansion, and a flat diaphragm, which is why it is sometimes referred to as wet lung syndrome. Mild cardiomegaly and pleural effusions may also be present. Pulmonary function studies reveal that pulmonary function in infants with TTN is compatible with airway obstruction and gas trapping. The FRC is normal or reduced, and thoracic gas volumes are usually increased, suggesting that some of the gas in the lungs is not in communication with the airways.

Diagnosis and Treatment

Because TTN is similar in initial clinical presentation to conditions such as RDS, group B streptococcal pneumonia, and persistent pulmonary hypertension of the newborn (PPHN), it is usually diagnosed after these disorders have been ruled out. The respiratory distress seen with TTN usually resolves after 24 hours of oxygen therapy, whereas in RDS the infant generally requires longer support. Although the chest radiograph of an infant with RDS will demonstrate hypoaeration and a reticulogranular pattern, that of an infant with TTN may appear as a flattened diaphragm, bulging intercostal spaces, and perihilar streaking. Because the symptoms and radiographs of an infant with TTN are also similar to those of an infant with neonatal sepsis and pneumonia, the infant should be evaluated for infection, which would include looking for an elevated white blood cell count. A broad-spectrum antibiotic may be administered until a differential diagnosis is made.[48]

Oxygen Therapy and Continuous Positive Airway Pressure

The objectives of treatment of TTN are to maintain adequate oxygenation and ventilation.[48] Supplemental oxygen via oxygen hood (usually <40%) is indicated when signs of respiratory distress are present.[53] The distress, hypoxemia, and mild respiratory acidosis usually resolve within 12 to 24 hours, with the infant frequently breathing room air by 48 hours of age. CPAP levels of 3 to 5 cm H_2O may be needed when higher FIO_2 levels are required. The infant's position is changed frequently to prevent further retention of pulmonary fluid. Bottle feedings are postponed until the tachypnea resolves to prevent aspiration.

Mechanical Ventilation

Occasionally an infant with TTN will require mechanical ventilation for respiratory failure. This usually occurs in the preterm infant who is unable to exert sufficient transpleural pressure to clear the alveoli of fluid. Low ventilator settings are used with a minimal pressure or normal tidal volume of 3 to 4 ml/kg to maintain adequate ventilation, PEEP of 3 to 4 cm H_2O, and intermittent mandatory ventilation of 15 to 20 breaths per minute. Weaning is fairly rapid, with ventilatory support rarely needed for more than 24 hours.

NEONATAL PNEUMONIA

Pneumonia presents one of the most serious challenges in neonatal care, with the tiny, immature lung being a common site of infection. Pneumonia occurs in more than 10% of the infants in a neonatal intensive care unit, with premature infants affected more often than term infants.[49] Infections may be acquired in utero (transplacental), during delivery (perinatal), or postnatally in the nursery.[49] Certain groups of mothers seem to have a higher incidence of infection, including those of lower socioeconomic status, those who are teenagers, and those who are sexually active. The severity of the disease course and subsequent level of treatment vary widely and often depend on the particular organism responsible for infection. Pneumonias are classified as either early-onset (infants <7 days of age) or late-onset infections (infants >7 days of age), based on the manifestation and clinical symptoms. Late-onset infections are often easier to treat and are usually less devastating to the infant.[54-56]

Etiology and Pathophysiology

Pneumonia in the newborn is often associated with the development of hyaline membranes.[49] Atelectasis is a result of damage to the alveolar capillary membrane and leakage of proteins into the alveolus. This effluent disturbs the surface properties of pulmonary surfactant, which is why neonatal pneumonia is often indistinguishable from surfactant-deficient RDS.[57] An inflammatory response may occur, followed by partial obstruction of terminal bronchioles and even pneumothorax. An interstitial pneumonitis may develop, as may necrosis of the lung and pulmonary hemorrhage. Box 27-3 lists organisms that are generally associated with pneumonia in the neonate.

Modes of Transmission
Transplacental Pneumonia

Transplacental or congenital pneumonia involves widespread infection that is transmitted to the fetus across the placenta, causing significant distress or even death

Box 27-3	Pathogens Often Responsible for Pneumonia in Neonates Acquired Transplacentally

- Listeria monocytogenes
- *Haemophilus influenzae*
- *Mycobacterium tuberculosis*
- *Treponema pallidum*
- *Toxoplasma*
- Syphilis
- Rubella
- Varicella zoster
- Cytomegalovirus
- Herpes simplex virus
- Human immunodeficiency virus
- Pneumonia Acquired during Labor and Delivery
- Group B β-hemolytic *Streptococcus*
- *Klebsiella*
- *Escherichia coli*
- *Chlamydia trachomatis*
- Nosocomial Pneumonia Acquired after Delivery
- Pseudomonas
- *Serratia marcescens*
- *Staphylococcus aureus*
- *Staphylococcus epidermidis*
- *Klebsiella*
- *Candida albicans*
- Respiratory syncytial virus
- Cytomegalovirus
- Herpes simplex virus

either in utero or at birth. It is more often a result of a maternal viral infection than of a maternal bacterial infection during pregnancy.

Perinatal Pneumonia

Most pneumonias seen in the newborn are a result of infection acquired during labor and delivery. The infant can contract pneumonia through contaminated amniotic fluid, which may be aspirated, or by extended exposure to bacteria that may be in the vaginal tract. This type of "ascending vertical transmission" of bacteria is a result of heavy colonization of the maternal genitourinary tract. PROM greater than 12 to 24 hours before delivery poses a significant chance of the infant's contracting bacteria and is thought to be one of the greatest predisposing factors to neonatal pneumonia.[58-61]

Group B *Streptococcus* has emerged as a predominant pathogen in neonatal pneumonia and presents a serious threat to the newborn. Obstetric complications have been implicated in 50% to 80% of infants with early onset of group B streptococcal pneumonia, indicating intrauterine infection; this infection occurs most often in very low–birth-weight infants. Early-onset pneumonia from group B *Streptococcus* may progress rapidly to shock

or death, and mortality is high (20% to 50%) regardless of treatment. When the onset of group B streptococcal disease is later (2 to 3 weeks after birth), the infant may present with meningitis rather than pneumonia, the pathogen is usually a different strain of the organism, and there is a more optimistic prognosis.[54,58-61]

Postnatal Pneumonia

Nosocomial pneumonia acquired in the postnatal period, also known as horizontal transmission, can be caused by numerous sources. In the treatment of neonates, certain invasive lines (e.g., umbilical catheters, intravenous lines) as well as intubation and respiratory equipment can be avenues for infection. Cross-contamination of bacteria or viruses within the hospital setting is unfortunately a risk with the neonatal patient, especially if there is a large patient-to-caregiver ratio. Careful screening of visitors and extensive care in hand washing and other protective infection control measures should be undertaken to protect these particularly susceptible neonates. Some of the organisms responsible for postnatal pneumonia are airborne, whereas others are spread by contact. Many can be fatal to the neonate, whose immune system is not fully developed.

Complications

Careful management requires frequent assessment for signs of complications that may accompany prematurity, sepsis, and treatment interventions. These include the risk of IVH, air leaks, and necrotizing enterocolitis, as well as the development of BPD if mechanical ventilation is required for extended periods. These infants can suffer significant neurologic damage and developmental delay, or they may have totally normal capabilities. In some cases, however, the impairment may have occurred in utero, and severe neurologic problems or even death may be imminent.

Morbidity and mortality associated with neonatal pneumonia depend on the organism and the ability to successfully treat the infant and keep complications to a minimum. The key to treatment in these infants would seem to be early intervention and aggressive therapy; however, in some infants, especially those with early-onset group B streptococcal pneumonia, the disease process is often fulminative and unresponsive to therapy.

Clinical Presentation

The infant who has acquired transplacental pneumonia may be in noticeable distress at birth or within 6 to 12 hours later. If the infant has aspirated bacteria or otherwise acquired pneumonia during delivery or in the postnatal period, the initial symptoms may not be present until several days later. The infant may have a history of fetal tachycardia with low Apgar scores and often requires some type of supplemental oxygen or even resuscitation at birth.

The chest radiograph may show a diffuse granular pattern with widespread bilateral involvement, especially if the infant acquired the infection in utero. If aspiration of contaminated amniotic fluid has occurred, the chest radiograph may appear as an aspiration pneumonitis with patchy infiltrates. When an infection is acquired postnatally, the radiographic findings often change from normal to severely abnormal over the first few days. Depending on the severity of the disease process and required treatment, pleural effusions, pulmonary edema, pneumatoceles, cardiomegaly, and evidence of barotrauma may be seen. ABG values reveal hypoxemia that is refractory to oxygen therapy and hypercarbia that responds poorly to ventilatory efforts. Metabolic acidosis may develop as infection becomes more severe. Box 27-4 lists clinical signs and symptoms in the infant with neonatal pneumonia.

Box 27-4	Clinical Manifestations and Complications of Neonatal Pneumonia

- Respiratory distress
- Tachypnea
- Cyanosis   *more hypoxia →*
- Grunting   *PP HN*
- Nasal flaring
- Retractions
- Apnea
- Poor peripheral perfusion
- Tachycardia
- Lethargy
- Temperature instability
- Abdominal distention
- Excessive jaundice
- Asphyxia
- Septic shock
- Persistent fetal circulation
- Pulmonary hemorrhage
- Pulmonary edema
- Myocardial insufficiency
- Pleural effusion
- Hypotension
- Disseminating intravascular coagulation
- Hypoxemia
- Hypercarbia
- Respiratory acidosis
- Metabolic acidosis
- Barotrauma
- Intraventricular hemorrhage
- Bronchopulmonary dysplasia
- Necrotizing enterocolitis

Diagnosis and Treatment

Several factors should alert the health care provider to the possibility of neonatal pneumonia—namely, a history of maternal infection or fever, toxemia, premature labor, PROM, malodorous or stained amniotic fluid, lesions of the vagina or placenta, and frequent digital examinations of the cervix.[25] Anytime neonatal pneumonia is suspected, appropriate laboratory diagnostic tests should be performed, such as cultures of blood, urine, and cerebrospinal fluid. Newborns with pneumonia often have an abnormal white blood cell count along with tracheal or gastric aspirates that provide evidence of infection. These test results can help in making a definitive diagnosis of pneumonia.

The normal course of treatment in neonatal pneumonia is relatively straightforward, regardless of the pathogen, and includes appropriate antibiotic or antiviral therapy, oxygenation, adequate ventilation, and pharmacologic support. To prevent rapid deterioration, early intervention, aggressive management, and continuous monitoring are required, especially in the infant with early-onset group B streptococcal disease.

Pharmacologic Support

Many physicians believe that PROM, or the onset of premature labor in and of itself, is often the first sign of infection and should be treated as such, with broad-spectrum antibiotic therapy instituted immediately. This has been shown to be effective in improving the outcome in certain disease processes, especially infection with group B *Streptococcus*. Whenever neonatal pneumonia is suspected, broad-spectrum antibiotics are given for at least 72 hours, or until definitive culture results are obtained. If results prove that infection is present, antibiotics are continued for 14 to 21 days. It is often thought that the bacteria itself may be the cause of prematurity that leads to RDS, which is why the infant with RDS is often treated empirically with antibiotics. Infants with pneumonia may require vasopressor support and intravascular volume replacement to maintain circulation. Blood transfusions may also be necessary in the course of treatment, especially if the infant is having frequent ABG and laboratory assessments.

Antiviral agents (e.g., ribavirin, acyclovir) may be administered in infants with pneumonia of viral origin. In the case of some viral pathogens that are congenitally transmitted, such as cytomegalovirus and rubella, irreversible damage to the central nervous system has already occurred and there is little therapy available to reverse it.

Mechanical Ventilation

The infant with cyanosis, hypoxemia, and hypercarbia may require mechanical ventilation to maintain oxygenation. The most critically ill infants may need extreme ventilator settings with high PIP, rate, and oxygen levels. ABG values and transcutaneous monitors, or pulse oximetry, or both, are used to monitor the patient's respiratory status.

Extracorporeal Membrane Oxygenation

Near-term and term infants who are unresponsive to conventional ventilation and other supportive measures may benefit from extracorporeal membrane oxygenation (ECMO).[62] Improved rates of survival have been reported in this group.

MECONIUM ASPIRATION SYNDROME

Meconium is the green-tinged bowel content of an infant, which is usually passed within 48 hours after delivery. Although it seems impossible, this substance of tarry consistency is sterile and composed of swallowed amniotic fluid, salts, mucus, bile, and other cellular debris.[63] In and of itself, meconium is harmless; however, if in utero the infant passes meconium into the amniotic fluid, it may cause serious airway obstruction, air trapping, and enhanced growth of bacteria. Furthermore, contents of the meconium can compete with surfactant components for adsorption to the alveolar surface, and enzymes in meconium can break down certain surfactant components.[64] Thus it becomes a life-threatening entity that must be dealt with immediately.

Meconium staining of the amniotic fluid at the time of delivery occurs in 8% to 15% of all infants delivered, with approximately 5% of these infants acquiring meconium aspiration syndrome (MAS). Approximately 30% of the infants in whom MAS develops will require mechanical ventilation, at least 11% will experience pneumothorax, and more than 4% will die.[65] Because meconium passage into the amniotic fluid requires strong peristalsis and anal sphincter tone, which is not common in preterm infants, MAS rarely occurs in infants of less than 36 weeks' gestational age.[66] The longer a pregnancy is allowed to continue past 42 weeks, the greater the chances are of the passage of meconium.

Etiology and Pathophysiology

Fetal passage of meconium has long been accepted as a sign of intrauterine stress or hypoxia. Theoretically, the infant becomes hypoxic in utero (possibly because of cord or fetal head compression or prolonged labor), which exhausts oxygen reserves, causing a vagal response, relaxed anal sphincter tone, and passage of meconium into the amniotic fluid. The normal intrauterine activity of the neonate involves the movement of small amounts (1 to 5 ml) of amniotic fluid into and out of the upper airways. The potential of aspiration is always present, but chances are increased with hypoxia or stress because of greater respiratory effort and possibly gasping respirations in utero. Even more damaging is the aspiration that occurs after delivery of the chest when expansion allows the fluid or meconium, or both, to be dispersed even farther into the infant's lungs.[67]

After delivery, the normal pulmonary mechanisms are hindered and the clinical picture varies drastically. The amount and viscosity or dilution of the meconium present may significantly affect the degree of obstruction that occurs. If the infant has a large amount of thick meconium within the airways at the time of delivery, complete bronchiole obstruction with subsequent alveolar collapse will result. The more typical picture, however, is that of smaller amounts of meconium within amniotic fluid, causing a ball-valve effect because of partial obstruction of the airways. The airways dilate on inspiration, whereas air remains trapped behind the obstruction during expiration, causing hyperinflation and greatly predisposing the infant to air leaks. Inflammation of the airways and secretion production (a normal body response to a foreign substance within the lungs) also occurs, and a chemical pneumonitis often develops.[68,69] Studies have also suggested that meconium hinders surfactant, which may lead to atelectasis and decreased pulmonary compliance.[64,70]

It has been suggested that intrauterine hypoxia not only stimulates the passage of meconium but also causes restructuring of the pulmonary vascular bed. The profound hypoxia may result in pulmonary vasoconstriction, which may be the reason that many infants with MAS quickly develop PPHN.[71] Figure 27-1 summarizes the pathophysiologic events that occur with the passage of meconium and MAS.

Complications

Complications of MAS are widespread and depend on the severity of the disease and the level of treatment necessary for survival. Barotrauma or air leak syndrome is always a risk with positive-pressure ventilation, especially in the infant with MAS in which the ball-valve effect produces air trapping. Because the infant is at significant risk for air leaks, frequent chest films should be obtained so that prompt treatment can be instituted. The patient should be closely monitored for sudden deterioration, which could be indicative of tension pneumothorax. Immediate needle aspiration of the air or insertion of a chest tube, or both, may be indicated.

Another serious complication in MAS is increased intracranial pressure. Because the cranium is a fixed cavity, volume capacity is limited. Venous drainage is inhibited by the increased intrathoracic pressures, creating a potential for elevated intracranial pressure. The neonate with unstable vasculature who is already compromised

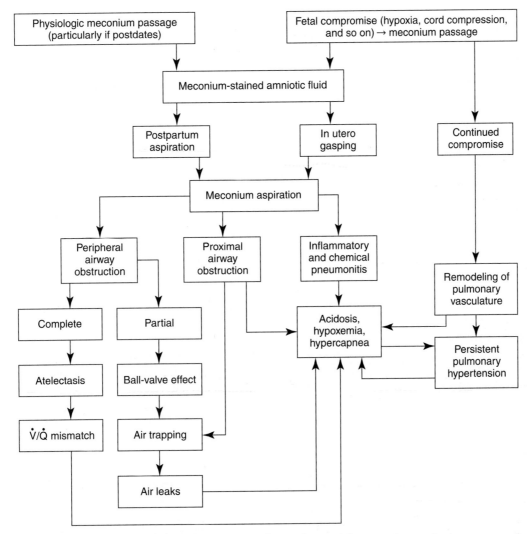

FIGURE 27-1 Pathophysiology of the passage of meconium and the meconium aspiration syndrome. (Redrawn from Wiswell TE, Bent RC: Meconium staining and the meconium aspiration syndrome, *Pediatr Clin North Am* 1993; 40:957; modified from Bacsik RD: Meconium aspiration system, *Pediatr Clin North Am* 1977; 24:467.)

may be predisposed to a higher incidence of IVH, and frequent ultrasonography of the head is performed to monitor for this complication.

Outcome

The outcome in infants with MAS has drastically changed over the past 25 years.[72] Passage of meconium was previously associated with imminent fetal mortality. However, with new techniques at delivery aimed at prevention of further aspiration, as well as the careful administration of resuscitative measures, many more infants survive today and do well. Some infants with MAS experience delayed neurologic function and cerebral palsy.[73,74] When managed properly, however, the majority of these infants do mature with normal neurologic development. Survivors of MAS often acquire chronic respiratory disease, including BPD.[72,75] Another

common occurrence is spontaneous wheezing or exercise-induced bronchospasm, with a large component of obstructive airway disease found years later. As technology expands and new modalities are more accessible, the incidence of long-term chronic problems may lessen.

Clinical Presentation

The infant with MAS is usually a term or postterm infant who has been delivered through meconium-stained fluid (often referred to as pea soup) and has already experienced significant intrauterine stress or hypoxia. The history may include prolonged labor, breech delivery, and ominous fetal heart rate monitor tracings such as late decelerations or nonvariability.

On completion of delivery, the physical examination often reveals a mature infant with yellowish skin, nails, and cord, as well as the postmature signs of peeling skin and long fingernails. The umbilical cord may lack or have very little Wharton's jelly. Depending on the extent of stress or hypoxia, the infant is depressed at birth with low Apgar scores; however, some infants have 1-minute Apgar scores of 5 or more. The infant quickly exhibits signs of respiratory distress, including cyanosis, gasping respirations, grunting, retractions, nasal flaring, and tachypnea. The respiratory distress is often related to the viscosity of the meconium, with a thicker meconium causing more respiratory symptoms.[67,76] Auscultation of the chest reveals rales as well as areas of significantly diminished aeration, with the anteroposterior diameter of the chest often increased. The infant may or may not appear to need immediate intervention, depending on the severity of the aspiration and the degree of hypoxia.

ABG analysis indicates hypoxemia in infants with mild MAS having a normal pH and normal or decreased $PaCO_2$ resulting from the increased respiratory effort. The infant may also have significant metabolic acidosis depending on the severity of the hypoxia before birth. The infant with moderate to severe MAS has increasing hypoxemia and hypercarbia. A combination of respiratory and metabolic acidosis eventually develops as the infant is unable to overcome the obstructive and inflammatory processes. This progresses to the point of respiratory failure and severe hypoxemia, which alerts the physician to the probability of PPHN.[77]

The radiographic appearance varies according to the severity of the disease and complications. The typical chest radiograph shows patchy areas of atelectasis due to obstruction, as well as hyperexpansion from air trapping. There is usually widespread involvement, with no particular area of the lungs being affected more. The radiograph of the infant with severe MAS may reveal total bilateral opacity with only large bronchi distinguishable. Pulmonary air leaks, including pulmonary interstitial emphysema, pneumothorax, and pneumomediastinum, may also be found. The chest radiograph of the infant with MAS is similar to that of an infant with pneumonia, especially when a bacterial infection develops.[78]

Diagnosis and Treatment

Although the majority of infants are normal, MAS is suggested whenever there is meconium staining of the amniotic fluid. The diagnosis of MAS is generally made whenever meconium is visualized at the vocal cords and the infant has clinical signs of respiratory distress, including hypoxemia, hypercarbia, and a characteristic chest radiographic pattern.

Intrapartum Intervention

Some fetuses may be assessed as "at risk" for MAS, including those with oligohydramnios, abnormal fetal heart rate tracings, and thick, meconium-stained amni-

otic fluids.[66] A promising intrapartum intervention for these infants is amnioinfusion.[79,80] It is believed that by infusing fluid into the mother's uterus, the uterine fluid volume may either dilute the meconium or alleviate compression of the cord and prevent gasping.

Suctioning

Although no prevention has been found for MAS, prompt intervention in the delivery room can make a drastic difference in the outcome. To prevent aspiration into the lungs, pharyngeal suction should be performed when the infant's head is delivered and before delivery of the thorax (before the first breath is taken). A bulb syringe may be used; however, an 8 or 10 French flexible suction catheter may be more effective in removing thick meconium. Regardless of the thickness of meconium, infants who are vigorous at birth with adequate tone and respiratory effort and heart rate greater than 100 beats per minute may not require immediate intubation. These infants should be observed for signs of respiratory distress before deciding on intubation.[80] Infants who are depressed at birth with poor tone and absent or gasping respirations should have the trachea cleared of meconium. Once the infant is intubated, the endotracheal tube should be used as a suction catheter with 80 to 100 cm H_2O negative pressure applied as the tube is withdrawn. Suction catheters inserted into the endotracheal tube are too small to aspirate thick meconium and may become clogged, delaying removal. More than one pass may be needed to clear the trachea of meconium. Ventilation and oxygenation according to established neonatal resuscitation guidelines should be carried out after suctioning. Saline lavage may be used to dilute the meconium while the infant continues to be intubated. All infants born with meconium-stained amniotic fluid should be closely monitored.[81-84]

Mechanical Ventilation

In spite of early intervention with thorough suctioning, some infants will still acquire MAS.[85] The infant who presents with meconium-stained amniotic fluid and progresses to a state of worsening respiratory distress and hypoxemia should be intubated and mechanically ventilated. This infant is a management challenge. Sedation and paralysis are often required for effective ventilation. Optimal ventilator parameters are a combination of PIP, PEEP, inspiratory time, and flow rates that result in the lowest mean airway pressure possible to provide adequate oxygenation and ventilation. Ventilator parameters range from a gentle ventilation with higher $PaCO_2$s and lower PaO_2s to more aggressive techniques with the $PaCO_2$ at 25 to 30 mm Hg and a "high-normal" PaO_2.[86] Aggressive ventilation may affect hemodynamics, prompting worsening of blood gases. This may lead to higher ventilator settings with little clinical improvement.

Other therapies associated with the treatment of neonates with MAS include sedation, alkalosis with bicarbonate or tromethamine (Tham), paralytic agents, minimal stimulation, and chest physiotherapy and suctioning.[87]

High-Frequency Ventilation

HFV has been used in MAS in the hope that the lower pressures and higher frequencies will prove advantageous.[88] Benefits may include less barotrauma, increased mobilization of secretions, maintenance of respiratory alkalosis, and fewer chronic changes. However, the high airway resistance and obstructive nature of MAS may hinder the effectiveness of HFOV. Oxygenation is not necessarily improved with the use of either conventional ventilation or HFV.

Emerging Clinical Treatments

Because surfactant within the lung may be hindered by the presence of meconium, surfactant replacement therapy can be considered as a treatment for MAS (see Chapter 16).[88,89] Surfactant administration seems to reduce severity of respiratory symptoms and reduces progression of the disease and may reduce the need for ECMO.[90] Some infants with MAS will progress to the point of developing severe hypoxemia and respiratory failure, exacerbating pulmonary hypertension.[91] Liquid ventilation with perfluorocarbon may be beneficial in MAS by washing out meconium, improving surface tension and ventilation-perfusion mismatch (see Chapter 22). Animal models have shown some promising results.[92,93]

PERSISTENT PULMONARY HYPERTENSION OF THE NEWBORN

PPHN is a clinical syndrome characterized by severely increased PVR with right-to-left shunting and alterations in pulmonary vasoreactivity. It occurs most often in infants who are term or postterm and is associated with several underlying neonatal clinical conditions, including MAS, RDS, and birth asphyxia; however, it may also be idiopathic with no known cause. Because of the persistent right-to-left fetal shunts (i.e., PDA, foramen ovale) and lack of a known cause, idiopathic pulmonary hypertension of the newborn was formerly known as persistent fetal circulation. The term *persistent* was added to reflect the pathophysiology of the disease.[51,94]

Etiology and Pathophysiology

PPHN may be caused by many factors that are classified as primary or secondary. Primary causes deal with anatomic malformation (e.g., alveolar capillary dysplasia, pulmonary hypoplasia), genetic differences in pulmonary smooth muscle development, chronic intrauterine stress, intrauterine closure of the ductus arteriosus, and abnormal levels of vasoactive agents (i.e., increased vasoconstrictors, decreased vasodilators). Secondary causes are associated with underlying disease processes, such as MAS, congenital heart disease, infection, polycythemia, and upper airway obstruction.[51] Box 27-5 lists factors frequently associated with PPHN.

Box 27-5	Factors Associated With Persistent Pulmonary Hypertension of the Newborn

FETAL FACTORS
- Intrauterine stress
- Hypoxia
- Acidosis
- Placental vascular abnormalities
- Maternal Factors
- Diabetes
- Hypoxia
- Cesarean section

PHARMACOLOGIC FACTORS
- Prostaglandins
- Indomethacin
- Salicylate
- Phenytoin

PULMONARY FACTORS
- Pneumonia
- Meconium aspiration
- Pulmonary hypoplasia
- Diaphragmatic hernia
- Respiratory distress syndrome

- Transient tachypnea of the newborn
- Lobar emphysema

HEMATOLOGIC FACTORS
- Increased hematocrit
- Maternal-fetal blood loss
- Abruptio placentae
- Placenta previa
- Acute blood loss
- Polycythemia

CARDIOVASCULAR FACTORS
- Systemic hypotension
- Congenital heart disease
- Shock

OTHER FACTORS
- Central nervous system disorders
- Neuromuscular disease
- Hypoglycemia
- Hypocalcemia
- Septicemia

In fetal life, the placenta functions as the organ for gas exchange. This function is facilitated by both the shunting of the blood through the foramen ovale and the hypoxic pulmonary arteriole vasoconstriction, which causes the blood to bypass the lungs and move toward the placenta. At birth, the umbilical cord is cut and the lungs make the transition to becoming the organ for gas exchange. With the first postnatal breaths, PVR decreases dramatically. By 24 hours of life, 80% of the total decrease in PVR has occurred, with the remaining reduction taking place over the next 2 weeks of life. The reduction in PVR is in response to

1. increases in PaO_2 and pH
2. air expanding the lung, and
3. release of vasoactive substances, including prostaglandins, bradykinin, and endogenous nitric oxide production.[95]

In infants with PPHN, this decrease in PVR either fails to occur or is reversed by pulmonary vascular hyperreactivity to irritating stimuli. However, pulmonary hypertension caused by irritating stimuli is not reversed simply by removing the stimulus. Infants with PPHN may have a muscular thickening of the small pulmonary arteries, which results in increased stiffness of the vascular bed and reduced alveolar expansion.[96,97]

Complications and Outcome

The mortality rate for infants with PPHN ranges from 20% to 40%, with an increase in survival seen when nitric oxide or ECMO is used. Approximately 12% to 32% of patients with PPHN suffer from neurologic problems, including impaired neurologic development and neurosensory hearing loss. Seizures, cerebral infarction, and IVH have all been documented in PPHN survivors. BPD is also a risk in patients who require ventilatory assistance with high FIO_2 levels, high rates, and high pressures. The underlying disorder, as well as the management of the patient, contributes to patient outcome.[98]

Clinical Presentation

The infant with PPHN usually presents within the first 12 hours of life with cyanosis, tachypnea, and hypoxia that are refractory to oxygen therapy, and signs of respiratory distress, including retractions, grunting, and nasal flaring.[94,99] ABG assessment reveals hypoxemia. Infants may hyperventilate owing to the persistent hypoxemia. Hypocalcemia and hypoglycemia may develop rapidly as well. A right-to-left shunt through a PDA or the foramen ovale, or both, may be present, along with tricuspid and pulmonic valve regurgitation.[100]

The chest radiograph varies depending on the associated disorder. Early chest radiographs are often clear, with minimal evidence of respiratory involvement, which is often perplexing in light of the severe cyanosis and respiratory distress the infant exhibits. Idiopathic and asphyxic PPHN may show well-expanded or hyperexpanded lungs with diminished vascularity, whereas PPHN resulting from pulmonary disorders (e.g., MAS, RDS, TTN) reveals abnormal pulmonary findings characteristic of that particular disorder. Cardiomegaly may be evident and develops as a result of the increased right ventricular afterload caused by the pulmonary hypertension.

Diagnosis

The differential diagnosis of PPHN includes RDS, lung disease, and congenital heart disease. Various tests may be used to assist in the diagnosis. Classic tests to assess PPHN evaluate the response in PaO_2 to hyperoxia and hyperoxia-hyperventilation. To confirm PPHN, the PaO_2 should not increase appreciably with hyperoxia alone, but PaO_2 will usually rise above 100 mm Hg if the infant is hyperventilated until a $PaCO_2$ of 20 to 25 mm Hg is attained. Now, however, because of the known risk of oxidative injury and the potential for low $PaCO_2$ levels to reduce cerebral blood flow, these tests are no longer considered safe. The current tests used to confirm PPHN are Preductal-Postductal PaO_2 Comparison and/or Doppler Flow Studies and Cardiac Catheterization.

Preductal-Postductal PaO_2 Comparison

A PaO_2 measurement from the right radial artery is compared with that from the umbilical artery, or a transcutaneous PaO_2 measurement from the right arm is compared with that from the abdomen. Right-to-left shunting is demonstrated if the preductal sample is more than 20 mm Hg greater than the simultaneous postductal sample. However, a normal test result (difference in preductal and postductal samples <20 mm Hg) does not rule out PPHN. An abnormal test result can also occur in infants with some congenital heart defects.

Doppler Flow Studies and Cardiac Catheterization

Shunts through the foramen ovale and a PDA can be observed with cardiac ultrasound studies. Pulmonary artery pressure may be measured by means of pulmonary artery catheterization, with infants having PPHN demonstrating elevated pressures.[101]

Treatment

Treatment for PPHN is relatively straightforward. Mechanical ventilation is used to recruit the lung, usually with high-frequency ventilation, and surfactant therapy can be used if a secondary cause such as MAS is suspected. Acidosis should be avoided by maintaining a base deficit of 0, without raising pH beyond the normal range. Cardiac output is maintained with the appropriate volume and pressor therapies. Pulmonary vasodilatation is achieved with iNO therapy. Infants that do not respond to this treatment paradigm are candidates for ECMO.

High-Frequency Ventilation

HFV is frequently used to ventilate infants with PPHN. Retrospective studies indicate that there is no difference in mortality, incidence of air leaks, or BPD between high-frequency jet ventilation and conventionally ventilated groups. Some reports suggest, however, that high-frequency oscillatory ventilation may improve the outcome in PPHN.[100,102,103]

Nitric Oxide Therapy

Having been recognized in the late 1980s as a potent pulmonary vasodilator, inhaled nitric oxide (iNO) is being successfully used in the treatment of PPHN.[104-112] Specialized ventilator systems such as the INOvent (INO Therapeutics, LLC, Clinton, NJ) contribute controlled quantities of nitric oxide gas to the inspiratory gas mixture delivered to the infant by a mechanical ventilator. A number of large randomized, controlled studies have shown that low doses such as 20 ppm iNO improve outcomes and reduce the need for extreme measures such as ECMO.[104,105,113] Some infants have benefited from a combination of high-frequency oscillatory ventilation and nitric oxide.[104] Echocardiographic measurements have shown a decrease in PVR, in right-to-left shunting, and in tricuspid insufficiency and an increase in pulmonary blood flow and PaO_2.[111] Weaning from iNO therapy needs to be done with care to avoid rebound increases in PVR.[104,107] Box 27-6 lists clinical conditions that may benefit from nitric oxide therapy (see Chapter 23).[114-119]

Extracorporeal Membrane Oxygenation

ECMO is being used in some centers for neonates with severe PPHN who are not responsive to less invasive

Box 27-6	Conditions That May Benefit From Nitric Oxide Therapy

- Persistent pulmonary hypertension of the newborn
- Hypoxic pulmonary hypertension
- Methacholine-induced bronchoconstriction
- Septic shock
- Pulmonary hypertension before and after cardiac surgery
- Adult respiratory distress syndrome
- High-altitude pulmonary edema

therapies; with studies indicating an increase in survival from 20% to 83%[120,121] (see Chapter 24). ECMO is generally considered for infants that are refractory to iNO therapy.

APNEA OF PREMATURITY

Apnea of prematurity is perhaps the most common form of infant apnea and is a significant cause of morbidity and mortality in premature infants.[122] Apnea of prematurity is defined as a cessation of breathing effort greater than 20 seconds in duration, or any respiratory pause that is long enough for signs of bradycardia or cyanosis, or both, to appear in an infant younger than 37 weeks' gestation.[123] Approximately 75% of premature infants weighing less than 1250 g and more than 25% of those weighing more than 1500 g suffer from severe apnea. Neurologic immaturity and the degree of maturity of pulmonary stretch reflexes and the ventilatory response to carbon dioxide may be better predictors of the risk for apneic spells than chronologic age.[124]

Etiology and Pathophysiology

There are two types of apnea related to the degree of asphyxia. Primary apnea occurs after a rapid increase in respiratory rate and depth. The infant can usually be manually stimulated to begin breathing again. If allowed to continue, the infant then suffers approximately 1 minute of apnea followed by several minutes of gasping. This apneic episode can progress to a secondary stage in which resuscitation is required to reestablish respiration. Approximately 30% of all premature infants suffer from this secondary form, which lasts for more than 30 seconds and is associated with a drop in oxygen saturation. Secondary apnea may also be accompanied by bradycardia and hypotension. Benign periodic breathing is frequently seen in young infants, and may be distinguished from apnea by its characteristic cycle of short pauses in respiration followed by an increased respiratory rate.[125]

Premature infants are believed to be susceptible to apneic episodes because of immature afferent input from chemoreceptors, lung and airway receptors, and the central nervous system. Sleep may be a factor in apnea and periodic breathing. Nearly 80% of a preterm infant's time is spent sleeping, with approximately 90% of a sleep cycle spent in rapid-eye-movement (REM) sleep in which there is respiratory depression. However, only 50% of a full-term infant's sleep is spent in REM sleep. Also, the infant's very compliant rib cage is less compliant during REM sleep, which may result in decreased lung volumes. Box 27-7 lists factors that are believed to trigger apneic spells in infants.[126-130]

Although in most infants with apnea the episodes gradually decrease in both frequency and severity as they mature, there is a questionably higher incidence of

Box 27-7	Factors Associated With Apnea in Infants

SYSTEMIC PROCESSES
- Sepsis
- Group B *Streptococcus*
- Respiratory syncytial virus
- Hypothermia
- Hypoglycemia
- Hyponatremia
- Hypocalcemia

PULMONARY DISEASE
- Pneumonia
- Respiratory distress syndrome

CARDIAC DISEASE
- Left-to-right shunt
- Congestive heart failure
- Patent ductus arteriosus closure

NEUROLOGIC DISEASE
- Seizures
- Meningitis
- Intracranial hemorrhage

GASTROINTESTINAL DISEASE
- Botulism
- Gastroesophageal reflux
- Abnormal coordination of swallowing

- Reflexes
- Hiccups
- Vagal response to bowel movement
- Suctioning of nasopharynx and trachea
- Stimulation of laryngeal chemoreceptors

CONTROL OF VENTILATION
- Rapid-eye-movement sleep
- Depressed response to hypoxia
- Depressed response to hypercarbia
- Congenital central hypoventilation (Ondine's curse)
- Environmental Conditions
- Ambient temperature changes
- Position
- Head flexion

DRUG DEPRESSION
- Sedatives
- Analgesics
- Prostaglandins

ANATOMIC ABNORMALITIES
- Micrognathia
- Macroglossia
- Choanal atresia
- Temporomandibular ankylosis

Modified from Leistner HL: Apnea in infants and children. In Zimmerman SS, Gildea J, editors: *Critical care pediatrics*. Philadelphia. WB Saunders, 1985.

sudden infant death syndrome associated with neonatal apnea. If results from polysomnography or sleep testing show persistent abnormalities of respiration, the infant may be discharged on a home apnea-bradycardia monitor (see Chapters 11, 32, and 46).

Clinical Presentation

Infants with apnea invariably respond with bradycardia. Other initial symptoms include snoring, choking, and mouth breathing, although some infants exhibit no signs of respiratory distress. There may be changes in muscle tone, skin color (cyanosis or pallor), and respiratory pattern.

Diagnosis and Treatment

Infants with frequent apnea should have routine screening tests that include a chest radiograph, ABG analysis, electrocardiogram and Holter monitoring, complete blood cell count, and electrolyte determination. Blood, urine, and cerebrospinal fluid cultures should be performed if infection is believed to be a contributing factor and all other causes are ruled out. Close monitoring to evaluate possible causes of the apnea should focus on respiratory rate and pattern, heart rate, circumstances preceding the apneic episode, associated bradycardia, skin color, muscle tone,

and termination of the episode (whether spontaneous, with stimulation, or with resuscitation).

Once the underlying cause for the apnea has been determined, the treatment focuses on preventing further episodes from occurring. This begins with monitoring and treatment of ineffective respiration before it degenerates to apnea. The infant may benefit from tactile stimulation only; however, if the apnea persists, ventilation with oxygen is initiated with bag and mask. To reduce the risk of retinopathy of prematurity, the infant should be ventilated only with the FIO_2 needed to maintain adequate oxygen saturation. Upright positioning; small, frequent feedings of thickened formula; temperature stability; or a combination of these factors may be helpful in prevention. Frequently, a low FIO_2 of 0.23 to 0.25 is effective in decreasing apneic episodes. With prolonged episodes, a low dose of a methylxanthine derivative, such as caffeine, theophylline, or doxapram, has been initiated to stimulate respiration.[131] Because gastroesophageal reflux may be exacerbated by xanthine therapy, it should be ruled out before xanthines are administered. Oscillating water beds or "bump" beds may be used to stimulate respiration in the infant. A bump bed can be constructed by connecting a rubber glove to a pressure ventilator or intermittent positive-pressure breathing machine with a respiratory rate and inspiratory pressure set. The glove is placed under the infant's mattress pad, and the periodic inflation-deflation of the glove will bump the infant and, it is hoped, stimulate respirations. Current studies have not been adequate to determine the effectiveness of kinesthetic stimulation compared with other treatments.[132] With current minimal stimulation and developmental care guidelines for premature infants, this method is discouraged in most nurseries.

ASSESSMENT QUESTIONS

1. A 25-week gestation newborn appears cyanotic and with ABG analysis indicating hypoxia and hypercarbia. The infant has severe chest wall retractions with inspiratory effort. The amniotic fluid appeared normal at birth. What is most likely the cause of respiratory distress?
   A. Surfactant deficiency
   B. Meconium aspiration syndrome
   C. Pneumonia
   D. Bronchopulmonary dysplasia

2. An infant diagnosed with RDS subsequent to lung prematurity is receiving oxygen therapy with an FIO_2 of 0.8 and NCPAP set at 10 cmH$_2$O. The infant is experiencing progressive hypercarbia and apnic episodes are appearing prolonged. The next logical course of action is to
   A. Increase the FIO_2 by 0.1 and look for improvements in ABG parameters
   B. Start iNO therapy to improve the lung V:Q ratio
   C. Increase NCPAP to 12 cmH$_2$O and refit the nasal prongs
   D. Intubate the infant and begin mechanical ventilation

3. A full-term infant is delivered via cesarean section and demonstrates mild symptoms of RDS including cyanosis, tachypnea, and nasal flaring. APGAR scores are good and chest radiographs show hyperexpansion and perihilar streaking. Which situation most likely fits this case?
   A. This infant is in the "honeymoon" period and is expected to develop more severe RDS.
   B. This infant has TTN and will likely recover completely by 72 hrs.
   C. This infant is in the early stages of pneumonia and should be started on broad-spectrum antibiotics.
   D. This infant likely has elevated PVR and a hyperoxia test should be performed to confirm PPHN.

4. A 4-day-old infant, born at 27 weeks' gestation, develops recurrent symptoms of RDS. The infant had been removed from mechanical ventilation and extubated at day 3, and was receiving NCPAP with an FIO_2 of 0.4 when lung function acutely worsened. Chest radiographs show a

widespread, diffuse granular pattern and analysis of arterial blood samples from the umbilical line demonstrates that oxygen saturation is refractory to increase in FIO_2. The most likely cause for these recurrent symptoms of RDS is:
   A. Progressive periods of apnea
   B. Patent ductus arteriosus
   C. Meconium aspiration syndrome
   D. Postnatal pneumonia

5. A newborn infant begins to develop symptoms of respiratory distress at 5 days of life. A cerebrospinal fluid culture tests positive for B streptococcus infection. Which mode(s) of transmission is most likely the cause of the infection?
   A. Transplacental or perinatal
   B. Transplacental only
   C. Perinatal or postnatal
   D. Postnatal only

6. Which condition would be most critical in leading the caregiver to anticipate MAS?
   A. Desaturation refractory to oxygen therapy
   B. Yellowish-green colored amniotic fluid
   C. Distinct chest wall retractions with inspiratory efforts
   D. Cyanosis and nasal flaring

7. Which fetal assessments may suggest that, when born, an infant will be at risk for MAS?
   A. Fetal oligohydramnios
   B. Abnormal fetal heart rate tracings
   C. Both A and B
   D. Neither A nor B

8. PPHN can be associated with which underlying pulmonary disorders?
   A. MAS
   B. RDS
   C. None (idiopathic)
   D. All of the above

9. A full-term newborn diagnosed with PPHN is refractory to oxygen therapy and mechanical ventilation. Which would be the next logical therapy to try?
   A. High-frequency ventilation
   B. Volume therapy
   C. iNO therapy
   D. All would be have potential benefits

10. A newborn at 34 weeks' gestation is experiencing brief periods of apnea, which result in bradycardia and cyanosis. Blood and cerebrospinal fluid cultures test negative for infection. Which intervention(s) can help reduce the incidence of apneic episodes?
    A. Upright positioning
    B. Temperature stability
    C. Low FIO_2 of 0.23 to 0.25
    D. All of the above

References

1. Miller JM, Fanaroff AA, Martin RJ: Other pulmonary problems. In Fanaroff AA, Martin RJ, editors: *Neonatal-perinatal medicine diseases of the fetus and infant*, ed 5, vol 2, St Louis. Mosby; 1992. pp 834-861.

2. American Lung Association: American Lung Association State of Lung Disease in Diverse Communities: 2007. Available online at: www.lungusa.org/site/pp.asp?c=dvLUK900E&b=308853

3. U.S. Department of Health and Human Services: Press release (P10–33), Washington, DC, July 26, 1989.

4. Hansen T, Corbert A: Disorders of the transition. In Taeusch HW, Ballard RA, Avery ME, editors: *Schaffer and Avery's diseases of the newborn*, ed 6, Philadelphia, WB Saunders; 1991.

5. Kliegman RM, Behrman RE: Disturbances of organ systems. In Behrman RE et al, editors: *Textbook of pediatrics*, ed 14, Philadelphia, WB Saunders, 1992.

6. Graven SN, Misenheimer HR: Respiratory distress syndrome and the high risk mother, *Am J Dis Child* 1965;109:489.

7. Usher RH, Allen AC, McLean FH: Risk of respiratory distress syndrome related to gestational age, route of delivery and maternal diabetes, *Am J Obstet Gynecol* 1971;111:826.

8. Avery ME, Mead J: Surface properties in relation to atelectasis and hyaline membrane disease, *Am J Dis Child* 1959;97:517.

9. Stahlman M et al: Six-year follow-up of clinical hyaline membrane disease, *Pediatr Clin North Am* 1973;20:433.

10. Rooney SA: The surfactant system and lung phospholipid biochemistry, *Am Rev Respir Dis* 1985;131:439.

11. Meyrick B, Reid L: Ultrastructure of alveolar lining and its development. In Hodson WA, editor: *Development of the lung*, New York. Marcel Dekker; 1977. pp 135-214.

12. Clements JA, King RJ: Composition of surface-active material. In Crystal RG, editor: *The biochemical basis of pulmonary function*, New York. Marcel Dekker; 1976. pp 363-387.

13. Hawgood S, Clements JA: Pulmonary surfactant and its apoproteins, *J Clin Invest* 1990;86:1.

14. Boyden EA: Development and growth of the airways. In Hodson WA, editor: *Development of the lung*, New York, Marcel Dekker; 1972. pp 3-36.

15. Hislop AA, Wigglesworth JS, Desai R: Alveolar development in the human fetus and infant, *Early Hum Dev* 1986;13:1.

16. Stark AR, Frantz ID III: Respiratory distress syndrome, *Pediatr Clin North Am* 1986;33:533.

17. Nelson NM et al: Pulmonary function in the newborn infant, the alveolar-arterial oxygen gradient, *J Appl Physiol* 1963;18:534.

18. Murdock AI, Swyer PR: The contribution to venous admixture by shunting through the ductus arteriosus in infants with respiratory distress syndrome of the newborn, *Biol Neonate* 1968;13:194.

19. Verma RP: Respiratory distress syndrome of the newborn infant, *Obstet Gynecol Surv* 1995;50:542-555.

20. Jobe AH, Ikegami M: Mechanisms initiating lung injury in the preterm, *Early Hum Dev* 1998;53:81-94.

21. Jobe AH, Ikegami M: Prevention of bronchopulmonary dysplasia: *Curr Opin Pediatr* 2001;13:124-129.

22. Lee WL, Slutsky AS: Ventilator-Induced Lung Injury and Recommendations for Mechanical Ventilation of Patients with ARDS: *Semin Respir Crit Care Med* 2001;22:269-280.

23. Mannino FL, Gluck L: The management of respiratory distress syndrome. In Thibeault DW, Gregoary GA, editors: *Neonatal pulmonary care*, Reading, Mass, Addison-Wesley; 1979. pp 261-276.

24. Avery ME et al: Is chronic lung disease in low birth-weight infants preventable? A survey of eight centers, *Pediatrics* 1987;79:26.

25. Lebourges F et al: Pulmonary function in infancy and in childhood following mechanical ventilation in the neonatal period, *Pediatr Pulmonol* 1990;9:34.

26. Bhutani VK et al: Pulmonary mechanics and energetics in preterm infants who had respiratory distress syndrome treated with synthetic surfactant, *J Pediatr* 1992;120:S18.

27. Miller TL et al: MMP and TIMP expression profiles in tracheal aspirates do not adequately reflect tracheal or lung tissue profiles in neonatal respiratory distress: Observations from an animal model, *Pediatr Crit Care Med* (In Press).

28. Davis GM, Bureau MA: Pulmonary and chest wall mechanics in the control of respiration in the newborn, *Clin Perinatol* 1987;14:551.

29. Escobedo MB: Hyaline membrane disease. In Schreiner RL, Kisling JA, editors: *Practical neonatal respiratory care*, New York, Raven Press; 1982. pp 87-103.

30. Whitfield CR, Sproule WD: Prediction of neonatal respiratory distress, *Lancet* 1972;1:382.

31. Lemons JA, Jaffe RB: Amniotic fluid lecithin/sphingomyelin ratio in the diagnosis of hyaline membrane disease, *Am J Obstet Gynecol* 1973;115:233.

32. Hallman M et al: Phosphatidylinositol and phosphatidylglycerol in amniotic fluid: indices of lung maturity, *Am J Obstet Gynecol* 1976;125:613.

33. Clements JA et al: Assessment of the risk of the respiratory distress syndrome by a rapid test for surfactant in amniotic fluid, *N Engl J Med* 1972;286:1077.

34. Ballard PL: Hormonal regulation of pulmonary surfactant, *Endocr Rev* 1989;10:165.

35. Pramanik AK, Holtzman RB, Merritt TA: Surfactant replacement therapy for pulmonary diseases, *Pediatr Clin North Am* 1993;40:913.

36. Long W et al: Effects of two rescue doses of a synthetic surfactant on mortality rate and survival without bronchopulmonary dysplasia in 700- to 1350-gram infants with respiratory distress syndrome, *J Pediatr* 1991;118:595.

37. Gaillard EA, Cooke RW, Shaw NJ: Improved survival and neurodevelopmental outcome after prolonged ventilation in preterm neonates who have received antenatal steroids and surfactant, *Arch Dis Child Fetal Neonatal* 2001;84(3):F194-F196.

38. Davis JM: Role of oxidant injury in the pathogenesis of neonatal lung disease, *Acta Paediatr Suppl* 2002;91:23-25.

39. Gittermann MK et al: Early nasal continuous positive airway pressure treatment reduces the need for intubation in very low birth weight infants, *Eur J Pediatr* 1996;56:384-388.

40. Kamper J: Early nasal continuous positive airway pressure and minimal handling in the treatment of very-low birthweight infants, *Biol Neonate* 1999;76(suppl 1):22-28.

41. Alba J et al: Efficacy of surfactant therapy in infants managed with CPAP, *Pediatr Pulmonol* 1995;20:172-176.

42. Schimmel MS, Hammerman C: Early nasal continuous positive airway pressure with or without prophylactic surfactant therapy in the premature infant with respiratory distress syndrome, *Pediatr Radiol* 2000;30: 713-714.

43. Soll RF, Morley CJ: Prophylactic versus selective use of surfactant in preventing morbidity and mortality in preterm infants (Cochrane Review), *Cochrane Database Syst Rev*2001;2:CD000510.

44. Miller TL, Shaffer TH, Greenspan JS: Pulmonary function evaluation in the critically ill neonate. In Askins DF, editor: *Acute Respiratory Care of the Neonate*, ed 4, Neonatal Network, 2005.

45. Hummler H et al: Influence of different methods of synchronized mechanical ventilation on ventilation, gas exchange, patient effort, and blood pressure fluctuations in premature neonates, *Pediatr Pulmonol* 1996;22:305-313.

46. Green TP et al: Prophylactic furosemide in severe respiratory distress syndrome: blinded prospective study, *J Pediatr* 1988;112:605.

47. Greenough A et al: Routine daily chest radiographs in ventilated, very low birthweight infants, *Eur J Pediatr* 2001;160:147-149.

48. Avery ME, Gatewood OB, Brumley G: Transient tachypnea of the newborn, *Am J Dis Child* 1966;111:380.

49. Whitsett JA et al: Acute respiratory disorders. In Avery GE, Fletcher MA, MacDonald MG, editors: *Neonatology*, ed 4, Philadelphia, JB Lippincott, 1994.

50. Tudehope DI, Smith MH: Is transient tachypnoea of the newborn always a benign condition. *Aust Paediatr J* 1979;15:160.

51. Levin DL: Idiopathic persistent pulmonary hypertension of the newborn. In Rudolph AM, Hoffman JIE, Rudolph CD, editors: *Rudolph's pediatrics*, ed 19, Norwalk, Conn, Appleton & Lange, 1991.

52. Gross TL, Sokol RJ, Kwong MS: Transient tachypnea of the newborn: the relationship to preterm delivery and significant neonatal morbidity, *Am J Obstet Gynecol* 1983;14:236.

53. Bucciarelli RL et al: Persistence of fetal cardiopulmonary circulation: manifestation of transient tachypnea of the newborn, *Pediatrics* 1976;58:192.

54. Battaglia FC, Rosenberg AA: The newborn infant. In Groothuis JRet al, editors: *Current pediatric diagnosis & treatment*, Norwalk, Conn, Appleton & Lange, 1993.

55. Durand DJ, Gleason CA: Respiratory complications. In Keith LG, Witter FR, editors: *Textbook of prematurity*, Boston, Little, Brown, 1993.

56. Pursley DM, Richardson DK: Management of the sick newborn. In Graef JW, editor: *Manual of pediatric therapeutics*, ed 5, Boston, Little Brown, 1994.

57. Rudiger M et al: Disturbed surface properties in preterm infants with pneumonia, *Biol Neonate* 2001;79:73-78.

58. Corbet A, Hansen T: Neonatal pneumonias. In Avery ME, Ballard RA, Taeusch AW: *Schaffer and Avery's diseases of the newborn*, ed 6, Philadelphia, WB Saunders, 1991.

59. Nelson RM: Group B *Streptococcus* (GBS). In Behrman RE et al, editors: *Textbook of pediatrics*, ed 14, Philadelphia, WB Saunders, 1992.

60. Adams WG et al: Outbreak of early onset group B streptococcal sepsis, *Pediatr Infect Dis J* 1993;12:565.

61. Tooley WH: Neonatal pneumonia due to beta-hemolytic *Streptococcus* group B. In Rudolph AM, editor: *Rudolph's pediatrics*, ed 19, Norwalk, Conn, Appleton & Lange, 1991.

62. Hocker JR, Simpson PM, Rabalais GP: Extracorporeal membrane oxygenation and early-onset group B streptococcal sepsis, *Pediatrics* 1992;89:1.

63. Goetzman BW: Meconium aspiration, *Am J Dis Child* 1992;146:1282.

64. Schrama AJ et al: Phospholipase A2 is present in meconium and inhibits the activity of pulmonary surfactant: an in vitro study, Acta Paediatr 2001;90:412-416.

65. Wiswell TE, Tuggle JM, Turner BS: Meconium aspiration syndrome: have we made a difference? *Pediatrics* 1990;85:715.

66. Wiswell TE, Bent RC: Meconium staining and the meconium aspiration syndrome, *Pediatr Clin North Am* 1993;40:955.

67. Rossi EM et al: Meconium aspiration syndrome: intrapartum and neonatal attributes, *Am J Obstet Gynecol* 1989;161:1106.

68. Tyler DC, Murphy J, Cheney FW: Mechanical and chemical damage to lung tissue caused by meconium aspiration, *Pediatrics* 1978;62:454.

69. Wiswell TE et al: Management of a piglet model of the meconium aspiration syndrome with high frequency or conventional ventilation, *Am J Dis Child* 1992;146:1287.

70. Moses D et al: Inhibition of pulmonary surfactant by meconium, *Am J Obstet Gynecol* 1991;104:758.

71. Perlman EJ, Moore GW, Hutchins GM: The pulmonary vasculature in meconium aspiration, *Hum Pathol* 1989;20:701.

72. Swaminathan S et al: Long-term pulmonary sequelae of meconium aspiration syndrome, *J Pediatr* 1989;114:356.

73. Nelson KB: Relationship of intrapartum and delivery room events to long-term neurologic outcome, *Clin Perinatol* 1989;16:995.

74. Altshuler G, Hyde S: Meconium-induced vasocontraction: a potential cause of cerebral and other fetal hypoperfusion and of poor pregnancy outcome, *J Child Neurol* 1989;4:137.

75. MacFarlane PI, Heaf DP: Pulmonary function in children after neonatal meconium aspiration syndrome, *Arch Dis Child* 1988;63:368.

76. Dooley SL et al: Meconium below the vocal cords at delivery: correlation with intrapartum events, *Am J Obstet Gynecol* 1985;153:767.

77. Mitchell J et al: Meconium aspiration and fetal acidosis, *Obstet Gynecol* 1985;65:352.

78. Yeh TF et al: Roentgenographic findings in infants with meconium aspiration syndrome, *JAMA* 1979;242:60.

79. Henleigh P, Loots M: Complications associated with amnioinfusion for meconium, *Am J Obstet Gynecol* 1991;164:317.

80. Wiswell TE et al: Delivery room management of the apparently vigorous meconium-stained neonates: results of the multi-center, international collaborative trial, *Pediatrics* 2000;105:1-17.

81. American Academy of Pediatrics and American College of Obstetricians and Gynecologists: *Guidelines for perinatal care*, Evanston, Ill, AAP/ACOG, 1983;p 69.

82. Hageman JR et al: Delivery room management of meconium staining of the amniotic fluid and the development of meconium aspiration syndrome, *J Perinatol* 1988;8:127.

83. Linder N et al: Need for endotracheal intubation and suction in meconium-stained neonates, *J Pediatr* 1988;112:613.

84. Kresch MJ, Brion LP, Fleischman AR: Delivery room management of meconium-stained neonates, *J Perinatol* 1991;11:46.

85. Davis RO et al: Fatal meconium aspiration syndrome despite airway management considered appropriate, *Am J Obstet Gynecol* 1985;151:731.

86. Vidyasagar D et al: Assisted ventilation in infants with meconium aspiration syndrome, *Pediatrics* 1975;56:208.

87. Wiswell TE: Advances in the treatment of the meconium aspiration syndrome, *Acta Paediatr Suppl* 2001;436:28-30.

88. Wiswell TE et al: Surfactant therapy and high-frequency jet ventilation in the management of a piglet model of the meconium aspiration syndrome, *Pediatr Res* 1994;36:494-500.

89. Findlay RD, Taeusch HW, Walther FJ: Surfactant replacement therapy for meconium aspiration syndrome, *Pediatrics* 1996;97:48-52.

90. Soll RF, Dargaville P: Surfactant for meconium aspiration syndrome in full term infants, *Cochrane Database Syst Rev* 2000;(2):CD002054.

91. Koumbourlis AC, Mutich RL, Moyoyama EK: Contribution of airway hyperresponsiveness to lower airway obstruction after extracorporeal membrane oxygenation for meconium aspiration syndrome, *Crit Care Med* 1995;23:749-754.

92. Barrington KJ et al: Partial liquid ventilation with and without inhaled nitric oxide in a newborn piglet model of meconium aspiration, *Am J Respir Crit Care Med* 1999;160:1922-1927.

93. Shaffer TH et al: Liquid ventilation: effects on pulmonary function in distressed meconium-stained lambs, *Pediatr Res* 1984;18:47.

94. Levin DL et al: Persistent pulmonary hypertension of the newborn infant, *J Pediatr* 1976;89:626.

95. Loeb AL et al: Endothelium-derived relaxing factor in cultured cells, *Hypertension* 1987;9:186.

96. Stevens DC, Schreiner RL: Persistent fetal circulation. In Schreiner RL, Kisling JA, editors: *Practical neonatal respiratory care*, New York, Raven Press, 1982.

97. Geggel RL, Reid L: The structural basis of PPHN, *Clin Perinatol* 1984;11:525.

98. Dworetz AR et al: Survival of infants with persistent pulmonary hypertension without extracorporeal membrane oxygenation, *Pediatrics* 1989;84:1.

99. Drummond WH, Peckham GJ, Fox WW: The clinical profile of the newborn with persistent pulmonary hypertension: observations in 19 affected neonates, *Clin Pediatr* 1977;16:335.

100. Walsh-Sukys MC: Persistent pulmonary hypertension of the newborn: The black box revisited, *Clin Perinatol* 1993;20:127.

101. Peckman GJ, Fox WW: Physiologic factors affecting pulmonary artery pressure in infants with persistent pulmonary hypertension, *J Pediatr* 1978;93:1005.

102. Kohelet D et al: High-frequency oscillation in the rescue of infants with persistent pulmonary hypertension, *Crit Care Med* 1988;16:510.

103. Carlo WA et al: High-frequency jet ventilation in neonatal pulmonary hypertension, *Am J Dis Child* 1989;143:233.

104. Kinsella JP, Abman SH: Inhaled nitric oxide: current and future uses in neonates, *Semin Perinatol* 2000;24:387-395.

105. Clark RH et al: Low-dose nitric oxide therapy for persistent pulmonary hypertension of the newborn. Clinical Inhaled Nitric Oxide Research Group, *N Engl J Med* 2000;342: 469-74.

106. Roberts JD: Inhaled nitric oxide for treatment of pulmonary hypertension in the newborn and infant, *Crit Care Med* 1993;21:S374.

107. Oriot D et al: Paradoxical effect of inhaled nitric oxide in a newborn with pulmonary hypertension, *Lancet* 1993;342:364.

108. Davidson D: NO bandwagon, yet: inhaled nitric oxide (NO) for neonatal pulmonary hypertension, *Am Rev Respir Dis* 1993;147:1078.

109. Kinsella JP, Abman SH: Inhalational nitric oxide therapy for persistent pulmonary hypertension of the newborn, *Pediatrics* 1993;91:997.

110. Kinsella JP et al: Selective and sustained pulmonary vasodilation with inhaled nitric oxide therapy in a child with idiopathic pulmonary hypertension, *J Pediatr* 1993;122:803.

111. Roberts JD Jr et al: Inhaled nitric oxide reverses pulmonary vasoconstriction in the hypoxic and acidotic newborn, *Circ Res* 1993;72:246.

112. Moncada S et al: Nitric oxide: physiology, pathophysiology, and pharmacology, *Pharmacol Rev* 1991;43:109.

113. Davidson D et al: Inhaled nitric oxide for the early treatment of persistent pulmonary hypertension of the term newborn: a randomized, double-masked, placebo- controlled, dose-response, multicenter study. The I-NO/PPHN Study Group, *Pediatrics* 1998;101:325-34.

114. Wessel DL: Inhaled nitric oxide for the treatment of pulmonary hypertension before and after cardiopulmonary bypass, *Crit Care Med* 1993;21:S344.

115. Rich GF et al: Inhaled nitric oxide: selective pulmonary vasodilation in cardiac surgical patients, *Anesthesiology* 1993;78:1028.

116. Gibaldi M: What is nitric oxide and why are so many people studying it. *J Clin Pharmacol* 1993;33:488.

117. Weitzberg E et al: Nitric oxide inhalation attenuates pulmonary hypertension and improves gas exchange in endotoxin shock, *Eur J Pharmacol* 1993;233:85.

118. Bone RC: A new therapy for the adult respiratory distress syndrome, *N Engl J Med* 1993;328:431.

119. Bouchet M et al: Safety requirements for use of inhaled nitric oxide in neonates, *Lancet* 1993;341:968.

120. O'Rourke PP et al: Extracorporeal membrane oxygenation and conventional medical therapy in neonates with persistent pulmonary hypertension of the newborn: a prospective randomized study, *Pediatrics* 1989;84:957.

121. Roberts JD, Shaul PW: Advances in the treatment of persistent pulmonary hypertension of the newborn, *Pediatr Clin North Am* 1993;40:983.

122. Thach BT: Apnea and the sudden infant death syndrome. In Saunders NA, Sullivan CE, editors: *Sleep and breathing*, ed 2, New York, Marcel Dekker; 1994. pp 649-671.

123. Keens TG, Ward SLD: Apnea spells, sudden death, and the role of the apnea monitor, *Pediatr Clin North Am* 1993;40:897.

124. Gerhardt T, Banclari E: Apnea of prematurity: lung function and regulation of breathing, *Pediatrics* 1984;74:58.

125. Toney SB: Apnea. In Fleischer GR, Ludwig S, editors: *Textbook of pediatric emergency medicine*, ed 3, Baltimore, Williams & Wilkins, 1993.

126. Leistner HL: Apnea in infants and children. In Zimmerman S, Gildea J, editors: *Critical care pediatrics*, Philadelphia, WB Saunders, 1985.

127. Martin RJ, Miller MB, Carlo WA: Pathogenesis of apnea in preterm infants, *J Pediatr* 1986;109:733.

128. Rigatto H, Brady JP: Periodic breathing and apnea in preterm infants: I. Hypoxia as a primary event, *Pediatrics* 1972;50:219.

129. Brouillette RT : Hiccups in infants: characteristics and effects on ventilation, *J Pediatr* 1980;96:219.

130. Menon A, Schefft G, Thach BT: Apnea associated with regurgitation in infants, *J Pediatr* 1985;106:625.

131. Aranda JV, Thurman T: Methylxanthines in apnea of prematurity, *Clin Perinatol* 1979;6:87.

132. Osborn DA, Henderson-Smart DJ: Kinesthetic stimulation versus theophylline for apnea in preterm infants. (Cochrane Review). In *The Cochrane Library, Issue 2*. Oxford. Update Software, 2001.

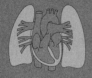

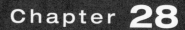

Chapter 28

Surgical Disorders in Childhood That Affect Respiratory Care

SCOTT KECKLER • KURT P. SCHROPP

OUTLINE

Choanal Atresia
Macroglossia
Mandibular Hypoplasia
Esophageal Atresia and Tracheoesophageal Fistula
Congenital Diaphragmatic Hernia
Chest Wall Malformations
    Pectus Excavatum
    Pectus Carinatum
    Asphyxiating Thoracic Dystrophy
    Scoliosis and Kyphoscoliosis

Lung Bud Anomalies
    Incidence
    Clinical Correlation
    Bronchogenic Cyst
    Congenital Cystic Adenomatoid Malformation
    Pulmonary Sequestration
    Congenital Lobar Emphysema
    Follow-up
Gastroschisis/Omphalocele
Necrotizing Enterocolitis

LEARNING OBJECTIVES

After reading this chapter the reader will be able to:

- Discuss the anatomy and pathophysiology of the various congenital anomalies and surgical conditions in newborns and infants.
- Recognize and manage an infant in distress resulting from choanal atresia or other upper airway anomalies.
- Recognize and manage the potential sequelae of upper airway obstruction from upper airway anomalies.
- Discuss the anatomy and pathophysiology of esophageal atresia with or without a tracheal fistula.

- Recognize and manage the signs and symptoms of esophageal atresia with or without a tracheal fistula.
- Discuss the development, anatomy, and pathophysiology of congenital diaphragmatic hernia.
- Recognize and perform the steps related to emergency management of an infant in distress resulting from congenital diaphragmatic hernia.
- Discuss the development, anatomy, and management of the problems associated with chest wall malformations.
- Discuss the anatomy, diagnosis, and management of the infant with lung bud anomalies and pulmonary cystic malformations.

Knowledge of the anatomy and pathophysiology of various congenital anomalies and acquired conditions in childhood is crucial to the proper respiratory care of these patients. Many times the respiratory therapist (RT) will be the first caregiver to recognize that a pathologic condition exists and may be able to make the preliminary diagnosis. This early knowledge can improve respiratory care, especially in emergent situations.

This chapter focuses on the anatomic and physiologic characteristics of the most common congenital anomalies treated by surgery and focuses on the some of the new and sometimes controversial treatments.

CHOANAL ATRESIA

A newborn infant is an obligate nasal breather, so the presence of complete nasal obstruction by choanal atresia results in immediate respiratory distress and possible death by asphyxia. During the newborn's first breaths, the tongue becomes directly associated with the hard and soft palates, creating a vacuum. An oral airway should be inserted and maintained to relieve the airway obstruction.

The exact embryologic malformation causing choanal atresia is unknown; however, certain theories now point to a failure of mesodermal flow to reach preordained positions in the facial process. Any abnormalities in this flow would affect the normal penetration of the nasal pits and the thinning that allows breakthrough at the anterior choana.[1]

Choanal atresia occurs in approximately 1 in 700 live births, with females affected 2:1 over males. Unilateral choanal atresia is twice as common as bilateral choanal atresia. The majority of these atresias are due to bony obstruction or obliteration of the nasal apertures at either the anterior or posterior nasal choana. Fifty percent of patients with choanal atresia have associated congenital anomalies that are either craniofacial or part of a cluster of defects known by the acronym **CHARGE** (colobomas, congenital heart defects, choanal atresia, retarded development, genital hyperplasia, and ear anomalies). Choanal atresia is frequently associated with isolated congenital heart defects.

The clinical presentation of choanal atresia may be severe, with immediate respiratory distress that requires intubation or an oral airway. Unilateral atresia, which may present as a unilateral mucoid discharge, may not cause acute respiratory distress. Alternatively, bilateral atresia or a secondarily obstructed unilateral atresia may present with a pattern of cyanosis cycling with momentary relief from obstruction. The neonate struggles to breathe normally and creates a vacuum between the tongue and the palate, resulting in obstruction and cyanosis. At the point of complete obstruction there is a cry of distress, and the mouth opens to allow relief.

An 8 French catheter is the best diagnostic tool for atresia in the newborn intensive care unit. If the catheter fails to pass through the nose into the oropharynx, choanal atresia should be suspected. The neonate is stabilized by immediately inserting an oral airway. Secondary anomalies should then be sought, and a facial computed tomographic scan with coronal projections, and possibly endoscopy, should be performed to delineate the anomaly. The ultimate management is surgical correction. However, appropriate respiratory care must be provided preoperatively to ensure that the oral or orotracheal airway is maintained until the infant can be brought to the operating room.

The surgical procedure addresses the required perforation of the atresia to establish and maintain adequate choanae. The timing and surgical approach depends on coincidental medical problems; however, infants weighing more than 1.5 kg may be operated on by either the transpalatal or the transnasal route. Recently, endoscopic repair with powered instrumentation has become more popular. However, many feel that this more modern technique is no better than the puncture, dilatation, and stenting technique that has been the gold standard.[2] There are risks and benefits with each procedure; however, the direct visual access afforded by the transpalatal route is preferred by many surgeons.[3] Once the repair is performed, a standard folded endotracheal tube is used to stent the choanae in a U configuration. A 4-mm tube is usually selected for a full-term neonate, and a 3.5-mm tube is used for a premature infant.[4] A suction catheter is measured so that it passes through the end of the stent into the nasopharynx. The catheter is passed through each side of the stent to prevent obstruction. The stent is mobilized every 4 hours to reduce the risk of stenosis and retard granulation tissue formation. Prophylactic antibiotics and steroid drops are given, and the stent is usually removed with the patient under general anesthesia. Continuing respiratory problems due to nasal congestion may be expected for 3 to 4 weeks postoperatively.

The prognosis following reconstruction is excellent and generally without complication; the most significant complication is restenosis of the choanae. This is managed by repeated dilatations of the choanae under endoscopic visualization with replacement of the stent. Rarely tracheostomy or long-term intubation may be required when choanal atresia is complicated by reconstructive maneuvers for other craniofacial abnormalities.

MACROGLOSSIA

Macroglossia, or a greatly enlarged tongue, causes respiratory distress by pharyngeal obstruction. Macroglossia can be associated with other disorders such as the

Beckwith-Wiedemann and Down syndromes, or it may be due to congenital lymphangioma or hemangioma. The diagnosis is relatively straightforward, and polysomnography and pulse oximetry are used to evaluate the extent to which macroglossia affects respiratory function.

Treatment for macroglossia should be individualized, depending on the severity of respiratory obstruction and etiology. For isolated macroglossia, prone positioning usually relieves mild cases. More severe cases may require one of the many surgical techniques to reduce tongue size.[5] Lymphangiomas and small hemangiomas of the tongue may require excision, and large congenital hemangiomas frequently respond to systemic corticosteroid or interferon therapy. Chronic hypoxia and CO_2 retention are frequent sequelae of macroglossia and require close follow-up. Immediate intubation may be necessary along with tracheostomy to temporize for reduction surgery.

MANDIBULAR HYPOPLASIA

Mandibular hypoplasia, or micrognathia, is generally found in conjunction with various other anomalies in conditions such as the Pierre Robin syndrome or Treacher Collins syndrome. The Pierre Robin syndrome is the most common of these associations, but the pathophysiology of respiratory distress associated with micrognathia is identical in the other disorders.

The primary features of the Pierre Robin syndrome include micrognathia, glossoptosis (or posterior displacement of the tongue), and cleft palate. These features result in pharyngeal obstruction and respiratory distress. If left untreated, infants with respiratory complications such as airway obstruction, cor pulmonale, and pulmonary hypertension have a mortality rate approaching 30%. Other complications of the Pierre Robin syndrome are failure to thrive, malnutrition, chronic hypoxia, and pneumonia. Recent polysomnographic studies using oximetry have demonstrated that hypoxia and CO_2 retention can occur without overt signs of airway obstruction.[6] Close monitoring and a complete evaluation must be performed before and for a time after therapy has been instituted.

Treatment for patients with micrognathia includes positioning, an intraoral or nasopharyngeal airway, and surgical procedures. Prone positioning combined with supplemental oxygen administration and carefully supervised feedings has been useful in treating mild forms of micrognathia. Intraoral and nasopharyngeal tubes or prostheses have been used in treating mild to moderate forms of micrognathia, but feeding difficulties limit the usefulness of these techniques. Surgical procedures designed to hold the tongue forward have

been advocated for symptomatic and severe forms of the disorder. These procedures include suture transfixion, creation of lip-tongue adhesion with sutures, and various sling procedures. The most severe cases may require tracheostomy. All of these treatments are designed to "buy time," as these disorders gradually improve with facial growth.

Great care must be used in treating these patients, and may fiberoptic assistance may be required for intubation. Patients with Treacher Collins Syndrome may be extremely difficult not only to intubate but to mask if there are temporal mandibular joint abnormalities.[7]

ESOPHAGEAL ATRESIA AND TRACHEOESOPHAGEAL FISTULA

Esophageal atresia and tracheoesophageal fistula represent a clinical spectrum of different malformations. The most essential elements of their pathophysiology are the blockage of the passage of saliva or food by esophageal atresia and the aspiration of either salivary contents or gastric secretions through a fistula between the trachea and esophagus.

Esophageal atresia and associated tracheoesophageal fistula result from an unknown in utero malformation that is one of the better-characterized embryologic foregut anomalies. Separation of the dorsal foregut from the ventral trachea begins distally at the carinal area and progresses proximally. If these two structures remain fused during this process, tracheoesophageal anomalies occur as atresias, fistulas, or laryngotracheal clefts. Different embryonic studies have focused on the "ingrowth" of the epithelial ridge in this area, which must be uninterrupted for complete tracheoesophageal formation. For unknown reasons, this constellation of tracheal and esophageal abnormalities may be associated with other midline vertebral, anal, cardiac, and renal or peripheral limb anomalies, which are known by the acronym the VACTERL (vertebral, anal, cardiac, tracheal, esophageal, renal, limb) syndrome.[8]

Tracheoesophageal fistula and esophageal atresia have been anatomically classified to describe the presence or absence of esophageal atresia and whether there is an associated fistula (Figure 28-1). This has important management as well as operative significance.[9] The most common combination of lesions is esophageal atresia associated with a distal tracheoesophageal fistula (see Figure 28-1, A). More than 85% of patients will present with this form of the anomaly, which results in a blind-ending upper esophageal pouch of variable length associated with a fistula from the lower trachea or main stem bronchi that leads into the distal esophagus. The second most common anomaly occurs in 5% of patients

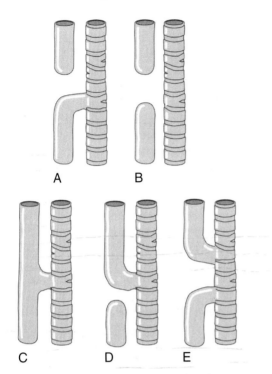

FIGURE 28-1 Five anatomic classifications describing tracheoesophageal fistula and esophageal atresia. **A,** Esophageal atresia with a distal tracheoesophageal fistula. **B,** Isolated esophageal atresia with a long gap of missing esophagus between proximal and distal esophageal pouches. **C,** Tracheoesophageal fistula without esophageal atresia, "*H*-type." **D,** Esophageal atresia with proximal fistula. **E,** Esophageal atresia with both proximal and distal tracheoesophageal fistulas.

as isolated esophageal atresia with a proximal blind-ending pouch and a "long gap" of missing esophagus above a small distal esophageal pouch (see Figure 28-1, *B*). In 3% of patients, esophageal atresia may be associated with a proximal and distal tracheoesophageal fistula. In addition, there is the isolated tracheoesophageal fistula that presents without atresia and usually occurs in the lower cervical or upper thoracic area. This is known as the *H*-type fistula. Finally, the fifth group represents 1% of patients who present with esophageal atresia with an isolated proximal fistula in the same configuration as seen with the isolated *H*-type fistula. In this condition, there is a "long gap" and then a small distal esophageal pouch with no distal tracheoesophageal fistula.

Drooling is the first symptom in the majority of newborns with esophageal atresia. The first feedings result in choking, coughing, and episodes of cyanosis. The respiratory distress may be severe and progressive, which should prompt an immediate work-up for esophageal atresia. If esophageal atresia is suspected, a stiff nasogastric tube is introduced until resistance is met. The tube is connected to constant suction and irrigated with 1 to 2 ml of saline at frequent intervals.

Esophageal atresia with tracheoesophageal fistula occurs in 1 in 3000 births with an equal male and female distribution. Because of the obstruction to amniotic fluid during fetal swallowing, polyhydramnios may be part of the perinatal history. The postnatal presentation of each type of anomaly varies significantly with the lesion and consequences of obstruction or aspiration. An isolated tracheoesophageal fistula may present as late as early adulthood with subtle symptoms of wheezing and recurrent respiratory infections. For infants with larger fistulas, choking and coughing episodes will be frequent. Significant abdominal distention caused by excessive air moving from the respiratory tract to the gastrointestinal tract through a patent fistula may also be a presenting symptom. Auscultation of the chest may reveal murmurs from concomitant congenital heart disease or decreased breath sounds caused by atelectasis or pneumonitis.

Chest and abdominal radiographs are critical to the diagnosis. Several important radiographic findings are specific for esophageal atresia. The course and end-point of the nasogastric tube confirms obstruction of the proximal esophagus by atresia and determines the relative position of the upper esophageal pouch. The lung fields must be examined to determine the presence of parenchymal changes resulting from aspiration. Changes in mediastinal structures give an early indication of congenital heart disease, and a careful search is made for the aortic arch to determine its left- or right-sided position. This is extremely important for surgical management because it directs the surgeon to an operative site away from the arch.

The next most important finding is the presence or absence of a gastric bubble. Proximal atresia with evidence of air in the gastrointestinal tract indicates a distal tracheoesophageal fistula, the most common form of the anomaly. A proximal obstruction without evidence of gas distally most likely indicates the presence of esophageal atresia with or without smaller fistulas. Other studies that aid in the diagnosis of related congenital anomalies include an echocardiogram, a renal ultrasound, and a vertebral spine film. The echocardiogram needs to be done preoperatively not only to identify heart defects but to help identify the aortic arch.

Once the diagnosis is made, the overall clinical condition of the infant dictates the timing of repair.[10] For patients who present with severe respiratory distress and low birth weight, mechanical ventilation is essential.[11] It may be necessary to perform an emergency procedure to divide a persistent distal tracheoesophageal fistula if delivered tidal volume is compromised and respiratory failure progresses. Operative maneuvers that allow placement of balloon catheters in the fistula or stapling of the distal esophagus have been described. The traditional approach is a right thoracotomy with an extrapleural dissection for direct separation and closure of the fistula and trachea. With improved antibiotics many surgeons have changed to a transpleural approach, worrying less about an empyema. Once that is accomplished, a primary anastomosis of the esophagus can be performed in larger, more stable babies.

The last few years has seen a great increase in the number of tracheoesophageal fistula repairs with minimally invasive surgery. It is hypothesized that there will be a better cosmetic result than with thoracotomy and also decreased scoliosis and pain. In a recent multi-institutional study of 104 neonates with attempted repair with minimally invasive surgery, only 4.8% were converted to an open surgery. There was an 11.5% leak rate and 31.7 % late stricture rate.[12] Long-term follow-up is needed to decide if this difficult surgery will replace the "gold standard" thoracotomy.

In esophageal atresia, the ability to successfully perform esophageal anastomoses has been life-saving.[13] The most significant complication of primary esophageal anastomosis is stricture or recurrent fistula formation. These complications have important implications for postoperative respiratory care. Even infants with successful anastomoses have persistent respiratory problems. With or without complications, postoperative respiratory symptoms have been noted in up to 50% of patients. Complications range from apnea and bradycardia to aspiration, recurrent pneumonia, and even respiratory arrest.[14] The largest single cause of persistent respiratory disease is gastroesophageal reflux from either esophageal dysmotility or an abnormal lower esophageal sphincter. Infants with reflux have recurrent aspiration pneumonias that must be treated medically; however, many of these infants require further operative management with some form of gastroesophageal fundoplication.

Another large group born with esophageal atresia, with or without tracheoesophageal fistula, has persistent tracheomalacia.[15] This is a much more difficult group of patients to manage. For those with tracheomalacia with even the slightest esophageal stricture formation, however, dilatation of the anastomotic stricture may alleviate much of the respiratory compromise. It is possible that recurrent fistulas or an undiscovered proximal fistula may be the source of persistent wheezing and respiratory difficulty. These fistulas can be diagnosed and defined with the use of a barium esophagogram with direct pressure injection at different levels of the esophagus.

With precise preoperative, perioperative, and postoperative management, the survival rate in infants with esophageal atresia has now approached greater than 95%. The respiratory care during each phase must be tailored with an understanding of the pathophysiology of each malformation and its related complications.

CONGENITAL DIAPHRAGMATIC HERNIA

The diaphragm forms when the pleura and the peritoneum fuse during the eighth week of embryonic life. During closure the pleuroperitoneal canals may remain open. These canals are located on the posteriorlateral portions of the diaphragm, and if they fail to fuse abdominal contents may herniate into the chest cavity.[16] The resulting defect is termed a Bochdalek's hernia and is more common on the left side (90%). The defect ranges is size from 2 to 3 mm to complete absence of the diaphragm. The herniated contents cause compression of the developing ipsilateral lung bud. The contralateral side may be compressed as well from shift of the mediastinum (Figure 28-2). The lung tissue is hypoplastic including the pulmonary vasculature, even on the contralateral side. Histologic studies demonstrate increased musculature in the media of the arterioles. After birth hypoxia, hypercapnia, and acidosis develop causing constriction of the arterioles. This constriction exacerbates pulmonary hypertension and persistent fetal circulation.

Infants with congenital diaphragmatic hernia (CDH) usually develop respiratory distress shortly after birth. The diagnosis of CDH is confirmed by chest radiography but is suggested in a tachypneic newborn with a scaphoid abdomen. After diagnosis resuscitation is immediately begun. The aim is to prevent hypoxia, hypercapnia, and acidosis [17] and includes the following steps:

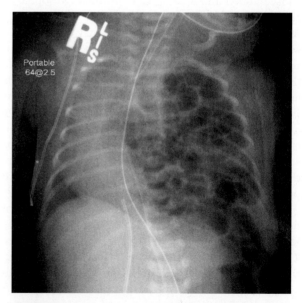

FIGURE 28-2 Radiograph of a left-sided congenital diaphragmatic hernia. Note shift of the mediastinum to the right.

1. A large orogastric tube is placed to decompress the gastrointestinal tract.
2. Bag mask ventilation is avoided in order to keep the gut in the chest from becoming distended and causing tension pneumothorax physiology.
3. An endotracheal tube is inserted and the infant is placed on mechanical ventilation avoiding high airway pressures.
4. Barotrauma may be avoided by using high-frequency oscillatory ventilation.
5. Maintaining alkalosis reduces the amount of pulmonary vasospasm. Traditionally $PaCO_2$ values were kept between 25 and 30 mm Hg. But recently a protocol of "permissive hypercapnia" with increased $PaCO_2$s and decreased pHs seems to be safe.
6. If a pneumothorax is seen, chest tube placement is indicated. The pneumothorax is seen on the contralateral side and results from excessive ventilation pressures.

Operative repair of the hernia does not reverse pulmonary hypertension or hypoplasia. The timing of operative repair has evolved from immediate repair to delayed repair. Multiple studies have shown better outcomes by allowing the infant to stabilize and adapt to postnatal life.[18] Surgical repair decreases thoracic wall compliance, further strengthening the argument for the delayed operative approach.[19] A transabdominal approach is the standard technique for repair. If small, the defect is repaired with permanent sutures alone. Larger defects may require a prosthetic patch. After surgical repair, air may remain in the ipsilateral pleural cavity. The expanding lung does not completely fill the cavity, so technically a pneumothorax does not exist. The normal placement of a chest tube to suction may be detrimental so it is used for gravity drainage only. Too rapid a shift of the mediastinum and contralateral lung may cause lung rupture or obstruct the vascular structures.

Following operative repair, most infants remain intubated for several days. Low-volume strategies are continued. Elevated pulmonary vascular resistance may develop 8 to 24 hours postoperatively. This elevation will worsen right to left shunting causing hypoxia and acidosis. Multiple modalities are used to decrease the amount of pulmonary artery vasospasm. Tolazoline, an adrenergic blocker, has been used in the past but side effects including fluid retention and hypotension limit the use. The inotrope dopamine when used at higher concentrations (10 mcg/kg/min) causes vasoconstriction. Raising systemic vascular resistance will tend to reverse the right to left shunt. High doses of dopamine will also cause vasoconstriction of the gut which is already at high risk for ischemia. Nitric oxide (NO) is a potent pulmonary vasodilator and its use in pulmonary hypertension has been established.[20] A large, randomized clinical trial using inhaled NO for infants with CDH did not reduce mortality or the need for extracorporeal membrane oxygenation (ECMO).[21] NO may be of benefit further along in the clinical course.

ECMO has probably increased the survival rates in neonates with CDH. This modality is often used to stabilize patients before surgery.[22] In recent years the use of ECMO for patients with CDH has decreased as different ventilator modalities including high-frequency oscillatory ventilation (HFOV) are increasingly utilized. The use of ECMO at a large pediatric hospital was analyzed. The number of patients on ECMO had decreased as the number of alternate therapies had increased. Nitric oxide, HFOV, and surfactant were the main alternatives. While the number of ECMO patients had decreased, the run time for each patient had increased.[23]

Experimental surgical treatments for CDH have been developed as well. Fetal intervention to include in utero repair of CDH was first performed in 1990.[24] Surgical techniques have been refined but survival has not increased. Currently no indications exist for in utero repair of CDH. With improved technique of fetal surgery this modality has been used for another surgical intervention, tracheal occlusion (TO). Experimental studies have shown reduced pulmonary hypoplasia with TO.[22] This procedure is currently performed at a few specialized centers with long-term results unknown at this time.

CHEST WALL MALFORMATIONS

A wide spectrum of chest wall malformations is seen in children. These can range from mild deformities that have primarily cosmetic implications and the attendant impact on self-esteem to severe deformities with high morbidity and mortality.

Pectus Excavatum

Pectus excavatum is the most common disorder of the chest wall, comprising almost 90% of chest wall deformities. The defect may range for small, deep deformities to large, shallow deformities. The term *funnel chest* has often been applied. Deformity of the cartilaginous ends of the rib causes an inward curve of the sternum. This inward curve will decrease the anteroposterior diameter of the chest, causing compression of the underlying structures. Familial cases have been reported; however, most are sporadic.[25] A male-to-female ratio of 4:1 is reported in the literature.[26] Connective tissue disorders are also associated with pectus excavatum; Marfan's syndrome and Ehlers-Danlos syndrome are seen in 3% and 2.2% of patients, respectively.[27]

Most defects are noted in infancy and progress with the child. Neonates may present with chest wall retraction during respiration due to the pliability of the chest wall. This has been termed "pseudopectus excavatum" and often disappears at 6 months of age. During infancy the defect often has no symptoms, but as the chest wall becomes more rigid and activity is increased symptoms often develop. With a decreased AP diameter of the chest the lungs are not able to fully expand; therefore, exercise capacity decreases. The heart is often displaced reducing ventricular filling, further decreasing exercise tolerance. Arrhythmias are another sequela of the altered chest wall diameter. Significant psychosocial effects are seen in these patients. Causative factors of exercise intolerance and embarrassment in front of peers when the shirt is removed, contribute to low self-esteem. Surgical repair has been shown to alleviate these effects.[28]

The age to undertake surgical correction had been debated in the literature. Repairing the defect at too early an age may limit chest wall mechanics and growth.[29] As children progress through puberty cartilage ossifies. The ossification of chest wall cartilage will make more extensive procedures necessary in the future. Secondary scoliosis may also develop if the defect is not repaired. Although a consensus has not been reached, most symptomatic children should be repaired between 7 to 14 years of age. The standard open approach for repair of pectus excavatum was described in 1912 but was modified 1949 by Ravitch.[30] This repair involves a transverse incision along the inframammary crease with exposure and resection of the involved cartilages. The sternum is then elevated and a strut is left in place. Within the last 15 years a minimally invasive approach pioneered by Nuss has been developed.[31] Bilateral incisions are made on the lateral chest and a retrosternal bar is passed between the sternum and the heart. The bar is then rotated 180 degrees, forcing the sternum anteriorly. The bar is left in place with annual follow-up appointments documenting growth and activity level. Most bars are left in an average of three years then removed. Overall results are excellent and the morbidity of an open repair is avoided. The major disadvantage seems to be that the immediate postoperative pain is worse than with the open procedure.

Pectus Carinatum

This defect, which accounts for 5% of chest wall deformities, is the opposite of pectus excavatum. Pectus carinatum is usually seen later in life around a growth spurt. The protrusion is most commonly located on the lower sternum. Since the sternum is protruded, the underlying structures are not compressed. The primary complaint is cosmetic. Surgical repair involves costochondral resection and sternotomy.[32] Results are excellent with rare recurrence.

Asphyxiating Thoracic Dystrophy

Asphyxiating thoracic dystrophy, also known as Jeune's syndrome, is a rare genetic disorder with an autosomal recessive inheritance pattern. This disorder is an osteochondrodystrophy that may have mild to severe expressions. The chest cavity is decreased in both the anteroposterior and superior and inferior orientations. Pulmonary development is often blunted due to the decreased cavity size, and postpartum the lungs are not able to fully expand. Multiple associated defects, including polydactyly, hypoplastic iliac wings, and fixed clavicles, may be seen.[33]

Recent surgical advances using prosthetic titanium ribs and expansion thoracoplasty have met with success[34]. The technique involves anterior and posterior rib osteotomies in ribs 3 to 9. This creates a mobilized segment that is then attached to the titanium prosthesis, which has been anchored to the 2nd and 10th ribs. The procedure is done in two stages three months apart. Every 6 months the devices are expanded.

Scoliosis and Kyphoscoliosis

In their severest forms scoliosis and kyphoscoliosis may lead to secondary chest wall deformities. The resulting chest wall deformity will decrease lung capacity.

LUNG BUD ANOMALIES

The term *lung bud anomaly* broadly describes four pathologic entities in a spectrum of parenchymal disease: bronchogenic cyst, congenital cystic adenomatoid malformation, pulmonary sequestration, and congenital lobar emphysema. The pathogenesis of these anomalies is poorly understood, but some speculation can be made based on known embryologic sequences.[35,36] In early fetal development a tube of endodermal epithelium, the cellular covering of all body cavities, is present along the entire longitudinal axis of the fetus. This tube, the primordial gastrointestinal tract, is referred to as the primitive foregut. At approximately 3 weeks of gestation, a small groove appears in the floor of the primitive foregut, near the oral end of the fetus (Figure 28-3). The groove develops into a ridge, and the ridge branches into two blind pouches at its distal end. This ridge eventually develops into the trachea, and the thickenings are referred to as lung buds; the entire ridge with the lung buds will eventually migrate away from the main epithelial tube, thus separating the early pulmonary system from the esophagus.

As these endodermal structures develop, their blood supply is formed from primitive tributaries to the aorta—the fourth and sixth aortic arches. The lung derives its blood supply from two distinct sources: (1) the pulmonary artery (sixth arch), which brings oxygen-poor

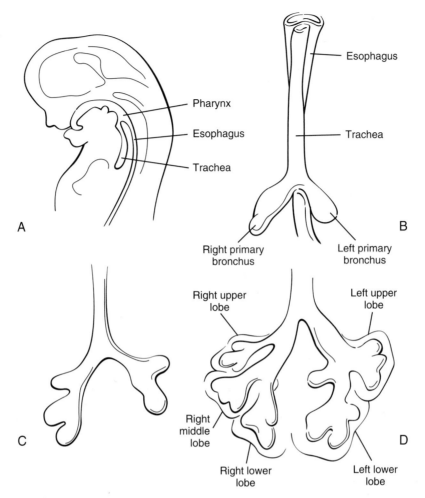

FIGURE 28-3 Developmental anatomy of the lung. The pulmonary tree develops from a common tube with the esophagus **(A).** By 3 weeks of gestation, the trachea (anterior) is separate from the esophagus. Two blind pouches that represent the left and right lung buds have appeared at the distal end of the primitive pulmonary system **(B).** Further dichotomous branching of the main bronchi results in the main lobes of each lung **(C and D).**

blood from systemic veins for oxygenation, and (2) the bronchial arteries (direct branches of the arch), which bring oxygen-rich blood to the parenchyma of the lung for nutritive purposes.

The budding part of the tube is composed of endoderm, a multipotential tissue in the embryo that forms the "business end" of each organ (e.g., the alveoli of the lungs, the mucosa of the gastrointestinal tract, the nephron of the kidney). The lung buds grow into the mesoderm, which is also a multipotential tissue that forms, in each organ, the connective tissue and the important supporting framework, including the blood vessels.

The interaction between these tissues is important in the development of each organ. In the primitive pulmonary system, the bud-forming endoderm induces important changes in the surrounding mesoderm that lead to a cohesive, functioning organ. Knowledge of these processes may help to explain how each anomaly occurs. For example, if both lung buds fail to form, the fetus would have bilateral pulmonary agenesis, which is incompatible with life; however, unilateral pulmonary agenesis is survivable. If the longitudinal groove with its attached buds fails to completely separate from the epithelial tube, a laryngoesophageal cleft or tracheoesophageal fistula may result. Although the exact nature of the developmental cause behind each anomaly is unclear, I will speculate as to the embryologic defect underlying the four lesions that compose lung bud anomalies as each anomaly is discussed.

Incidence

As a group, these entities are considered uncommon but not rare. Many factors make a precise assessment of the incidence extremely difficult. Some cystic pulmonary disease may result from barotrauma, rather than having a congenital origin. Asymptomatic patients may be uncounted because sequestrations may be silent for many years and become evident only during clinical investigation for unrelated complaints. Congenital lobar emphysema has been thought to resolve spontaneously, which may result in an underestimate of its true incidence.

Clinical Correlation

Although these lung bud anomalies have different histopathology, there are patterns in clinical presentation common to all. The presentation seems to follow two distinct patterns: (1) the condition becomes obvious in the early newborn period and is manifested by respiratory distress and (2) the condition occurs later in childhood and is characterized by repeated infections.

Newborns may be identified in the delivery room if the lesion is so large that immediate respiratory distress and circulatory compromise result. A cyst or emphysematous lobe can obstruct blood flow to the right side of the heart, causing edema that results in a "hydropic" appearance.

In many cases, the distress is not readily apparent but is characterized by a progressive course of intermittent tachypnea over the first few days or weeks. During this period a chest radiograph may be taken and the diagnosis suggested based on location and character of the lesion. In lobar emphysema, there is a hyperlucent lobe with a surrounding zone of atelectasis. The atelectasis may be interpreted as pneumonia, and the hyperlucent abnormal lung is accordingly misinterpreted as normal compensatory hyperinflation. Intubation and hyperventilation in this situation could be disastrous. An emphysematous lobe will expand preferentially according to the law of Laplace. As it enlarges and pressure in the chest rises from the expanding mass, blood return to the thoracic cavity becomes impaired. As the infant's condition worsens, the clinician may mistake the emphysematous lobe for a pneumothorax because of its similar clinical behavior—a shift of the mediastinum to the opposite side and hyperresonance on the affected side. A chest tube inserted into this lobe may considerably worsen the situation.

An important aspect of the differential diagnosis includes a consideration that a "multilocular cyst" may actually be air-filled loops of bowel from a CDH. Auscultation for bowel sounds may help to differentiate these two problems, as will decompression of the bowel loops with a nasogastric tube (pulmonary cysts will not decompress). In some cases, an upper gastrointestinal series may be necessary to differentiate these conditions.

Presentation in the newborn is due to a mass effect in the small thoracic space. Bronchogenic cysts and cystic adenomatoid malformations do not have direct communications with the bronchial tree, but air can still enter these cysts through the pores of Kohn. Some cysts contain tissue so immature that they lack these pores, and air entry is not possible. These lesions, lacking a way for air to enter, are not likely to expand abruptly in the newborn period. Cysts with pores or emphysematous lobes, however, will enlarge with ventilation and can present under tension. Should a cyst rupture, the lesion may present mimicking a pneumothorax. This is rare and less frequent than a pneumothorax caused by insertion of a chest tube into an intact cyst. As a cyst or lobe enlarges, it may directly compress the trachea, a major bronchus, or the vena cava. Even without direct compression of these structures, the pressure rise within the thorax can cause mediastinal deviation with its attendant consequences of decreased venous return. Presentation in the newborn period with tension may require emergency thoracotomy and resection.

After infancy, the most common presentation is with repeated or prolonged episodes of pneumonia despite adequate antibiotic coverage. The infectious course arises because the contents of the cyst do not communicate with the tracheobronchial tree, allowing bacteria and debris to accumulate in the cyst. This material cannot be cleared and acts as a nidus for infection, which often spreads to adjacent healthy tissue and lymph nodes in the hilum of the involved lung. Thus, a small infected cyst can result in pneumonia with fever and purulent cough. Although antibiotics are helpful, they are not curative and the underlying cause, that is, the cyst, must be resected to prevent recurrence of pulmonary infections.

The indolent course of this process may result in these children undergoing extensive diagnostic evaluation before the correct diagnosis is reached. There are usually numerous radiographs that, in retrospect, implicate a particular lobe. An ultrasound may have been obtained to evaluate cystic-appearing structures. Computed tomography or magnetic resonance imaging may have been used to elucidate airway anatomy and tissue density in the hope of securing a cause for frequent pneumonias. A child may have also undergone bronchoscopy to rule out aspiration of a foreign body. Bronchoscopy, however, has limited usefulness for the patient whose lung bud anomaly has already been diagnosed and could be dangerous if it causes complete obstruction of a lobe that previously was only partially obstructed. The diagnosis should be suspected when a febrile, septic child has a tube thoracostomy performed for drainage of a postpneumonic empyema and the cavity occupied by the now-drained fluid does not collapse, indicating an infected cyst, rather than an empyema. Serial chest radiographs are the most valuable source of information in reaching the diagnosis.

Resection of the infected cyst is curative. Preoperative treatment with antibiotics is important. In patients with severe sepsis, initial simple drainage of the cavity may be required for temporary palliation, allowing time for optimal preparation of the patient before definitive surgery.

As prenatal ultrasound has improved in the last decade, it has become apparent that many of these lesions identified prenatally become smaller or completely disappear. Controversy, therefore, exists as to the nonemergent treatment of these lesions, especially the small, asymptomatic abnormalities.[37] The correct treatment of these incidentally discovered lesions will evolve as they as they are more frequently treated at a later stage or nonoperatively.

Bronchogenic Cyst

The bronchogenic cyst may be thought of as a lung bud cyst, with endoderm that differentiates into respiratory epithelium but without normal bronchial components. It is therefore nonfunctional. These cysts can be located either within the thoracic cavity or outside it. When intrathoracic, the cyst can be in the bronchial wall, the pleura, the mediastinum, or the parenchyma of the lung itself. Ten percent of mediastinal masses are bronchogenic cysts. They are commonly located in the retrocarinal region (Figure 28-4, A). When intrapulmonary, they are usually on the right and may be multiple or multilocular (Figure 28-4, B).

The diagnosis of a bronchogenic cyst may be apparent radiologically in the newborn with respiratory distress where the radiograph reveals a circular or ovoid mass with smooth edges. Similarly, the radiograph can suggest the diagnosis in an older child who presents with stridor, wheezing, or recurrent pneumonia.

Treatment of bronchogenic cysts is surgical excision. The extent of resection will depend on the location of the cyst and any associated inflammatory conditions.

A unilocular cyst can usually be enucleated or removed by wedge resection and be an ideal case for a minimally invasive thoracoscopy. Lobectomy is performed in the exceptional case. A pneumonectomy is rarely needed.[38]

Congenital Cystic Adenomatoid Malformation

Congenital cystic adenomatoid malformation (CCAM), originally described in 1949,[38] has been recognized more frequently in recent years. In this lesion, differentiation of mesenchymal tissue appears to stop at the bronchial stage, before cartilage develops. The lesion is a hamartoma, that is, a disorganized overgrowth of embryonal tissue. This lesion reflects a failure of the inductive process, discussed earlier.

The morphologic appearance of this lesion may be of a single large cavitary cyst (type I), multiple small cysts (type II), or a solid mass (type III). The CCAM may be multilobular and bilateral, but it is most commonly located in the left lung. The clinical presentation and radiographic diagnosis are similar to those of a bronchogenic cyst. The surgical treatment usually requires a lobectomy and occasionally a pneumonectomy. Unlike a bronchogenic cyst, this lesion cannot usually be enucleated. Unless there is unusually extensive or bilateral disease, the postoperative course is smooth and the prognosis is excellent. Larger lesions, however, may be associated with pulmonary hypoplasia, hypertension, hydrops fetalis, and myocardiopathy. These features, depending on their magnitude, are associated with a severe prognosis. CCAMs are occasionally severe enough to warrant prenatal intervention ranging from thoracoamniotic shunt to fetal thoracotomy.[39]

Pulmonary Sequestration

Sequestrations are foci of mature lung tissue separate from the rest of the tracheobronchial tree, with concomitant failure of separation of the pulmonary and

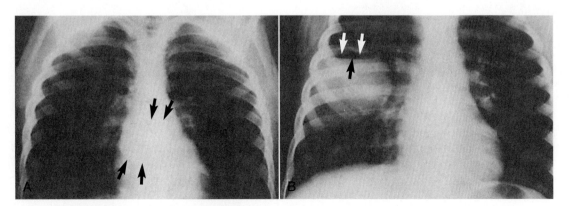

FIGURE 28-4 Bronchogenic cysts. **A,** Note the smooth border of the round, retrocarinal mass on this radiograph *(arrows).* **B,** Chest radiograph demonstrates an intraparenchymal mass that has become infected. Note the air-fluid level *(arrows).* This cyst is located on the right, which is typical of intraparenchymal bronchogenic cysts.

systemic circulations. The tissue may be either nonaerated or aerated through collateral channels (i.e., pores of Kohn), albeit with poor gas exchange. The sequestration typically has a systemic arterial blood supply (Figure 28-5). In intrapulmonary sequestrations the venous drainage is usually into the pulmonary veins; in extrapulmonary sequestrations the drainage is into systemic veins (azygos or hemiazygos vein, inferior vena cava, or right atrium). The extrapulmonary variety has a separate pleural envelope and may lie below the diaphragm. The defect in development may be caused by migration of an accessory lung bud before separation of the systemic and pulmonary circulations. Sequestrations are most commonly located in the left lower lobe region.

The patient with a sequestration may present with a variety of clinical symptoms, including a large shunt, a heart murmur, and heart failure.[40] A large, nonfunctional intrathoracic mass can present as obstructive respiratory signs such as wheezing and tachypnea. A common presentation is a recurrent febrile course with an occult infected sequestration.

The diagnosis of pulmonary sequestration can be elusive. A space-occupying lesion with or without an air-fluid level is often seen on a plain chest radiograph.[41] If a sequestration is suspected, an arteriogram can be diagnostic and help define the arterial anatomy, which is crucial to successful resection. The systemic arterial supply may arise directly from the aorta, at times even through the diaphragm from the intraabdominal

aorta. Injury or inadvertent division of this vessel without proper control may result in a hemorrhagic catastrophe. An upper gastrointestinal contrast study may reveal a fistulous connection to the intestinal tract.

Radionuclide lung scanning may reveal an unventilated but perfused mass in the chest. Finally, computed tomography can demonstrate extrathoracic lesions, and magnetic resonance imaging can visualize any abnormal blood supply. Resection of the mass is curative. Resection of the extrapulmonary variety is usually an easy thoracoscopic procedure, with the major risk being losing control of the systemic vessel.

Congenital Lobar Emphysema

Congenital lobar emphysema is an overdistention of one lobe of the lung, usually one of the upper lobes.[42] The lobe becomes distended because air enters but cannot exit, often owing to obstruction of a segmental or lobar bronchus. Alternatively, there may be a defect in the cartilage so that increases in parenchymal pressure during expiration cause the bronchus to collapse.[43] This results in airway obstruction and air trapping. Additionally, an aberrant artery or vascular ring may compress the bronchus during expiration. Regardless of the cause, the lobe becomes progressively more distended, eventually causing obstruction to air entry at the main bronchus or trachea and obstruction of venous return to the right atrium. These two conditions, separately or together, may constitute a surgical emergency.

The radiographic appearance may be confusing. Normal lung in proximity to the diseased lung tissue may be collapsed and appear atelectatic or consolidated (Figure 28-6). Thus, the child with respiratory distress

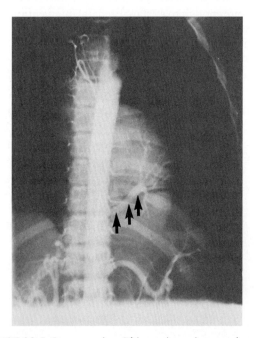

FIGURE 28-5 Sequestration. This aortic angiogram shows the segment of lung above the diaphragm that is supplied by a vessel from below the diaphragm *(arrows)*. The splenic and hepatic branches of the celiac axis are seen below.

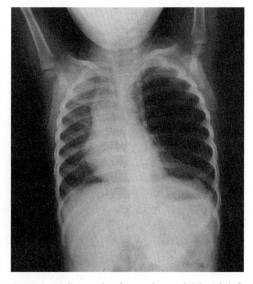

FIGURE 28-6 Radiograph of a newborn child with left-sided congenital lobar emphysema.

and such a radiograph may be thought to have pneumonia, with the real diagnosis unsuspected. Recognition of this lesion is critical early in the symptomatic course because of the general tendency to hyperventilate a child in respiratory distress. In the case of lobar emphysema, such a maneuver would hasten circulatory collapse by rapidly overdistending the affected lobe. Without a confirmatory radiograph, a chest tube may be inadvertently inserted into the emphysematous lobe with disastrous consequences. Resection of the lobe is curative.

Follow-up

Children tolerate these operations remarkably well. Postoperatively, the patient will have a chest tube that is usually removed within a few days of the operation but may have no tubes at all if the procedure was done thoracoscopically. Analgesics are important so that the child will breathe deeply and open atelectatic areas. For children too young to understand the use of incentive spirometry, instructing them to take the kind of deep breath required before blowing soap bubbles or spinning a windmill will achieve the same effect. Patient-controlled anesthesia in the older child, intrapleural or epidural anesthesia, intercostal blocks, and intravenous morphine are all important postoperative pain control strategies. Adequate analgesia also permits chest physical therapy, which is crucial in the recovery process.[44] Recovery is usually rapid, and normal growth is to be expected. When the child has an isolated lung bud anomaly, the prognosis is excellent. For bilateral or extensive disease, or when there are associated cardiac or genetic anomalies, the prognosis may be worse and is related mostly to the degree of parenchymal involvement or the associated anomaly.

GASTROSCHISIS/ OMPHALOCELE

The development of the abdominal wall and gastrointestinal tract come from three embryonic folds—cephalic, caudal, and lateral—composed of splanchnic and somatic tissue. If these folds fail to develop normally, a defect is seen in the abdominal wall.[45] The two most common defects are omphalocele and gastroschisis.

When the lateral folds fail to fuse, an omphalocele will develop. This defect is always at the umbilicus and covered by a peritoneal sac although this sac may rupture to expose the viscera (Figure 28-7). Omphalocele occurs early during fetal development, at the time of organogenesis, so other defects are commonly seen. These defects include cardiac, sternal, hindgut, and bladder defects with cardiac being the most common. Approximately one third of patients will have trisomy 13, 18, or 21. Diagnosis is often made during prenatal visits with ultrasonography. Elevated levels of alpha

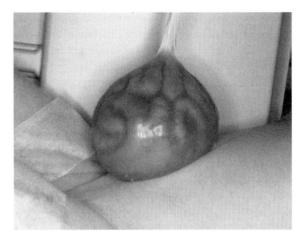

FIGURE 28-7 Baby with moderate-sized omphalocele.

fetoprotein in the maternal serum and amniotic fluid are often times present.[46] After delivery the gastrointestinal tract should be decompressed with nasogastric suction as well as digital rectal examination to assist with meconium passage. Small to medium defects are often repaired primarily. After reduction and repair, pressure parameters such as airway and intragastric should be monitored. Larger defects may require a staged repair. The first stage uses Silastic sheets or a spring-loaded silo to reduce the size of the sac to the fascial level and thereby permit definitive closure.[47] The defect may include the liver, which should be handled with care to prevent liver laceration or hepatic vein injury. The incidence of omphalocele has decreased recently as more of these fetuses are aborted.

Gastroschisis is thought to develop when the umbilical coelom fails to form. The expanding gut cannot be contained in the peritoneal cavity and herniates to the right of the umbilicus[45] (Figure 28-8). The right umbilical vein reabsorbs leaving a weakness in the abdominal wall allowing herniation. Gastroschisis has been reported on the left

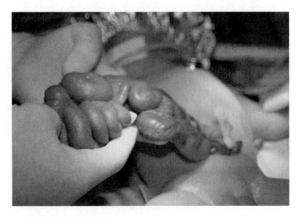

FIGURE 28-8 Typical appearance of bowel in a patient with gastroschisis.

side but is extremely rare. This anomaly develops later in gestation than does omphalocele, so associated defects are not usually seen with the exception of intestinal atresias, which occur in 15% of patients.[48] The herniated viscera are not covered by peritoneum so this defect should be repaired early. After delivery the gastrointestinal tract should be decompressed as in the case of omphalocele. Since the viscera are exposed, the infant should be placed in a sterile bowel bag up to the axillae to prevent evaporative fluid losses and to protect the bowel. Operative repair is aimed at reducing the viscera and closing the defect. Often this may be done primarily. In other cases the abdominal contents may be too distended to achieve primary closure. In these instances a Silastic spring-loaded silo is placed over the intestines (Figure 28-9). The spring-loaded portion is placed in the abdominal cavity and sutured to the skin. Sequential tightening of the sac reduces the viscera until they are contained within the abdominal cavity, which then allows definitive closure.

Recent reports in the literature have described different methods for closure of the abdominal wall defect. Bianchi and colleges developed a method of reducing the abdominal contents without anesthesia in the neonatal intensive care unit. This technique avoids the complications of tracheal intubation and mechanical ventilation. The extent and the rate of reduction are monitored using the awake infant's reactions.[49] A sutureless closure has been reported by Sandler et al.[50] In this technique the eviscerated contents are reduced until they can be contained within the abdominal cavity and the defect is closed with the umbilical cord. Tegaderm dressings are then applied. The authors report

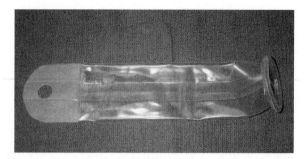

FIGURE 28-9 Spring-loaded silo.

better cosmetic outcome with the umbilicus in the natural position. The technique's simplicity is another advantage as this can be performed at the bedside.

NECROTIZING ENTEROCOLITIS

Necrotizing enterocolitis (NEC) is primarily a disease of premature infants, who account for approximately 90% of cases.[51] The cause of NEC is multifactorial with ischemia and necrotic tissue being the result. The introduction of enteral feeds to the premature gut is thought to be the initial inciting factor. Neutrophils are released followed by inflammatory mediators that contribute to tissue injury. Specific mediators include platelet activating factor, tumor necrosis factor, and NO.[52] Inflammatory mediators also increase the release of acute phase proteins from the liver. Enteral bacteria also play a role, most likely an opportunistic one.

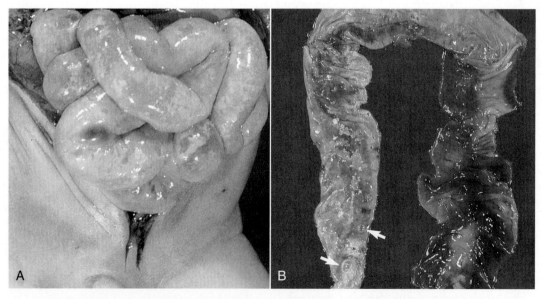

FIGURE 28-10 A, Postmortem examination in a severe case of necrotizing enterocolitis shows the entire small bowel is markedly distended with a perilously thin wall (usually this implies impending perforation). **B,** The congested portion of the ileum corresponds to areas of hemorrhagic infarction and transmural necrosis microscopically. Submucosal gas bubbles can be seen in several areas *(arrows).*

Infants with NEC will present with abdominal distension, intolerance to feeds, rectal bleeding, and abdominal wall erythema. Laboratory values include thrombocytopenia, neutropenia, and metabolic acidosis. Severe acidosis may require intubation and mechanical ventilation. The diagnosis is confirmed radiographically. Distended loops will be seen and pneumatosis intestinalis is pathognomic. Air may be seen in the portal system as well. Pneumoperitoneum confirms a perforated viscus necessitating operation.

Treatment of NEC is nonoperative in the majority of cases. Fluid resuscitation, antibiotics (ampicillin, gentamicin, clindamycin), and nasogastric decompression are the mainstays of therapy. Eighty percent of patients will not require surgery. The management of severe NEC has evolved over the last 20 years. Ein and associates[53] reported their experience with peritoneal drainage using local anesthesia. Their technique involves insertion of a Penrose drain most often in the right lower quadrant. In 32% of patients this was the definitive management. In this study drainage was used in infants weighing less than 1500 g and provided a stabilizing modality for seriously ill neonates. Peritoneal drainage was used for weighing less than 1500 g with severe NEC by Morgan et al. They reported 62% of patients requiring no laparotomy.[54] Infants with documented perforation and who are stable are taken to surgery for laparotomy (Figure 28-10). The operative approach is to preserve the maximal amount of bowel. Stricture formation is commonly seen in NEC patients, with the colon being the most common site. The overall survival for NEC is between 60% and 70%. Infants with NEC and very low birth weight who require surgery have neurodevelopmental delays when compared to equal weight infants without NEC.[52]

ASSESSMENT QUESTIONS

See Evolve Resources for the answers.

1. An infant brought to the NICU presents with cyanosis and upper airway obstruction relieved by crying with improvement in color. Suspecting choanal atresia, the best action is to
   A. Insert an 8 French suction catheter to verify the diagnosis
   B. Insert an oral airway
   C. Start nasal continuous positive airway pressure
   D. Provide heated humidity
   E. Stimulate the infant to induce crying
2. Complications related to chronic upper airway obstruction from anatomic malformations result in which of the following?
   I. Chronic hypoxia and CO_2 retention
   II. Pulmonary hypertension and cor pulmonale
   III. Hyperventilation and acidosis
   IV. Failure to thrive
   V. Congestive heart failure
   A. I, III
   B. I, II, IV
   C. I, II, III, V
   D. II, III, IV
   E. II, IV, V
3. The most common tracheoesophageal fistula and esophageal atresia lesion is classified as which type?
   A. Esophageal atresia with a long gap
   B. Esophageal atresia with distal tracheoesophageal fistula
   C. *H*-type tracheoesophageal fistula
   D. Esophageal atresia with proximal fistula
   E. Esophageal atresia with proximal and distal tracheoesophageal fistulas

ASSESSMENT QUESTIONS—cont'd

4. A drooling newborn infant with polyhydramnios in utero and suspected kidney and cardiac anomalies is admitted to the NICU and presents with coughing, respiratory distress, and cyanosis during feedings. The most likely diagnosis is
   A. Gastroschisis
   B. Tetralogy of Fallot
   C. Pulmonary sequestration
   D. Esophageal atresia with tracheoesophageal fistula
   E. Choanal atresia
5. Which of the following are true concerning a congenital diaphragmatic hernia (CDH)?
   I. Pulmonary hypoplasia is present in both lungs.
   II. Persistent pulmonary hypertension is the main complication.
   III. Surgical correction results in complete reversal of the respiratory distress.
   IV. CDH formation is a defect that occurs very early in gestational age.
   V. The right lung (contralateral side) is not usually affected.
   A. I, II, IV
   B. I, III, IV, V
   C. I, IV, V
   D. II, III, IV, V
   E. II, III, V
6. A 3200-g term infant male is born to a healthy mother. Apgar scores are 7 and 5 with the infant gasping and heart rate decreasing to 90. Physical exam reveals cyanosis, a scaphoid abdomen, and visible tracheal deviation to the right. Considering this information the ONLY appropriate action would be to
   A. Get a blood gas
   B. Bag mask ventilate

ASSESSMENT QUESTIONS—cont'd

   C. Suction and stimulate vigorously
   D. Insert an oral suction catheter to vent the stomach
   E. Vigorously stimulate and give 100% O_2 blow-by

7. Considering a likely diagnosis of congenital diaphragmatic hernia, which would be appropriate decision concerning ventilator strategy(s)?
   A. Hypoxic gases
   B. Rapid rate and low pressures
   C. High pressure and long inflation times
   D. Slow rate and short inflation times
   E. Low pressure with high peep

8. A female infant was born with a large gastroschisis anomaly. The reduction surgery will most likely affect the respiratory system by causing
   A. An increase in airway resistance.
   B. A decrease in pulmonary compliance.
   C. A decrease in transpulmonary pressure.
   D. An increase in the respiratory time constant.
   E. B and D.

9. When comparing gastroschisis and omphalocele, which of the following is true?
   A. They are both full thickness defects of the abdominal wall.
   B. They are both commonly associated with other anomalies.
   C. Omphalocele is a midline defect, while a gastroschisis is a lateral wall defect.
   D. An omphalocele is covered by epidermal tissue.
   E. Gastroschisis requires surgical reductions that frequently must be performed in several stages, while omphalocele is completed in a single surgery.

10. Although the lung bud anomalies have different histopathology, clinical presentation usually
   A. Becomes obvious in the early newborn period and is manifested by respiratory distress
   B. Becomes obvious in the early newborn period and is manifested by recurrent pulmonary infections
   C. Develops later in childhood and is characterized by severe respiratory distress
   D. Remains undetected until adolescence or early adulthood
   E. Presents as severe respiratory distress requiring mechanical ventilation

References

1. Hengerer AS, Strome M: Choanal atresia: A new embryologic theory and its influence in surgical management, *Laryngoscope* 1982;92:913.
2. Gujrathi CS et al: Management of bilateral choanal atresia in the neonate: an institutional review, *Int J Pediatr Otorhinolaryngol* 2004;68:399.
3. Tneogaray T, Dawson S: Practical management of congenital choanal atresia, *Plast Reconstr Surg* 1981;72:634.
4. Cotton RT, Stith JA: Choanal atresia in current therapy in otolaryngology. In Gates GA, ed: *Head and neck surgery*, vol 3, Philadelphia, BC Decker; 1987.
5. Wang J, Goodger NM, Pogrel MA: The role of tongue reduction, *Oral Surg Oral Med Oral Pathol Oral Radiol Endod* 2003;95:269.
6. Freed G et al: Polysomnographic indications for surgical intervention in Pierre Robin sequence: Acute airway management and follow-up studies after repair and take-down of tongue-lip adhesion, *Cleft Palate J* 1988;25:151.
7. Nargozian C: The airway in patients with craniofacial abnormalities, *Pediatic Anesthesia* 2004;14:53.
8. Quan L, Smith DW: The VATER association: Vertebral defects, anal atresia, T-E fistula with esophageal atresia, radial and renal dysplasia: A spectrum of associated defects, *J Pediatr* 1973;104:7.
9. Aschcraft KW, Holder TM: The story of esophageal atresia and tracheoesophageal fistula, *Surgery* 1969;65:332.
10. Weber TR, Smith W, Grosfeld JL: Surgical experience in infants with the VATER association, *J Pediatr Surg* 1980;15:849.
11. Templeton JM et al: Management of esophageal atresia and tracheoesophageal fistula in the neonate with severe respiratory distress syndrome, *J Pediatr Surg* 1985;20:394.
12. Holcomb GW III et al.: Thoracoscopic repair of esophageal atresia and tracheoesophageal fistula: a multi-institutional analysis, *Ann Surg* 2005;242:422.
13. Randolph JG, Newman KD, Anderson KD: Current results in repair of esophageal atresia with tracheoesophageal fistula using physiologic status as a guide to therapy, *Ann Surg* 1989;209:524.
14. Delius RE, Wheatly MJ, Coran AG: Etiology and management of respiratory complications after repair of esophageal atresia with tracheoesophageal fistula, *Surgery* 1992,112.527.
15. Davies MRQ, Cywes S: The flaccid trachea and tracheoesophageal congenital anomalies, *J Pediatr Surg* 1978;13:363.
16. Skandalakis JE, Gray SW, Ricketts RR: The diaphragm. In Skandalakis JL, Gray SW, editors: Embryology for Surgeons, ed 2, Baltimore, Williams and Wilkins; 1994. pp 491–493.
17. Cartlidge PH, Mann NP, Kapila L: Preoperative stabilization in congenital diaphragmatic hernia, *Arch Dis Child* 1986;61:1226
18. Breaux CW, Rouse TM, Cain WS: Improvement in survival of patients with congenital diaphragmatic hernia utilizing a strategy of delayed repair after medical and/or extracorporeal membrane oxygenation stabilization, *J Pediatr Surg* 1991;26:333.
19. Sakai H et al: Effect of surgical repair on respiratory mechanics in congenital diaphragmatic hernia, *J Pediatr* 1987;111:432.
20. Kinsella JP, Abman SH: Inhaled nitric oxide therapy for persistent pulmonary hypertension of the newborn, *Pediatrics* 1993;91:997.
21. The Neonatal Inhaled Nitric Oxide Group (NINOS): Inhaled nitric oxide and hypoxic respiratory failure in infants with congenital diaphragmatic hernia, *Pediatrics* 1997;99:838.

22. Arensman RM, Bambini MD, Chiu B: Congenital diaphragmatic hernia and eventration. In Ashcraft KW, Holcomb III GW, Murphy JP, editors: *Pediatric surgery*, ed 4, Philadelphia, Saunders; 2005. pp 304–323.

23. Wilson JM et al: ECMO in evolution: The impact of changing patient demographics and alternative therapies on ECMO, *J Pediatr Surg* 1996;31:1116.

24. Harrison MR et al. Correction of congenital diaphragmatic hernia in utero, V: Initial clinical experience *J Pediatr Surg* 1990;25:47.

25. Ravitch MM: *Congenital deformities of the chest wall and their operative correction*, Philadelphia, WB Saunders; 1977.

26. Shamberger RC: Congenital chest wall deformities. In *Pediatric surgery*, ed 5, Philadelphia, Elsevier; 1998. pp 787–817.

27. Nuss, D et al: Congenital chest wall deformities. In Ashcraft KW, Holcomb III GW, Murphy JP, editors: *Pediatric surgery*, ed 4, Philadelphia, Saunders; 2005. pp 245–263.

28. Lawson ML et al: A pilot study of the impact of surgical repair on disease-specific quality of life among patients with pectus excavatum, *J Pediatr Surg* 2003;38:916.

29. Haller JA et al: Chest wall constriction after too extensive and too early operations for pectus excavatum, *Ann Thorac Surg* 61:1996;1618.

30. Ravitch MM: The operative treatment of pectus excavatum, *Ann Surg* 1949;129:429.

31. Nuss D et al: A 10-year review of a minimally invasive technique for the correction of pectus excavatum, *J Pediatr Surg* 1998;33:545.

32. Ravitch MM: The operative correction of pectus carinatum (pigeon breast), *Ann Surg* 1960;151:705.

33. Oberklaid F et al: Asphyxiating thoracic dysplasia *Arch Dis Child* 1977;52:758.

34. Campbell RM, Hell-Vocke AK: Growth of the thoracic spine in congenital scoliosis after expansion thoracoplasty, *J Bone Joint Surg Am* 2003;85:409.

35. Ferguson TB: Congenital lesions of the lungs and emphysema. In Sabiston DC, Spencer FC, editors: *Gibbon's surgery of the chest*, ed 4. Philadelphia. WB Saunders; 1983.

36. Skandalakis JE, Gray SW, editors: *Embryology for surgeons: the embryological basis for the treatment of congenital defects*, Baltimore. Williams & Wilkins; 1994.

37. Laberge JM, Puligandla P, Flageole H: Asymptomatic congenital lung malformations, *Semin Pediatr Surg* 2005;14:16.

38. Haller JA Jr et al: Surgical management of lung bud anomalies: lobar emphysema, bronchogenic cyst, cystic adenomatoid malformation, and intralobar pulmonary sequestration. *Ann Thorac Surg* 1979; 28:33.

39. Wilson RD, Hedrick HL, Liechty KW, et al.: Cystic adenomatoid malformation of the lung: review of genetics, prenatal diagnosis, and in utero treatment, *Am J Med Genet A* 2006 15;140:151.

40. Levine MM et al: Pulmonary sequestration causing congestive heart failure in infancy: a report of two cases and review of the literature, *Ann Thorac Surg* 1982;34:581.

41. John PR, Beasley SW, Mayne V: Pulmonary sequestration and related disorders: a clinico-radiological review of 41 cases, *Pediatr Radiol* 1989;20:4.

42. Hendren HW, McKee D: Lobar emphysema of infancy, *J Pediatr Surg* 1966;1:24.

43. Murray GF: Congenital lobar emphysema (collective review), *Surg Gynecol Obstet* 1967;124:611.

44. McIlvaine WB, Chang JHT, Jones M: The effective use of intrapleural bupivacaine for analgesia after thoracic and subcostal incisions in children, *J Pediatr Surg* 1988;23:1184.

45. Skandalakis JE et al: Anterior body wall. In Skandalakis JL, Gray SW, editors: *Embryology for surgeons*, ed 2, Baltimore, Williams and Wilkins: 1994. pp 540–593.

46. Touloukian RJ, Hobbins JC: Maternal ultrasonography in the antenatal diagnosis of surgically correctable fetal abnormalities, *J Pediatr Surg* 1980;15:373.

47. Klein MD: Congenital abdominal wall defects, In Ashcraft KW, Holcomb III GW, Murphy JP, editors: *Pediatric surgery*, ed 4, Philadelphia, Saunders; 2005. pp 659–669.

48. Snyder CL et al: Management of intestinal atresia in patients with gastroschisis, *J Pediatr Surg* 2001;36:1542.

49. Bianchi A, Dickson AP, Alizai NK: Elective delayed midgut reduction-no anesthesia for Gastroschisis: Selection and conversion criteria, *J Pediatr Surg* 2002;37:1334.

50. Sandler A et al: A "plastic" sutureless abdominal wall closure in gastroschisis, *J Pediatr Surg* 2004;39:738.

51. Kliegman RM, Fanaroff AA: Neonatal necrotizing enterocolitis: A nine-year experience, *Am J Dis Child* 1981;135:603.

52. St Peter SD, Ostlie DJ: Necrotizing enterocolitis. In Ashcraft KW, Holcomb III GW, Murphy JP, editors: *Pediatric surgery*, ed 4, Philadelphia, Saunders; 2005. pp 461–476.

53. Ein SH et al: A 13-year experience with peritoneal drainage under local anesthesia for necrotizing enterocolitis perforation, *J Pediatr Surg* 1990;25:1034.

54. Morgan LJ, Shochat SJ, Hartman GE: Peritoneal drainage as primary management of perforated NEC in the very low birth weight infant, *J Pediatr Surg* 1994;29:310.

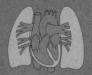

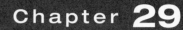
Chapter **29**

Neonatal Complications of Respiratory Care

CHARLES L. PAXSON, JR

OUTLINE

Clinical Presentations of Chronic Lung Disease
 Wilson-Mikity Syndrome
 Pulmonary Insufficiency in Prematurity
 Classic Bronchopulmonary Dysplasia
 The "New" BPD
Diagnosis of Chronic Lung Disease
Pathophysiology
 Surfactant Deficiency/Inactivation
 Oxidative Stress (Oxygen Toxicity)
 Inflammation/Infection
 Mechanical Ventilation (Barotrauma)
 Barotrauma and Air Block Syndromes
Treatment of Chronic Lung Disease
 Temperature
 Oxygenation
 Surfactant Replacement
 Resuscitation and Ventilation
 Tracheobronchial Injury
 Inflammation

Patent Ductus Arteriosus
Infection/Antibiotics
Fluids/Electrolytes
Pharmacology
Nutrition
Gastroesophageal Reflux
Stimulation/Pain
Social Issues
Retinopathy of Prematurity
 Pathophysiology
 Clinical Presentation
 Treatment
Intraventricular Hemorrhage
 Pathophysiology
 Clinical Presentation
 Treatment
 Complications
 Prevention

LEARNING OBJECTIVES

After reading this chapter, the reader will be able to:
- Differentiate the types of neonatal chronic lung diseases
- Discuss the pathophysiology and risk factors for each type of chronic lung disease
- Apply patient management methods to help prevent or minimize the risk for chronic lung disease
- Manage the newborn patient in the treatment of chronic lung disease
- Discuss the pathophysiology and risk factors of retinopathy of the newborn and understand

how to prevent or minimize the risk for this disease
- Discuss the treatments for retinopathy as they relate to stage and severity
- Discuss the pathophysiology, various risk factors, and how they are related to preventing or minimizing the risk for intraventricular hemorrhage
- Discuss the treatments for intraventricular hemorrhage as they relate to grade and severity

498

Of the numerous complications of respiratory care, the continuing spectrum of chronic lung disease (CLD), retinopathy of prematurity (ROP), and intraventricular hemorrhage (IVH) are the foci of this chapter. As with any health care problem, prevention should always be the initial goal of the clinician. For newborn infants, this means avoiding preterm delivery. An anticipated ill preterm infant should be delivered in a hospital that has some type of special care nursery (NICU). This NICU should be staffed with highly trained physicians, nurses, and respiratory therapists.

CLINICAL PRESENTATIONS OF CHRONIC LUNG DISEASE

Physicians providing neonatal care find it difficult to know which complications are unavoidable, and which result from the inability to properly use certain life-saving therapies. Recognizing this, the wise physician will avoid unproven therapies and begin to use the newest therapies only after they have been properly prospectively investigated.

Today's new drug or therapy may be tomorrow's calamity.

Some degree of lung disease may occur in preterm infants younger than 30 weeks' gestation even if the infant has not been exposed to oxygen or mechanical ventilation. It seems reasonable to consider several variants of chronic newborn lung disease as entities occurring within a continuing broad spectrum of one illness. Insults we inadvertently deliver may produce different complications depending upon the stage of lung development when the insult occurs. Ironically, while ventilation and oxygen usage probably are two factors involved in producing CLD, without these two therapeutic modalities some preterm infants would not survive.

Wilson-Mikity Syndrome

In 1960, Wilson and Mikity described preterm infants with diffuse lung infiltrates appearing at 10 to 30 days.[1] These five preterm infants had respiratory distress in the first days of life, which appeared to resolve. Then, 1 to 5 weeks later, the tachypnea and cyanosis returned. Radiologically, there were diffuse pulmonary infiltrates that in some infants changed to a cystic emphysematous pattern. The sickest infants developed heart failure and died. In Wilson-Mikity survivors, pulmonary function testing showed flow rates to be significantly lower than in other preterm infants.[2,3]

In 1969 Hodgman et al described 34 more babies as the Wilson-Mikity syndrome.[4] Most of the infants had a transient respiratory illness that ended by 48 hours of life. All but 3 of these infants received supplemental oxygen but 12 infants subsequently expired[4] (Figure 29-1).

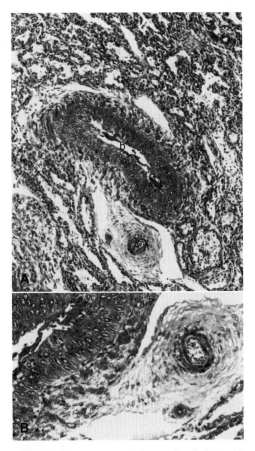

FIGURE 29-1 **A,** An autopsy specimen of an infant with Wilson-Mikity syndrome. Note the markedly overinflated pulmonary lobules alternating with areas of atelectasis. **B,** A positive print Diazo replication from a similar autopsy specimen.

Pulmonary Insufficiency in Prematurity

Some preterm infants weighing less than 1200 gm have normal lung function in the first 2 days, but then undergo a deterioration of lung function by day 7. Burnard et al described this condition in 1965 before the widespread use of mechanical ventilators. The amount of oxygen and quantity of positive-pressure ventilation were not mentioned in their article.[5] Subsequent investigators labeled this condition chronic pulmonary insufficiency of prematurity (CPIP). These infants frequently become apneic and require supplemental oxygen but chest radiographs are normal. In the 1970s, the mortality rate for infants with CPIP approached 20%. With current standards of care, all these infants survive.[6]

Classic Bronchopulmonary Dysplasia

In the early 1960s, mechanical ventilators were not commonly used. NICU personnel would hand-ventilate ill infants for days and weeks. Unfortunately, most of the smaller infants died. In the late 1960s, many infants survived because of the combined use of oxygen and mechanical ventilation. Some survivors developed a chronic lung disorder, which Northway et al termed bronchopulmonary dysplasia (BPD).[7] BPD has four stages, with each stage having an identifiable clinical, radiologic, and pathologic pattern (Table 29-1). Diagnosis of BPD was made by recognizing any one of these stages.[8] Other infants, such as those suffering from hypoplastic lungs (Potters syndrome, congenital diaphragmatic hernia), may have a pulmonary x-ray picture similar to that of BPD. In addition to their hypoplastic lungs, they have muscularized distal pulmonary arterioles, which results in severe pulmonary hypertension.[9]

The "New" BPD

Surfactant use and other improvements in newborn care have altered the pathologic and clinical picture of infants with lung disease.[10-15] Infants much smaller than the 2.3 kg mean birth weight of those reported by Northway et al are surviving. These survivors exhibit findings Coalson has described as the "New" BPD. These infants can exhibit clinical hyperinflation or cystic emphysema similar to patients with BPD. However pathology specimens show they have large, simplified alveolar structures and variable interstitial cellularity (Figures 29-2 and 29-3).[13] "New BPD" infants may come from mothers with chorioamnionitis, and all have been

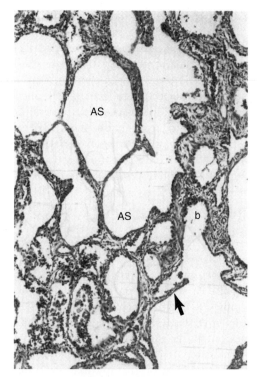

FIGURE 29-2 This biopsy specimen was taken from a 7-month-old infant born at 26-27 weeks GA. Notice thinning of the distal airspaces (AS), and the impairment in alveolization. Note the variation in the interstitial fibroproliferation and the unevenly expanded airspaces. The bronchiole (b) branches into the alveolar duct area, which shows a thickened alveolar septum as denoted by the black arrow (H & E; x110).

TABLE 29-1			
Radiologic Staging of Classic Bronchopulmonary Dysplasia, With Pathologic Correlates			
Radiologic Stage	**Patient Age (Days)**	**Radiologic Description**	**Pathologic Description**
I	2-3	Granular pattern Air bronchograms Small lung volume	Atelectasis Hyaline membranes Lymphatic dilation
II	4-10	Opacification	Necrosis and repair of alveolar epithelium Persistent hyaline membranes Emphysematous coalescence of alveoli and bronchiolar necrosis
III	10-20	Small areas of lucency alternating with areas of irregular density	Resisting airway injury to alveolar epithelium Groups of emphysematous alveoli with atelectasis of surrounding alveoli Interstitial edema and septal thickening Bronchiolar mucosal metaplasia and hyperplasia with marked mucus secretions
IV	Beyond 30 days	Enlargement of lucent areas alternating with thinner strands of radiodensity	Emphysematous

Data from Northway WH et al: Pulmonary disease following respiratory therapy of hyaline membrane disease, *N Engl J Med* 1967;276:357; and Edwards PK et al: Radiographic-pathologic correlation in bronchopulmonary dysplasia, *J Pediatr* 1979;95:835.

treated with oxygen and mechanical ventilation. Many of these infants suffer from complications of patent ductus arteriosus (PDA) and sepsis.[16-21] They all have a persistent oxygen requirement, and chest x-rays demonstrate a hazy or hyperinflated appearance, and occasionally cystic emphysema.

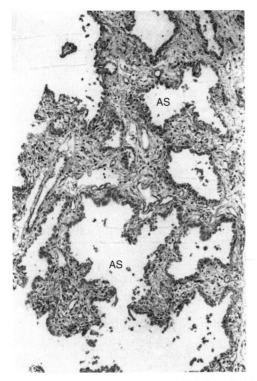

FIGURE 29-3 This section was taken at autopsy from an infant born at 25 weeks GA, who expired at 2.5 months age. Note the saccular walls showing interstitial fibroproliferation and the centrally placed dilated vessels (v). The unevenly sized airspaces (AS) show no alveoli (H&E stain x110).

DIAGNOSIS OF CHRONIC LUNG DISEASE

It is logical for the clinician to consider all these respiratory problems as a continuing spectrum of one disorder. Each infant exhibits a unique clinical variation in the spectrum produced by an insult at some distinct point in lung maturation. Each infant may exhibit some diagnostic abnormality, or they may have none. Some clinicians now define CLD as a condition occurring in an infant who required oxygen or mechanical ventilation and continues to require oxygen at 36 weeks gestational age.

The Vermont Oxford network is a collaborative effort of health care professionals dedicated to the improvement of care for the ill newborn infant. In 2007, participating hospitals and their physicians reported data on 91,417 newborns, including 52,889 infants weighing 501 to 1500 gm at birth. 50,765 of these infants received surfactant and 89% were given oxygen. Of these infants, 26% were diagnosed as having CLD.[22]

PATHOPHYSIOLOGY

Surfactant Deficiency/Inactivation

Surfactant is a phospholipid-protein mixture stored intracellularly in lamellar bodies and eventually secreted by lung alveolar type II cells. This layered mixture reduces surface tension inside alveolar ducts, alveoli, and terminal bronchioles. Without active surfactant to decrease surface tension, a small alveolus would lose its air to a larger one and collapse. This could lead to eventual rupture of the larger alveolus. However, if adequate surfactant layers are present, turbulent gas exchange is prevented, and both alveoli are kept stable, open, and functioning (Figure 29-4).

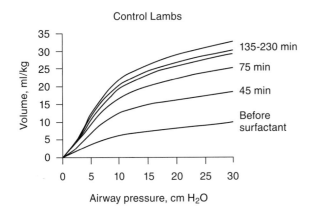

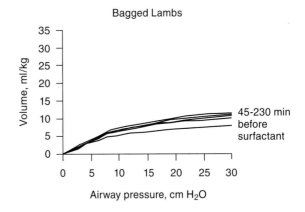

FIGURE 29-4 In the figure on the left, control lambs are given surfactant and then bagged. As the airway pressures increase, the lung volumes increase accordingly. In the figure on the right, the bagged lambs fail to respond to the surfactant and as the airway pressures increase, there is no increase in lung volumes. If the pressures would continue to go up, the lungs would presumably rupture.

Pulmonary surfactant is primarily composed of phosphatidyl lipid compounds: 10% PG (phosphatidylglycerol), 32 % unsaturated PC (phosphatidylcholine), and 36% DPPC (dipalmitoylphosphatidylcholine); and ~10 % proteins. Most of the surfactant deficiencies in the newborn period are lipid deficiencies occurring in preterm infants. These infants have not matured enough to produce an adequate supply of PG, PC, or DPPC. Lipid deficiencies can also occur in near-term or term cases of asphyxia and maternal diabetes.

Normal lamellar body formation requires the transport of protein ABCA3. Surfactant proteins B and C (SP-B and SP-C) help spread the surfactant lipids evenly inside the alveolus. Deficiencies in ABCA3, SP-B, and SP-C have all been reported. Deficiency of ABCA3 protein is the most common, followed by deficiencies of SP-B protein.[23-26] Unfortunately, without a lung transplant, these infants expire as they do not respond to artificial surfactant.

Inactivation or physiologic disappearance of surfactant may also lead to CLD. Meconium, blood, albumin, and oxidative stress inactivate surfactant. Fibrinogen and fibrin monomers also inactivate surfactant by sequestering the apoproteins.[27-33] Some newborns fail to respond to surfactant administration. The mechanisms of these failures are not clear; they may result from some unique timing event in lung maturation or from the type or degree of insult incurred (e.g., oxidative stress).[34-36] Surfactant failures may result from improper resuscitation techniques. Animal studies have shown that only a few ventilation breaths can compromise ability of the lung to respond to artificial surfactant[37] (see Figure 29-4).

Oxidative Stress (Oxygen Toxicity)

Bonikos et al and others have demonstrated that oxygen exposure without ventilation causes anatomic lung damage in mice, rats, rabbits, and preterm baboons.[38-42] These anatomic changes are similar to those noted in the BPD infants described by Northway et al.[7] Davis et al proved that newborn piglets exposed to 100% oxygen with or without ventilation develop significant lung injuries. Davis concluded that hyperoxia alone causes more significant lung damage than does ventilation.[43] This hyperoxic damage is most likely caused by cytotoxic oxygen metabolites, which include superoxide, peroxide, and hydroxyl radicals as well as hydrogen peroxide and singlet oxygen. Adult lungs have intact antioxidant systems capable of detoxifying all of these radicals[44-47] (Table 29-2). Unfortunately, the development of adult-level concentrations of the enzymes (superoxide dismutase, catalase, and glutathione peroxidase) does not occur until late in gestation.[48-49] Therefore, in early human gestation oxidative stress leads to radical-induced lung injury. Infants delivered closer to term have increased levels of these enzymes and more resistance to hyperoxic insults. Nonenzymatic antioxidants (ceruloplasmin and vitamins A, E, and C) have been given to preterm rats, lambs, and humans. Unfortunately, none of these compounds have been proven efficacious and safe for clinical use.[50-53]

Inflammation/Infection

Oxidative stress and mechanical ventilation both lead to inflammation. The neutrophil is the most prevalent cell in the alveolar washings of infants with respiratory distress syndrome (RDS). With resolution of RDS or mild lung disease, the neutrophil numbers decrease.

TABLE 29-2		
Antioxidant Protective Mechanisms		
Reactive O$_2$ Species	**Antioxidant Enzymes**	**Cell Components Attacked by Reactive O$_2$ Species**
O$_2^-$ superoxide radical	$O_2^- + O_2^- + 2H^+ \xrightarrow{(SOD)} O_2 + H_2O_2$	Lipids: peroxidation of unsaturated fatty acids in cell membranes
H$_2$O$_2$ hydrogen peroxide	$2H_2O_2 \xrightarrow[(GP)]{(CAT)} O_2 + 2H_2O$	Proteins: Oxidation of sulfhydryl-containing enzymes (enzyme inactivation)
ROO peroxide radical	$2ROO\cdot + 2H^+ \xrightarrow{(GP)} 2ROH + O_2$	Carbohydrates: depolymerization of polysaccharides
^{1}O$_2$ singlet oxygen	scavenged by ß-carotene	Nucleic acids: base hydroxylation cross-linkage, scission of DNA strands
OH hydroxyl radical	scavenged by vitamin E (GSH)	(Also, inhibition of protein, nucleotide, fatty acid biosynthesis)

The table demonstrates the effect of antioxidant enzymes in reducing cytotoxic reactive oxygen species. SOD = superoxide dismutase; CAT = catalase; GP = glutathione peroxidase; GSH k = glutathione. ROH is nontoxic lipid alcohol. Table is from Frank L, and IR Sosenko: Development of lung antioxidant enzyme system in late gestation: Possible implications for the prematurely born infant, *J Pediatr* 1987;110:11.

If the infant develops CLD, however, the neutrophil numbers persist. Some authors feel that inflammation is the major pathway participating in lung damage.[54-55]

Infants may be born preterm following maternal urinary tract infection or chorioamnionitis. A multivariate analysis by Cooke demonstrated that bacterial sepsis was more frequent in infants developing CLD.[56] Bacterial organisms are not commonly identified, but when one is, it may be *E. coli, Ureaplasma,* or *Mycoplasma* species. Sometimes these infants have pneumonia, generalized sepsis, or no signs of infection at all.[57]

Mechanical Ventilation (Barotrauma)

Barotrauma is a nonspecific term used by some authors when considering effects of mechanical ventilation on the human lung. Some authors have proven ventilation alone produces adverse sequelae even in the absence of increased inspired oxygen. As discussed, ventilation may prevent normal surfactant rescue and also prevent normal alveolar development.[37,58-60] One would expect pressure applied to a very immature lung (23 weeks gestational age [GA]) to produce a respiratory complication uniquely different from that observed when the same pressure is applied to a more mature lung (36 weeks GA). The severity and type of lung damage observed may in fact depend on the stage of lung development (immaturity), surfactant activity, and magnitude of the applied ventilation pressure. Van Marter et al performed multivariate logistic regression analyses on a number of specific respiratory care practices at medical centers in New York and Boston. After adjusting for baseline risk, most of the risk of CLD was explained by the initiation of mechanical ventilation. CLD risk was elevated for maximum peak inspiratory pressures above 25.[61]

Barotrauma and Air Block Syndromes

In the normal newborn lung, surfactant layers coat the inside of the alveoli, the alveolar ducts, and the terminal bronchioles. These layers reduce the surface tension and thereby reduce the inspiratory pressure required to deliver a normal tidal volume. This minimizes stress on the delicate alveolar walls (Figure 29-5).

If surfactant is absent or inactivated, some alveoli, ducts, or bronchioles may collapse while others become overdistended and rupture.[62] The air may rupture into the interstitial lung tissue (pulmonary interstitial emphysema [PIE]), directly into the pleural space (pneumothorax), or may travel the path of the perivascular sheath around the arteriole at the rupture site causing a pneumoperitoneum, pneumomediastinum, or pneumopericardium (Figure 29-6).

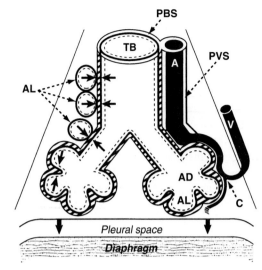

FIGURE 29-5 Normal acinus. Surfactant *(broken lines)* lines the alveoli (AL), alveolar ducts (AD), and respiratory bronchioles. Alveoli are open and have a pressure equal and opposite to the airway pressure *(small arrows)*. The transseptal pressure in the alveoli is zero, with equal pressures on both sides of the septa *(small arrows)*. The pulmonary artery (A) runs with the airway and ends in capillaries (C) before continuing as a vein (V) in periacinar connective tissue. The terminal bronchiole (TB) is surrounded by a peribronchiolar space (PBS), and the artery is surrounded by a perivascular space (PVS).

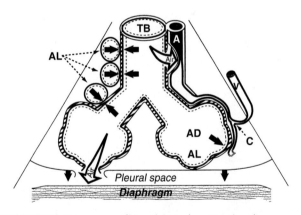

FIGURE 29-6 Lung overdistention and rupture in a lung with inadequate or inactivated surfactant. The excessive inspiratory volume has overdistended the small airway and alveoli. The larger acinar airway is protected by an equally large pressure and volume in the surrounding alveoli *(AL, solid arrows)*. However, in areas where the alveolar and bronchiolar pressures are not balanced there is a rupture of the wall *(open large arrows)*. The interstitial air can compress arteries (A) and lead to the air-block syndrome with decreased perfusion to the capillaries (C) and veins (V). Air can move in the perivascular space to the mediastinum or break into the pleural space to form a pneumothorax.

PIE could dissect through lung tissue to the pleura resulting in blebs or a pneumothorax. PIE is space occupying and increases interstitial pressure. This decreases lung compliance and requires the clinician to use even higher mechanical inspiratory pressures to maintain normal gas exchange and prevent hypoxemia and hypercarbia. In small immature infants, airways may balloon out and become deformed by the increased positive inspiratory pressure (PIP). This damages the elastic and collagen templates necessary for normal lung development. Diffuse bilateral PIE in infants younger than 32 weeks usually occurs to those with lower Apgar scores and higher oxygen and airway pressure requirements during the first week of life.[63-64] In more mature infants of 32 to 40 weeks gestation, PIE is less common because the small airway connective tissues of elastin and collagen are more developed.

Pneumothorax

Pneumothorax occurs in 5% of babies 501 to 1500 gm birth weight.[22] It may occur in the first hours of life or anytime during mechanical ventilation. "Spontaneous" pneumothorax may occur after asphyxia, meconium aspiration, or in infants with congenital cardiac anomalies.[65] Clinically, tachypnea, hypoxemia, or hypercarbia should lead to suspicion of pneumothorax. With a "tension" pneumothorax, apical pulse and heart sounds are shifted away from the side of the pneumothorax. The chest is transilluminated with a focused bright light and the air collection will "light up." Some ventilators may show a decrease in compliance and tidal volume at set pressures. Diagnosis is confirmed by an emergency chest x-ray or a "hissing" sound as air escapes from the chest following thoracotomy. Caution must be exercised not to confuse skin folds with a pneumothorax. If simultaneous hypotension and bradycardia are present, cardiopulmonary collapse or death is imminent, and treatment cannot await chest x-rays. A skilled nurse or physician must insert a needle or catheter into the chest to release the air until a chest tube can be placed under aseptic conditions.

Pneumomediastinum

Pneumomediastinum may follow alveolar rupture or airway perforation from a traumatic intubation. It is rare in infants younger than 34 weeks gestation. Physical examination could reveal muffled heart sounds, or chest x-rays could reveal the pneumomediastinal air anterior to the heart. The air collection usually disappears in 1 to 2 days, but surgical intervention might be needed. Subcutaneous emphysema could occur if the air moves into cervical subcutaneous tissue.

Pneumopericardium and Pneumoperitoneum

Surfactant use has made these two entities rare, but they may result from ruptured alveoli and air passage down perivascular sheaths. Pressure from inside the pericardial sac may give rise to cardiac tamponade, and a skilled physician must remove this air tension immediately. Sudden onset of cyanosis (drop in transcutaneous oxygen levels), bradycardia, or hypotension may be signs of pneumopericardium or cardiac tamponade. Chest radiographs show gas surrounding and under the inferior surface of the heart. Patients with pneumopericardium require rapid skilled therapy or they will die.[66]

Pneumoperitoneum (free air in the peritoneal cavity) resulting from lung disease must be differentiated from a pneumoperitoneum resulting from a GI perforation. A skilled pediatric surgeon can help the neonatologist in differentiating these diagnoses.[67] (Figure 29-7).

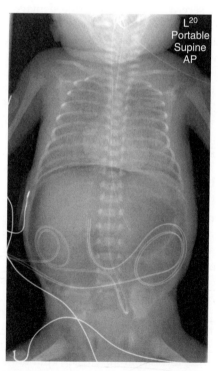

FIGURE 29-7 Chest and abdominal radiograph of an 825-gm infant with respiratory distress syndrome. The chest has a "ground-glass" appearance typical for RDS. The thin dark area just beneath the diaphragm and all around the periphery of the abdomen is free air (a pneumoperitoneum) from a ruptured intestine. The perforation required immediate surgery, and the infant survived.

TREATMENT OF CHRONIC LUNG DISEASE

Temperature

Temperature support of the ill infant is the initial step in preventing CLD. In the delivery room and in the NICU, attention is given to all the mechanisms by which babies lose heat (conduction, convection, evaporation, and radiation). It has long been known that cold stress inhibits surfactant production. All infants should be kept warm, and given proprioceptive stimuli—ideally gentle flexion of one hip joint. Infants below 1500 grams BW are placed in a plastic body bag and then taken to the NICU and placed upon a radiant warmer bed for observation and placement of indwelling vascular catheters. Larger infants are dried off and cared for in a similar manner. Very few newborn infants need to be bathed in the first day of life.

Oxygenation

Oxidative stress occurs if newborns are hyperoxic or too immature for antioxidant enzymes to function. When oxidative stress occurs, two molecules of antioxidant-reduced glutathione bind together and inactivate toxic free radicals. This produces an increase in measurable oxidized glutathione, which proves that oxidative stress has occurred.[68-71]

Historically, hypoxic newborns have been resuscitated at birth with protocols including 100% oxygen. Vento et al compared 526 infants resuscitated with 100% oxygen to 304 infants resuscitated with room air.[72] The infants given 100% oxygen had elevated levels of oxidized glutathione and required longer to establish a normal breathing pattern. No advantage resulted from 100% oxygen resuscitation. Vento has shown oxidative stress can last up to one month.

Temesvari et al have shown impaired neurologic outcome in newborn piglets resuscitated with 100% oxygen compared with air.[73] The method of using 100% oxygen to resuscitate a hypoxic infant exposes the infant to further oxidative stress and reperfusion injuries.[74-78] Nearly 2200 infants have been in studies comparing room air with 100% oxygen resuscitation. Meta-analysis have shown that infants resuscitated at birth with room air have less oxidative stress, a more rapid establishment of normal breathing, and a reduction in reperfusion damage to major organs (brain, heart, and kidneys).[79-87]

Increasing antioxidant intake could offset newborn oxidative stress. Unfortunately no IV or dietary compounds have been proven safe for prolonged usage. Even with much-studied vitamin E (alpha-tocopherol), plasma measurements are unreliable, and prolonged dosage of vitamin E has been involved with an increased incidence of sepsis and necrotizing enterocolitis.[88-89]

Surfactant Replacement

Suresh and Soll stated that no newborn therapy has been studied as extensively as surfactant replacement. More than 400 trials have evaluated efficacy and safety of surfactant use.[90] Use of surfactant leads to an improvement in oxygenation and stimulation of an infant's endogenous surfactant production.[91]

Several different products have been studied, and new products are evaluated every 2 to 4 years. Currently used surfactants are lipid extracts of animal lungs. Surfactant is instilled into the infant's airway via an endotracheal tube (ET tube). Surfactant coats the inner lining of the alveoli and acts to stabilize them. Smaller alveoli are kept open and prevented from giving up gases to other alveoli. Larger alveoli are prevented from becoming overdistended and rupturing (see Figure 29-5).

Many studies have evaluated the dosage and timing of surfactant administration. Most infants need a second or third dose. Ideally, preterm infants should be born in the hospital where NICU care can be given. However, if infants are not born in a hospital with a NICU, they can be transported there and given surfactant on arrival at the NICU. In a study of 6039 infants, there was no difference in mortality or pneumothorax comparing surfactant given in the delivery room versus giving it after 2 hours of age.[92] In our experience, surfactant is effective when instilled as late as 9 hours of life.[93]

Resuscitation and Ventilation

Immediately after delivery, while the infant is being dried and stimulated, a transcutaneous oxygenation sensor is placed on the right wrist or right thorax to allow a preductal oxygen assessment (SpO_2 or TcO_2). This is an estimation of the infant's blood gas status and not a replacement for a preductal arterial blood gas. Clinicians must remember the preductal arterial blood gas is the "gold standard" for evaluating oxygenation and acid-base status of the ill infant. In healthy term infants, SpO_2 rises to 90% by 5 minutes of age, but no comparable values for preterm infants are available.[94-95] Transcutaneous pCO_2 monitors may be used to estimate the infant's pCO_2.

Correct placement of the ET tube is made by visualizing the tube tip passing through the moving vocal folds; listening to the right thorax; or by use of a colorimetric CO_2 detector. Remember that small infants may not move enough air to produce a change in the CO_2 detector. Some infants require initial continuous positive airway pressure (CPAP), which can be applied by a facial apparatus. Most term asphyxiated babies can be resuscitated with 21% oxygen. Preterm infants may require 25% to 30% oxygen.[72,79,80,96] If the preductal pulse oximeter reads below 90%, or the infant remains cyanotic, 40% oxygen should be given. If the arterial blood gas value prompts ET tube placement, surfactant should be given per manufacturer's instructions. Some clinicians advocate giving surfactant via the ET tube, removing the tube, and applying facial CPAP. However, this may place the infant at risk of airway trauma if the ET is subsequently needed for mechanical ventilation. It is preferable to leave the ET tube in place 4 to 6 hours or until ventilatory needs can be more precisely determined. Ventilation should be initiated with low peak inspiratory pressures or tidal volumes, but enough support must be given to keep the blood gas pCO_2 between 35 and 45 mm Hg. Ventilation should continue only with enough oxygen to keep blood gas pO_2 between 60 and 80 mm Hg, or the preductal SpO_2 between 85% and 95%. Minimal use of oxygen will reduce oxidative stress. Arterial blood gas values are obtained from an indwelling arterial catheter every 6 to 8 hours once the infant appears stable. These samples can be drawn and sent to the laboratory; or a closed loop system (e.g., VIA-LVM device), which allows bloodless sampling every 6 minutes could also be used (viamedical.com). Continuous SpO_2 are estimates of blood values, but if no indwelling radial or umbilical arterial line is in place, periodic checks of arterial blood gases must be made. Congenital cardiac disease must be a consideration for infants not responding to respiratory care.

We usually begin conventional ventilation through a 3.0 ET tube when PaO_2s are below 60 in 40% oxygen. PIP and positive end-expiratory pressure (PEEP) are adjusted to keep pCO_2s normal (35-45). For a 1500-gm infant with RDS we usually begin ventilation with pressures of 18/4, a rate of 60, and an I/E time of 0.35 seconds. Changes are made as clinically indicated by the arterial blood gas analyses. Changes in ventilator rates are initially preferred over changes in peak inspiratory pressures. Mistakes made with changes in rates are not harmful. Mistakes made with increases in peak inspiratory pressures can be harmful and difficult to correct.

Infants who do not respond to surfactant treatment and conventional ventilation should have a trial of high-frequency ventilation (HFV). Use of HFV requires that the infant be adequately hydrated. Chest x-rays must be obtained every 3 to 4 hours to evaluate for a silent pneumothorax. Infants who do not respond to HFV rescue may need extracorporeal membrane oxygenation (ECMO).

No clinical studies have shown the superiority of either conventional ventilation or HFV as an initial therapy. We begin mechanical ventilation with a conventional ventilator because of the slight increase in incidence of pneumothorax and neurologic sequelae reported with HFV.

Tracheobronchial Injury

The most highly skilled personnel should be available for anticipated delivery of an ill newborn. Considerable experience is required in decision making and, when necessary, in the placement of an ET tube and indwelling catheters. If resuscitation is not performed by a skilled clinician in a calm, controlled environment, vocal folds can be sheared away and ruptures of the tracheobronchial tree occur. Experience in adults suggests that if an intubation rupture occurs, conventional conservative management, not surgical repair, is best.[117]

Prolonged mechanical ventilation can result in chronic injury to the upper airways. This is unusual, but when it occurs, the upper airways collapse during expiration. Diagnosis can be made by viewing the enlarged tracheal diameter on chest radiograph, or by observing dynamic airway collapse on the flow-volume loops. PEEP will support the airways during expiration, and tracheotomy is only needed in the most severe situation. It will take many months for these lesions to recover.[118]

Inflammation

It has been postulated that the common pathway to CLD from oxidative stress and ventilation is the inflammatory response. Work in animals has suggested that using medications to decrease inflammation might decrease lung or brain injury. Studies have not given reproducible results applicable to preterm humans.[97-98]

Patent Ductus Arteriosus

A PDA might complicate the course of CLD. PDA or persistent pulmonary hypertension should be suspected when a differential SpO_2 from the right arm and left arm (or leg) is greater than 20 mm Hg, or when surfactant gives no immediate improvement. Fluids should be restricted, and pharmacologic closure of the PDA considered. NeoProfen (Ibuprofen lysine) is the "new" drug for PDA closure, but it is no more effective than indomethacin, and use of NeoProfen has resulted in a higher incidence of CLD.[99] If PDA ligation is required, it can be safely performed by a skilled surgeon in the NICU.

Infection/Antibiotics

Any infant with a respiratory rate greater than 60 breaths/minute at 1 hour of age[100] or later must be considered septic and a blood culture be obtained. Once that culture has been drawn, IV antibiotics consisting of Ampicillin and an aminoglycoside should be given. We start with Ampicillin and Gentamicin. Therapy is continued for 2 to 3 days until a sterile culture is reported. Initial therapy with Cefotaxime is avoided because initial empiric usage of that drug has been associated with some deaths.[101] Signs of infection that appear during later CLD treatment prompt a repeat blood culture, a urine culture, and a spinal tap. At that point, assume a nosocomial infection with staphylococcal organisms and begin Vancomycin. Additional diagnostic parameters (e.g., white blood cell count ratios or CRP greater than 5 mm Hg) may occasionally be of help.[14,22,23,30,33] If the platelet count has dropped, we consider Candida sepsis and begin an antifungal medication.

Fluids/Electrolytes

Fluids for the first 24 hours should be dextrose 5% for infants below 1500 gm. Begin IV fluids at 60 to 80 ml/kg/day and adjust the IV rate to keep blood sugars and urine output normal. Normal blood sugar is 60-80 mg/dl and urine output is a wide range of 0.5 to 5 ml/kg/hour. Electrolytes should be obtained at 12 and 24 hours, and electrolytes added to the fluids as indicated.

Ill infants should be kept NPO and receive intravenous hyperalimentation fluids (TPN) by 24 to 48 hours of age. If "air block" or hyponatremia occurs, measurements of urine and serum osmolality (specific gravity), and urine sodium should be determined to evaluate for SIADH (syndrome of inappropriate antidiuretic hormone secretion).[102]

Strict attention must be given to acid-base balance. Ventilator changes and fluid adjustments should be to correct acidosis. We no longer recommend or use bicarbonate infusions as standard care in cardiopulmonary arrests or with metabolic acidosis. Only the rare neonate with severe kidney disease may benefit from bicarbonate.[103]

Systemic blood pressure should be constantly monitored via an indwelling arterial catheter or an appropriately sized limb cuff. If the infant develops hypotension or urine output decreases dramatically, normal saline or lactated ringers; and dopamine should be given to maintain systemic pressure and cerebral blood flow.[104] If blood pressure is still low following fluid and dopamine, an evaluation of circulating blood volume should be made. Technetium or 51Cr-labeled RBC blood volume could be determined, and an appropriate amount of blood infused.[105-108] Albumin infusions are controversial. Albumin leaves the vascular space rapidly after infusion, can lead to IVH, and produces no better results than saline infusions.[109] If the infant is receiving mechanical ventilation, transfusions should be given to keep peripheral hematocrit above 40 to prevent grade IV IVH.[110-111]

Pharmacology

Pharmacologic agents given to the newborn infant must be judiciously selected. Far too many infants receive mixtures of drugs for which interaction information is entirely unknown. Clinicians must daily remind themselves of the unique pathophysiology of neonatal illnesses. One infant might respond to a medication, but another will not. If a drug is prescribed, its efficacy must be evaluated.

Many investigators have evaluated using postnatal steroids to decrease the incidence of CLD. The desire to use steroids is understandable because of their mediating role in inflammation. However, steroid usage has produced inconsistent results: patient selection, dosage, mechanism of action, and short and long term side effects all remain to be properly evaluated.[112]

Studies in both animals and humans suggest inhaled nitric oxide (iNO) may prove to be useful. It inhibits endothelial dysfunction and reverses pulmonary hypertension and bronchoconstriction. iNO also results in increased alveolar counts in developing lungs, improves lung growth, and improves the outcome in preterm infants receiving mechanical ventilation.[113,114]

Nutrition

It is difficult to provide adequate nutrition for the preterm infant. Some animal studies suggest that starvation causes increased sensitivity to oxidative stress.[115] In the first few days of life, ill infants should receive TPN. If an indwelling umbilical arterial catheter was placed for blood sampling, it must be removed before gavage feedings are started.

Gastroesophageal Reflux

For some unknown reason, gastroesophageal reflux (GER) is fairly common in CLD. Bedside nurses detect this when attempting feedings. Diagnosis should be confirmed with an acid-reflux, barium swallow, or video swallow test. A trial of antireflux meds may be given, but the diagnostic tests must be repeated to ensure drug efficacy. Some clinicians believe thickened feedings are helpful. In the most severe cases, the pediatric surgeon will have to be consulted and a fundal plication considered.

Stimulation/Pain

Infants should be kept in a cycling light/dark environment with minimal noise. Medications are given for any procedures causing pain.

Social Issues

Dealing with a chronic childhood illness can be frustrating for any parent. Parents must be given all the facts of their baby's status and as much emotional support as possible. Notice must be taken of those parents who might tend toward child abuse.[116]

RETINOPATHY OF PREMATURITY

Retinopathy of prematurity (ROP) is a disease first described in 1942 as retrolental fibroplasia (RLF). By the late 1980s, the term RLF was replaced by ROP. As currently diagnosed, ROP is disordered vascularization and fibrovascular changes occurring in the retinas of preterm infants. ROP is more prevalent in smaller premature infants. The incidence among infants with a birth weight of less than 750 gm was reported as 90% in 1991.[119] In 2007, VON data reported that 36% of infants with birth weights between 501 and 1500 gm exhibited ROP (35,528 infants).[22]

Pathophysiology

Vascularization of a normal retina occurs as vessels grow from the optic disc peripherally. Complete retinal vessel development is attained at 40 to 42 weeks after conception. ROP is a disruption of this normal vascularization process. Originally it was thought that ROP was caused exclusively by excessive oxygen and hyperoxemia. Although hyperoxia may play a role, it is not the sole cause of ROP. In fact, infants with cyanotic congenital heart disease with relative hypoxemia may develop ROP.[120] Other factors, including hypercarbia, anemia, or copper deficiencies have been suggested as etiologic factors[121-129] (Box 29-1).

It has been suggested that fluctuating PO_2s or PCO_2s following vasoconstrictive injury might predispose the retina to disturbances in growth factors—e.g., vascular endothelial growth factor (VEGF). VEGF stimulus might produce an uncontrolled neovascularization and lead to scarring, retinal retraction, or retinal detachment.[130]

Clinical Presentation

ROP is detected during scheduled screening exams of preterm infants by pediatric ophthalmologists. Screening is usually done in infants born at less than 32 GA who have lived 4 to 6 weeks. The goal is to identify ROP so treatment can be undertaken at the appropriate time. Examinations done earlier than 32 weeks GA usually identify only immature retinas that will need repeat examinations. Screening is repeated every 1 to 2 weeks until the retinal vascularization has extended into zone 3 and the risk for "threshold disease" is gone (Figure 29-8). So-called threshold disease is that degree of ROP for which intervention is generally performed.

ROP is diagnosed and staged by the description of retinal fibrovascular changes outlined by the International Committee for the Classification of ROP criteria.[131-132] Disease changes are described by location (zone I, II, or III), extent (number of clock hours involved), and severity. Stage 1 is minimal severity with abnormal vessel branching leading up to the line demarcating the avascular retina anteriorly from the vascular retina posteriorly. Stage 2 is diagnosed by observing a ridge arising in the region of the demarcation line. In stage 3, neovascularization extends from the ridge into the vitreous. Stage 4 includes at least partial retinal detachment. Stage 5 consists of funnel-shaped total retinal detachments.

Plus disease is diagnosed when a standard photograph reveals a predefined amount of venous dilatation and arteriolar tortuosity of the posterior retinal vessels in a minimum of two quadrants. *Pre-plus disease* exists when tortuosity does not quite reach the photographic definition of plus disease.

ROP generally develops in the several weeks before term and reaches peak severity at about 40 weeks GA. Most cases of ROP regress over time. Cases that fail to regress may result in permanent retinal scarring. Scarring and remodeling of the retina may result in a wide range of minimal to severe vision deficits. If severe, permanent retinal scarring occurs, and the infant will have cicatricial retraction leading to retinal detachment.

Treatment

The "threshold" for ROP is defined as disease in either zone I or II, and stage 3 or greater covering 5 contiguous, or 8 total clock hours. Once this threshold has been reached, indirect laser therapy is performed for ablation of the diseased portions of the retina. Other interventions proposed to limit the extent of the disease have included light reduction, vitamin E, and oxygen supplementation. Light reduction has failed to show any benefit, and vitamin E studies have yielded mixed

Box 29-1	Factors Associated With Retinopathy of Prematurity

- Preterm Birth (low birth weight)
- Respiratory distress syndrome
- Mechanical ventilation
- Chorioamnionitis
- Apnea of prematurity
- Exchange transfusion
- Oxidative stress
- Surfactant deficiency
- Mg and Cu deficiencies
- Hypoxia and acidosis
- Pneumonia/Sepsis
- Chronic lung disease
- Surgical PDA closure
- Hypercarbia
- Apnea
- Anemia
- IVH

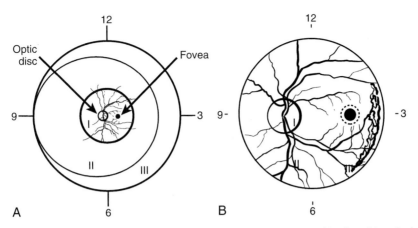

FIGURE 29-8 A, Chart illustrating zones and clock hour orientation used in describing the location and extent of retinopathy of prematurity (ROP) lesions. **B,** Diagrammatic representation of early ROP lesion with line of demarcation. This lesion could be described as zone 1, stage 1, extending 3 clock hours (2 to 5 o'clock). The vessels are usually not significantly tortuous nor increased in stage 1 lesions.

results.[127,133] It seems paradoxical to suggest oxygen supplementation for treatment of ROP. However, this might improve outcome by stabilizing oxygen delivery to the injured areas of retina, thereby limiting the overproduction of VEGF growth factors.[134-135] A test of this hypothesis found a modest reduction in ROP progression when SpO_2 levels were maintained at 96% to 99%, but this came with a worsening of the CLD. It may be reasonable to use supplemental oxygen during the time ROP development is most likely (after 32 weeks postconception), but *such care should be limited to prospective investigations* by skilled ophthalmologists and neonatologists.[136-139] Complications of ROP from mild visual loss to total blindness demonstrate that our ability to prevent ROP remains limited.

INTRAVENTRICULAR HEMORRHAGE

One of the most devastating problems in the newborn is brain damage from perinatal or postnatal hypoxic-ischemic insults which lead to IVH or periventricular leukomalacia (PVL). IVH begins along the bases of the lateral ventricles in the subependymal germinal matrix, and the bleeding may rupture into the ventricular cavities. The germinal matrix is a highly cellular gelatinous matrix filled with fragile blood vessels.[140-141] The smallest preterm infants may suffer IVH or PVL or both. With advancing GA, the germinal matrix gets smaller until nearly disappearing by 36 weeks GA, so more mature infants may suffer from PVL, but not always IVH. IVH or PVL may result in severe long-term neurodevelopmental sequelae. Even with improved survival rates of the smallest infants, no reduction in IVH/PVL or subsequent

disabilities has occurred.[142-143] In hospitals participating in the VON network, no significant reduction in incidence of IVH/PVL was reported from 1990 to 2007. In that period, 396,995 babies were followed with birth weights between 501 and 1500 gm. The average yearly incidence of IVH/PVL was 26% (24.9% to 27.7%).[22]

Pathophysiology

Pathogenesis of IVH/PVL is multifactorial. Under normal circumstances in healthy newborn infants, cerebral blood flow (CBF) is protected by a process termed autoregulation. If autoregulation is intact, systemic pressure may fall or rise, but nothing adverse happens to CBF. If autoregulation is absent, any factor adversely affecting systemic pressure puts the brain at risk of ischemia or hemorrhage because of the pressure-passive status of the CBF.[144-145]

At least one study has shown that CBF is markedly decreased in infants subsequently developing IVH.[146] Some factors reported to alter CBF and put the infant at risk of IVH/PVL are: hypotension, hypoplastic left heart syndrome, PDA (with retrograde cerebral diastolic flow), thrombocytopenia, pneumothorax, hypoxemia, hypercarbia, hypocarbia, bicarbonate infusions, umbilical arterial catheter blood withdrawal, ET suctioning, and mechanical ventilation.[147-159]

PVL may occur with or without IVH. Pathogenesis of PVL has been summarized by Volpe as resulting from three interacting problems. They are:
1. A maturation-dependent impairment in regulation of CBF
2. A vulnerability to insults of immature periventricular white matter
3. An exquisite vulnerability of the oligodendroglial precursor cells to free radical toxicity[160]

Clinical Presentation

The occurrence of IVH may be diagnosed in utero or in the NICU after delivery.[161] Onset of symptoms may be in the first 6 hours of life in a tiny infant delivered vaginally, or onset may occur later in the first week.[162] IVH may be a catastrophic event, with dramatic neurologic, respiratory, or cardiovascular signs. In contrast, IVH may be a silent event, heralded by minimal changes in patient movement, tone, or responsiveness. One of the most helpful signs of significant IVH is an abrupt drop in hematocrit.[163] Failure of hematocrit values to rise following a packed RBC may also signal the diagnosis. With acute onset and massive bleeding, severe hypoxemia and bradycardia may be life threatening.

IVH is frequently diagnosed in the NICU by cranial ultrasound examination (HUS). MRI evaluations could be performed, but the infant would have to leave the NICU and be subjected to cold stress. After IVH occurs, bleeding is graded according to a standard system. Papile et al's work gave us a good scale to grade IVHs from 1 (least severe) to 4 (most severe).[164-165] Grade 1 hemorrhages leave blood within the subependymal germinal matrix area. In contrast, grade 4 hemorrhages include extension of bleeding into the ventricle, distorting ventricular anatomy and extending into the parenchyma of the brain. Most IVHs occur after day 1, and HUSs are performed thereafter. Clinicians used to believe that a small preterm infant with a normal HUS would be normal. We now know that close follow-up is required of all infants weighing less than 1000 gm because even those with a normal HUS can have abnormal mental developmental indices or cerebral palsy.[166]

Treatment

Care of babies suffering from IVH is mainly supportive. Blood loss and hypoxemia must be corrected. If seizure symptoms occur, an EEG is done and phenobarbital ordered.[167] Bedside HUS may be required to follow the course of the illness. About 20% of the most severe IVHs may require ventriculoperitoneal shunting for hydrocephalus.[168]

Complications

Prognosis after IVH/PVL correlates roughly with the extent of the primary lesion,[164] but may also be affected by the presence of CLD or ROP. Approximately 13% of patients with grade I or II IVH have neurodevelopmental disability noted during long-term follow-up.[139] Infants with grade III or IV IVH have a 36% incidence of significant neurologic sequelae.

Babies with the most extensive intraparenchymal bleeding will suffer the most severe sequelae. The most common form of disability is a contralateral hemiparesis, or some other form of paresis or spasticity termed "cerebral palsy." Learning disabilities or visual difficulties may also occur. Mortality corresponds roughly with the grade and extent of the lesion. Approximately 50% of babies with a grade 4 hemorrhage die shortly after the hemorrhage occurs.[142,143,159,169]

The course of a patient surviving with IVH may be complicated by posthemorrhagic hydrocephalus. This results because blood clots obstruct normal CSF flow. Progressive hydrocephalus and ventricular dilation may require placement of a ventriculoperitoneal shunt. When a complicating factor (e.g., nosocomial infection) or a high fluid protein level precludes definitive shunt placement, a subcutaneous reservoir is placed. This reservoir is drained daily until the infection has been treated and previously high protein levels become low enough to allow a definitive shunt to be placed.

Prevention

Many postnatal therapies have been evaluated to reduce IVH incidence or severity. Some of the therapies evaluated were phenobarbital, ethamsylate, vitamin E, and indomethacin. Indomethacin might help an individual patient by closing a large PDA; however, indomethacin prophylaxis for PDAs has not been shown to alter the incidence of CLD, ROP, IVH, or mortality.[170]

The association between hypercarbia and IVH has been recognized for decades. Kaiser et al suggested that hypercarbia causes loss of CBF autoregulation, and then fluctuations in systemic blood pressure are transmitted to the CBF causing IVH.[171] Keeping pCO_2s, CBF, and cerebral oxygenation normal seems wise. Infants receiving ventilation should have transfusions to keep their hematocrits higher than 46% to prevent IVH.[111] Particular care should be taken to avoid any factor producing fluctuations in systemic blood pressure. Hypoxemia, hypercarbia, hypocarbia, pneumothorax, suctioning ET tubes, and other nursing maneuvers have been suggested as factors disrupting cerebral blood flow.

Numerous authors have studied IVH in animal models. Mice, dogs, cats, and baboons have all been used.[172-173] Of all animal models studied, the beagle puppy model produces a pattern of IVH most like that of the preterm human.[174-176]

Some physicians have advocated using the adult technique of permitting pCO_2s to become elevated (permissive hypercapnia). The postulation is that minimal ventilator settings allowing elevated pCO_2s will decrease barotrauma. This works in adults with ARDS, but it does not work in newborn infants. Use of this permissive hypercapnic technique could lead to a subset of infants with elevated pCO_2, as well as altered CBF and IVH. Whenever possible, infants should have pCO_2s kept normal (35-45).

ASSESSMENT QUESTIONS

See Evolve Resources for the answers.

1. How is chronic lung disease (CLD) defined in an infant?
   A. Persistent infiltrates and emphysema-like changes on chest x-ray ✓
   B. Requiring oxygen and any form of positive pressure support upon discharge
   C. High levels of vitamin E and A as markers of CLD and greater than 1 liter of oxygen at 40 weeks
   D. Requiring oxygen or mechanical ventilation, and continuing to require oxygen at 36 weeks gestational age
   E. Six sequential radiographic stages culminating in CLD

2. Which of the following statements are true about the cause of CLD in the newborn?
   A. Results from oxygen use during the newborn period
   B. Results from positive pressure ventilation during the newborn period ✓
   C. Depends on the severity of surfactant dysfunction
   D. A and B
   E. A, B, and C

3. What is an important component to preventing oxidative stress in the treatment of CLD in the newborn?
   A. Administering high dose beta carotene
   B. Resuscitating with a minimum F_{IO_2} at birth ✓
   C. Includes administration of vitamin E ✓
   D. B and C
   E. A, B, and C

4. Which of the following are true about the development of CLD of the newborn?
   I. Oxidative stress and mechanical ventilation lead to inflammation. ✓
   II. Neutrophils are prevalent in infants with RDS but decrease as RDS resolves.
   III. Neutrophil degranulation prevents surfactant production.
   IV. Neutrophils are prevalent despite the resolution of RDS.
   V. Vitamin E enhances the protective of lamellar bodies. ✓
   A. I, III, IV
   B. II, III, V
   C. III, IV, V
   D. I, II, IV
   E. II, III, IV, V

5. Which of the following may be used to reduce mortality and morbidity associated with RDS leading to chronic lung disease?
   I. Nasal CPAP therapy ✓

ASSESSMENT QUESTIONS—cont'd

   II. Surfactant replacement ✓
   III. Corticosteroid therapy ✓
   IV. Inhaled nitric oxide
   V. Extracorporeal membrane oxygenation
   A. II, IV
   B. II, IV, V
   C. I, III, V
   D. III, IV, V
   E. I, II, IV

6. What does the diagnosis of retinopathy of prematurity include?
   A. Staging the retinal vascular change
   B. Timing the rate of vascular change in clock hours
   C. A description of the location and extent of the retinal vascular change ✓
   D. A, B, and C
   E. A and C

7. Treatment to reverse the effects of retinopathy of prematurity consists of
   A. Laser ablation of the affected vascular area
   B. Administration of vitamin E and limiting light exposure
   C. Supplemental oxygen
   D. None of the above
   E. A, B, and C

8. What is the most important cause of intraventricular hemorrhage?
   A. Positive pressure ventilation ✓
   B. Hypoxemia and respiratory failure
   C. Lack of autoregulation and resulting fluctuations in cerebral blood flow
   D. Intravascular administration of glucose and other nutrients
   E. Administration of medications used to close a patent ductus arteriosus

9. Which procedure is performed to diagnose intraventricular hemorrhage?
   A. An echocardiogram
   B. A pericardiocentesis
   C. A spinal tap
   D. A head ultrasound
   E. Blood cultures

10. A 30-week GA newborn has been on the ventilator for 9 weeks with $PaCO_2$ values around 60 and PaO_2 values around 60, despite increased ventilator settings. Chest x-rays reveal atelectasis, hyperlucencies, cystic changes, hyperinflation, and mild cardiomegaly. The most likely diagnosis is which of the following?
   A. Cystic fibrosis
   B. Bronchopulmonary dysplasia
   C. Bacterial pneumonitis
   D. Pulmonary interstitial emphysema
   E. Meconium aspiration

References

1. Wilson G, Mikity VG: A new form of respiratory disease in premature infants, *Am J Dis Child* 1960;99:489.
2. Swyer PR et al: The pulmonary syndrome of Wilson and Mikity, *Pediatrics* 1965;36:374.
3. Coates AL et al: Long-term sequelae of the Wilson-Mikity syndrome, *J Pediatr* 1978;92:247.
4. Hodgman JE et al: Chronic respiratory distress in the premature infant, *Pediatrics* 1969;44:179.
5. Burnard ED et al: Pulmonary insufficiency in prematurity, *Aust Paediatr J* 1965;1:12.
6. Krauss AN et al: Chronic pulmonary insufficiency of prematurity, *Pediatrics* 1975;55:55.
7. Northway WH et al: Pulmonary disease following respiratory therapy of hyaline membrane disease, *N Engl J Med* 1967;276:357.
8. Edwards DK et al: Radiographic-pathologic correlation in bronchopulmonary dysplasia, *J Pediatr* 1979;95:835.
9. Miniati D: Pulmonary vascular remodeling, *Semin Pediatr Surg* 2007;16:80.
10. Coalson JJ et al: Decreased alveolarization in baboon survivors with bronchopulmonary dysplasia, *Am J Respir Crit Care Med* 1995;152:640.
11. Charafeddine et al: Atypical chronic lung disease patterns in neonates, *Peds* 1999;103:759.
12. Coalson JJ: Pathology of chronic lung disease of early infancy. In Bland RD, Coalson JJ, editors: *Chronic lung disease in early infancy*. New York: Marcel Dekker; 2000.
13. Coalson JJ: Pathology of bronchopulmonary dysplasia, *Semin Perinatol* 2006;30:179.
14. Jobe AH: The new BPD, *NeoReviews* 2006;7:e531.
15. Coalson JJ Pathology of new bronchopulmonary dysplasia, *Semin Neonatol* 2003;8:73.
16. Goldenberg, RL et al: Intrauterine infection and pre-term delivery, *N Engl J Med* 2000;342: 1500.
17. Kallapur SG et al: Vascular changes following intra-amniotic endotoxin in preterm lamb lungs, *Am J Physiol Lung Cell Mol Physiol* 2004,287.Ll178.
18. Moss MJM et al: Experimental intra-uterine *Ureaplasma* infection in sheep, *Am J Obstet Gynecol* 2005;192:1179.
19. Ikegami J, Jobe A: Postnatal lung inflammation increased by ventilation of preterm lambs exposed antenatally to *E. coli* endotoxin, *Pediatr Res* 2002;52:356.
20. Van Marter LJ et al: Chorioamnionitis, mechanical ventilation, and postnatal sepsis as modulators of chronic lung disease in preterm infants, *J Pediatr* 2002;140:171.
21. Young KC et al: The association between early tracheal colonization and bronchopulmonary dysplasia, *J Perinatol* 2005;25:403.
22. Horbar JD, Carpenter JH, Kenny M, editors: *Vermont Oxford Network 2007 very low birth weight database summary*. Burlington, Vt: Vermont Oxford Network. Burlington, Vermont.(1995-2005). *http://www.vtoxford.org*
23. Wegner, DJ et al: A major deletion in the surfactant protein B gene causing lethal respiratory distress, *Acta Pediatr* 2007;96:516.
24. Schulenin S et al: ABCA3 gene mutations in newborns with fatal surfactant deficiency, *N Engl J Med* 2004;350:296.
25. Cheong N et al: Functional and trafficking defects in ATP binding cassette A3 mutants associated with respiratory distress syndrome, *J Biol Chem* 2006;281:9791.
26. Hamvas A: Inherited surfactant protein-B deficiency and surfactant protein-C associated disease: Clinical features and evaluation, *Semin Perinatol* 2006;30:316.
27. Notter RH and Wang Z: Pulmonary surfactant: Physical chemistry, physiology, and replacement, *Rev Chem Engineering* 1997;4:1.
28. Torresin M et al: Exogenous surfactant kinetics in infants RDS: A novel method with stable isotopes, *Am J Resp Crit Care Med* 2000;161:1584.
29. Gunther A et al: Surfactant alteration and replacement in acute respiratory distress syndrome, *Respir Res* 2001;2:353.
30. Warriner HE et al: A concentration dependent mechanism by which serum albumin inactivates replacement lung surfactants, *Biophys J* 2002;82:835.
31. Holm, BA et al: A biophysical mechanism by which plasma proteins inhibit lung surfactant activity, *Chem Phys Lipids* 1988;49:49.
32. Moses, D et al: inhibition of pulmonary surfactant function by meconium, *Am J Obstet Gynecol* 1991;164:477.
33. Seeger W et al: Alteration of surfactant function due to protein leakage: Special interaction with fibrin monomer, *J Appl Physiol* 1985;58:326.
34. Rodriguez-Capote K et al: Reactive oxygen species inactivation of surfactant involves structural and functional alterations to surfactant proteins SP-B and SP-C, *Biophys J* 2006;90: 2808.
35. Gunther A et al: Cleavage of surfactant-incorporating fibrin by different fibrinolytic agents: Kinetics of lysis and rescue of surface activity, *Am J Respir Cell Mol Biol* 1999;21:738.
36. Gilliard N et al: Exposure of the hydrophobic components of porcine lung surfactant to oxidant stress alters surface tension properties, *J Clin Invest* 1994; 93:2608.
37. Bjorklund J et al: Manual ventilation with a few large breaths at birth compromises the therapeutic effect of subsequent surfactant replacement in immature lambs, *Pediatr Res* 1997;42:348.
38. Bonikos DS et al: Oxygen toxicity in the newborn: The effect of chronic continuous 100 percent oxygen on the lungs of newborn mice, *Am J Patrol* 1976;85:623.
39. Deems RA et al: Oxygen toxicity in the premature baboon with hyaline membrane disease, *Am Rev Respir Dis* 1987;136:677.
40. Rendell SH et al: Neonatal hyperoxia alters the pulmonary alveolar and capillary structure of 40-day-old rats, *Am J Patho* 1990; 136:1259.
41. Lorenzo A V: The pre term rabbit: A model for the study of acute and chronic effects of premature birth, *Pediat Res* 1985;19:201.
42. Hershenson MB et al: Hyperoxia-induced airway remodeling in immature rats, *Am Rev Respir Dis* 1992;146:1294.
43. Davis JM et al: Differentiate effects of oxygen and barotrauma on lung injury in the neonatal piglet, *Pediatr Pulmonol* 1991;10:157.
44. Huber GL, Drath DB: Pulmonary oxygen toxicity. In: Gilbert, DL, editor: *Oxygen and living processes: An interdisciplinary approach*. New York: Springer-Verlag; 1988.
45. Frank L, Massaro D: Oxygen toxicity, *Am J Med* 1980;69:117.
46. Freeman EA et al: Hyperoxia increases oxygen radical production in rat lung homogenates, *Arch Biochem Biophys* 1982;216:477.
47. Fridovich I: Oxygen radicals, hydrogen peroxide, and oxygen toxicity. In Prior WA, editor: *Free radicals in biology*, vol 1. New York: Academic Press; 1976.

48. Frank L, Sosenko IR: Development of lung antioxidant enzyme system in late gestation: Possible implications for the prematurely born infant, *J Pediatr* 1987;110:11.

49. Walther FJ et al: Ontogeny of antioxidant enzymes in the fetal lamb lung, *Exp Lung Res* 1991;17:39.

50. Rosenfeld W et al: Prevention of bronchopulmonary dysplasia by administration of bovine superoxide dismutase in preterm infants with respiratory distress syndrome, *J Pediatr* 1984;105:781.

51. Tanswell AK, Freeman BA: Liposome-entrapped antioxidant enzymes prevent lethal O_2 toxicity in the newborn rat, *J Appl Physiol* 1987; 63:347.

52. Frank L: Antioxidants, nutrition and bronchopulmonary dysplasia, *Clin Perinatol* 1992;19:541.

53. Shenai JP et al: Clinical trial of vitamin A supplementation in infants susceptible to bronchopulmonary dysplasia, *J Pediatr* 1987;111: 269.

54. Pierce MR, Bancalari E The role of inflammation in the pathogenesis of bronchopulmonary dysplasia, *Pediatr Pulmonol* 1995;19:371.

55. Arnon S et al: Pulmonary inflammatory cells in ventilated preterm infants: Effect of surfactant treatment, *Arch Dis Child* 1993;69:44.

56. Cook RWI: Factors associated with chronic lung disease in preterm infants, *Arch Dis Child* 1991;60:776.

57. Yoder BA et al: Effects of antenatal colonization with *ureaplasma urealyticum* on pulmonary disease in the immature baboon, *Pediatr Res* 2003;54:797.

58. Solca M et al: Management of the antenatal preterm fetal lung in the prevention of respiratory distress syndrome in lambs, *Biol Neonate* 1983;44:93.

59. Penn RB et al: Effect of ventilation on mechanical properties and pressure-flow relationships of immature airways, *Pediatr Res* 1988;23: 519.

60. Albertine KH et al: Chronic lung injury in preterm lambs: Disordered respiratory tract development, *Am J Respir Crit Care Med* 1999;159:945.

61. LJ Van Marter et al: Do Clinical markers of barotrauma and oxygen toxicity explain interhospital variation in rates of chronic lung disease? *Peds* 2000;105:1194.

62. Macklin MT, Macklin CC: Malignant interstitial emphysema of the lungs and mediastinum as an important occult complication in many respiratory diseases and other conditions: an interpretation of the clinical literature in the light of laboratory experiment, *Medicine* 1944; 23:281.

63. Verma RP et al: Risk factors and clinical outcomes of pulmonary interstitial emphysema in extremely low birth weight infants. *J Perinatol* 2006;26:197.

64. McAdams RM: Risk factors and clinical outcomes of pulmonary interstitial emphysema in extremely low birth weight infants, *J Perinatol* 2006;26:521.

65. Katar S et al: Symptomatic spontaneous pneumothorax in term newborns, *Pediatr Surg Int* 2006;22:755.

66. Mordue BC: A case report of the transport of an infant with a tension pneumopericardium, *Adv Neonatal Care* 2005;5:190.

67. Chiu B: To drain or not to drain: A single institution experience with neonatal intestinal perforation, *J Perinat Med* 2006;34:338.

68. Asensi M et al: Ratio of reduced to oxidized glutathione as indicator of oxidative stress status and DNA damage, *Methods Enzymol* 1999;299:267.

69. Schaeffer FQ, Buettner GR. Redox environment of the cell as viewed through the redox state of the glutathione disulfide/glutathione couple. *FRBM* 2001;30: 1191-1212.

70. Vento, M et al: Hyperoxia caused by resuscitation with pure oxygen may alter intracellular redox status b increasing oxidized glutathione in asphyxiated newly born infants, *Semin Perinatol* 2002;26:406.

71. de Zart et al: Biomarkers of free radical damage applications in experimental animals and in humans, *Free Radic Biol Med* 1999;26:202.

72. Vento M et al: Six years of experience with the use of room air for the resuscitation of asphyxiated newly born term infants, *Biol Neonate* 2001;79:261.

73. Temesvari P et al: Impaired early neurologic outcome in newborn piglets reoxygenated with 100% oxygen compared with room air after pneumothorax-induced asphyxia, *Pediatr Res* 2001;49:812.

74. Kutschke S et al: Hydrogen peroxide production in leukocytes during cerebral hypoxia and reoxygenation with 100% or 21% oxygen in newborn piglets, *Pediatr Res* 2001;49:834.

75. Collard CD et al: Pathophysiology, clinical manifestations, and prevention of ischemia-reperfusion injury, *Anesthesiology* 2001;94:1133.

76. Fellman V, Raivio K: Reperfusion injury as the mechanism of brain damage after perinatal asphyxia, *Pediatr Res* 1997;41:599.

77. Li C et al: Reactive species mechanisms of cellular hypoxia-reoxygenation injury, *Am J Physiol* 2002;282:C227.

78. Munkeby BH et al: Resuscitation with 100% O_2 increases cerebral injury in hypoxemic piglets, *Pediatr Res* 2004;56:783.

79. Vento M. et al: Resuscitation with room air instead of 100% oxygen prevents oxidative stress in moderately asphyxiated term neonates, *Pediatrics* 2001;107:642.

80. Saugstad OD et al: Resuscitation of depressed newborn infants with ambient air or pure oxygen: A meta-analysis, *Biol Neonate* 2005;87:27.

81. Vento M et al: Oxidative stress in asphyxiated term infants resuscitated with *100%* oxygen, *J Pediatr* 2003;142:240. (Published correction in 2003;142: 616)

82. Vento M et al: Room-air resuscitation causes less damage to heart and kidney than 100% oxygen, *Am J Respir Crit Care Med* 2005;172:1393.

83. Tyree MM et al: Impact of room air resuscitation on early growth response gene-1in a neonatal piglet model of cerebral hypoxic ischemia, *Pediatr Res* 2006;59:423.

84. Haase E et al: Resuscitation with 100% oxygen causes intestinal glutathione oxidation and reoxidation injury asphyxiated newborn piglets, *Ann Surg* 2004;240:364.

85. Dohlen G et al: Reoxygenation of hypoxic mice with 100% oxygen induces brain nuclear factor-kappa B, *Pediatr Res* 2005;58:941.

86. Richards JG et al: A dose-response study of graded reoxygenation on the carotid haemodynamics, matrix metalloproteinase-2 activities and amino acid concentrations in the brain of asphyxiated newborn piglets, *Resuscitation* 2006;69:319.

87. Haase E et al: Cardiac function, myocardial glutathione, and matrix metalloproteinase-2 levels in hypoxic newborn pigs reoxygenated by 21%, 50%, or 100% oxygen, *Shock* 2005;23:383.

88. L Johnson et al: Relationship of prolonged pharmacologic serum levels of vitamin E to incidence of sepsis and necrotizing enterocolitis in infants with birth weight 1,500 grams or less, *Pediatrics* 1985;75:619.

89. Jankov RP et al: Antioxidants as therapy in the newborn: some words of caution, *Pediatr Res* 2001;50:681.

90. Suresh GK, Soll RF: Overview of surfactant replacement trials, *Jrnl of Perinatol* 2005;25:Supplement 2 S40-S44.

91. Jan Erik H Bunt et al: Treatment with exogenous surfactant stimulates endogenous surfactant synthesis in premature infants with respiratory distress syndrome, *Crit Care Med* 2000;28:3383.

92. Horbar JD et al: Collaborative quality improvement to promote evidence based surfactant for preterm infants: a cluster randomized trial, *BMJ* 2004;329:1.

93. Costakos D, CL Paxson, et al: Surfactant therapy prior to the interhospital transport of preterm infants, *Am Jrnl of Perinatol* 1996;13:309.

94. Saugstad OD: Oxygen saturations immediately after birth, *J Pediatr* 2006;148:569.

95. Kamlin CO et al: Oxygen saturation in healthy infants immediately after birth, *J Pediatr* 2006;148:585.

96. Saugstad OD et al: Response to resuscitation of the newborn: early prognostic variables, *Acta Paediatr* 2005;94:890.

97. Eun B et al: Pentoxifylline attenuates hypoxic-ischemic brain injury in immature rats *Pediatr Res* 2000;47:73.

98. Asikainen TM et al: Improved lung growth and function through hypoxia-inducible factor in primate chronic lung disease of prematurity, *FASEB J* 2006;20:1698.

99. Ohlsson A et al: Ibuprofen for the treatment of PDA in preterm and/or low birth weight infants, *Cochrane Database Syst Rev* 2005;19:CDOO3481.

100. Desmond MM: Clinical transitional behavior of the newly born infant, *Pediatr Clin North Am* 1966; 13:656.

101. RH Clark et al: Empiric use of ampicillin and cefotaxime, compared with ampicillin and gentamicin, for neonates at risk for sepsis is associated with an increased risk of neonatal death, *Pediatrics* 2006;117:67.

102. Paxson C et al: Syndrome of inappropriate ADH secretion in neonates with lung disease, *Jrnl of Peds* 1977;91:459.

103. JL Aschner, RL Poland: Sodium bicarbonate: basically useless therapy, *Peds* 2008;122:831.

104. Munro MJ et al: Hypotensive extremely low birth weight infants have reduced cerebral blood flow, *Pediatrics* 2004;114:591.

105. Paxson C: Neonatal shock, *Am Jrnl Diseases Child* 1978;132:509.

106. Paxson C: Collection and use of autologous fetal blood, *Am Jrnl Obstet Gyn* 1979;134:708.

107. Quaife MA, Dirksen JW, Paxson C: RBC volume in preterm neonates, *Clin Nuclear Med* 1981;6:476.

108. Dirksen J, Quaife MD, Paxson C: Evaluation and testing of in vitro labeled technetium (Tc-99m) RBC in two animal models for neonatal RBC volume determinations, *Pediatr Res* 1981;15:905.

109. MJ Oca et al: Randomized trial of normal saline versus 5% albumin for the treatment of neonatal hypotension, *J Perinatology* 2003;23:473.

110. Bell E et al: Randomized trial of liberal versus restrictive guidelines for RBC transfusion in preterm infants, *Pediatrics* 2005;115:1685.

111. Bell E (editorial): Transfusion thresholds for preterm infants: How low should we go? *Jrnl Peds* 2006;149:287.

112. Watterberg KL: Postnatal steroids for BPD: Where are we now? *Jrl Peds* 2007;150:327.

113. McCurnin DLC et al: Inhaled NO improves early pulmonary function and modifies lung growth and elastin deposition in a baboon model of neonatal chronic lung disease, *Am J Physiol Lung Cell Mol Physiol* 2005;288:L450.

114. Ballard RA et al: Improved outcome with inhaled nitric oxide in preterm infants mechanically ventilated at 7-21 days of age, *N Engl J Med* 2006;355:1.

115. Massaro D et al: Calorie-related rapid onset of alveolar loss, regeneration, and changes in mouse lung gene expression, *Am J Physiol Lung Cell Mol Physiol* 2004;286:L896.

116. ten Bensel R, Paxson C: Child abuse following neonatal separation, *Jrnl of Peds* 1977;90:490.

117. Conti M et al: Management of post intubation tracheobronchial ruptures, *Chest* 2006;130:412.

118. Bhutani VK et al: Acquired tracheomegaly in very preterm neonates, *Am J Dis Child* 1986;140:449.

119. Palmer EA et al: Incidence and early course of retinopathy of prematurity: The Cryotherapy for Retinopathy of Prematurity Cooperative Group, *Ophthalmology* 1991;98:1628.

120. Johns KJ et al: Retinopathy of prematurity in infants with cyanotic congenital heart disease, *Am J Dis Child* 1991;145:200.

121. Holmes JM et al: Carbon dioxide-induced retinopathy in the neonatal rat, *Curr Eye Res* 1998;17:608.

122. Holmes JM et al: The effect of raised inspired carbon dioxide on developing rat retinal vasculature exposed to elevated oxygen, *Curr Eye Res* 1994;13:779.

123. Shohat M: Retinopathy of prematurity: Incidence and risk factors, *Pediatrics* 1983;72:59.

124. Organisciak DT et al: Retinal light damage in rats exposed to intermittent light: comparison with continuous light exposure, *Invest Ophthalmol Vis Sci* 1989;30:795.

125. Glass P: Light and the developing retina, *Doc Ophthalmol* 1990;74:195

126. Kabra NS et al: Neurosensory impairment after surgical closure of patent ductus arteriosus in extremely low birth weight infants: results from the trial of indomethacin prophylaxis in preterms, *Jrnl Pediatr* 2007;150:229.

127. Reynolds JD et al: Lack of efficacy of light reduction in preventing retinopathy of prematurity: Light Reduction in Retinopathy of Prematurity (LIGHT -ROP) Cooperative Group, *N Engl J Med* 1998;338:1572.

128. Teoh SL et al: Duration of oxygen therapy and exchange transfusion as risk factors associated with retinopathy of prematurity in very low birthweight infants, *Eye* 1997;9:733.

129. Caddell JL: Hypothesis: The possible role of magnesium and copper deficiency in retinopathy of prematurity, *Magnes Res* 1995;8:261.

130. Robbins SG et al: Evidence for upregulation and redistribution of vascular endothelial growth factor (VEGF) receptors flt-1 and flk-1 in the oxygen-injured rat retina, *Growth Factors* 1998;16:1.

131. International Committee for the Classification of ROP: An international classification of retinopathy of prematurity: II. The classification of retinal detachment; International Committee for the

Classification of the Late Stages of Retinopathy of Prematurity [published erratum appears in *Arch Ophthalmol* 1987; 105:1498]. *Arch Ophthalmol* 1987;105:906.

132. International Committee for the Classification of ROP: The international classification of retinopathy of prematurity revisited, *Arch Ophthalmol* 2005;123:991.

133. Raju TN et al: Vitamin E prophylaxis to reduce retinopathy of prematurity: a reappraisal of published trials, *J Pediatr* 1997;131:844.

134. Alon T et al: Vascular endothelial growth factor acts as a survival factor for newly formed retinal vessels and has implications for retinopathy of prematurity, *Nat Med* 1995;1:1024.

135. Stone J et al: Roles of vascular endothelial growth factor and astrocyte degeneration in the genesis of retinopathy of prematurity, *Invest Ophthalmol Vis Sci* 1996;37:290.

136. Gaynon MW et al: Supplemental oxygen may decrease progression of prethreshold disease to threshold retinopathy of prematurity, *J Perinatol* 1997;17:434.

137. Supplemental therapeutic oxygen for prethreshold retinopathy of prematurity (STOP-ROP), randomized controlled trial. I: primary outcomes, *Pediatrics* 2000;105:295.

138. Hay WW Jr, Bell EF: Oxygen therapy, oxygen toxicity, and the STOP-ROP trial, *Pediatrics* 2000;105:424.

139. Early Treatment for ROP Cooperative Group. Revised indications for the treatment of ROP: results of the early treatment for ROP randomized trial, *Arch Ophthalmol* 2003;121:1684.

140. Ment LR et al: Germinal matrix microvascular maturation correlates inversely with the risk period for neonatal intraventricular hemorrhage. *Brain Res Dev Brain Res* 1995;84:142-149.

141. Kuban KC, Gilles FH: Human telencephalic angiogenesis, *Ann Neurol* 1985;17:539.

142. Wilson-Costello D et al: Improved survival rates with increased neurodevelopmental disability for extremely low birth weight infants in the 1990s, *Pediatrics* 2005;115:997.

143. Patra K et al: Grades I-II intraventricular hemorrhage in extremely low birth weight infants: Effects on neurodevelopment, *J Pediatr* 2006;149:169.

144. Greisen G: Autoregulation of cerebral blood flow in newborn babies, *Early Hum Dev* 2005;81:423.

145. Boylan GB et al: Dynamic cerebral autoregulation in sick newborn infants, *Pediatr Res* 2000;48:12.

146. Meek JH et al: Low cerebral blood flow is a risk factor for severe intraventricular hemorrhage, *Arch Dis Child Fetal Neonatal Ed* 1999;81:F15.

147. Lou HC et al: Pressure passive cerebral blood flow and breakdown of the blood-brain barrier in experimental fetal asphyxia, *Acta Paediatr Scand* 1979;68:57.

148. Pryds O: Control of cerebral circulation in the high-risk neonate, *Ann Neurol* 1991;30:321.

149. Miall-Allen VM et al: Blood pressure fluctuation and intraventricular hemorrhage in the preterm infant of less than 31 weeks' gestation [see comments], *Pediatrics* 1989;83:657.

150. Perlman JM et al: Fluctuating cerebral blood-flow velocity in respiratory-distress syndrome: Relation to the development of intraventricular hemorrhage, *N Engl J Med* 1983;309:204.

151. Lott JW, Conner GK, Phillips JB: Umbilical artery catheter blood sampling alters cerebral blood flow velocity in preterm infants, *J Perinatol* 1996;16:341.

152. Fabres J et al: Both extremes of arterial carbon dioxide pressure and the magnitude of fluctuations in arterial carbon dioxide pressure are associated with severe intraventricular hemorrhage in preterm infants, *Pediatrics* 2007;119:299.

153. Evans N, Kluckow M: Early ductal shunting and intraventricular haemorrhage in ventilated preterm infants, *Arch Dis Child Fetal Neonatal Ed* 1996;75:F183.

154. Amato M et al: Coagulation abnormalities in low birth weight infants with peri-intraventricular hemorrhage, *Neuropediatrics* 1988;19:154.

155. O'Shea TM et al: Perinatal events and the risk of intraparenchymal echodensity in very-low-birthweight neonates, *Paediatr Perinatal Epidemiol* 1998;12:408.

156. Hill A et al: Relationship of pneumothorax to occurrence of intraventricular hemorrhage in the premature newborn, *Pediatrics* 1982;69:144.

157. Tamura M et al: Comparison of the incidence of intracranial hemorrhage following conventional mechanical ventilation and high frequency oscillation in beagle puppies, *Acta Paediatr Jpn* 1992;34:398.

158. Cheung PY et al: Rescue high frequency oscillatory ventilation for preterm infants: neurodevelopmental outcome and its prediction, *Biol Neon* 1997;71:282.

159. Vohr BR et al: Neurodevelopmental outcomes of extremely low birth weight infants <32 weeks gestation between 1993 and 1998, *Pediatrics* 2005;116:635.

160. Volpe JJ: Neurobiology of periventricular leukomalacia in the premature infant, *Pediatr Res* 2001;50:553.

161. Huang YF et al: Fetal intracranial hemorrhage (fetal stroke) report of four antenatally diagnosed cases and review of the literature, *Taiwan J Obstet Gynecol* 2006;45:135.

162. Osborn DA: Hemodynamic and antecedent risk factors of early and late periventricular/intraventricular hemorrhage in premature infants, *Pediatrics* 2003;112:33.

163. Lazzara A et al: Clinical predictability of intraventricular hemorrhage in preterm infants. *Pediatrics* 1980;65:30.

164. Papile LA et al: Incidence and evolution of subependymal and intraventricular hemorrhage: a study of infants with birth weights less than 1,500 gm, *J Pediatr* 1978;92:529.

165. Dolfin T et al: Incidence, severity, and timing of subependymal and intraventricular hemorrhages in preterm infants born in a perinatal unit as detected by serial real-time ultrasound, *Pediatrics* 1983;71:541.

166. Laptook AR et al: Adverse neurodevelopmental outcomes among extremely low birth weight infants with a normal head ultrasound: prevalence and antecedents, *Pediatrics* 2005;115:673.

167. Clancy RR: Prolonged electroencephalogram monitoring of seizures and their treatment, *Clin Perinatol* 2006;33:649.

168. Murphy BP: Posthaemorrhagic ventricular dilatation in the premature infant: Natural history and predictors of outcome, *Arch Dis Child Fetal Neonatal Ed* 2002;87:37.

169. Papile LA, Munsick-Bruno G, Schaefer A: Relationship of cerebral intraventricular hemorrhage and early childhood neurologic handicaps, *J Pediatr* 1983;103:273.

170. Cordero L et al: Indomethacin prophylaxis or expectant treatment of patent ductus arteriosus in extremely low birth weight infants? *J Perinatol* 2007;27:158.

171. Kaiser et al: The effects of hypercapnia on cerebral autoregulation in ventilated very low birth weight infants, *Pediatr Res* 2005;58:931.

172. Balasubramaniam J, Del Bigio MR: Animal models of germinal matrix hemorrhage, *J Child Neurol* 2006;21:365.

173. Pryds A et al: Cerebral pressure autoregulation and vasoreactivity in the newborn, *Pediatr Res* 2005;57:294.

174. Ment LR et al: Beagle puppy model of perinatal cerebral insults: Cerebral blood flow changes and intraventricular hemorrhage evoked by hypoxemia, *J. Neurosurg* 1986;65:847.

175. Ment LR et al: Beagle puppy model: Effect of superoxide dismutase on cerebral blood flow and prostaglandins, *J Neurosurg* 1985;62:563.

176. Ment LR et al: Beagle puppy model of perinatal cerebral infarction: Acute changes in cerebral blood flow and metabolism during hemorrhagic hypotension, *J Neurosurg* 1985;63:441.

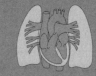

Chapter 30

Congenital Cardiac Defects

JOHN SALYER • TEODOR D. BUTIU • DAVID N. CROTWELL

LEARNING OBJECTIVES

After reading this chapter the reader will be able to:
- Describe normal cardiac anatomy and blood flow in newborns
- Describe the normal transition from intrauterine to extrauterine blood flow
- Describe the various sites of shunting of blood from systemic to pulmonary circulation
- Understand the basic classification schemes for congenital cardiac defects
- Explain the 12 most common congenital cardiac defects
- Recognize the various causes of changes in pulmonary vascular resistance

- Describe the importance of balancing pulmonary and systemic blood flow (Q_p/Q_s) associated with various defects
- Recommend ventilator strategies commonly used with various congenital cardiac defects
- Describe the clinical indications for subambient oxygen therapy and hypercarbic inhaled gas therapy in the treatment of certain types of congenital cardiac defects
- Recommend and understand the limitations of various types of physiologic monitoring necessary for the care of patients with congenital cardiac defects

517

There are over 35,000 infants born yearly in the United States with significant congenital heart disease. Approximately one third of these will undergo palliative or corrective surgery in their first year of life.[1] As recently as the turn of the 20th century, conventional medical wisdom held that many congenital cardiac anomalies were incompatible with life and that little could be done to ameliorate their effects. Since then, there have been enormous advances in the diagnosis and treatment of congenital cardiac disease.[2,3] There are now a wide variety of surgical and pharmacologic interventions for these defects, which have resulted in improvements in outcomes that would have seemed miraculous to the clinicians from the beginning of the previous century. It is estimated that 150,000 adults in the U.S. are now living with some form of complex congenital heart disease.[4] Respiratory therapists have played a large role in the perioperative care of these patients. Congenital cardiac disease occurs in about 10 in 1000 live births.[5] Almost all diagnosis and treatment of newborns with congenital cardiac defects occurs in highly specialized centers, usually tertiary pediatric academic medical centers.

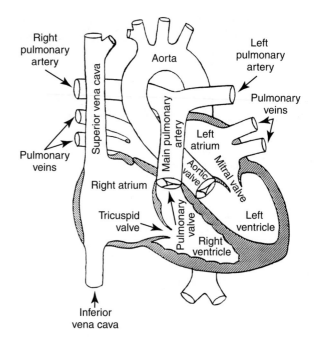

FIGURE 30-1 Anatomy of the normal heart and great vessels.

CARDIOPULMONARY ANATOMY AND PHYSIOLOGY

Knowledge of blood flow during fetal circulation, changes that occur at birth (see Chapter 2), circulation of a normal heart, persistent fetal circulation, and the importance of the ductus arteriosus is essential to understanding the treatment and management of congenital cardiac anomalies.

Anatomy and Blood Flow of the Normal Heart

The normal heart can be thought of conceptually as a pump consisting of four chambers (Figures 30-1 and 30-2). The right atrium (RA) receives blood from all parts of the body through three veins:

1. the superior vena cava brings blood from parts of the body superior to the heart.
2. the inferior vena cava brings blood from parts of the body inferior to the heart.
3. the coronary sinus drains blood from most of the vessels supplying the heart.

The RA then delivers the blood into the right ventricle (RV), which pumps it into the main pulmonary artery. This artery divides into a right and a left pulmonary artery, each of which carries blood to the lungs. In the lungs, carbon dioxide diffuses out of the blood and oxygen diffuses in. This oxygenated blood is then returned to the heart through four pulmonary veins that empty into the left atrium (LA), from which the

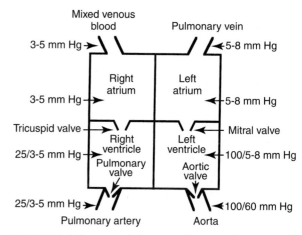

FIGURE 30-2 Pressure of the normal heart and great vessels of the older child.

blood is pumped into the left ventricle (LV). The blood is then pumped from the LV into the aorta and from there to all other parts of the systemic circulation.

The size of each chamber of the heart varies according to its function. The RA, which must collect blood coming from nearly all parts of the body, is slightly larger than the LA, which receives blood only from the lungs. The thickness of the chamber walls also varies. The atria are thin walled because they need only enough cardiac muscle to create pressure adequate to deliver the blood into the ventricles. This is relatively easy because at the same time that the atria contract, the ventricles relax (diastole). The RV has a thicker layer of myocardium than does the atria because it must overcome pulmonary vascular resistance (PVR). The LV has the thickest walls because it must pump blood at higher pressures through thousands of miles of vessels in the head, trunk, and extremities. Atrioventricular (AV) valves lie between the atria and the ventricles. The right AV valve is also called the tricuspid valve because it consists of three flaps, or cusps. The left AV valve has two flaps and is called the bicuspid or mitral valve. Both arteries that exit the heart have a semilunar valve that prevents blood from flowing back into the heart. The pulmonary semilunar valve lies in the opening where the pulmonary artery leaves the RV. The aortic semilunar valve is situated at the opening between the LV and the aorta. Like the AV valves, the semilunar valves permit blood to flow in one direction only, in this case from the ventricles into the arteries.

Adaptation to Extrauterine Life

Once the umbilical vessels are clamped, the low-pressure system of the placenta is removed from the fetal circulation (Figure 30-3). As the lungs inflate and gas exchange occurs, the increase in Pao_2 causes dilatation of the pulmonary vascular bed, resulting in a reduction in PVR. Pressures in the right side of the heart decrease and pressures in the left side increase. During this time, the pressure in the aorta increases

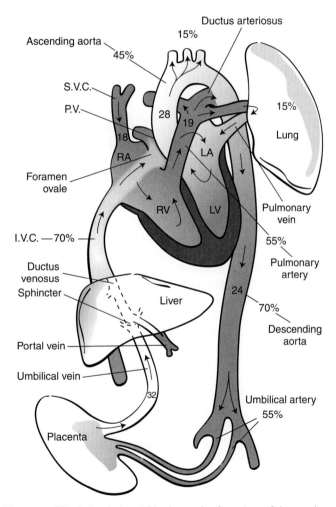

FIGURE 30-3 Diagram of fetal circulation. This shows the four sites of shunt: placenta, ductus venosus, foramen ovale, and ductus arteriosus. Intravascular shading is in proportion to oxygen saturation, with the lightest shading representing the highest Po_2. The numerical value inside the chamber or vessel is the Po_2 for that site in mm Hg. The percentages outside the vascular structures represent the relative flows in major tributaries and outlets for the two ventricles. The combined output of the two ventricles represents 100%. a, Artery, IVC, inferior vena cava, LA., left atrium, LV, left ventricle, PV, pulmonary vein, RA, right atrium, RV, right ventricle, SVC, superior vena cava, v, vein.

and becomes greater than the pressure in the pulmonary artery, thus decreasing the amount of shunting through the ductus arteriosus and foramen ovale. During the immediate postnatal period, these two shunts may not close completely. Closure of the ductus arteriosus usually occurs within the first 24 hours to 2 weeks of life, except in the premature infant in whom musculature of the ductus arteriosus may not be well developed and its ability to constrict is limited. The PVR will be lower than the systemic vascular resistance (SVR) and blood will flow into the lungs from the systemic circulation (left to right). The ductus arteriosus may not close completely in some postterm infants (e.g., in meconium aspiration). These patients may experience very high PVR, and blood will then flow from right to left through the ductus arteriosus from the pulmonary circulation to the systemic circulation, bypassing the lungs. Because the foramen ovale flap allows blood to flow only from right to left, it closes when the pressures in the LA become greater than those in the RA. If the foramen ovale lacks a flaplike structure or has a defective one, the opening begins to function as an atrial septal defect (ASD). The pressures in the various chambers of a normal heart and great vessels of the older child can be seen in Figure 30-2.

CLASSIFICATION OF CARDIAC ANOMALIES

In discussions of congenital cardiac anomalies, two categories have typically been used to classify these lesions—cyanotic and acyanotic—referring to whether the principal direction of extrapulmonary shunting is right to left (cyanotic) or left to right (acyanotic). However, patients with right-to-left shunting do not always actually clinically manifest cyanosis, whereas some patients with left-to-right shunting may well be cyanotic. Within these two categories, numerous subcategories have been recognized: cyanosis as the outstanding physical feature, cyanosis with moderate respiratory distress, and cyanosis with low cardiac output. For simplicity, this chapter separates the anomalies into the two categories describing the shunting of blood: left-to-right shunts (increased pulmonary blood flow) and right-to-left shunts (decreased pulmonary blood flow). When possible, the description, radiographic findings, presurgical management, surgical repair, and postsurgical management are discussed for each cardiac anomaly.

In congenital cardiac disease with a right-to-left shunt (often termed *cyanotic cardiac defect*), desaturated systemic venous blood is shunted from right to left within the heart (extrapulmonary), bypassing the lungs and entering the systemic arterial circulation. Central cyanosis is a frequent finding that leads to the early diagnosis of many of these lesions. In congenital cardiac disease with a left-to-right shunt (often termed *acyanotic cardiac defect*), oxygenated blood is shunted from left to right within the heart, mixing with deoxygenated blood. Even though there is a mixing of oxygenated and deoxygenated blood, these infants often initially appear pink and healthy. The left-to-right shunt often results in increased pulmonary blood flow as well as increased PVR. With both types of shunts, there are several lesions that depend on a patent ductus arteriosus (PDA) for adequate pulmonary and systemic blood flow. These anomalies are also called ductal-dependent lesions because spontaneous closure of the ductus arteriosus can prove catastrophic (e.g., severe coarctation of the aorta, hypoplastic left heart syndrome, Tetralogy of Fallot with pulmonary atresia). Often, acyanotic infants are discharged home with their condition undiagnosed, with symptoms developing as the ductus arteriosus begins to close 12 to 48 hours later.

CONGENITAL CARDIAC ANOMALIES

Patent Ductus Arteriosus

During fetal life, the ductus arteriosus allows most of the right ventricular output to bypass the lungs and be shunted from right to left from the pulmonary artery to the aorta. Within hours to days after birth, the ductus arteriosus closes spontaneously as a result of hormonal, chemical, and blood gas changes. However, it may not constrict but remains open in some infants, especially those born prematurely. After birth, as the PVR falls, the pressure in the aorta is higher than that in the pulmonary artery and the direction of blood flow through the PDA reverses. The blood flow is now from left-to-right from the aorta to the pulmonary artery, causing an increase in pulmonary blood flow (Figure 30-4). The constrictor response of the ductus arteriosus to oxygen and the dilator effect of prostaglandin E_2 are functions of gestational age; hence, the greater the prematurity, the more delayed the ductal closure. Delayed closure of the ductus arteriosus may be associated with respiratory distress syndrome and prematurity. PDA is one of the most common cardiac defects seen in neonatal intensive care units. The delay in spontaneous closure of the ductus is inversely related to gestational age and incidence varies from 20% in premature infants greater than 32 weeks' gestation up to 60% in those less than 28 weeks' gestation.[6]

If a PDA is suspected, the presence of ductal shunting can be confirmed by looking for a difference in oxygenation of preductal versus postductal blood. This can

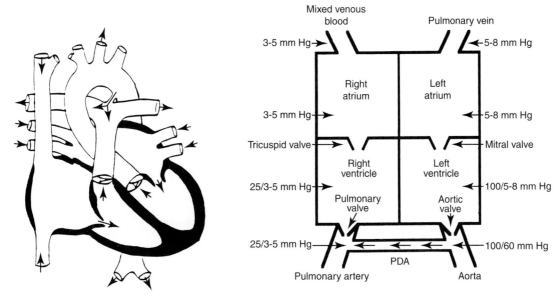

FIGURE 30-4 Patent ductus arteriosus. Communication between the pulmonary artery and the aorta.

be done by obtaining preductal (right radial or temporal artery) and postductal (umbilical artery) blood gases. A Pao_2 differential of > 15 mm Hg is considered indicative of significant ductal shunting.[7,8] This assessment can also be done noninvasively with preductal (right hand) and postductal (left hand or lower extremities) pulse oximetry readings. A pulse oximetry difference of > 5 % is suggestive of ductal shunting.

In numerous congenital cardiac defects it is imperative for survival that a PDA be present to provide either systemic or pulmonary blood flow. In these defects all attempts, pharmacologic or surgical, will be made to maintain the PDA.

Even an isolated PDA in the absence of other congenital cardiac defects can eventually lead to congestive heart failure and pulmonary hypertension due to pulmonary overcirculation. These patients often experience deterioration in lung mechanics and gas exchange, which can complicate ventilation and weaning in infants requiring mechanical ventilation. Although a PDA may close spontaneously at any time, it is unlikely that this will occur after the patient is 1 year of age. Chest radiographic findings are usually normal, but in extreme cases in which congestive heart failure develops, there may be enlarged pulmonary vascular markings. The definitive diagnosis of PDA is typically made with echocardiography.

Medical management of the PDA includes maintaining euvolemia, keeping the hemoglobin level at the high end of the normal, and providing indomethacin treatment, which is most effective if given in the first day after birth.[9] A single dose of indomethacin (0.2 mg/kg iv)

given in the first 24 hours after delivery can be effective in preventing clinical symptoms associated with PDA.[10] Many variations in the dosage regimens of indomethacin have been reported. Usually the treatment is given over a 48-hour period. With 0.1 to 0.2 mg/kg iv doses serious side effects are uncommon—except oliguria and dilutional hyponatremia, which may necessitate interruption of a full course of treatment.

Digoxin does not seem to play an important role in the treatment since the contractility of myocardium is increased rather than reduced in infants with PDA.

Addition of PEEP in mechanically ventilated patients seems to be beneficial by decreasing the left-to-right shunting through ductus arteriosus and consequently increasing the systemic blood flow.[11]

Surgical repair of a PDA before the 10th day of life has been reported to reduce the duration of ventilatory support and hospital stays and result in lower morbidity. Practice varies considerably, but the most common approach involves a trial of indomethacin followed within a few days by surgical repair if symptoms persist. The surgery can now be performed with low morbidity and mortality in the intensive care unit. Postoperative ventilatory support is not often necessary except in those patients who required it preoperatively. Normal arterial blood gas and pulse oximetry measurements can be expected.

Atrial Septal Defect

An ASD is a communication between the right and left atria (Figure 30-5). Several anatomic types result in a defect of the lower or upper sections of the septum, including:

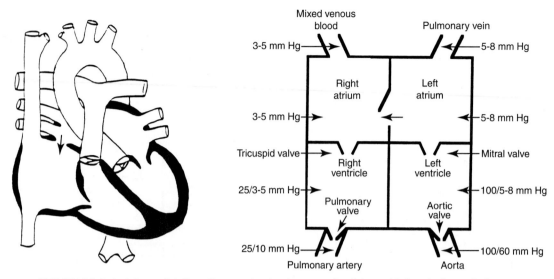

FIGURE 30-5 Atrial septal defect. Communication between the right and left atria through the septum.

1. an incompetent foramen ovale that allows regurgitation between the atria
2. a developmental defect in the septum itself, or
3. failure of development in the endocardial cushion area.

As a consequence, there are three types of ASD; primum ASD in the lower part of the septum (30% of ASDs), secundum ASD in the central portion of the septum (50% to 70% of ASDs), and sinus venosus defect in the proximity of SVC or IVC connection to the right atrium (10% of ASDs). Blood flow is usually shunted from left to right through the ASD, with an increase in pulmonary blood flow occurring. This rarely produces congestive heart failure in children, although the RV may become hypertrophic because of the increased blood flow. Although symptoms have been reported in the neonatal period, most of these patients remain asymptomatic until school age, with only approximately 8% having their conditions identified before they are 2 years old.[12] Minimally invasive surgical repairs are now being done successfully in the cardiac catheterization laboratory, replacing open chest procedures that were previously necessary for ASDs and ventricular septal defects (VSDs).[13,14] Chest radiographic findings are usually normal, but in extreme cases in which congestive heart failure develops there may be enlarged pulmonary vascular markings and cardiomegaly. The timing of the decision to proceed with repair of both ASDs and VSDs depends largely on the degree of pulmonary overcirculation and resultant pulmonary hypertension.

If open chest surgical repair is indicated, the defect is closed during cardiopulmonary bypass, usually by a simple suture. If the defect is large enough, a tailored patch is sewn into the septum. Postsurgical management often includes mechanical ventilation, during which blood gas and pulse oximetry measurements can be expected to be normal.

Ventricular Septal Defect

A VSD is a communication between the right and left ventricles (Figure 30-6). It may be a single small hole, multiple holes or a hole large enough to make the ventricular septum almost completely absent. The location can be anywhere along the ventricular septum. In about 10% of infants with VSD, other anomalies are also present. Approximately 20% of all patients with congenital cardiac anomalies have a VSD as the only lesion. The majority of the blood flow is shunted from left to right, because the resistance of the pulmonary vascular bed is relatively low compared to systemic vascular resistance. Shunting typically occurs during ventricular systole.

The shunt may be large and result in congestive heart failure and pulmonary hypertension. If the VSD is small, the heart may appear normal on the chest radiograph. If the VSD is large, the cardiac silhouette will be enlarged and the pulmonary vascular markings increased, as seen in infants with congestive heart failure. A left-to-right shunt may increase pulmonary blood flow to the point that the increased pressure and volume result in thickening and fibrosis of the pulmonary arterioles. This causes permanent damage to the pulmonary vascular bed, resulting in irreversible pulmonary hypertension and/or congestive heart failure. Resistance in the pulmonary system may become greater than that in the systemic circulation, and the left-to-right shunt is reversed to a right-to-left shunt. This is called Eisenmenger

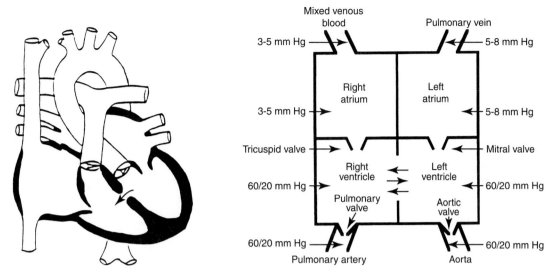

FIGURE 30-6 Ventricular septal defect. Communication between the right and left ventricles through the septum.

syndrome and is rarely seen in children today because most defects are corrected before irreversible damage can occur. These patients have noncompliant lungs and experience difficulty breathing.

The majority of small VSDs close spontaneously within the first and second years of life, and in most cases no intervention is necessary. If medical management is mandated, it usually includes digoxin and furosemide. The decision to proceed from medical management to surgical repair varies considerably among patients. Typically, patients in whom medical management fails exhibit poor growth, repeated pulmonary infections, and ultimately pulmonary hypertension. The Pao$_2$ and Sao$_2$ will be in the low end of the normal range depending on the degree of mixing across the ventricular wall.

Pulmonary banding is sometimes performed to help direct the cardiac blood flow by narrowing the diameter of the pulmonary artery and thus increasing resistance to blood flow. It consists of tightly wrapping a Dacron or polytetrafluoroethylene (Teflon) strip around the pulmonary artery and decreasing the degree of left-to-right shunting. This is a relatively simple palliative procedure that does not correct the defect itself. It is often performed when an infant or child's condition is too unstable or the child is too small for the corrective repair to be undertaken. The banding allows the child to grow and the condition to stabilize before open-heart surgery is performed. If total repair is indicated, the defect is closed during cardiopulmonary bypass, usually by suturing. If the defect is large, a tailored patch is sewn to the septum. If the patient has undergone previous pulmonary banding, the band is removed at this time as well. Brief postoperative mechanical ventilation is used in most patients. Normal arterial blood gas and pulse oximetry measurements can be expected.

Atrioventricular (AV) Canal Defect

The term *AV canal* refers to an anomaly in which there is incomplete development of the septa between both the atria and the ventricles and a common AV valve that takes origin from both atria (Figure 30-7). Simply stated, there is a large ASD and a VSD with deformed and many times incompetent mitral and tricuspid valves, resulting in a large "hole" that allows the blood to mix among any of the heart chambers. The defect has a "scooped-out" appearance, hence the term *canal*. There are varying degrees of AV canal, but all involve a mixing of atrial and ventricular blood. There is a large left-to-right shunt, resulting in increased pulmonary blood flow. AV canal anomalies are one of the most common types of heart disease present in infants with Down syndrome (Trisomy 21).[15]

Chest radiography usually reveals cardiomegaly with increased pulmonary vascular markings and congestive heart failure. The presurgical management of a newborn with an AV canal defect is designed to optimize heart function. Sometimes many months pass before surgery is required. Pulse oximetry values may remain low (75% to 90%) because of venous admixing and left-to-right shunting but appear to be tolerated well by most of these patients. Supplemental oxygen may be given, but this should be carried out judiciously to minimize pulmonary vascular dilation, which might increase pulmonary blood flow, causing pulmonary vascular engorgement.

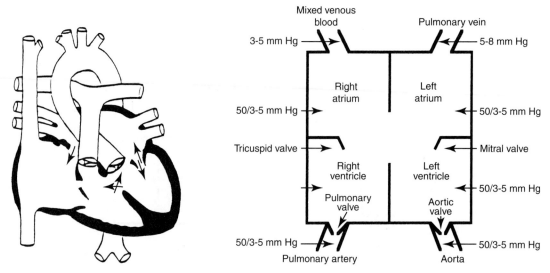

FIGURE 30-7 Atrioventricular canal defect. Incomplete development of the atrial and ventricular septa, which allows complete cardiac mixing of blood.

There are divergent opinions regarding the best surgical approach to managing AV canal defects. Banding of the pulmonary artery (PA banding) to increase PVR and thus decrease pulmonary blood flow has been the procedure of choice because of its simplicity, but it should be used only if there is no significant mitral valve regurgitation. This procedure lessens congestive heart failure but does nothing for the defect itself (i.e., it is palliative), giving the infant time to become stabilized and gain weight before future repairs. A complete surgical repair can be performed without banding of the pulmonary artery, and is now the preferred approach. The atrial and ventricular septa are closed with a patch or with whatever part of the septum is available. The common AV valve (tricuspid and mitral) is divided and reconstructed on the newly constructed septum. Rebuilding the common valve and making two valves tends to be the most difficult part of the procedure and can result in a leaky or deformed mitral valve. Care is taken to avoid deep sutures near the coronary sinus during the valve repairs in order to avoid disruption of AV conduction. Patients with Down syndrome tend to be repaired earlier because of their propensity to develop early severe pulmonary hypertension.

Postoperative management varies, depending on the surgical procedure performed. If pulmonary artery banding is performed, the mixing of oxygenated and deoxygenated blood will continue; therefore, lower Pao_2 (40 to 60 mm Hg) and Sao_2 (75% to 85% at sea level) values should be expected. If a complete repair is performed, normal arterial oxygenation can be anticipated. Because of the complexity of the septal repairs performed, there can be some residual mixing among chambers

of the heart and mitral and tricuspid valve regurgitation. Whenever the septa are surgically repaired, there can be a disruption of the conductive system; therefore, these patients usually have pacing wires placed for the postoperative treatment of possible arrhythmias. Postoperatively there is a high incidence of pulmonary hypertension, which can contribute to immediate postoperative mortality.[16]

LEFT VENTRICULAR OUTFLOW TRACT OBSTRUCTION

Aortic Stenosis

Left ventricular outflow tract obstructions include a number of conditions that cause a physical impediment to the ejection of blood from the left ventricle. They include valvular aortic stenosis, coarctation of the aorta, hypoplastic aortic arch, and interrupted aortic arch. Valvular aortic stenosis is a narrowing located below (subvalvular), at (valvular), or above (supravalvular) the aortic valve (Figure 30-8). The degree of clinical manifestation of impaired cardiac function is related to the severity of the stenosis. The myocardium is always hypertrophied, with the ventricle overdistended to varying degrees. If left ventricular pressures are great enough, congestive heart failure may result. Occasionally, left atrial pressures and the resulting distention can cause blood to flow from left to right through the foramen ovale.

The chest radiograph reveals findings similar to those of an infant in congestive heart failure. The heart is usually enlarged. The pulmonary vessels appear enlarged on chest x-ray because of pulmonary venous congestion.

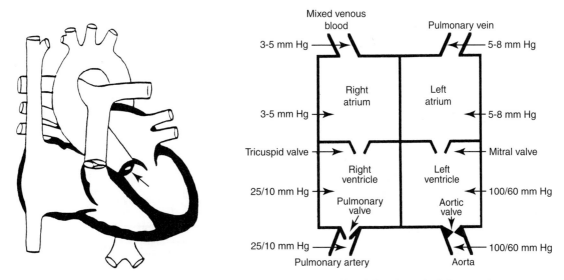

Mixed venous blood

Pulmonary vein

3-5 mm Hg

5-8 mm Hg

Right atrium

Left atrium

3-5 mm Hg

5-8 mm Hg

Tricuspid valve

Mitral valve

Right ventricle

Left ventricle

25/10 mm Hg

100/60 mm Hg

Pulmonary valve

Aortic valve

25/10 mm Hg

100/60 mm Hg

Pulmonary artery

Aorta

FIGURE 30-8 Aortic stenosis. Outflow obstruction of the aorta, impeding blood flow from the left ventricle.

Infants with aortic stenosis are rarely symptomatic in the first month of life. If they are symptomatic, it generally indicates that they are critically ill and that cardiac output is extremely low. These infants are likely to die unless surgery is performed rapidly. Ventilatory support is necessary to relieve acidosis, cyanosis, and the respiratory distress that often accompanies this defect. These patients are often ductal dependent, with systemic circulation depending on blood flow through the ductus arteriosus. Although supplemental oxygen is most likely indicated, it should be given judiciously to limit the vasodilatory effects of oxygen on the pulmonary vasculature and the constricting effect on the ductus arteriosus. The most important aspect of presurgical management of symptomatic aortic stenosis is the use of prostaglandin E_1 to minimize ductal constriction. Dosages range from 0.05 to 0.1 µg/kg/min. Inotropic support is sometimes needed for the treatment of congestive heart failure.

Infants with congestive heart failure from severe aortic stenosis are in urgent need of surgery. Children with less severe aortic stenosis translated into peak systolic pressure gradient of 50 to 80 mm Hg may be operated on an elective basis. Surgery is indicated in patients with symptoms (chest pain, syncope) even with a systolic pressure gradient slightly < 50 mm Hg. Closed aortic valvotomy by cardiac catheterization without cardiopulmonary bypass may be performed in sick infants. Under cardiopulmonary bypass the following surgical procedures may be performed, depending on the anatomy; aortic valvuloplasty, replacement with an artificial valve, replacement with pulmonary valve autograph (Ross Procedure), excision of the membrane for subvalvular aortic stenosis, or widening of the stenotic area using a synthetic patch for supravalvular aortic stenosis. Normal arterial blood and pulse oximetry values can be expected. Attention must be paid to limiting systemic blood pressure postoperatively to avoid putting excessive strain on the repair site. Aortic valvular insufficiency may occur after repair of the stenosis and replacement of the valve may be required later in life.

Coarctation of the Aorta

Coarctation of the aorta is defined as severe narrowing of the aortic lumen in the area of the aortic arch, almost always adjacent to the ductus arteriosus, resulting in decreased blood flow distal to the obstruction (Figure 30-9). This narrowing causes an increased left ventricular pressure and workload. As an isolated anomaly, this defect is the fifth or sixth most commonly occurring congenital cardiac anomaly. The mortality rate for coarctation of the aorta is < 5% and the mortality rate for concomitant repair of coarctation of aorta associated with VSD is < 10%. During fetal life, coarctation results in an increase in left ventricular outflow resistance compared with right ventricular outflow resistance. Although it is normal for the RV to do more work than the LV in utero, this difference is exaggerated in coarctation, and can result RV hypertrophy during early infancy. If the coarctation is not identified and repaired and the ductus arteriosus is closed, LV hypertrophy may develop in older children.

The location of the coarctation may be either preductal or postductal. A preductal narrowing (the more serious defect) is frequently associated with other cardiac anomalies such as aortic stenosis and VSD. In the postductal type, there is a pressure gradient between the proximal and distal (with respect to the coarctation)

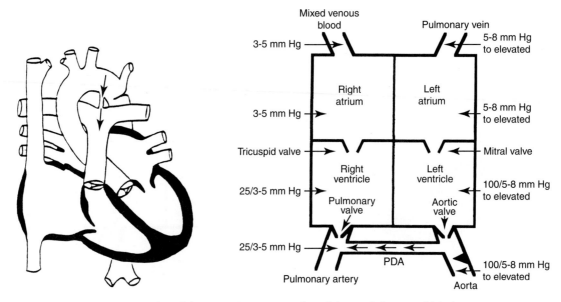

FIGURE 30-9 Coarctation of the aorta. Severe narrowing of the aortic lumen, which decreases blood flow through the aorta. A patent ductus arteriosus is often present to allow pulmonary blood flow when the coarctation is severe. PDA, Patent ductus arteriosus.

portions of the aorta during fetal life, which is a strong stimulus for the development of collateral circulation. This allows continued systemic blood flow even after ductal closure. In the preductal type of coarctation, during fetal life, with the ductus open, the descending aorta is perfused by the RV through the ductal right-to-left shunt. In this type of lesion, it is less likely that collateral circulatory pathways will develop. Thus, when the ductus arteriosus begins to constrict after birth, there can be a sudden decrease in perfusion of the descending aorta, with possible resulting circulatory shock and renal shutdown.

Radiographically, in symptomatic patients the heart is enlarged and there is pulmonary vascular congestion. Symptomatic patients often present with dyspnea, tachypnea, and irritability. Hypertension is often seen in the upper extremities; thus, blood pressure should be measured in both upper and lower extremities. Blood pressure differential between upper and lower extremities may only become apparent after the start of inotropic support in patients with shock.

The most important preoperative treatment is the use of prostaglandin E_1 to minimize ductal constriction until surgical correction can be achieved. This has significantly improved the outcome in these patients. The presurgical management may also include inotropic agents and diuretics for treatment of cardiac failure. Ventilator management is sometimes necessary for patients in shock. Surgery is usually postponed until later in the first year of life if cardiac failure can be controlled medically and an adequate weight gain sustained.

A variety of surgical procedures are used, including:
1. excision of the coarctated segment of aorta with an end-to-end anastomosis of the cut ends
2. tubular graft bypass of the coarctation
3. patch aortoplasty (to enlarge the area) using a longitudinal incision through the coarctation with a patch on the open vessel. This patch is either synthetic or fashioned from an excised portion of the patient's subclavian artery.

There may continue to be a gradient between upper and lower extremity blood pressures after surgery (residual coarctation). A systolic pressure gradient is < 20 mm Hg in the presence of adequate lower body perfusion (including renal perfusion) is generally considered acceptable. Postoperative management usually includes a short period of mechanical ventilation. Normal blood gas and pulse oximetry values can be expected. Rebound or paradoxical systemic hypertension is sometimes present and may require treatment and is thought to be caused by various derangements of the blood pressure mediation system. This postoperative problem is less common in patients younger than 5 years of age.

Hypoplastic Left Heart Syndrome

Hypoplastic left heart syndrome is a continuum which can affect all left sided cardiac structures from the mitral valve to the aortic arch[17] (Figure 30-10). This continuum is characterized by hypoplasia of the LV and includes atresia or critical stenosis of the aortic or mitral valves and hypoplasia of the ascending aorta and aortic arch. Shunting of blood can occur at two sites in different directions, and

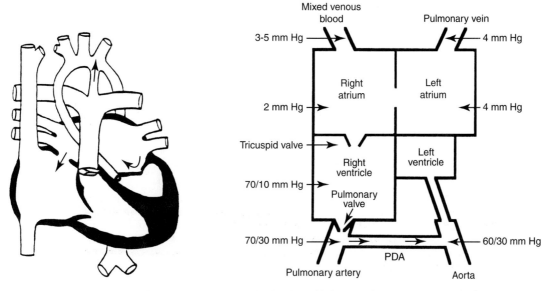

FIGURE 30-10 Hypoplastic left ventricle. Underdeveloped left ventricle and severe narrowing of the ascending aorta. It may include mitral atresia (pictured here), lack of the mitral valve, aortic atresia, or lack of the aorta, or a combination. A patent ductus arteriosus is necessary for systemic blood flow. PDA, Patent ductus arteriosus.

these directions can change depending on the balance of pulmonary and systemic resistances. Because there is little or no output from the LV, the pulmonary venous blood returning to the LA must pass through the foramen ovale to the RA. This site of shunting is left to right. The entire systemic output is supplied by means of right-to-left flow through the PDA. When the ductus arteriosus narrows postnatally, there is severe impairment of cardiac output, producing circulatory shock and metabolic acidosis. Without treatment, death usually occurs in the first month of life. Occasionally, the infants live for many weeks if the PDA and patent foramen ovale opening are large. In 15% of patients there may also be an atrial septal defect as well. Chest radiography reveals a moderately to markedly enlarged heart with increased pulmonary vascular markings due to pulmonary edema. The heart may also have a globular shape.

Preoperatively, prostaglandin E_1 is given immediately to maintain ductal patency. The difference between systemic and pulmonary vascular resistance must be carefully balanced. Without this balance, these patients are at high risk for pulmonary overcirculation and systemic and coronary hypoperfusion. This balance is managed by increasing pulmonary vascular resistance, relative to systemic, by using two different interventions. One of these is the administration of subambient oxygen concentrations ($F_{IO_2} < 0.21$). This relative hypoxemia increases the pulmonary vascular resistance. The F_{IO_2} is usually kept in the 0.17 to 0.21 range in order to keep systemic oxygen saturations 70% to 80%.

The other technique is called hypercarbic therapy. The goal of this therapy is to create elevated Pa_{CO_2} levels, which in turn produce a respiratory acidosis. The resulting decrease in pH increases pulmonary vascular resistance. A target pH of 7.20 is generally used, but it may range from 7.15 to 7.30. There are several ways to increase Pa_{CO_2}. These include: 1) addition of mechanical dead space to the ventilator circuit, 2) Pa_{CO_2} reductions in minute ventilation, 3) increases in inhaled CO_2 concentrations by adding CO_2 to the inspired gas in the ventilator circuit. Exhaled CO_2 is typically targeted with an $F_{I}CO_2$ of 2% to 5% using a specific type of end-tidal CO_2 monitor.[18] Subambient oxygen therapy can be used in patients who are intubated or not, whereas hypercarbic therapy can only be effectively administered to intubated, heavily sedated, or paralyzed patients where the minute ventilation and exact inspired gas concentrations can be controlled.

As recently as 1986 this defect was not considered reparable and the only treatment offered was comfort care. Since patients with hypoplastic left heart syndrome have no functional left ventricle, the systemic and pulmonary blood flow is provided by the right ventricle. There are three phases of surgical repair. The goal of each successive surgical intervention is to provide the growing patient with an appropriate balance between systemic and pulmonary blood. The decision to perform these surgeries is based on measurements of oxygenation and ratio of pulmonary to cardiac blood flow (Q_p/Q_s).

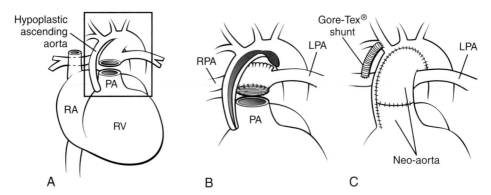

FIGURE 30-11 The Norwood procedure. **A,** The heart with aortic atresia and a hypoplastic ascending aorta and aortic arch are shown. The main pulmonary artery (PA) is transected. **B,** The distal PA is closed with a patch. An incision that extends around the aortic arch to the level of the ductus is made in the ascending aorta. The ductus is ligated. **C,** A modified right Blalock-Taussig shunt is created between the right subclavian artery and the right PA (RPA) as the sole source of pulmonary blood flow. By the use of an aorta or PA allograft (shaded area), the main PA is anastomosed to the aorta and the aortic arch to create a large arterial trunk. The procedure to widen the atrial communication is not shown. LPA, Left pulmonary artery, RA, right atrium, RV, right ventricle.

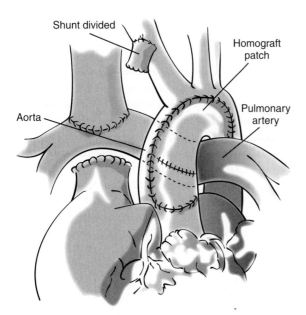

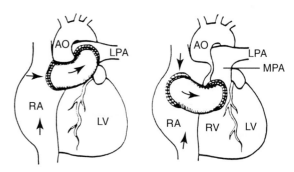

FIGURE 30-13 Fontan procedure. Blood from the right atrium is routed to the left or main pulmonary artery using a baffle, which may contain a fenestration or pop-off valve to allow blood flow to enter the ventricle in the presence of high pulmonary artery pressures. AO, Aorta; LPA, left pulmonary artery; RA, right atrium; LV, left ventricle; MPA, main pulmonary artery; RV, right ventricle.

FIGURE 30-12 Bidirectional Glenn shunt. The divided right superior vena cava has been anastomosed at the previous site of the distal anastomosis of the modified right Blalock shunt.

The goal of the first phase, the Norwood procedure (Figure 30-11), is to reconstruct the aorta and to provide pulmonary blood flow either through a modified Blalock-Taussig shunt or right ventricular to pulmonary artery conduit (RV-PA) conduit. The second phase (called the Glenn procedure) (Figure 30-12) is to remove the BT shunt or RV-PA conduit and connect the superior vena cava (SVC) directly to the pulmonary artery. The third phase of the repair, called the Fontan procedure (Figure 30-13), is to connect the right atrium to the pulmonary artery. Phase one is typically done soon after birth. Phase two is done when the child outgrows the BT shunt (or RV-PA conduit), and phase three is done when the child needs more pulmonary blood flow than the SVC alone can provide. There are several different approaches to surgical correction in phase one:
1. Classic Norwood procedure (see Figure 30-11)
2. Norwood-Sano procedure[19] (Figure 30-14) and
3. Hybrid procedure.

These three approaches use a variety of surgical corrections, which are explained in Figure 30-15. These corrections include PA banding, modified BT shunt,

RV-PA conduit, atrial septostomy, PDA ligation, and reconstruction of the aortic arch. PA banding reduces pulmonary blood flow by constricting the size of the pulmonary artery. The modified BT shunt connects the right or left subclavian artery to the pulmonary artery using a synthetic shunt. The RV-PA conduit replaces the normal connection of the right ventricle to the pulmonary artery. This is necessary when the right ventricle is connected to newly constructed aorta because the normal connection from the RV to the PA has been used to connect to the aorta.

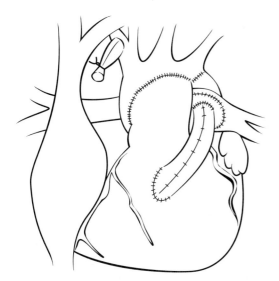

FIGURE 30-14 The Sano shunt.

The Norwood corrections require the patient to undergo cardiopulmonary bypass during surgery. The Hybrid procedure does not require bypass and thus is used on children too sick to tolerate cardiopulmonary bypass. Although this approach is less invasive initially, these patients will still have to have an aortic reconstruction, which is just postponed until phase two.

Postoperative management focuses on maintaining hemodynamic stability by controlling PVR and optimizing systemic perfusion. Ventilatory management is an important aspect of care, and F_{IO_2} management is very important in controlling PVR in patients who have had a classic Norwood procedure. It may be necessary to use specific ventilatory techniques that induce (or maintain) a high PVR (e.g. subambient or hypercarbic therapy). Hyperventilation should be avoided, since it can reduce PVR. A helpful convention is the "rule of forties," which seeks to keep arterial blood gases in the following range: Pa_{O_2} approximately 40 mm Hg, and Pa_{CO_2} approximately 40 mm Hg. Because suctioning changes hemodynamics and PVR and may even cause an irreversible decline in the patient's condition, it is performed sparingly, especially in classic Norwood repairs.

Over recent years ventilator management has become less complex due to the advent of the Norwood-Sano procedure, which typically produces less postoperative hemodynamic instability.

For second and third phase repairs (Glenn and Fontan procedures), a low-rate, high–tidal volume approach is

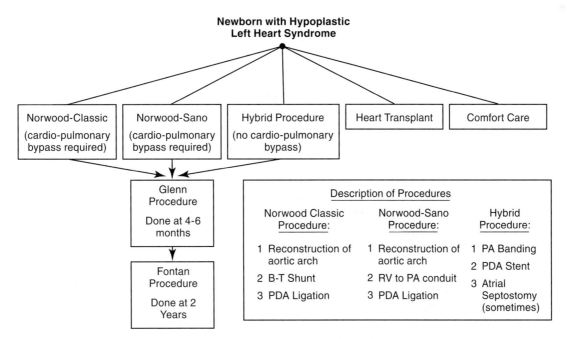

FIGURE 30-15 Sequence of procedures for the treatment of hypoplastic left heart syndrome.

recommended. This allows for the longest expiratory phase possible, which keeps mean intrathoracic pressure low, thus improving venous drainage from the SVC/IVC into the pulmonary arteries. Early extubation is also recommended because spontaneous breathing and the resulting negative intrathoracic pressure, promotes better pulmonary blood flow by improved venous drainage from the SVC/IVC into the pulmonary arteries. Some centers have had success using negative pressure ventilators and were able to wean patients from traditional mechanical ventilation earlier.

For the Glenn procedure there are published studies describing improved systemic oxygenation after hypoventilation-induced hypercarbia. "The likely mechanism for this effect is that hypoventilation-induced hypercarbia decreases cerebral vascular resistance, thus increasing cerebral, superior vena caval and pulmonary blood flow," which then creates improved venous return from the SVC to the pulmonary artery.[20]

Total Anomalous Pulmonary Venous Return

Anomalies involving aberrant connections between the pulmonary venous drainage and the systemic circulation can occur in a variety of ways. The common feature is pulmonary veins that have no connection with the LA and drain either directly or indirectly into the RA (Figure 30-16). This results in mixing of pulmonary and systemic blood returning to the RA as well as increased pressures and volume in the right side of the

heart. A simplified classification of total anomalous pulmonary venous return (TAPVR) lists the four common anomalies as

1. supracardiac, in which the common pulmonary vein drains into the superior vena cava through a vertical vein that runs above the heart
2. cardiac, in which the common pulmonary vein empties into the coronary sinus
3. infracardiac, in which the common pulmonary vein drains to the portal vein, ductus venosus, hepatic vein, or inferior vena cava
4. mixed type.

Preoperatively, the chest radiograph in TAPVR is relatively normal, although there can be increased pulmonary vascular markings in infants with severe obstruction. Occasionally, the dilated accessory venous channels to the superior vena cava can be seen on the anteroposterior film. Intubation and mechanical ventilation for acidosis, cyanosis, and ventilatory failure are not uncommon. PEEP is often used for the management of pulmonary edema. Because of the venous admixture and the right-to-left shunt across the ASD, the Pao_2 and $Paco_2$ will be nearly equal to 40 mm Hg (rule of forties) and arterial oxygen saturations are typically 75%. Symptoms of congestive heart failure are treated with inotropic agents and diuretics. Balloon atrial septostomy may be performed at the time of preoperative cardiac catheterization to enlarge the ASD.

All patients with TAPVR must have corrective surgery. The goal of the various corrective procedures is to

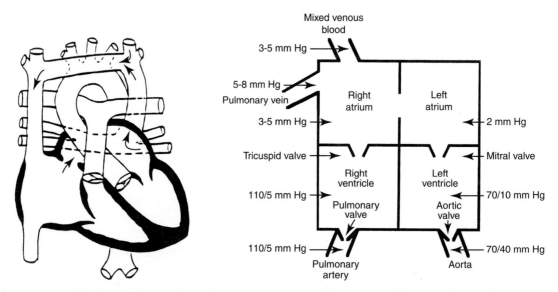

FIGURE 30-16 Total anomalous pulmonary venous return. Pulmonary venous return is routed to the right atrium instead of the left atrium. Pulmonary drainage can be routed (1) above the heart (supracardiac), as pictured here; (2) through the heart (cardiac); (3) through the portal vein, ductus venosus, hepatic vein, or inferior vena cava (infracardiac); or (4) through the diaphragm or esophageal hiatus (subdiaphragmatic).

redirect pulmonary venous return to the LA. The defect may be associated with pulmonary venous obstruction. This is more frequently encountered with the infracardiac type of lesions. Typically, surgical correction is done soon after diagnosis, even in the newborn period, especially when there is heart failure that may or may not be associated with pulmonary venous obstruction.

Postoperative mechanical ventilation is universally indicated in all of the repairs. The infracardiac repair requires extensive revision and is the most unstable of all anomalies because of the higher risk of pulmonary vein obstruction. Normal arterial blood gas and pulse oximetry values can be expected after all repairs. Pulmonary edema may occur, requiring prolonged ventilatory support with PEEP. There are considerable fluctuations in pulmonary artery pressure in some patients in the immediate postoperative period. These patients can exhibit episodes of paroxysmal pulmonary hypertension that can be severe and life threatening. This may require aggressive treatment with pulmonary vasodilatory interventions.

Tetralogy of Fallot

Tetralogy of Fallot is one of a class of anomalies called *conotruncal,* a term referring to the site of the developmental derangement that leads to the lesion. Others in this family of anomalies include truncus arteriosus and transposition of the great arteries. Tetralogy of Fallot consists of four concomitant conditions (Figure 30-17):
1. overriding aorta
2. pulmonary stenosis

3. VSD
4. right ventricular hypertrophy

Depending on the severity of the pulmonary stenosis, the magnitude of the shunt through the VSD will vary. With mild stenosis, the shunt may be from left to right, with the infant being acyanotic. However, the majority of infants with tetralogy of Fallot present with pronounced pulmonary stenosis, resulting in a right-to-left shunt that produces significant cyanosis and arterial oxygen saturations as low as 60%. The infant may be mildly cyanotic at birth (while the ductus arteriosus is open); however, after the ductus arteriosus constricts the child becomes more cyanotic and hypoxemic. Infants with extreme cases of tetralogy of Fallot may present with pulmonary atresia or pulmonary stenosis that is so severe that they are totally dependent on blood flow through the PDA. These infants are severely cyanotic at birth and require emergency surgery to provide pulmonary blood flow once the ductus arteriosus closes. Prostaglandin E_1 is administered to maintain a PDA until surgery or cardiac catheterization can be performed. Chest radiography often reveals a classic "boot-shaped" appearance of the heart. This is caused by a narrow mediastinum and the effect of sustained pulmonary outflow obstruction, which result in right ventricular hypertrophy. In 25% of cases the aortic arch is on the right side.

Because of the presence of a large VSD, the pressures equalize in both ventricles. The relative amounts of blood flow to the pulmonary versus systemic vasculatures are directly related to the degree of pulmonary

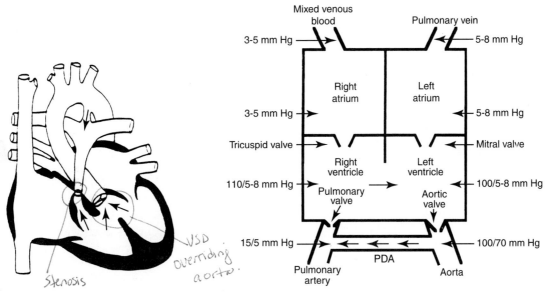

FIGURE 30-17 Tetralogy of Fallot. Overriding aorta, pulmonary artery stenosis, right atrial hypertrophy, and a ventricular septal defect. A patent ductus arteriosus is often present to allow pulmonary blood flow if pulmonary stenosis is severe. PDA, Patent ductus arteriosus.

stenosis and SVR. A slight change in any of these factors can dramatically change the hemodynamics and constrict the pulmonary outflow tract. These changes are sometimes manifested in spells of profound cyanosis, often referred to as "tet" spells. Tet spells occur most commonly in infants 2 to 4 months of age and are characterized by

1. hyperpnea or exaggerated, deep spontaneous breathing
2. irritability and prolonged crying
3. increasing cyanosis
4. decreased intensity of the heart murmur
5. fainting

Otherwise benign phenomena such as defecating, crying, or feeding can precipitate tet spells by increasing the right-to-left shunt. The resulting hypoxemia can increase the PVR, which causes even more right-to-left shunt, which then causes more profound hypoxemia. Thus a vicious cycle is created from which escape may be difficult. Patients with tetralogy of Fallot are often slow to recover from these potentially catastrophic events, which should be avoided by minimizing interventions such as suctioning, handling, and manipulating the ventilatory circuit or airway. Box 30-1 lists steps that may be used to break the cycle of a tet spell.

Preoperative intubation and assisted mechanical ventilation may be necessary because of the degree of cyanosis, acidosis, and recurring tet spells. Prostaglandin E_1 is

given to minimize PDA closure and to ensure adequate pulmonary blood flow by reducing PVR. Because of the venous admixture, the PaO_2 values will be approximately 40 mm Hg and the SaO_2 will be approximately to 75%, but this can vary.

Surgical repair involves a number of procedures. Symptomatic or cyanotic infants with favorable anatomy of the right ventricular outflow tract may have primary corrective repair at any time after 3 to 4 months of age. Some centers perform primary repair in even younger infants, including newborns.

Corrective repair of Tetralogy of Fallot consists of widening of the right ventricular outflow tract that involves resection of the infundibular tissue and placement of a patch, reconstruction of the stenotic pulmonary artery, and closing of the VSD. Corrective surgery is done under cardiopulmonary bypass. If the pulmonary stenosis or the right ventricular outflow tract is severely obstructed, a systemic-to-pulmonary connection is accomplished to increase blood flow to the lungs and to promote enlargement of the pulmonary arteries. This is usually a Blalock-Taussig shunt from the subclavian artery to the pulmonary artery. There are several variations of shunts that allow systemic arterial blood to flow to the lungs. It is beyond the scope of this chapter to offer detailed description of these variations.

Postoperative ventilatory support is always required after repair of Tetralogy of Fallot. It is particularly important for the clinician to know which repair is used when caring for these patients postoperatively. If the pulmonary stenosis is repaired through dilation or reconstruction of the infundibular tissue and the VSD is closed, normal arterial blood gas and saturation values can be expected. When the repair involves a right ventriculotomy and/or resection of the infundibular tissues, derangement of cardiac conduction system may occur. This is why most of these patients will have atrial and ventricular pacing wires placed during surgery. A common postoperative complication is junctional atrial tachycardia.

Truncus Arteriosus

Truncus arteriosus is a defect in which a single great artery arises from the ventricles of the heart supplying the coronary, pulmonary, and systemic arteries (Figure 30-18). A large VSD allows total mixing of blood from the two ventricles, making the heart function as a single ventricle. The truncal valve usually resembles a normal aortic valve. This defect occurs in <1 % of all infants with congenital cardiac defects. The balance between PVR and SVR affects oxygenation and cardiac output. If PVR decreases relative to SVR, there is an increase in blood flow to the lungs through the truncus, decreasing systemic cardiac output. Pulmonary vascular engorgement

---

| Box 30-1 | Treatment of TET Spells |

- Hold the child in the knee-chest position. This may trap venous blood in the legs and decrease the systemic venous return as well as calm the child.
- Administer morphine sulfate. This will suppress the respiratory center and abolish hyperpnea. (The hyperpnea decreases intrathoracic pressure and may increase venous return to the chest.) It will also chemically mediate pulmonary artery dilation directly, which allows more blood flow through the patent ductus arteriosus and increases pulmonary blood flow and oxygenation.
- Administer oxygen. This will improve oxygenation and decrease pulmonary vascular resistance.
- Administer sodium bicarbonate for acidosis. This will minimize the resultant pulmonary artery constriction.
- Administer propranolol (Inderal). Although the mechanism of action is not clear, this may reduce pulmonary artery spasms or act peripherally by stabilizing vascular reactivity of the systemic arteries, thereby preventing a sudden decrease in systemic vascular resistance.
- Administer vasoconstrictors. These may raise systemic vascular resistance should it suddenly drop.

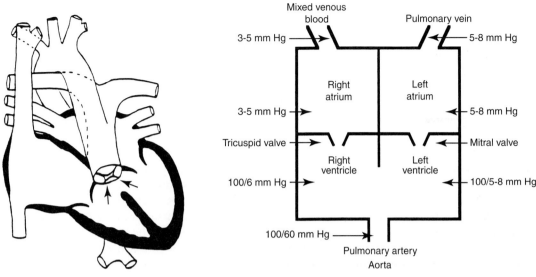

FIGURE 30-18 Truncus arteriosus. A single great artery arises from the ventricles carrying both pulmonary and systemic blood flow.

may then occur. If SVR decreases, blood flow will be shunted from right to left and bypass the lungs, resulting in severe hypoxemia and acidosis.

The heart is enlarged on chest radiography because of dilation of the LA and LV. The pulmonary vascular markings are increased, and there may be symptoms of congestive heart failure. A right aortic arch is present in about one fourth of the cases. Intubation and ventilation are usually required because of the unstable hemodynamics of the pulmonary and systemic vascular circulation, which causes hypoxemia and acidosis. Because of the degree of venous admixture, the rule of forties is also used for blood gas management. Like the other conotruncal anomalies described, extreme care must be used with oxygen therapy, and subambient FIO_2 may be employed. The symptoms of congestive heart failure are treated with inotropic agents and diuretics.

Palliative pulmonary artery banding may be performed in newborns presenting with congestive heart failure or in infants who might not survive the surgical procedure required for total repair due to their age and overall clinical condition. Unfortunately, banding of these arteries has been associated with high mortality and may also deform the pulmonary artery so that later correction is difficult.

A palliative pulmonary artery banding may be done as a bridge to complete corrective surgery, although early repair of the defect is recommended. If a pulmonary banding is performed, mixing of deoxygenated and oxygenated blood will continue. Pao_2 is acceptable at 40 mm Hg, and Sao_2 should be at approximately 75%. Corrective surgery is referred to as a Rastelli procedure

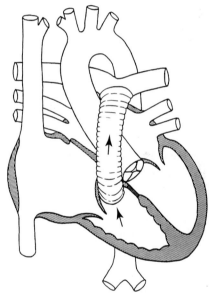

FIGURE 30-19 Modified Rastelli procedure. Blood is routed from the right ventricle to the pulmonary artery using a conduit, and the ventricular septal defect is closed.

(Figure 30-19). The right and left pulmonary arteries are separated off the main truncus along with a cuff of tissue. The truncus is patched in the places from which the pulmonary arteries have been removed. A valve-bearing conduit is attached from the RV to the pulmonary arteries. The VSD is then closed; the truncus will then act as the aorta. Postoperative mechanical ventilation is always required. If corrective repair is performed, normal arterial blood gas and pulse oximetry values can be expected. Because of the extensive repair, there are often problems with hemodynamic instability that require inotropic support.

Complete Transposition of the Great Arteries

In complete transposition of the great arteries, the positions of the aorta and the pulmonary artery are reversed. The aorta arises from the RV, and the pulmonary artery arises from the LV (Figure 30-20). Basically, the two circulations are in parallel (separate) instead of in series with each other. The systemic venous blood passes through the right heart chambers and then to the body without flowing through the lungs. The pulmonary venous blood traverses the left side of the heart and then returns to the lungs. Survival depends on mixing between the two separate circuits. In the immediate postnatal period, shunting through a PDA and the foramen ovale is usually sufficient. This bidirectional shunting from aorta to pulmonary artery and LA to RA improves mixing and prevents severe cyanosis. However, as the ductus arteriosus closes, the shunting at this level is eliminated and the only site of mixing becomes the foramen ovale. This mixing is usually inadequate, resulting in severe hypoxemia, acidosis, and eventually death if it is not corrected. Approximately 5% of all infants born with congenital cardiac disease have transposition of the great arteries.[21] The chest radiograph is usually normal for a newborn except that the malposition of the great arteries is seen. This malposition is often described as "egg-shaped or egg-on-side." After a few hours to days, pulmonary vascular enlargement and cardiomegaly may be seen.

Prostaglandin E_1 is used immediately after diagnosis to maintain ductal patency because continued survival depends on it. Intubation and ventilation are usually required because of hypoxemia, acidosis, and prostaglandin induced apnea episodes. Oxygen is given judiciously to help maintain the appropriate balance between pulmonary and systemic blood flow. Because there is considerable venous admixture, the rule of forties is used for oxygenation management. These patients usually have a small ASD; however, in some cases it needs to be larger, and a balloon atrial septostomy (also called Rashkind procedure) is performed during cardiac catheterization. This procedure includes advancing a balloon-tipped catheter from the RA through the foramen ovale into the LA. The balloon is inflated and rapidly and forcefully withdrawn to create a large ASD. This ensures adequate mixing between the two atria until corrective surgery can be performed.

Definitive surgical repair can be done by switching the right- and left-sided structures at the level of the great arteries (arterial switch operation, Figure 30-21), at the atrial level (Mustard operation, Figure 30-22), or at the ventricular level (Rastelli procedures Figure 30-23). Nowadays, the most commonly used procedure is the arterial switch, also called the Jatene operation. It is indicated in infants with good left ventricular function, enabling them to have normal systemic output.[49] Left ventricular function can be improved before the repair by performing a banding of the pulmonary artery. This increase in PVR will recondition the left ventricle in preparation for the arterial switch, after

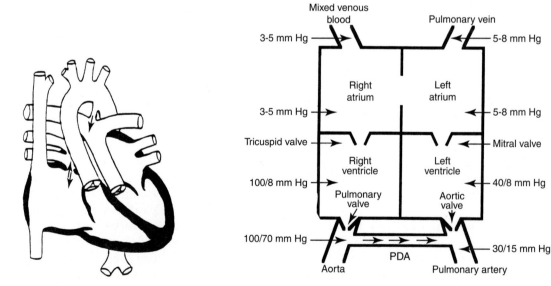

FIGURE 30-20 Transposition of the great arteries. The aorta arises from the right ventricle, and the pulmonary artery arises from the left ventricle. A patent ductus arteriosus is necessary to allow pulmonary blood flow. PDA, Patent ductus arteriosus.

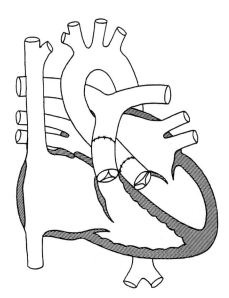

FIGURE 30-21 Arterial switch. The pulmonary artery and aorta are separated from their respective origins and reattached to provide normal pulmonary and aortic blood flow.

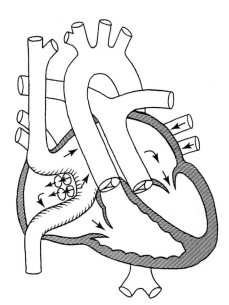

FIGURE 30-22 Mustard procedure. The atrial septum is removed, and a conduit is placed inside the atria. Blood from the right atrium is directed to the mitral valve, into the left ventricle, out the pulmonary artery, and then to the lungs. Blood from the pulmonary veins is directed from the left atrium by a baffle to the tricuspid valve. It then flows into the right ventricle and out the aorta.

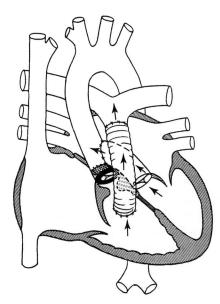

FIGURE 30-23 Rastelli procedure. Blood is routed from the right ventricle to the pulmonary artery through the ventricular septal defect using a conduit. The pulmonary artery is separated and is anastomosed to the aorta.

which the left ventricle must be able to provide all systemic cardiac output. However, deciding which procedure to perform is based on many other factors. In the arterial switch the main trunks of the pulmonary artery and the aorta are cut (transected) just above their respective origins on the heart. The portion of the pulmonary artery still attached to the LV is then anastomosed to the cut section of the aorta. The portion of the aorta still attached to the RV is anastomosed to the cut section of the pulmonary artery. Because the coronary arteries arise off the section of the aorta remaining attached to the RV, they must be excised from the aorta and implanted into the section of the pulmonary artery that remains attached to the LV so that they may carry oxygenated blood to the myocardium.

In the Mustard procedure, blood is routed from the RA to the left side of the heart using the atrial septum. Pulmonary venous blood is routed to the right side of the heart using a baffle (see Figure 30-22). Both of the baffles are sutured in place, thus hindering blood flow from the RA into the RV and flow from the LA into the LV. Functionally, this results in a switching of the circulations at the level of the atria. This procedure is associated with more early and late complications.

In the Rastelli procedure (see Figure 30-23), redirection of the pulmonary and systemic blood flow is carried out at the ventricular level, in comparison with the atrial level in the Mustard procedure. This procedure is selected if the infant also has a VSD. A conduit is placed between the right ventricle and the pulmonary artery that allows deoxygenated blood to enter the pulmonary system. The VSD is repaired is such a fashion as to keep the aorta open only to the left ventricle. Thus, the pulmonary venous blood flows from the LA into the LV, and then into the aorta, providing systemic circulation. After this repair, there will no mixing of pulmonary and systemic circulations. This procedure is associated with fewer complications than the Mustard, but requires the replacement of the conduit as the child grows.

Because of the obvious hemodynamic problems associated with transposition of the great arteries, these patients will likely be unstable and require inotropic support and mechanical ventilation. Normal arterial blood gas and pulse oximetry values can be expected postoperatively.

Hypoplastic Right Ventricle

Hypoplastic right ventricle is caused by a tricuspid atresia and/or pulmonary atresia (Figure 30-24). With tricuspid atresia, the tricuspid valve does not form and thus there is no blood flow between the RA and RV. The only way for blood to leave the RA is through an ASD or patent foramen ovale. The systemic and pulmonary venous blood enters and mixes in the LA, then empties into the LV. A VSD allows blood to flow back into the RV, but only a small amount, if any, is pumped to the pulmonary system. A PDA must be present to facilitate additional pulmonary blood flow.

Pulmonary atresia obstructs the outflow of the RV and may be located at, or slightly distal to, the pulmonary valve. The left side of the heart receives blood from the right side of the heart through an ASD or patent foramen ovale. There may be a VSD, although it is unusual. There is no blood flow from the RV to the pulmonary system; thus, a PDA must be present to support life.

The chest radiograph reveals a heart that may be normal to slightly enlarged. There are decreased pulmonary vascular markings and a concave main pulmonary artery. The LV can be slightly enlarged, giving the overall heart a boot-shaped appearance. An enlarged RA may also be noted.

Preoperative management includes the administration of prostaglandin E_1, given immediately to maintain ductal patency. Mechanical ventilation is usually required for hypoxemia, acidosis, and prostaglandin-induced apneic episodes. Oxygen therapy is used judiciously to help maintain the balance between pulmonary and systemic blood glow. Because there is total venous admixing, Pao_2 and $Paco_2$ values are kept near 40 mm Hg and Sao_2 is maintained at approximately 75%. A balloon atrial septostomy may be performed during cardiac catheterization if there is the need to improve the right-to-left shunt.

A variety of surgical repairs can be performed, depending on the severity of the hypoplastic RV and whether tricuspid or pulmonary atresia is involved. These repairs are performed in stages to allow patient growth and stabilization between the surgeries.

In the first stage, a Blalock-Taussig shunt is performed to create a systemic to pulmonary communication used to offset the effect of ductal closure. In the second stage, a bidirectional Glenn procedure is performed to enhance pulmonary blood flow and reduce hypoxemia (Figure 30-25). In this procedure, the superior vena cava is separated from the RA and is

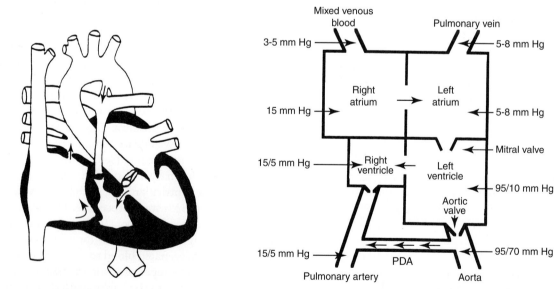

FIGURE 30-24 Hypoplastic right ventricle. This results from either lack of a tricuspid valve, as pictured here, or pulmonary atresia. An atrial septal defect or patent foramen ovale is necessary for right atrial outflow of blood. A patent ductus arteriosus is necessary to allow pulmonary blood flow. PDA, Patent ductus arteriosus.

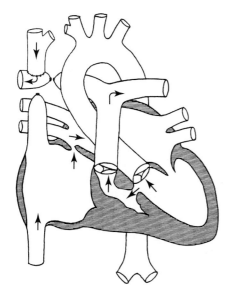

FIGURE 30-25 Glenn procedure for hypoplastic right ventricle. The superior vena cava is separated from the right atrium, and the proximal end of the superior vena cava is sewn to the right pulmonary artery. The right pulmonary artery is separated from the main pulmonary artery.

anastomosed to the right pulmonary artery. This procedure allows the venous return from the head and upper extremities to flow directly into the pulmonary circulation. The venous return from the inferior vena cava will enter the RA and flow to the LA to mix with oxygenated pulmonary venous return. Fontan procedure is performed as the third stage of surgical correction.

Postoperative management of the first stage of surgical repair includes limiting oxygen administration, instituting the rule of forties for blood gas measurement, and providing inotropic support for cardiovascular instability. Management after the Fontan procedure was discussed earlier.

CLINICAL MONITORING OF PATIENTS WITH CARDIAC ANOMALIES

Blood Pressure

A wide array of physiologic monitoring capabilities are available to the clinician caring for the patient with congenital cardiac anomalies. The development of indwelling plastic catheters, combined with computerized signal processing, has made sophisticated monitoring of hemodynamic variables commonplace. The systemic arterial and central venous blood pressures are typically monitored continuously. It is also possible to monitor pulmonary arterial and left atrial blood pressures, but this is done less frequently and varies from hospital to hospital and according to the type of lesion.

The measurement of systemic arterial blood pressure is very important but it represents only one of many cardiovascular system variables. Diastolic blood pressure is essential to coronary perfusion.

In assessing the contractile properties of the cardiac muscle, it is important to specify the degree of tension on the muscle when it begins to contract (the *preload*) and to specify the force opposing ventricular ejection (the *afterload*). For cardiac contraction, the *preload* is usually estimated by end-diastolic volume and/or end-diastolic pressure. The most important component of the *afterload* is the pressure in the artery leading from the ventricles.[22]

Pulse pressure (the difference between systolic and diastolic pressures) generally decreases in the presence of hypovolemia. It may increase in patients with a Blalock-Taussig shunt because of "run-off" phenomenon. During diastole the blood flows from the systemic to the pulmonary circulation through the B-T shunt.

Central venous pressure reflects the preload (within certain limits). There are conditions where CVP is elevated but preload is not. Cardiac tamponade or high mean airway pressures (in ventilated patients) can be transmitted to the large veins (IVC and SVC) and thus CVP readings can be falsely high. Preload is better assessed through the measurement of pulmonary artery and capillary wedge pressures through right heart or pulmonary artery catheters. These catheters also allow reliable sampling of true mixed venous blood. Samples of venous blood from the superior or inferior vena cava can have differing amounts of oxygen extracted from them because they have circulated through parts of the body with widely different oxygen demands. The blood from coronary sinus has a high degree of oxygen extraction because of the high demands of the myocardium. Thus, a mixed venous blood sample should be obtained from the right atrium. The insertion of a right heart or pulmonary artery catheter (as opposed to a central venous line) is therefore necessary to get a sample of true mixed venous blood. The mixed venous oxygen saturation is usually required to compute certain cardiovascular variables.

Pulse Oximetry

Pulse oximetry has become a de facto standard for noninvasive monitoring of oxygenation in critically ill patients, including those with congenital cardiac anomalies. Applications include the ongoing monitoring of systemic oxygenation and assessment of the degree of right-to-left shunting. In the presence of such shunting, there can be significant differences in oxygen saturation in the preductal and postductal arterial circulation. Placing one pulse oximeter (SpO_2) on a right upper extremity (preductal) and concomitantly placing a probe on any other extremity (postductal) can assess the difference. Right-to-left shunting is suspected if the Spo_2 gradient is > 5% to 10%. Some clinicians do not support measurement of postductal blood in the left arm, believing that there may be incomplete mixing of preductal and postductal blood by the time the flow traverses the origin of the left subclavian artery. Hence, there may be a disproportionately large amount of preductal (e.g., oxygenated) blood in the left upper extremity. In such a case, a significant shunt may be masked. Under certain conditions the pulse oximeter can produce very unreliable readings. Spo_2 accuracy is known to deteriorate during periods of profound desaturation, motion, and low peripheral perfusion. Some brands of oximeters perform much better than others under these conditions as a result of their improved signal-processing capabilities[23,24,25] and there is a growing body of evidence that improved oximeter performance combined with oxygen management protocols can improve processes and outcomes of care.[26,27,28]

End-Tidal Carbon Dioxide

The monitoring of $ETco_2$ can be useful in assessing adequacy of ventilation, cardiac function, pulmonary blood flow, as well as airway patency. Minute ventilation is inversely proportional to $ETco_2$ and thus the monitor can detect changes in ventilation. The gradient between $ETco_2$ and $Paco_2$ is normally approximately 2 to 5 mm Hg. Increases in this gradient can be caused by decreases in pulmonary perfusion which can be caused by relatively low intravascular volume status or decreases in cardiac function. Some clinicians tend to believe that an increasing gradient is indicative of monitor malfunction and sometimes fail to recognize changes in cardiac function and pulmonary blood flow as the cause. The monitoring technology is remarkably reliable and increasing gradients are rarely a result of a loss of calibration or other equipment malfunction. An increasing P_{ET}-aCO_2 gradient can be caused by cardiac failure or noncardiogenic derangements in the ventilation perfusion relationship in the lung. Thompson and Jaffe present an excellent set of capnographic waveforms demonstrating various conditions and the diagnostic value of the capnometer.[29]

A huge decrease or loss of the $ETco_2$ signal can indicate a loss of the artificial airway. If the patient's exhaled gas is not going through the endotracheal tube (e.g., during esophageal intubation), the $ETco_2$ will be near zero. One limitation of the use of $ETco_2$ is the presence of a large airway leak, since much of the exhaled gas may not pass through the $ETco_2$ sensor, and true end-tidal gas may not be sampled. $ETco_2$ measurements can be plotted graphically over time. This is called capnography.

Changes in ventilation and cardiac function can be readily identified by changes in the aspect of the waveform of $ETco_2$ plotted over time. It is also now possible to monitor $ETco_2$, flow, pressure, and volume of gas at the airway simultaneously with the same instrument. This allows for the plotting of $ETco_2$ versus exhaled volume. This is termed volumetric capnography and is now being studied for its ability to help predict successful extubation in cardiac surgery patients.

RESPIRATORY CARE OF PATIENTS WITH CARDIAC ANOMALIES

Interventions Affecting Vascular Resistance

The pulmonary and systemic vasculatures are defined as low- and high-resistance systems, respectively. In congenital cardiac anomalies, the balance between PVR and SVR heavily influences the balance between pulmonary and cardiac blood flow. This is represented by the ratio of pulmonary to cardiac blood flow (Q_P/Q_S) which influences oxygenation, cardiac output, and patient survival. The normal value for Q_P/Q_S is approximately 1. Abnormal shunting of blood between the pulmonary and vascular systems occurs from the system with the highest resistance to the system with the lowest. There are many treatments and interventions that can affect PVR. These are listed in Box 30-2.

Box 30-2	Interventions That Affect PVR

INCREASE
- ↓ pH
  - ↓ Ve to ↑ $Paco_2$ ≥ 45mm Hg
  - ↑ Inhaled CO_2 to ↓ pH
- ↓FIQ < 0–21 pRN
- ↑ - MAP
  - ↑ PiP, ↑ Peep, ↑ F, ↑ Freq - ↑ I:E Ratio
- Treatment ≤ × Adrenergic Agents
  - Dopamine—High Dose
  - EPI
  - Norepi
  - Phenylephrine

DECREASE
- ↑ pH
  - ↑ Ve to ↓ V $Paco_2$ to < 45mm Hg
- ↑ Fio_2
- ↓ PEEP
- ↓ MAP
- Pharmacol
  - pGE 1
  - iNO
  - Prostacyclin

Ventilator Management

In general, the preoperative and postoperative ventilator management of patients with congenital cardiac anomalies is not demonstrably different from that in most other ventilated populations, with some important exceptions. The most important aspect of the management of these patients is the potential effect of changes in ventilatory parameters on PVR. Thus, a goal of ventilatory support is to minimize variations in oxygenation and acid-base status that might otherwise cause fluctuations in PVR and SVR.

Although the debate continues about the utility of volume versus pressure modes of ventilation, knowing the tidal volume being delivered and maintaining its stability are essential ingredients in ventilator management. There is some evidence that delivering a given tidal volume with a decelerating flow profile results in improved oxygenation, improved gas distribution, and reduced work of breathing when compared with the similar tidal volumes delivered with a constant flow.[30,31,32,33] Decelerating flow profiles can also result in higher mean airway pressures while having lower peak inspiratory pressures. In the presence of rapidly changing time constants in the lung (due to reactive airway disease or accumulation of secretions), tidal volumes may vary considerably when pressure control modes are used. This potential variation in tidal volumes can be avoided with the use of dual control modes of ventilation, such as pressure-regulated volume control, where a targeted tidal volume is achieved, using a decelerating flow profile. Breath-to-breath variations in peak airway pressure are acceptable, but should be kept within certain adjustable limits. This is the most commonly used mode in our postoperative cardiac surgery patients. Tidal volumes are typically kept in the 6 to 8 ml/kg range, although occasionally volumes are increased to 10 ml/kg, depending on disease. As an example, in postoperative bidirectional Glenn repairs some people prefer to use larger tidal volumes and lower rates to allow for longer expiratory times, while keeping the same minute ventilation. The rationale is that pressures created within the thorax through the airways can be transmitted to the alveolar capillaries, causing a mechanical impediment to blood flow through the capillary bed with the resultant increase in PVR. Thus, keeping inspiratory time short and expiratory time long minimizes the effect of this pressure transmission.

Extubation criteria for the post surgical management of most cardiac surgery patients include:

1. intact cough
2. ability to clear the airway
3. adequate oxygenation with the F_{IO_2} less than or equal to 0.4
4. normalized Pa_{CO_2} in the presence of age-adjusted normal spontaneous respiratory rates
5. cardiovascular stability
6. adequate cardiac output.

Early extubation in the postoperative period is a general goal for most of these patients, especially after Glenn and Fontan procedures. One reason is that spontaneous ventilation promotes improved pulmonary blood flow because negative intrathoracic pressure is created during inspiration. Early extubation also reduces the risk of lower respiratory tract infection and accidental extubation, both of which are known risks of mechanical ventilation. Early extubation has been studied in recent years and been shown to be possible and advantageous in this population.[34,35,36] There is large variation in the reported length of ventilation after cardiac surgery. Cray and colleagues report a median length of postoperative ventilation of 5 hours[37] in a series of 102 pediatric cardiac surgery patients with a mean age of 4.8 years. Fischer et al report a series of 272 infants with a median age of 1.3 years that had median time to extubation of 3 days.[38] Variation this large is hard to explain. It might be a result of differences in age and disease severity in the population. Cray and colleagues used a standardized postoperative weaning and extubation protocol, which is more than likely the reason for their much shorter length of ventilation.

One of the risks of early extubation is the need for reintubation, which is also called extubation failure. In the general PICU population, extubation failure has been reported to occur in $\approx 5\%$ of patients.[39] When studied in pediatric and neonatal cardiac surgery patients, extubation failure has been reported between 10% and 25% of patients.[40,41] However, when early extubation was studied in a controlled fashion, extubation failure rates are reported as low as 2.7%.[27]

Inhaled Nitric Oxide Therapy

The use of inhaled nitric oxide in the perioperative management of patients with congenital cardiac disease has become widespread and is typically a response to pulmonary hypertensive crises or a treatment for imbalances between PVR and SVR. Patient selection and assessment of efficacy is different in this population than in other populations where the gas can be used to treat hypoxemic respiratory failure. The decision to initiate this therapy is based not only on measurements of oxygenation, such as oxygenation index or Pa_{O_2} to F_{IO_2} ratio, but also on echocardiographic findings and/or pulmonary artery pressures directly measured with a pulmonary artery catheter.

Subambient Oxygen Therapy

The preoperative stability of patients with certain types of cardiac lesions is often depends partially on maintaining an elevated PVR. FIO_2 of less than 0.21 may be administered to patients with ductal-dependent lesions to limit the pulmonary vasodilatory effect of oxygen, thus maintaining a high PVR. This prevents pulmonary overcirculation and helps to balance pulmonary and systemic blood flow.

FIO_2 is decreased to < 0.21 by blending additional amounts of nitrogen into the inhaled gas. This is achieved using a specially modified external blender system, where pure nitrogen is attached to the oxygen inlet of the external blender (Figure 30-26). The outflow of this external blender is then attached to the air inlet of the ventilator. The ventilator FIO_2 control is left at 0.21 and the external blender then controls the FIO_2. When the control knob on the external blender is turned up, the FIO_2 delivered to the patient *decreases*. Since this setup requires using a blender in a fashion that it is not designed for, special care must be taken to avoid the potential of a misapplication. It is possible to give the pure nitrogen in this setup if the external blender control knob is turned all the way up. For safety purposes, therefore, you must use a continuous oxygen analyzer in line with high and low alarms. In some hospitals this procedure is done infrequently and thus prone to setup errors. It is advisable to have two clinicians check this setup before attaching it to a patient.

Typically, a targeted SpO_2 is achieved by titrating the FIO_2, which may range as low as 0.16 to 0.17. Targeted SpO_2 usually is kept 75% to 85%.

Some hospitals also use subambient oxygen therapy in nonintubated patients, using the same blender setup attached to a hood.

Hypercarbic Therapy

Another method of increasing PVR and thus balancing pulmonary and systemic blood flows is the use of elevated levels of $FICO_2$.[42,43] Whereas adding nitrogen to the inhaled gas reduces available oxygen, increasing $FICO_2$ directly increases $PaCO_2$ and thus decreases pH. This induced acidosis causes an increase in PVR. Clinical goals of this therapy are more complex than those for subambient oxygen therapy. Typically, one goal is to keep the pH between 7.20 and 7.25. Saturations of 75% to 85% are an indirect indication that the therapy is effective, although sometimes it is acceptable to have higher saturations if systemic perfusion is adequate. To evaluate systemic perfusion we can use serum lactate levels, capillary refill time, and urinary output. Unlike subambient therapy, which decreases SaO_2, SvO_2 and cerebral oxygenation, hypercarbic therapy has been shown to actually increase cerebral blood flow and oxygenation due to cerebral vasodilation. In a spontaneously breathing patient elevated CO_2 levels will result in increased minute ventilation. Thus this therapy should only be used in patients who are intubated and heavily sedated or paralyzed.

Chatburn and Anderson describe a method for delivering elevated levels of $FICO_2$ by using a specially modified air-oxygen mixer.[44] We achieve this by bleeding CO_2

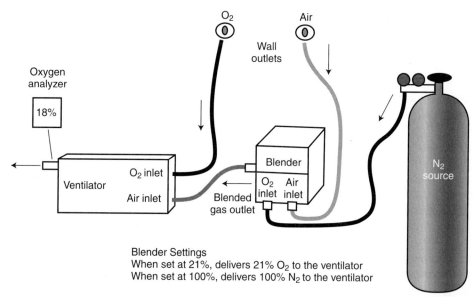

FIGURE 30-26 Schematic representation of the equipment used for administration of subambient oxygen levels through a ventilator.

into the ventilator circuit. However, $FICO_2$ must be carefully measured on the inspiratory side of the ventilator circuit. This can be achieved using a capnometer that can have its display changed to read in percent CO_2. The use of this capnometer allows the use of high and low $FICO_2$ alarms. This is a very important safety consideration in this therapy. Bleeding gas into the circuit allows for the potential for dangerously high $FICO_2$ levels.

There are no studies assessing the long-term developmental outcome of patients who have received subambient oxygen or hypercarbic therapy. Subambient oxygen therapy has the potential advantage of not requiring patients to be intubated while awaiting surgery. Hypercarbic therapy has the theoretical benefit of increased cerebral blood flow and oxygenation.

ASSESSMENT QUESTIONS

See Evolve Resources for the answers.

1. Normal transition to extrauterine life depends on the pulmonary vascular system
   A. Remaining in a steady state of balance with the hepatic blood flow
   B. Changing from a low pulmonary vascular resistance to a high pulmonary vascular resistance
   C. Changing from a high pulmonary vascular resistance to a low pulmonary vascular resistance.
   D. Maintaining a patent ductus arteriosus.
2. Which of the following affects pulmonary vascular resistance?
   A. Changes in Pao_2
   B. Changes in $Paco_2$
   C. Changes in pH
   D. All of the above
   E. None of the above
3. What are the two categories that have typically been used to classify congenital cardiac defects?
   A. Right-sided versus left-sided
   B. Atrial versus ventricular
   C. Cyanotic versus acyanotic
   D. Simple versus complex
   E. Above versus below the diaphragm
4. The patent ductus arteriosus connects which two vessels?
   A. Superior vena cava and the pulmonary artery
   B. Aorta to the pulmonary artery
   C. Pulmonary artery and the pulmonary vein
   D. Coronary arteries and the aortic arch
   E. Ductus venosus to the right atrium

ASSESSMENT QUESTIONS—cont'd

5. What is the therapeutic goal of subambient oxygen therapy?
   A. Increase the pulmonary vascular resistance
   B. Balance blood flow between the vena cava and the right atrium
   C. Decrease pulmonary vascular resistance
   D. Increase diastolic blood pressure
6. The purpose of managing pulmonary vascular resistance in the presence of cardiac defects is to ensure the desired balance between systemic and pulmonary blood flow.
   A. True
   B. False
7. Tetralogy of Fallot consists of which four concomitant conditions:
   I. Truncus arteriosus
   II. Left ventricular hypertrophy
   III. Right ventricular hypertrophy
   IV. Overriding aorta
   V. Interrupted aortic arch
   VI. Pulmonary stenosis
   VII. Ventricular septal defect
   VIII. Right ventricular outflow tract obstruction
   a. I, II, III, V
   b. III, IV, VI, VII
   c. V, VI, VII, VIII
8. In complete transposition of the great arteries, the aorta and the pulmonary artery circulation run in series.
   A. True
   B. False
9. For which condition is a ventilator strategy utilizing larger tidal volumes, lower rates, and shorter inspiratory times typically used?
   A. Unrepaired truncus arteriosus
   B. Total anomalous venous return
   C. Situs inversus
   D. Bidirectional Glenn
10. Increasing gradients between $ETco_2$ and $Paco_2$ in patients with congenital cardiac defects are often the result of:
    A. Loss of calibration
    B. Ventilation-perfusion mismatching
    C. Equipment malfunction

References

1. Shillingford AJ, Wernovsky GG: Academic performance and behavioral difficulties after neonatal and infant heart surgery, *Pediatr Clin N Am* 2001;51:1625.
2. Chang AC: Pediatric cardiac intensive care: current state of the art and beyond the millennium, *Curr Opin Pediatr* 2000;12:238.

3. Gersony WM: Major advances in pediatric cardiology in the 20th century: II. Therapeutics, *J Pediatr* 2001;139:328.

4. Warnes CA et al: Task force I: the changing profile of congenital heart disease in adult life, *J Am Coll Cardiol* 2001;37:1170.

5. Halliday HL, McClure BG, Reid M: Cardiovascular problems. In Halliday HL, editor: *Handbook of neonatal intensive care,*. Philadelphia. WB Saunders, 1998; pp 277-297.

6. Wyllie J: Treatment of patent ductus arteriosus, *Seminars in Neonatology* 2003;8:425.

7. Schumacher RE, Donn SM: Persistent pulmonary hypertension of the newborn. In Sinha SK, Donn SM, editors: *Manual of neonatal respiratory care*, Armonk, NY: Futura; 1999. pp 281-287.

8. Fluck RR: Congenital cardiovascular disorders. In Aloan CA, Hill TV, editors: *Respiratory care of the newborn and child*, Philadelphia: Lippincott-Raven; 1997. pp 223-249.

9. Schmidt B et al: Long term effects of indomethacin prophylaxis in extremely low birth weight infants, *N Engl J Med* 2001;344:1966.

10. Kruger E, Mellander M, Bratton D, Cotton R: Prevention of symptomatic patent ductus arteriosus with a single dose of indomethacin, *J Pediatr* 1987;111:749.

11. Cotton RB, Lindstrom DP: Effects of positive-end-expiratory pressure on right ventricular output in lambs with hyaline membrane disease, *Acta Paediatr Scand* 1980;69:603.

12. Holzer R, Hijazi ZM: Interventional approach to congenital heart disease, *Curr Opin Cardiol* 2004;19:84.

13. Black MD: Minimally invasive repair of atrial septal defects, *Ann Thorac Surg* 1998;65:765.

14. Burke RP: Minimally invasive techniques for congenital heart surgery, *Semin Thorac Cardiovasc Surg* 1997;9:337.

15. Welke KF, Komanapalli C, Shen I, Ungerleider RM. Advances in congenital heart surgery. *Curr Opin Pediatr.* 2005 Oct;17(5):574-578.

16. Pozzi M et al: Atrioventricular septal defects: analysis of short and medicum term results, *J Thorac Cardiovasc Surg* 1991;101:138.

17. Theilen U, Shekerdemian L: The intensive care of infants with Hypoplastic left heart syndrome, *Arch Dis Child Fetal Neonatal Ed* 2005;90:F97.

18. Tabbutt S et al: Impact of inspired gas mixtures on preoperative infants with hypoplastic left heart syndrome during controlled ventilation, *Circulation* 2001;104:(12 suppl 1):I159.

19. Sano S et al: Right ventricle-pulmonary artery shunt in first-stage palliation of hypoplastic left heart syndrome, *J Thorac Cardiovasc Surg,* 2003;126:504.

20. Bradley, SM, Simsic JM, Mulvihill DM: Hypoventilation improves oxygenation after bidirectional superior cavopulmonary connection, *J Thorac Cardiovasc Surg* 2003;126;1033.

21. Park MK: Cyanotic congenital heart defects. In: *Pediatric cardiology for practitioners*, ed 4, St. Louis: Mosby; 2002. pp174-240.

22. Guyton AC, Hall JE: *Textbook of medical physiology*, ed 11,. Philadelphia: Saunders; 2006. p 111.

23. Irita K et al: Performance evaluation of a new pulse oximeter during mild hypothermic cardiopulmonary bypass, *Anesth Analg* 2003;96:11.

24. Malviya S et al: False alarms and sensitivity of conventional pulse oximetry versus the Masimo SET(tm)

technology in the pediatric postanesthesia care unit, *Anesth Analg* 2000;90:1336.

25. Torres A Jr et al: Pulse oximetry in children with congenital heart disease: effects of cardiopulmonary bypass and cyanosis, *J Intensive Care Med* 2004;19:229.

26. Salyer JW: Neonatal and Pediatric Pulse Oximetry, *Respir Care* 2003;48:386.

27. Durbin CG Jr, Rostow SK: More reliable oximetry reduces the frequency of arterial blood gas analyses and hastens oxygen weaning after cardiac surgery: a prospective, randomized trial of the clinical impact of a new technology, *Crit Care Med* 2002;30:1735.

28. Chow LC, Wright KW, Sola A: Can changes in clinical practice decrease the incidence of severe retinopathy of prematurity in very low birth weight infants? *Pediatrics* 2003;111:339.

29. Thompson JE, Jaffe MB: Capnographic waveforms in the mechanically ventilated patient, *Respir Care* 2005;50:100.

30. Wong PW et al: The effect of varying inspiratory flow waveforms on pulmonary mechanics in critically ill patients, *J Crit Care* 2000;15:133.

31. Kocis KC et al: Pressure-regulated volume control versus volume control ventilation in infants after surgery for congenital heart disease *Pediatr Cardiol* 2001;22:233.

32. Kallet RH et al: The effects of pressure control versus volume control assisted ventilation on patient work of breathing in acute lung injury and acute respiratory distress syndrome *Respir Care* 2000;45:1085.

33. Davis K Jr, Branson RD, Campbell RS, Porembka DT: Comparison of volume control and pressure control ventilation: Is flow waveform the difference? *J Trauma* 1996;41:808.

34. Kloth RL, Baum VC: Very early extubation in children after cardiac surgery, *Crit Care Med* 2002;30:787.

35. Davis S, Worley S, Mee RBB, Harrison AM. Factors associated with early extubation after cardiac surgery in young children. *Pediatr Crit Care Med* 2004;5:63-68.

36. Vricella LA et al: Ultra fast track in elective congenital cardiac surgery, *Ann Thorac Surg* 2000;69:865.

37. Cray SH et al: Early tracheal extubation after paediatric cardiac surgery: the use of propofol to supplement low-dose opioid anaesthesia, *Paeditr Anesthes* 2001;11:465.

38. Fischer JE, Allen P, Fanconi S: Delay of extubation in neonates and children after cardiac surgery: impact of ventilator-associated pneumonia, *Intensive Care Med* 2000;26:942.

39. Baisch SD, Wheeler WB, Kurachek SC, Cornfield DN: Extubation failure in pediatric intensive care incidence and outcomes, Pediatr Crit Care Med.2005;6:312.

40. Harrison AM et al: Failed extubation after cardiac surgery in young children: prevalence, pathogenesis, and risk factors, *Pediatr Crit Care Med* 2002;3:148.

41. Heinle JS, Diaz LK Fox LS: Early extubation after cardiac operations in neonates and young infants, *J Thoracic Cardiovasc Surg* 1997;114:1101.

42. Tabbut S et al: Impact of Inspired Gas Mixtures on Preoperative Infants With Hypoplastic Left Heart Syndrome During Controlled Ventilation, *Circulation* 2004;104:I-159.

43. Jobes DR et al: Carbon dioxide prevents pulmonary over-circulation in hypoplastic left heart syndrome. *Ann Thorac Surg* 1992;54:150.

44. Chatburn RL et al: Controlling carbon dioxide delivery during mechanical ventilation, *Respiratory Care* 1994;39:1039.

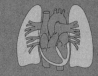

Chapter 31

Sudden Infant Death Syndrome and Pediatric Sleep Disorders

PEARL YU

LEARNING OBJECTIVES

After reading this chapter the reader will be able to:
- Discuss sudden infant death syndrome (SIDS) and apparent life-threatening events (ALTE)
- Describe normal control of breathing and heart rate
- Interpret sleep studies and parameters that are measured in a sleep study
- Describe normal sleep development

- Define apnea and review the different apnea types
- State the incidence of obstructive sleep apnea (OSA) and snoring in children
- Appraise the sequelae of untreated OSA in children
- Select treatments for OSA
- Explain the role of home cardiorespiratory monitors

Sudden infant death syndrome (SIDS), also referred to as "crib death," is a major disorder associated with sleep during the first year of life. It is the leading cause of death in infants between 1 week and 1 year of age, affecting more than 5,000 infants in the United States each year. SIDS is best defined as the sudden and unexpected death of an infant for which sufficient cause cannot be found by a death scene investigation, review of the history, and a postmortem examination. As this definition implies, it is a diagnosis of exclusion: there are no findings on autopsy that are entirely specific for SIDS.

Because of the breadth of the definition and the lack of specific postmortem lesions, it is probable that SIDS has multiple causes.[1]

Closely linked to any discussion of SIDS is the phenomenon of apparent life-threatening events. An apparent life-threatening event (ALTE) is defined by the American Thoracic Society as "an episode of apnea, color change (pallor, cyanosis, or erythema), and hypotonia that the observer believes to be life-threatening to the infant and for which some intervention (stimulation, shaking, and/or cardiorespiratory resuscitation) is felt to be required."[2] Although the relationship between ALTE and SIDS is poorly understood, many believe that ALTE may indicate a risk for cardiorespiratory instability, which could lead to death.

SIDS almost always takes place when the infant is presumed to have been asleep, either during the day or night. However, more than 70% of its victims are found in the early morning hours after the nighttime sleep.[3] SIDS is widely considered to have a developmental component because infants in the first month of life are generally spared. The incidence then peaks in infants from 2 to 4 months of life, which coincides with significant changes known to occur in sleep organization and in the modulation of brainstem centers involved in respiratory and arousal state control by the forebrain.[4] Crib death is uncommon after infants are 6 months old, with 90% of SIDS victims affected in the first 6 months of life. It is rare after the first birthday. This particular pattern of incidence is unique to SIDS (Figure 31-1).

There are many risk factors for SIDS, most of which cannot be easily eliminated (Box 31-1). However, there are several risk factors that lend themselves to intervention:

1. prone positioning
2. maternal smoking
3. bottle-feeding

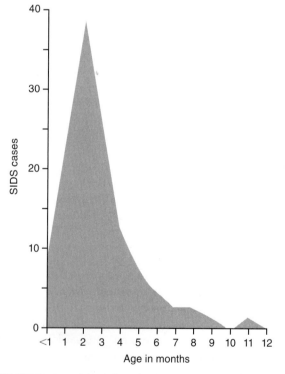

40

30

20

10

0

SIDS cases

<1 1 2 3 4 5 6 7 8 9 10 11 12
Age in months

FIGURE 31-1 Sudden infant death syndrome (SIDS) deaths in Maryland in 1985. Note the peak at 2 months of age and a decrease after 6 months of age.

Box 31-1

Risk Factors for Sudden Infant Death Syndrome
- Male sex
- African-American race
- Teenaged mother
- Exposure to opioids and cocaine in utero
- Anemia during pregnancy
- Late or no prenatal care
- Bottle-feeding
- Prematurity
- Low birth weight
- Prone position
- Winter season

Historically, numerous international epidemiologic studies pointed to an increased risk of SIDS when infants are put to sleep in the prone position.[5-7] A U.S. study confirmed this relationship, although the relative risk of prone versus supine posture in this study was lower than it had been in the foreign studies. Many mechanisms have been proposed to explain the relationship to sleep position, but most have not been tested or have not withstood critical examination. One hypothesis is that a subgroup of prone-positioned infants actually "burrow" their faces into their bedding rather than keep their heads turned to one side. These infants are theorized to die because of suffocation or rebreathing of carbon dioxide.[8] An analysis of one supine-sleeping campaign in Norway published in 1998 showed that the SIDS rate dropped from 3.5 deaths per 1000 live births to 0.3 deaths per 1000 live births 4 years after an intervention program designed to avoid prone sleeping.[5] Similar public education campaigns to inform parents about the risk factors associated with SIDS in the United States have yielded a clear decline in the incidence of SIDS. These risk factors include prone and side infant sleeping positions, exposure of infants to cigarette smoke, and potentially hazardous crib-related sleeping environments.[9]

Maternal cigarette smoking during pregnancy is associated with increased risk in a dose-dependent fashion: the more cigarettes smoked, the greater the risk.[10] This dose dependency suggests a relationship between a factor that may be causing SIDS and prenatal maternal cigarette smoking. In addition, there is evidence that postnatal exposure to cigarette smoke (passive smoking) further increases the risk. Some studies have found breastfeeding to be partly protective against SIDS, but other studies have found no effect. Any beneficial effect may be related to the fact that breastfed babies have fewer infections than do bottle-fed babies because infections may increase the risk for SIDS.

NORMAL CONTROL OF BREATHING AND HEART RATE

Much of the control of breathing resides in the most primitive part of the brain, the brainstem. It is there that the central rhythm generator (CRG) is postulated to exist, and information flows from the peripheral chemoreceptors and the mechanoreceptors to the brainstem, modulating the output from the CRG. The presence of an "off switch" mechanism is also postulated because phrenic nerve output to the diaphragm is absent during expiration. The off switch terminates inspiration by inhibition of the CRG. Input from higher centers of the brain, such as the cortex, is also integrated within the brainstem. Hence, the ability to voluntarily control breathing also exists.

Control of the heart rate occurs primarily through the autonomic nervous system, which is divided into sympathetic and parasympathetic branches. Sympathetic stimulation of the heart increases heart rate, whereas parasympathetic stimulation decreases the heart rate. The vagus nerve is the parasympathetic conduit from nuclei (ambiguous nuclei and tractus solitarius) in the brainstem to the heart. "Vagal" stimuli such as coughing, choking, or expiring against a closed glottis (the Valsalva maneuver) can induce bradycardia. The bradycardia that follows obstructive apnea may also be vagally mediated.

ETIOLOGY

The importance of the brainstem in the control of breathing and possibly SIDS is further supported by the fact that apnea in premature infants is associated with immaturity of the brainstem. Premature infants with apnea have prolonged brainstem conduction times for auditory-evoked responses compared with premature infants without apnea. Also, some SIDS victims have gliosis (representing scarring) of cellular bodies in the medulla oblongata, specifically in the area of the arcuate nucleus that controls respiratory and cardiac function.[11,12]

Although the specific neuronal dysfunction that leads to both central apnea and periodic breathing has yet to be determined, it appears that factors in the maturation of central chemoreceptors and mechanoreceptors play a pivotal role in the alterations of respiratory drive in preterm infants. Some preterm infants exhibit an unexpected and paradoxical decrease in ventilatory response to increases in carbon dioxide values. Also, preterm infants often respond to a fall in inspired oxygen concentrations with a transient increase in ventilation followed by a return to baseline or even a depression of ventilation. The diminution of respiratory drive during hypercarbia and the biphasic response to hypoxia can potentially predispose a vulnerable child to apnea and its sequelae.[13]

As intriguing as these hypotheses may be, the precise cause of SIDS is not known. SIDS may have several causes, but all are likely to be related to a developmental immaturity or malfunction of the brain leading to either cardiac or respiratory death.

TESTS TO ASSESS RISK OF SUDDEN INFANT DEATH SYNDROME

There is no test that accurately predicts risk for SIDS, perhaps because it has multiple causes and because most tests are performed weeks or months before death, during a period of life in which the infant is undergoing rapid change. The pneumocardiogram is a two- to four-channel recording usually consisting of transthoracic impedance (chest movements) and heart rate, as well as oxygen saturation data and an air flow channel in the more sophisticated models (Figure 31-2). It is usually performed overnight in a controlled but unattended setting. Its value is markedly diminished because it provides limited ability to differentiate between central and obstructive apnea and does not provide thorough information regarding the severity and physiologic consequences of the breathing disturbance. It is widely accepted that the pneumocardiogram is not effective at screening for risk of SIDS.[14]

Polysomnography (PSG) performed according to the standards accepted by the American Thoracic Society[2] provides the clinician with a more thorough evaluation of pediatric sleep and breathing disorders than a pneumocardiogram. PSG for cardiopulmonary indications includes simultaneous recording of physiologic variables, including sleep state, respiration, cardiac rhythm, muscle activity, gas exchange, and snoring data (Figure 31-3). The personnel in attendance during PSG are trained to evaluate and document behavioral and physiologic changes as well as quality of sleep. Thus a more accurate diagnosis of obstructive sleep apnea is possible with PSG, in contrast to the lack of this capability in the limited-channel pneumocardiogram (Figure 31-4).

Although PSG is not always indicated after an uncomplicated ALTE, it may be helpful to define the frequency of type of apnea and the extent of cardiac, blood gas, and sleep alterations in certain infants with apnea or an ALTE. PSG is especially useful for the detection of occult hypoxemia. Test results may also suggest the further direction of the workup; for example, if abnormal amounts of obstructive apnea are noted, consultation with an otolaryngologist may be indicated. In addition, data acquired from these studies are often helpful in the later interpretation of waveforms from home memory

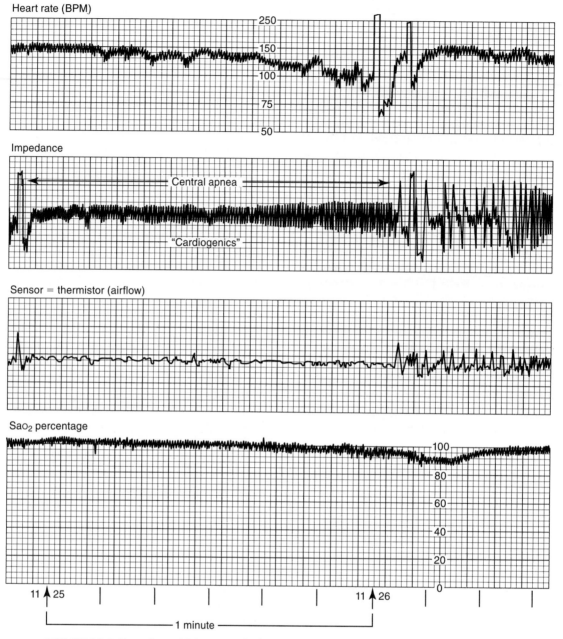

FIGURE 31-2 Four-channel Edentec study that captured a 1-minute-long central apneic episode in a premature infant. Cardiogenics refers to the artifactual detection of heart beats by the impedance channel; these signals occur with each heart beat and thus are not breaths. The Sao$_2$ percentage channel displays oxygen saturation data with a superimposed pulse waveform. BPM, Beats per minute.

monitors. However, the major concern after an ALTE episode is the related risk of recurrent events or death.

POLYSOMNOGRAPHIC PARAMETERS

Data used for the staging of infant sleep include the combined measurement of the electroencephalogram (EEG) to record brain activity, the electrooculogram (EOG) to record bilateral eye movements, and the electromyogram (EMG) to record facial and intercostal muscle tone. The placement of the EEG leads is based on the international "10-20" electrode placement system. EEG placement for scoring sleep in children is similar to that used in an adult population. Electrodes are placed at A1, A2, O1, O2, C3, and C4, and sleep stage is determined by the monopolar derivation C3/A2 or C4/A1. However, because of the special criteria used to

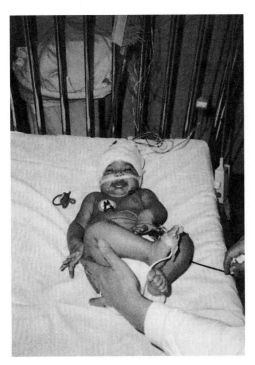

FIGURE 31-3 This patient is nearly ready for polysomnography. The head is wrapped with gauze to protect the scalp electroencephalogram (EEG) electrodes. An electrode to detect movements of the left eye is also covered by gauze, although monitoring bilateral eye movements using two separate electrodes is standard. Tape below the nostrils will hold the thermistor and the CO_2 cannula in place. A transcutaneous oxygen electrode sits on the right side of the upper chest, and an electrocardiographic electrode is opposite it. Stretching across the abdomen is a strain gauge to detect breathing efforts. An oxygen saturation sensor is attached to the right foot.

define sleep states in infants younger than 6 months old and the unique EEG features for this population, an extended EEG montage, or PSG channel derivation, is preferred. This extended montage should include bilateral EEG electrodes utilizing bipolar channels to more accurately evaluate the EEG of the two hemispheres of the brain. EEG features specific to infants, such as tracé alternant and "brushes," as well as certain epileptiform activity, can provide useful information regarding the maturity of the brain and alert clinicians to potential problems in brain activity. Additionally, certain normal features of the infant EEG, such as rudimentary sleep spindles, are better seen using an extended EEG montage that includes frontal leads.

The accurate scoring of sleep stages also requires bilateral EOG sensors to monitor the rapid eye movements that normally occur in rapid-eye-movement (REM) sleep and the slow eye movements that occur with the onset of sleep. An EMG recording of facial muscle tone assists the clinician in more accurately determining the presence of REM sleep when skeletal muscle tone, particularly the muscles of the face, is normally inhibited.

To comprehensively assess the adequacy of ventilation and identify and differentiate between central and obstructive apnea and its severity, PSGs should also include movements of the chest wall and abdomen, air flow at the nose and mouth, transcutaneous oxygen saturation data (with validating pulse wave from the monitor), and end-tidal carbon dioxide ($ETco_2$) measures. A pulse waveform is necessary to assess the reliability of oxygenation data because oxygen saturation monitors can yield artifactual data at times when the infant is feeding or moving. Capnography, a graphic representation of $ETco_2$, is recommended because it can assess both air flow and ventilation simultaneously. Calibrated $ETco_2$ measurements can effectively detect possible CO_2 retention associated with apnea or prolonged hypoventilation.

A standard PSG also includes additional parameters that can provide important information relevant to the patient's electrophysiologic status. An electrocardiogram (ECG) monitors cardiac rate and rhythm and is useful in evaluating the consequences of breathing disorders on the heart. Inductive plethysmography involving the placement of bands around the rib cage and abdomen detects respiratory effort as well as phase relationship allowing for differentiation between central versus obstructive apnea. A PSG can include EMG of the anterior tibialis muscles to identify periodic limb leg movement disorders, although these disorders are rare in infants and leg EMGs are not routinely monitored in children unless clinically indicated.

To assess for the presence of gastroesophageal reflux and its potential cardiorespiratory consequences, continuous esophageal pH measurement can be done in conjunction with PSG. Video recording with sound is recommended because it provides invaluable information on sleep behavior, snoring, respiratory effort, and sleep positions associated with a particular respiratory pattern. Finally, PSG on infants should be monitored by a trained technologist who ensures the integrity of the recording, provides descriptions regarding unusual events or behaviors, and makes notations on the recording regarding physiologic changes such as snoring and color changes such as cyanosis, pallor, and erythema. Polysomnographic technologists working with this age group must be certified in pediatric cardiopulmonary resuscitation (CPR).

LABORATORY SUPERVISION

A pediatrician with training and experience in pediatric respiratory disorders and/or sleep medicine should be responsible for supervision of a sleep laboratory whose

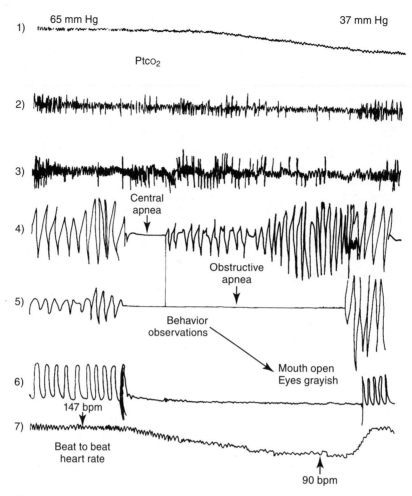

FIGURE 31-4 Thirty-seven-second mixed apnea recorded during polysomnography. Channel 1 shows a drop in transcutaneous oxygen tension from 65 to 37 mm Hg over the 1 minute of this recording. Channel 4 depicts breathing movements, and channels 5 and 6 depict nasal air flow. Note the onset of central apnea, as indicated on channel 4, followed by obstructive apnea, as channels 5 and 6 show no air flow despite breathing movements in channel 4. Pt co_2, Transcutaneous oxygen; bpm, beats per minute.

primary activity is performing PSG in infants and children with cardiorespiratory disorders. If this is not possible, it is recommended that a pediatrician with expertise in pediatric pulmonology, neonatology, neurology, or pediatric sleep medicine oversee laboratory operations related to children. A pediatric specialist can ensure that the PSG is performed, scored, and interpreted appropriately for the age and condition of the child.

SETTING

Children should be studied in a dedicated pediatric facility with a laboratory decor that is both age appropriate and nonthreatening. If a separate pediatric laboratory is not available, an area of the laboratory should be dedicated for children. Accommodations for a parent to sleep near the child are recommended because

immediate parental access to the child is often necessary to reduce fear and anxiety and provide ordinary child care while the study is in progress. It is sometimes helpful to use videocassette recorders and provide stickers to toddlers and older children for distraction and to obtain compliance during the setup. Safe and comfortable bedding is necessary when performing PSG on infants and children. Mattresses should be firm and made of material that is easy to clean and disinfect if soiled.

PERSONNEL

A pediatric sleep laboratory should be staffed with personnel trained to deal with children and their parents or guardians. Because PSG evaluation can be seen as stressful, particularly in this age group, laboratory personnel should have knowledge of childhood behavior and developmental stages to effectively deal with children and provide medical information in a nonthreatening manner. Because of the differences in the sleep characteristics of children as compared with adolescents and adults, only qualified individuals who know the unique characteristics of sleep breathing in children of different ages should evaluate the PSG.[2]

NORMAL SLEEP DEVELOPMENT

Neonates cycle through REM and non-REM (NREM) sleep differently than an older child or adult.[15] In the first few months of life, they have not yet become fully entrained to a day-night cycle and more of the control of sleep is internal. Full-term infants can spend as much as 50% of their total sleep time in REM sleep. At this age, this is referred to as "active sleep."[16] The infant often enters the sleep cycle in REM. By about 6 months of age, as sleep cycling approaches the adult mode, sleep state progression matures and NREM sleep typically precedes REM sleep. Breathing abnormalities, including obstructive sleep apnea syndrome (OSAS), may be exacerbated or only seen in REM sleep. For this reason, sleep staging is an important aspect of PSG evaluation to assess the sleep-state dependence of breathing abnormalities and to ensure that all stages have been documented during the study.[2]

Normally, brief arousals occur as the sleeper transitions between each stage of sleep, usually without a return to full wakefulness.[17,18] These endogenous transitional arousals are common as sleep begins to differentiate in the REM and NREM progression of the

infant both quantitatively and qualitatively as the child matures. As an individual transitions to REM through the lighter phases of NREM sleep during the night, a continuum of behaviors including stretching, brief vocalizing, crying, or changing of position is common. Arousals during PSG are scored because these may also be consequences of abnormal breathing events during sleep. However, there is the suggestion that apnea in children may not always be terminated with frank cortical arousal.[2]

APNEA

Apnea is best defined as the absence of air flow at the nostrils and mouth. The three main categories of apnea are central, obstructive, and mixed. Central apnea occurs when respiratory effort ceases; there is no chest movement and hence no air flow (Figure 31-5). Diagnosis of central apnea must take into account a multitude of factors. It is ordinarily significant when it exceeds 20 seconds in duration. Because infants normally have a more rapid baseline respiratory rate and a reduced respiratory reserve, and therefore less protection from hypoxia, shorter central events can be more clinically significant in this age group. Central apnea can yield significant physiologic compromise such as bradycardia or color change associated with declining oxyhemoglobin levels.

For infants, central sleep apnea must be distinguished from other causes for respiratory pauses, including the more common periodic breathing pattern and the obligatory respiratory pauses that follow a deep yawn or sigh. Although a rare cause of central apnea, seizures will also change the respiratory pattern seen on a tracing.

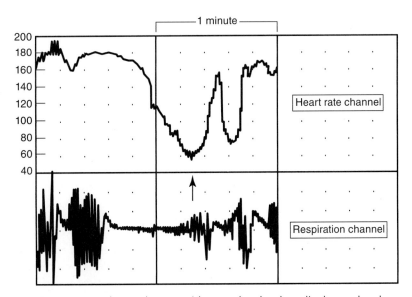

FIGURE 31-5 Forty-second central apnea with secondary bradycardia detected and recorded by a Corometrics 500-E memory monitor.

In the more severe cases, central apneas can be treated with medication. The presence of frequent central sleep apnea is a usual cause for respiratory monitoring during sleep. Premature infants are at increased risk for central apneas. Central apnea accounts for 10% to 25% of all apnea in premature infants.[13]

In children, OSAS is a disorder of breathing during sleep characterized by prolonged partial upper airway obstruction (hypopnea) and/or intermittent complete obstruction (apnea) that disrupt normal ventilation during sleep and normal sleep patterns. Clinically, obstructive apnea is the lack or diminution of air flow despite the continuation of respiratory efforts. The obstruction can be functional or anatomic. When obstruction is present, respiratory efforts continue and tugging or retraction of the skin can be seen. OSAS accounts for only 10% to 20% of all apneas in preterm infants.[13] It has been estimated that 7% to 15%[19-24] of children snore regularly, with an estimated prevalence of OSAS of 1% to 3% in 2- to 8-year-old children.[19,20,24,25] Most affected children breathe normally while awake. However, a minority with marked upper airway obstruction also have noisy, mildly labored breathing while awake.

Obstruction lasting 10 seconds or longer is regarded as significant in adults. For some children, however, durations of obstruction shorter than 10 seconds are important. Thus some physicians have suggested using a criterion of two respiratory cycles in duration, whereas others have suggested 6 or 8 seconds as durations indicating significant upper airway obstruction during childhood. In some infants with clinically significant OSAS, little or no snoring may be heard by the caregiver, unlike the clinical manifestations of OSAS in older children and adults.[2]

Obstructions can be caused by the presence of an anatomic abnormality, neurologic condition, or medical condition. Reduction of the airway size leads to increased respiratory effort, which can create negative airway pressure and paradoxically worsen the obstruction. The most common anatomic factors leading to OSAS include large tonsils or adenoids, obesity, micrognathia (small jaw), or other anatomic anomalies. Muscular hypotonia is one of the most common neurologic factors contributing to OSAS. Normal muscle tone inhibition during REM sleep can change respiratory patterns with more breath-to-breath variability increasing the risk of full or partial airway obstruction. Hypotonia can be commonly seen in Down syndrome, muscular dystrophy, and other genetic disorders. Allergies or even mild upper respiratory tract infections can serve to swell mucous membranes and thereby contribute to obstruction. Some of the less common risk factors include laryngomalacia, pharyngeal flap surgery, sickle cell disease, structural malformations of the brainstem, and certain metabolic and genetic disorders.

Complications

Apneas and hypopneas lead to a drop in oxygen saturations and an increase in blood carbon dioxide and often will cause a full or partial arousal pattern in sleep EEG tracings. When these events occur multiple times at night, there are several anticipated effects. The presence of frequent arousals leads to fragmented, inefficient, and insufficient sleep. This can lead to increased daytime sleepiness, as well as hyperactive behavior.[26,27] In young children, this can result in increased time sleeping and more behavioral difficulties.[23] In older children, this sleepiness is often manifested by behavioral changes and poor school performance (in appropriately aged children). All children are at risk for cardiac and pulmonary effects of recurrent hypoxia and hypercarbia. These can lead to *cor pulmonale*, a condition in which the blood pressure in the vessels of the lung is increased and the right side of the heart enlarges in order to compensate. With time, these abnormalities can become irreversible.

Treatment

Adenoidal and tonsillar enlargement account for most cases of pediatric obstructive sleep apnea. Removal of the adenoids and/or tonsils usually provides a cure in those instances. Older children may also benefit from nasal continuous positive airway pressure (NCPAP), which is also commonly used in adults. NCPAP acts as a splint to prevent collapse of the pharyngeal tissues. Because a range of pressures may be therapeutic, NCPAP must be titrated to the patient. Usually this is done an overnight polysomnogram to obtain a precise titration. The major drawbacks to NCPAP are poor patient tolerance and poor compliance. Children will often benefit from the opportunity to become acclimated to the mask, and behavioral support may improve compliance. If the obstruction is severe and unresponsive to other interventions, tracheostomy may be necessary.

Mixed sleep apnea is the combination of central and obstructive apnea, with the central component usually followed by obstruction (see Figure 31-4). Because of this, therapies that are effective for central apnea are also effective in treating mixed apnea. For example, during infancy, medications can be used to treat both forms of apnea.

In the normal neonate, particularly the premature infant, breathing can be irregular. Periodic breathing is defined as a series of three or more apneic events of at least 3 seconds duration, separated by less than 20 seconds of uninterrupted breathing. Apnea is considered a more serious condition because the respiratory pause lasts longer and is frequently associated with more significant decreases in heart rate below 80 beats per minute and declining oxyhemoglobin values. Although periodic breathing is usually considered benign, for very small infants even short apneic pauses can cause significant bradycardia and oxygen desaturations.

Periodic breathing can occur during wakefulness, active sleep (REM), and quiet sleep (NREM), but its prevalence is increased in active sleep. In quiet sleep, periodic breathing becomes regular—that is, breathing and apneic intervals are of similar duration. In active sleep, the frequency of respirations and subsequently periodic breathing becomes irregular. The most well-defined periodic breathing observable in small infants is in quiet sleep during the EEG pattern known as tracé alternant, commonly seen in infants younger than 44 weeks' conceptional age.[28] Tracé alternant is an episodic EEG pattern in which complex bursts of moderate- to high-amplitude slow waves are superimposed on a continuous background of polymorphic theta and faster rhythms.[29]

All types of apnea are seen in the neonatal intensive care unit (NICU) and at home in the first year of life, although obstructive apnea is less common in infants. The causes of apnea in the NICU are numerous. The most important include apnea of prematurity (idiopathic), gastroesophageal reflux, hypoxia, anemia, and intraventricular hemorrhage. Sedative drugs passed to the infant during labor and delivery, or later through breast milk, can also lead to apnea.

Apnea during infancy at home can be a component of an ALTE. These episodes were often referred to as "near miss" SIDS in the past. Those that require vigorous stimulation or CPR are severe ALTEs and demand special attention because there is an increased risk of subsequent death. Episodes that occur while the infant is awake are more likely to be associated with gastroesophageal reflux, seizures, incoordination of swallowing and breathing during feedings, and crying with breath-holding.[30] In contrast to the neonate in the NICU and the infant at home, the older child is predominately affected by OSAS.

HOME CARDIORESPIRATORY MONITORS

Because apnea and/or respiratory instability have been the most prominent hypotheses for several decades, cardiorespiratory monitors (also called apnea monitors) are frequently prescribed for high-risk infants. Recordings of a small number of SIDS deaths, however, show that bradycardia is present for several minutes before the advent of central apnea.[31] The cause of this bradycardia then becomes the crucial issue. It may be secondary to hypoxemia after apnea.

One of the consequences of our uncertainty about the cause or causes of SIDS is that a rational approach to prevention is difficult. Cardiorespiratory monitors theoretically should be useful in prevention of either cardiac or respiratory death, but the efficacy of these devices has not been scientifically proved or disproved, and monitored infants have died despite quick parental response to the alarm.[31] Conversely, there are hundreds of anecdotal reports that infants have been saved after a caregiver is alerted by a monitor alarm.

Cardiorespiratory monitors for use at home have two immediate purposes: they alert the caregiver to a cardiorespiratory abnormality, and they are diagnostic devices.[32] Ultimately, they are intended to prevent death. The standard monitor in the United States is an impedance-type monitor that detects chest movements and ECG tracings through electrodes placed on the chest. The monitors contain alarms for conditions such as apnea, tachypnea, bradycardia, tachycardia, and sometimes oxygen desaturation. The settings at which each alarm may ring are typically adjustable. Because the monitors detect chest wall movement, they are not as sensitive for obstructive apneas, since chest wall movements may continue through the apnea.[33]

Many alarms can record data in memory for later downloading and analysis. In this manner, the conditions leading up to an alarm can be evaluated for clinical significance and "false alarms" eliminated. Often, alarms will be programmed to save data recorded just before, during, and after an alarm (Figure 31-6). However, the alarm memory will also indicate the total recording time, which is a useful gauge of parental compliance with monitoring. Ensuring compliance may be important because some studies suggest that the majority of infant deaths with prescribed monitors occur during periods of noncompliance or inappropriate use.[34,35] Hence, encouraging parents to use the monitor is vital.

False alarms are often apnea alarms for which the monitor fails to detect the breathing movements that are actually present. Inspection of the recorded waveforms may show a complete lack of breathing movements but without any associated change in the heart rate or oxygen saturation. The presence of the ECG allows confirmation of bradycardia and recognition of some arrhythmias. This is how the monitor functions as a diagnostic device.

Several studies have shown that false apnea alarms and loose lead alarms can be frequent and can substantially outnumber true alarms.[34,35] False alarms can be reduced by attention to electrode placement so that the electrodes "see" maximal chest or abdominal wall movements. This often means that parents must be properly trained in lead placement. However, there will always be

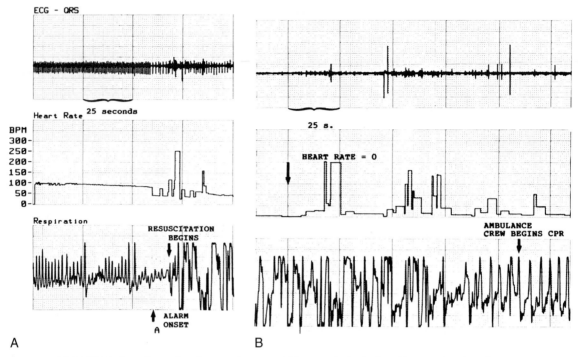

FIGURE 31-6 A, Recording from patient over 100 seconds, including 62 seconds of prealarm data. At the beginning of the prealarm phase, the heart rate is already low at 100 beats per minute. Subsequently, there is a slow but steady drop in heart rate to 80 beats per minute, followed by an abrupt drop to 40 beats per minute 2 seconds before the bradycardia alarm. A resuscitation artifact can be seen 6.5 seconds after alarm onset. **B,** Recording over 150 seconds shows the heart rate falling to 0 beats per minute as parental resuscitation efforts continue. The heart rate then increases to an apparent rate of 250 beats per minute, but the ECG channel *(top panel)* shows artifact. Toward the end of this tracing, resuscitation becomes much more rhythmic after the arrival of the ambulance crew. No central apnea is seen in either **A** or **B**, because the resuscitation efforts would obscure this. ECG, Electrocardiogram; CPR, cardiopulmonary resuscitation.

some false alarms. Appropriate attention to the monitor settings can help eliminate false alarms set off by patient crying or movement.

It is essential that parents and other caretakers be fully trained in how to respond to an alarm. This includes being able to distinguish a false alarm from a true event and to be prepared to administer CPR if necessary. CPR is a complex skill that we expect parents to be able to perform effectively at a time when they are worried or panicked. In fact, there is evidence that parents forget CPR training within a matter of weeks.[36] Affording the parents the opportunity to have repeated CPR training sessions may be lifesaving because many repeat ALTEs are signaled by a home monitor within weeks after discharge from the hospital.

Monitors are traditionally intended only for infants in various high-risk groups, which include those with severe ALTEs and preterm infants who continue to have apneas and bradycardias as discharge from the NICU approaches. As monitoring is begun it is often helpful to have clear clinical criteria for the discontinuation of

monitoring at a later date. Monitoring is often perceived by families as an important safety net, and it can often be difficult to stop monitoring even when the clinical indications for monitoring are no longer present. Because parents are understandably often incorrect in their assessment of alarms, it follows that discontinuation is much easier and surer when the infant is on a memory-equipped monitor.

The time of hospital discharge is an emotionally taxing time for parents. The anxiety produced by having a child on a monitor at home is magnified by the likelihood that parents' sleep will be more disrupted to attend to false alarms during the night. A support system composed of personnel from the monitor supply company and medical professionals responsible for the infant's care can lessen this burden.[37] The most important criterion for the discontinuation of a home apnea monitor is the absence of any significant events for 2 consecutive months. A significant real event is a real alarm for which the infant, in the judgment of the clinician, required stimulation.

For Assessment Questions, please see Evolve Student Resources. To access, http://evolve.elsevier.com/walsh/perinatal/contentupdates.

References

1. Tildon JT, Meny RG, O'Brien J: Sudden infant death syndrome. In Dulbecco R, editor: *Encyclopedia of human biology,* San Diego: Academic Press, 1991. pp 315-322.
2. Loughlin GL et al: Standards and indications for cardiopulmonary sleep studies in children: official statement of the American Thoracic Society adopted by the ATS board of directors, July 1995, *Am J Respir Care Med* 1996;153:866.
3. National Commission on Sleep Disorders Research: *Report of the National Commission on Sleep Disorders,* Department of Health and Human Services publication, no 92, vol 1, Washington, DC: US Government Printing Office, 1992.
4. Glotzbach S, Ariagno R, Harper R: Sleep and the sudden infant death syndrome. In Ferber R, Kryger M, editors: *Principles and practice of sleep medicine in the child,* Philadelphia: WB Saunders, 1995. p 231.
5. Skadberg BT, Morild I, Markstad T: Abandoning prone sleeping: effect on the risk of sudden infant death syndrome, *J Pediatr* 1998;132:340.
6. Mitchell EA et al for the New Zealand Cot Death Study: Changing infant's sleep position increases risk of sudden infant death syndrome. *Arch Pediatr Adolesc Med* 1999;153:1136.
7. Oyen N, Markestad T, Skaerven R: Combined effects of sleeping position and prenatal risk factors in sudden infant death syndrome: the Nordic Epidemiological SIDS Study, *Pediatrics* 1997;100:613.
8. Kemp JS et al: Positional ventilatory impairment in a serial study of 23 SIDS cases, *Pediatr Res* 1992; 31:360A.
9. Carroll JL, Siska ES: SIDS: Counseling parents to reduce the risk, *Am Fam Physician* 1998;57:1566.
10. Haglund B, Cnattingius S: Cigarette smoking as a risk factor for sudden infant death syndrome: a population-based study, *Am J Public Health* 1990;80:29.
11. Kinney HC et al: Reactive gliosis in the medulla oblongata of victims of the sudden infant death syndrome, *Pediatrics* 1983;72:181.
12. Panigrahy A et al: Decreased kainate receptor binding in the arcuate nucleus of the sudden infant death syndrome, *J Neuropathol Exp Neurol* 1997;56:1253.
13. Miller MJ, Martin RJ: Pathophysiology of apnea of prematurity. In Polin RA, Fox WW, editors: *Fetal and neonatal physiology,* Philadelphia: WB Saunders, 1998. pp 1129-1143.
14. National Institutes of Health: Consensus development conference on infantile apnea and home monitoring, 1986, *Pediatrics* 1987;79:292.
15. Anders T: Developmental course of nighttime sleep-wake patterns in full-term and premature infants during the first year of life, *Sleep* 1985;8:173.
16. Parks JD: *Sleep and its disorders,* London: WB Saunders, 1985. pp 4-70.

17. Hauri PJ: *Current concepts: Sleep disorders,* Kalamazoo, Mich: The Upjohn Company, 1992.
18. Kleitman N: *Sleep and wakefulness,* Chicago: University of Chicago Press, 1963. (Original work published in 1939) (Midway reprint edition, pp 122-127).
19. Ali NJ, Pitson D, Stradling JR: Snoring, sleep disturbance and behaviour in 4-5 year olds. *Arch Dis Child,* 1993;68:360.
20. Gislason T, Benediktsdottir B. Snoring, apneic episodes, and nocturnal hypoxemia among children 6 months to 6-years-old, *Chest* 1995;107:963.
21. Owen GO, Canter RJ, Robinson A: Snoring, apnea and ENT symptoms in the paediatric community, *Clin Otolaryngol Allied Sci* 1996;21:130.
22. Ferreira AM, Clemente V, Gozal D, et al. Snoring in Portuguese primary school children, *Pediatrics.* 2000;106(5). Available at: pediatrics.org/cgi/content/full/106/5/e64.
23. O'Brien LM et al. Sleep and neurobehavioral characteristics in 5-7 year old hyperactive children, *Pediatrics.* 2003;111:554.
24. Klaus CJ et al. Neurobehavioral Implications of Habitual Snoring in Children, *Pediatrics* 2004;114;44.
25. Redline S et al: Risk factors for sleep-disordered breathing in children: Associations with obesity, race, and respiratory problems, *Am J Respir Crit Care Med* 1999;59:1527.
26. Owens J: The ADHD and sleep conundrum: A review, *Developmental and Behavioral Pediatrics* 2005;26:312.
27. Gozal D: Sleep-disordered breathing and school performance in children, *Pediatrics* 1998;102:616.
28. Rigatto H: Control of breathing during sleep in the fetus and neonate. In Ferber R, Kryger M, editors: *Principles and practice of sleep medicine in the child,* Philadelphia: WB Saunders, 1995. p 35.
29. Pedley TA, Lombroso C, Hanley R: Introduction to neonatal electroencephalography: Interpretation, *Am J EEG Technol* 1981;21:15.
30. Spitzer AR et al: Awake apnea associated with gastroesophageal reflux: a specific clinical syndrome, *J Pediatr* 1984;104:200.
31. Kelly DH, Pathak A, Meny R: Sudden severe bradycardia in infancy, *Pediatr Pulmonol* 1991;10:199.
32. Meny RG et al: Sudden infant death and home monitors, *Am J Dis Child* 1988;142:1037.
33. Ward SLD et al: Sudden infant death syndrome in infants evaluated by apnea programs in California, *Pediatrics* 1986; 7:451.
34. Weese-Mayer DE et al: Assessing validity of infant monitor alarms with event recording, *J Pediatr* 1989;115:701.
35. Nathanson I, O'Donnell J, Commins MF: Cardiorespiratory patterns during alarms in infants using apnea/bradycardia monitors, *Am J Dis Child* 1989; 143:476.
36. Berardi C et al: CPR skill retention in caregivers of high risk home monitored infants, *Pediatr Pulmonol* 1991;11:369.
37. Ahmann E, Wulff L, Meny RG: Home apnea monitoring and disruptions in family life: a multidimensional controlled study, *Am J Public Health* 1992;82:719.

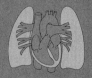

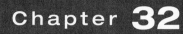

Chapter 32

Pediatric Airway Disorders and Parenchymal Lung Diseases

BRIAN K. WALSH • NICO VEHSE

OUTLINE

LEARNING OBJECTIVES

After reading this chapter the reader will be able to:
- Identify and name upper and lower airway disorders
- Recognize the signs of severe or complete airway obstructions that require interventions

- Describe the basic treatment of each of the airway disorders and parenchymal lung diseases
- Discuss the different types, and therefore the etiology, of pneumonia

THE PEDIATRIC AIRWAY

Airway disorders may cause severe and, at times, sudden threats to a child's life. The special susceptibility of children to disorders of the airways stems from several factors. Congenital abnormalities of airway structures tend to cause difficulties early in life. Even when normal anatomy is present, the relatively small size of the pediatric airway puts children at a distinct disadvantage. The inherently narrow trachea, bronchi, and bronchioles can become critically compromised by minimal swelling of the respiratory mucosal lining or by the presence of foreign objects. Children are at increased risk for such narrowing or obstruction because of their susceptibility to respiratory infections and their tendency to engage in risky behaviors, such as placing small objects in their mouths.

In comparison to the adult, once a child's airway becomes narrowed or obstructed, the pediatric respiratory system is less able to cope with the resulting ventilation abnormality. In the event of complete airway obstruction, children undergo rapid onset of hypoxia, with its resultant neurologic damage or death. Respiratory events are the major reason for cardiac arrest in children. The rapidity of this oxygen desaturation is in part caused by the child's small functional residual capacity and dependency on dynamic compliance combined with an overall increased metabolic rate. Essentially there is minimal oxygen reserve available to supply the child's oxygen requirement. This combination of increased susceptibility to and decreased ability to cope with airway compromise helps explain why children suffer so frequently from airway disorders.

Upper Airway

Many unique aspects of anatomy must be understood to appropriately support and intervene on behalf of a child during respiratory illness. The upper airway consists of all structures connecting the mouth and nose with the glottis. This includes the nose, nasal choanae, nasopharynx, mouth, oropharynx, and structures of the larynx (Figure 32-1). When compared with that of the adult, the anatomy of the infant's airway contains several differences and functional limitations.

The epiglottis is long, floppy, and angled away from the tracheal axis. It shrouds the laryngeal opening because of poor support by the surrounding tissues. Structurally, the infant's larynx is positioned higher in the neck (near C3-4) than is an adult's larynx (at C4-5). Because of this superior location, the tongue base tends to "hide" the larynx from view during direct laryngoscopy. The cricoid cartilage is a nonexpandable cartilaginous ring that is normally the only complete ring of cartilage in the airway. In the pediatric airway, it is the

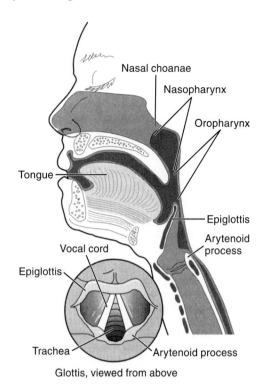

FIGURE 32-1 Normal upper airway structures.

larynx's narrowest portion. With this reduced and fixed dimension, an endotracheal tube may pass through the vocal cords and yet not proceed to the subglottic trachea. This already narrowed portion of the airway becomes severely narrowed by even small amounts of edema that develop with diseases such as laryngotracheobronchitis (LTB) or trauma (e.g., endotracheal intubation).

Infants are considered obligate nose breathers until 3 to 6 months of age. Immaturity of coordination between respiration and oropharyngeal motor activity accounts partly for obligate nasal breathing. Also, the infant's tongue is closer to the roof of the mouth and makes mouth breathing difficult. Because the large tongue and small mouth make air passage through the mouth impossible, except when crying, patency of the nasopharynx is critical in an infant.

The upper airway and lung do not complete development until approximately 8 years of age. The immature cartilage found in the infant's trachea and bronchi is soft and highly compressible. When the supporting cartilage is excessively flexible, the diagnosis of laryngomalacia or tracheomalacia is applied.

Lower Airway

The trachea divides into the mainstem bronchi, which in turn divide into smaller divisions called subsegmental bronchi. This repeated division continues in the adult to 23 generations (divisions) of smaller and smaller air passages, creating a huge surface area for gas exchange.

At birth, however, the infant has only 16 to 17 generations of airways. The terminal generation of airways, the respiratory bronchioles, are present in relatively small numbers, resulting in a small transectional area for gas exchange in the infant. This is in part compensated for by fetal hemoglobin, which has an oxygen affinity superior to adult hemoglobin. Because of the developmentally small airway cross-sectional area, small amounts of inflammation at the level of the respiratory bronchioles can result in severe respiratory embarrassment. In young children, the respiratory bronchioles are commonly attacked by viruses, such as respiratory syncytial virus (RSV), resulting in respiratory failure. The same infection will have little or no respiratory effect on an adult or older child with a larger number of terminal airways.

AIRWAY OBSTRUCTION

Obstruction of the upper or lower airway of a child may lead to life-threatening hypoxia and/or hypercarbia. With the high risk of morbidity comes the need to identify the etiology, recognize the clinical signs and symptoms, and choose the diagnostic methods for and treatment of the many causes of airway obstruction.

Radiographic evaluation of the upper airways includes both frontal anteroposterior and lateral views of the head and neck. When performed at the proper angle and exposure, these films are helpful in evaluating the site of upper airway obstruction (Figure 32-2).

Fearing the unfamiliar surroundings of a hospital or clinic, a child may wiggle and scream, further increasing respiratory effort. To be successful in what could be a very difficult examination, the practitioner must proceed with slow and deliberate movement in a kind and gentle manner. However, this does not guarantee cooperation from a frightened and ill child.

The narrow airway of the child makes even a small obstruction significant, leading to a marked increase in respiratory effort. Obvious clinical signs of impaired respiratory function are tachypnea, nasal flaring, retractions, cyanosis, and a change in mental state, including a reduced level of consciousness or increased agitation. As a rule, tachypnea and nasal flaring alone suggest a less severe, but earlier sign of obstruction than the presence of deep retractions. However, if obstruction is severe with prolonged respiratory distress, the child may be exhausted and only able to exhibit nasal flaring. In infants the exhaustion of respiratory muscle leads to decreased dynamic compliance and ineffective respiration, since they have a relatively soft rib cage leading to increased chest wall compliance. The child's mental state may range from fearful and agitated to lethargic or even unconscious. A child with mild hypoxia tends to have increased levels of agitation, whereas the child with increasing hypoxemia and hypercarbia becomes more lethargic.

Auscultation of the child's upper airway (over the trachea) and the lower airway (over the thorax) is vital to determine the extent of air movement and obstruction.

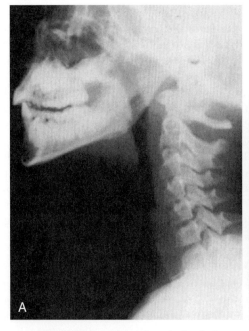
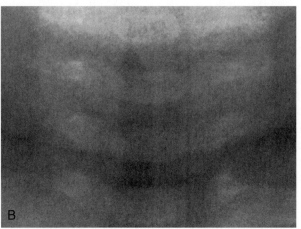

FIGURE 32-2 Normal cervical soft tissue radiographs. **A,** Lateral view shows a thin epiglottis. **B,** Anteroposterior view illustrates the "shoulders" appearance of the subglottic trachea.

Some sounds, such as stridor, may be so prominent that they are audible from outside the patient's room! Stridor is a coarse, vibrating noise generated by airway soft tissue that typically occurs in the presence of narrowed or obstructed upper airway (extra thoracic). Extrathoracic obstruction of the trachea causes stridor during inspiration. The deeply negative intrathoracic pressure causes the pressure inside the trachea to fall and allows the higher atmospheric pressure (outside the trachea) to collapse the trachea or larynx. This results in the 'crowing' sound of stridor. During exhalation, the positive intraairway pressure forces the airway open and eliminates the stridor (Figure 32-3). When airway narrowing is intrathoracic, stridor is present during a forced exhalation. The positive intrathoracic pressure that occurs with exhalation causes the circumferential tracheal cartilage, and hence the trachea, to collapse. During inspiration, stridor from an intrathoracic airway obstruction is minimized by the radially outward tracheal traction caused by negative intrathoracic pressures.

Auscultation of air movement during inspiration and expiration aids in determining the severity and location of the obstruction. The pitch of the stridor can be used to assess improvement or worsening of the obstruction. Low-pitched sounds signify mild obstruction, whereas a higher pitch indicates that the child is in more distress and is attempting to generate a higher air flow rate. Sounds heard on inspiration but not expiration may indicate a "ball valve" obstruction and an accompanying risk for a pneumothorax. Absence of air movement constitutes a true emergency.

UPPER AIRWAY DISORDERS

Supralaryngeal Obstruction

Common causes of obstruction above the larynx include congenital lesions, acute inflammatory disorders, and disorders related to abnormal supralaryngeal tissue or airway tone or both (e.g., obstructive apnea).

Choanal Atresia

Choanal atresia, the stenosis or absence of the nasal passages (choanae), typically presents in the immediate postnatal period. The infant presents with severe respiratory distress that appears to lessen with crying,

when the infant manages to exchange air through the mouth, and is exacerbated again once the crying stops. Occasionally, the condition is discovered when attempting to nasally suction the infant and a size 5 or 6 catheter cannot be passed through the nares in to the oropharynx for a distance of at least 32 mm. Insertion of an oral airway provides temporary relief of the obstruction but does not preclude early surgical intervention.

Pierre Robin Syndrome

Other congenital anomalies that present similarly include masses that obstruct the nasopharynx, such as encephaloceles (an outpouching of the brain into the airway) and dermoid cysts. Infants with Pierre Robin syndrome have extremely small mandibles and a small oropharynx that causes the tongue to occlude the airway. The respiratory distress is not relieved by crying. Treatment includes temporary insertion of oral or nasal airways, placement of the infant in a prone position, and surgical repair. See Clinical Scenario 1.

CLINICAL SCENARIO 1

You are called to the delivery room for a term infant delivery complicated by maternal fever. The infant is delivered via spontaneous vaginal delivery with the umbilical cord around the neck. The obstetrician performs superficial nose and mouth suctioning with a bulb syringe and untangles the umbilical cord from the newborn's neck. The infant is handed to you and no spontaneous respiration is noted under the warmer. You dry the infant and provide stimulation. The infant cries and turns pink. After a few seconds the infant calms down and exhibits respiratory distress relieved by crying.

- What is your differential diagnosis and how do you assess the infant?

Deep Neck Infections

Deep neck infections are feared complications of upper respiratory and upper gastrointestinal tract infections. Aerobic and anaerobic pathogens are the common cause. They can become rapidly severe, causing airway obstruction, aspiration, and rapidly spread to adjoining anatomical structures (such as the mediastinum).

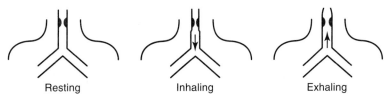

Resting   Inhaling   Exhaling

FIGURE 32-3 Obstruction of the upper (extrathoracic) airway. Dynamic motion during the respiratory cycle causes accentuated narrowing during inspiration, resulting in stridor.

Antibiotic treatment, airway protection, and surgical intervention are necessary. Peritonsillar and retropharyngeal abscesses are very common examples of these infections and need to be differentiated from simple tonsillar enlargement.

Tonsillar Enlargement

The child with an acute illness characterized by fever and sore throat may develop swelling of the oropharyngeal tissues. Inflammation and swelling can progress to airway obstruction. Tonsillitis, or *streptococcal pharyngitis,* presents as exudative pharyngitis and cervical adenopathy. However, the presence of a cough and nasal congestion increases the likelihood that the infection is viral. A throat culture or rapid streptococcal antigen test is obtained to identify the causative organism. Therapy is routinely restricted to antibiotics unless the swelling is severe.

Peritonsillar Abscess

This abscess commonly forms unilaterally around the tonsillar tissue. It causes unilateral swelling and protrusion of the affected tonsil into the oropharynx with classical deviation of the uvula to the unaffected side. Patients commonly complain about trismus (difficulty opening their mouth), sore throat, torticollis, and muffled or hoarse voice. The diagnosis is made clinically and by culture, if in doubt a frontal anteroposterior and lateral views of the head and neck can aid in the diagnosis. The most likely organism would be *Streptococcus pyogenes* (group A streptococcus) or *Staphylococcus aureus.*

Retropharyngeal Abscess

Retropharyngeal abscess commonly occurs in children younger than 3 years of age and can cause obstruction from forward displacement of the posterior pharyngeal wall. Infectious agents involved are group A *Streptococcus, Staphylococcus aureus,* and, occasionally, anaerobic bacteria. The child often presents with a sore throat, fever, dysphagia, and voice changes. The voice sounds as if the child is attempting to speak without moving the tongue while maximally expanding the oropharyngeal airway. This is described as "hot potato voice." A lateral neck radiograph is obtained to determine the tissue thickness surrounding the abscess. Visualization of the posterior pharynx may reveal a displaced retropharynx. Surgical drainage is the preferred treatment, along with administration of appropriate antibiotics based on culture results of the aspirated material.

Obstructive Apnea

Children with a chronic history of noisy snoring and air flow loss, in spite of active chest wall movement, are likely suffering from obstructive apnea. Abnormally large adenoids or tonsils with or without abnormal positioning of the airway tissues are likely causes of obstruction. During sleep, the airway muscular tone is decreased, resulting in more severe airway obstruction. Typically, the child with a neuromuscular disorder, such as cerebral palsy, enlarged tonsils and adenoids, or morbid obesity, is at risk for developing obstructive apnea. An electrocardiogram is obtained if nocturnal hypoxia with right ventricular hypertrophy is suspected. Sedation is usually avoided because it exacerbates airway obstruction. Surgery may relieve the obstruction in a child who has not 'outgrown' the obstruction. Weight loss is often beneficial in obese children. In the interim, nasal continuous positive airway pressure can noninvasively ameliorate the disorder. See Clinical Scenario 2.

CLINICAL SCENARIO 2

A 14-year-old female presents to the emergency room complaining of sore throat, fever, and dysphagia. She has no prior health issues and no known sick contact. She says she had been well the day before and noticed her symptoms on awakening in the morning. Physical findings include a mild stridor on auscultation over both apical lung fields and over the trachea. Inspection of the retropharynx is complicated by the patient not being able to open her mouth, but you can see the uvula is being displaced to the left. She also has problems rotating her head to the left.
- What is the most likely diagnosis and what would be your next step in diagnosis?
- What is the treatment?

Periglottic Obstruction

Obstruction of the airway at or just below the level of the glottis typically presents as high-pitched stridor. This region is relatively fixed in diameter because the noncompliant cartilage surrounding the glottis does not "balloon open" to allow air passage around the obstruction, as easily occurs in the more pliable tissues of the supralaryngeal airway. As a result, progressive obstruction of the periglottic area quickly leads to significant distress with both inspiratory and expiratory compromise. The most common causes of periglottic obstruction in the pediatric age group are infectious, with epiglottitis and LTB representing important causes of respiratory morbidity for this patient population.

Congenital lesions that present as periglottic obstruction are rare and include laryngeal webs and cysts and subglottic hemangioma. Vocal cord paralysis may be congenital or iatrogenic, caused by birth trauma or inadvertent surgical injury to the recurrent laryngeal nerve. Subglottic stenosis may also be congenital or acquired secondary to local trauma after intubation.

A more common and benign congenital cause of upper airway obstruction is laryngomalacia. In this condition the epiglottis and arytenoid processes are oversized and floppy, causing collapse into the glottis during vigorous breathing. High-pitched stridor is noted during the neonatal period but tends to disappear by the child's first or second birthday.

Epiglottitis

Epiglottitis is a life-threatening infection that affects both children and adults.[1] It results from bacterial invasion of the soft tissues of the larynx, causing inflammation of the supraglottic structures. This leads to sudden, marked swelling of the epiglottis and surrounding tissues and may result in complete airway obstruction and death. Historically, epiglottitis has been a disease of childhood, with little prodrome, and rarely recurs. In contrast, adult symptoms are more nonspecific and often clouded by coexistent diseases.

Incidence and Etiology

The most common organism causing epiglottitis has been *Haemophilus influenzae* type B. Before widespread vaccinations with *H. influenzae* type B vaccine, bacterial epiglottitis was a fairly common pediatric illness, seen most often in children younger than 6 years of age. With the advent of widespread vaccination in 1985, the incidence has decreased by over 95%. Despite the vaccinations and reduced incidence, *H. influenzae* type B still causes 75% of epiglottitis episodes.[2] Although the vaccination program has profoundly reduced the incidence of epiglottitis, multiple isolated cases have occurred in patients with a complete vaccination history.[3] With the initiation of the vaccination program, patients with epiglottitis now tend to be older, with non–*H. influenzae*

type B, principally group A β-hemolytic *Streptococcus,* being the infecting organism. Primary group A β-hemolytic streptococcal epiglottitis can develop as a rare complication of varicella in an otherwise normal host. Noninfectious causes of epiglottitis in children include thermal epiglottitis from aspiration of hot liquid and traumatic epiglottitis from repeated intubation attempts or a blind finger sweep to remove a foreign body from the airway.

Signs and Symptoms

Onset of bacterial epiglottitis is usually abrupt and associated with high fever; severe sore throat; dysphagia with drooling; cough, progressing rapidly over a few hours to stridor; muffled ("hot potato") voice without hoarseness; air hunger; and cyanosis. Suprasternal, substernal, and intercostal retractions, along with nasal flaring, bradypnea, and dyspnea, are frequently displayed. The child assumes a characteristic position of sitting upright with the chin thrust forward and with the neck hyperextended (sniffing position) in a tripod position. The streptococcal variant of epiglottitis may be associated with a longer prodrome lasting more than 24 hours.[4]

Diagnosis

Diagnosis of epiglottitis must be assumed based on the clinical presentation. Table 32-1 lists the clinical characteristics used in the differential diagnoses for epiglottitis and LTB. Because manipulation or agitation of the child with epiglottitis can trigger complete upper airway obstruction, unnecessary diagnostic procedures are avoided (e.g., arterial blood gas analysis, chest radiography) and every attempt made to maintain a nonthreatening atmosphere for the child. Until controlled

---

TABLE 32-1

Differential Diagnosis of Laryngotracheobronchitis and Epiglottitis

	below cords Laryngotracheobronchitis	Epiglottitis *above cord*
Age	3 mo–3 yr	2–6 yr
Cause	Viral (parainfluenza, RSV)	Bacterial (*Haemophilus influenzae,* type B)
History	Gradual onset (2–3 days)	Acute onset (few hours)
	Previous cold symptoms	Complaint of sore throat
Symptoms	Stridor	Stridor
	Barking cough	Minimal cough
	Fever variable	High fever
	Hoarse voice	Muffled voice
	No position preferred	Prefers sitting upright with chin forward
	Retractions	Retractions
	Irritable	Drooling
	Does not appear acutely ill	Anxiety
		Appears acutely ill
Radiographic findings	Subglottic narrowing	Swollen epiglottis (thumb sign)

RSV, Respiratory syncytial virus.

intubation can be achieved (conducted under general anesthesia with a pediatrician, otolaryngologist, and anesthesiologist present), attempts to directly visualize the epiglottis, draw blood, insert intravenous lines, or lay the child flat for an examination are avoided. Instead, allow the child to assume a position of comfort with 'blow-by' oxygen therapy provided if necessary. If the clinical history and physical appearance of the child are only mildly suggestive of epiglottitis, more detailed examination or neck radiographs (Figure 32-4), or both, are helpful in confirming the diagnosis.

Treatment

Establishment of a stable, artificial airway is the first priority in the treatment of epiglottitis. Placement of an endotracheal tube (ETT) under general anesthesia is a safe way to provide a secure, temporary artificial airway. Because there is considerable swelling to the upper airway structures, an ETT one size smaller than the predicted size (based on age) is typically used. Dramatic improvement in respiratory distress is expected after intubation, which bypasses the site of obstruction. Once the ETT is inserted, it must remain in place during the 12 to 48 hours required for the inflamed tissue to shrink in response to therapy.

Treatment of infectious epiglottitis is relatively short, with a 2-day course of ceftriaxone as effective as 5 days of chloramphenicol. This may be adjusted based on patient response and on the results of culture and sensitivity reports from blood and epiglottis swab specimens taken at the time of intubation. Close nursing supervision, constant use of arm restraints, along with continuously infused sedatives may suffice to prevent attempts at self-extubation. Mechanical ventilation may be needed for a short time if heavy sedation is required.

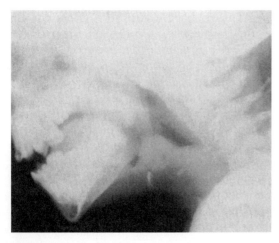

FIGURE 32-4 Epiglottitis. The lateral neck radiograph illustrates the distorted, thumb-shaped epiglottic shadow.

Extubation is usually considered within 24 hours when signs of toxicity (e.g., fever) diminish and when an air leak at 20 cm H_2O pressure develops around the ETT. Traumatic epiglottitis often takes several days longer for complete recovery. The physician may choose to directly visualize the epiglottis (by direct laryngoscopy or bronchoscopy) before attempting extubation to ensure adequate tissue shrinkage has occurred. The child is closely monitored for the return of stridor and other signs of respiratory distress for 12 to 24 hours after extubation.

Laryngotracheobronchitis
Incidence and Etiology

LTB, also known as croup, is the most common cause of airway obstruction in children between 6 months and 6 years of age. Typically, it presents in the fall and winter. Parainfluenza virus 1 is the most common cause, resulting in biennial epidemics in the United States during October through February of odd-numbered years. Other much less common infectious causes include influenza viruses, RSV, herpes simplex virus, and *Mycoplasma pneumoniae*.

The viral infection causes a mucosal edema and exudate formation in the glottic and subglottic areas, involving the airways from the larynx to the bronchus, hence the name laryngotracheobronchitis. The edema develops over several days, and the resultant airway narrowing becomes severe enough to cause various degrees of airway obstruction. Obstruction is more severe during inspiration, owing to the deeply negative airway pressures needed to inspire against the edematous airway. Average hospital admission rate for LTB is more than 40,000 children per year, resulting in an annual cost of $190 million, with approximately 91% of the children younger than 5 years of age.[1]

Signs and Symptoms

The child with LTB presents with a gradual prodrome of low-grade fever, malaise, rhinorrhea, and hoarse voice. Over several days, the illness progresses to inspiratory stridor and a 'barky' cough, often described as sounding like the bark of a seal. Physical examination reveals nasal flaring, nasal congestion, use of accessory muscles, and suprasternal, subcostal, and intercostal retractions that along with the stridor become worse when the child is agitated.

Estimating the severity of the disease can be difficult. The illness usually occurs during cold seasons. Transporting an ill child in moderate distress in an automobile with cold ambient air commonly results in the child being virtually symptom-free on arrival in the emergency department. Inhalation of the cold air reduces the swelling and rapidly reduces the respiratory distress.

TABLE 32-2		
Croup Scoring System		
Indicators of Severity	**Findings**	**Croup Score**
Inspiratory stridor	None	0
	At rest, with stethoscope	1
	At rest, without stethoscope	2
Retractions	None	0
	Mild	1
	Moderate	2
	Severe	3
Air entry	Normal	0
	Decreased	1
	Severely decreased	2
Cyanosis	None	0
	With agitation	4
	At rest	5
Level of consciousness	Normal	0
	Altered mental status	5

From Westley CR, Cotton EK, Brooks JG: Nebulized racemic epinephrine by IPPB for the treatment of croup: a double-blind study, *Am J Dis Child* 1978;132:484.

More recent attempts to quantify LTB severity have centered around the presence of pulsus paradoxus[5] and the Croup Score developed by Westley (Table 32-2).[6]

Diagnosis

A lateral neck radiograph, sometimes obtained to help differentiate the disease from epiglottitis, demonstrates a large retropharyngeal air shadow without epiglottic swelling. The anteroposterior chest radiograph reveals the classic 'steeple sign,' a sharply sloped, wedge-shaped, linear narrowing of the trachea. This demonstrates the subglottic tracheal edema that extends from the larynx to the thoracic trachea (Figure 32-5).

Treatment

Treatment of mild cases of LTB is largely supportive—ensuring temperature control, adequate hydration, and humidification of inspired air. Techniques to cool the airway have traditionally used humidified air with water particles large enough to 'rain out' onto the upper airway and tracheal mucosa. Cool mist tents (croup tents) were designed to provide continuous humidified air to the trachea. Little, if any, proof of effectiveness exists on the use of this form of humidification, although anecdotes about its effectiveness are common.

If increasing respiratory effort, irritability, and inability to engage in play or eating develop, hospitalization may be indicated. Hospital care for the child with LTB is largely symptomatic and centers on careful

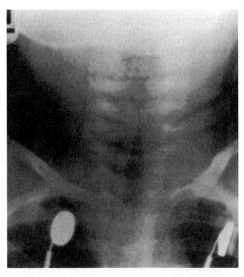

FIGURE 32-5 Laryngotracheobronchitis. The anteroposterior neck radiograph reveals steeply angled subglottic walls ("steeple sign").

monitoring for advancing respiratory compromise. Regular assessment of the respiratory rate, degree of retractions, mental status, and air exchange is essential. Oxygen saturation monitoring is useful, but generally desaturation is a late finding. Children requiring an F_{IO_2} of more than 0.35 are watched closely for evidence of impending respiratory failure.

Nebulized racemic epinephrine is used to induce vasoconstriction of the upper airway. With the use of a 2.2% solution, 0.5 to 1.0 ml of medication is diluted to a 3.0 ml volume with normal saline and given by inhalation with a face mask over a period of approximately 10 minutes. The aerosols are often begun in an emergency department and the child evaluated for their effectiveness. A reduction in airway edema usually occurs within 10 to 20 minutes, with a gradual reduction of its effect over 2 hours. Although the aerosols may be given as frequently as every 30 minutes, the potential side effects from cardiovascular stimulation and the implied severity of respiratory distress should limit such use to an intensive care unit setting. Reports of a 'rebound' effect from persistent use of the racemic epinephrine restricted its use to inpatient settings until recently.[7,8] Today, patients are treated with dexamethasone and racemic epinephrine and discharged from the emergency department to home if they are free of intercostal retractions and stridor after a 2-hour waiting period.[9]

Recommendations for adrenocorticosteroid therapy in patients with LTB have had a long and complicated course. Original proof of effectiveness came with the combined analysis of many studies (metaanalyses) that demonstrated effectiveness of a single dose of dexamethasone at 0.6 mg/kg given intramuscularly. More recent studies have compared inhaled corticosteroids to oral systemic corticosteroids, with and without inhaled racemic epinephrine. Administration of oral dexamethasone at 0.6 mg/kg has been recommended as the least expensive and least invasive means by which to lower hospitalization rates.[7,8]

Endotracheal intubation may be necessary if the child becomes exhausted or severe respiratory distress develops. To avoid traumatizing the inflamed subglottic tissue, the ETT should be at least 1 mm smaller in diameter than that estimated for the child's age. As with epiglottitis, dramatic improvement in respiratory distress is expected after intubation. Attempts at extubation can be made if an air leak develops around the ETT at pressures under 20 to 30 cm H_2O. The child is closely monitored in the 4 to 12 hours after extubation for the return of stridor.

Traumatic and Postoperative Laryngotracheobronchitis

Airway obstruction may occur as a sequela of endotracheal intubation. Even the most carefully placed ETT can result in significant injury to the tracheal lining. The cilia in the trachea are easily damaged, especially with aggressive suctioning procedures. Excessively large endotracheal tubes lead to necrosis of the tracheal mucosa. An ETT leak of 20 to 25 cm H_2O is recommended to minimize the pressure the ETT applies against the surface of the trachea near the cricoid ring. The value of this leak has been called into question in studies in which the presence of an ETT leak was found to be less predictive of postextubation LTB than the duration of intubation.[10]

Historically, noncuffed endotracheal tubes have been used in children younger than 8 years of age. This practice began several decades ago when low-volume, high-pressure endotracheal tubes used during anesthesia became overdistended when nitrous oxide diffused into the ETT cuff, resulting in pressure-related injury to the trachea. The safety of cuffed endotracheal tubes has since been reevaluated in several studies.

In one study when this was done, 99% of the patients had a minimal leak with no increase in the incidence of postextubation LTB when compared with patients using a noncuffed ETT.[11]

Direct airway injury from suctioning induces scar tissue and granuloma development that will result in varying degrees of airway obstruction. Granulomas have developed even after very brief periods of endotracheal intubation in infants.[12]

Children who exhibit postextubation stridor are treated with racemic epinephrine per inhalation, using the same dosage of medication as when treating LTB. Dexamethasone is also given at 0.5 mg/kg intravenously (maximum dose 10 mg), repeated every 6 hours for two doses. See Clinical Scenario 3.

CLINICAL SCENARIO 3

A 2-year-old girl arrives in the emergency room intubated with a 4.0 ETT by EMS. The mother states the toddler had been ill for several days with a runny nose, fever, and a cough. The night before the mother had noted that the girl was breathing 'funny' and had a barking cough. This morning she refused her bottle, had increased difficulty breathing, and was very irritable. She has had multiple episodes of vomiting with coughing, but no diarrhea. After consulting her pediatrician by phone, she had been advised to call an ambulance and have the child transported to the hospital. EMS reports to have found the toddler in respiratory distress and altered mental state. Marked stridor was audible and the O_2 saturation was measured at 58%. The infant was sedated and paralyzed; the intubation with the 4.0 ETT was extremely difficult and required multiple attempts.
- What is your differential diagnosis?
- What treatment should you recommend?
- What complications should you expect?

LOWER AIRWAY DISORDERS

Bacterial Tracheitis

Bacterial tracheitis is a medical emergency that can result in complete airway obstruction and death. Patients typically have an antecedent upper respiratory infection or LTB-like symptoms for several days before presentation with severe airway obstruction. Although the slow progression of the disease closely resembles LTB, the fever, toxic appearance, and elevated white blood cell count with an increased percentage of premature white cell forms (bands) all suggest the likelihood of a bacterial disease. Neck and chest radiographs reveal narrowing of a subglottic airway with irregular mucosal surface, without evidence of epiglottic swelling.[1]

Bacterial tracheitis responds poorly to racemic epinephrine and typically requires the placement of an artificial airway to manage the copious tracheal secretions. Treatment includes antibiotics to cover for S. aureus, H. influenzae, and S. pneumoniae. The disease resolves more slowly than epiglottitis, requiring nearly a week before extubation is attempted.

Obstruction of the Trachea and Major Bronchi

Tracheal narrowing produces either expiratory or biphasic (inspiratory and expiratory) wheezing. The degree and flexibility of the airway narrowing will determine the severity of the wheeze. Because the trachea serves as the final conduit for the removal of secretions, lesions in this area may result in pooling of mucus with rhonchi audible during auscultation. The abnormalities are heard radiating throughout the chest but are best appreciated over the sternal area. It is often difficult to discern where the wheezes or rhonchi originate in a small child. Wheezes or rhonchi that remain equal in pitch across all regions of the chest but are heard loudest around the sternum most likely have originated in the trachea. Larger bronchial lesions produce similar manifestations but are more localized to the side of the lesion.

Tracheomalacia

Tracheomalacia is a condition of dynamic tracheal collapse caused by abnormal shape and flexibility of the tracheal cartilage rings. The abnormality can affect either a small section or the entire length of the trachea. Although often idiopathic in origin, there may be identifiable extrinsic causes that have led to tracheal wall softening. Common injurious events include neonatal ventilation with high pressures, chronic trauma to the trachea from a malpositioned ETT or aggressive endotracheal suctioning, and external compressive structures, such as a vascular ring.

In most cases of tracheomalacia the infant or child presents with chronic wheezing that becomes more severe with vigorous breathing. Fortunately, the abnormality tends to improve with time as the child's airway grows, and little intervention is necessary. Severe tracheomalacia may result in complete obstruction and profound episodic hypoxemia, especially during forced exhalation. Repeated airway collapse during exhalation leads to increasingly severe lung hyperinflation. Because exhalation is impaired by airway collapse, once the lung is completely inflated air movement is no longer possible. This scenario is most often seen in older infants with a history of prolonged positive-pressure ventilation and severe bronchopulmonary dysplasia (BPD). During severe agitation, these infants become cyanotic and even bradycardic, with little or no air movement in spite of increased respiratory effort.

Treatment options are few, mostly unsatisfactory, and include prolonged continuous positive airway pressure or ventilatory support with a tracheostomy tube in place to distend or 'splint open' the airways. For milder cases, chronic sedation may avoid the episodic agitation that leads to the airway obstruction.

Congenital Tracheal or Bronchial Stenosis

Like tracheomalacia, congenital tracheal or bronchial stenosis may involve extensive or short lengths of the involved airway. The severity of symptoms depends on the degree and length of the stenosis. A common cause of stenosis in the newborn is the formation of a vascular ring. This occurs in infants with congenital malformation of the great vessels of the heart, usually a double aortic arch. With this malformation, the aorta wraps around both the esophagus and trachea. Infants can present with feeding difficulties and uncontrollable wheezing. Surgical correction of the defect can reduce symptoms, although the residual presence of focal tracheomalacia may cause respiratory symptoms to persist postoperatively.

Tracheal stenosis results from complied or nearly complied rings of cartilage. They present as segmental stenosis anywhere in the tracheobronchial tree or as generalized stenosis/hypoplasia. Funnel-shaped lesions are associated with pulmonary artery sling. This is a very rare anomaly and outcome has recently been improved through new surgical techniques.

Intraluminal Obstruction

An acquired cause of airway narrowing is the development of intraluminal obstruction. In the child, foreign body obstruction is encountered more frequently than the adult problem of endobronchial tumor. Infectious agents (e.g., *Mycobacterium tuberculosis*) or a neoplasm, classically Hodgkin's lymphoma, may cause lymphadenopathy that compresses the airway. The other differential diagnosis to consider is cardiomegaly in patients with congenital heart defects, which especially can compress the left main bronchus due to its anatomical relation to the heart. The diffuse, chronic wheeze associated with these disorders is often confused with asthma. Endobronchial compression is suspected in an infant or child with persistent wheezing that does not respond to bronchodilator therapy. Diagnostic studies to differentiate the cause of wheezing in these patients include barium swallow (for evidence of a vascular ring), bronchoscopy, and computerized tomography of the chest. Treatment of intrinsic tracheal and major airway obstruction is frequently surgical and is directed at widening the narrowed area. Additionally, treatment of the primary cause for the lymphadenopathy, such as Hodgkin's lymphoma, is critical.

Foreign Body Aspiration
Incidence

A leading cause of accidental death in the toddler is foreign body aspiration. The degree of respiratory sequelae depends on the nature of the material aspirated, whereas the severity of neurologic sequelae depends on the duration of ventilatory compromise. Mobile infants and toddlers are at particularly high risk by virtue of their tendency to place objects in their mouths. Inappropriate toys for a child's age may have loose parts, whereas certain foods (e.g., nuts, Vienna sausages, hot dogs) are just the right size to become lodged in a child's airway. The preferred location for small enough objects is the right middle lobe bronchi, which has the most direct and straight connection to the trachea. If the child is neurologically intact, these aspirations commonly occur if the child is straddled or falls while harboring such objects in or near the mouth.

Signs and Symptoms

Signs and symptoms of foreign body aspiration vary with the location of impaction and the degree of airway obstruction. They can range from unilateral wheezing or recurrent pneumonia, as when peanuts or popcorn obstruct the smaller airways, to immediate occlusion of the upper airway with complete absence of air movement and rapid death from suffocation, as seen in hot dog or balloon aspiration fatalities. It is not necessary for the foreign body to be in the trachea: a big enough object stuck in the esophagus can elicit very similar symptoms of respiratory distress.

Diagnosis

The cause of the obstruction and adequacy of ventilation should be quickly determined. A thorough history of the circumstances surrounding the onset of symptoms helps determine whether this is a foreign body aspiration or an infectious process. However, a complete history is frequently difficult to obtain. Examiners must determine, first and foremost, the adequacy of ventilation, followed by the location of the obstruction. Children with sudden onset of wheezing, particularly if wheezing has never occurred before and is unilateral in nature, raise suspicions of foreign body aspiration.

Anteroposterior and lateral neck/chest radiographs are useful if the object is radiopaque. Although the appearance of a radiopaque foreign body on a radiograph is striking, many aspirated materials, such as peanuts and carrots, cannot be detected in this fashion (Figure 32-6). Foreign body aspiration usually occurs at the laryngeal level. Deviation in the airway shape may indicate a foreign body not otherwise visible. Recurrent pneumonia in the same lobe is also suspicious. Asymmetric lung hyperinflation can result from a ball-valve effect of foreign material localized in a major bronchus. This defect is most often apparent on an expiratory film (Figure 32-7).[13] Comparison between an expiratory and inspiratory film can also yield the diagnosis, but depends greatly on the cooperation of the child.

Fiberoptic laryngoscopy or bronchoscopy is helpful in both finding and retrieving the foreign body. Such procedures are best done in an OR setting and with a rigged bronchoscope. Pulse oximetry is used to determine the need for supplemental oxygen. Arterial blood gas analysis is indicated if hypercarbia is suspected in the child with severe obstruction.

Treatment

Therapy employed will vary with the severity of the obstruction. If the child is well oxygenated and ventilated, a controlled therapeutic bronchoscopy or laryngoscopy with appropriate anesthesia is preferred. When foreign body aspiration is suspected and respiratory symptoms are acute, urgent bronchoscopy with removal

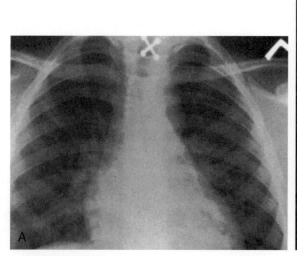
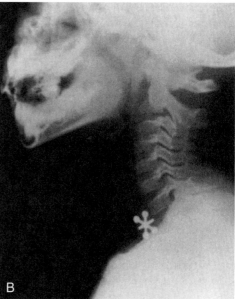

FIGURE 32-6 Foreign body obstruction. Posteroanterior **(A)** and lateral **(B)** chest radiographs reveal an esophageal foreign body that caused respiratory distress from posterior pressure on the trachea.

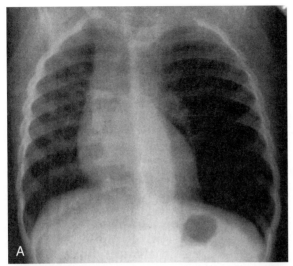

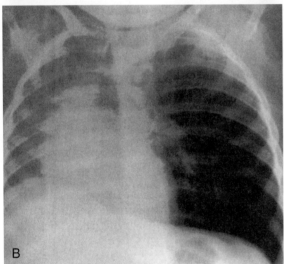

FIGURE 32-7 Foreign body aspiration. Asymmetric lung volumes **(A),** accentuated during exhalation **(B),** indicate an obstructing ball-valve type of lesion in the left bronchus.

of the object is necessary. Even if the child appears to be stable, movement of the object to a more critical area can result in sudden clinical deterioration. The child with complete obstruction may require emergent crico-thyrotomy to establish a patent airway.

Pediatric Advanced Life Support (2005) guidelines state that signs of severe or complete airway obstructions that require intervention are:
- inability to speak or cry audibly
- weak, ineffective cough
- high-pitched sound or no sound during inhalation
- increased difficulty breathing with distress
- cyanosis
- universal chocking sign (thumb and index finger clutching neck)

No interventions should be taken if the child can cough forcefully or speak. In this case one should stay with the child monitoring the situation and providing emotional support. The intervention described below addresses the classical, everyday foreign body obstruction scenario. In a hospital setting the situation may be different and more likely related to a causes or complications of medical treatment. In those cases trouble-shooting equipment and suctioning of the airway should be the first line of action.

Once the obstruction is relieved, some children will be discharged as soon as they recover from anesthesia. In others, resolution of symptoms may be delayed. Airway edema may develop and require corticosteroid therapy along with careful monitoring to ensure that a progressive obstruction does not ensue. Reactive granulation tissue at the site of impaction along with postobstructive infection may take some time to resolve. A second bronchoscopy may be required because of reaccumulation of secretions.

If intubation and mechanical ventilation is indicated, the ventilation strategies often include synchronized intermittent mandatory ventilation (SIMV), pressure support, or volume support. Remembering that these children usually have normal lung function, the Fio_2 and minute ventilation requirements are low and are set to obtain normal arterial blood gas values. Once patency of the airway is ensured, mechanical ventilation is weaned. Secondary infection and prolonged intubation are occasional complications.

Atelectasis
Etiology and Pathophysiology

Atelectasis is collapsed lung parenchyma and is best compared to a wet sponge that fails to reinflate after being compressed. Many processes can cause atelectasis. Internal or parenchymal disorders that are characterized by an inadequate tidal volume, loss of lung compliance (e.g., acute respiratory distress syndrome), airway obstruction (e.g., mucus plugging), and increased elastance of lung tissue can all result in atelectasis. External forces also lead to compression of lung parenchyma, with the reduction in lung volume resulting in atelectasis. These include chest wall disorders (e.g., kyphosis, flail chest), accumulation of pleural fluid, obesity, and abdominal ascites.

The right middle lobe, which has the poorest collateral air circulation and smallest bronchial opening of the major lung segments, is particularly prone to mucus plugging and collapse. Intubated patients, particularly young infants, have a propensity toward right upper lobe collapse. This is most likely related to their supine positioning and tendency toward obstruction of the right upper lobe bronchus (the most proximal of all the lobar bronchi) by a migrating ETT. Postoperative patients are at particular risk of atelectasis because of an ineffective cough, impaired mucus transport, and the effect of anesthesia. Surfactant deficiency may occur in the child after smoke inhalation or lung contusion, resulting in various degrees of lung collapse. Tracheobronchial suctioning has also been related to atelectasis in children and is believed to result from the negative pressure that the airway is exposed to during the suctioning process.

Signs and Symptoms

Clinical presentation will vary with the cause and severity of the lung volume loss. Clinical history may reveal slow regression of activity and deterioration of pulmonary function, as may be seen with a slowly growing pleural tumor. Conversely, the patient may experience rapid-onset dyspnea and cyanosis from a foreign body aspiration that occludes a large bronchus, leading to airway collapse.

Patients with enough atelectasis to create a severe ventilation/perfusion $\dot{V}/\dot{Q}$ mismatch exhibit clinical symptoms of cyanosis, tachypnea, nasal flaring, retractions, and grunting. The patient may complain of chest pain on deep inspiration if the pleura is inflamed or there is accompanying pneumothorax.[14]

Arterial blood gas analysis reveals low oxygen saturations, manifesting low $\dot{V}/\dot{Q}$ ratios. The $Paco_2$ levels often remain normal in the presence of atelectasis, owing to the rapid diffusion characteristics of CO_2 and close regulation of the $Paco_2$ by an altering respiratory rate.

Diagnosis

Although atelectasis is most often found on a chest radiograph, it may first be suspected during a physical examination. Decreased breath sounds, increased tactile fremitus, tracheal deviation, and an elevated diaphragm may indicate atelectasis; however, many patients with atelectasis are asymptomatic on physical examination. Diagnosis is confirmed with evidence of volume loss on a chest radiograph (Figure 32-8).

Treatment

Treatment of atelectasis is aimed at removing the cause and depends on the individual patient's clinical course. Drainage of pleural fluid or removal of external compressors will allow the lung to reexpand. If the cause is airway obstruction, bronchoscopy or good pulmonary hygiene, including aerosolized bronchodilators and chest physiotherapy, will facilitate returned airway patency. In the intubated patient, the use of continuous distending pressure may reverse and prevent further lung collapse.[15] Early mobilization and position changes in postoperative patients, along with encouragement in coughing and deep breathing (e.g., incentive spirometry), are techniques used to prevent and often treat atelectasis.

Bronchiectasis
Etiology and Pathophysiology

Bronchiectasis is defined as irreversible dilation of the bronchial tree. Typically, the segmental and subsegmental bronchi become irregularly shaped and dilated,

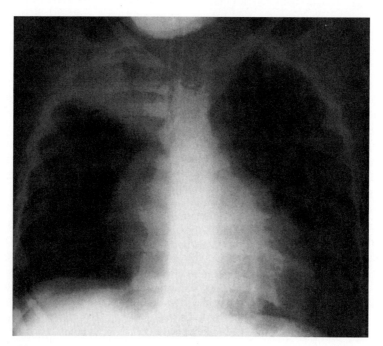

FIGURE 32-8 Anteroposterior chest radiograph with right upper lobe atelectasis.

leading to a loss of the typical funnel configuration that allows smooth central flow of secretions. Additionally, ciliary activity in the area of the dilation is inadequate and further contributes to the difficulty in mobilizing secretions. The secretions become infected as they pool. The lower lobes, particularly the left lower lobe, are most frequently involved.

A small number of patients may have congenital bronchiectasis in which there is a defect in the development of bronchial cartilage or there is developmental failure of the elastic and muscular tissues of the trachea and main bronchi. Most patients 'acquire' the disease, and bronchiectasis develops as a result of airway obstruction or chronic infection. Causes include bronchial obstruction (e.g., foreign body aspiration, mediastinal mass), infections (e.g., measles, pertussis, pneumonia), Kartagener syndrome, and cystic fibrosis (CF).

Signs and Symptoms

Bronchiectasis may occur acutely after an infection or have a more insidious onset in patients suffering from chronic pulmonary diseases such as CF or reflux and aspiration. Patients experience chronic cough, often productive of copious amounts of thick purulent sputum that has a three-layered appearance if left standing for some time, and only occasional hemoptysis. Pulmonary infections are common, with recurrent fever and foul-smelling breath or sputum. Dyspnea on exertion and clubbing of the digits may manifest in some cases. The lower lobes, particularly the left lower lobe, are most frequently involved.

Diagnosis

Bronchiectasis may be suspected on the basis of the clinical history and physical examination. Plain chest radiographs are seldom normal but alone are not definitive in diagnosing the disease. The abnormal pattern of bronchiectasis is seen most strikingly during bronchography.[16] However, this is rarely performed today. Instead, computed tomographic scanning is used to confirm the diagnosis (Figure 32-9). Pulmonary function may be abnormal, with spirometry demonstrating an obstructive pattern. A combined obstructive and restrictive disease pattern may be present in the more severe cases.[17]

Treatment

Medical management depends on the severity of the disease. Chest physiotherapy, including postural drainage and percussion, along with adequate hydration is performed to improve the mobilization of pulmonary secretions. Newer concepts favor the idea that low mucus salinity rather than underhydration contributes to mucus retention. This may explain the success and increased use of nebulized hypertonic saline in these patients.

Antibiotic therapy is given orally, by nebulization (i.e., tobramycin), or by the intravenous route. The choice of antibiotic is based on the results of the individual patient's sputum culture results. Blind use of broad-spectrum antibiotics in this chronic disease may lead to more resistant colonization.[18] The improved empiric use of intravenous antibiotic and new mucous clearing medications and treatments in CF patients has improved the outcome in this particular disease.

In those cases in which the child suffers severe illness (i.e., failure to thrive, severe hemoptysis) in spite of antibiotic therapy and chest physiotherapy, surgical resection of the bronchiectatic section of lung may be considered. Patients with the disease localized to only one or two lobes are considered better candidates for surgical intervention.[19,20] See Clinical Scenario 4.

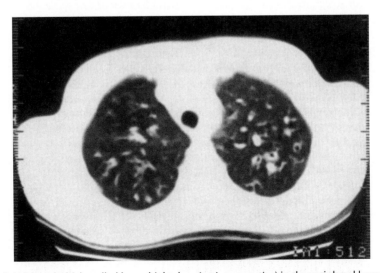

FIGURE 32-9 Widened, thick-walled bronchial tubes (*cut in cross section*) in the peripheral lung zones.

A 3½-year-old male is admitted to the ICU after heart surgery. He was on cardiopulmonary bypass for 190 minutes and the operation went well. In the ICU he is sedated and ventilated. A chest x-ray and cultures are obtained on day one post-op for fever. The chest x-ray shows consolidation of the left lower lobe and it remains the same over the next days. All cultures are negative and he is successfully extubated on post-op day 4. The chest x-rays remain unchanged and the decision for bronchoscopy is made. Before the bronchoscopy the plan is to reintubate the child. He is paralyzed and his baseline O_2 saturation remains at 75% to 79% under bag-mask ventilation. An ETT is placed under good visualization of the vocal cords, but his O_2 saturations fall to 60% to 65% with minimal chest rise and increased resistance to bagging. He is extubated and it is not possible to bag-mask ventilate him. His O_2 saturations continue to drop and after a second intubation attempt with good visualization of the vocal cords he goes in to cardiac arrest.

- What is your differential diagnosis?
- What are your actions?

Acute Bronchiolitis
Etiology and Pathophysiology

The term *acute bronchiolitis* is applied to a condition in infants in which a viral respiratory tract infection results in clinical symptoms of small airway obstruction.[21,22] In the majority of infants with bronchiolitis, the causative organism is respiratory syncytial virus (RSV).[23]

RSV is a highly contagious virus and has its greatest impact on young infants. Infants younger than 6 months of age are at particular risk of severe infection, with the peak incidence for hospitalization occurring between 2 and 6 months of age.[24] Although most cases are mild and do not require hospital admission, epidemics of the infection occurring between December and March result in nearly 100,000 hospitalizations in the United States each year.[25] Postmortem evaluation of infants with severe bronchiolitis reveals obstructed airway lumina from impacted cellular debris. In vitro studies suggest that an intense inflammatory response occurs in the infant's airways and may contribute to increased mucus secretion and transudation of fluid into the airways and airway walls.[26]

Incidence

Acute bronchiolitis is seen most often in infants who are younger than 1 year of age, were born prematurely, live in a crowded environment, attend day care facilities, and are exposed to passive smoke.[24] Bronchiolitis with RSV infection is particularly devastating to infants with certain at-risk conditions, including premature birth, chronic lung disease (e.g., BPD, CF), congenital heart disease (especially those with pulmonary hypertension), and immunodeficiencies.[27] These infants are at risk of respiratory failure and death.

Signs and Symptoms

Physical findings vary considerably with the patient's age. Infants (younger than 1 year of age) develop coryza, cough, respiratory distress, wheezing, and tachypnea. The symptoms of infection usually peak around 48 to 72 hours and a previously healthy infant can progress from what was thought to be a simple cold to severe respiratory distress during that time. In contrast, the principal symptoms in children older than 2 years of age are profound nasal congestion and productive cough. Chest auscultation reveals diffuse, coarse, 'sticky' rales (Velcro rales), which may be accompanied by wheezes. A chest radiograph typically reveals intense lung hyperinflation with flattened hemidiaphragms (obstructive), with occasional films showing evidence of collapse or consolidation (Figure 32-10).

Severe, life-threatening apnea is a common symptom in the very young infant with bronchiolitis, especially in those with cardiorespiratory disease or a history of premature birth or apnea. An infant may also be agitated and have difficulty feeding as a consequence of hypoxia. This may lead to dehydration as well as respiratory failure. Development of cyanosis usually heralds impending respiratory failure. Arterial P_{CO_2} rising above 45 mm Hg despite tachypnea indicates impending respiratory failure and respiratory support needs to be prepared, including intubation.

Diagnosis

Clinical diagnosis of acute viral bronchiolitis is confirmed by identifying the RSV or other respiratory virus. Nasopharyngeal aspirate or nasal lavage provides samples of the virus. Diagnosis is based on the clinical presentation and the results of viral culture and antigen detection assays (i.e., enzyme-linked immunosorbent assays).[28]

Treatment

Treatment of bronchiolitis is largely supportive, along with careful monitoring. The infection is self-limiting in many patients, and hospitalization is not necessary if symptoms are mild. The infant is monitored for apnea, hypoxia, and dehydration. Care is taken to provide adequate feedings and prevent further respiratory distress.

The decision to hospitalize a child with bronchiolitis involves a multifactorial assessment of the risk factors, clinical symptoms, age, and familial resources. Supportive care with supplemental oxygen, intravenous hydration

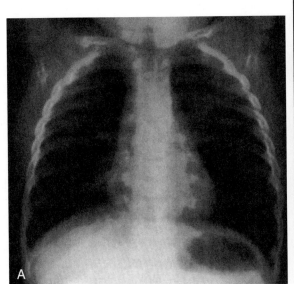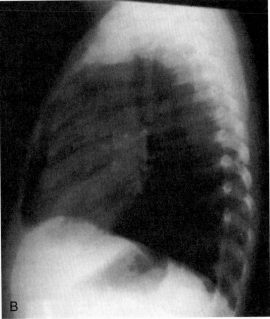

FIGURE 32-10 Severe bronchiolitis. Posterior (A) and lateral (B) chest radiographs reveal flattening of the diaphragm and widening of the anteroposterior diameter, which is indicative of severe air trapping. Perihilar markings are accentuated.

if needed, and close clinical monitoring is essential. In most cases, low flow oxygen therapy (hood or nasal cannula) is sufficient to reduce the hypoxia and respiratory distress. Patients with recurrent apnea or respiratory failure may need intubation and mechanical ventilation. Continuous monitoring with pulse oximetry is essential, as well as arterial blood gas analysis for those patients in whom respiratory failure is suspected. Mild yet persistent hypoxia (Spo$_2$88% to 92%) despite oxygen therapy can be an ominous sign of impending respiratory failure as the patient could be moving from the obstructive (improved functional residual capacity) to the restrictive (atelectasis) phase of disease. In practice it is very important to ensure patent nares, especially if nasal canula is used, since RSV typically generates copious amounts of nasal secretions. This is best achieved by frequent and efficient suction of the nares.

Infants with tachypnea, agitation, and cough are at risk of dehydration. In many moderate to severe cases they stop eating as they cannot correlate the sequence of suck, swallow, and breathe at high respiratory rates. This is a frequent concern in those patients who experience vomiting with the cough. Intravenous fluids or frequent small-volume feedings are both routes to consider when fluid intake is poor.

Although the role of bronchodilators in the management of bronchiolitis is controversial, there is some evidence that they are effective. In some studies, albuterol brought significant short-term improvement in clinical scores but was not found to reduce admission rates or

decrease the length of hospitalization.[29] Ipratropium bromide and theophylline have not proven to be beneficial as bronchodilators in the treatment of bronchiolitis.[30,31] Despite the evidence of airway inflammation, use of systemic or inhaled corticosteroids early in the symptomatic phase of the disease does not tend to improve outcome.[32] However, inhaled corticosteroids are sometimes given to reduce short-term morbidity when there is delayed recovery. It is questionable if these interventions are successful in infants and children with a tendency to have recurrent wheezing or asthma in the future or if the children with treatment success have some other unknown underlying respiratory physiology and/or chemistry variety.

Ribavirin, a broad-spectrum virustatic agent, continues to play a contentious role in the treatment of bronchiolitis. It is administered as an aerosol and delivered to the patient, through either an oxygen hood or a ventilator circuit, for 12 to 18 hours per day. Although early studies proclaimed its benefits, concerns remain about its safety, cost, and efficacy. Reported side effects are uncommon; however, precautions are taken to minimize exposure to hospital personnel and family.[33] Ribavirin is expensive to use, and there is no convincing evidence that its use aids in reducing morbidity or mortality.[34-36] Studies that have concluded that there is a reduction in the morbidity and mortality rate among high-risk patients have been criticized, with many centers suggesting that the improvement was caused by improved supportive care rather than the antiviral therapy.[37] For those who support the use of ribavirin, the majority consider it most beneficial in treating extremely ill patients, immune compromised, and those requiring mechanical ventilation. Today the role of ribavirin remains controversial and its use varies significantly among clinicians.

If the patient requires mechanical ventilation, surfactant replacement therapy may be a consideration. Multicenter trials with animal and synthetic surfactants are being conducted to test this hypothesis. Currently this is an off label indication and is reserved for the most severe patients.

RSV spreads rapidly and is transmitted through touch, with the virus able to survive on hands and other surfaces (e.g., bed rails, toys). RSV prevention is accomplished by strict avoidance of other infected children and careful attention to hand washing. Disease prevention in high-risk patients (e.g., those with BPD or premature birth) can best be accomplished by passive immunization with immune serum globulin (RSV-IGIV). This passive immunity decreases the incidence of RSV hospitalization by 40% to 65% and decreases the number of hospital days by 50% to 60%.[29,38] Strict avoidance of air pollutants, especially cigarette smoke, assists in the long-term recovery from bronchiolitis.

Prognosis

The mortality rate of infants in high-risk groups is much improved over the past several years. Recurrence of bronchiolitis episodes is seen in some patients; however, subsequent infections are usually much less severe. Studies have indicated that many patients have recurrent cough and wheezing several years after RSV infection. An increase in bronchial responsiveness is often found later in childhood.[23]

Primary Ciliary Dyskinesia
Etiology and Pathophysiology

Normal cilia beat in a coordinated fashion, effectively propelling overlying mucus in one direction out of the airway. The upper and lower respiratory tract is cleared of secretions, inhaled particles, and bacteria. Without the forward thrust of the cilia and coordinated ciliary beating, mucus transport is slowed and there is an accumulation of particles, secretions, and bacteria in the dependent portions of the lungs.

In 1933, Kartagener described a unique clinical triad of situs inversus, chronic sinusitis, and bronchiectasis. This became known as Kartagener syndrome. Subsequent studies found that these patients had defects in the ultrastructure of the cilia that line the mucous membranes of the sinus cavities, lungs, and nose. The syndrome was initially called immotile cilia syndrome. However, further studies have demonstrated that the cilia in patients with this syndrome are not always immotile but often have uncoordinated or ineffective cilia motility.[39] The term *primary ciliary dyskinesia* (PCD) is used increasingly today.

Signs and Symptoms

Chronic cough, often productive, is the most common presenting feature of PCD. It is most apparent early in the morning and with sleep and exercise. Although the mucopurulent sputum initially clears with antibiotic therapy, with age the patient develops increasingly severe airway obstruction. Physical findings include persistent crackles, although wheezing is relatively uncommon. A chest radiograph may reveal lung hyperinflation and changes consistent with bronchiectasis.

Upper respiratory tract infections are common. Persistent nasal congestion, a common presenting feature, may progress to chronic nasal drainage with radiographic evidence of sinusitis. Chronic otitis media, with or without chronic effusions, frequently occurs and requires prolonged use of transtympanic ventilation tubes.[39]

A right-to-left reversal of the position of the heart and intestinal structures, known as situs inversus, is seen in approximately 50% of the patients with PCD. Isolated dextrocardia may also be found. The accepted explanation for the association of situs inversus with the ciliary defect is that normal rotation of chest and abdominal organs depends on properly functioning embryonic cilia during closure of the thoracic and abdominal cavities. Because similar functional defects are found in both mucosal cilia and sperm flagella, the abnormal cilia motility affects male fertility and males are nearly always sterile.

Diagnosis

Diagnosis can be made rapidly by microscopic evaluation for ciliary motility in specimens taken from paranasal sinuses, nose, or tracheal mucosa. Light and electron microscopy of bronchial mucosal cells reveal abnormal cilia numbers with abnormal ciliary structures. Patients with PCD have defects in the dynein arms, radial spokes, and nexin links. Cilia with an inadequate number of out-dynein arms may be immotile or may have some disorganized rigid movement.[40] Absence of radial spokes and alteration in the figuration of the microtubules in the cilia are other ciliary ultrastructural changes.[41]

Treatment

Treatment of PCD focuses on reducing the volume of pooled respiratory secretions in the lung. Chest physiotherapy for airway clearance is essential and is used with exercise and aerosolized β_2-agonists. Children with PCD have evidence of obstructive pulmonary disease. The obstruction is best minimized by exercise before physiotherapy, instead of relying on β_2-agonist therapy.[42] Because cough is one of the few mechanisms available for removing secretions, antitussive therapy is contraindicated.

Nebulized recombinant human DNase (Pulmozyme) is indicated for treatment of cystic fibrosis. It reduces sputum viscosity, improves pulmonary function, and results in a small reduction in acute respiratory exacerbations. It has been found to be beneficial in the treatment of PCD. Aerosolized or intravenous antibiotics directed by bacterial antibiotic sensitivities, in combination with CPT and Pulmozyme therapy, are believed to reduce the progression of obstructive pulmonary disease. Although rarely necessary, surgical excision of the pulmonary segments is considered when suppurative disease is poorly controlled and localized to a single area.

PNEUMONIA

Lower respiratory tract infections are a leading cause of morbidity and mortality in the pediatric population. They most often affect children younger than 2 years of age. These children typically experience the greatest number of complications. At the University of North Carolina at Chapel Hill, Denny and Clyde monitored the number of patients treated for pneumonia in their outpatient clinic.[43] Their results trace the incidence and cause of pneumonia in specific age groups (Figure 32-11).

Gram-positive cocci, particularly group B *Streptococcus* and *S. aureus,* along with gram-negative enteric bacilli, are the source of most neonatal pneumonias. Children between 1 month and 5 years of age are the most frequent victims of viral pneumonia. RSV and parainfluenza viruses types 1, 2, and 3, along with adenovirus, are the most common infectious viral agents. However,

Chlamydia pneumoniae, H. influenzae, S. pneumoniae, and *S. aureus* are occasional bacterial agents in this age group. *S. pneumoniae* is the major cause of bacterial pneumonia in children older than 5 years, whereas *M. pneumoniae* and *C. pneumoniae* are more common in school-age children and young adults. Box 32-1 lists the infectious causes of pneumonia in the pediatric population.

Viral Pneumonia
Respiratory Syncytial Virus

Nearly 80% of all pneumonias in the pediatric population have a viral etiology, with RSV occurring most often. RSV commonly affects children younger than 2 years old, although it has been found in older immunocompromised children or in children with chronic lung disease. Outbreaks occur annually during the

Box 32-1	Infectious Causes of Pneumonia

VIRUSES
- Respiratory syncytial virus
- Parainfluenza types 1, 2, and 3
- Influenza virus
- Adenovirus
- Rhinovirus
- Cytomegalovirus
- Epstein-Barr virus
- Herpes simplex virus

MYCOPLASMA
- Mycoplasma pneumoniae
- Ureaplasma *urealyticum*

BACTERIA
- *Streptococcus pneumoniae*
- *Haemophilus influenzae*
- *Staphylococcus aureus*
- *Streptococcus agalactiae*
- *Legionella pneumophila*
- *Mycobacterium tuberculosis*

PROTOZOA
Pneumocystis *carinii*

FUNGI
- Histoplasma capsulatum
- Coccidioides immitis
- Candida spp.
- Blastomyces dermatitidis
- Cryptococcus *neoformans*

RICKETTSIAE
- *Coxiella* burnetii *(Q fever)*

CHLAMYDIA
- Chlamydia pneumoniae
- Chlamydia trachomatis
- Chlamydia *psittaci*

PARASITES
- *Ascaris* lumbricoides

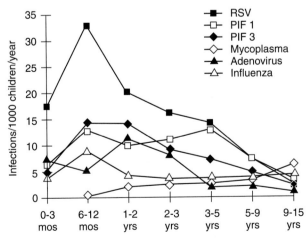

FIGURE 32-11 Etiology of pediatric lower respiratory tract infection in Chapel Hill, NC by age during an 11-year period.

winter and are rarely seen during the spring and summer. RSV often causes bronchiolitis, but pneumonia can develop.[44]

The first symptoms noted are usually coryza and nasal congestion, followed by cough, fever, and malaise. Retractions, nasal flaring, tachypnea, wheezes, and rhonchi are common. The chest radiograph typically shows hyperinflated lungs with patchy infiltrates and/or atelectasis (most often involving the right upper lobe). Dehydration can develop as a result of tachypnea, cough, and decreased feeding.

Diagnosis is confirmed with rapid immunofluorescent detection of RSV antigen in nasal washings or enzyme-linked immunosorbent assays of nasal secretions. Test methods are relatively inexpensive.

Aerosolized ribavirin is an antiviral agent that may be used to treat the infection; however, its use remains controversial. Hypoxemia and hypercarbia are complications of RSV pneumonia and may mandate supplemental oxygen for an extended period. Supportive care is aimed at monitoring the severity with pulse oximetry and arterial blood gas analysis. Patients may experience progressive hypoxemia and respiratory failure, necessitating intubation and mechanical ventilation. There may be further progression to advanced respiratory failure, in spite of maximal ventilatory support. Those patients may require extracorporeal membrane oxygenation (ECMO). Patients thought to have a less than 20% chance of survival without ECMO have a nearly 60% chance of survival with ECMO.[45]

Parainfluenza Virus Types 1, 2, and 3

The parainfluenza viruses are the second-most common cause of LTB and pneumonia. Type 3 is the most common cause in children younger than 5 years of age and occurs year round with no seasonal peak. Clinical presentation is similar to that described for RSV. Chest radiographs typically reveal patchy or interstitial infiltrates. Diagnosis is confirmed with rapid antigen testing or viral isolation from a nasal washing. Therapy is supportive, with supplemental oxygen and additional hydration provided as needed. Parainfluenza virus is not to be confused with influenza virus, which has a very narrow seasonal peak.

Influenza Virus

Although influenza virus may cause pneumonia, it occurs predominantly in the very young and very old patient. Yearly epidemics occur during the late winter and early spring. Clinical symptoms consist of rapidly developing fever, malaise, and myalgia. Duration of the illness is usually shorter than that of RSV and the parainfluenza viruses. Although rarely occurring, a rapid pneumonia may result in death within 2 days of onset.

Diagnosis and treatment are similar to that of RSV and parainfluenza virus infections. Vaccines are provided annually and are recommended for those high-risk children with chronic cardiopulmonary and immunologic disorders. Chest radiographs typically reveal interstitial or patchy alveolar infiltrates.

Adenovirus

Although it occurs year round, adenoviral pneumonia is most often seen in the late summer and early fall. It occurs most often in children younger than 2 years of age. It is easily confused with bacterial illnesses because it mimics their symptomatology: rapid onset, high fever, leukocytosis, and chest radiograph consistent with pneumonia. Additional findings may include lymphadenopathy and conjunctivitis. A chest radiograph reveals patchy or interstitial infiltrates.

Certain adenoviral types (i.e., 3, 7, 21) are associated with a high mortality rate owing to the overwhelming sepsis and cardiovascular collapse that occurs. Diagnosis is confirmed with rapid antigen testing or viral isolation from a nasal washing. Therapy is supportive, and no specific treatment is available. Close monitoring for bacterial superinfection is suggested.

New viruses are being isolated and their implications will become clearer over time. One example is the human metapneumovirus, identified in 2001.

Bacterial Pneumonia
Incidence

Although the incidence of bacterial pneumonia is less than that of viral pneumonia, it has a higher mortality rate. It may occur as a secondary problem to a primary viral pneumonia, as is often seen with pneumonia from influenza virus. Certain other factors known to increase the risk of bacterial pneumonia include compromised immune function, recurrent aspiration from gastroesophageal reflux, malnutrition, day-care attendance or school-aged sibling, exposure to passive cigarette smoke, and congenital abnormalities of the airway (e.g., tracheoesophageal fistula). Bacterial pneumonia is seen throughout the year, with a peak incidence in the winter and early spring.

Etiology

Bacterial agents that cause pneumonia vary considerably throughout the pediatric age group. In the neonatal patient, the offending bacteria are most often contaminates from the mother's genital tract and include group B *Streptococcus, Escherichia coli, Listeria monocytogenes,* and *C. trachomatis*.[46] Infants older than 4 to 6 weeks of age tend to develop pneumonia from *S. pneumoniae, H. influenzae,* and *S. aureus*. Less likely organisms include *Bordetella pertussis, M. pneumoniae,* and *C. pneumoniae.*

Bacterial pneumonia develops when the intrinsic host defenses are decreased, either by another disease process (e.g., viral infection) or when the anatomic protective mechanisms are destroyed (e.g., primary ciliary dyskinesia). Therefore, any microorganism colonizing the upper respiratory tract has the potential to cause pneumonia if it evades these defenses.

Signs and Symptoms

There are no symptoms that distinguish a bacterial pneumonia from a viral pneumonia in children, although children with bacterial pneumonia tend to present with more severe symptoms of fever and distress. Prodromal symptoms are often nonpulmonary and include headache, fever, malaise, and abdominal pain. Productive cough, with sputum often swallowed, and chest pain during inspiration (pleuritic pain) are common complaints. Physical examination usually reveals nasal flaring, accessory muscle use, intercostal and subcostal retractions, tachypnea, and shallow breathing. Crackles, decreased breath sounds, increased fremitus, and dullness to percussion are often found during auscultation and examination of the chest.[47]

Diagnosis

The chest radiograph is an important diagnostic tool when evaluating a child with suspected bacterial pneumonia. Although bacterial pneumonia is commonly manifested as an alveolar consolidation, lobar and interstitial infiltrates are often found as well as pleural effusion. It has been suggested that certain radiographic findings vary among the various bacterial agents involved and may help determine the etiology.[48,49]

An elevated total band count (>1500 total bands) is common in the presence of bacterial pneumonia. Increased C-reactive protein levels and erythrocyte sedimentation rates provide supporting, albeit not specific, evidence of inflammation. Blood culture is the most helpful test to give absolute confirmation of bacterial disease, but it is only positive in 25% of patients with S. pneumoniae pneumonia and 33% of patients with S. aureus pneumonia. Similarly, the latex particle agglutination and countercurrent immunoelectrophoresis studies are insensitive in most cases of pneumonia. When pleural fluid is present in significant quantities, sampling for Gram stain and culture will yield specific bacterial diagnosis in 65% to 80% of the patients. Bronchoalveolar lavage fluid obtained during a bronchoscopy can be used for atypical presentations. Lung tissue may be obtained for culture through an open-lung biopsy, transthoracic needle aspiration biopsy, or percutaneous lung puncture.

Precise microbiologic diagnosis is not always obtained even though bacterial pneumonia is suspected.

There are several reasons why clinicians may take an empirical approach to treatment. Many of the diagnostic procedures are much too invasive for any but the sickest patients. Some procedures use instruments (e.g., bronchoscope, suction catheter) that pass through the contaminated pharynx or upper airway. Although it is difficult to obtain a sputum specimen in children younger than 8 years of age, when it is obtained the flora in the upper airway contaminates the sputum, making the etiologic diagnosis questionable.

Treatment

Standard initial treatment of bacterial pneumonia varies considerably according to the patient's age and immunologic status, time of year, and local antibiotic sensitivity patterns. The need for hospitalization is often determined by the severity of the symptoms. When the cause is identified, antimicrobial therapy is determined and is usually given for 7 to 14 days by the parenteral route, although the clinical symptoms and history of underlying disease often guide empirical therapy. Neonatal pneumonia is routinely treated with intravenous antibiotics. The patient is monitored with pulse oximetry and arterial blood gas analysis when indicated. Supplemental oxygen is provided if hypoxia occurs and mechanical ventilation is provided if there is respiratory failure. The role of chest physiotherapy in the treatment of pneumonia is debated, with some clinicians doubting its efficacy.

Streptococcus pneumoniae

The most common cause of bacterial pneumonia is the pneumococcus.[50] The clinical picture differs with age. The infant presents initially with a sudden fever and diarrhea or vomiting. Signs of respiratory distress, including nasal flaring, tachypnea, grunting, and retractions, appear along with restlessness and cyanosis. The classic clinical presentation of the older child is that of rapid-onset respiratory distress, high fever, shaking chills, headache, pleuritic pain, and cough with rust-colored sputum. The chest radiograph usually reveals lobar or segmental alveolar consolidation, which may be accompanied by a pleural effusion or empyema. Sputum reveals sheets of gram-positive diplococci and many white blood cells. The clinical diagnosis can be made based on these findings. However, in reality the clinical presentation is rarely this clear and treatment of suspected bacterial pneumonia includes pneumococcal coverage.

Pneumococcal pneumonia can be rapidly fatal without appropriate therapy. Penicillin is the antibiotic of choice; erythromycin is used in the penicillin-allergic individual. Although penicillin resistance in the United States is rare, it is increasingly common in Europe and Africa. Therefore, treatment should be guided by antibiotic susceptibilities when an organism is recovered. Other antibiotics that have successful activity against *S. pneumoniae* include cephalosporins, chloramphenicol, clindamycin, and vancomycin.

Haemophilus influenzae

Before the use of vaccination against serotype b, this gram-negative rod was a frequent cause of pneumonia in children. Infection occurs most often in children younger than 5 years of age. The chest radiograph is highly variable and can exhibit any pattern from a bronchiolitic-type picture with hyperinflation to patchy infiltrates to segmental or lobar consolidation. Pleural effusion is present in about one third of the patients. Positive blood culture results or positive results on urine antigen screens confirm diagnosis. Empirical therapy is usually with a cephalosporin. Other potentially therapeutic drugs effective against all *H. influenzae* isolates include trimethoprim-sulfamethoxazole, clarithromycin, azithromycin, chloramphenicol, and amoxicillin/clavulanate.

Staphylococcus aureus

Pneumonia caused by *S. aureus* ('staph') is a virulent, aggressive disease that can be rapidly fatal, particularly in infants younger than 1 year of age. This organism is commonly found on the skin and mucosa, with 20% to 30% of the population carrying bacteria in the nose. Pneumonia is frequently seen in debilitated patients who often have associated skin infections. It is common to have a history of an antecedent viral infection, particularly influenza.[50]

The severity of clinical symptoms varies, with the typical presentation being an upper respiratory tract infection, fever, cough, and respiratory distress. The clinical course in the neonate is often rapidly progressive and is associated with a high mortality rate shortly after the onset of symptoms. The chest radiograph usually reveals large consolidation that can progress rapidly to a 'whiteout' of the lung. Pleural effusion and empyema as well as a pneumothorax often complicate the clinical picture. While resolving, areas of consolidation often progress to pneumatoceles, which are round, air-filled areas of lung destruction that are easily visible on the radiograph. The pneumatoceles may contain fluid and change rapidly in number and size, leading to a mediastinal shift.

Diagnosis is by positive blood, skin abscess, or pleural fluid culture results. Therapy is with antistaphylococcal penicillins such as nafcillin and oxacillin. Susceptibility testing is imperative to exclude the possibility of methicillin-resistant *S. aureus* spreading throughout the general community, which requires treatment with vancomycin.

Atypical Pneumonia

The major pathogens of pneumonia that are commonly missed by the tests listed previously cause 'atypical' pneumonia. In the neonate, those agents include the uncommon viral diseases of rubella, varicella-zoster, and cytomegalovirus and the even rarer nonbacterial agents of *Toxoplasma*, *Treponema pallidum*, and *C. trachomatis*. In the older child, *M. pneumoniae*, *C. pneumoniae*, and *M. tuberculosis* cause atypical pneumonia.

Mycoplasma pneumoniae

M. pneumoniae commonly causes a community-acquired pneumonia that is seen year-round but peaks in the late summer and early fall. Although it occurs in all age groups, it is most often a disease of school-aged children and young adults.[51]

The incubation period is 2 to 3 weeks, and it presents as a viral upper respiratory infection. Clinical onset is insidious, with a gradual development of malaise, fever, and cough, which are the most prominent symptoms. Cough is nonproductive or productive with blood-tinged sputum. Chills, pharyngitis, headache, nausea, vomiting, diarrhea, and chest pain are also associated with this infection. Crackles are heard most often during auscultation, with occasional wheezing, although there may be no abnormal findings at the beginning of the illness. The clinical and radiographic findings are often out of proportion with the clinical severity; hence the common lay description of 'walking pneumonia' is often applied to this infection. The chest radiograph usually reveals bronchopneumonia with patchy infiltrates.[52,53] The complete blood cell count is usually normal; however, a cold hemagglutinin assay with titers of 1:64 is highly suggestive of infection with *M. pneumoniae*.

Without treatment, the illness resolves in 2 to 4 weeks. Oral erythromycin for 10 to 14 days provides optimal therapy and the patient usually becomes afebrile within 48 hours. Azithromycin has also shown efficacy and is widely used as a 5–day therapy course.[54]

Chlamydia pneumoniae

Infected respiratory droplets most likely transmit *C. pneumoniae*. Primary infection occurs most often in school-aged children and young adults.[55] Only a small portion of patients infected are clinically symptomatic, yet some patients experience severe illness leading to death. Most infections with *C. pneumoniae* are mild and commonly coincide with other bacterial pathogens. Illness is characterized by pharyngitis, followed several days later with cough. Fever is often present early in the illness but does not persist. Wheezing is frequently heard on auscultation. In fact, this infection has a strong correlation with recent-onset asthma.[56,57]

Host factors appear to influence the severity of this illness. Immunocompromised patients with the acquired immunodeficiency syndrome, malignancy, primary immune deficits, and sickle cell disease may have severe or frequent infections. *C. pneumoniae* is a frequent cause of acute chest syndrome in children with sickle cell disease and may also act as a trigger for acute asthma.[58]

C. pneumoniae is difficult to isolate, even in tissue culture, and requires special handling of the culture sample. Because of the long delay in serologic diagnosis, empirical antibiotic therapy is commonly employed. Infection with *C. pneumoniae* is treated with tetracycline or erythromycin for 10 to 14 days, although a prolonged course of 21 days is not uncommon.

Ventilator-Associated Pneumonia

A patient who is receiving mechanical ventilatory support is at risk of developing pneumonia. New onset of pulmonary infiltrates can occur, stemming from a multitude of causes including atelectasis, infection, spontaneous or catheter-related pulmonary emboli, or acute lung injury. The pathogenesis appears to involve the microaspiration of oropharyngeal organisms. Clinical and radiographic criteria for diagnosing ventilator-associated pneumonia are unreliable.

The development of ventilator-associated pneumonia (VAP) increases hospitalization stay by 30% but does not change mortality rates. In pediatric patients undergoing mechanical ventilation, polymicrobial aerobic and anaerobic floras are isolated from pulmonary specimens. Predominant aerobic bacteria are *Pseudomonas aeruginosa* and *Klebsiella pneumoniae;* the predominant anaerobic bacteria are *Prevotella, Porphyromonas, Peptostreptococcus, Fusobacterium,* and *Bacteroides fragilis.*[59]

To better establish the diagnosis of VAP, Gram stain of bronchoalveolar lavage fluid is obtained through a fiberoptic bronchoscope. Bronchoalveolar lavage fluid is considered positive for VAP when the following conditions occur:

1. polymorphonuclear neutrophils are greater than 25 per optic field at a magnification times 100
2. squamous epithelial cells are less than 1%; and
3. one or more microorganisms are seen per optic field at a magnification of 1:1000.

Gram stain of bronchoalveolar lavage fluid is 77% sensitive and 87% specific with a positive predictive value of 71% and a negative predictive value of 90%.[60] Although bronchoalveolar lavage samples acquired through bronchoscopy are used to diagnose VAP, quantitative cultures of endotracheal aspirates are easier and less expensive to obtain. Persistence of significant numbers of pathogens in quantitative cultures of endotracheal aspirates occurred in 82% of the samples. This quantitative culture of endotracheal aspirates is reproducible and may be useful in the diagnosis of VAP.[61]

Multiple forms of therapy have been attempted to minimize the risk of developing VAP, including routine hand washing, closed airway suctioning, elevating the head of bed, frequent humidifier and ventilator tubing changes, heat and moisture exchangers instead of a heated water humidifier, and heated wire circuits. Some studies suggest that the use of heat and moisture exchangers is a cost-effective clinical practice associated with fewer late-onset hospital-acquired VAPs and results in improved resource allocation and utilization.[62] However, other studies conclude their use does not affect the frequency of VAP and could potentially lead to mucus hardening.[63] Decreasing the frequency of ventilator circuit changes from three times per week to once per week had no adverse effect on the overall rate of VAP, thus prompting institutions to change ventilator circuits as needed and convincing the majority of experts that the ventilator has nothing to do with VAP.[64] If fact, some experts are calling for a name change suggesting that this phenomena be call endotracheal tube-associated pneumonia (EAP) as it appears that the ETT has more to do with VAP than the ventilator. Scheduled changes in antibiotic class for empirical treatment of VAP have been demonstrated to lower the incidence of bacteremia associated with antibiotic-resistant gram-negative bacteria.

TUBERCULOSIS

Incidence and Etiology

Tuberculosis (TB) is the most frequent infectious cause of death throughout the world. Although the frequency declined in the 1980s and early 1990s, the disease is again increasing in incidence and severity.[65,66] It is a chronic bacterial disease caused by infection with *M. tuberculosis.* This organism is a very hearty and virulent bacterium that resists inactivation by drying, heat, and sunlight. Patients infected with *M. tuberculosis* are usually medically underserved, poverty stricken, or immunocompromised. Most children do not develop clinical disease unless disease resistance declines, owing to malnutrition, fatigue, or chronic illness.[67]

Transmission

Transmission is airborne, occurring through the inhalation of viable respiratory droplets in an enclosed space (e.g., room, hospital). The pathogen is rapidly killed by ultraviolet light in the outside air. The household contact for an infant or child is usually an adult; rarely is there child-to-child transmission. The incubation period lasts from 2 to 10 weeks, at which time a skin test becomes positive, manifesting a delayed-type hypersensitivity (Box 32-2).

Box 32-2	Cut-off Size of Induration for Positive Mantoux Tuberculin Skin Test

=5 MM
- Contacts of infectious cases
- Abnormal chest radiograph
- HIV-infected and other immunosuppressed patients

=10 MM
- Foreign-born persons from areas of high prevalence
- Low-income populations
- Residents of prisons, nursing homes, institutions
- Intravenous drug users
- Other medical risk factors
- Health care workers
- Locally identified high-risk populations
- Infants

=15 MM
- No risk factors

HIV, Human immunodeficiency virus.
Modified from Starke JR, Jacobs RF, Jereb J: Resurgence of tuberculosis in children, *J Pediatr* 1992;120:839.

Signs and Symptoms

Most infants and children who become infected with *M. tuberculosis* never develop TB and remain asymptomatic. They may continue with few if any clinical symptoms or may manifest nonspecific signs of fever, weight loss, and failure to thrive. Most patients develop cough and wheezing, with crackles and rhonchi heard in some cases. Chest radiography in these individuals reveals focal or diffuse infiltrates. Many cases of pulmonary infection with *M. tuberculosis* are caused by reactivation and are characterized by focal findings on chest radiography in a patient with chronic respiratory and systemic symptoms.

Diagnosis

Diagnosis in the adult is based on identification of stains of gastric or respiratory washings that have bacteria uniquely resistant to acid decoloration ('acid fast'). In children, owing to the low number of bacilli, 3 consecutive days of gastric washings may increase the sensitivity of this test. More commonly, the diagnosis of TB is based on a positive skin test (Mantoux skin test) in a patient with an appropriate clinical picture and radiographic findings.[67,68] Proper interpretation of these skin tests is critical and is based on the probability of disease using a combination of risk factors, clinical findings, and the size of induration resulting from the skin test (see Box 32-2). Differential diagnosis includes asthma, foreign body aspiration, tumors, sarcoidosis, and all pulmonary pathogens.

Treatment

Treatment of TB in children focuses on early diagnosis, identification of the primary case that spread the disease to the child, and long-term antituberculosis medications. For the patient with active disease, multiple medications are indicated for an extended period. These include isoniazid, rifampin, pyrazinamide, and ethambutol. Corticosteroid therapy can be safely used in conjunction with antituberculosis drug therapy to lower the inflammatory response to the infection, reduce the size of enlarged lymph nodes, and accelerate the resorption of fluid when a large pleural effusion has developed. See Clinical Scenario 5.

CLINICAL SCENARIO 5

A 13-month-old former 24-week gestation premature infant with resolving BPD is brought to his pediatrician for a 2-day history of decreased appetite, runny nose, and increased cough. It is February and the toddler is due for his repeat Synergist vaccination in 4 days. His O$_2$ saturation, vitals, and exam are unremarkable and the decision is made to discharge him home with close follow up. Two days later his O$_2$ requirement is up to 1 L/min O$_2$ via nasal cannula (from 0.25 L/min O2 via nasal cannula) and he exhibits increased respiratory distress. O$_2$ saturation is decreased to 80% and he is afebrile. He is admitted to the hospital with decreased PO intake and respiratory distress. A rapid RSV test is positive and his chest x-ray shows infiltrates in the right middle lobe and the left upper lobe.
- What is your diagnosis and treatment?

RSV infections demonstrate the difficulty of distinguishing between bacterial and viral pneumonias. In the case of a child with underlying lung disease, such as BPD, this may lead to a more conservative and widespread use of antibiotics. There are multiple studies in the recent literature establishing the importance of neutrophils in many respiratory diseases, including RSV bronchilitis [69,70] and attempts to use Bronchial Aveleory Lavage (BAL) samples and cell count as a clinical marker in conjunction with cultures.[71] They demonstrated the predominance of neutrophils in viral infections of the airway and other lung diseases.[72,73] More interesting is the observation that neutrophilic inflammation can be correlated to the extent of lung injury.[74] Currently we lack a medical treatment targeting neutrophils in the airway, but the development of such treatements is underway. It remains to be seen how effective they might be in the treatment of RSV, bronchiolitis, and similar pulmonary diseases associated with neutrophilc inflammation and if BAL examination has a future value in the routine testing of pediatric patients with lung diseases.

SICKLE CELL DISEASE

Incidence and Etiology

Sickle cell disease is an autosomal recessively inherited disorder of the hemoglobin structure and is the most common inherited disease of the African-American population. Defective hemoglobin S converts from a soluble hemoglobin molecule contained in the red cells to a gelatinous state in the presence of low oxygen, low pH, rapid temperature changes, or hypernatremic dehydration. This gelatinous state causes the red cells to 'sickle,' resulting in a variety of complications including acute chest syndrome, cardiomegaly and left ventricular failure, splenectomy, and renal disease. Pulmonary complications are the primary cause of illness and death in patients with sickle cell disease.[75,76]

Pathophysiology

A complex interaction between the abnormal cells and vascular endothelium results in a hypercoagulable state. Recent reports indicate that high levels of endothelin-1, an endothelial-derived vasoactive mediator, are present during a vasoactive crisis. An abnormality of the vascular endothelium may contribute to the development of acute chest syndrome. The red blood cells are more rigid, resulting in increased viscosity of blood, which causes plugging of the blood vessels.

The pulmonary effects that occur most often in patients with sickle cell disease include pneumonia, acute chest syndrome, pulmonary vascular injury, pulmonary infarction, and sickle cell chronic lung disease. Bacterial pneumonia is a frequent cause for hospitalization, and pulmonary vascular injury can cause sudden death if the occlusion is in a large vessel.

Signs and Symptoms

Acute chest syndrome is the leading cause of death in sickle cell disease and presents as pleuritic or chest wall pain and dyspnea. The chest radiograph often reveals pulmonary infiltrates, frequently located in the lower lobes, as well as atelectasis and pleural effusion. Young children, aged 2 to 4 years old, who present with acute chest syndrome have fever, cough, and a negative physical examination, with little or no pain. Adults are often afebrile, complaining of severe dyspnea, chills, and severe pain along the ribs, sternum, abdomen, and back.[77]

Reports in the 1970s suggested that sickle cell disease was caused by a bacterial infection; however, more recent studies suggest that bacterial infection is found in only 3% to 14% of patients, whereas *Mycoplasma* and/or *Chlamydia* infections are found in approximately 15%. Children younger than 5 years of age tend to have a milder disease course that is usually triggered by infection. Risk of death is four times higher in adults with acute chest

syndrome than in children and most likely related to the higher incidence of fat embolism from bone marrow infarction. Aplastic crisis in young children with sickle cell disease is typically associated with acute human parvovirus B19 infection. Infection with this pathogen may also be related to acute chest syndrome.[78]

Pneumonia and pulmonary infarction can occur simultaneously and are sometimes difficult to differentiate. Fever and chills are seen more often with pneumonia, with fever resolving slowly. Acute pulmonary symptoms with tachypnea and pleuritic chest pain are more suggestive of pulmonary infarction. In some cases, pneumonia causes hypoxemia that leads to pulmonary infarction.[79]

Sickle cell chronic lung disease occurs most often during the teenage years and may develop after multiple episodes of acute chest syndrome. Hypoxemia is present as a result of pulmonary fibrosis and a reduction in diffusion and pulmonary perfusion. Parenchymal lung injury and an increase in pulmonary vascular resistance cause progressive dyspnea and cor pulmonale. Diffuse interstitial markings and edema are common findings on the chest radiograph.[76,78,80]

Treatment

Empirical therapy includes antibiotics for gram-positive encapsulated organisms of *Streptococcus, Staphylococcus,* and *Salmonella.* Erythromycin is used to provide coverage for the pathogens *M. pneumoniae* and *C. pneumoniae.* Antibiotics are quickly instituted because the infections, especially a pneumococcal pneumonia, can become life threatening.[79]

Adequate hydration is an essential therapeutic modality and is used cautiously to avoid pulmonary edema. Red blood cell transfusions are provided to improve the hemoglobin's ability to transport oxygen and reduce the incidence of acute chest syndrome, myocardial ischemia, and sickle cell chronic lung disease. Aerosolized bronchodilators for bronchiole constriction, incentive spirometry, and adequate pain control can be important adjuvants. Supplemental oxygen is used when indicated, but depending on the case can foster additional sickling. In cases of impending respiratory failure, mechanical ventilation is instituted.[81,82] Successful treatment of acute chest syndrome with venovenous ECMO is reported in patients experiencing life-threatening acute chest syndrome despite maximum conventional ventilation support.[83]

A new experimental approach is to treat acute chest syndrome with inhaled nitric oxide. This idea is based on an abnormality discovered in the nitric oxide metabolism in sickle cell patients. The theory is that the nitiric oxide might prevent the adhesion of sickle erythrocytes to the endothelial. At this time it is under clinical investigation and used only in those settings.

Prevention
Acute Chest Syndrome

The treatment of recurrent acute chest syndrome is aimed at preventing repeated vascular and parenchymal insults, which constitute the greatest risk for the development of sickle cell chronic lung disease. Chronic transfusion programs aim to decrease the sickle cell amount to less than 30%, a level that will prevent recurrence of acute chest syndrome. The risks involved are transfusion-associated infections and iron overload. Hydroxyurea was shown to be clinically effective in reducing acute chest syndrome recurrence and vaso-occlusive crises by 50%, but the long-term effects of this treatment are uncertain and frequent peripheral blood count monitoring is necessary. Antibiotic prophylaxis with penicillin is recommended for patients between 4 months of age to 3 years of age, as well as routine polyvalent pneumococcal vaccine for children and adults.

RECURRENT ASPIRATION SYNDROME

Etiology

Neurologically impaired patients, those with abnormal anatomy of the gastrointestinal tract or airways, and patients with gastroesophageal reflux are often diagnosed with recurrent aspiration syndrome. The patient aspirates respiratory secretions and/or stomach contents. The low pH of the stomach contents results in a chemical pneumonitis and inflammatory response in the airways. The patients and their families suffer through multiple hospitalizations for pneumonia and airway hyperreactivity. Children who are treated for frequent asthma exacerbations, yet have negative responses to allergens, benefit from evaluation for recurrent aspiration. Infants with gastroesophageal reflux are at particular risk for pneumonia.[84]

Diagnosis

Diagnosis is based on clinical and radiographic findings. Barium swallow may reveal a tracheoesophageal fistula or other malformation that requires surgical intervention. Bronchoscopy with bronchoalveolar lavage can reveal pathogens normally found in the gastrointestinal tract as well as provide visual confirmation of inflamed airways.[85]

Treatment

The cause and severity of the disease determine treatment. Fundoplication, a surgical tightening of the gastroesophageal junction, may alleviate gastroesophageal reflux. Appropriate antibiotic coverage is necessary to control infection. Inhaled corticosteroids are indicated to control and reduce the airway damage that occurs from chronic inflammation. Prevention of recurrent aspiration is paramount to obtaining a long-term, positive outcome. Prognosis in uncontrolled recurrent aspiration syndrome is guarded, owing to the chronic reinjury of the respiratory parenchyma.[86] Respiratory and cardiac insufficiency may develop over time. Accurate and early diagnosis, prevention, and prophylaxis may reduce the severity of the injury and improve the patient's quality of life.

ASSESSMENT QUESTIONS

See Evolve Resources for the answers.

1. Where do you find the narrowest portion of the pediatric airway that may compromise endotracheal intubation?
   A. Vocal cords
   B. Oro-pharynx
   C. Cricoid cartilage
   D. Epiglottis
   E. Trachea
2. What is not a sign of respiratory distress in an infant?
   A. Nasal flaring
   B. Retractions
   C. Irritability
   D. Lethargy
   E. Crying
3. A child presents with high fever; severe sore throat; dysphagia with drooling; cough, progressing rapidly over a few hours to stridor; muffled ('hot potato') voice without hoarseness; air hunger; and cyanosis. Severe intercostal retractions, along with nasal flaring, bradypnea, and dyspnea, are present. The child assumes a characteristic position of sitting upright with the chin thrust forward and with the neck hyperextended in a tripod position. Bacterial epiglottitis is suspected. What is the next necessary action?
   A. Visualize the upper airway
   B. Upper airway radiographic imaging
   C. Call supporting services
   D. Lay the child flat and provide flow by oxygen
   E. Secure an intravenous line for sedation
4. What is the right estimated ETT size for a 6–year-old male, using a cuffed ETT?
   A. 4
   B. 4.5
   C. 5
   D. 5.5
   E. 6

ASSESSMENT QUESTIONS—cont'd

5. You are in a restaurant and the child at the table next to you starts to cough violently. He is 5 years old and was eating French fries when he suddenly turned red, started to cough, and fell to the floor. His parents are nervously patting his back and try to lift him up from the floor. What intervention needs to be done?
   A. Perform the Heimlich maneuver
   B. Open his airway with the tongue-jaw-lift
   C. Finger swipe the oro-pharynx
   D. Leave the child on the floor and monitor
   E. Push the parents out of the way and perform efficient back blows

6. What is a bronchiectasis?
   A. Irreversible dilation of the bronchial tree
   B. Puss accumulation in the airway
   C. The airway immediately placed before an emphysema
   D. Only found in cystic fibrosis patients
   E. Restrictive lung disease

7. Which infant is especially at risk for severe or life-threatening RSV bronchiolitis infections: BPD, premature infant, congenital cardiac disease, immune-compromised children, oncology patient?
   A. Immune-compromised patient
   B. History of prematurity
   C. Congenital heart defect
   D. BPD
   E. All the above

8. What combination of pneumonia to causative pathogen is incorrect?
   A. Viral pneumonia; parainfluenza virus types 3
   B. Bacterial pneumonia; *Escherichia coli*
   C. Atypical pneumonia; *Mycoplasma pneumoniae*
   D. Bacterial pneumonia; *Streptococcus pneumoniae*
   E. Atypical pneumonia; MRSA

9. Which signs suggest acute chest syndrome in a patient with sickle cell disease?
   A. Fever
   B. Rib pain
   C. Pleuritic pain
   D. Tachypnea
   E. All except B

10. The major culprit for ventilator-associated pneumonia (VAP) appears to be what?
    A. Ventilator tubing
    B. Ventilator circuit
    C. Endotracheal tube
    D. Droplet transfection from hospital personal
    E. Routine antibiotic usage

References

1. Grad R: Acute infections producing upper airway obstruction. In Chernick V, Boat TF, Kendig EL, editors: *Disorders of the respiratory tract in children*. Philadelphia. WB Saunders, 1998; pp 447-461.
2. Frantz TD, Rasgon BM: Acute epiglottitis: changing epidemiologic patterns, *Otolaryngol Head Neck Surg* 1993;109:457
3. Breukels MA et al: Invasive infection with Haemophilus influenzae type B in spite of complete vaccination, *Ned Tijdschr Geneeskd* 1998;142:586.
4. Lacroix J et al: Group A streptococcal supraglottitis, *J Pediatr* 1986;109:20.
5. Steele DW et al: Pulsus paradoxus: an objective measure of severity in croup, *Am J Respir Crit Care Med* 1998;157:331.
6. Westley CR, Cotton EK, Brooks JG: Nebulized racemic epinephrine by IPPB for the treatment of croup: a double-blind study, *Am J Dis Child* 1978;132:484.
7. Super DM et al: A prospective randomized double-blind study to evaluate the effect of dexamethasone in acute laryngotracheitis, *J Pediatr* 1989;115:323.
8. Kairys SW, Olmstead EM, O'Connor GT: Steroid treatment of laryngotracheitis: a meta-analysis of the evidence from randomized trials, *Pediatrics* 1989;83:683.
9. Rizos JD et al: The disposition of children with croup treated with racemic epinephrine and dexamethasone in the emergency department, *J Emerg Med* 1998;16:535.
10. Khalil SN et al: Absence or presence of a leak around tracheal tube may not affect postoperative croup in children, *Paediatr Anaesth* 1998;8:393.
11. Khine HH et al: Comparison of cuffed and uncuffed endotracheal tubes in young children during general anesthesia, *Anesthesiology* 1997;86:627.
12. Kelly SM, April MM, Tunkel DE: Obstructing laryngeal granuloma after brief endotracheal intubation in neonates, *Otolaryngol Head Neck Surg* 1996;115:138.
13. Kenna MA, Bluestone CD: Foreign bodies in the air and food passages, *Pediatr Rev* 1988;10:25.
14. Johnson NT, Pierson DJ: The spectrum of pulmonary atelectasis: pathophysiology, diagnosis, and therapy, *Respir Care* 1986;31:1107.
15. Duncan SR et al: Nasal continuous positive airway pressure in atelectasis, *Chest* 1987;92:621.
16. Westcott JL: Bronchiectasis, *Radiol Clin North Am* 1991;29:1031.
17. Ferkol TW, Davis PB: Bronchiectasis and bronchiolitis obliterans. In Taussig LM, Landau LI, editors: *Pediatric respiratory medicine*, St Louis: Mosby, 1999; pp 784-792.
18. Barker AF, Bardana EJ: Bronchiectasis: update of an orphan disease, *Am Rev Respir Dis* 1988;137:969.
19. Wilson JF, Decker AM: The surgical management of childhood bronchiectasis: a review of 96 consecutive pulmonary resections in children with nontuberculous bronchiectasis, *Ann Surg* 1982;195:354.
20. Annest LS, Kratz JM, Crawford FA: Current results of treatment of bronchiectasis, *J Thorac Cardiovasc Surg* 1982;83:546.
21. Balck-Payne C: Bronchiolitis. In Hilman BC, editor: *Pediatric respiratory disease, diagnosis and treatment.* Philadelphia: WB Saunders; 1993. pp 205-217.

22. Wohl MEB: Bronchiolitis. In Chernick V, Boat TF, Kendig EL, editors: *Disorders of the respiratory tract in children.* Philadelphia. WB Saunders, 1998; pp 473-484.

23. Everard ML: Acute bronchiolitis and pneumonia in infancy resulting from the respiratory syncytial virus. In Taussig LM, Landau LI, editors: *Pediatric respiratory medicine*, St Louis: Mosby; 1999. pp 580-595.

24. Sandritter TL, Kraus DM: Respiratory syncytial virus-immunoglobulin intravenous (RSV-IGIV) for respiratory syncytial viral infections: I, *J Pediatr Health Care* 1997;11:284.

25. Levy BT, Graber MA: Respiratory syncytial virus infection in infants and young children, *J Fam Pract* 1997;45:473.

26. Everard ML et al: Analysis of cells obtained by bronchial lavage of infants with respiratory syncytial virus infection, *Arch Dis Child* 1994; 71:428-432.

27. American Academy of Pediatrics Committee on Infectious Disease: Use of ribavirin in the treatment of respiratory syncytial virus infection, *Pediatrics* 1993;92:501.

28. Hughes JH, Mann DR, Hamparian VV: Detection of respiratory syncytial virus in clinical specimens by viral culture, direct and indirect immunofluorescence and enzyme immunoassay, *J Clin Microbiol* 1988;26:588.

29. Klassen TP: Recent advances in the treatment of bronchiolitis and laryngitis, *Pediatr Clin North Am* 1997;44:249.

30. Wang EEL et al: Bronchodilators for treatment of mild bronchiolitis: a factorial randomized trial, *Arch Dis Child* 1992;67:289.

31. Schena JA, Crone RK, Thompson JE: Theophylline therapy in bronchiolitis, *Crit Care Med* 1984;12:225.

32. Roosevelt G et al: Dexamethasone in bronchiolitis: a randomised controlled trial, *Lancet* 1996;348:292.

33. Fackler JC et al: Precautions in the use of ribavirin at the Children's Hospital, *N Engl J Med* 1990;322:634.

34. Moler FW et al: Effectiveness of ribavirin in otherwise well infants with respiratory syncytial virus-associated respiratory failure, *J Pediatr* 1996;128:422.

35. De Boeck K, Moens M, Schuddinck L: Early ribavirin treatment did not prevent disease in high-bronchopulmonary dysplasia patients with respiratory syncytial virus infection, *Pediatr Pulmonol* 1996;21:343.

36. Randolph AG, Wang EE: Ribavirin for respiratory syncytial virus lowers respiratory tract infection *Arch Pediatr Adolesc Med* 1996;150:942.

37. Groothuis JR et al: Early ribaviri treatment of respiratory syncytial viral infection in high-risk children, *J Pediatr* 1990;117:792.

38. Wandstrat TL: Respiratory syncytial virus immune globulin intravenous, *Ann Pharmacother* 1997;31:83.

39. Leigh MW: Primary ciliary dyskinesia. In Chernick V, Boat TF, Kendig EL, editors: *Disorders of the respiratory tract in children.* Philadelphia: WB Saunders: 1998. pp 819-826.

40. Pedersen M, Mygind N: Ciliary motility in the 'immotile cilia syndrome,' *Br J Dis Chest* 1980;74:239.

41. Boat TF, Carson JL: Ciliary dysmorphology and dysfunction-primary or acquired, *N Engl J Med* 1990;323:1681.

42. Phillips GE et al: Airway response of children with primary ciliary dyskinesia to exercise and beta2-agonist challenge, *Eur Respir J* 1998;11:1389.

43. Denny FW, Clyde WA: Acute lower respiratory tract infections in nonhospitalized children, *J Pediatr* 1986;108:635.

44. Glezen WP: Viral pneumonia. In Chernick V, Boat TF, Kendig EL, editors: *Disorders of the respiratory tract in children*, Philadelphia: WB Saunders: 1998. pp 518-525.

45. ECMO Registry of the Extracorporeal Life Support Organization (ELSO), Ann Arbor, Mich, July 1998.

46. Correa AG, Starke JR: Bacterial pneumonias. In Chernick V, Boat TF, Kendig EL, editors: *Disorders of the respiratory tract in children*, Philadelphia: WB Saunders: 1998. pp 485-502.

47. Chin TW, Nussbaum E, Marks M: Bacterial pneumonia. In Hilman BC, editor: *Pediatric respiratory disease, diagnosis, and treatment*, Philadelphia: WB Saunders; 1993. pp 271-281.

48. Swischuk LE, Hayden CK Jr: Viral vs. bacterial pulmonary infections in children (is roentgenographic differentiation possible?), *Pediatr Radiol* 1986;16:278.

49. Overall J: Is it bacterial or viral? Laboratory differentiation, *Pediatr Rev* 1993;14:251.

50. Miller MA, Ben-Ami T, Daum RS: Bacterial pneumonia in neonates and older children. In Taussig LM, Landau LI, editors: *Pediatric respiratory medicine*, St Louis: Mosby: 1999. pp 595-664.

51. Murphy SM, Florman AL: Lung defenses against infection: a clinical correlation, *Pediatrics* 1983;72:1.

52. Fernaldl GW: Infections of the respiratory tract due to Mycoplasma pneumoniae. In Chernick V, Boat TF, Kendig EL, editors: *Disorders of the respiratory tract in children*, Philadelphia: WB Saunders; 1998. pp 526-531.

53. Hailen M: Mycoplasma pneumoniae infections. In Hilman BC, editor: *Pediatric respiratory disease, diagnosis, and treatment*, Philadelphia: WB Saunders; 1993. pp 282-284.

54. Shehab Z: Mycoplasma infections. In Taussig LM, Landau LI, editors: *Pediatric respiratory medicine*, St Louis: Mosby; 1999. pp 737-742.

55. Thom DH et al: *Chlamydia pneumoniae* strain TWAR, *Mycoplasma pneumoniae*, and viral infections in acute respiratory disease in a university student health clinic population, *Am J Epidemiol* 1990;132:248.

56. Atmar RL, Greenberg SB: Pneumonia caused by *Mycoplasma pneumoniae* and the TWAR agent, *Semin Respir Infect* 1989;4:19.

57. Hahn DL, Dodge RW, Golubjatnikov R: Association of Chlamydia pneumoniae (strain TWAR) infection with wheezing, asthmatic bronchitis, and adult-onset asthma, *JAMA* 1991;266:225.

58. Hammerschlag MR: *Chlamydia trachomatis* and *Chlamydia pneumoniae* infections. In Chernick V, Boat TF, Kendig EL, editors: *Disorders of the respiratory tract in children*, Philadelphia: WB Saunders; 1998. pp 978-987.

59. Brook I: Pneumonia in mechanically ventilated children, *Scand J Infect Dis* 1995;27:619.

60. Prekates A et al: The diagnostic value of Gram stain of bronchoalveolar lavage samples in patients with suspected ventilator-associated pneumonia, *Scand J Infect Dis* 1998;30:43.

61. Bergmans DC et al: Reproducibility of quantitative cultures of endotracheal aspirates from mechanically ventilated patients, *J Clin Microbiol* 1997;35:796.

62. Kirton OC et al: A prospective, randomized comparison of an in-line heat moisture exchange filter and

heated wire humidifiers: rates of ventilator-associated early-onset (community-acquired) or late-onset (hospital-acquired) pneumonia and incidence of endotracheal tube occlusion, *Chest* 1997;112:1055.

63. Boots RJ et al: Clinical utility of hygroscopic heat and moisture exchangers in intensive care patients, *Crit Care Med* 1997;25:1707.

64. Long MN et al: Prospective, randomized study of ventilator-associated pneumonia in patients with one versus three ventilator circuit changes per week, *Infect Control Hosp Epidemiol* 1996;17:14.

65. Centers for Disease Control and Prevention: Tuberculosis morbidity — United States, 1997, *Morb Mortal Wkly Rep* 1998;47:253.

66. Nahmias AJ et al: Older and newer challenges of tuberculosis in children, *Pediatr Pulmonol Suppl* 1995;11:28.

67. Inselman LS, Kendig EL: Tuberculosis. In Chernick V, Boat TF, Kendig EL, editors: *Disorders of the respiratory tract in children*, Philadelphia: WB Saunders; 1998. pp 883-919.

68. American Academy of Pediatrics Committee on Infectious Diseases: Update on tuberculosis skin testing of children, *Pediatrics* 1996;97:282.

69. Emboriadou M et al: Human neutrophil elastase in RSV bronchiolitis, *Ann Clin Lab Sci* 2007;37:79.

70. McNamara PS et al: Bronchoalveolar lavage cellularity in infants with severe respiratory syncytial virus bronchiolitis, *Arch Dis Child* 2003;88:922.

71. Chang AB et al: A bronchoscopic scoring system for airway secretions—airway cellularity and microbiological validation, *Pediatr Pulmonol* 2006;41:887.

72. Simpson JL et al: Innate immune activation in neutrophilic asthma and bronchiectasis, *Thorax* 2007;62:211.

73. Sarafidis K et al: Evidence of early systemic activation and transendothelial migration of neutrophils in neonates with severe respiratory distress syndrome, *Pediatr Pulmonol* 2001;31:214.

74. Hussain N et al: Neutrophil apoptosis during the development and resolution of oleic acid-induced acute lung injury in the rat, *Am J Respir Cell Mol Biol* 1998;19:867.

75. Nickerson BG: The lung in sickle cell disease. In Chernick V, Boat TF, Kendig EL, editors: *Disorders of the respiratory tract in children*, Philadelphia.: WB Saunders; 1998. pp 1117-1122.

76. Smith JA: Cardiopulmonary manifestations of sickle cell disease in childhood, *Semin Roentgenol* 1987;22:160.

77. Sprinkle RH et al: Acute chest syndrome in children with sickle cell disease: a retrospective analysis of 100 hospitalized cases, *Am J Pediatr Hematol Oncol* 1986;812:105.

78. Weil JV et al: Pathogenesis of lung disease in sickle hemoglobinopathies, *Am Rev Respir Dis* 1993;148:249.

79. Barrett-Connor E: Pneumonia and pulmonary infarction in sickle cell anemia, *JAMA* 1973;224:997.

80. Powars D et al: Sickle cell chronic lung disease: prior morbidity and the risk of pulmonary failure, *Medicine* 1988;67:66.

81. Bunn HF: Pathogenesis and treatment of sickle cell disease, *N Engl J Med* 1997;337:762.

82. Collins FS, Orringer EP: Pulmonary hypertension and cor pulmonale in the sickle hemoglobinopathies, *Am J Med* 1982;73:814.

83. Pelidis MA et al: Successful treatment of life-threatening acute chest syndrome of sickle cell disease with veno- venous extracorporeal membrane oxygenation, *J Pediatr Hematol Oncol* 1997;19:459.

84. Orenstein SR, Orenstein DM: Gastroesophageal reflux and respiratory disease in children, *J Pediatr* 1988;112:847.

85. Meyers WF et al: Value of tests for evaluation of gastroesophageal reflux in children, *J Pediatr Surg* 1985;20:515.

86. Blister A, Krespi YP, Oppenheimer RW: Surgical management of aspiration, *Otolaryngol Clin North Am* 1988;2:743.

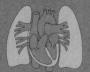

Chapter 33

Asthma

THOMAS J. KALLSTROM • MARIDEE JONES

LEARNING OBJECTIVES

After reading this chapter the reader will be able to:
- Explain the pathophysiology of asthma
- Treat asthma from an evidence-based approach
- Identify the five components of asthma
- Explain how to improve the efficacy of the medications we use to treat asthma

Asthma is the most common chronic childhood disease, affecting more than 20.5 million persons, 6.5 million of whom are children. Approximately 7.7% of children in the United States have asthma. It is the most common reason for pediatric hospitalizations and the most common cause of absence from school. Hospitalization rates have remained stable over the past 10 years but this has not been consistent through all childhood age groups. The highest incidence of asthma occurs in children 4 years of age or younger.[1] While the number of asthma patients has climbed, the death rate is decreasing. Improvements in the science behind asthma care have led to increased awareness among patients and physicians about the disease's underlying causes, but widespread misunderstanding still exists. A survey called *Children and Asthma in America* found

582

that most respondents incorrectly believed that only the symptoms of the disease should be treated as opposed to the underlying cause of the disease. Ninety-three percent of the respondents could not correctly identify inflammation as an underlying cause of asthma attacks, and 90% of the respondents we unable to identify airway constriction as the other main cause (http://www.asthmainamerica.com/widespread.html).

To improve awareness of the causes and treatments of asthma in America, the National Lung Heart and Blood Institute's (NHLBI's) National Asthma Education and Prevention Program (NAEPP) in 1991 released its first set of asthma management guidelines referred to as the Expert Panel Report.[2] This was followed by Expert Panel Report II in 1997[3] and an update of the report on selected items in 2002.[4] In 2007 they released the Expert Panel Report III, which is available to caregivers and patients. The report provides guidelines for management of asthma based on the expert panel review with an emphasis on evidence-based practice of medicine.[5]

PATHOGENESIS OF ASTHMA

Definition

Asthma is defined as a chronic inflammatory disorder of the airways. Many cells and cellular elements play a role in the disease, in particular, mast cells, eosinophils, T lymphocytes, IgE, macrophages, neutrophils, and epithelial cells. In susceptible individuals, this inflammation causes recurrent episodes of wheezing, chest tightness, breathlessness, and coughing, especially at night or in the early morning. These episodes are usually associated with widespread but variable airflow obstruction that is often reversible either spontaneously or with treatment. The inflammation also causes an associated increase in the existing bronchial hyperresponsiveness to a variety of stimuli. A number of factors can play a role in the development of inflammation, including exposure to viruses, allergens, and other occupational irritants. The growing awareness that asthma is not a homogeneous disorder has important implications for how asthma will be diagnosed and managed in the future.

Pathophysiology

Asthma is characterized by chronic airway inflammation, bronchial hyperresponsiveness, and hypersecretion of mucus. Airway obstruction is the consequence of these pathologic mechanisms. There are six significant components to airway obstruction:

1. Inflammation
2. Acute bronchoconstriction
3. Airway edema
4. Mucous plugging
5. Airway hyperresponsiveness
6. Airway remodeling

The obstruction can result in increasingly difficult air entry, air trapping, atelectasis, ventilation-perfusion abnormalities, hypoxia, and hypercarbia. Approaches to therapy are directed toward blocking the inflammation as well as preventing and relieving airway hyperresponsiveness and remodeling.

Airway Inflammation

Our understanding of the pathogenesis of airway inflammation in asthma continues to grow as the function and interaction of inflammatory mediators are revealed. Inflammation results from the introduction and or/activation of specific mediators in the airway. In adult asthma there is evidence that inflammatory findings (e.g., eosinophilic airway inflammation, hypergranulation of mast cells, increased IgE levels, and increased allergic response) are due in part to an inappropriate activation of the CD4+ T cells that result in release of inflammatory cytokines.

In some individuals, primarily adults with asthma, neutrophils appear to be the primary mediator of cytokine release and inflammation. These individuals appear to be less responsive to steroids and bronchodilators and are more likely to experience remodeling of their airways. No matter what the underlying pathology is, inflammation and the resulting swelling of airway mucosa can affect the airway caliber and decreases airflow. We now know that airway inflammation is persistent and that early intervention with anti-inflammatory medications may help to slow the course of the disease, but any successful response usually requires weeks to achieve and in some instances may be incomplete.[6]

The Path of Inflammation in Allergic Asthma

Asthma has been shown to be predominately allergic in nature with 80% of children and more than 50% of adults with asthma.[7] IgE has been identified as a key molecule in mediating allergic asthma. Total serum IgE levels have been shown to have a close association with self-reported asthma.[7]

Allergic disease starts with a sensitization phase in which an allergen on the airway mucosa is processed by an antigen-presenting cell (APC), such as a dendritic cell. The dendritic cell travels to regional lymph nodes and acts as a key antigen-presenting cell, causing the release of interleukins that cause the naïve T cell to differentiate into a Th2 cell. The Th2 cell then releases IL-4, which enhances the production of IgE by stimulating B cells to differentiate into IgE. IL-4 also stimulates the differentiation of more naïve T cells to Th2 to further this process. IgE binds to high- and low-affinity receptors on mast cells, basophils, and eosinophils. These cells contain inflammatory mediators. The IgE produced is specifically sensitive to the allergen (antigen) that started the process. When the allergen is reintroduced into the system, (on mucosa or in the bloodstream), it will bind to the IgE attached to mast cells, eosinophils, and basophils. This will result in cross-linking that causes a calcium influx and resulting degranulation that releases the inflammatory mediators within the cells that cause allergy and asthma symptoms.[8]

There are three phases of inflammation. The first phase involves the preformed mediators that are released with degranulation: histamine, heparin, tryptase. These mediators result in airway smooth muscle contraction, vasodilation, increased vascular permeability, and mucous secretion. The resulting injury to airway cells attracts other mediators such as cytokines (leukotrienes, IL4,5,13, TNF alpha, and eosinophils, to name a few) resulting in a late phase that occurs 4 to 8 hours after the immediate response. Persistent inflammation can lead to a remodeling phase that results in airway smooth muscle hypertrophy, hyperplasia, increased angiogenesis, and collagen deposition.[9] This last phase will result in a decline in lung function and irreversible obstructive lung disease.

The Definition and Role of T Cells: The Th1/Th2 Paradigm

T helper cells, Th1 and Th2, cross-regulate each other and regulate immune responses. There continues to be considerable interest in the role of immune responses in airway inflammation. It has become clear that a bias toward the production of Th2 cells results in increased atopy and asthma. Th2 cells produce IL-4, which enhances IgE synthesis; IL-5, which stimulates eosinophil production; IL-9, which increases mast cell production; and IL-13, which increases mucous production and airway hyper-responsiveness. Th1 cells produce interferon-y and IL-2, which aid in defense of infection. It is believed that a newborn is skewed towards a Th2 response through exposure to infections and other environmental stimuli. When the Th2 response triggers, the Th1 response is activated and a balance between the Th1 and Th2 responses occurs.[10] The "Hygiene Hypothesis" suggests that due to immunizations and increased use of antibiotics, children are not exposed to the stimuli to drive the Th1 response, and the cytokine pattern then favors the Th2 response in susceptible individuals, which will cause the production of more IgE and thus atopy and risk for asthma.

Airway Hyperresponsiveness

Hyperresponsiveness is an exaggerated broncho constricting response to stimuli. The level of hyperresponsiveness is often correlated with the severity of constriction created by a bronchoprovocation test (such as a methacholine challenge). Exposure to certain allergens causes an IgE-dependent release of mediators from the mast cell. These mediators include histamine, tryptase, leukotrienes, and prostaglandins. They directly contract airway smooth muscle, giving rise to acute bronchoconstriction or airway hyperresponsiveness. Other "triggers" of airflow obstruction include aspirin and nonsteroidal antiinflammatory drugs, exercise, cold air, irritants, gastroesophageal reflux, respiratory infections, and psychological stress. When reduction of airway inflammation is achieved, better control of asthma should be expected.

Airway remodeling is the permanent structural change that occurs in the airway. It is associated with progressive loss of lung function and may not be prevented by of fully reversible by current therapeutic interventions.[11] The process of repair and remodeling in the airway are not well understood, but it is certain that these processes are key to explaining why asthma remains persistent and in some cases resistant to therapy. Features of airway remodeling include inflammation, mucous hypersecretion, subepithelial fibrosis, airway smooth muscle hypertrophy, and angiogenesis.[5] Inflammatory mediators stimulate hyperplasia of mucous glands resulting in more and chronic mucous production. The excessive mucus secretion and plugging of the airway may act to reduce the diameter of the airway and further limit airflow. Activation of inflammatory mediators also results in increased vascular permeability and leakage with activation of structural cells such as epithelial tissue, mucous glands, and blood vessels. Repeated inflammatory episodes result in airway mucosa thickening and eventual fibrosis.

RISK FACTORS FOR DEVELOPMENT OF ASTHMA IN CHILDREN

Asthma is a dynamic disease. Its progression will vary over time regardless of the age of the patient. Although the etiology of asthma is not well defined, there appear to be risk factors associated with the its onset and persistence. Asthma is more prevalent in prepubescent boys but more common in girls after puberty. It is more frequent among inner city and African-American and Hispanic children in the United States; however, there is disagreement as to whether racial and ethnic background is a risk factor or if poverty has the greater impact. Currently available data from genetic studies of asthma suggest a strong genetic component. However, the exact mode of inheritance is unknown. Low–birth-weight infants as well as children born to young mothers or mothers who smoke during pregnancy tend to have an increased incidence of asthma. Other theories have emerged to suggest that asthma develops in children when there is a predominant T2 cell response (as opposed to a predominant T1 cell response) when exposed to various triggers. It has been proposed that this shift results from early exposure to certain viruses and/or the lack of exposure to early childhood diseases, as well as from the overuse of antibiotics.

Allergic Response—Atopy

Atopy seems to be the strongest identifiable predisposing factor for developing asthma, with atopic dermatitis often preceding its onset. Infants who become sensitized to food allergens early in life have an increased risk for developing asthma. The majority of children with asthma are atopic, but not all atopic children develop asthma. Inhaled allergens are thought to be the most important factor in the onset of asthma in the child predisposed to atopy.

Environmental Triggers

There are several significant indoor environmental triggers. Once an aggravating agent is identified, it is essential that that the household undergo intervention that could remediate or eliminate it. If the child is sensitive to warm-blooded animals, the suggested interventions include the removal of the pet from the home or, if this is not possible, to keep the bedroom door closed so that the animal does not have access to the child's room.

Tobacco smoke is closely linked with increased asthma prevalence and morbidity and therefore it is important that the patient and others who live in the household refrain from smoking. Smoking cessation measures are suggested. If there are smokers in the home, it is important that all smoking take place outside the home.

Cockroach exposure is another concern that impacts patients who live in the inner city.[12] Cockroach antigens are commonly found in the bedrooms of children who are sensitized. It is important that the family practice a routine that includes not leaving food exposed or the garage opened. Poison baits, boric acid, and traps are also important tools that can reduce or eliminate the cockroach problem. Of course in using these interventions it is important to make sure that the child not be able to access baits or poisons.

Molds are another common trigger in the home. Once identified it is essential the mold be cleaned out

and the area dried. This can be a particular problem in humid environments or where there are plumbing leaks that are left unattended.

House-dust mites are another trigger. To manage this problem it is recommended that the mattresses and pillow be encased with an allergen-impermeable cover. It also is advisable that the bedding be washed in water that is warmer than 130°F. Other suggested steps would be to reduce humidity in the home to less than 40%, remove carpeting from the bedroom, avoid lying on upholstered furniture, and do not carpet over concrete flooring. It is important to not expose stuffed toys to dust but rather keep them covered and consider frequent washing as well. It appears that exposure to any environmental allergen, if it is intense and persistent, may lead to sensitization in atopic children and then be associated with chronic asthma.

Much research has been devoted to the relationship between wheezing illnesses in infants and the development of asthma. Respiratory syncytial virus is the most common viral respiratory tract pathogen isolated from infants who wheeze. Many of these infants with severe infection with respiratory syncytial virus develop recurrent wheezing and asthma later in life.

NATIONAL ASTHMA EDUCATION AND PREVENTION PROGRAM GUIDELINES

Purpose

The National Asthma Education and Prevention Program (NAEPP) was formed by the National Institutes of Health in the late 1980s to assist in the promotion of asthma education to the public, the health care professional, and the patient. The most significant undertaking of this organization has been the development and dissemination of the *Expert Panel Report 3: Guidelines for the Diagnosis and Management of Asthma,* also known as "The Asthma Guidelines." Because of ongoing changes in the diagnosis and treatment of asthma, particularly in the pharmacologic care, an updated set of guidelines has been published every 5 years. The recommendations in the latest version are also evidence based, which allows for a document that has been under the scrutiny of the Expert Panel. All sets of guidelines have been written by a science-based committee of experts from all medical disciplines, all based in the United States.

The stated purpose of the guidelines is to serve as a comprehensive tool in the diagnosis and management of asthma. The NAEPP states that the report, which is not an official regulatory document, should serve as a guide, and that a patient's specific history must be considered when implementing its guidelines. In spite of

Box 33-1   Goals of Asthma Management

1. Prevent chronic asthma symptoms and minimize asthma exacerbations, using the least aggressive therapy that is sufficient.
2. Maintain normal activity levels including exercise and other physical activities; avoid missing school activities.
3. Maintain normal or near-normal pulmonary function.
4. Prevent recurrent asthma exacerbations and minimize the need for emergency department visits or hospitalizations.
5. Provide optimal pharmacotherapy with minimal or no adverse effects.
6. Meet patient's and family's expectations of and satisfaction with asthma care received.

massive public promotion directed to the medical community, the response has to the report has been mixed. Disagreement by primary care physicians with components of the guidelines has often led to poor compliance, whereas still other physicians remain unfamiliar with the guidelines. Asthma specialists tend to be more familiar with the guidelines and receptive their use. Getting the guidelines into the hands of all providers who interact with asthma patients and influencing them to utilize the guidelines to guide therapy remains the goal of the NAEPP. It is also essential that the clinician, patient, and family members understand and abide by the goals of optimal management (Box 33-1).

DIAGNOSIS

Children who present with chronic or episodic cough, wheezing, difficulty breathing, or chest tightness may have asthma. The diagnosis of asthma cannot be established until alternative diagnoses are excluded. There should be evidence of airflow obstruction that is at least partially reversible and episodic symptoms of airflow limitation or airway hyperresponsiveness. The NAEPP guidelines recommend a detailed medical history, physical examination, and spirometry to determine reversible disease. It is also important to determine the severity, control, and responsiveness to therapy to determine the patient's current asthma status. Once a diagnosis has been made, it is important that the clinician use methods (e.g., testing for allergies and determining IgE levels) to identify precipitating factors.

Medical History

A detailed medical history is essential in identifying the symptoms, triggers, and severity of asthma. A diagnostic history includes recurrent wheezing, chest tightness, shortness of breath, and cough, with nocturnal symptoms being common. Symptoms that occur or worsen with various stimuli (e.g., allergens, respiratory infections, emotional expressions, menses, viral infection, exercise, weather changes) or follow a seasonal pattern are highly suggestive of asthma.

A thorough history includes descriptions and frequency of previous exacerbations, hospitalizations, number of emergency department visits or unscheduled office visits, amount of school missed because of symptoms, and response to previous therapy. It is also important to determine if symptoms are episodic or persistent. A history of allergic disorders (including family history), premature birth, and sinus and respiratory infections is often linked to asthma.

Physical Examination

A physical examination of the upper respiratory tract, chest, and skin is essential for the diagnosis of asthma, as well as to rule out another disorder. However, examinations may be completely normal between acute exacerbations, and the medical history is a stronger factor in supporting a diagnosis of asthma. Symptomatic children may present with audible wheezing and prolonged expiration, cough, increased nasal secretions, hyperexpansion of the thorax, retractions, use of accessory muscles, and tachypnea. Examination of the upper airways may show evidence of allergic disease (e.g., allergic shiners, edematous nasal mucosa, postnasal drip). Atopic dermatitis is typical in the presentation of asthma; however, digital clubbing is rarely found in asthma and raises the suspicion of cystic fibrosis. Many physical examination findings lead to consideration of a diagnosis other than asthma.

Pulmonary Function Testing

Pulmonary function testing is used to help confirm the diagnosis of asthma, estimate the severity of airway inflammation, and follow the response to changes in therapy.[13] Because all pulmonary function tests are essentially effort dependent, children must be old enough to correctly perform the test and provide maximum effort. Some children can perform an acceptable expiratory maneuver at 4 years of age, whereas others are unable to accomplish this until they are 7 or 8 years of age. If effort and/or technique is poor, results are not helpful in diagnosis or treatment of asthma and should not be used.

Typical spirometry measurements in the diagnosis of asthma include the total volume of air exhaled forcefully from a maximal inhalation (forced vital capacity, FVC), the volume of air exhaled during the first second of the FVC (forced expiratory volume in 1 second, FEV_1), and the FEV_1/FVC ratio. Other measurements, including the flow in the middle portion of the FVC

(FEF_{25-75}), are often reported. The FEF_{25-75} is also known as the maximum midexpiratory flow. It is sensitive to small changes in airway caliber and also decreases with increasing obstructive disease; however, it is highly variable. Airway obstruction is indicated when the FEV_1 is less than 80% of the predicted value and FEV_1/FVC values are less than 65% (or below the lower limit of normal).

The diagnosis of asthma requires that the airway obstruction be reversible. Spirometry measurements are performed before and after inhalation of a short-acting bronchodilator (e.g., albuterol). Significant reversibility is established when there is a greater than 12% increase in the postbronchodilator FEV_1 measurement.[14]

Pulmonary function tests are performed at the time of initial diagnosis and after treatment has been initiated or changed. It is also performed periodically to document optimal pulmonary function values. If the patient demonstrates deterioration in pulmonary status, additional testing is warranted. It is recommended that children who require long-term control medication for asthma are capable of performing the tests have pulmonary function tests performed at least annually.

Bronchoprovocational Challenges

Airway responsiveness can be assessed using pharmacologic (histamine, methacholine) and nonpharmacologic (exercise, cold air hyperventilation) challenges. Methacholine and histamine are the most common pharmacologic agents used for bronchoprovocational challenge. The challenge is performed in a medical facility with a physician and resuscitative equipment present.

Methacholine Challenge

During a methacholine challenge, carefully increased doses of methacholine are nebulized and delivered directly to the patient through a face mask or mouthpiece. The patient's FEV_1 is measured after inhalation of each concentration until there is a 20% decrease in the FEV_1 or until all nine concentrations have been delivered. A 20% decrease in the FEV_1 is considered a positive challenge. This demonstrates the presence of bronchial hyperresponsiveness and is highly associated with asthma. When the test is completed, the bronchoconstriction may be relieved with inhalation of a quick-relief bronchodilator.

Methacholine challenge is safe and reproducible in children. However, it is recommended that the patient's FEV_1 be greater than 70% predicted before performing the challenge.[15] Patients with well-documented asthma should not be challenged. A negative bronchoprovocational challenge may be useful in ruling out asthma.

Exercise Challenge

Exercise tolerance tests are performed using a variety of forms of exercise, including treadmill running, free running, and bicycle ergometry. Most children are exercised until their heart rate reaches at least 170 beats per minute or more than 85% of the predicted maximum heart rate for their sex and age for 5 to 8 minutes. The FEV_1 is measured immediately after and at 5-minute intervals for 20 to 30 minutes after exercise has stopped. A decrease in the FEV_1 of 15% or more from the pretest baseline indicates a positive response and exercise-induced bronchospasm (EIB).[16] When comparing the results of exercise challenge with the pharmacologic challenges, exercise testing has been observed to be less sensitive and a poorer screening test for bronchial hyperresponsiveness.[17]

Differential Diagnosis

Asthma is the most common cause of recurrent or persistent wheezing, cough, and dyspnea in children. However, several diseases and conditions produce similar signs and symptoms and may simulate an asthma exacerbation. Whether it is the first exacerbation for the child or further assessment of the "difficult-to-manage" asthmatic, other causes of wheezing and airway obstruction must be considered. This is of particular importance in the infant and young child whose small airways are more easily obstructed.[18] The differential diagnosis of conditions that cause wheezing and airway obstruction varies with the age of the child. A thorough history, including response to prior treatment, physical examination, and data from additional tests, can help differentiate other disorders. Box 33-2 lists respiratory conditions that can present with asthmalike symptoms.

MANAGEMENT OF ASTHMA

After the diagnosis of asthma has been made, the NAEPP guidelines suggest a stepwise approach to classifying the severity of asthma and initiating treatment. For classifications beyond mild asthma, daily control medication is recommended and the amount of medication is increased, described as a "step up," as the need for treatment increases. When the asthma is under control, the amount of medication is decreased and described as a "step down." The treatment prescribed is determined by classification of disease severity. Although asthma morbidity and mortality has increased in the United States, for most children with asthma proper disease management helps to provide a normal lifestyle.

The pharmacologic management of asthma requires the use of long-term control and short-term relief medications. Identification, avoidance, and control of factors that worsen asthma symptoms are as essential to

Box 33-2	Respiratory Conditions That Mimic Asthma

- Upper airway disorders
- Allergic rhinitis and sinusitis
- Vocal cord dysfunction
- Tonsillar/adenoid hypertrophy
- Laryngeal web
- Laryngeal papillomatosis
- Laryngotracheomalacia
- Tracheobronchomalacia
- Tracheoesophageal fistula
- Subglottic stenosis
- Tracheal stenosis
- Bronchial stenosis
- Vascular ring
- Enlarged lymph nodes or tumor
- Foreign body aspiration
- Lower airway disorders
- Acute viral bronchiolitis
- Bronchiolitis obliterans
- Bronchopulmonary dysplasia
- Cystic fibrosis
- Primary ciliary dyskinesia
- Mediastinal cysts or tumors
- Pulmonary embolism
- Aspiration syndromes
- Aspiration bronchitis
- Aspiration pneumonia
- Gastroesophageal reflux
- Hypersensitivity pneumonitis
- Allergic bronchopulmonary aspergillosis
- Cardiac disease
- Large left-to-right shunts
- Congestive heart failure
- Cardiomyopathy
- Myocarditis
- Hysterical symptoms
- Psychogenic cough
- Hyperventilation syndrome

asthma management as the use of medication. The regular monitoring and assessment of asthma severity have been proven to aid in control of the disease. Finally, management of a chronic illness such as asthma requires patient and family involvement in developing a treatment plan and in understanding the illness.

Pharmacologic Therapy
Long-Term Control Medications
Pharmacologic management involves using medications to control and relieve symptoms. Any medication that is taken to provide ongoing control of asthma is classified as a long-term control medication. Long-term control medications are taken daily to achieve and maintain control of persistent asthma.

Antiinflammatory agents. Antiinflammatory agents are still considered the most effective long-term treatment for chronic inflammation in asthma. They block late phase reaction to allergens, reduce airway hyperresponsiveness, and inhibit antiinflammatory cell migration and activation.[5] They are considered first-line antiinflammatory agents for children with mild to moderate asthma. Although the potency of their antiinflammatory activity is less documented than that of inhaled corticosteroids, they have few adverse effects.[19]

Inhaled corticosteroids are the most consistently effective controller medication for asthma and are considered first-line therapy for its treatment. Their advantage over oral corticosteroids is that they are clinically effective without having significant side effects. Oral corticosteroid-dependent patients have been able to decrease or discontinue their use of oral corticosteroids when appropriate inhaled corticosteroid therapy is initiated.

Although there is much less risk of developing adverse events with inhaled compared with systemic corticosteroids, the potential for side effects remains. Dysphonia, voice change, reflex cough, and oral candidiasis occur most often with higher doses, although these manifestations can occur at any dose. Use of spacers or holding chambers along with rinsing after inhalation may reduce these effects. Questions remain about the clinical significance of all side effects, particularly concern regarding growth suppression in children. Until more data are obtained, the NAEPP guidelines recommend that children be maintained on the lowest dose of inhaled corticosteroid tolerated with close monitoring of linear growth and development.

Systemic or oral corticosteroids are often required during an asthma exacerbation. However, daily or every-other-day use, along with high doses of an inhaled corticosteroid, is necessary in some patients with very severe disease. The side effects of long-term, regular use of systemic corticosteroids are significant and are listed in Box 33-3. Once asthma control is achieved, efforts are made to wean the patient from oral corticosteroids.

Long-acting β2-agonists. Salmeterol and formoterol are long-acting inhaled β_2-agonists (LABAs) available in the United States. Salmeterol is available alone as a dry-powder discus. It is also available in a dry-powder discus in combination with the corticosteroid fluticasone. Formoterol is available in a dry-powder inhaler device alone and as combination therapy and most recently in a liquid form for nebulization. The biggest difference between the two long-acting bronchodilators is their onset of action. Salmeterol can take from 30 minutes to 90 minutes to have peak effect while formoterol begins to work in 3 to 5 minutes. Evidence on the use of LABAs in asthma has demonstrated that the addition

Box 33-3 — Side Effects of Long-Term Use of Systemic Corticosteroids

- Adrenal suppression
- Growth suppression
- Muscle myopathy
- Aseptic hip necrosis
- Hyperglycemia
- Increased risk of infection
- Skin atrophy and striae
- Psychological disturbances
- Easy bruising
- Fluid retention
- Hypertension
- Osteoporosis
- Peptic ulcer
- Cataracts
- Acne
- Weight gain
- Obesity
- Hirsutism
- Glaucoma
- "Moon" facies
- "Buffalo hump"

of LABAs to treatment of asthma not well controlled on low- or medium-dose inhaled corticosteroids improves lung function and decreases symptoms more effectively than the use of ICS therapy alone.[5] Concerns were raised regarding the use of these medications when a large clinical trial comparing daily salmeterol with placebo added to usual asthma therapy demonstrated an increased risk of asthma-related deaths in those on salmeterol.[20] This resulted in the FDA placing a black box warning on all asthma mediations containing an LABA. These studies resulted in the Expert Panel-3 recommending that the option of increasing the ICS dose be given equal weight to the decision to add an LABA for uncontrolled asthma symptoms. It is also not recommended that LABAs be used in the treatment of acute asthma symptoms or as monotherapy for long-term control.

Methylxanthines. Although theophylline was at one time a prominent component of daily asthma treatment, its role has changed dramatically over the past 10 years. It is listed as an alternative, but not preferred, adjunct therapy to ICS. With the current focus on anti-inflammatory therapy for asthma, along with its narrow therapeutic window and need for close monitoring of serum levels, theophylline has limited use in the pharmacologic management of asthma in children.

Leukotriene modifiers. Leukotrienes are potent proinflammatory mediators that promote bronchospasm, mucus production, and airway edema. Leukotriene modifiers are the first new class of medicines for asthma treatment in 20 years. Leukotriene action is modified by agents that either inhibit production of the leukotrienes or block their action. These agents are still relatively new, and studies are needed to determine their role in pediatric asthma care.

Zileuton is the only approved agent that inhibits the production of the leukotrienes; however, suggested dosing is four times daily and there have been reports of elevated results of liver function tests in patients taking the medication. Therefore it has a limited role in pediatric asthma care. The Expert Panel Report recommends that this classification of medication be considered as an alternative but not a preferred therapy in the management of mild persistent asthma. It does recommend its use as an adjunct therapy with inhaled corticosteroids for patients 12 years of age and over.[5]

Cromolyn sodium and nedocromil. Stabilized mast cells can interfere with chloride channel function. They are used as alternative, but not preferred. They can also be used as preventive treatment before exercise or unavoidable exposure to known allergens.[5]

Immunomodulators. Omalizumab, the only drug that specifically binds circulating IgE, is indicated for the moderate to severe asthmatic over 12 years of age with a positive skin test or positive in vitro test for aeroallergens, a quantitative IgE level between 30 and 700 IU/L and who is not controlled on ICS therapy. Omalizumab is dosed based on the quantitative IgE level and the person's weight. Injections of 150 to 375 mg are given subcutaneously 1 to 2 times monthly. Omalizumab can significantly reduce exacerbations in the patient with atopic asthma.[21]

Quick-relief Medications

Medications in the quick-relief category are short-acting β_2-agonists, anticholinergic agents, and systemic corticosteroids. These medications are used to relieve acute airway obstruction. All patients with asthma need a quick-relief medication, preferably a short-acting β_2-agonist, to take as needed for acute symptoms.

Short-acting β-agonists. With a rapid onset of action of 5 to 15 minutes and a 4- to 6-hour duration of action, these agents are the treatment of choice for acute episodes of bronchospasm. They are often referred to as "rescue" medications and are most effective when inhaled. They are used only on an as-needed basis and not as part of the regularly scheduled medication regimen. Increased use of these agents, particularly using more than one canister per month, is an indication of inadequate asthma control and increasing severity. The most common side effects are tremor, palpitations, and tachycardia. Although acute respiratory symptoms are relieved, short-acting β_2-agonists have no antiinflammatory action. They are used to prevent EIB.

Anticholinergics. Ipratropium bromide is the anticholinergic agent approved for use in the United States. It is available alone in a metered-dose inhaler and nebulizer formulation. Given alone, it is a less potent bronchodilator than short-acting β_2-agonists. The combination of ipratropium bromide and albuterol is marketed in a metered-dose inhaler and a nebulizer unit-dose preparation.

Systemic corticosteroids. Patients with acute exacerbations often receive 3- to 10-day bursts of prednisone or methylprednisolone. The bursts are primarily used to hasten recovery and prevent recurrence of symptoms. The dose of corticosteroid is tapered as symptoms resolve. However, if the symptoms return within 1 month or if the bursts are frequently required, changes are likely required in the long-term control medication regimen.

Delivery Systems

Asthma medications are usually given through inhalation in an aerosol form. The medications are administered by a metered-dose inhaler, by a dry-powder inhaler, or by nebulization. The majority of propellants that power the metered-dose inhalers utilize chlorofluorocarbons, chemicals that have been found to contribute to depletion of the ozone. Manufacturers of metered-dose inhalers are actively replacing propellants in accordance with the Montreal Protocol timelines.

Spacers and valved holding chambers are simple, inexpensive tools that have been developed to use with metered-dose inhalers. Their purpose is threefold:
1. to slow aerosol velocity
2. to minimize particle impaction in the oropharynx
3. to enhance deposition in the lower respiratory tract.

Their use in children is recommended to reduce the problem of coordinating actuation of the metered-dose inhaler with the inhalation. Studies have demonstrated that the decrease in pharyngeal deposition results in improved drug efficacy and reduction in local side effects. It is imperative that patients along with parents or caregivers are instructed in the proper use of all inhalers, nebulizers, masks, and spacers or valved holding chambers.

Control of Asthma Triggers

Most children with asthma have an allergic component to their disease. If asthma is to be managed adequately, the allergens and irritants that worsen symptoms must be identified and controlled. The most common allergens implicated in chronic asthma are listed in Box 33-4. Exposure to allergens and irritants may significantly increase bronchial hyperresponsiveness, whereas reduced exposure to allergens can decrease asthma symptoms.

Box 33-4	Allergens Associated With Asthma

- House dust mite
- Pet allergen
- Cat
- Dog
- Guinea pig
- Rabbit
- Rodent
- Rat
- Mouse
- Cockroach
- Indoor mold
- *Aspergillus*
- *Penicillium*
- Outdoor mold
- *Alternaria*
- *Cladosporium*

Identification of Allergens

Because childhood asthma is often exacerbated by allergen exposure, it is helpful to identify the allergens. Allergy skin testing, along with a thorough history and physical examination, is one method an allergist uses to determine which allergens may be aggravating a child's asthma. Another common test used to determine what allergens are responsible for allergic disease is the radioallergosorbent (RAST) test.

Avoidance and Control Measures

It is nearly impossible for a child with asthma to avoid exposure to all offending allergens and irritants. But it is possible to minimize exposure to them. This begins with teaching the child and family to recognize the triggers and use measures to control and avoid them. Box 33-5 lists control measures for environmental factors that often exacerbate asthma in children.

Role of Immunotherapy

Allergen avoidance can produce changes in asthma disease activity and bronchial hyperresponsiveness, but often there are no practical means for avoiding exposure to all allergens. Allergen immunotherapy, or "allergy shots," should be considered for asthma patients when
1. there is clear evidence of a relationship between asthma symptoms and allergen exposure
2. the patient is symptomatic during a major portion of the year
3. symptoms are difficult to control with pharmacologic therapy.

The value of immunotherapy in children with asthma remains controversial.[22,23] Evidence suggests that it can

Box 33-5 — Environmental Control Measures

HOUSE DUST MITE
- Kill with hot water (>130°F) and dry cleaning
- Enforce bedroom dust control
- Encase pillows, mattresses, and box springs in zippered allergen-impermeable covers
- Wash sheets and blankets weekly in hot water
- Replace wool bedding with cotton or synthetics
- Avoid feather or down bedding
- Remove stuffed toys, wall hangings, and other "dust-catchers"
- Hot-water wash or freeze stuffed toys weekly
- Vacuum/dust weekly wearing mask; vacuum with double-thick bag and HEPA filter
- Keep heat, ventilation, and air conditioner filters clean
- Remove carpeting; wash rugs; avoid heavy curtains and blinds
- Keep clothing in closets with doors closed
- Clean with damp cloths
- Reduce indoor humidity
- Replace upholstered furniture with wood, vinyl, or leather

ANIMAL DANDER
- Remove animal from house or restrict animal to washable area (may take 4 to 6 months to remove cat allergen)
- Banish animal from bedroom
- Close bedroom door and vents
- Use HEPA or electrostatic filter in bedroom
- Remove carpets and minimize upholstered furniture and other allergen reservoirs

COCKROACH
- Hire professional exterminator
- Use poison baits
- Store food and garbage in sealed containers
- Perform meticulous regular cleaning
- Eat only in kitchen/dining room

INDOOR MOLD
- Kitchen, bathroom, and basement are most common sites
- Leaky pipes, shower curtains, refrigerator drip pans, garbage pails, and window edgings are major sources
- Wrap plumbing to eliminate condensation
- Use commercial fungicides and bleach solution
- Reduce humidity to less than 45% with dehumidifiers, air conditioning, and increased ventilation
- Avoid humidifiers and vaporizers
- Close windows, especially in bedroom
- Remove moldy items
- Repair water leaks
- Dry clothing/shoes before placing in closet
- Limit houseplants and remove them from bedroom
- Avoid live Christmas trees

NONALLERGEN IRRITANTS
- Avoid tobacco smoke and passive smoke in the home and closed car
- Avoid wood stoves, kerosene heaters, cleaning products, and perfumes

be safely given to children with asthma and that life-threatening reactions are uncommon when the process is prescribed and supervised by an appropriately trained physician. However, the risk of anaphylaxis remains and the injections must be administered in a health care facility where personnel, medication, and emergency equipment are immediately available to treat a systemic reaction. The patient waits 20 to 30 minutes after each injection because this is the interval of highest risk for a systemic reaction. It is also suggested that the immunotherapy be delayed when the child has an acute illness or asthma exacerbation. Allergen immunotherapy is typically given every 7 to 28 days for 3 to 5 years, with a positive effect often seen within 1 year of therapy.

Peak Flow Monitoring

Using a peak flow meter to monitor peak expiratory flow rates (PEFR) is an important tool in asthma management when it is accompanied by a written action plan. It can be performed in children as young as 3 to 4 years old. Monitoring assists children and parents or caregivers in recognizing changes in respiratory status, affording them the chance to make necessary interventions.

Peak Flow Meter

The peak flow meter is a comparatively inexpensive monitoring tool that measures the PEFR (Figure 33-1). It is used only for ongoing monitoring and not to diagnose asthma. Different brands of peak flow meters are available, and it is possible to get a slightly different peak flow value when using a different meter. Because there is variation between different brands, it is important to use the same peak flow meter or model for long-term monitoring.[24] Box 33-6 lists the steps in performing a peak flow maneuver. Patients are asked to bring their peak flow meter to their physician's office to check the

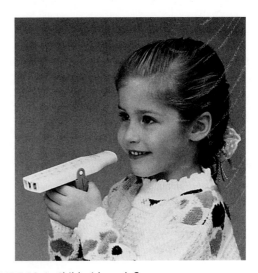

FIGURE 33-1 Child with peak flow meter.

Box 33-6	How To Use a Peak Flow Meter

1. Make sure the meter reads zero or the indicator is at the bottom of the numbered scale.
2. Stand up (unless there is a physical disability). Remove any food or gum from your mouth.
3. Take as deep a breath as possible, filling your lungs completely.
4. Place the meter in your mouth, behind your teeth, and close your lips around the mouthpiece. Do not let your tongue block the mouthpiece.
5. Blow out as hard and as fast as you can in a single blow. Do not cough into the meter.
6. The force of your breath moves the indicator on the peak flow meter. The number opposite the indicator is your peak flow.
7. Write down the peak flow number obtained.
8. Repeat the steps two additional times. Record the highest of the three attempts (not the average) in your diary or on your peak flow chart.

Box 33-7	Traffic Light Zone System

- Green Zone: Peak expiratory flow is greater than 80% of personal best number
- Good control of asthma is indicated.
- Patient is relatively symptom-free.
- Quick-relief medication is not indicated.
- Long-term–control medication is only medication indicated.
- If peak flow is constantly in the Green Zone with minimal variation, the physician may consider changing or decreasing daily medication.

YELLOW ZONE: PEAK EXPIRATORY FLOW IS 50% TO 80% OF PERSONAL BEST NUMBER
- "Cautious" zone; asthma is worsening.
- There is less than optimal control of asthma.
- Asthma symptoms may be increased, with awakening at night.
- Quick-relief medication is needed (usually a short-acting β2-agonist).
- Increase in daily maintenance therapy may be needed.

RED ZONE: PEAK EXPIRATORY FLOW IS LESS THAN 50% OF PERSONAL BEST NUMBER
- "Danger" zone; exacerbation is severe.
- Asthma is poorly controlled.
- Asthma symptoms are serious and possibly life threatening.
- Immediate intervention is required (usually a short-acting β2-agonist).
- Depending on physician's direction and patient's response to quick-relief medication, patient may be directed to seek emergency care.

accuracy of the meter as well as to recheck for proper technique. When a quick-relief medication is taken because of an increase in asthma symptoms, it is suggested that a peak flow reading be obtained before and after taking the medication.

Peak Flow Diary

Keeping a diary or chart of the readings is for many patients an important part of their treatment plan. Graphs for plotting peak flows are often included with the peak flow meter and can be photocopied for additional use. With daily peak flow monitoring, a patient may see a drop in the peak flow before severe symptoms are felt and may begin early treatment or seek medical help. This may prevent asthma exacerbations from occurring or lessen the seriousness of an episode by medicating at the first sign of low peak flow readings. The physician reviews the peak flow diary at each office visit.

Personal Best Reading

There are predicted "normal" peak flow values that are determined by height, age, gender, and race. However, it is necessary to determine a child's "personal best" peak flow reading. This is defined as simply the highest or best measurement obtained when the patient is free of symptoms and asthma is under control. To determine the personal best reading, the patient records peak flow readings at least once a day for 2 to 3 weeks. The best peak flow reading will usually occur in the early afternoon.

Peak Flow Zone System

Once a patient's personal best peak flow has been established, every effort is made to maintain the peak flow values within 80% of this number. One peak flow monitoring system uses a zone system to indicate asthma severity and to guide a patient to an appropriate response. As illustrated in Box 33-7, green, yellow, and red zones are established. The zones are broad guidelines designed to simplify asthma management.

Asthma Action Plan

The physician provides a written management plan, or action plan (Figure 33-2), with information that the patient can immediately refer to should the patient become symptomatic. No action plan should be developed without the physician's input. Based on the patient's current peak flow reading and the personal best number, the plan provides the patient with appropriate actions to take when the peak flow values drop. Included are detailed instructions specifying when to begin quick-relief medications, when to increase daily medications, and when to contact a physician or seek emergency care. Also identified are the specific medications to be given, the route of administration, the

Name: _____ No. _____
Date: _____

ASTHMA ACTION PLAN USING YOUR PEAK FLOW READINGS

Know your zone. Measure your peak flow every _____ and anytime you need to know your zone.

GREEN ZONE: You are in the **GREEN** zone if your reading is at least _____ (>80% personal best).
       Green zone means GO. No sign of cough, wheeze, or chest tightness.

Take these medications daily: How much   When to take

1. _____   _____   _____
2. _____   _____   _____
3. _____   _____   _____
4. _____   _____   _____
5. _____   _____   _____

Take ___ puffs of _____ before you exercise, if needed for exercise-induced asthma.

YELLOW ZONES: (50%-80% of personal best). You may have increased asthma symptoms,
       awakening at night with asthma, or inability to do your normal activities.

    HIGH YELLOW ZONE: Your peak flow is between _____ and _____.
- Take _____ puffs of _____ (quick relief medicine) or an updraft treatment. * Repeat every _____ hours until in the Green zone.
- Take _____ puffs of _____ (antiinflammatory medicine). Repeat every _____ hours until in the Green zone. Then return to your Green zone dose.

    LOW YELLOW ZONE: Your peak flow is between _____ and _____. Follow this plan if the peak flow does not reach **High** Yellow Zone within 15 minutes after taking inhaled quick-relief medicine or updraft treatment, or drops back into Low Yellow Zone within 4 hours.
- Continue _____ puffs of _____ (quick relief medicine) or an updraft treatment every _____ hours.*
- Add oral steroids** _____. Continue _____ mg/day for _____ days or till in Green Zone for 24 hours.
- Contact your doctor to report persistent low readings or use of oral steroids.

**If your condition does not improve within 2 days after starting oral steroids, contact your doctor again.

RED ZONE: Your peak flow reading is below _____. (< 50% personal best).
       Red zone means STOP. Your asthma symptoms are serious.
- Take _____ puffs of _____ (quick relief medicine) or an updraft treatment.*
- Take oral steroids _____ mg immediately
- If your peak flow does **not** reach the **low yellow zone** in 15 minutes after taking your quick-relief medicine or drops back into the Red zone in 4 hours, contact your doctor or go to the emergency room.

---

*Always measure your peak flow 15 minutes after taking your quick-relief medicine.

FIGURE 33-2 Example of an asthma action plan.

dose to be administered, and the frequency of dosing. Reminders to recheck the peak flow reading are included. It is helpful to have the physician's name and phone number on the plan along with the phone number of a close relative or neighbor.

Patients are instructed to take the action plan and peak flow meter with them when traveling. If the patient attends school, a copy of the plan is provided for the school to be used by the teacher or school nurse in the event of an exacerbation or to prevent EIB while at school.

Patient and Family Education

For any asthma disease management program to be successful there must be an active partnership between patients, their families, and health care providers. This partnership is critical when the patient has a chronic disease such as asthma. Patient and family education begins at diagnosis and is a continual process, with the ultimate goal being to improve self-management.

It is unlikely that the patient's physician has the time to devote to a complete regimen of education; therefore, all members of the health care team need to work together to reinforce the same message. It is recommended that clinicians teach patients and families the essential information concerning the disease process, medication skills, self-monitoring techniques, and environmental controls.

A successful partnership keeps the lines of communication open. Asking open-ended questions can lead to the patient and family being freer in discussing concerns, fears, and expectations regarding asthma care. Perception of the disease and beliefs about treatment are influenced by earlier experience with the disease, education, personality characteristics, socioeconomic and cultural background, and the available support systems.[25] It is important to be sensitive to the cultural background of the patient and family. Ethnic beliefs can often affect the way the patient and family view asthma and its treatment. For example, some cultures view an illness as either a "hot" or a "cold" disease. Many in the Hispanic population believe that asthma should be treated with a "hot" remedy such as hot tea. Often there is no harm in the belief; however, there may be times when the clinician must intercede in the interest of patient safety.

Asthma Disease Process

Key points concerning the disease process include a basic understanding of what asthma is and what can trigger asthma episodes. Often drawings of a normal airway contrasted to that of one with asthma helps patients visualize what is occurring in their own lungs.

Medication Skills

It is imperative that patients (depending on age) and families understand the names of their medication, proper dosing, when and how to take each medication, and the side effects of each. Providing written instructions for each medication assists in understanding and adherence to the treatment regimen. Proper inhaler technique is taught and then reviewed at each subsequent physician visit. It is stressed that the long-term control medications are preventive in nature and are to be taken even if the patient is symptom free. Patients often discontinue use of their controller medications, only to develop an asthma exacerbation within 3 to 4 weeks.

Identification and Control of Triggers

Patients and their families need information to discern what triggers their asthma as well as ways to avoid the triggers. Although all triggers may not be totally avoidable, the patient and family are urged to take all necessary measures to avoid them and learn to monitor which variables influence their symptoms.

Self-Monitoring Techniques

Patients must learn to monitor and recognize signs and symptoms of worsening asthma. Education in the proper use of a peak flow meter and how to follow an asthma action plan is an essential component of asthma education. Reinforcing appropriate behavior includes reviewing peak flow monitoring, inhaler technique, and implementation of the action plan. Review of the action plan at each visit has been shown to improve patient compliance and decrease the chance for confusion.

MANAGING ASTHMA EXACERBATIONS IN THE EMERGENCY DEPARTMENT

Patients presenting to the emergency department have often had previous emergency admissions and hospitalizations for treatment of severe asthma. Often these patients have no primary care physician and rely on symptomatic control and emergency departments as their primary source of medical care. Along with inadequate use of corticosteroids, these characteristics are associated with an increased risk for fatal asthma.[26]

Assessment

The intensity and progression of the asthma exacerbation can vary and will determine the intensity of treatment in the emergency department. It is essential that a primary classification of severity be determined in the emergency department. On admission, a physical examination is performed along with measurement of oxygenation and air flow. A pulse oximeter is used to measure oxygen saturation. Continuous monitoring of oxygen with a pulse oximeter is crucial in order to prevent desaturation.

A peak flow meter or spirometer can provide assessment of the severity of airway obstruction from inflammation and bronchospasm. If a child who normally uses a peak flow meter is unable to perform the maneuver during an attack, severe air flow obstruction is considered and intensive medical therapy is indicated. Peak flow measurements are taken before and 5 to 15 minutes after β_2-agonist therapy.

β_2-Agonists

One of the first lines of therapy is with β_2-agonist agents, such as albuterol or levalbuterol. The EPR-3 recommends that the patient receive three treatments given every 20 to 30 minutes by either nebulization or MDI. If there is an inadequate response to this, continuous nebulization of albuterol may be initiated. In severe exacerbation the addition of ipratropium bromide to β_2-agonists should be considered. Adverse effects typically seen with the use of β_2-agonists, such as tremor, tachycardia, and nervousness, are often pronounced, and some patients may not want to take the treatment because of this response.[27]

Corticosteroids

It is critical that corticosteroids be given to treat the inflammation that occurs during an acute exacerbation. Early treatment, which may include the use of intravenous corticosteroids, is effective in preventing an increase in the severity of symptoms and may avoid hospitalization and relapses.[28] Because intravenous lines are uncomfortable and can be difficult to place in a child, studies have investigated the use of oral corticosteroids in the emergency setting.[29,30] If the child cannot adequately be given oral then corticosteroids, the intravenous route should be considered. Consideration of other adjunct interventions in severe exacerbation should be considered as well. These include intravenous magnesium sulfate or heliox.[5]

HOSPITALIZATION AND RESPIRATORY FAILURE

Regardless of the care given in the emergency department, some children will not respond adequately and will require hospitalization. Criteria for hospitalization vary; however, continuing deterioration or failure to improve with therapy is an indication for intensive monitoring and treatment. Box 33-8 lists criteria considered for hospitalization.

Intubation

If all attempts to reverse bronchospasm and improve air flow are futile, careful consideration is given to intubation and mechanical ventilation. Diligent patient monitoring is essential, and immediate steps are taken once the patient demonstrates respiratory muscle fatigue or failure.

It is best to intubate on a semielective basis rather than in an emergent situation, and the clinician most experienced in managing pediatric airways should perform it. Intubation is attempted only under controlled settings with continuous cardiorespiratory monitoring and resuscitation equipment and medication available. Once intubated and stabilized, the patient is monitored in a pediatric intensive care unit, which may mean transporting the child to another medical facility.

Mechanical Ventilation

After intubation, the child is mechanically ventilated with low tidal volumes without positive end-expiratory pressure (PEEP) because the lungs are hyperinflated and there is a degree of auto-PEEP present. The mode of ventilation and set respiratory rate is determined according to the patient's degree of sedation, peak inspiratory pressures generated, oxygenation, and acceptable levels of $Paco_2$. Initially the Fio_2 is 1.0, with the goal to decrease the level to 0.5 or less when able. Ventilation with permissive hypercapnia is allowed with an inspiratory-to-expiratory ratio that allows for adequate exhalation.

All patients receiving mechanical ventilation are at risk of complications, including auto-PEEP, air trapping, pneumothorax, hypotension, adult respiratory distress syndrome, and death. The child with asthma is especially prone to such problems because of the high degree of airway resistance and the need for high inspiratory pressures.

EXERCISE-INDUCED BRONCHOSPASM

Sometimes referred to as exercise-induced asthma, EIB begins during exercise and tends to reach its peak 5 to 10 minutes after the child has ceased activity. It may take another 20 to 30 minutes for symptoms to spontaneously resolve. EIB is caused by a loss of heat and/or water from the child's airway during exercise. This is often caused by hyperventilation of cool or dry air.

The prevalence of EIB has been reported to vary from 40% to 90% in children with asthma, with greater prevalence in those children with severe asthma. Absenteeism from school and poverty has been associated with findings of EIB. Early detection of EIB in school-aged children through screening could facilitate early treatment, enhance exercise-related activities, and possibly decrease the number of school absences. Notifying day care personnel, schoolteachers, and coaches that a child has EIB can alert them to monitor symptoms and may elicit a more effective response should symptoms occur.

The diagnosis of EIB is based on a history that is compatible with asthma symptoms that occur with or directly after exercise. An exercise challenge can be performed to confirm the diagnosis.

The management of these episodes is generally of a preventive nature. Recommended treatment is inhalation

---

Box 33-8	Criteria for Hospitalization

- Poor response to 4 hours of bronchodilator therapy
- Previous visit to emergency department within 24 hours
- Hospitalization with asthma within the past year
- Previous hospitalization with admission to intensive care unit
- History of mechanical ventilation for asthma
- Poor access to medical care
- Recent increase in need for oral corticosteroids

of a β_2-agonist, cromolyn sodium, nedocromil, or salmeterol, given 5 to 60 minutes before exercise, preferably closer to the start of exercise if possible. Providing a 5- to 10-minute "warm-up" period before any exercise is recommended as well. An increase or change in long-term control medications may be appropriate in some children with EIB. Outdoor activities may need to be adjusted if conditions are unfavorable. This is particularly important if the pollen, weed, or mold count is elevated. Extreme cold and windy weather are also circumstances that may call for more caution to ensure that asthma symptoms do not develop during the activities. Efforts to prevent EIB require open communication with the schoolteacher and coach to allow premedication by the student athlete under a physician's guidance.

ASTHMA AT SCHOOL

One third of those with asthma in the United States are younger than 18 years of age. Dealing with asthma while at school can present problems for the child, the parent, and the school personnel. Asthma symptoms can interfere with many activities that the school-aged child desires to pursue. It is the leading cause of school absences, with an average of more than 10 days per year missed. The child with severe asthma may miss more than 30 days per year. An obvious conclusion drawn from these statistics is that missing school may result in poor academic achievement, inability to participate in school activities, and low self-esteem. The goal of the school-aged child with asthma is to keep symptoms under control and participate fully in the physical and extracurricular activities the school system may offer.

Various organizations provide resources to aid in the care of children with asthma in the school systems. The American Association for Respiratory Care offers a program that involves direct education of school administrators, teachers, and students. Called Peak Performance USA, it is available to all members upon request. The educational interventions can address each particular school because not all schools have similar needs or programs. Another similar school intervention is available through the American Lung Association. A child-centered, school-based asthma education program has been associated with an increase in knowledge of asthma, improvement in skills for peak flow meter and inhaler use, and a reduction in the severity of asthma symptoms.[31]

School personnel, including teachers, coaches, and nurses, need to be familiar with the early warning signs of an impending asthma attack and what to do if the symptoms are present. It is recommended that a copy of the child's asthma action plan be kept at the school and that the teacher and school nurse be familiar with the plan. Unfortunately, many school systems do not employ a nurse dedicated to each individual school. Therefore there are occasions when the nurse is not available and other school personnel may need to provide care for the child. It is essential that the asthma action plan, peak flow meter, and rescue medications be readily accessible to school staff.

Parents can take a proactive role by determining how "asthma friendly" the school's environment is for their child. Some key questions to ask are listed in Box 33-9. The school building can present a hostile environment for children with asthma. There are numerous potential triggers found in most schools, including dust mites, mold, cockroaches, chalk dust, birds, rodents, animal dander, and strong odors (e.g., paint, chemicals, perfumes, pesticides). Therefore it is essential that these irritants be minimized or eliminated so that the child with asthma can attend school without risking further complications.

Box 33-9   Is Your School Asthma Friendly?

- Does the school have a "NO SMOKING" policy for all personnel, including teachers and custodial staff?
- Does the school maintain clean indoor air quality? How is this ensured?
- Is there a school nurse available at the school at all times? If not, how often is she/he there? Is she/he trained in pediatric asthma care?
- Can children with asthma take prescribed medications at school? Can they carry their rescue medications on their person? Must the medications be kept in a locked location?
- Does the school have an emergency plan for treating a child with a severe asthma episode?
- Does the school staff know the early warning signs of an asthma episode? Do they know the possible side effects of asthma medications and how they may impact the student's performance at school?
- Are students encouraged to participate in school activities and sports, regardless of having asthma?
- Are less strenuous activities provided if a recent exacerbation precludes full participation?
- Do teachers and coaches understand that exercise, especially that in cold air, can trigger asthma?
- Is the school staff provided opportunities to learn about asthma and allergies?
- Is there a copy of the asthma action plan in each student's classroom?
- Do school personnel understand that asthma is not an emotional or psychological disease but that strong emotions can trigger an acute episode?

ASTHMA CAMPS

In recent years we have seen a growth in the number of asthma camps for children. These camps offer children with asthma the opportunity to spend time with other children who have the same disorder. This type of experience can be priceless. The camps are structured to assist children in recognizing symptoms and how to respond to them, with particular attention given to use of an asthma action plan. Identification of triggers and avoidance techniques are discussed as well. The proper use of medication delivery devices and peak flow meters is also reinforced.

Positive effects from attending camp include a reduction in the rate of post-camp hospitalizations, school absenteeism, and emergency department visits. [32,33] The camps are usually operated with a team approach that includes physicians, respiratory therapists, social workers, and nurses.

ASSESSMENT QUESTIONS

See Evolve Resources for Answers.

1. The incidence of asthma has done what over the past 10 years?
   A. Remained stable
   B. Increased
   C. Decreased
   D. Decreased in incidence but increased in severity
2. When gathering information about a patient's medical history it is essential to include
   A. Recurrent wheezing or chest tightness
   B. Shortness of breath and cough
   C. Nocturnal symptoms
   D. All of the above
3. Dust mites are better controlled in what environment?
   A. Less relative humidity
   B. When bedding is washed in hot water >130°F
   C. When pillows and mattress are enclosed in zippered allergen-impermeable covers
   D. All of the above
4. When educating a patient or family member it is always essential to remember to
   A. Not ask open-ended questions
   B. Ask open-ended questions
   C. Try not to maintain eye contact for long periods of time
   D. Avoid questions that deal with a patient's expectations of their asthma management

ASSESSMENT QUESTIONS—cont'd

5. The purpose of a spacer is to slow aerosol velocity, to minimize particle impaction in the oropharynx, and to
   A. Enhance deposition in the lower respiratory tract
   B. Allow for larger particles
   C. Decrease the size of the particles
   D. Change aerosol particles to vapor, thus allowing better delivery of medication
6. Omalizumab is generally dosed for patients with IgE levels between
   A. 30 and 1500 IU/L
   B. 30 and 700 IU/L
   C. 500 and 1200 IU/L
   D. 3000 and 5500 IU/L
7. What is the best way to manage cockroaches?
   A. Removing carpeting
   B. Boric acid
   C. Acetic acid
   D. Bleach
8. Triggers of airflow obstruction include
   A. Aspirin and nonsteroidal antiinflammatory drugs, exercise, cold air, irritants, gastroesophageal reflux, respiratory infections, and psychological stress
   B. Aspirin, exercise, cold air, gastroesophageal reflux, respiratory infections, and excessive use of LABA
   C. Respiratory infections, cold or warm air, psychological stress, aspirin, exercise, and antiinflammatory drugs
9. In adult asthma, the inflammatory findings such as eosinophilic airway inflammation, hypergranulation of mast cells, increased IgE levels, and increased allergic response are due in part to an inappropriate activation of
   A. CD4+T cells
   B. IL-4
   C. T cells
   D. Th2 cells
10. What are the five components of asthma?
    A. Inflammation, acute bronchoconstriction, airway edema, mucous plugging, airway hyperresponsiveness, and wheezing
    B. Inflammation, acute bronchoconstriction, airway edema, mucous plugging, airway hyperresponsiveness, and airway remodeling
    C. Inflammation, acute bronchoconstriction, airway edema, mucous plugging, airway hyperresponsiveness, and increased levels of nitric oxide
    D. Inflammation, acute bronchoconstriction, airway edema, mucous plugging, airway hyperresponsiveness, and an allergic presentation

References

1. National Center for Heath Statistics, Centers for Disease Control and Prevention: *Asthma prevalence, heath care use and mortality*: United States, 2003-05.

2. National Asthma Education Program; National Heart, Lung, and Blood Institute: *Guidelines for the diagnosis and management of asthma: Expert Panel report.* NIH publication No. 91-3642. Bethesda, Md. National Institutes of Health, 1991.

3. National Asthma Education and Prevention Program; National Heart, Lung, and Blood Institute: *Guidelines for the diagnosis and management of asthma: expert panel report 2.* NIH publication No. 97-4051 Bethesda, Md. National Institutes of Health, 1997.

4. EPR-Update 2002. *Expert Panel Report: Guidelines for the diagnosis and management of asthma. Update on selected topics 2002 (EPR-Update 2002).* NIH Publication No. 02-5074. Bethesda, MD, U.S. Department of Health and Human Services; National Institutes of Health; National Heart, Lung, and Blood Institute, National Asthma Education and Prevention Program.

5. EPR-3. Expert Panel Report 3: Guidelines for the Diagnosis and Management of Asthma (EPR-3) NIH Publication. Bethesda, MD, U.S. Department of Health and Human Services; National Institutes of Health; National Heart, Lung, and Blood Institute; National Asthma Education and Prevention Program, 2007

6. Bateman ED et al; GOAL Investigators Group: Can guideline defined asthma control be achieved? The Gaining Optimal Asthma Control Study, *Am J Respir Crit Care I* 2004;170:836.

7. Burrows Johansson and Lundahl, 2001, Curr Allergy Asthma Rep, 1, 89-90 et al., 1989, N Engl J Med, 320, 271-7.

8. Platts-Mills TA: Allergen avoidance in the treatment of asthma and rhinitis, *N Engl J Med* 2003;349:207.

9. Vignola AM: Effects of inhaled corticosteroids, leukotriene receptor antagonists, or both, plus long-acting beta2-agonists on asthma pathophysiology: a review of the evidence, *Drugs* 2003;63(Suppl 2):35.

10. Eder W, Ege MJ, von Mutius E: The "hygiene hypothesis": The asthma epidemic, *N Engl J Med* 2006;355:2226.

11. Holgate ST, Polosa R: The mechanisms, diagnosis, and management of severe asthma in the development of early childhood asthma, *Pediatrics* 1985;75:859.

12. Huss K et al: House dust mite exposure is strong risk factors for positive allergy skin test responses in the Childhood Asthma Management Program, *J Allergy Clin Immunol* 2001;107:48.

13. Voter KZ, McBride JT: Pulmonary function testing in childhood asthma, *Immunol Allergy Clin North Am* 1998;18:133.

14. American Thoracic Society: Standardization of spirometry—1994 update, *Am J Respir Crit Care Med* 1995;152:1107.

15. Williams PV: Inhalation bronchoprovocation in children, *Immunol Allergy Clin North Am* 1998;18:149.

16. Custovic A et al: Exercise testing revisited: The response to exercise in normal and atopic children, *Chest* 1994;105:1127.

17. Zwiebel AH: Bronchoprovocation testing, *Immunol Allergy Clin North Am* 1999;19:63.

18. Milgrom H, Wood RP, Ingram D: Respiratory conditions that mimic asthma, *Immunol Allergy Clin North Am* 1998;18:113.

19. Shapiro GG: Management of pediatric asthma: Care by the specialist *Immunol Allergy Clin North Am* 1998;18:1.

20. Nelson HS et al SMART STUDY GROUP: The salmeterol multicenter asthma research trial: A comparison of usual pharmacotherapy for asthma or usual pharmacotherapy plus salmeterol, *Chest* 200;129:15.

21. Busse WW. Anti-immunoglobulin E (omalizumab) therapy in allergic asthma, *Am J Respir Crit Care Med* 2001;164:S12.

22. Giovane AL et al: A three-year double-blind placebo-controlled study with specific oral immunotherapy to *Dermatophagoides:* Evidence of safety and efficacy in paediatric patients, *Clin Exp Allergy* 1994;24:53.

23. Adkinson NF Jr et al: A controlled trial of immunotherapy for asthma in allergic children, *N Engl J Med* 1997;336:324.

24. Jackson AC: Accuracy, reproducibility, and variability of portable peak flow meters, *Chest* 1995;107:648.

25. Ponte CM: Education of the patient with asthma, *Immunol Allergy Clin North Am* 1999;19:161.

26. Dales RE et al: Asthma management preceding an emergency department visit, *Arch Intern Med* 1995; 152:2041.

27. White M, Sander N: Asthma from the perspective of the patient, *J Allergy Clin Immunol* 1999;104:S47.

28. Tal A, Levy N, Bearman JE: Methylprednisolone therapy for acute asthma in infants and toddlers: a controlled clinical trial, *Pediatrics* 1990;86:350.

29. Barnett PL, Caputo GL, Baskin M: Intravenous vs. oral corticosteroids in the management of acute asthma in children, *Ann Emerg Med* 1997;29:212.

30. Scarfone RJ et al: Controlled trial of oral prednisone in the emergency department treatment of children with acute asthma, *Pediatrics* 1993;92:513.

31. Christianson S et al: Evaluation of a school-based asthma education program for inner-city children, *J Allergy Clin Immunol* 1997;100:613.

32. Kelly CS et al: Outcomes analysis of a summer camp, *J Asthma* 1998; 35:165.

33. Menng A et al: Asthma day camp, *MCN Am J Matern Child Nurs* 1998;23:300.

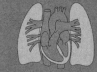

Chapter 34

Cystic Fibrosis

BRUCE M. SCHNAPF

OUTLINE

Genetics
Diagnosis
  Sweat Test
  CFTR Gene Analysis
  Nasal Electrical Potential Difference
  Newborn Screening
Pulmonary Disease
  Mucus Production and Airway Obstruction
  Bacterial Infection
  Airway Inflammation
  Clinical Presentation

Treatment of Pulmonary Disease
  Secretion Clearance
  Aerosol Therapy
  Antibiotic Therapy
  Oxygen Therapy
  Lung Transplantation
Other Clinical Manifestations
  Upper Airway Disorders
  Gastrointestinal Disorders
  Hepatobiliary Disorders
Prognosis

LEARNING OBJECTIVES

After reading this chapter the reader will be able to:
- Identify how the diagnosis of cystic fibrosis is made
- Describe the lung pathophysiology of cystic fibrosis
- Review treatment interventions that enhance airway clearance with cystic fibrosis
- Review various pharmacologic interventions used in treating cystic fibrosis

- Describe the potential risks and benefits of lung transplantation in cystic fibrosis
- Evaluate common clinical manifestations of cystic fibrosis other than lung disease
- Discuss common upper airway disorders commonly described in patients with cystic fibrosis
- Discuss the overall prognosis of patients with cystic fibrosis

Cystic fibrosis (CF) is the most common lethal autosomal recessive genetic disease in Caucasians and affects over 30,000 individuals in the United States. It is a chronic disorder with primary manifestations in the respiratory, digestive, and reproductive systems. Other complications of CF include diabetes mellitus, cirrhosis, sinusitis, and nasal polyposis. The disease was referred to in German folklore over 1000 years ago; it was in 1938, however, that Anderson first described the fibrocystic changes seen in the pancreas and used the term *cystic fibrosis of the pancreas*.[1]

The disease is characterized primarily by the following:
- Chronic obstruction and infection of the airways;
- Exocrine pancreatic insufficiency, with its consequences of maldigestion and small bowel obstruction
- Elevated sweat chloride concentration.

CF has an incidence of 1 in 3200 newborns in the United States.[2] It is less common in Hispanics (1 in 9500), African-Americans (1 in 17,000), and Asians (1 in 90,000).[3]

CF is marked by wide variability in the frequency and severity of clinical manifestations and complications.

Some children die in infancy, whereas others with CF live beyond their 40s and 50s. The median survival age has increased to about 35 years.[4] In the United States, about 40% of all patients with CF are older than 18 years of age, of which 90% are high school (or equivalent) graduates and 30% have attained a 4-year college degree. In nearly 70% of cases, the diagnosis is established before 1 year of age, usually within the first several months of life.[5] Approximately 7% of newly diagnosed patients are adults.

GENETICS

The cause of CF is a defect in a single gene on chromosome 7. The gene, which was cloned in 1989, encodes a membrane protein called the cystic fibrosis transmembrane conductance regulator (CFTR).[6] CFTR functions as a cyclic adenosine monophosphate-regulated chloride channel. It normally helps control the flow of ions and substrates across the apical surface of cell membranes lining the airways, intestines, vas deferens, biliary tree, sweat ducts, and pancreatic ducts.[7] CFTR dysfunction alters ion permeability of the cell membrane and creates an imbalance of ions and water in the intracellular areas.[3] When the chloride ion cannot be transported by CFTR, there is an insufficient secretion of fluid and inadequate hydration, which, in turn, alters the physical and chemical properties of secretions. The dehydration results in thickened secretions that plug the airways and ducts, impaired mucociliary clearance, and dysfunction of several organs, including the pancreas, liver, gallbladder, reproductive organs, and sweat glands.[6] Mucosal obstruction of exocrine glands is the chief contributor to morbidity and mortality in patients with CF.

It has been suggested that the CFTR defect may reduce the resistance of epithelial cells to bacterial pathogens.[8] This concept provides an explanation for the chronic bacterial colonization observed in the lungs of CF patients. The combination of airway obstruction, caused by mucous plugging, and persistent infection results in recurrent episodes of lung damage, including bronchiectasis.

CF is inherited as an autosomal recessive disease with mutations in the CFTR gene.[6] Both parents of a child with CF are carriers of the CFTR gene; they carry both a normal CFTR allele and a mutated CFTR allele. These couples have a 1 in 4 chance of having a child with CF who inherits the mutated CFTR allele from both parents. There are 2 chances in 4 that their child will inherit one normal and one mutated CFTR allele and be a carrier. And there is 1 chance in 4 that they will have a normal child. Siblings of an individual with CF have about a 7 in 10 chance of being a carrier, whereas first cousins of a patient with CF have about a 1 in 120 chance of having

the disease.[9] There is a family history in only 17% of newly diagnosed patients.

Based on incidence figures, it is estimated that 4% of Caucasians in the United States are carriers (heterozygotes) of the CFTR gene. Heterozygotes have no recognizable clinical symptoms, although an increased incidence of airway reactivity has been reported in CF carriers, suggesting a subtle abnormality of autonomic function.[10]

Box 34-1   Clinical Presentations Indicating Evaluation for Cystic Fibrosis

RESPIRATORY
- Persistent wheezing
- Chronic cough
- Frequent thick sputum production
- Recurrent respiratory infections
  - colds
  - bronchitis
  - pneumonia
- Respiratory infection with pathogens common to cystic fibrosis
  - *Staphylococcus aureus*
  - *Pseudomonas aeruginosa*
  - *Haemophilus influenzae*
  - *Burkholderia cepacia*
- Persistent abnormal chest radiograph
- Nasal polyps
- Parasinusitis
- Clubbing of nailbeds

GASTROINTESTINAL
- Failure to thrive
- Frequent, greasy, foul-smelling stools
- Voracious appetite
- Formula/milk intolerance
- Rectal prolapse
- Meconium ileus
- Meconium peritonitis
- Distal intestinal obstruction syndrome
- Pancreatic insufficiency
- Pancreatitis

HEPATOBILIARY
- Hepatomegaly
- Focal biliary cirrhosis
- Prolonged neonatal jaundice
- Cholelithiasis

REPRODUCTIVE
- Obstructive azoospermia

NUTRITIONAL DEFICITS
- Fat-soluble vitamin deficiency (vitamins A, D, E, K)
- Hypoproteinemia, with or without edema
- Hypochloremic metabolic alkalosis

DIAGNOSIS

The diagnosis of CF is made at a median age of 6 months.[4] The diagnosis of CF is suspected based on the presence of one or more distinguishing phenotypic features or a family history of the disease. Box 34-1 lists clinical presentations that are reasons to consider an evaluation for CF. Even though the disease occurs most often in the Caucasian population, it is considered in the differential diagnosis of patients with diverse racial backgrounds who present with these features. A diagnosis of CF requires positive laboratory testing along with a history or clinical conditions consistent with CF (Box 34-2).[11]

Sweat Test

The standard for diagnosis of CF is the sweat test. Normal secretion and resorption of chloride in the sweat gland are dependent on CFTR. In CF, there is production of hypertonic sweat containing high concentrations of sodium and chloride. A sweat chloride concentration greater than 60 mEq/L on two separate occasions confirms the diagnosis of CF. A concentration between 40 and 60 mEq/L is considered a borderline range, and the diagnosis is supported by having other evidence of CFTR dysfunction or clinical symptoms consistent with CF. Normal adults occasionally have elevated sweat chloride concentrations.

Proper testing must be performed by the quantitative pilocarpine iontophoresis (Gibson-Cooke or Westcor macroduct methods) sweat test in a laboratory with experienced personnel and established quality control. The sweat is obtained by stimulating the skin on the forearm with pilocarpine iontophoresis (Figure 34-1).[12] Technical error can result in false negative and false positive results. In addition to inadequate sweat collected, malnutrition, edema, and hypoalbuminemia can result in a false negative result. Therefore, patients with clinical features of CF but normal or borderline sweat test results should have a repeat sweat test performed in a center that is very experienced with this procedure.[13] Conditions that can produce false-positive results (i.e., elevated sweat chloride level in a child without CF) include evaporation, adrenal insufficiency, and hypothyroidism.[14]

CFTR Gene Analysis

A diagnosis of CF can be confirmed when there is evidence of two mutated CFTR alleles. Over 1600 mutations have been identified (reviewed March 16, 2008) and are listed on a website (http://www.genet.sickkids.on.ca/cftr/). The most common mutation in CF is the ΔF508.[15] There are individuals who possess the CFTR mutations but do not have the typical

Box 34-2	Diagnosis of Cystic Fibrosis

At least one item from each of the following categories must be present:

LABORATORY TESTING
Sweat chloride level >60 mEq/L
or
Two CFTR mutations identified
or
Abnormal ion transport across nasal epithelia

HISTORY OR CONDITION
Clinical evidence of cystic fibrosis
or
Sibling with cystic fibrosis
or
Positive newborn screening for cystic fibrosis

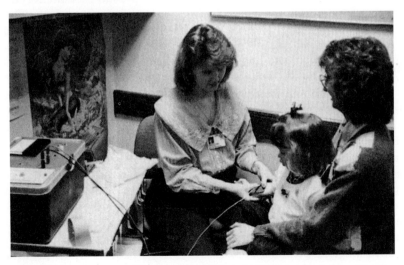

FIGURE 34-1 Sweat test being performed. The child is held in her mother's lap while electrodes are positioned on her forearm to stimulate the skin to produce sweat.

clinical presentations of CF. The CF phenotype-genotype correlation is complex and variable. As a general rule, the severity of disease correlates with influence of the gene mutation on CFTR function as a chloride channel.

Nasal Electrical Potential Difference

Measuring the difference in voltage potentials across the nasal epithelium is a newer method used in the diagnosis of CF. Certain alterations in the nasal potential differences are characteristic of CF and can be used to identify some patients with CF.[16] The availability of this analysis remains limited. Interpretation of this measurement requires in-depth knowledge of ion transport physiology.

Newborn Screening

Although not done routinely, there are a number of centers that provide newborn screening for CF.[17] In 2008, more than 40 states began newborn screening for cystic fibrosis. The most common method is measurement of serum immunoreactive trypsinogen obtained from a heel-stick blood sample. Elevated levels of serum trypsinogen are associated with pancreatic insufficiency and CF. There is increasing evidence of the benefit of early diagnosis of CF, which may lead to an increase in the use of such screening programs. In October 15, 2004, the Centers for Disease Control and Prevention released recommendations on the screening of newborns for cystic fibrosis and is available online at http://www.cdc.gov/mmwr/preview/mmwrhtml/rr5313a1.htm. When an infant has a positive newborn screen for CF, a referral takes place to the regional CF Center where an evaluation and a quantitative sweat test is performed. Interpretation of the sweat test in an infant is as follows: > 30 mEQ/L is possible for a CF diagnosis, 40 – 60 mEQ/L is probably positive, and > 60 mEQ/L is diagnostic for CF.

PULMONARY DISEASE

Although CF is a disorder involving multiple organs, pulmonary disease accounts for much of the morbidity and is the cause of death in more than 90% of all cases.[4] As a result of CFTR dysfunction, there is abnormal water and electrolyte transport across the respiratory epithelium. This in turn leads to the typical features of CF: thick tenacious mucus, impaired secretion clearance, mucous plugging of the airways, chronic bacterial infection, and airway inflammation. Severity of lung disease varies. Some patients have little or no respiratory compromise and slow progression of symptoms over time, whereas others have severe lung disease with a rapid change in lung function and infection. Pulmonary disease is usually heralded by the onset of a nonproductive cough that evolves into a loose, productive cough with purulent secretions.

Mucus Production and Airway Obstruction

The lungs of a newborn with CF are histologically normal at birth.[18] However, airway dysfunction begins during the first year of life, with the earliest pathologic change being thickened mucus and plugging of the submucosal gland ducts in the large airways.[19] These changes appear to precede infection and inflammation.[20]

Goblet cells and submucosal glands are the predominant secretory structures of normal airways. In the CF patient, there is an increased number of goblet cells and hypertrophy of submucosal glands, which leads to an increase in secretions and sputum production. Airway secretions are relatively dehydrated and viscous. Thick and viscid mucus is such a common feature that at one time the disease was referred to as "mucoviscidosis."

Mucociliary clearance is variable in CF, with some patients having severe impairment whereas others have normal clearance. The reduction in clearance is believed to be caused by the increased volume of respiratory secretions and the abnormally thick mucus. Studies have shown the cilia from CF patients to be normal, although chronic inflammation may result in a loss of ciliated cells.[21]

Bacterial Infection

In time there is colonization of CF airways with various bacteria. Initially, *Staphylococcus aureus* and *Haemophilus influenzae* appear, with *S. aureus* reaching maximum prevalence at ages 6 to 17 years and *H. influenzae* peaking at 2 to 5 years of age.[9] *S. aureus* may be found in 40% of children and adolescents, and nontypable *H. influenzae*, found in 15%.

A distinctive feature of cystic fibrosis is the increased susceptibility to respiratory infection with *P. aeruginosa*.[22] By 18 years of age, about 80% of patients in the United States have developed a *Pseudomonas* infection.[9] Initial colonization is with nonmucoid strains of *Pseudomonas*, often occurring during a staphylococcal infection. However, more than 80% of patients with advanced lung disease shelter mucoid strains of *Pseudomonas* that are heavy slime producers.[23] It is believed that a marked decline in lung function is caused by the mucoid phenotype of *P. aeruginosa*. The mucoid strains are rarely found in other diseases and prompt investigation for CF when discovered. Once there is colonization of the airways, *Pseudomonas* is difficult to eradicate, in spite of aggressive antibiotic therapy.[24] However, it does tend to remain localized to the respiratory tract.

Infection with *Burkholderia cepacia* occurs in about 4% of CF patients.[4] It was identified as an important pathogen in CF in the early 1980s. This hardy organism is resistant to aminoglycosides and possibly all antibiotics.

Infection may result in an acute necrotizing pneumonia and septic shock. Once colonization occurs, there is the possibility of catastrophic deterioration and a poorer prognosis for survival. It is often transmitted either directly or indirectly by person-to-person transmission, with risk factors including hospitalization and having a colonized sibling.[25] The emergence of *B. cepacia* has profoundly affected infection control policies and has caused a change in activities and visitation among CF patients. Total segregation of colonized patients to different hospital floors or rooms and separate clinic visits is practiced. Most CF isolates are genomovar II or III, the latter of which appears to be associated with a more rapid clinical deterioration.

Patients with CF who do not respond to antimicrobial agents may have colonization of other organisms. These include viruses, atypical mycobacteria, *Klebsiella* organisms, *Aspergillus* species, and *Stenotrophomonas maltophilia*.

The bacterial load, accompanied by the destructive attempts of the immune system to eradicate the infection, results in progressive damage to the airway wall and accumulation of thicker, more caustic sputum within the scarred airways. Severe obstruction of the airway results, and the CF patient eventually develops bronchiectasis and respiratory failure.

Airway Inflammation

Inflammation of the airways is a major component of CF and may occur early in the disease process. Recent studies of bronchoalveolar lavage fluid from infants suggest that airway inflammation is present in those as young as 4 weeks old, likely occurring before infection.[26] An abundance of neutrophils and the enzyme neutrophil elastase may be responsible for the airway destruction and inflammatory response found in the lungs of CF patients.[27]

Clinical Presentation

Nearly half of all patients with CF are diagnosed as a result of pulmonary symptoms.[28] The diagnosis of CF should be considered in every patient who presents with chronic or recurrent lower respiratory tract disorders, including bronchitis, bronchiectasis, pneumonia, and refractory asthma. Children with CF have frequent pulmonary exacerbations, with the most consistent feature being a chronic cough. The cough may be dry and hacking, or it can be paroxysmal with the patient gagging, choking, or even vomiting during coughing episodes. Sputum often becomes mucopurulent and difficult to expectorate. Other symptoms include tachypnea, retractions, dyspnea, and use of accessory muscles. Occasionally, patients will present with hemoptysis and fever. Wheezing, crackles, rhonchi, and decreased air exchange are common findings during auscultation of the chest.

The chest radiograph initially shows hyperinflation with flattened diaphragms secondary to air trapping (Figure 34-2). Mucous plugging and bronchial wall thickening are also seen. Diffuse fibrosis and bronchiectasis

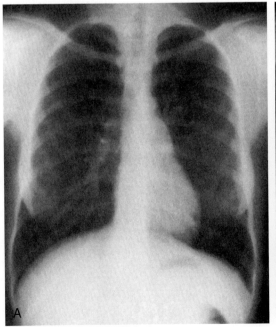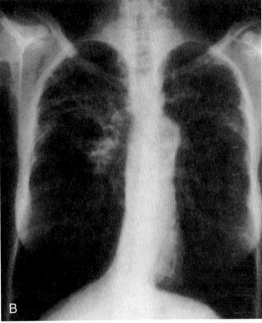

FIGURE 34-2 Cystic fibrosis. Chest radiographs from a patient at ages 14 years **(A)** and 22 years **(B)** illustrating the changes of advancing disease.

are found predominantly in the upper lobes. However, over time all lung fields are involved. Pneumothorax occurs most often in older patients with more advanced disease and is a result of rupture of subpleural blebs. The recurrence rate is high at 50% to 70%.[29] The progressive lung disease and chronic hypoxemia lead to an increase in pulmonary vascular resistance, pulmonary hypertension, and cor pulmonale. As cor pulmonale progresses, the electrocardiogram shows thickening in the wall and enlargement of the right ventricle.

Pulmonary function testing initially demonstrates air flow obstruction. As the disease progresses, both a restrictive and an obstructive pattern can be seen, along with a decrease in air flow. About 50% of patients with CF have a positive methacholine challenge test, which indicates airway hyperreactivity. Digital clubbing and pulmonary hypertrophic osteoarthropathy are universal findings in CF patients with advanced pulmonary disease. Pulmonary exacerbations of CF vary in severity and are usually defined by subjective symptoms. Although there is no clear definition of a CF exacerbation, most are associated with the characteristics found in Box 34-3.

TREATMENT OF PULMONARY DISEASE

Treatment of the pulmonary manifestations of CF focuses on routine therapy aimed at physically removing thickened mucus from the airways and pharmacologic control of infection with the aggressive use of antibiotics.

Box 34-3	Signs and Symptoms of a Pulmonary Exacerbation in Cystic Fibrosis

- Increased cough
- Increased sputum production
- Change in sputum appearance
- Hemoptysis
- Dyspnea
- Tachypnea
- Increased chest congestion
- Change in findings of chest physical examination
- Decrease in oxygen saturation
- Change in chest radiograph
- Deterioration in pulmonary function
- Fever
- Weight loss
- Decreased appetite
- Increased fatigue
- Decreased exercise tolerance

Secretion Clearance

Airway clearance techniques are used to assist in the removal of bronchial secretions and are recommended at the first indication of lung involvement. Patients with minimal symptoms may only require one treatment session per day, whereas others with a greater volume of thick secretions may need three or more sessions per day. Postural drainage, manual or mechanical percussion, vibration, and assisted coughing have proven to be beneficial in removing secretions. Physical activity and exercise programs have been shown to augment airway clearance.

Several alternative methods have been developed. These include active cycle breathing, forced expiratory technique, positive expiratory pressure (PEP) therapy, autogenic drainage, high frequency chest wall oscillation, the Flutter, and the intrapulmonary percussive device. The "huff" and autogenic drainage method are breathing techniques that improve ventilation and maximize the effectiveness of a cough. The PEP valve provides a distending pressure to the airways and, when combined with breathing maneuvers, allows for enhanced mucus clearance. The Flutter is a pipe-shaped hand-held device that contains a stainless steel ball. During expiration, the ball oscillates, causing oscillatory waves to be transmitted to the lower airways, shearing secretions from the airway walls. High-frequency chest wall oscillations are also helpful in shearing mucus from the airway wall. However, it is not effort dependent like the Flutter and PEP devices. A detailed discussion of the techniques and devices is provided in Chapter 14. Studies have compared various outcomes, including peak flow rates, sputum production, pulmonary function values, and oximetry, among different airway clearance techniques.[30-36] However, controversy remains concerning the advantage of one form over another. The addition of these new modalities has provided patients with more options when developing a program that best fits their lifestyle. This may improve treatment adherence and be more efficacious overall.

Aerosol Therapy

Aerosol therapy in CF patients includes bronchodilators, mucolytic agents, antiinflammatory agents, hydrating agents, proteolytic agents, and antibiotics. Administration is through various devices, depending on the patient's clinical status and the specific agent being used.

Bronchodilators

Airway hyperreactivity is common in the majority of patients with CF.[37] Inhalation of a bronchodilator followed with an airway clearance technique is the most common treatment regimen used routinely between exacerbations. Medications used most often include ß2-agonists, such as Albuterol, and the anticholinergic agent ipratropium bromide. The medication is delivered with either a metered-dose inhaler or a nebulizer. Although bronchodilators are routinely used, their responsiveness has been shown to be variable in CF patients.[38,39] Most patients with CF demonstrate an improvement in lung function after inhalation of a bronchodilator.[40] Occasionally, a patient worsens after bronchodilator therapy.[41] Air flow may decrease or hyperinflation may increase as a result of smooth muscle relaxation and a decrease in airway elasticity. In these patients, treatment with ipratropium bromide has resulted in significant improvement in pulmonary function, especially in adult patients.[42] Some patients respond better to combination therapy using albuterol and/or ipratropium bromide.[43]

Mucolytic Agents

The sputum of CF patients is not only more abundant but also has abnormal viscosity. This is believed to be caused by increased glycoprotein sulfation and the high concentrations of DNA released from dead neutrophils.[44] Although used for many years, most mucolytic agents, including N-acetylcysteine, are not effective in the treatment of CF.

Recombinant DNase (rhDNase) has been developed to reduce the viscosity of purulent CF sputum.[45] The synthetically produced rhDNase breaks up the thickened mucus by disrupting the long, sticky DNA molecules. Studies have demonstrated that the lung function of CF patients with mild to moderate pulmonary disease improved after they received aerosolized rhDNase. A reduction in the use of antibiotics for respiratory infections has also occurred after treatment.[46] Voice alteration is the only significant side effect and resolves when the medication is discontinued.

There has been renewed interest in the use of nebulized 7% hypertonic saline to facilitate airway clearance.[47] Because hypertonic saline causes bronchospasm in some patients, it is generally recommended to premedicate with a ß2-agonist. In general, it was found to be an inexpensive, safe, effective additional therapy in CF patients with stable lung function. Its use has been associated with a modest improvement in lung function and reduced frequency of pulmonary exacerbations.[48,49] A 7% hypertonic saline kit is available from the Cystic Fibrosis Pharmacy website.[50]

Antiinflammatory Agents

Because inflammation of the airways is responsible for a large part of the pulmonary symptoms in CF, it seems logical to consider antiinflammatory agents as part of the treatment regimen. Systemic corticosteroids have been shown in clinical trials to improve lung function; however, side effects are serious and include growth suppression and increased susceptibility to osteoporosis and cataracts.[51] Studies have reported using inhaled corticosteroids in CF with improvement in lung function and respiratory symptoms, but the studies had small sample sizes.[52,53] Ibuprofen has been studied as well, demonstrating ability to slow the progression of lung disease. However, specific dosing and close pharmacokinetic monitoring is required when using this medication.[54]

Amiloride

A characteristic of CF airways is an excessive absorption of sodium and water across the epithelium. It is believed that this abnormality is linked to the CFTR gene mutation. Amiloride is a sodium channel blocker normally used as a diuretic. It is given as an aerosol to CF patients in an attempt to improve sputum viscosity and increase secretion clearance by inhibiting the abnormal sodium absorption.[55] Studies suggest that it reduces the rate of deterioration of lung function and improves mucociliary and cough clearance.

Antibiotic Therapy

Aerosolized antibiotics such as TOBI™ are frequently used as chronic suppressive therapy to treat patients infected with P. aeruginosa to prolong the time between pulmonary exacerbations and to slow the progression of lung function decline.[56] A Cochrane review of inhaled tobramycin for CF concluded that aerosolized antipseudomonal antibiotics improved lung function.[57] A unit dose of 300mg/5ml is considered standard. It is given twice a day for 28-day cycles every other month. Inhaled colistin is also available for use.[58] In addition, inhaled aztreonam is being assessed as another potentially useful inhaled antibiotic against CF lung disease. However, the main focus in the treatment of pulmonary symptoms continues to be secretion removal and antibiotic therapy. Because the airway infection cannot be eradicated, the goal of antibiotic therapy in the treatment of CF is suppression of the infecting organism to a level at which clinical symptoms are minimal.[9] There has been recent interest in the use of oral azithromycin as prolonged therapy because of an antiinflammatory effect it achieves by decreasing cytokine production.

Antibiotic Selection

Antibiotic therapy is usually given for 2 weeks during pulmonary exacerbations. Antibiotics can be administered orally, by nebulization, or intravenously. The choice of antibiotic is based on results of the individual patient's sputum or throat culture and the sensitivity profile of the specific organisms. If handled properly, the sputum culture accurately reflects infection in the lungs. Agents known to be particularly effective against *S. aureus* and *Pseudomonas* species are usually chosen. For patients infected with *P. aeruginosa,* combination therapy with a ß-lactam and an aminoglycoside is administered. Ciprofloxacin is a common choice for an oral antibiotic. Therapy can be extended to cover *S. aureus* if it is also present in the sputum. Because of abnormal pharmacokinetics of most antibiotics in CF patients, a higher than normal dose is usually required to achieve therapeutic levels.[9]

Hospitalization

Advances in providing stable venous access have allowed the intravenous administration of antibiotics at home, with the patient continuing school or work activities.[59] Criteria for proceeding with hospitalization and intravenous therapy include severe illness but also moderate illness that is unresponsive to home therapy, or even mild illness complicated by growth failure. If a patient does not respond to outpatient management, hospitalization is recommended with a 10- to 21-day course of intensive antibiotic therapy. Hospitalization for a pulmonary exacerbation also includes aggressive treatment to remove secretions.

Oxygen Therapy

With disease progression, CF patients often develop hypoxemia, especially at night and with exercise. Oxygen saturations initially drop to less than 90% during acute exacerbations, then chronically during sleep, and then throughout the day. Supplemental oxygen is provided to reduce the hypoxemia and pulmonary hypertension, which can lead to development of cor pulmonale.

Unlike other pediatric patients, CF patients with advanced disease, particularly those with a baseline $Paco_2$ elevation, may convert from the normal CO_2-driven respiratory pattern to one triggered primarily by hypoxia. Supplemental oxygen, given in excess, can result in significant respiratory drive suppression. Therefore, in CF patients with more severe disease, oxygen flow rates and FiO_2 levels are initially targeted to maintain saturation in the 90% to 95% range only.

Lung Transplantation

Patients with severe CF, who are at significant risk of dying from their disease within 2 years, are increasingly being considered for lung transplantation. There has been no evidence of the redevelopment of CF in the transplanted lungs, but new problems related to lung rejection and opportunistic infection in patients receiving immunosuppressive agents can occur. Although more than 100 CF patients undergo a lung or heart-lung transplant each year, each year patients succumb

to the disease while waiting for donor organs. Rate of decline of FEV_1 as well as worsening of clinical status are key factors in determining the timing of referral for lung transplantation. In addition, the median regional waiting period for donor lungs for patients with CF may assist in the timing of referral. Chapter 25 provides a thorough discussion of lung transplantation.

OTHER CLINICAL MANIFESTATIONS

Although pulmonary compromise is the main factor that limits longevity in CF patients, there are a number of other systems affected by the disease. Certain conditions can prompt consideration of the diagnosis of CF. The more common conditions include meconium ileus, prolonged neonatal jaundice, rectal prolapse, and failure to thrive.

Upper Airway Disorders

Nearly all patients with CF have sinusitis, most often involving the maxillary and ethmoidal sinuses. It is often difficult to control in spite of oral and intravenous antibiotic therapy. The abnormally thick mucus that is characteristic of CF occludes the sinus passages and prevents drainage.[60] These patients also have a high incidence of nasal polyps, occurring most often in the older child and adolescent.[61] More than half of the patients who require surgical removal of the polyps experience a recurrence. A diagnosis of CF is suspected in children who present with sinusitis and nasal polyposis.

Gastrointestinal Disorders
Pancreatic Insufficiency

More than 90% of patients with CF have pancreatic insufficiency. CFTR dysfunction results in insufficient secretion of pancreatic fluid, which causes plugging and obstruction of the pancreatic ducts. Siblings with CF often share similar degrees of pancreatic insufficiency.[62,63] Symptoms are controlled with supplementation of pancreatic enzymes. A small number of CF patients have pancreatic sufficiency and do not require pancreatic enzyme supplements. These patients often have lower sweat chloride values, better lung function, and lower incidence of *Pseudomonas* colonization and are often diagnosed with CF at an older age. Overall prognosis is usually better, but occasional episodes of pancreatitis occur and there is continued risk of the development of pancreatic insufficiency. Therapy is individualized and supplements are taken each time the patient eats. Infants require supplements with any type of milk, including breast milk, and children require them with all snacks and meals.

Failure of the pancreas to produce sufficient enzymes results in malabsorption of fat and protein.

The presence of steatorrhea, which is excessive loss of fat in the stool, is often the first indication of CF. These children frequently produce bulky, foul-smelling, oily stools and may experience rectal prolapse. Complaints of constipation or stomach cramps, especially after eating, can lead to a decrease in appetite and oral intake. Infants often present with failure to thrive, failing to gain weight in spite of a voracious appetite. Other clinical consequences include hypoproteinemia with or without edema and deficiency of vitamins A, D, E, and K.

The incidence of diabetes mellitus is much greater in children with CF than in the general pediatric population.[63] As fibrosis of the pancreas progresses, endocrine function is affected and CF-related diabetes (CFRD) develops. At 10 years of age, there is an increasing incidence of CFRD.[4] This is associated with a 2.5-fold increase relative risk of morbidity and mortality. Weight loss is usually the first symptom. Initiation of insulin therapy has been associated with increased body mass and improved lung function.

Meconium Ileus and Distal Intestinal Obstruction Syndrome

Failure to secrete water into the gut is a result of CFTR dysfunction. Abnormal intestinal electrolyte and water transport can lead to a number of disorders. The earliest clinical manifestation of CF may be meconium ileus.[5] Occurring at birth, nearly every full-term infant who has meconium ileus is considered to have CF until proven otherwise. Presentation includes abdominal distention, vomiting, and abdominal radiograph showing distended loops of bowel with gas bubbles trapped among meconium, giving a ground-glass appearance. With an incidence higher in older patients, distal intestinal obstruction syndrome occurs when the thick, sticky stool of the CF patient adheres to the bowel wall and obstructs the small intestine and colon. Only rarely is this seen in a patient with pancreatic sufficiency.

Rectal Prolapse

Episodes of rectal prolapse are related to malnutrition, abnormal stool (e.g., diarrhea, constipation), and paroxysmal coughing. Onset rarely occurs after 5 years of age.[64] The association with CF is so common that a sweat test is indicated in any child presenting with rectal prolapse.

Gastroesophageal Reflux Disease

Patients with CF often experience heartburn and gastric reflux, especially those with advanced pulmonary disease.[65] This may be the result of frequent coughing, obstructive lung disease with hyperinflation, and increased abdominal pressure. Treatment includes dietary restrictions and medication with antacids and histamine-2 blockers.

Hepatobiliary Disorders

The hepatobiliary manifestations of CF occur less frequently than the gastrointestinal disorders. Serious complications are uncommon before adolescence. Cirrhosis and portal hypertension are the most common hepatic disorders that occur in CF patients, although only 2% to 4% of patients with CF develop any apparent liver disease.[66] Prolonged neonatal jaundice may occur in neonates with CF and raises the suspicion of a diagnosis of CF.

Gallbladder abnormalities are quite common in CF patients.[67] Microgallbladder is the most common biliary tract disorder. It is believed that mucus obstruction of the cystic duct results in atrophy of the gallbladder. Most patients are asymptomatic. The incidence of abnormalities increases with age, with gallstones occurring quite frequently in patients with pancreatic insufficiency. Cholecystectomy is considered in patients who are symptomatic.

PROGNOSIS

Advances in the management of CF, especially the pulmonary manifestations, have led to a more favorable prognosis. Today the median survival is about 35 years.[5] This is a long stride from the life expectancy of less than 1 year when CF was described by Anderson in the late 1930s.[1] Although patients with CF continue to survive longer, some children still succumb to the disease before reaching adulthood, in spite of advances in diagnostic techniques and treatment. We know that various factors influence a patient's prognosis, including the progression of pulmonary disease, the involvement of other organ systems, nutritional status, and environment. Investigations and projects that affect these factors will make a difference in the lives of many children. The respiratory therapist is an essential member of the CF multidisciplinary care team delivering direct care to hospitalized patients. In addition, the therapist assesses, teaches, and periodically reviews the most effective airway clearance technique for each patient.

ASSESSMENT QUESTIONS

See Evolve Resources for the answers.

1. Which of the following is *not* true regarding the diagnosing cystic fibrosis?
   A. The sweat chloride test result is greater than 60 mEq/L.
   B. CF gene mutation analyses are not helpful when offering a diagnosis of CF.
   C. Nasal electrical potential difference may assist in the diagnosis of CF.

    D. There is a family history with signs of respiratory distress and malnutrition.

    E. None of the above

2. The increased production in the viscous airway secretions of a patient with CF are caused by all of the following, except:

    A. Decreased ciliary function

    B. Increased goblet cells

    C. Hypertrophied submucosal glands

    D. Both A and C

3. CF is characterized by which of the following sequlae?

    A. Chronic airway obstruction

    B. Pancreatic insufficiency

    C. Liver and gallbladder insufficiencies

    D. All of the above

4. The *most* common bacterial pathogens in an individual with CF include the following, except

    A. *Staph aureus*

    B. *Pseudomonas Aeruginosa*

    C. *Burkholderia cepacia*

    D. Salmonella

    E. *Hemophilus influenzae*

5. Which of the following airway clearance methods is useful in CF management?

    A. Flutter

    B. Positive expiratory pressure therapy

    C. Autogenic drainage

    D. High-frequency chest wall oscillations

    E. All of the above

6. Which of the following are prophylactic medications useful in CF lung disease?

    A. Albuterol

    B. Ipratropium Bromide

    C. Tobramycin (TOBI)

    D. 7% hypertonic saline

    E. All of the above.

7. The chest x-ray of a patient with cystic fibrosis can have all of the following, except

    A. Hyperinflation with flattened diaphragms

    B. Diffuse fibrosis and bronchiectasis

    C. Blebs and pneumothoraces

    D. Left ventricular hypertrophy

    E. Cors pulmonale

8. Patients with severe chronic forms of CF should only be given oxygen to maintain saturations between 90% to 95% for which of the following reasons?

    A. To eliminate drying of secretions

    B. To eliminate CO_2 retention

    C. To preserve hypoxic drive

    D. Both B and C

9. Today, the median survival rate for CF is _____ years.

    A. 10

    B. 15

    C. 25

    D. 36

10. The most common upper airway problems encountered by children with CF include

    A. Nasal polyps

    B. Sinusitis

    C. Croup

    D. Subglottic stenosis

    E. Both A and B

REFERENCES

1. Anderson DH: Cystic fibrosis of the pancreas and its relation to celiac disease: a clinical and pathological study, *Am J Dis Child* 1938;56:344.

2. Hamosh A et al: Comparison of the clinical manifestations of cystic fibrosis in African-Americans and Caucasians, *J Pediatr* 1998;132:255.

3. Welsh MJ et al: Cystic fibrosis. In Scriver CR et al, editors: *The metabolic and molecular basis of inherited disease*, ed 7, New York. McGraw-Hill, 1995; pp 3799–3879.

4. Cystic Fibrosis Foundation: *Cystic Fibrosis Foundation patient registry 2003 annual data report*. Bethesda, Md, 2004.

5. FitzSimmons SC: The changing epidemiology of cystic fibrosis, *J Pediatr* 1993;122:1.

6. Riordan JR et al: Identification of the cystic fibrosis gene: Cloning and characterization of complementary DNA, *Science* 1989;245:1066.

7. Cutting GR: Cystic fibrosis. In Rimoin DL, Connor JM, Pyeritz RD, editors: *Emery and Rimoin's principles and practice of medical genetics*, London. Churchill Livingstone, 1997; p 2685.

8. Smith JJ et al: Cystic fibrosis airway epithelia fail to kill bacteria because of abnormal airway surface fluid, *Cell* 1996;85:229.

9. Davis PB: Cystic fibrosis, *Pediatr Rev* 2001;22:257.

10. Davis PB: Autonomic and airway reactivity in obligate heterozygotes for cystic fibrosis, *Am Rev Respir Dis* 1984;129:911.

11. Rosenstein B, Cutting GR: Diagnosis of cystic fibrosis: a consensus statement, *J Pediatr* 1998;132:589.

12. LeGrys VA: Sweat testing for the diagnosis of cystic fibrosis: practical consideration, *J Pediatr* 1996; 129:892.

13. MacLean W, Tripp R: Cystic fibrosis with edema and falsely negative sweat test, *J Pediatr* 1973;83:85.

14. Wood RE, Boat TF, Doershuk CF: Cystic fibrosis, *Am Rev Respir Dis* 1996;833.

15. Worldwide survey of the delta F508 mutation-report from the cystic fibrosis genetic analysis consortium, *Am J Hum Genet* 1990;47:354.

16. Boat TF et al: *The diagnosis of cystic fibrosis*. Bethesda, Md. Cystic Fibrosis Foundation, 1998.

17. Wilcken B: Newborn screening for cystic fibrosis: its evolution and a review of the current situation, *Screening* 1993;2:43.

18. Chow C, Landau L, Taussig L: Bronchial mucous glands in the newborn with cystic fibrosis, *Eur J Pediatr* 1982;139:240.

19. Lamb D, Reid L: The tracheobronchial submucosal glands in cystic fibrosis: a qualitative and quantitative histochemical study, *Br J Dis Chest* 1972;66:240.

20. Zuelzer W, Newton W: The pathogenesis of fibrocystic disease of the pancreas: a study of 36 cases with special reference to the pulmonary lesions, *Pediatrics* 1949;4:53.

21. Katz SM, Holsclaw DS Jr: Ultrastructural features of respiratory cilia in cystic fibrosis, *Am J Clin Pathol* 1980;73:682.

22. Thomassen MJ, Demko CA, Doershuk CF: Cystic fibrosis: a review of pulmonary infections and interventions, *Pediatr Pulmonol* 1987;3:334.

23. Kerem E et al: Pulmonary function and clinical course in patients with cystic fibrosis after pulmonary colonization with *Pseudomonas aeruginosa*, *J Pediatr* 1990;116: 714.

24. Goldman DA, Klinger JD: *Pseudomonas aeruginosa*: biology, mechanisms of virulence, epidemiology, *J Pediatr* 1986;108:806.

25. Tablan OC et al: Colonization of the respiratory tract with *Pseudomonas cepacia* in cystic fibrosis risk factors and outcomes, *Chest* 1987;91:527.

26. Khan T et al: Early pulmonary inflammation in infants with cystic fibrosis, *Am J Respir Crit Care Med* 1995;151:1075.

27. Suter S et al: Granulocyte neutral proteases and *Pseudomonas* elastase as possible causes of airway damage in patients with cystic fibrosis, *J Infect Dis* 1984;149:523.

28. Wistrak BJ, Meyer CM, Cotton RT: Cystic fibrosis presenting with sinus disease in children, *Am J Dis Child* 1993;147:258.

29. Spector M, Stern R: Pneumothorax in cystic fibrosis: a 26-year experience, *Ann Thorac Surg* 1989;47:204.

30. Desmond K et al: Immediate and long-term effects of chest physiotherapy in patients with cystic fibrosis, *J Pediatr* 1983;103:538.

31. deBoeck C, Zinman R: Cough versus chest physiotherapy: a comparison of the acute effects on pulmonary function in patients with cystic fibrosis, *Am Rev Respir Dis* 1984;129:182.

32. vanderSchans C et al: Effect of positive expiratory pressure breathing in patients with cystic fibrosis, *Thorax* 1991;46:252.

33. Burnett M et al: Comparative efficacy of manual chest physiotherapy and a high frequency chest compression vest in inpatient treatment of cystic fibrosis, *Am Rev Respir Dis* 1993;147:A30.

34. Warwick W, Hansen L: The long-term effect of high-frequency chest compression therapy on pulmonary complications of cystic fibrosis, *Pediatr Pulmonol* 1991;11:265.

35. Konstan M, Stern R, Doershuk C: Efficacy of the Flutter device for airway mucus clearance in patients with cystic fibrosis, *J Pediatr* 1994;124:689.

36. Zach M, Purrer B, Oberwaldner B: Effect of swimming on forced expiration and sputum clearance in cystic fibrosis, *Lancet* 1981;2:1201.

37. Eggleston P et al: Airway hyperreactivity in cystic fibrosis: clinical correlates and possible effects on the course of disease, *Chest* 1988;94:360.

38. Pattishall EN: Longitudinal response of pulmonary function to bronchodilators in cystic fibrosis, *Pediatr Pulmonol* 1990;9:80.

39. Kattan M et al: Response to aerosol salbutamol, SCH 1000, and placebo in cystic fibrosis, *Thorax* 1980;35:531.

40. Hordvik NL et al: The effects of albuterol on the lung function of hospitalized patients with cystic fibrosis, *Am J Respir Crit Care Med* 1996;154:156.

41. Zach MS et al: Bronchodilators increase airway instability in cystic fibrosis. *Am Rev Respir Dis* 1985;131:537–543.

42. Weintraub SJ, Eschenbacher WL: The inhaled bronchodilators ipratropium bromide and metaproterenol in adults with CF, *Chest* 1989;95:861.

43. Sanchez I, Holbrow J, Chernick V: Acute bronchodilator response to a combination of beta-adrenergic and anticholinergic agents in patients with cystic fibrosis, *J Pediatr* 1992;120:486.

44. Lethem MI et al: The origin of DNA associated with mucus glycoproteins in cystic fibrosis sputum, *Eur Respir J* 1990;3:19.

45. Shak S et al: Recombinant human DNase I (rhDnase) greatly reduces the viscosity of cystic fibrosis sputum, *Pediatr Pulmonol* 1990;5:S173.

46. Fuchs H et al: Effect of aerosolized recombinant DNase on exacerbations of respiratory symptoms and on pulmonary function in patients with cystic fibrosis, *N Engl J Med* 1994;331:637.

47. Robinson M et al: Effect of hypertonic saline, amiloride, and cough on mucociliary clearance in patients with cystic fibrosis, *Am J Respir Crit Care Med* 1996;153:1503.

48. Elkins MR et al: A controlled trial of long-term inhaled hypertonic saline in patients with cystic fibrosis, *N Engl J Med* 2006;354:229.

49. Donaldson SH et al: Mucus clearance and lung function in cystic fibrosis with hypertonic saline, *New Engl J Med* 2006;354:241.

50. www.cff.org/cf_services_pharmacy

51. Eigen H et al: CF Foundation Prednisone Trial Group: a multicenter study of alternate-day prednisone therapy in patients with cystic fibrosis, *J Pediatr* 1995;126:515.

52. vanHaren E et al: The effects of inhaled corticosteroid budesonide on lung function and bronchial hyperresponsiveness in adult patients with cystic fibrosis, *Am Rev Respir Dis* 1994;149:A667.

53. Nikolaizik W, Schonl M: Pilot study to assess the effect of inhaled corticosteroids on lung function in patients with cystic fibrosis, *J Pediatr* 1996;128:271.

54. Konstan MW et al: Effect of high-dose ibuprofen in patients with cystic fibrosis, *N Engl J Med* 1995;332:848.

55. Knowles MR et al: A pilot study of aerosolized amiloride for the treatment of lung disease in cystic fibrosis, *N Engl J Med* 1990;322:1189.

56. Ramsey BW et al: Intermittent administration of inhaled tobramycin in patients with cystic fibrosis, *N Engl J Med* 1999;340:23.

57. Ryan G et al. Nebulised anti-pseudomonal antibiotics for cystic fibrosis, *Cochrane Database Syst Rev* 2003;CD001021.

58. Jensen T: Colistin inhalation therapy in cystic fibrosis patients with chronic *Pseudomonas aeruginosa* lung infection, *J Antimicrob Chemother* 1987;19:831.

59. Donati MA, Guenette G, Auerbach H: Prospective controlled study of home and hospital therapy of cystic fibrosis pulmonary disease, *J Pediatr* 1987;111:28.
60. Ramsey B, Richardson M: Impact of sinusitis in cystic fibrosis, *J Allergy Clin Immunol* 1992;90:547.
61. Drake-Lee A, Morgan D: Nasal polyps and sinusitis in children with cystic fibrosis, *J Laryngol Otol* 1989;103:753.
62. Corey M et al: Familial concordance of pancreatic function in cystic fibrosis, *J Pediatr* 1989;115:273.
63. Moran A et al: Pancreatic endocrine function in cystic fibrosis, *J Pediatr* 1991;118:15.
64. Stern RC et al: Treatment and prognosis of rectal prolapse in cystic fibrosis, *Gastroenterology* 1982;82:707.
65. Scott RB, O'Loughlin EV, Gall DG: Gastroesophageal reflux in patients with cystic fibrosis, *J Pediatr* 1985;106:223.
66. Scott-Jupp R, Lama M, Tanner MS: Prevalence of liver disease in cystic fibrosis, *Arch Dis Child* 1991;66:698–701.
67. Stern RC, Rothstein FC, Doershuk CF: Treatment and prognosis of symptomatic gallbladder disease in patients with cystic fibrosis, *J Pediatr Gastroenterol Nutr* 1986;5:35.

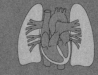

Chapter 35

Acute Respiratory Distress Syndrome

IRA CHEIFETZ • JENNIFER L. TURI

OUTLINE

Definition
Etiology
Prevalence
Clinical Course
    Stage of ARDS
    Mortality
Pathology and Role of Immunomodulators
    Pathology/Pathophysiology
    Immunomodulators

Pulmonary Mechanics
Treatment/Ventilatory Support
    Positive End-expiratory Pressure
    Low Tidal Volume Ventilation
    Gas Exchange Goals
    Permissive Hypercapnia
Adjunct Therapies
Summary

LEARNING OBJECTIVES

After reading this chapter the reader will be able to:
- Define the criteria to diagnose acute lung injury and acute respiratory distress syndrome
- Describe the pathophysiology of acute respiratory distress syndrome

- Explain the clinical approach to the management of the patient with acute lung injury

Acute respiratory distress syndrome (ARDS) represents an acute lung injury characterized by pulmonary edema secondary to the disruption of the alveolar-capillary membrane, hypoxemia, and widespread infiltrates on a chest radiograph that can occur after a wide variety of pulmonary and nonpulmonary insults. Pulmonary edema in the absence of heart failure was initially described almost a century ago. These conditions were originally known by the inciting injury rather than the overall clinical manifestation and included such names as shock lung, noncardiogenic pulmonary edema, and traumatic wet lung.[1,2] In 1967, Ashbaugh and colleagues[3] recognized ARDS as a constellation of pathophysiologic findings that were precipitated by a wide variety of insults, highlighting ARDS as a final common pathway initiated by local or systemic insults.

DEFINITION

In 1994, the American-European Consensus Conference on ARDS (the Consensus) was charged to formally define ARDS, provide uniformity and clarity in diagnosis, and facilitate comparison of clinical investigations.[4] The simplest clinical definition of ARDS is a diffuse, hypoxemic acute lung injury. Radiographically, there are bilateral areas of consolidation with air bronchograms that reflect alveolar filling and atelectasis (Figure 35-1).

611

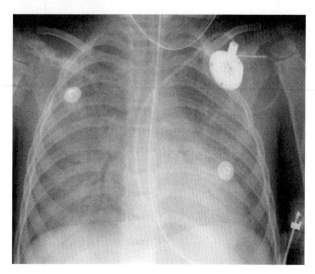

FIGURE 35-1 Chest radiograph of a patient with ARDS. Note the infiltrates in all five lobes, the air bronchograms that appear due to areas of consolidation, and the loss of lung volume.

Clinically, the patient demonstrates moderate to severe respiratory failure, hypoxemia, and decreased pulmonary compliance. The Consensus specifically defines ARDS as follows:[4]

1. Acute onset of respiratory symptoms
2. Frontal chest radiograph with bilateral infiltrates
3. $Pao_2/ Fio_2 \leq 200$ mm Hg
4. No clinical evidence of left atrial hypertension as defined by a pulmonary capillary wedge pressure less than 18 mm Hg, if measured.

Furthermore, the Consensus included a return from the use of *adult* respiratory distress syndrome back to *acute* respiratory distress syndrome to acknowledge that infants, children, and adults may be affected by the same pathophysiologic mechanisms.[4]

The Consensus also recommended that a new designation "acute lung injury (ALI)" be defined as "a syndrome of inflammation and increased permeability that is associated with a constellation of clinical, radiographic and physiologic abnormalities."[4] Clinically, ALI was defined by the acute onset of bilateral infiltrates on a chest radiograph without evidence of elevated left atrial pressure and a Pao_2/ Fio_2 (P/F ratio) of less than 300.

One of the limitations of the P/F ratio to differentiate patients with ARDS versus ALI is that mechanical ventilator support (specifically mean airway pressure) is not considered. An alternative objective scoring system utilized in the clinical setting is the oxygenation index (OI):[5-9]

$$OI = (P\overline{aw} \times Fio_2)/Pao_2 \times 100$$

where Paw is the mean airway pressure, Fio_2 is the fraction of inspired oxygen, and Pao_2 is the arterial oxygen tension. The OI equation accounts not only for the ratio of admin-

istered Fio_2 to arterial oxygenation but also the mean airway pressure. OI has been correlated with outcome, can be objectively used to define entry for clinical studies or response criteria for various clinical studies, and can describe criteria for more highly invasive therapies such as extracorporeal membrane oxygenation (ECMO).[5-9]

ETIOLOGY

ALI and ARDS can be incited by numerous insults that both directly and indirectly affect the lung via the generation of inflammatory mediators. Direct pulmonary insults include pneumonia, aspiration, chest trauma, and smoke inhalation. Indirect lung injury may be the result of generalized systemic conditions, such as sepsis, closed head injury, multitrauma, transfusion reactions, and hemorrhagic shock. While numerous insults may generate an inflammatory response, innate genetic differences regulate immune responses of the lungs and are important in pathogenesis.[10]

PREVALENCE

The lack of universally accepted diagnostic criteria and the diversity of underlying causes make it difficult to determine the true prevalence of ARDS. Depending on the diagnostic criteria, there may be as many as 150,000 cases of adult ARDS per year in the United States.[11] Several studies agree that of all adult intensive care unit admissions approximately 7% of patients meet the Consensus ARDS diagnosis criteria.[4,12-15] A European study (ALIVE)[15] involving 78 ICUs from 9 countries in which all patients (n = 5457) were admitted to one of the participating units for at least 4 hours during a 2-month study period reported that 7.4% had, or developed, ALI/ARDS. However, this study noted considerable variations in the occurrence of ALI/ARDS among countries ranging from 1.7% to 19.5%.[16] This study indicates that although diagnostic criteria may be the same, interpretation and/or true prevalence of ARDS does vary between countries and possibly within countries.

The prevalence of pediatric ARDS is less certain but does appear to be lower than for adult patients.[17] Davis *et al* published data from a single-institution study reporting that ARDS was present in 2.7% of pediatric intensive care unit admissions and accounted for 8% of patient days.[18] Goh *et al* reported a prevalence of 4.3% in pediatric patients.[19]

CLINICAL COURSE

Respiratory distress and failure are clinical diagnoses of a pulmonary system that is no longer capable of providing normal gas exchange. The term *respiratory distress* indicates that compensatory mechanisms are being utilized by the patient to preserve adequate gas exchange. *Respiratory failure* is a late clinical finding resulting from the failure of these compensatory mechanisms.

Respiratory failure indicates the need for an artificial airway and/or mechanical respiratory support. The main function of the respiratory system is to provide adequate oxygenation and carbon dioxide elimination. In the setting of acute respiratory failure, the lungs are unable to preserve adequate gas exchange. Subsequently, tissue oxygen delivery can be impaired resulting in anaerobic metabolism and lactic acid formation and/or ventilation can be inadequate resulting in hypercapnia and a potentially worsening acidosis. In patients with ARDS, impairment of oxygenation is an early finding, while impairment of ventilation occurs much later in the disease process.

Respiratory disease, especially in infants and young children, can rapidly progress from respiratory distress to the acute onset of respiratory failure and significant impairment in gas exchange. Although respiratory failure is classically described by arterial blood gas values (Pao_2 less than 60 mm Hg and/or $PaCO_2$ greater than 50 mm Hg), it is best recognized as a clinical syndrome of the progression of the physical signs and symptoms of respiratory distress. Infants and young children are particularly prone to developing respiratory distress and failure due to:

(a) a smaller caliber of airways resulting in a greater resistance to air flow,

(b) an increased chest wall compliance, which can cause paradoxical breathing and restrict lung capacitance due to chest wall retractions as may occur with forceful inspiratory effort, and/or

(c) a greater propensity for rapid fatigue of the respiratory muscles and the diaphragm.

However, the progression of respiratory failure to ARDS is more likely to occur in adult patients as indicated by the prevalence data.

Stages of ARDS

The clinical course of ARDS is characterized by distinct clinical, radiographic and pathologic manifestations.[20] The first stage consists of acute injury to the lung tissue, directly or indirectly. Clinically, patients may display mild tachypnea and dyspnea and tend to have normal radiographic findings. The second stage, or latent period, lasts a variable period of time after the acute injury. During this time the patient may appear clinically stable, but begins to develop early signs of pulmonary injury or insufficiency manifested by hyperventilation with hypocarbia and a respiratory alkalosis. The chest radiograph may remain clear or may begin to demonstrate a fine reticular pattern related to the development of pulmonary interstitial fluid.[21-22]

The third stage, acute respiratory failure, is heralded by the rapid onset of respiratory failure with hypoxemia refractory to supplemental oxygen. Diffuse pulmonary edema and worsening compliance cause significant atelectasis and intrapulmonary shunting. Clinically, patients develop rapid, shallow tachypnea with increased work of breathing. The physical signs of respiratory failure will vary with age and include subcostal and supraclavicular retractions, grunting (i.e., an attempt to generate an increased intrinsic positive end-expiratory pressure [PEEP]), nasal flaring, and head bobbing. Lung examination usually reveals diffuse crackles on auscultation. Radiographically, there are bilateral areas of consolidation with air bronchograms that reflect alveolar filling and atelectasis (see Figure 35-1).[21-22] A significant percentage of these patients will require endotracheal intubation and mechanical ventilation with the application of PEEP. However, noninvasive ventilation may be an alternative for a subgroup of patients.

Mortality

Most studies indicate that mortality associated with ARDS is due to nonrespiratory causes (i.e., die with, rather than of, ARDS). Montgomery et al reported that only 16% of deaths were caused by respiratory failure.[23] In most cases, early death (within 72 hours) was caused by the underlying illness or injury, whereas late death (beyond 72 hours) was caused by infection. More than 10 years later, Ferring and Vincent reported similar findings.[24] In a series of 129 patients with ARDS, 67 (25%) died. Fifty percent of these patients died of sepsis/multiple organ failure (MOF), 16% of respiratory failure, 15% of cardiac failure/arrhythmia, 10% of neurologic failure, and 8% of other causes. Bersten et al reported that respiratory failure contributed to death in only 24% of ARDS patients and was the only cause of death in 9% of the population studied.[14]

Mortality for patients requiring mechanical ventilation varies widely depending on the clinical condition requiring ventilatory support. For otherwise healthy infants and children with acute, self-limited conditions, mortality rates approach 0%. Patients with severe ARDS may have mortality rates that range between 15% and 60% depending on the data reviewed. Mortality has classically been described as between 40% and 70%.[1] Mechanically ventilated patients with multiorgan system failure and/or severe immunodeficiency have a mortality rate that may exceed 90%. Recent studies suggest mortality from ARDS is declining; however, the reason behind this overall improvement is not clear. Except for low tidal volume ventilation, no single intervention for ARDS has been clearly shown to decrease mortality.[25] One report described 133 pediatric patients with severe hypoxic respiratory failure who had a mortality rate of only 13%.[26] A more recent report of 328 pediatric intensive care unit admissions for ALI/ARDS had a mortality rate of 22%.[27] This prospective evaluation additionally demonstrated that, as in adults, pneumonia, sepsis, and aspiration are the most common causes of ALI and ARDS in children.

PATHOLOGY AND ROLE OF IMMUNOMODULATORS

Pathology/Pathophysiology

The clinical stages of ARDS coincide with three pathologic stages, namely the Exudative Stage, the Proliferative Stage, and the Fibrotic Stage. The Exudative Stage is marked by the development of diffuse injury to the alveolar-capillary membrane. Influx of inflammatory cells and mediators destroy type I pneumocytes, resulting in sloughing of these cells, and subsequent formation of a protein-rich hyaline membrane on the denuded basement membrane. Furthermore, activation of the endothelium and leukocytes results in barrier dysfunction and the formation of microthrombi within the vasculature, which contributes to the propagation of acute lung injury and alterations in pulmonary vascular tone. Disruption of both the epithelial and endothelial surfaces of the alveolar-capillary membrane significantly increases permeability and results in flooding of the alveoli with proteinaceous fluid.

The loss of the alveolar-capillary integrity and the subsequent development of pulmonary edema in both the interstitial and alveolar spaces are due to both altered capillary permeability and oncotic gradients early in the disease process and to increases in pulmonary vascular resistance in later stages of ARDS. Pulmonary compliance is significantly worsened by the presence of edema and can result in widespread atelectasis. Pulmonary compliance is further impacted by the inactivation of surfactant that results from the presence of plasma protein, such as fibrin, and inflammatory mediators, such as proteinases, in the alveolar space.[28,29] The development of microthrombi within the pulmonary vasculature together with the release of numerous vasoactive mediators from inflammatory cells and the activated endothelium contributes to the development of pulmonary hypertension and further contributes to the ventilation/perfusion abnormalities characteristic of ARDS. The degree of epithelial injury and the subsequent ability to clear edema fluid, as well as the reversibility of pulmonary hypertension, are important predictors of outcome in ARDS.[30,31]

The Proliferative Stage occurs 1 to 3 weeks after the initiation of injury and is characterized by an attempt to repair the disrupted epithelium. This involves the proliferation of type II pneumocytes to replace type I cells on the denuded basement membrane and to begin to replace surfactant. While the turnover of type II cells is typically low, it accelerates after acute lung injury, and these cells may differentiate abnormally.[32,33] Epithelial repair requires not only the close coordination of numerous growth factors but also an intact basement membrane to provide a platform for cell adhesion and migration.[10] Inflammatory cells continue to be recruited to phagocytose hyaline membrane and debris, which provides a framework for the elaboration of fibrous tissue.[34] Alternatively, fibroblasts proliferate to convert hemorrhagic exudates into cellular granulation tissue.

The ability of the lung to recover depends on the presence of functional epithelium to clear the alveolar fluid and the body's ability to attenuate the inflammatory process. If lung injury and inflammation persist, the patient may develop severe physiologic abnormalities and may progress to the Fibrotic Stage of ARDS. This injury can be seen as early as 5 to 7 days after the onset of disease, although this is more definitive after several weeks. Histologically, the alveolar space becomes filled with mesenchymal cells, and lung tissue is replaced by collagenous tissue.[35] In addition, there is increased evidence of angiogenesis. Vascular changes occur throughout the later stages of ARDS with obliteration of small precapillary vessels and an increase in the medial thickness of intraacinar pulmonary arteries. Overall, these changes markedly decrease the available surface area for gas exchange and result in intractable respiratory failure or chronic lung disease, potentially requiring prolonged ventilator support. Treatment strategies seek to avoid this final, intractable stage of ARDS.

Immunomodulators

Numerous mediators of inflammation are implicated in the pathogenesis of ARDS (Box 35-1).[36] It is unclear, however, whether some of these mediators directly cause ARDS or are a secondary product of the inflammation resulting from lung injury. Direct lung injury from aspiration or smoke inhalation, for example, may result in inflammation and the release of inflammatory cytokines that augment microvascular permeability. Regardless of whether inflammatory mediators are primarily or secondarily involved in the pathogenesis of ARDS, they are clearly complex contributors to its development. The effects of mediators and inflammatory cells involved in ARDS, as well as those of their regulatory molecules, are tightly interwoven and ultimately result in a balance between pro- and antiinflammatory and pro- and antiedematous factors.[37] While inflammatory mediators could themselves disrupt the capillary-alveolar membrane, they may also create effects that keep the inflammatory response in check. This may account for the lack

Box 35-1	Possible Contributors to the Development of ARDS

- Polymorphonuclear leukocytes
- Macrophages
- Monocytes
- Platelets
- Lymphocytes
- Fibroblasts
- Bacterial toxins (endotoxin, teichoic acids, toxic shock syndrome toxin-1)
- Oxygen free radicals
- Tumor necrosis factor-α
- Interleukins
- Prostaglandins
- Thromboxane
- Leukotrienes
- Serotonin
- Free fatty acids
- Histamine
- Activated complement
- Proteases
- Platelet-activating factor
- Fibrin-platelet microthrombi
- Fibrin degradation products
- Thromboplastin (tissue factor)
- Hageman factor (factor XII)
- Bradykinin
- α_1-Antitrypsin deficiency
- Pulmonary fibrosis

From Willson DF et al: Calf's lung surfactant extract in acute hypoxemic respiratory failure in children. *Crit Care Med* 1996; 24:1316-1322.

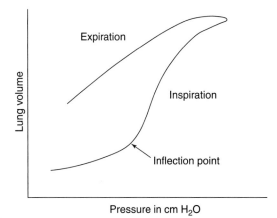

FIGURE 35-2 Representation of the pressure-volume (compliance) loop in ARDS. Below the inflection point is the pressure at which the alveoli begin to collapse, leading to loss of lung volume, or FRC.

of success of pharmacologic inhibitors to decrease the mortality associated with ARDS. Research efforts continue to investigate potential ways to more effectively modulate the inflammatory response during ARDS.[36-38]

PULMONARY MECHANICS

ARDS alters pulmonary mechanics in several ways. The loss of surfactant function, coupled with the development of edema around and within the alveoli, leads to alveolar collapse. The result is a decrease in lung compliance, lung volume, and functional residual capacity. This is associated with a large intrapulmonary shunt fraction $\dot{Q}_s/\dot{Q}_p$ that contributes to the significant hypoxemia associated with ARDS.

During ARDS, marked hysteresis of the pressure-volume loop occurs, such that significantly higher transpulmonary pressures are necessary to achieve a given lung volume on inspiration than on expiration. The point on the pressure-volume loop where the shape changes from concave to exponential is known as the lower inflection point. It reflects the pressure point at which alveoli begin to open and is located above functional residual capacity

(Figure 35-2). This suggests that many gas exchange units will collapse at normal transpulmonary pressures in acutely injured lungs and may need significant PEEP to maintain patency during expiration.

Finally, lung injury and areas of involvement in ARDS are heterogeneous and not uniform through all lung units. Some areas of the lung, typically in the dependent regions, are grossly affected. Other regions of the lung, typically in the nondependent regions, may be relatively unaffected.[39] This creates varying areas of compliance within the lung itself. Dependent regions are generally fluid filled, atelectatic, and noncompliant. Nondependent areas are relatively normal and, thus, at risk for overdistention (i.e., volutrauma) and/or barotrauma during mechanical ventilation.

TREATMENT/VENTILATORY SUPPORT

Management of the patient with respiratory distress or failure includes an assessment of airway, breathing, and circulation ("ABCs"). Prompt cardiopulmonary resuscitation is vital to restoring adequate systemic oxygen delivery. Identification and targeted therapy for the underlying etiology and elimination of any potential source for exacerbation of the disease is a critical first step in treatment.

The goal in the treatment of ARDS is to treat the underlying disease (if possible), achieve adequate (but not necessarily optimal) tissue oxygenation, and avoid complications. All ARDS patients require supplemental oxygen, and most require mechanical ventilation. Tissue oxygenation is provided by ensuring adequate cardiac output and hemoglobin levels. Overhydration could augment pulmonary edema, so fluids should be carefully titrated and monitored to normalize volume and maintain cardiac output. Antibiotics are used to treat pneumonia and sepsis. Adequate nutrition should be provided to optimize caloric intake.

Every patient with ARDS is hypoxemic by definition. Prolonged administration of high concentrations of oxygen can damage the lungs, owing to the formation of highly reactive oxygen free radicals. Human and animal studies suggest that a prolonged FIO_2 greater than 0.60 should be avoided to prevent oxygen-induced pulmonary damage.[40] However, the exact FIO_2 cutoff for oxygen toxicity in the ARDS patient remains unknown and may be less than 0.60.

Positive End-expiratory Pressure

The mainstay in treating ARDS is the administration of PEEP. No gas exchange will occur in atelectatic or fluid-filled alveoli. PEEP helps maintain alveolar patency and restore functional residual capacity. PEEP also maintains the transthoracic pressure above the point at which additional alveoli will collapse during expiration. PEEP is typically increased to a level that allows adequate oxygenation as defined by an arterial oxygen saturation (Sao_2) of 85% or greater at an acceptable FIO_2 of 0.60 or less. It should be noted that the minimal acceptable arterial oxygen saturation remains very controversial. A PEEP level of 10 to 15 cm H_2O, or even higher, may be required to achieve adequate oxygenation. However, as PEEP levels exceed 12 to 15 cm H_2O, the increase in intrathoracic pressure may adversely affect cardiac output, primarily by decreasing systemic venous return.[41] As PEEP is increased, the ARDS patient should be monitored for a decrease in cardiac output with a decrease in peripheral perfusion. In most cases, a decrease in cardiac output can be compensated for by intravascular volume loading and possibly inotropic support.[42,43]

A study by the ARDS Network investigated the optimal PEEP-FIO_2 strategy for adult patients with ARDS.[44] The results of this prospective, randomized, multicenter study indicate that in adult ARDS patients who are ventilated with 6 ml/kg tidal volumes and an end-inspiratory plateau pressure of less than 30 cm H_2O, a "moderately high" or "very high" PEEP strategy produced similar survival rates. It must be noted that this study investigated two relatively aggressive PEEP strategies. The implication of this ARDS Network study is that once appropriate PEEP is applied to maintain the lungs at an ideal lung volume, a further increase in PEEP in an attempt to reduce the FIO_2 does not lead to an improved outcome.

Low Tidal Volume Ventilation

Ventilation is achieved through a combination of respiratory rate, tidal volume, and inspiratory time.

Historically, ventilator tidal volumes between 10 and 15 ml/kg were used for patients with ARDS. Because the remaining compliant lung volume in a patient with ARDS is significantly reduced, these tidal volumes often required inflation pressures that resulted in pulmonary overdistention and lung injury.[45-50]

The ARDS Network reported in the *New England Journal of Medicine* in 2000 that in adult patients with acute lung injury and ARDS, low tidal volume mechanical ventilation (6 ml/kg) decreased mortality by 22% and increased the number of ventilator-free days as compared to a more traditional tidal volume (12 ml/kg).[25] The mortality rate was 31.0% in the low tidal volume group and 39.8% ($p = 0.007$) in the higher tidal volume group. Additionally, the plateau pressure (Pplat) was significantly decreased in the low tidal volume group as compared to the control group.

Although still unproven, these results are likely applicable to infants and children with acute lung injury and acute respiratory distress syndrome. Until a similar large-scale, prospective, randomized trial is accomplished in pediatrics, it seems reasonable to utilize the low tidal volume guideline. It should be emphasized that the low tidal volume ventilation strategy was studied in patients with acute lung injury, and it remains uncertain whether larger tidal volumes can be safely used in pediatric and adult populations with more normal lung function.

Before the ARDS Network low tidal volume study, several studies offered conflicting results on this topic. Amato et al concluded that a lung protective ventilation strategy was associated with a significant decrease in mortality at 28 days but was not associated with a higher rate of survival to hospital discharge.[51] A major limitation in the application of the results of this study is the high mortality rate in the control group (71%). In contrast, the next article in the same issue of the *New England Journal of Medicine* was a report by Stewart et al that concluded that a low tidal volume strategy does not reduce mortality for adult patients with ARDS.[52]

The apparently conflicting results from the low tidal volume studies by Amato, Stewart, and the ARDS Network become more consistent when considering the plateau pressures utilized. In the ARDS Network study, the protocol was designed to maintain plateau pressure less than 50 cm H_2O in the control group and less than 30 cm H_2O in the low tidal volume group.[25] The results indicate that in the low tidal volume group Pplat remained ≤ 26 cm H_2O throughout the first week of ventilation; while in the control group Pplat ranged from 33 ± 9 to 37 ± 9 cm H_2O over the first week. In the Amato study, Pplat remained less than 32 cm H_2O for the protective ventilation group; in the control group Pplat ranged from 34.4 ± 1.9 to 37.8 ± 1.2 cm H_2O over the first 7 days of ventilation.[51] Of interest, the study by Stewart et al revealed no improvement with mortality with low tidal volume ventilation; however, in both groups the Pplat was maintained less than 29 cm H_2O throughout the study.[52] This finding is similar to the study by Brochard et al, which also failed to demonstrate improved survival with low tidal volume ventilation.[53] For both groups, Pplat was maintained at less than 32 cm H_2O throughout the first week of ventilation.

Thus, the data support the conclusion that for adult patients with ARDS, the Pplat should be limited to less than approximately 32 cm H_2O to improve outcome. The applicability of this conclusion to pediatric ARDS patients requires investigation. It is very possible that the "critical" limit on plateau pressure for infants and children will be less than 32 cm H_2O and may vary with patient age/size.

It must be stressed that although the ARDS Network study indicates that a 6 ml/kg tidal volume led to improved mortality as compared to a 12 ml/kg tidal volume, the tidal volume associated with the least mortality may lie somewhere between 6 and 12 ml/kg (or possibly even less than 6 ml/kg). Lastly, it should be stressed that most previous ARDS trials have been based on a "magic bullet" strategy in which a single intervention is studied. Mortality from ARDS has improved over the past decade without ever truly finding the "magic bullet." Most likely, the improvements in the care of ARDS patients have been multifactorial. Although difficult, future clinical studies should investigate a combination of therapies to further decrease mortality from ARDS.

Multiple modes of mechanical ventilation are currently used in clinical practice to provide respiratory support for patients with acute lung injury and acute respiratory distress syndrome. To date, no data exist to determine the ventilatory mode which provides the greatest benefit and the least risk to an individual patient. Prospective, randomized, multicenter studies for mechanical ventilation and ARDS are limited. For most clinical questions, data are extrapolated from studies in the adult population.

Gas Exchange Goals

Improved oxygenation is not correlated with improved outcomes. This was best demonstrated in the ARDS Network low tidal volume study, in which the control (12 ml/kg) group demonstrated improved oxygenation for the first 72 hours of ventilation.[25] If this study had been designed as an acute gas exchange study, the conclusion would have been false and mortality for ARDS could have increased. This lack of association between oxygenation and survival has been demonstrated in multiple other studies.[54-57] Timmons et al demonstrated no correlation between oxygenation or ventilation in

survivors or nonsurvivors of pediatric ARDS.[17] Dobyns et al showed that, in acute hypoxic respiratory failure in children, although oxygenation improved with inhaled nitric oxide, there was no difference in mortality.[54] Improved oxygenation without a significant improvement in survival was also demonstrated in a follow-up study of inhaled nitric oxide in combination with high-frequency oscillatory ventilation.[55]

Permissive Hypercapnia

A logical consequence of low tidal volume ventilation is hypercapnia. Limiting the peak inspiratory pressure by reducing the tidal volume may decrease minute ventilation and result in hypercapnia. The exact degree of respiratory acidosis that can be safely tolerated remains controversial. However, most undesirable effects are reversible and mostly minor with respiratory acidosis when pH is greater than approximately 7.20.[58]

It should be noted that a Cochrane review of the large, multicenter low tidal volume studies of ARDS was unable to reach a firm conclusion on the implications of permissive hypercapnia.[57] This review noted confounding variables on the role of permissive hypercapnia in the management of acute lung injury. It should be noted that these low tidal volume studies were not designed to address the specific question of hypercapnia. However, the medical literature does support the beneficial role of permissive hypercapnia in ALI/ARDS. Limited evidence does suggest that low-volume, pressure-limited ventilation with permissive hypercapnia may improve outcome in both adults and pediatric patients with ARDS.[26,59,60] In a 10-year study, Milberg et al reported a positive association between permissive hypercapnia and outcomes.[61] Recent data from a laboratory model of ischemia-reperfusion acute lung injury indicate that hypercapnic acidosis is protective and that buffering of the hypercapnic acidosis attenuates its protective effects.[62]

ADJUNCT THERAPIES

Some patients are unable to achieve acceptable therapeutic goals while avoiding oxygen toxicity or an intolerably high peak inspiratory pressure with conventional ventilator strategies. Two of the more commonly used therapeutic modalities for treating patients with ARDS are high-frequency ventilation and ECMO.[63-70] These topics are presented in detail in Chapters 21 and 24.

Other potential adjunct therapies include trials of corticosteroids, inhaled nitric oxide, and surfactant replacement. Although one small study suggests that corticosteroids may improve outcome in patients who progress into the late fibrotic fourth stage, large prospective trials have shown that corticosteroids fail to improve outcome and may be harmful in certain patients.[71-73] Studies of inhaled nitric oxide for pediatric ALI/ARDS have demonstrated improved oxygenation acutely, but this improvement in gas exchange has not translated into improved survival.[54,55,74] A recent publication by Willson et al reported that exogenous surfactant (Calfactant) acutely improved oxygenation and significantly decreased mortality in infants and children with acute lung injury.[75] This study revealed no significant decrease in duration of mechanical ventilation, length of PICU admission, or length of hospital stay. Despite promising results of prone positioning from investigations in adults with ARDS, a study of prone positioning for pediatric acute lung injury was recently closed for futility. This prospective, randomized, multicenter study by Curley et al revealed no change in mortality with prone positioning.[56]

SUMMARY

Acute lung injury and acute respiratory distress syndrome represent a spectrum of clinical disease of varying pulmonary and nonpulmonary etiologies. Although much has been learned about the pathophysiology of lung injury over the past 2 decades, the only treatment strategy that has been proven to improve clinical outcome is low tidal volume ventilation. However, it should be noted that even in the years before the publication of the low tidal volume ventilation data, overall survival rates for adult and pediatric ARDS patients had been slowly increasing. Future clinical investigations are likely to study combined therapeutic strategies as opposed to focusing on discovering the single "magic bullet."

ASSESSMENT QUESTIONS

See Evolve Resources for the answers.

1. Which of the following Pao_2 / Fio_2 values define acute respiratory distress syndrome (ARDS)?
   A. ≤ 100
   B. ≤ 200
   C. ≤ 250
   D. ≤ 300
2. Oxygenation Index (OI) is defined as
   A. (mean airway pressure × Fio_2)/Pao_2 × 100
   B. (peak inspiratory pressure × Fio_2)/Pao_2 × 100
   C. (mean airway pressure × Pao_2)/Fio_2 × 100
   D. Pao_2/ Fio_2

ASSESSMENT QUESTIONS—cont'd

3. Which one of the following is not one of the three pathologic stages of ARDS?
   A. Exudative Stage
   B. Proliferative Stage
   C. Fibrotic Stage
   D. Edematous Stage
4. Which of the following treatment strategies for acute lung injury in adult patients has been demonstrated to improve mortality?
   A. Prone positioning
   B. Inhaled nitric oxide
   C. Low positive end-expiratory pressure
   D. Low tidal volume ventilation
5. The overall goal(s) in the treatment of ARDS include
   A. Treatment of the underlying disease
   B. Achieve adequate tissue oxygenation
   C. Minimize ventilator induced lung injury
   D. All of the above
6. The criteria used to define ARDS include
   A. Hypoxemia
   B. Bilateral pulmonary infiltrates
   C. Abscess of left heart failure
   D. All of the above
7. Which of the following adjunct therapies has been associated with a decrease in mortality in *pediatric* patients with acute lung injury?
   A. Permissive hypercapnia
   B. Permissive hypoxemia
   C. Exogenous surfactant administration
   D. Low tidal volume ventilation
8. Which of the following characteristics of infants and young children (as compared to older children and adults) causes this population to be particularly prone to respiratory failure?
   A. Small caliber airways
   B. Increased chest wall compliance
   C. Greater propensity for rapid fatigue of respiratory muscles
   D. All of the above
9. The most common immediate cause of death in patients with ARDS is
   A. Failure of gas exchange
   B. Multiorgan system failure
   C. Renal failure
   D. Cardiac failure
10. Which of the following is generally the latest clinical finding in patients with ARDS?
    A. Hypoxemia
    B. Decreased pulmonary compliance
    C. Increased work of breathing
    D. Hypercapnia

References

1. Fackler JC et al: Acute respiratory distress syndrome. In Rogers MC, editor: *Textbook of pediatric intensive care*. Baltimore. Williams & Wilkins, 1996.
2. Bernard GR: Acute Respiratory Distress Syndrome A Historical Perspective, *Am J Respir Crit Care Med* 2005;172:798.
3. Ashbaugh DG et al: Acute respiratory distress in adults, *Lancet* 1967;2:319.
4. Bernard GR et al: The American-European Consensus Conference on ARDS, *Am J Respir Crit Care Med* 1994;149:818.
5. Rivera RA, Butt W, Shann F: Predictors of mortality in children with respiratory failure: possible indications for ECMO. *Anaesth Intensive Care* 1990;18:385.
6. Durand M et al: Oxygenation index in patients with meconium aspiration: conventional and extracorporeal membrane oxygenation therapy, *Crit Care Med* 1990;18:373.
7. Monchi M et al: Early predictive factors in survival in the acute respiratory distress syndrome, *Am J Resp Crit Care Med* 1998;158:1076.
8. Mehta S et al: High frequency oscillatory ventilation in adults, *Chest* 2004;126:518.
9. Petrou S et al: Cost effectiveness analysis of neonatal extracorporeal membrane oxygenation based on four year results from the UK Collaborative ECMO Trial, *Arch Dis Child* 2004;89:263.
10. Piantadosi CA, Schwartz DA: The Acute Respiratory Distress Syndrome, *Ann Intern Med* 2004;141:460.
11. National Heart and Lung Institute, National Institutes of Health: *Respiratory distress syndromes: Task force on problems, research approaches, needs*. DHEW publication No. (NIH) 73-432. Washington, DC. US Government Printing Office, 1972; pp 165–180.
12. Monchi M et al: Early predictive factors of survival in the acute respiratory distress syndrome, *Am J Respir Crit Care Med* 1998;158: 1076.
13. Roupie E et al: Prevalence, etiologies and outcome of the acute respiratory distress syndrome among hypoxemic ventilated patients, *Intensive Care Med* 1999;25:920.
14. Bersten AD et al: Incidence and mortality of acute lung injury and the acute respiratory distress syndrome in three Australian States, *Am J Respir Crit Care Med* 2002;165:443.
15. Brun-Buisson C et al: The European Survey of acute lung injury and ARDS: Preliminary results of the ALIVE study. Abstr. *Intensive Care Med* 2000;26 (Suppl 3): 617.
16. Minelli C et al: Variability between countries in the occurrence of ALI and ARDS: Preliminary results of the ALIVE European Study, Abstr. *Intensive Care Med* 2000;26 (Suppl 3): 329.
17. Timmons OD, Havens PL, Fackler JC: Predicting death in pediatric patients with acute respiratory failure, *Chest* 1995;108:789.
18. Davis SL, Furman DP, Costarino AJ: Adult respiratory distress syndrome in children: associated diseases, clinical course, and predictors of death, *J Pediatr* 1993;123:35.
19. Goh AY et al: Incidence of acute respiratory distress syndrome: A comparison of two definitions. *Arch Dis Child* 1998;79:256.
20. Ware LB, Matthay MA: Medical Progress: The Acute Respiratory Distress Syndrome, *New Engl J Med* 2000: 342:1334.
21. Aberle DR, Brown K: Radiologic considerations in the adult respiratory distress syndrome, *Clin Chest Med* 1990;11:737.
22. Effman EL et al: Adult respiratory distress syndrome in children, *Radiology* 1985;157:69.
23. Montgomery BA et al: Causes of mortality in patients with the adult respiratory distress syndrome, *Am Rev Respir Dis* 1985;132:485.
24. Ferring M, Vincent JL: Is outcome from ARDS related to the severity of respiratory failure? *Eur Respir J* 1997;10:1297.
25. ARDS Network: Ventilation with lower tidal volumes as compared with traditional tidal volumes for acute lung injury and the acute respiratory distress syndrome, *N Engl J Med* 2000;342:1301.
26. Fackler JC et al: ECMO for ARDS: Stopping a randomized clinical trial, *Am J Respir Crit Care Med* 1997;155:A504.
27. Flori HR et al: Pediatric acute lung injury: Prospective evaluation of risk factors associated with mortality, *Am J Respir Crit Care Med* 2005;171:995.
28. Lewis JF et al: Altered alveolar surfactant is an early marker of acute lung injury in septic adult sheep, *Am J Resp Crit Care Med* 1994;150:123.
29. Seeger W et al: Alveolar surfactant and adult respiratory distress syndrome: pathogenetic role and therapeutic prospects, *Clin Invest* 1993;71:177.
30. Matthay MA: Intact epithelial barrier function is critical for the resolution of alveolar edema in humans, *Am Rev Respir Dis* 1990;142:1250.
31. Ware LB, Matthay MA: Alveolar fluid clearance is impaired in the majority of patients with acute lung injury and the acute respiratory distress syndrome, *Am J Resp Crit Care Med* 2001;163:1376.
32. Berthiaume Y et al: Treatment of adult respiratory distress syndrome: Plea for rescue therapy of the alveolar epithelium, *Thorax* 1999;54:150.
33. Tanswell AK et al: Limited division of low-density adult rat type II pneumocytes in serum-free culture, *Am J Physiol* 1991;260:L395.
34. Bitterman PB. Pathogenesis of fibrosis in acute lung injury, *Am J Med* 1992;92:39S.
35. Kuhn C et al: An immunohistochemical study of architectural remodeling and connective tissue synthesis in pulmonary fibrosis, *Am Rev Respir Dis* 1989;140:1693.
36. Ranieri VM et al: Effect of mechanical ventilation on inflammatory mediators in patients with acute respiratory distress syndrome: A randomized controlled trial, *JAMA* 1999;282:54.
37. Matthay MA Zimmerman GA: Acute lung injury and the acute respiratory distress syndrome four decades of inquire into pathogenesis and rational management, *Am J Resp Cell Molec Biol* 2005;33:319.
38. Rinaldo JE, Christman JW: Mechanisms and mediators of the adult respiratory distress syndrome, *Clin Chest Med* 1990;11:621.
39. Gattinoni L, Pesenti A: ARDS: The nonhomogenous lung: facts and hypothesis, *Intensive Crit Care Dig* 1987;61:1.
40. Jenkinson SG: Oxygen toxicity, *New Horizons* 1993;1:504.
41. Mitaka C et al: Two-dimensional echocardiographic evaluation of inferior vena cava, right ventricle, and

left ventricle during positive-pressure ventilation with varying levels of positive end-expiratory pressure, *Crit Care Med* 1989;17:205.

42. Mohsenifar Z et al: Relationship between O_2 delivery and O_2 consumption in adult respiratory distress syndrome, *Chest* 1983;84:267.

43. Pollack MM, Fields AI, Holbrook PR: Cardiopulmonary parameters during high PEEP in children. *Crit Care Med* 1980;8:372.

44. Brower RG et al: Higher versus lower positive end-expiratory pressure in patients with acute respiratory distress syndrome, *New Eng J Med* 2004;351:327.

45. Tsuno K et al: Histopathologic pulmonary changes from mechanical ventilation at high peak airway pressures, *Am Rev Respir Dis* 1991;143:1115.

46. Webb HH, Tierney DF: Experimental pulmonary edema due to intermittent positive- pressure ventilation with high inflation pressures: protection by positive end-expiratory pressure, *Am Rev Respir Dis* 1974;110:556.

47. Dreyfuss D et al: Intermittent positive-pressure hyperventilation with high inflation pressures produces pulmonary microvascular injury in rats, *Am Rev Respir Dis* 1985;132:880.

48. Kolobow T et al: Severe impairment in lung function induced by high peak airway pressure during mechanical ventilation: an experimental study, *Am Rev Respir Dis* 1987;135:312.

49. Corbridge TC et al: Adverse effects of large tidal volume and low PEEP in canine acid aspiration, *Am Rev Respir Dis* 1990;142:311.

50. Parker JC et al: Lung edema caused by high peak inspiratory pressures in dogs: role of increased microvascular filtration pressure and permeability, *Am Rev Respir Dis* 1990;142:321.

51. Amato MB et al: Effect of a protective-ventilation strategy on mortality in the acute respiratory distress syndrome, *N Engl J Med* 1998;338:347.

52. Stewart TE et al: Evaluation of a ventilation strategy to prevent barotrauma in patients at high risk for acute respiratory distress syndrome, *N Engl J Med* 1998;338:355.

53. Brochard L et al: Tidal volume reduction for prevention of ventilator-induced lung injury in acute respiratory distress syndrome, *Am J Resp Crit Care Med* 1998;158:1831.

54. Dobyns EL et al: Multicenter randomized controlled trial of the effects of inhaled nitric oxide therapy on gas exchange in children with acute hypoxemic respiratory failure, *J Pediatr* 1999;134:406.

55. Dobyns EL et al: Interactive effects of high-frequency oscillatory ventilation and inhaled nitric oxide in acute hypoxemic respiratory failure in pediatrics, *Crit Care Med* 2002;30:2425.

56. Curley MA et al: Effect of prone positioning on clinical outcomes in children with acute lung injury: A randomized clinical trial, *JAMA* 2005;294:229.

57. Petrucci N, Iacovelli W: Ventilation with lower tidal volumes versus traditional tidal volumes for acute lung injury and acute respiratory distress syndrome, *Cochrane Database of Systematic Reviews*. Most recent update: February 25, 2004.

58. Feihl F, Perret C: Permissive hypercapnia: how permissive should we be? *Am J Respir Crit Care Med* 1994;150:1722.

59. Hickling KG, Henderson SJ, Jackson R: Low mortality associated with low volume pressure-limited ventilation with permissive hypercapnia in severe adult respiratory distress syndrome, *Intensive Care Med* 1990;16:372.

60. Hickling KG et al: Low mortality rate in adult respiratory distress syndrome using low-volume, pressure-limited ventilation with permissive hypercapnia: A prospective study, *Crit Care Med* 1994;22:1568.

61. Milberg JA et al: Improved survival in patients with acute respiratory distress syndrome, *JAMA* 1995; 273:306.

62. Laffey JG et al: Buffering hypercapnic acidosis worsens acute lung injury, *Am J Resp Crit Care Med* 2000;161:141.

63. Arnold JH et al: Prospective, randomized comparison of high-frequency oscillatory ventilation and conventional ventilation in pediatric respiratory failure. *Crit Care Med* 1994;22:1530-1539.

64. Green TP et al: The impact of extracorporeal membrane oxygenation on survival in pediatric patients with acute respiratory failure, *Crit Care Med* 1996;24:323.

65. Kinsella JP et al: High-frequency oscillatory ventilation versus intermittent mandatory ventilation: Early hemodynamic effects in the premature baboon with hyaline membrane disease, *Pediatr Res* 1991;29:160.

66. Clark RH et al: Prospective randomized comparison of high-frequency oscillatory and conventional ventilation in respiratory distress syndrome, *Pediatrics* 1992;89:5.

67. Froese AB: High-frequency oscillatory ventilation for adult respiratory distress syndrome: Let's get it right this time! *Crit Care Med* 1997;25:906.

68. Arnold JH et al: High frequency oscillatory ventilation in pediatric respiratory failure: A multicenter experience, *Crit Care Med* 2000;28:3913.

69. Derdak S et al: High-frequency oscillatory ventilation for acute respiratory distress syndrome in adults: a randomized, controlled trial, *Am J Respir Crit Care Med* 2002;166:801.

70. Petrous S, Edwards L: Cost effectiveness analysis of neonatal extracorporeal membrane oxygenation based on four year results from the UK Collaborative ECMO Trial, *Arch Dis Child Fetal Neonatal Ed* 2004;89:F2633.

71. Meduri GU, Chinn A: Fibroproliferation in late adult respiratory distress syndrome: response to corticosteroid rescue treatment, *Chest* 1994;105(3 suppl):127S.

72. Bernard GR et al: High-dose corticosteroids in patients with the adult respiratory distress syndrome, *N Engl J Med* 1987;317:1565.

73. Bone RC et al: A controlled clinical trial of high-dose methylprednisolone in the treatment of severe sepsis and septic shock, *N Engl J Med* 1987;317:653.

74. Abman S et al: Acute effects of inhaled nitric oxide in children with severe hypoxemic respiratory failure, *J Pediatr* 1994;124:881.

75. Willson DF, et al: Effect of exogenous surfactant (Calfactant) in pediatric acute lung injury: A randomized controlled trial. *JAMA* 2005;293:470.

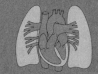

Chapter 36

Shock and Anaphylaxis

CYNTHIA L. GIBSON • ANTHONY D. SLONIM

LEARNING OBJECTIVES

After reading this chapter the reader will be able to:
- Explain the pathophysiologic changes of shock in the critically ill child
- Describe the classification schema used in pediatric shock and the methods to assess, monitor, and treat this disorder

- Appraise anaphylaxis in pediatric patients including its pathology, presentation, and treatment

SHOCK

Shock is a syndrome that results from widespread reduction in effective tissue perfusion leading to cellular dysfunction and organ failure. This reduction results in an imbalance between the *supply* of essential nutrients, oxygen, and substrate to the organ and the metabolic *demand* of that organ. The child's response involves a number of compensatory mechanisms that aim to restore balance to the deranged organ system. The clinician's role is to provide early identification of the etiology, treat the underlying pathologic process, and provide support to maintain the functioning of the organs throughout the period of treatment and rehabilitation (Figure 36-1).

Physiologic Changes

There are several physiologic mechanisms that lead to shock including a global reduction in systemic perfusion from low cardiac output, maldistribution of blood flow, or a defect of substrate utilization at the cellular level.[1] The primary goal of therapy for shock is to maintain an adequate cardiac output so the tissues are continually supplied with an oxygen-rich environment. The supply of essential nutrients to the tissues of an organ depends on the amount of blood the organ receives, the amount of oxygen and nutrients contained in the blood, and the ability of the tissues to utilize the substrate supplied. Regardless of the type of shock described, the basics of supplying nutrients from a systemic point of view are the same.

621

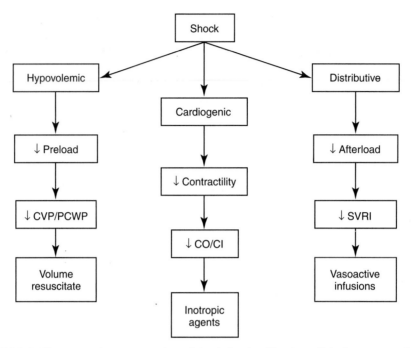

FIGURE 36-1 Diagrammatic representation of shock, its classification, clinical measures of altered stroke volume, and treatment strategies. CVP, Central venous pressure; PCWP, pulmonary capillary wedge pressure; CI, cardiac index; CO, cardiac output; SVRI, systemic vascular resistance index.

At the cellular level, the availability and use of oxygen is linked to energy production. Shock produces cellular dysfunction by several mechanisms: cellular ischemia, the production of inflammatory mediators, and direct free radical injury.[1] When oxygen delivery is inadequate, the cells shift to a less efficient method of producing energy known as anaerobic metabolism.[2] This shift leads to the production of lactic acid and an anion gap metabolic acidosis. The manifestations of this acidosis can produce symptoms that affect the entire organism. Acidosis can have multiple effects on cellular function and overall organ dysfunction. Acidosis causes a reduction in cardiac myocyte and vascular smooth muscle responsiveness to catecholamines. In addition, oxygen delivery, oxygen consumption, and end organ dysfunction are affected by these deranged metabolic functions.[3]

Cardiac Output

In physiologic terms, the cardiac output is the amount of blood pumped from the heart to the organs and tissues of the body. It can be expressed mathematically as liters of blood pumped per minute.[4] Children are different from each other in terms of their size, so all hemodynamic measurements must be corrected for these differences. When the cardiac output is corrected for size, the cardiac index (cardiac output divided by body surface area) is derived.[5] In children, normal values for the cardiac index are in the range of 3.3 to $6.0\,L/min/m^2$.[2,6] A cardiac index of $< 2.0\,L/min/m^2$ has been associated with an increase in mortality.[2]

The cardiac output is determined by the heart rate and the stroke volume.[1,2,7] The heart rate is simply how fast the heart beats per minute and the stroke volume is the amount of blood pumped out of the heart with each mechanical beat. Three components contribute to the stroke volume: preload, inotropy, and afterload.[1,8] Another representation of cardiac output, which represents "blood flow," can be characterized as the change in pressure (mean arterial pressure[MAP] – central venous pressure[CVP]) divided by resistance (systemic vascular resistance[SVR]). This relationship is mathematically expressed as (MAP – CVP)/SVR.[2,9]

Components of Stroke Volume

Preload is measured as the central venous pressure and is a representation of the amount of volume present in the heart and great vessels at rest. This volume exerts a pressure against the walls of the blood vessels in the vascular tree. Preload is dependent on adequate venous return. It increases as the intravascular volume increases and decreases when there is a reduction in intravascular volume. The Frank-Starling principle relates this central pressure to the initial stretch on the myocardial muscle fibers.[8] The stretch, and the resultant contractile ability, increases as this central pressure increases, up to a threshold limit determined by the individual's myocardial compliance. At this point, the contractile ability cannot increase further.

Inotropy is the term that characterizes the contractile state of the heart muscle. Inotropic problems may occur despite an adequate preload if the contractile state is compromised. Further, problems with contractility increase the susceptibility of the myocardium to increases in afterload.[2]

Afterload is a measure of the resistance or force against which the heart must pump. Resistance to the flow of blood in a vessel is proportional to the length of the vessel and the viscosity of the blood, and inversely proportional to the radius of the vessel to the fourth power.[1] The vessel's cross sectional area determines the vascular resistance and is highly dependent upon the arteriolar tone. The systemic vascular resistance index is expressed mathematically as the difference of the mean arterial pressure and the central venous pressure divided by the cardiac output and multiplied by a factor of 80, $SVRI = [(MAP - CVP)/CO] \times 80$. The diastolic blood pressure is a surrogate marker for the basal level of pressure present within the vascular system. As afterload increases, stroke volume decreases. Infants and children have a limited ability to increase stroke volume. As a result, they will attempt to compensate for a reduction in cardiac output by increasing their heart rate.[5] Tachycardia is one of the first signs of decreased peripheral perfusion in children. Hypotension is an unreliable and late finding of shock in children occurring when the child's compensatory mechanisms have already failed.[9,10]

Shock can be classified based upon the adequacy of the cardiac output or by one of its components: heart rate, preload, inotropy, or afterload.[11] This schema also provides for therapeutic interventions targeted to the area of the circulatory system experiencing a problem (see Figure 36-1). In addition, each one of these physiologic parameters can be measured clinically in the child with shock, thereby allowing continuous monitoring and assessment of the response to therapeutic interventions.[5,7,9]

Nutrients and Oxygen in Blood

The cardiac output is responsible for transferring blood and nutrients from the heart to the tissues and organs and back again. The nutrients are carried in the blood by two physical methods.[12] First, some nutrients and oxygen are dissolved in the blood, accounting for a relatively small amount of oxygen transport. Second, nutrients and oxygen can be bound to red blood cells or macromolecules and "carried" by the cardiac output to the site of utilization. Oxygen delivery depends significantly on hemoglobin concentration.[9] The amount of oxygen bound to hemoglobin is described by the oxyhemoglobin dissociation curve and is affected by physical properties such as temperature and acidosis.[12] The contribution of each of these components is

Box 36-1	Formulas Used in the Calculation of Oxygen Content, Oxygen Delivery, and Oxygen Consumption

OXYGEN CONTENT

Cao_2 (ml/dl) = Amount of O_2 dissolved in blood + Amount bound to hemoglobin

Amount of O_2 dissolved (ml of O_2/ml of blood) = $0.003 \times Pao_2$ (mm Hg)

Amount bound = $1.34 \times$ Hemoglobin (g/dl) $\times$ % Oxygen saturation

OXYGEN DELIVERY

$Do_2 = O_2$ Content $\times$ Cardiac output

OXYGEN CONSUMPTION

$\dot{V}o_2$ (ml/min) = (Arterial – venous) O_2 Content $\times$ Cardiac output (ml/min)

0.003, A constant that represents the milliliters of oxygen dissolved in 100 ml of blood; *1.34*, a constant that represents the amount of oxygen that can be bound per gram of hemoglobin.

symbolized in a mathematical formula that represents the arterial oxygen content (Box 36-1).[12-14] The Clinical Scenario features an example that demonstrates how the mathematical formulas shown in Box 36-1 may be used to quantify oxygen transport. Once the oxygen content is calculated, it can be considered within the framework of the cardiac output.

Delivery of Blood to the Tissues

The cardiac output delivers oxygenated blood to the tissues on a global or systemic level.[8,12,15] Delivery of oxygenated blood, however, is only one part of this complex physiologic process. Oxygen delivery depends on oxygen carrying capacity (% hemoglobin), oxygen provided (oxygen bound to hemoglobin plus dissolved oxygen), and cardiac output.[2] Once oxygenated and nutrient-rich blood reaches the target organ, the organ must be able to utilize the substrates it receives.[15] There must be uptake of oxygen in the tissues and cells of the organ along with the exchange of organ byproducts that are then transported back to the lungs. A major component of these byproducts is carbon dioxide, which has a higher solubility in the blood than oxygen.[12]

Oxygen consumption is a measure of the amount of oxygen, or substrate, utilized by the organs of the body.[11] Comparing the amount of oxygen being supplied to the organs from the arterial circuit and the amount of oxygen remaining in the venous circuit after removal by the organs provides an estimate of how much is being consumed.[12,16,17] As cardiac output decreases and metabolic demands remain the same, the tissues will extract more oxygen to maintain the same consumption, but the oxygen returning to the

CLINICAL SCENARIO 36-1

Example of Use of Oxygen Content, Oxygen Delivery, and Oxygen Consumption Formulas in the Care of a 5-Year-Old Child in Shock

CASE EXAMPLE

A 5-year-old girl is in septic shock in the pediatric intensive care unit as a result of an overwhelming infection. She has a hemoglobin level of 10 g/dl, a cardiac output of 4.0 L/min, and arterial blood gas findings of pH 7.35; P_{CO_2}, 36 mm Hg; Pa_{O_2}, 85 mm Hg; HCO_3^-, 20 mEq/L; and a corresponding oxygen saturation of 95%. A mixed venous blood sample demonstrates pH, 7.32; P_{CO_2}, 34 mm Hg; Pa_{O_2}, 37 mm Hg; and an oxygen saturation of 62%. Calculate the oxygen content, delivery, and consumption as follows:

ARTERIAL OXYGEN CONTENT

Ca_{O_2} = Amount dissolved in blood + Amount bound to hemoglobin (arterial side)

Amount dissolved = $0.003 \times Pa_{O_2}$

Amount dissolved = 0.003×85 mm Hg = 0.255 or 0.255 ml of O_2 in 100 ml of blood

Amount bound = $1.34 \times$ Hemoglobin $\times$ % O_2 saturation

Amount bound = $1.34 \times 10 \times 0.95 = 12.73$ ml of oxygen per 100 ml of blood

$Ca_{O_2} = 0.255 + 12.73 = 12.99$ ml of O_2 per 100 ml of blood

MIXED VENOUS OXYGEN CONTENT

$C\bar{v}_{O_2}$ = Amount dissolved + Amount bound to hemoglobin (venous side) = $0.003 \times P\bar{v}_{O_2}$

Amount dissolved = $0.003 \times P\bar{v}_{O_2}$

Amount dissolved = 0.003×37 mm Hg = 0.115 or 0.115 ml of O_2 in 100 ml of blood

Amount bound = $1.34 \times$ Hemoglobin $\times$ % O_2 saturation

Amount bound = $1.34 \times 10 \times 0.62 = 8.31$ ml of O_2 per 100 ml of blood

$C\bar{v}_{O_2} = 0.115 + 8.31 = 8.425$ ml of O_2 per 100 ml of blood

OXYGEN DELIVERY

D_{O_2} = O_2 content $\times$ Cardiac output

$D_{O_2} = 12.99$ ml of O_2 per 100 ml of blood $\times$ 4000 ml/min

Arterial $D_{O_2} = 519.6$ ml/min

OXYGEN CONSUMPTION

$\dot{V}_{O_2}$ (ml/min) = (Arterial – venous) O_2 content $\times$ Cardiac output (ml/min)

$\dot{V}_{O_2}$ (ml/min) = (12.99 – 8.425) ml of O_2 per 100 ml of blood $\times$ 4000 ml/min = 182.6

---

heart in the venous circulation will be less.[2] In children oxygen consumption depends more on oxygen delivery than oxygen extraction.[9] Oxygen consumption > 200 mL/min/m² has been associated with improved survival.[2,9] The amount of nutrient consumed by the organs relative to delivery is referred to as the oxygen extraction.[15] Oxygen extraction is independent of supply for patients with shock. As shock worsens, organ

tissue perfusion decreases and the organ extracts fewer nutrients from the blood. This measure of the severity of shock has been associated with survival.[5] Regardless of the etiology of the shock, alterations in cellular metabolism, mitochondrial dysfunction, abnormal carbohydrate metabolism, and the failure of many energy-dependent enzyme reactions lead to difficulty with utilization of substrate at the cellular level and eventually cell death.[1] These changes in cellular oxygen utilization alter the consumption of oxygen in each of the organs, leading to organ dysfunction. Organ system dysfunction resulting from shock, if left untreated, ultimately leads to failure of multiple organ systems. The term *multiorgan dysfunction syndrome* (MODS) has been applied to this disseminated pathologic response.[1]

Metabolic Response

The body's response to poor tissue perfusion results in a number of metabolic responses. Many of the manifestations of shock represent the body's compensatory mechanisms, which attempt to maintain effective tissue perfusion and correct the abnormalities of shock. These responses attempt to maintain mean circulatory pressure, maximize cardiac output, redistribute perfusion to the most vital organs, and optimize the unloading of oxygen to the tissues.[1] The compensatory mechanisms are designed to autoregulate in the setting of hemodynamic or metabolic dysfunction.

The central nervous system releases adrenocorticotropic hormone in the setting of stress, which stimulates the adrenal glands to release cortisol. Adequate adrenocortical function is essential to survive critical illness, and most critically ill patients will exhibit elevated cortisol levels.[2,18] Many patients, however, exhibit a state of "relative" adrenal insufficiency because of an inadequate production of cortisol.[18] The sympathetic nervous system is regulated by arterial and cardiopulmonary baroreceptors and releases epinephrine and norepinephrine, which increase cardiac output by increasing heart rate and stroke volume. Cortisol assists the actions of these two catecholamines. Intrinsic vasoactives are released in response to increased metabolic activity and oxygen tension. The angiotensin/aldosterone–ADH/vasopressin system is activated to preserve intravascular volume.[2] Other vasodilators released locally and systemically include nitric oxide, prostacyclin, and kinins; vasoconstrictors include endothelin, renin, and oxygen free radicals. These substances affect the vascular tone, systemic vascular resistance, and therefore blood pressure.

The inflammatory response is a physiologic, homeostatic mechanism designed to respond to injury or infection. Inflammatory mediator release usually provides beneficial effects; however, in shock, the inflammatory response becomes unregulated.[1] The production of immune mediators is triggered by ischemic or hypoxic insults and produces further tissue injury. The systemic inflammatory response syndrome (SIRS) is the term used to describe the nonspecific inflammatory process that accompanies these insults.[10] The immune response leads to changes in T and B lymphocyte responses, activation of the complement cascade, activation of coagulation factors, and cytokine release (TNF and IL-6). These mediators exert their influence on the vasculature to produce inadequate perfusion or direct cellular injury.[1] All of these contribute to organ dysfunction and the eventual signs and symptoms the body may experience in shock.

Classification

There are four major types of shock and each type can be categorized by its effect on one of the components of stroke volume (preload, inotropy, or afterload) and cardiac output (see Figure 36-1). Using this paradigm, health care providers are able to identify the potential causes of shock based on the observed hemodynamic profile observed.[7] An understanding of cardiorespiratory interactions is useful not only for the diagnosis and classification of shock but also for the goals of monitoring its progress and the response to treatment.

Hypovolemic Shock

In children, hypovolemic shock is the most common type of shock and arises from a variety of different causes. Hypovolemia results from fluid or blood loss and is due to a decreased intravascular circulating volume leading to reduced filling pressure or preload.[1] The result is inadequate cardiac output[3]. When a sudden decrease in the intravascular volume becomes so severe that effective tissue perfusion cannot be maintained, hypovolemic shock is present.[14]

The causes of hypovolemic shock depend on what component (blood, fluid, or plasma) of the intravascular volume is lost. If red blood cells are lost from the vascular space, hemorrhagic shock is present.[14,19] Common examples of hemorrhagic shock include trauma, gastrointestinal bleeding, and bleeding resulting from a coagulopathy. Fluid and electrolyte losses may occur with vomiting and diarrhea in patients with gastroenteritis. This is a common cause of hypovolemic shock, especially in infants and young children.[13,14] Hypovolemia may also occur because of inadequate fluid intake. Infants who are abused or neglected or who have insufficient replacement to account for losses in warm climates fit into this category. Endocrine disorders, such as diabetic ketoacidosis, also contribute to this category.

Children with burns and nephrotic syndrome lose large amounts of plasma and ultimately experience hypovolemic shock if careful attention to rehydration is not maintained.[14] Plasma proteins provide a force known as oncotic pressure, which helps maintain the extracellular fluid within the intravascular space. When these proteins are lost, the fluid seeps into the interstitial space and the shock state is perpetuated.

Cardiogenic Shock

Cardiogenic shock is caused by a severe reduction in cardiac function resulting from direct myocardial damage or a mechanical abnormality of the heart affecting the cardiac output.[1] Cardiogenic shock occurs when low cardiac output results from a problem related to the heart rate, the contractile state (inotropy), or the afterload as the heart attempts to supply blood to the tissues of the body (see Figure 36-1).[20,21] An alteration in the heart rate outside the normal physiologic range, either too fast or too slow, can result in a reduction of the cardiac output. A slow heart rate occurs in children who experience hypoxia or heart block.[22] If the hypoxia and its concomitant bradycardia are not corrected quickly, cardiac output begins to fall and the child manifests poor perfusion and shock. Fast cardiac rhythms, such as ventricular or supraventricular tachycardia, may also reduce the cardiac output and ultimately affect organ perfusion.[20]

When inotropy of the heart is affected, either by an inflammatory process, such as myocarditis, or by an alteration in the contractile state of the muscle, as in cardiomyopathy, the stroke volume and cardiac output are compromised.[20] Additionally, increases in afterload because of valvular or muscular defects, or changes in the systemic resistance, such as in hypertensive emergencies, inhibit cardiac output by reducing stroke volume.[20] Compensatory responses can have deleterious effects in patients with cardiogenic shock. These mechanisms often perpetuate the shock due to further depression of the cardiac output. As contractility deteriorates and cardiac output decreases, systemic vascular resistance increases as a response to inflammatory mediators.[23] This causes an increase in afterload and further reduces the ability of the heart to pump effectively. Myocardial dysfunction is frequently a late manifestation of shock of any etiology.[23]

Obstructive Shock

Extracardiac obstructive shock results from obstruction to the flow in the cardiovascular circuit.[1] The common causes of this type of shock in children are coarctation of the aorta, tension pneumothorax, or pericardial tamponade. Each of these disorders can create an "obstruction" to flow. Supportive care with the administration of intravenous fluids may be of assistance in improving end organ perfusion until the etiology of the shock can be resolved.

Distributive Shock (Peripheral Vasodilation)

Distributive shock is characterized by vasodilatation of the vascular bed and a reduction in peripheral resistance, which leads to a relative decrease in preload (see Figure 36-1). Vasodilating substances act directly and indirectly on the cells of the blood vessels to create an enlargement of the intravascular potential space, a relative hypovolemia, and reduced tissue perfusion. Distributive shock has many potential causes. Sepsis is defined by a systemic inflammatory response (SIRS) with proven or suspected infection. Septic shock transpires when sepsis is accompanied by organ dysfunction.[10,24] Infectious microorganisms release endotoxins, which stimulate a number of inflammatory and immune mediators thereby perpetuating the shock state.[1,24] Septic shock is characterized by cardiac dysfunction and changes in peripheral vascular tone. The cardiac dysfunction can be manifested by systolic or diastolic dysfunction. Children with septic shock often exhibit a higher cardiac index than in other forms of shock.[2] Neurogenic shock originates from a neurologic insult such as a spinal cord contusion or transection. Anaphylactic shock results from antigen exposure and the release of mediators from an IgE antigen-antibody reaction.[25,26] Adrenal insufficiency is also included in this category because of a similar hemodynamic profile. Regardless of the type of distributive shock, the physiologic dysfunction is characterized by vasodilation with a reduced afterload and increased cardiac output.

Assessment

The approach to the child in shock begins with an evaluation of vital functions as expounded by the ABCs of resuscitation.[22] Maintenance of the airway and attention to oxygenation and ventilation are the initial priorities. The circulatory system is evaluated by the presence of a pulse. If a pulse is absent, cardiopulmonary resuscitation needs to be performed and cardiotonic medications consistent with advanced life support need to be administered.[22] The presence and quality of the pulse reflects systemic vascular tone as well as cardiac output. Vascular access should be rapidly obtained, and if there is difficulty with peripheral venous access, an intraosseous or central venous route should be used.[9]

Once the ABCs are established, attention can be directed to measuring vital signs and performing a secondary survey. Normal values for pulse, respiratory rate, and blood pressure are age dependent. The knowledge

of these age-related differences is essential to being able to care for any child.[10,27]

A brief and directed patient history and physical examination can be obtained at this point. It should be directed at determining a potential cause of the shock. In addition, obtain essential information regarding past medical history, especially a history of congenital heart disease, immunodeficiency, trauma, possible ingestion of toxic substances, medications, and allergies.

After assessment of vital signs, an evaluation of the systemic perfusion as a sign of the effectiveness of the cardiac output is completed. Capillary refill (the process of blanching the skin for several seconds and timing the return of blood flow to the blanched skin) is a quick, useful, and noninvasive test that provides important information regarding perfusion in the acute setting.[22] The normal capillary refill time should be less than 2 seconds and correlates with a cardiac index of $> 2.0 \, L/min/m^2$.[22] Prolongation of the capillary refill is considered a sign of inadequate tissue perfusion and impending shock. Assessment of the perfusion to the skin, the brain, and the kidney is often performed next because they are easy to perform and correlate better with hemodynamic measurements than capillary refill.[28]

Evaluation of the skin color and temperature is easily performed. The skin of children in shock may be pale, cyanotic, or mottled because of poor perfusion. Traditionally, practitioners have described two phases of septic shock.[2,9] In early septic shock the skin appears well perfused, warm, and pink. This occurs from the vasodilatation and increased cardiac output. Later in the course of shock, the cardiac output begins to fall. The skin during this period is likely to be cool, cyanotic, or mottled and represents a decrease in the amount of substrate reaching the skin. Further assessment of the skin may reveal petechiae, poor skin turgor, or skin rashes indicative of a coagulopathy, hypovolemia, or an infectious etiology.

Examining the child's level of awareness, orientation, and response to commands can assess perfusion to the child's brain. It is important to ensure that medications that might obscure the examination have not been given. Children in shock may show signs of agitation or restlessness. Alternatively, they may also have a mental status that is stuporous or comatose.

Monitoring urine production assesses perfusion of the child's visceral organs. If the child is making adequate urine (at least 1 ml/kg/hr), then the cardiac output to the kidneys, which produces renal blood flow and drives glomerular filtration, is considered adequate. Both the kidney and the brain have vasomotor autoregulation mechanisms that maintain blood flow and perfusion in shock until a critical point is reached and perfusion pressure falls below the ability of the organ to maintain adequate blood flow.[2,9] At this point, the shock is classified as decompensated shock. In decompensated shock, the blood pressure falls and the perfusion of end organs is compromised.

Laboratory values can often provide useful clues to the proper diagnosis and management of shock. Evaluation of the acid-base status including routine electrolytes and an arterial blood gas with the calculation of the anion gap are important first steps.[3] As shock progresses, a metabolic acidosis and an elevated lactate level may occur. Lactate is a measure of anaerobic metabolism but can also be elevated in many conditions in the absence of shock.[2]

Anemia, thrombocytopenia, and elevation of prothrombin time and partial thromboplastin times (PT/PTT) may identify a coagulopathy or disseminated intravascular coagulation (DIC). An elevated or reduced white blood cell count may indicate the presence of infection or an immunodeficiency. Elevated liver enzymes or creatinine may provide evidence about the extent of hypoperfusion to the liver and kidneys and potential for subsequent dysfunction in these organs. An electrocardiogram and a chest x-ray may offer valuable clues as the etiology of the shock is investigated.

Monitoring

The child in shock requires ongoing assessment, intervention, and reassessment. Attention to the effects of an intervention on vital signs and end organ perfusion must be continually observed. Children with fluid-responsive shock can be monitored with standard noninvasive methods. However, if the child fails to respond to fluid (e.g., >60 ml/kg), additional strategies for monitoring and maintaining equilibrium may need to be incorporated. In addition, if a treatment does not have its intended effect on restoring homeostasis, the therapeutic approach and underlying etiology need to be reconsidered.

A number of technologies are now available in the pediatric intensive care unit (PICU) for the assessment and monitoring of the child in shock. These techniques augment the information derived from the vital signs and physical examination. The arterial catheter, the CVP monitor, and the pulmonary artery catheter are three of the more common strategies employed to detect physiologic changes and to supplement the clinical assessment of the child in shock. Echocardiography can also be an important noninvasive technique that provides valuable information regarding cardiac structure and function as contributors to the shock state.[9]

Arterial Catheters

Because children maintain their blood pressure until late in the course of shock, blood pressure measurements become important adjuncts to understanding the condition of the child. Auscultatory methods for the measurement of the blood pressure may be unreliable in children. Electronic blood pressure cuff measurements are easier to use, more reliable, and are able to provide the mean arterial blood pressure in addition to the systolic and diastolic measurements.

The placement of a catheter in a peripheral or central artery can be performed for the monitoring of blood pressure on a continuous basis in the intensive care unit. Arterial catheterization can provide beat-to-beat monitoring of the blood pressure.[1] The shape and characteristics of the waveform provide additional information regarding the characteristics of the cardiac output, including volume, afterload, and contractility. Intense vasoconstriction or vasodilation may affect the distal amplification of the waveform obtained with a peripherally placed arterial catheter. Assessment of central systemic blood pressure is most reliable if measured at relatively central sites.[29] Placement of an arterial catheter also allows for the extraction of blood for arterial blood gas measurements without repetitive arterial punctures.

Central Venous Pressure Measurements

The placement of a catheter in the central venous system allows for an assessment of the volume status of the child with shock. The catheter, when attached to a continuous column of fluid and a pressure transducer, measures the downstream intravascular pressure, or CVP, in the right atrium. This intravascular pressure represents preload, one of the contributors to the stroke volume, which contributes to the cardiac output (see Figure 36-1). Because the left side of the heart receives its blood from the right side of the heart, the measurement of these right heart pressures is accepted as an alternative for the dynamics on the left side of the heart in the patient whose myocardial and pulmonary compliance is normal. If biventricular function is equal and pulmonary artery resistance is low, CVP measurements closely reflect pulmonary artery wedge pressure.[29] This information helps the provider to diagnose and treat the patient in shock. If the CVP is high in the setting of normal myocardial compliance, then the intravascular volume is adequate and may not be accounting for the reduction in cardiac output. The CVP may be elevated if the blood is unable to be ejected because of a failing myocardium. If the CVP is low, additional intravenous fluid needs to be given to improve the intravascular volume deficit being observed. A central venous catheter also provides easy access for blood sampling, measuring mixed venous oxygenation, and providing access for rapid fluid resuscitation and provision of inotropic medications, if necessary.

Pulmonary Artery (PA) Catheter Measurements

The use of a pulmonary artery (PA) catheter in children has been debated, but in children with fluid refractory and dopamine resistant shock, the PA catheter may provide additional information to make a more appropriate assessment of the hemodynamic status of the patient.[9,30] The use of PA catheters in children is supported by the American College of Critical Care Medicine for circumstances in which irreversible shock manifesting as poor perfusion, acidosis, and hypotension persists despite the use of therapies directed at the arterial blood pressure, CVP pressure, and oxygen saturation indices.[9]

The placement of the catheter allows direct measurements of hemodynamic parameters that contribute to stroke volume and cardiac output. CVP measurements can be taken from the pulmonary artery catheter (see Figure 36-1). In addition, the pulmonary capillary wedge pressure can measure downstream pressures from the left atrium, providing an indirect assessment of the preload to the left ventricle, which may be a more exact measure of preload when the myocardial or pulmonary compliance is abnormal.

Pressure measurements within the pulmonary artery allow for the identification of problems with the pulmonary vasculature or its reactivity as a contribution to shock. If the pulmonary vasculature is constricted, the movement of blood from the right side of the heart to the left side is restricted. Hence, the pulmonary artery catheter provides information regarding the left side of the heart as well as the interaction between the heart and lungs.

In addition to the measurements obtained directly from the catheter, a number of derived values provide information regarding the homeostatic function of the child. Systemic vascular resistance, a measure of afterload, can be calculated by measuring the pressure differences across the vascular bed of the heart and dividing by the cardiac output [(MAP − CVP)/CO].[9] Pulmonary vascular resistance, a measure of afterload as it affects only the right ventricle, can be calculated by considering only the output of the right ventricle. Oxygen delivery and consumption can be calculated by using the cardiac output measures.[2,5,6] Measurement of cardiac output and oxygen consumption has been proposed as being beneficial to patients with persistent shock because higher values have been associated with improved survival.[6] Calculating oxygen consumption and oxygen extraction can be performed by measuring the mixed venous oxygen saturation of blood

from the pulmonary artery. The normal mixed venous saturation ranges from 70% to 75%. Higher values may be obtained when the organ in unable to extract oxygen from the blood. This signifies a more severe stage of shock. If the saturation is less than 70%, inotropes and vasodilators can be used to improve cardiac output until the central venous saturation is > 70%.[2] From these values, extraction ratios and an analysis of the degree of shock can be calculated. Moreover, a physiologic approach to the treatment and management can be used.

Treatment

The goals of treatment for shock are to maintain adequate tissue perfusion, to avoid end-organ damage, and to treat the underlying primary process. Therapeutic strategies should enhance the delivery of oxygen and nutrients to the tissues, reduce the oxygen demand, and correct the metabolic abnormalities. Continuous monitoring of the patient's response to interventions is critical and may lead to redirection of therapies. Early aggressive therapy of shock, focused on maintaining blood pressure and oxygen delivery, improves the outcomes in critically ill children.[2]

Respiratory

Airway and breathing should be rigorously monitored and maintained for patients in shock. Endotracheal intubation with mechanical ventilation may reduce the work of breathing and optimize oxygen content. During intubation, induction agents, cardiotonic medications, and respiratory support modes must be chosen carefully so as not to worsen an already compromised cardiovascular status.

Vascular Volume

The rapid restoration of an adequate circulating blood volume is essential for a patient in shock regardless of the cause (see Figure 36-1).[29-32] Normal saline or lactated Ringer's solutions are the fluids of choice for initial resuscitation because they maintain intravascular volume.[1,2,9,31,32] The use of colloids, such as albumin or starch, to maintain intravascular volume has not demonstrated a beneficial effect on survival.[1,2,9] If there is evidence of anemia or suspected losses of blood, repletion of the intravascular volume with packed red blood cells should be performed.[2,9,10]

The initial administration of 20 ml/kg of fluid is recommended.[2,9,22,32] Reassessment of the patient's condition based on vital signs and end-organ perfusion helps to determine the need for additional fluid.[9] The administration of intravenous fluid will decrease the heart rate and increase the MAP and CVP. Carcillo and colleagues demonstrated that when the initial amount of volume resuscitation administered within the first hour was cumulatively greater than 40 ml/kg, the survival rates were improved.[28] Thus, both the amount of fluid and the rapidity of administration have outcome benefits. Rapid volume resuscitation restores intravascular volume and reduces the inflammatory response and coagulopathy that often accompany shock.[2] Large fluid deficits typically exist and initial volume resuscitation usually requires 40 to 60 ml/kg but can be as much as 200 ml/kg in some cases of septic shock.[2,9,33] Continued fluid losses and persistent hypovolemia due to capillary leak can persist despite fluid resuscitation. Ongoing fluid replacement is necessary to maintain adequate tissue perfusion, and large volumes may be required as vascular permeability results in peripheral and third space losses.[33] When total administered volumes of 60 ml/kg are reached, intravascular monitoring and initiation of vasoactive support should be considered.

The development of rales, a gallop rhythm, hepatomegaly, and increased work of breathing may all indicate worsening cardiovascular function leading to pulmonary edema because of the relationship to the Frank-Starling principle.[34] Additional aliquots of fluid may be contraindicated at this point.[20,30] In these instances, careful invasive monitoring with pulmonary artery catheters can provide valuable information and help guide further management.

Myocardial Function

Once the intravascular volume is optimized, manipulation of other components of cardiac output should be attempted (see Figure 36-1). If the heart rate is ineffective because it is too slow, rate enhancing drugs such as atropine, or pacing should be considered.[22] Bradycardia might be the primary manifestation of hypoxia in children; therefore, adequate ventilation and oxygenation should be achieved before primary efforts directed at correcting slow heart rates are undertaken.

Abnormalities in heart rate resulting in poor perfusion and shock should be addressed quickly. An unstable tachycardia manifested with hypotension or signs of shock should be treated with electrical therapy in the form of synchronized cardioversion or defibrillation.[22] Cardioversion synchronizes the delivery of the shock with the QRS complex to prevent deterioration to a more lethal arrhythmia and should be used in patients who have a palpable pulse. Defibrillation delivers a shock regardless of the timing of the cardiac cycle and is indicated in pulseless rhythms that have resulted in cardiovascular collapse.[22]

Inotropic dysfunction can result from an abnormality in any of the structures of the heart or the abnormal contractility of the cardiac myocytes. Initially, adequate

preload through the judicious use of fluid resuscitation to maintain stroke volume should be ensured. After preload has been restored, additional fluid may worsen the ability of the myocardium to maintain cardiac output, especially in cardiogenic shock. Hence, the support of the myocardium can then take place with inotropic agents that act by a number of different mechanisms and can be titrated to the appropriate clinical response including the achievement of appropriate MAP, CVP, and cardiac index to ensure adequate perfusion.[9,20] Inotropic agents are used to increase contractility and cardiac output. Dobutamine is a beta-1 adrenergic agonist with chronotropic and inotropic actions, as well as afterload reduction. Dopamine, the most frequently used inotrope, increases renal blood flow but also has vasoconstrictive properties at high doses due to release of norepinephrine. Epinephrine is a naturally circulating neurohormone that increases contractility during stress and shock.[2] At low dose, it provides inotropy but at higher doses increases peripheral vascular tone and acts as a vasopressor. Patients with heart failure and increased systemic vascular resistance may be harmed by these higher doses unless epinephrine is combined with an inodilator or vasodilator.[2] Norepinephrine is another common inotropic agent and is effective for dopamine-resistant shock. It is a strong vasoconstrictor even at low doses, but has better inotropic effects when combined with an inodilator.

Inodilators work through a different mechanism. These drugs enhance inotropy while simultaneously vasodilating and reducing afterload, making it easier for the heart to eject blood.[2,20] Phosphodiesterase inhibitors, such as milrinone, mediate inotropy and vasodilation by preventing hydrolysis of cAMP and therefore potentiate the effects of beta receptor stimulation in cardiac and vascular tissue.[9] Alone, these improve contractility and diastolic relaxation and also cause vasodilation of pulmonary and systemic arterial vasculature. When combined with inotropes, vasodilators, and vasopressors, the interaction provides even better contractility and relaxation.[2]

If the problem with inadequate cardiac function is related to elevations in afterload, vasodilators should be administered.[20] Vasodilators reduce pulmonary vascular resistance or systemic vascular resistance and thereby improve cardiac output by reducing afterload.[2] Nitroprusside is a systemic and pulmonary vasodilator. Nitroglycerin has dose-dependent effects on coronary artery vasodilation, pulmonary vasodilation, and systemic vasodilation that increase with increasing doses. Prostaglandins can also be used as vasodilators, especially in ductal-dependent congenital heart disease. The use of vasodilators should be titrated to reducing afterload without causing tachycardia or diastolic hypotension. In many circumstances, inotropic agents in combination with vasodilators may be useful.[2,9,22]

Peripheral Vascular Resistance

The peripheral vascular resistance represents afterload (see Figure 36-1). Blood pressure is sustained by the interaction of the cardiac output with the peripheral vascular resistance. If there is a reduction in afterload because of vasodilating mediators or inflammatory mediators, such as occurs in sepsis or anaphylaxis, increasing afterload as a treatment strategy should be considered once adequate preload has been restored. Vasopressors are the drugs of choice to increase afterload and blood pressure. Dopamine works through a dose-dependent response on sympathetic receptors. Epinephrine, norepinephrine, and phenylephrine have differential affinity for sympathetic nervous system receptors. Norepinephrine is effective for dopamine resistant shock. Phenylephrine is the drug of choice for tetralogy of Fallot spells because it increases systemic arterial vasoconstriction and thereby shunts blood to perfuse the lungs.[2] Vasopressors increase vascular tone, peripheral vascular resistance, and afterload and have inotropic effects. This helps to maintain perfusion to vital organs such as the brain, kidneys, and gastrointestinal tract.

Hematologic

In hemorrhagic shock or anemic shock, intravascular volume should be replaced with packed red blood cells. Mortality rates increase when hemoglobin levels are <6 mg/dl. Provision of blood improves circulating blood volume and increases the oxygen delivery and substrate to the tissues. Hemoglobin should be maintained within the normal range for age. It is believed hemoglobin levels should be maintained at a minimum of 10 g/dl.[9]

Coagulation abnormalities occur in all forms of shock. Activation of the coagulation cascade can lead to disseminated intravascular coagulation which results in thrombocytopenia, decreased fibrinogen, elevated fibrin split products, and microangiopathic hemolytic anemia.[1] In prolonged states of shock, thrombosis and hypofibrinolysis can occur. The rapid reversal of shock often prevents disseminated intravascular coagulation and bleeding.[2] When resuscitation is inadequate, the replacement of clotting factors may be beneficial. Vitamin K, fresh frozen plasma, cryoprecipitate, and platelet transfusions should correct most coagulopathies. Activated factor VII has been effective in reversing refractory hemorrhagic shock in many situations. Patients with hemo-

philia or von Willebrand's disease may need specific replacement therapy to control bleeding.

Endocrine

Maintaining metabolic and hormonal homeostasis is important in children with shock. Adrenal insufficiency is common in the intensive care setting and presents with low cardiac output and high systemic vascular resistance or with high cardiac output and low systemic vascular resistance.[2] Adrenal insufficiency should be considered in any child who is unresponsive to catecholamines and there is a possibility that adrenal dysfunction actually contributes to the development of catecholamine resistant shock.[18] This insufficiency has been associated with worsening of multiple organ failure and higher mortality.[18,35] Steroid replacement should be considered when a measured cortisol level is <18 mg/dl. Hydrocortisone has glucocorticoid and mineralocorticoid effects and should be given at either a "stress" dose of 2 mg/kg/day or a "shock" dose of 50 mg/kg/day during acute shock.[2,33]

Hypothyroidism may be present along with adrenal insufficiency, especially in children with an abnormality with the hypothalamic-pituitary axis or in children with trisomy 21. Thyroid hormone levels are low in children with septic shock compared to controls and should be expected in patients requiring epinephrine or norepinephrine.[2,36] Tri-iodothyronine is an effective inotropic agent and has been used to preserve myocardial function in neonates after cardiac surgery and in patients with low T3 levels.[2,37] Thyroid hormone replacement may be life-saving in certain shock situations.

Electrolyte abnormalities are common in the ICU and following their values is an important part of the evaluation and management of the shock patient. As patients are resuscitated with fluid, sodium values may become abnormal and need correcting or they may be part of the presenting signs of dehydration and hypovolemic shock. If kidney dysfunction is present, hyperkalemia may become an issue that contributes to cardiac dysfunction or arrhythmias. Hypocalcemia is a frequent, reversible contributor to cardiac dysfunction and should be treated to maintain normal ionized calcium levels. Increased intracellular calcium increases contractility, whereas decreased calcium leads to relaxation in cardiac and vascular smooth muscle cells.[2] Correction of electrolyte abnormalities is crucial in maintaining stability.

Hyperglycemia occurs as a result of glycogenolysis and gluconeogenesis mediated by increases in adrenocorticotropic hormone, glucocorticoids, glucagons, and catecholamines as well as decreases in insulin.[1] Hyperglycemia contributes to reduced immune system function and promotes microbial and fungal growth.

There is a decrease in morbidity and mortality when tight glucose control, with levels between 80 to 120 mg/dl, is maintained with the use of insulin. Insulin also helps resolve the anion gap metabolic acidosis that contributes to cellular dysfunction.[2] Hypoglycemia may be a presenting sign in shock and should be corrected to avoid neurologic complications.

Immunologic

Treatment with broad-spectrum antibiotics with activity against gram positive and gram negative organisms should be started as soon as septic shock is considered. The choice of antibiotics should be based on the suspected focus of infection[24] and the first doses should be given during the initial resuscitation. The choice of antibiotic can be narrowed once an organism is identified. Many cases of septic shock, especially in neutropenic patients, have negative cultures. Despite this, antibiotics are typically continued for up to 14 days. Early antifungal therapy should be considered in immunocompromised patients and in those who are unresponsive to antibacterial therapy.

Many studies are being performed to target the inflammatory and immune mediators that contribute to the systemic inflammatory response to shock in an attempt to downregulate the response. Activated protein C showed an improved outcome in septic patients but had an associated increase in the incidence of bleeding.[24,33,35,38] Other modulators being studied include endotoxin, tumor necrosis factor, interleukins, and platelet-activating factor, as well as contributors to the coagulation cascade.[24]

Nutritional Status

Nutritional support of the critically ill child has a role in maintaining stability, promoting healing, and improving the outcome from acute and chronic illness.[39,40] The goals of nutritional support are to promote these end points while simultaneously providing adequate metabolic substrate for the growth and development of the child.[39]

Assessment of the nutritional status of critically ill children begins with baseline growth charts and nutritional studies.[40] Measurement of proteins with rapid turnover such as prealbumin or transferrin helps identify the child experiencing an impairment of nutrition related to an illness.[40] Nitrogen balance is a useful tool to estimate the adequacy of nutrition. The catabolic state of illness leads to a loss of endogenous protein for energy production and places the child at risk of a bad outcome unless the amount of nutrients being supplied offsets the metabolic needs of the body. A child with a negative nitrogen balance is receiving inadequate nutritional supplementation and is at risk for malnutrition.

When the patient is unable to optimize nutritional intake to meet the metabolic demand, supplementation should take place. Either enteral or parenteral nutrition should begin as soon as cardiovascular stability is obtained. Early enteral nutrition appears to prevent gut mucosal atrophy and bacterial translocation.[24] Substantial work in the area of vitamins, trace elements, and immune-modifying nutritional agents is in progress.

Extracorporeal Membranous Oxygenation

Patients remaining in shock despite the supportive therapies may benefit from mechanical cardiac support, such as extracorporeal membranous oxygenation (ECMO). ECMO is highly effective for cardiogenic shock since it helps support the ailing heart, but is less successful in septic shock, except possibly refractory low cardiac output septic shock.[2] Patients may still require vasoactive agents for persistent hypotension but less inotropic support because the circuit provides inotropy.[9]

ANAPHYLAXIS

One type of distributive shock that results from peripheral vasodilation is anaphylactic shock. Anaphylactic shock occurs when a foreign antigen interacts with the body and elicits a systemic, immediate hypersensitivity reaction caused by immunoglobulin E–mediated release of mediators from tissue mast cells and circulating basophils.[40] A variety of substances can elicit these reactions.[25,41] Dibs and associates found that latex allergy, foods, drugs, and snake venom were the most common inciting agents in the pediatric population.[25] There are times, however, when a cause of anaphylaxis may not be found despite an exhaustive search.[26,42]

Pathology

After the introduction of an antigen into the body, either by an enteral or parenteral route, reaction with the IgE antibody on tissue mast cells or circulating basophils occurs. This evokes the release of a number of chemical mediators responsible for the clinical and hemodynamic symptom complex elicited. The activation of numerous immunologic and metabolic pathways occurs due to the release of mediators. A widespread inflammatory reaction invokes the many antiinflammatory cascades of the host to modify the response to the antigen. Histamine is one of the most prominent of the mediators and is in large part responsible for the clinical effects observed.[26] Histamine is believed to be responsible for the increase in airway resistance and the fall in partial pressure of oxygen due to its contractile action on the smooth muscle of the lung.[26] There is vasodilation and increased vascular permeability that produces a rapid loss of intra-vascular volume, which then stimulates the release of catecholamines. Initially systemic vascular resistance is reduced and cardiac output is increased; however, with prolonged shock these reverse and the decrease in pre-load and afterload leads to myocardial depression.

Presentation

The presentation of the child with anaphylaxis varies depending on the severity of symptoms. Some children may present with only a skin eruption or edema whereas other patients may present with respiratory compromise or cardiovascular collapse and shock characteristic of an overt anaphylactic episode.[26,41] The presentation with an urticarial rash or respiratory symptoms is much more common than a cardiovascular source of symptoms.[25,42] However, shock and cardiovascular collapse can occur without a preceding cutaneous manifestation.[26] Other presenting symptoms may include gastro-intestinal complaints or neurologic symptoms such as dizziness, headache, or syncope.

Symptoms may begin within 5 minutes of anti-gen presentation or may be delayed for several hours. If symptoms begin immediately on exposure, the reaction tends to be more severe and can be rapidly fatal. An episode may be biphasic, where symptoms can abate for several hours and then return. Attacks may also persist for several days and have multiple recurrences with asymptomatic periods in between.

Treatment

The rapid recognition and prompt initiation of therapy is essential. The treatment of anaphylactic shock can be divided into two major phases. First, as with any shock state, attention is directed to the ABCs. Airway compromise may be present and takes priority. Once the airway is secure, oxygenation and ventilation are assessed. There is often bronchospasm with concomitant wheezing. Providing oxygen will help ensure adequate oxygenation and the wheezing often abates with the administration of epinephrine for circulatory support. Epinephrine is the mainstay of therapy. Circulatory dysfunction and shock are the next most pressing issues. For circula-tory collapse, large volume infusions, as in other types of shock, help to restore the circulating blood volume. Hypotension can be severe and resistant to therapy. Circulatory support with repeated doses of epinephrine and a continuous epinephrine infusion help support the patient until the directed therapy can begin.[26,41]

Once the vital functions have been addressed, atten-tion should turn to combating the antigen exposure. If the antigen and route are known—for instance if a blood transfusion is being administered—limitation of the antigen exposure becomes the next priority.

Antihistamines should be given to counter the effect of the inciting mediator. A combination of H1 (diphen-hydramine) and H2 (ranitidine) inhibitors is superior to an H1 antagonist alone for resolution of symptoms.[26] Corticosteroids may have a role in anaphylaxis by improving the inflammatory response and may help alleviate late phase reactions. Aerosolized beta-adrenergic agents may be useful if the bronchospasm is unresponsive to epinephrine.[26]

SUMMARY

Shock is a life-threatening emergency. The child with shock experiences an insult that begins at the cellular level and extends to the level of the organized systems of the body. Shock is a complex state of failure of the circulatory system to supply adequate oxygen and other nutrients to tissues resulting in lactic acid production, cellular dysfunction and death, and subsequent organ dysfunction. An understanding of the physiology and the determinants of oxygen delivery is essential to dif-ferentiate the causes of shock and to formulate an approach for treatment. The oxygen content determines the amount of oxygen and nutrients contained within the blood. The oxygen delivery depends on the oxygen content and the cardiac output to deliver those nutri-ents to the tissues of the body. Oxygen extraction may represent one measure of an organ's viability.

Shock can be classified based on the impairment in cardiac output. Identifying the source of impairment as one related to heart rate or one of the contributors of stroke volume (preload, inotropy, or afterload) can assist in guiding therapy. Fast heart rates can be thera-peutically slowed and slow heart rates can be therapeu-tically raised to enhance cardiac output. If the problem is inadequate preload, fluid resuscitation is necessary. If the problem is inotropy, agents that enhance the contractile function of the heart can be administered. And if the problem is afterload, agents that increase the vascular tone can be given.

The diagnosis, evaluation, and management of shock often occur simultaneously, and early goal-directed therapy to maintain blood pressure and oxygen deliv-ery is essential to the outcome of the child. A rapid clinical evaluation is used to determine the possible eti-ologies. This is followed by an initiation of therapies that attempt to prevent irreversible damage of the cells and organs. Further assessment determines the patient's response to therapy and possible need for more invasive interventions or redirection of possible causes and treat-ment. Intensive care unit practitioners have the ability to measure and respond to physiologic changes on a con-tinuous and ongoing basis. This ultimately enhances the outcome of the child with shock regardless of the cause.

ASSESSMENT QUESTIONS

See Evolve Resources for the answers.

1. Which one of the following is not a type of shock?
   A. Hemorrhagic
   B. Obstructive
   C. Hypovolemic
   D. Cardiogenic
   E. Oliguric
2. Cardiac output is determined by all of the following except
   A. Afterload
   B. Inotropy
   C. Preload
   D. Heart rate
   E. Oxygen content
3. Which of the following is a correct statement about oxygen consumption?
   A. It depends on oxygen-carrying capacity.
   B. It can be measured directly from the pulmonary artery catheter
   C. It is a measure of the oxygen utilized by the body.
   D. Oxygen consumption increases as cardiac output decreases.
   E. Lower oxygen consumption has been associated with improved survival.
4. How would shock from a burn be classified?
   A. Distributive
   B. Obstructive
   C. Cardiogenic
   D. Hypovolemic
   E. Anaphylactic
5. What should initial assessment of a patient in shock include?
   A. Attention to ABCs
   B. Examination of mental status
   C. Brief, directed history
   D. Examination of the skin
   E. All of the above
6. What does a pulmonary artery catheter give information on?
   A. Systemic blood pressure
   B. Cerebral perfusion
   C. Peripheral vascular resistance
   D. Inotropy
   E. Left ventricular preload
7. Regardless of etiology, what is the first step in treatment of shock?
   A. Begin rapid fluid infusion
   B. Establish and maintain an airway
   C. Placement of a central line
   D. Start dopamine
   E. Give shock dose of steroids

ASSESSMENT QUESTIONS—cont'd

8. Which of the following enhances inotropy and vasodilates?
   A. Milrinone
   B. Dopamine
   C. Norepinephrine
   D. Dobutamine
   E. Phenylephrine
9. Which of the following are commonly seen as part of the shock state?
   A. Adrenal insufficiency
   B. Disseminated intravascular coagulation
   C. Electrolyte abnormalities
   D. Hyperglycemia
   E. All of the above
10. Symptoms from anaphylaxis may be
    A. Immediate
    B. Delayed
    C. Cutaneous
    D. Cardiovascular collapse
    E. All of the above

References

1. Parillo JE: Approach to the patient with shock. In Goldman, editor: *Cecil textbook of medicine*, ed 22. Philadelphia: WB Saunders; 2004. pp 608-626.
2. Carcillo JA et al: *Pediatric shock*. In Slonim and Pollack, editors: *Pediatric critical care medicine*, Philadelphia, Lippincott, Williams and Wilkins, in press.
3. Gauthier PM, Szerlip HM: Metabolic Acidosis in the intensive care unit, *Critical Care Clinics* 2002;18:289.
4. Ross J, Covell JW: Frameworks for analysis of ventricular and circulatory function: Integrated responses. In West JB, editor: *Best and Taylor's physiological basis of medical practice*, ed 12. Baltimore: Williams & Wilkins, 1990.
5. Pollack MM, Fields AI, Ruttimann UE: Sequential cardiopulmonary variables in infants and children in septic shock, *Crit Care Med* 1984;12:554.
6. Pollack MM, Fields AI, Ruttimann UE: Distributions of cardiopulmonary variables in pediatric survivors and nonsurvivors of septic shock, *Crit Care Med* 1985;13:454.
7. Hazinski MF: Shock in the pediatric patient, *Crit Care Nurs Clin North Am* 1990;2:309.
8. Ross J, section editor: The cardiac pump. In West JB, editors: *Best and Taylor's physiological basis of medical practice*, ed 12. Baltimore. Williams & Wilkins, 1990.
9. Carcillo JA Fields AI: Clinical practice parameters for hemodynamic support of pediatric and neonatal patients in septic shock, *Critical Care Medicine* 2002;30:1365.
10. Goldstein B et al: International pediatric sepsis consensus conference: definitions for sepsis and organ dysfunction in pediatrics, *Pediatric Critical Care Medicine* 2005:28.

11. Levy FH, O'Rourke PP: Topics in pediatric critical care. In Barnhart S, Czervinske M, editors: *Perinatal and pediatric respiratory care*, Philadelphia: WB Saunders, 1995.

12. West JB, section editor: Gas transport to the periphery. In West JB, editor: *Best and Taylor's physiological basis of medical practice*, ed 12, Baltimore: Williams & Wilkins, 1990.

13. Tobin JR, Wetzel RC: Shock and multi-organ system failure. In Rogers MC, Nichols DG, editors: *Textbook of pediatric intensive care*, ed 3, Baltimore: Williams & Wilkins, 1996.

14. Thomas NJ, Carcillo JA: Hypovolemic shock in pediatric patients, *New Horiz* 1998;6:120.

15. Ross J, section editor: Intracardiac and arterial pressures and the cardiac output: cardiac catheterization. In West JB, editor: *Best and Taylor's physiological basis of medical practice*, ed 12, Baltimore: Williams & Wilkins, 1990.

16. Seear M, Wensley D, MacNab A: Oxygen consumption-oxygen delivery relationship in children, *J Pediatr* 1993;123:208.

17. Carcillo JA, Cunnion RE: Septic shock, *Crit Care Clin* 1997;13:553.

18. Pizzarro CF et al: Absolute and relative adrenal insufficiency in children with septic shock, *Pediatric Critical Care* 2005;33:855.

19. Morgan WM, O'Neill JA: Hemorrhagic and obstructive shock in pediatric patients. *New Horiz* 1998; 6:150-154.

20. Bengur AR, Meliones JN: Cardiogenic shock, *New Horiz* 1998;6:139.

21. Feltes TF, Pignatelli R, Kleinert S: Quantitated left ventricular systolic mechanics in children with septic shock utilizing noninvasive wall stress analysis, *Crit Care Med* 1994; 22:1647.

22. Hazinski MF, editor: *PALS provider manual*, Dallas: American Heart Association, 2002.

23. Smith L, Hernan L: Shock states. In Fuhrman BP and Zimmerman JJ, editors: *Pediatric critical care*, ed 3, St. Louis: Mosby-Elsevier; 2006. pp 394-410.

24. Balk RA, Ely EW, Goyette RE: *Sepsis handbook*, Knoxville, Thomson Healthcare, Advanced Therapeutics Communications, 2004.

25. Dibs SD, Baker MD: Anaphylaxis in children: a 5-year experience, *Pediatrics* 1997;99:E7.

26. Lieberman P: Anaphylaxis and anaphylactoid reactions. In Middleton E et al, editors: *Allergy: principles and practice*, ed 6, St Louis: Mosby; 2003. pp 1497-1517.

27. Behrman RE, Kliegman RM, Jenson HB, editors: *Nelson's textbook of pediatrics*, ed 16, Philadelphia: WB Saunders, 2000.

28. Tibby SM, Hatherill M, Murdoch IA: Capillary refill and core-peripheral temperature gap as indicators of haemodynamic status in paediatric intensive care patients, *Arch Dis Child* 1999;80:163.

29. Evans JM et al: Principles of invasive monitoring. In Fuhrman BP and Zimmerman JJ, editors, *Pediatric critical care*, ed 3, St. Louis, Mosby-Elsevier; 2006. pp 251-264.

30. Ceneviva G et al: Hemodynamic support in fluid refractory pediatric septic shock, *Pediatrics* 1998;102:E19.

31. Carcillo JA, Davis AL, Zaritsky A: Role of early fluid resuscitation in pediatric septic shock, *JAMA* 1991;266:1242.

32. Kallen RJ, Lonergan JM: Fluid resuscitation of acute hypovolemic hypoperfusion states in pediatrics, *Pediatr Clin North Am* 1990;37:287.

33. Saladino RA, Management of septic shock in the pediatric emergency department in 2004, *Clin Ped Emerg Med* 5:20.

34. Ross J, Schmid-Schoenbein G: Dynamics of the peripheral circulation. In West JB, editor: *Best and Taylor's physiological basis of medical practice*, ed 12, Baltimore: Williams & Wilkins, 1991.

35. O'Brien JM, Abraham E: New approaches to the treatment of sepsis, *Clin Chest Med* 2003;24:521.

36. Yildizdas D et al: Thyroid hormone levels and their relationship to survival in children with bacterial sepsis and septic shock, *J Pediatr Endocrinol Metab* 2004;17:1435.

37. Bettendorf M et al: Tri-iodothyronine treatment in children after cardiac surgery in a double blind, randomized placebo controlled study, *Lancet* 2000 356:529.

38. Burns JP: Septic shock in the pediatric patient: pathogenesis and novel treatments, *Pediatric Emergency Care* 2003;19:112.

39. Curley MAQ, Castillo L: Nutrition and shock in pediatric patients, *New Horiz* 1998;6:212.

40. Schears GJ, Deutschman CS: Common nutritional issues in pediatric and adult critical care medicine, *Crit Care Clin* 1997;3:669.

41. Lieberman P: Specific and idiopathic anaphylaxis: Pathophysiology and treatment. In Bierman CW et al, editors: *Allergy, asthma, and immunology from infancy to adulthood*, ed 3, Philadelphia: WB Saunders; 1996. pp 297-319.

42. Novembre E et al: Anaphylaxis in children: Clinical and allergologic features, *Pediatrics* 1998;101:E8.

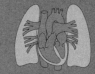

Chapter 37

Sepsis and Meningitis

JULIE LYNN FITZGERALD • TRACY KOOGLER

LEARNING OBJECTIVES

After reading this chapter the reader will be able to:
- Define sepsis, sepsis syndrome, severe sepsis, and septic shock
- Identify the most common pathogens by age and the appropriate empiric antibiotic choices for these pathogens
- Explain the pathophysiologic basis for sepsis

- Explain multiorgan system dysfunction syndrome (MODS) and discuss organ-specific supportive therapies
- Identify the most common pathogens by age and the appropriate empiric antibiotic choices for meningitis
- Explain the pathophysiology of meningitis
- Identify the complications of meningitis

Children with sepsis and bacterial meningitis are commonly encountered in the pediatric intensive care unit. Respiratory therapists play an important role in managing these complex and critically ill patients. Understanding and recognizing the etiology, presentation, therapy, and complications of these disease processes leads to improved outcomes for these potentially life-threatening clinical scenarios.

SEPSIS

Although once recognized as a severe systemic illness associated with bacteremia, sepsis is now understood to encompass a wide spectrum of clinical entities. Sepsis

syndrome may have bacterial or viral etiologies but can also be seen in the absence of documented infection, as in systemic inflammatory response syndrome (SIRS). To best manage patients with sepsis, one must be familiar with the various stages of sepsis and their definitions. Although there is some overlap between some of these terms (particularly between septic shock and severe sepsis), each is intended to define a particular patient population.

In 2005 an international pediatric sepsis conference provided a nomenclature for health care providers.[1] According to the conference, bacteremia and viremia are defined by a cultured confirmed presence of bacteria or viral particles in the blood. SIRS represents immune and inflammatory activity and a clinical syndrome of temperature abnormalities, leukocytosis or leucopenia, tachycardia, tachypnea, and hypotension. Sepsis is SIRS in the presence of a suspected or known infection. Severe sepsis is sepsis plus cardiovascular dysfunction, ARDS, or evidence of dysfunction in more than two organ systems. Patients with septic shock present with sepsis and cardiovascular dysfunction and/or collapse that responds to intravenous fluid therapy. Multiple organ dysfunction syndrome (MODS) presents as sepsis or SIRS in conjunction with any combination of disseminated intravascular coagulation, adult respiratory distress syndrome (ARDS), renal failure, and hepatobiliary dysfunction. Refractory septic shock does not improve with intravenous fluid therapy and requires the administration of vasoactive substances (Box 37-1).[2] In reviewing these definitions, it is also important to recognize that septic shock is a complex combination of hypovolemic, vasodilatory, and cardiogenic shock.

Epidemiology

There are few reliable pediatric studies defining the epidemiology of sepsis. Recent studies by Watson and colleagues at the University of Pittsburgh are perhaps the most comprehensive survey of pediatric septic shock, with an estimated incidence of 42,371 cases of severe sepsis in patients less than 20 years of age. The highest incidence was in neonates (5.2/1000) versus children 5 to 14 years of age (0.2/1,000). The overall mortality rate was 10.3% (4364 deaths annually nationwide). Of note, patients less than 1 year of age and patients with comorbidities had a higher mortality rate than patients 5 to 14 years old and patients without comorbidities.[3,4]

Box 37-1	Definition of Sepsis and Sepsis Syndrome in Pediatric Patients

Bacteremia: Culture-confirmed presence of live bacteria in blood

Sepsis: Evidence of infection with temperature changes, increased heart rate, increased respiratory rate, and leukocytosis or leucopenia

Sepsis syndrome: Sepsis plus at least one of the following: acute mental changes, decreased Pao_2, increased plasma lactate, or decreased urine output

Septic shock: Sepsis syndrome plus hypotension that responds to fluid therapy and/or drug therapy

Refractory septic shock: Sepsis syndrome plus hypotension for more than 1 hour that is not responsive to fluid and/or drug therapy and necessitates use of vasopressors

Multiple organ system failure: Any combination of disseminated intravascular coagulation, acute respiratory distress syndrome, renal failure, and hepatobiliary dysfunction

Modified from Jafari HS, McCracken GH Jr: Sepsis and septic shock: a review for clinicians, Pediatr Infect Dis J 1992;11:739.

Early onset neonatal sepsis (less than 3 days post-delivery) is associated with Group B *Streptococcus, Enterococcus,* and *Escherichia coli.* Late onset neonatal sepsis (more than 3 days postdelivery) is seen in conjunction with extended hospitalization, invasive devices, and colonization with hospital-acquired organisms. While coagulase negative *Staphylococcus* (CONS) is the most commonly identified organism, fungal organisms, gram-negative bacteria, and viruses have all been found to cause late onset neonatal disease.

The introduction of the *Haemophilus influenza* type B vaccine has virtually eradicated that pathogen as a cause of pediatric sepsis. *Streptococcus pneumoniae* and *Neisseria meningitis* are now leading causes of childhood sepsis with a growing number of cases of community-acquired Methicillin Resistant *Staphylococcus aureus* (MRSA). The increasing population of children with complex chronic diseases has also lead to an increased incidence of *Pseudomonas, Enterobacter,* and *Klebsiella* infections, many of which are multidrug resistant.

Group A *Streptococcus,* traditionally associated with impetigo and pharyngitis, has emerged as an aggressive pathogen leading to toxic shock syndrome, pneumonia with empyema, and septic shock, as well as necrotizing fasciitis. Patients may present with rapid onset septic shock and MODS with a generalized erythematous macular rash.

Although not often considered as a major category of pathogens, viruses play a nontrivial role in the etiology of sepsis. Respiratory syncytial virus (RSV), adenovirus, parainfluenza, and influenza can all cause rapid and refractory septic shock with MODS, especially in the very young patient, the immunocompromised, and the chronically ill child. Viral upper respiratory infection may also allow for bacterial superinfection and the subsequent development of sepsis.

Children with indwelling central venous catheters and peritoneal dialysis catheters, as well as transplant recipients and oncology patients, are all at an increased risk of sepsis due to coagulase negative Staphylococcus (CONS), fungi, and gram-negative bacteria.

Clinical Presentation and Differential Diagnosis

The signs and symptoms of sepsis are certainly not specific and can be quite varied depending on when in the disease course the patient is seen. Health care providers must consider other possible diagnoses when initially evaluating a patient with potential sepsis as it can often mimic other disease processes (Box 37-2).

Pathophysiology

The systemic response to infection is a complex balance mediated by proinflammatory and antiinflammatory

Box 37-2	Differential Diagnosis of the Septic Child

- Congenital heart disease
- Congestive heart failure
- Toxic ingestion
- Child abuse
- Severe anemia
- Cerebrospinal fluid shunt dysfunction
- Congenital adrenal hyperplasia
- Inborn errors of metabolism
- Cardiac arrhythmias
- Myocardial infarction
- Hypoglycemia
- Electrolyte disturbances

substances. The major components of sepsis and sepsis syndrome are:

1. infecting organisms leading to direct tissure damage and organ dysfunction
2. an excessive host inflammatory response
3. a failure of counterregulatory mechanisms.

A toxic stimulus, such as an infecting organism, triggers a release of cytokines (macrophage-derived peptides). Proinflammatory cytokines such as IL-1 and TNF enhance leukocyte adhesion to endothelial cells with the subsequent release of proteases. These cytokines trigger a cascade of inflammatory mediators such as thromboxanes, leukotrienes, prostaglandins, and clotting factors. TNF and IL-1 are responsible for the host febrile response as well. Myocardial depression seen in sepsis is thought to be secondary to the effects of TNF and IL-1. This response is mediated by the release of anti-inflammatory substances including IL-10, IL-4, corticosteroids, catecholamines, and prostaglandin E.[5] This inflammatory cascade leads to decreased systemic vascular resistance, increased vascular permeability, edema formation, ischemia, and capillary occlusion.

Nitric oxide (NO) has emerged as an important molecule in septic shock. As a free radical it plays a role in neurotransmission, bacterial killing, vasodilation, and signal transduction. NO is produced by nitric oxide synthase (NOS). The inducible form, iNOS, is expressed in response to bacterial products and cytokines. NO is responsible for pathologic vasodilatation, myocardial depression, and direct tissue injury seen in sepsis.[5,6]

The inflammatory cascade is closely linked to the coagulation system. The coagulation cascade is abnormally activated in sepsis creating disseminated intravascular coagulation (DIC). A consumptive coagulopathy, with alterations in fibrinolysis, and decreased anticoagulant activity, leads to a bleeding diathesis and microvascular thrombosis. There may also be a depletion of endogenous anticoagulants such as antithrombin III (AT-III), Protein C, and Protein S leading to increased clotting in the microvasculature.[7,8]

Organ Dysfunction and Management

The types and degree of organ dysfunction determine the treatments of sepsis. The major components of treatment include

1. restoration of intravascular volume
2. oxygen administration
3. vasoactive drugs to maintain cardiac output, vascular tone, and oxygen delivery
4. antimicrobial drugs, and
5. the removal of necrotic or purulent material.

Initial resuscitation begins with the "ABCs." Once an appropriate airway is established, aggressive volume resuscitation takes precedence to restore intravascular volume and cardiovascular stability, decrease oxygen consumption, and increase oxygen delivery to the periphery. This may require more than 60 cc/kg of isotonic non-dextrose containing fluid in the first hour alone.[9] Volume resuscitation is not limited by a specific number of cc/kg but rather to physiologic endpoints of decreasing heart rate, increased blood pressure, urine output, perfusion, and mentation.

Further cardiovascular support is necessary when the patient remains hypotensive despite aggressive volume resuscitation. Recall that sepsis is a combination of hypovolemic, cardiogenic, and vasodilatory shock. Dopamine, which provides inotropic support at low doses and increases vasomotor tone at high doses, is often used initially; however, other agents may be better options for cardiovascular support. Significant myocardial depression can result from cytokine release with a subsequent decrease in cardiac output and compensatory vasoconstriction or cold shock. This clinical scenario necessitates the addition of a direct inotrope such as epinephrine or dobutamine. Milrinone may be added to vasodilate and improve peripheral perfusion if the patient's blood pressure permits. Profound vasodilatation with bounding pulses and hypotension, or warm shock, responds best to norepinephrine or vasopressin.[10,11] The combination of vasoactive substances selected must be tailored to the individual patient and often requires frequent reevaluation and manipulation of medications. The physical exam—as well as invasive monitoring by arterial lines, central venous pressure transduction, mixed venous oxygen saturations, and rarely, pulmonary artery catheters—guides physicians' management of inotropic support. When inotropic and vasomotor support is maximized and hypotension persists, the only other salvage therapy available is extracorporeal membranous oxygenation (ECMO). This therapy is not widely available and the prognosis for patients who require this degree of hemodynamic support is poor.

Pulmonary dysfunction is a key element of sepsis. Respiratory system compliance is decreased with an increase in airway resistance. The patient is hypoxemic and tachypneic. Early intubation and mechanical ventilation decreases the work of breathing and oxygen consumption dramatically. Oxygen delivery can be significantly improved. Chest film findings can vary from mild pulmonary edema to complete airspace opacity as seen in ARDS. The adult literature clearly supports a mechanical ventilation strategy allowing hypercapnia and mild PEEP, although there are little pediatric data available at this time.[12]

Renal dysfunction occurs commonly in sepsis and can be polyuric, oliguric, or anuric. Patients may require hemodialysis for control of volume status, metabolic acidosis, and electrolyte abnormalities. The hemodynamically unstable patient on multiple inotropic agents may not tolerate conventional hemodialysis and may need continuous veno-venous hemodialysis (CVVH). Recent adult data have shown improved outcomes with CVVH and daily hemodialysis as opposed to thrice-weekly therapy in the intensive care setting.[13]

The septic patient may also present with endocrinologic derangements—most commonly abnormal glycemic control and adrenal insufficiency. Elevated blood glucose measurements are frequently encountered. Adult data strongly advocate tight glycemic control of both diabetic and nondiabetic patients between 80 and 120 gm/dl with an intravenous insulin drip.[14] Maintaining this level has been shown to lead to a significant decrease in morbidity and mortality in the ICU. Studies validating these data in pediatrics are not completed yet. Adrenal insufficiency is a controversial topic in pediatric critical care. While it has been well established that empiric high-dose steroid administration is harmful, hydrocortisone can be administered in physiologic doses if adrenal insufficiency is present. A test dose of adrenocorticotropic hormone is administered to evaluate the patient's adrenal function. Replacing glucocorticoids deficiencies appropriately can lead to a significant decrease in the amount of vasoactive substances required to maintain hemodynamic stability.[15]

Septic patients experience hematologic abnormalities including anemia, thrombocytopenia, and coagulopathy. Packed red blood cell transfusion may be used to improve arterial oxygen content and delivery as well as for volume expansion. For the bleeding patient or the patient in DIC, platelets, fresh frozen plasma, and cryoprecipitate may be necessary.

Activated Protein C, an important component of the coagulation cascade, has been shown in adult studies to have potential beneficial effects in the treatment of septic shock. A recent pediatric study was terminated early due to an unfavorable benefit-to-risk ratio. Therefore, activated protein C is not recommended for use in pediatric sepsis.[16]

Antimicrobial Therapy

Antimicrobial therapy remains a mainstay in a treatment of pediatric sepsis. Empiric antibiotic choices are determined based on the patient's age and the most likely pathogens. For the neonate, where infection with Group B Streptococcus (GBS), *E. coli*, and *Listeria* are commonly cultured, ampicillin, gentamicin, and cefotaxime are a standard antibiotic regimen. In infants 1 to 3 months old—where GBS, *N. meningitidis*, and *H. influenza* can be seen—ampicillin and cefotaxime, or ampicillin and ceftriaxone, or cefotaxime are used to treat *S. pneumoniae*, *S. aureus*, and *N. meningitidis*. A strong argument can be made for the empiric administration of vancomycin due to the increasing prevalence of beta-lactam and cephalosporin-resistant *S. pneumoniae* and *S. aureus* in the community (Table 37-1).[17] Vancomycin should routinely be administered to children of all ages who have indwelling central venous catheters in place. Immunocompromised patients should receive a broadened empiric regimen that includes vancomycin, gentamicin, and ceftazidime to cover for gram-negative organisms. Chronically ill children or children who reside in chronic care facilities are often colonized with resistant and unusual organisms. Therapy should be based on past culture data if they are available. In conjunction with empiric antibiotic therapy, abscesses should be drained quickly,

TABLE 37-1

Initial Antibiotic Regimens for Sepsis

Age	Organisms	Antibiotics
Neonatal	*Escherichia coli* Group B *Streptococcus* *Listeria monocytogenes*	Ampicillin and gentamicin or ampicillin and cefotaxime
1-3 months	Group B *Streptococcus* *Neisseria meningitidis* *Haemophilus influenzae* type B	Ampicillin and cefotaxime or ampicillin and ceftriaxone
3 months or older	*S. pneumoniae* *N. meningitidis* *H. influenzae* type B	Cefotaxime or ceftriaxone (*Note:* add vancomycin for suspected pneumococcus)

either percutaneously or surgically, and necrotic wounds should be aggressively débrided.

Overall, the diagnosis and management of the septic patient requires early recognition and therapy. With an aggressive and multifaceted treatment plan focused on early stabilization, outcomes for these critically ill infants and children can be optimized.[18]

MENINGITIS

Meningitis is an infection of the subarachnoid space and inflammation of the meninges due to bacteria and viral particles. Bacterial meningitis is most commonly the result of hematogenous spread although it can be due to direct invasion of the meninges with severe sinusitis. The spectrum of disease varies widely from a benign and self-limited process most often associated with viral meningitis to a severe illness with significant morbidity and mortality.[19]

Direct neuronal damage occurs secondary to endothelial damage and the release of toxic substances from activated neutrophils. This leads to cerebral edema formation and a subsequent increase in intracranial pressure.

The potential morbidities associated with bacterial meningitis include vision and hearing loss, seizures, hydrocephalus requiring ventriculoperitoneal shunting, and developmental delay.

Etiology

Bacterial agents that cause meningitis can be gram-negative or gram-positive organisms. Common infecting organisms vary according to the patient's age. In the neonate to the 3-month-old infant, the most commonly identified organism is GBS. It may have an early or late presentation. The early presentation is associated with prematurity and maternal obstetrical complications. Routinely obtaining vaginal cultures of expectant mothers and administering prophylactic antibiotics has significantly decreased the incidence of GBS meningitis. E. coli is the second most common pathogen in this age group. Galactosemia and urosepsis are often found in infants with E. coli meningitis. Listeria monocytogenes is a pathogen for infants 10 to 30 days old. Empiric antibiotic choices should include drugs with activity against this pathogen as well.

The most commonly encountered cause of viral meningitis in this age group is herpes simplex. Maternal infection and transmission may be undetected at the time of delivery if no skin lesions are present, especially if it is the primary infection for the mother. One must consider the addition of empiric acyclovir in this setting as well.

For infants and children older than 3 months of age, S. pneumoniae and N. meningitidis are the most common etiologies of bacterial meningitis. With the advent of the H. influenza type B vaccine, this pathogen has essentially been eliminated as a cause of meningitis. Enterovirus is the most common viral agent causing meningitis and encephalitis, mostly in the summer months.

Presentation

Newborns and infants often do not exhibit the classic signs and symptoms indicative of bacterial meningitis. Decreased activity, poor oral intake, and temperature abnormalities are often the only symptoms. A bulging fontanel is a late finding in bacterial meningitis. Classic meningeal signs are not seen in this age group. Children older than 1 year of age will exhibit the more classic signs and symptoms of meningitis such as altered mentation, nuchal rigidity, fever, vomiting, headache, photophobia, and seizures. N. meningitidis infection may also be associated with a rash, purpura fulminans. Bacterial meningitis may present as frank septic shock in all age groups, as has previously been described in this chapter. With more advanced stages of infection, coma, abnormal respiratory patterns such as Cheyne-Stokes respiration, cranial nerve dysfunction, and seizures can occur due to increasing intracranial pressure.

Diagnosis

The first step toward diagnosing bacterial meningitis is a high level of suspicion. A thorough history and physical exam are also crucial to making this diagnosis as physical findings may be subtle.

Definitive diagnosis is based on a cerebrospinal fluid (CSF) analysis in all age groups. Lumbar puncture is a benign procedure and should not be avoided when there is a suspicion of meningitis. CSF cell count, Gram stain and culture, glucose, and protein levels should be obtained. Additionally, perform a complete cell count, blood cultures, and urine analysis and culture. A hemodynamically unstable child or a child in significant respiratory distress should be stabilized before any attempt at lumbar puncture is made. Additionally, if a known coagulopathy exists, it should be corrected before a lumbar puncture. Stabilization of the patient should never delay the administration of antibiotics when bacterial meningitis is suspected, even if CSF has not been obtained. If focal neurologic findings are present, a CT scan of the head should be obtained to rule out the presence of a mass lesion before any attempts at lumbar puncture are made as herniation could occur in the presence of a mass.

Treatment

Treatment of bacterial meningitis is a combination of resuscitation and supportive care, antimicrobial therapy, and potentially antiinflammatory therapy.[20] Resuscitation and support, as always, consist of the ABCs, aggressive volume resuscitation, and maintaining a normal body temperature.

Early administration of antibiotics is based on the patient's age. For the neonate—where GBS, *E. coli,* and *Listeria* are the most common organisms—ampicillin, cefotaxime, and gentamicin are used routinely. Strong consideration should be given to the addition of acyclovir for the treatment of herpes simplex disease, where the morbidities can be equal to those of bacterial infection. Empiric treatment for the child older than 3 months of age should include ceftriaxone or cefotaxime plus high-dose vancomycin to cover for resistant *S. pneumoniae.*

There has been some interest in the administration of glucocorticoids to decrease the inflammatory response in bacterial meningitis. Pediatric studies have focused on children with *H. influenza* type B infection where steroids, were administered before antibiotics. Children who received dexamethasone before antimicrobial therapy had a decreased incidence of ataxia, hearing loss, seizure disorder, and focal neurologic deficits. These results have not been observed in bacterial meningitis due to other pathogens.[16-18] Administration of dexamethasone may also interfere with the diffusion of vancomycin across the blood-brain barrier. Therefore, it is not recommended to administer dexamethasone routinely in cases of suspected bacterial meningitis. There are no data to support its use in neonatal disease.

Complications

The complications of bacterial meningitis can have profound sequelae (Box 37-3). Cerebral edema is found in bacterial meningitis, leading to increased intracranial pressure, coma, fixed eye deviation, bradycardia, hypertension, and irregular respirations. Additionally, inflammation of the microvascular structures, as well as debris in the ventricular system, can lead to decreased reabsorption of CSF by the arachnoid villi and cause further increases in intracranial pressure. In the worst-case scenario, this cerebral edema can lead to herniation and resultant brain death.

Subdural empyema is associated with coma, increased intracranial pressure, seizures, and decorticate posturing. Confirmation of the diagnosis is made by CT scan of the head. Differentiation from subdural effusion may require subdural puncture in the critically ill child. This complication occurs more commonly when the source of meningitis is from direct invasion from the sinuses. It requires urgent surgical drainage. Rarely, bacterial meningitis can lead to brain abscesses causing focal neurologic findings and seizures. Brain abscesses also require surgical drainage.

Syndrome of inappropriate antidiuretic hormone (SIADH) is frequently seen with meningitis. These patients develop hyponatremia, hypo-osmolarity, and increased urinary sodium levels in the face of normal renal function. The treatment of this is fluid intake and occasionally the addition of oral sodium supplements or hypertonic saline.

In children with *N. meningitidis* infection, disseminated disease can lead to severe microvascular thrombosis of the extremities. This can result in the loss of digits of the hands and feet as well as the need for more aggressive amputations.

Outcomes

Early recognition, diagnosis, and treatment does not guarantee a favorable outcome in bacterial meningitis; however, aggressive treatment and attention to detail in the care of these patients may improve it. Long-term sequelae are related to the degree of neurologic damage and include hearing and vision deficits, seizures, and mental retardation.

SUMMARY

Despite advances in pediatric critical care, sepsis and meningitis continue to be significant causes of morbidity and mortality in the United States. Optimal care of these patients requires a team approach and meticulous attention to detail. With early diagnosis, aggressive resuscitation, and a multifaceted therapeutic approach, the best outcomes for these patients can be obtained.

Box 37-3	Complications of Bacterial Meningitis

- Seizure
- Septic arthritis
- Pericardial effusion
- Pneumonia/empyema
- Subdural effusion
- Syndrome of inappropriate secretion of antidiuretic hormone
- Cerebral edema
- Subdural empyema
- Brain abscess

ASSESSMENT QUESTIONS

See Evolve Resources for the answers.

1. What is systemic inflammatory response syndrome?
   A. Culture-proven presence of bacteria or viral particles in the blood
   B. Bacteremia plus ARDS, renal failure, and hepatic failure
   C. Immune and inflammatory reaction with temperature instability, abnormal WBC count, respiratory abnormalities, and hypotension
   D. Sepsis with MODS
2. What most commonly causes early onset neonatal sepsis?
   A. *H. influenza* type B
   B. Group B *Streptococcus*
   C. *E. coli*
   D. Herpes simplex virus
3. What are the major components of sepsis?
   A. Infecting organisms leading to direct tissue damage and organ dysfunction
   B. An excessive host inflammatory response
   C. A failure of counter-regulatory mechanisms
   D. All of the above
4. Which of the following is true regarding the cytokines activity is sepsis?
   A. TNF and IL-1 are proinflammatory molecules
   B. TNF and IL-1 are responsible for myocardial depression
   C. IL-10 and IL-4 mediate the proinflammatory response
   D. NO is a free radical that causes profound vasodilation
   E. All of the above
5. Which of the following is correct regarding the treatment of sepsis?
   A. Limited volume resuscitation improves outcome.
   B. Dopamine is the best initial vasoactive substance in the hypotensive patient.
   C. ECMO is a commonly used form of hemodynamic support.
   D. Activated Protein C is recommended for pediatric patients.
   E. Early empiric antimicrobial therapy is critical in the treatment of sepsis.
6. What should empiric antimicrobial therapy for a 5-year-old with presumed sepsis include?
   A. Ceftriaxone
   B. Vancomycin
   C. Ampicillin
   D. A and B
   E. A, B, and C

ASSESSMENT QUESTIONS—cont'd

7. Which patient group(s) have an increased risk of sepsis?
   A. Oncology patients
   B. Transplant patients
   C. Patients with chronic diseases
   D. Patients with indwelling central venous catheters
   E. All of the above
8. Which of the following are true regarding meningitis?
   A. Inflammation of the meninges is always due to bacterial infection.
   B. Meningitis does not cause cerebral edema.
   C. Bacterial meningitis is most often the result of hematogenous spread.
   D. There is little risk of chronic morbidity with bacterial meningitis.
   E. Bacteria, the cause of meningitis, are always gram-positive organisms.
9. What does the typical presentation of an infant with meningitis include?
   A. Lethargy
   B. Nuchal rigidity
   C. Poor oral intake
   D. A and B
   E. A and C
10. Which of the following is/are complications of bacterial meningitis?
   A. Vision loss
   B. Hearing loss
   C. Mental retardation
   D. Subdural empyema
   E. All of the above

References

1. Goldstein B et al: International pediatric sepsis consensus conference: Definitions for sepsis and organ dysfunction in pediatrics, *Pediatr Crit Care Med* 2005;6:1.
2. Jafari HS et al: Sepsis and septic shock: a review for clinicians, *Pediatr Infect Dis J* 1992;11:739.
3. Proulx F et al. Epidemiology of sepsis and multiple organ dysfunction syndrome in children' *Chest.* 1996;109:1033.
4. Watson RS et al: Severe sepsis in children: a U.S. epidemiologic study. *Crit Care Med* 2001;28:A46.
5. Dinarello CA: Proinflammatory and anti-inflammatory cytokines as mediators in the pathogenesis of septic shock, *Chest* 1997;112(supp):321S.
6. Cobb JP, Danner RL: Nitric oxide and septic shock, *JAMA* 1996;275:1192.
7. Salgado A et al: Inflammatory mediators and their influence on haemostasis, *Haemostasis* 1994;24:132.

8. Varvolet MG et al: Derangements of coagulation and fibrinolysis in critically ill patients with sepsis and septic shock, *Semin Thromb Hemost* 1998;24:33.

9. Carcillo JA. et al. Role of early fluid resuscitation in pediatric septic shock. *JAMA*. 1991;266:1243-1245.

10. Carcillo JA et al: Clinical practice parameters of hemodynamic support of pediatric and neonatal patients in septic shock, *Crit Care Med*. 2002; 30:1365.

11. Ceneviva G et al: Hemodynamic support in fluid-refractory pediatric septic shock, *Pediatrics* 1998;102:e19.

12. Amato MB et al: Beneficial effects of the "open lung approach" with low distending pressures in acute respiratory distress syndrome: a prospective randomized study on mechanical ventilation, *Am J Respir Crit Care Med* 1995;152:1935.

13. Kornecki A et al: Continuous renal replacement therapy for non-renal indication: experience in children, *Isr Med Assoc* 2002;4:345.

14. Van den Berghe G et al: Intensive insulin therapy in critically ill patients, *N Engl J Med* 2001;345:1359.

15. Annane D et al: Effect of treatment with low doses of hydrocortisone and fludrocortisones on mortality in patients with septic shock, *JAMA* 2002;288:862.

16. Bernard GR et al: Efficacy and safety of recombinant human activated protein C for severe sepsis, *N Engl J Med* 2001;344:699.

17. Gonzalez B et al: Severe Staphylococcal sepsis in adolescents in the era of community-acquired methicillin-resistant *Staphylococcus aureus*, *Pediatrics* 2005;115:3.

18. Martinot A et al: Sepsis in neonates and children: definitions, epidemiology, and outcome, *Pediatr Emerg Care* 1997;13:277.

19. Saez-Llorens X et al: Molecular pathophysiology of bacterial meningitis: current concepts and therapeutic implications, *J Pediatr* 1990;116:671.

20. Tunkel AR et al: Practice guidelines for the management of bacterial meningitis, *Clin Infect Dis* 2004;39:1267.

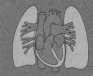

Chapter 38

Thermal and Inhalation Injury

RONALD P. MLCAK

OUTLINE

Thermal Injury
  Epidemiology
  Pathophysiology
  Management
Inhalation Injury
  Pathophysiology
  Evaluation of Injury

Management
Complications
Long-term Outcomes

LEARNING OBJECTIVES

After reading this chapter the reader will be able to:
- Discuss the epidemiology of thermal injury
- Recognize the four essential functions of normal skin that are necessary for survival
- Compare first-, second-, and third-degree burns
- Use the modified "rule of nines" chart to calculate the extent of burn injuries

- Discuss the basis management of thermal injury
- Discuss the incidence and pathophysiology of inhalation injury
- Describe the diagnosis of inhalation injury
- Discuss the management of inhalation injury
- Describe the long-term outcomes of patients with inhalation injury

THERMAL INJURY

Epidemiology

Modern care for the patient with thermal injury began in 1942, the year of the Coconut Grove Nightclub disaster in Boston in which fire claimed the lives of more than 400 people.[1] Since that time, the successful management of the patient with a severe burn has continued to be a challenge, particularly if the victim is a young child.

In the United States, thermal injury results in 60,000 hospitalizations and approximately 6000 deaths annually. About half of those deaths occur in children, accounting for only approximately 5% of pediatric burn injuries.[2-5] Mortality is highest in very young children and the elderly, with burn injury one of the three

leading causes of death in children. Less than 5% of pediatric thermal injuries are the result of chemical or electrical burns. Flame burns account for 10% to 15% of thermal injuries and when associated with smoke inhalation are the cause of most deaths. Scalding burns account for 75% to 80% of the thermal injuries among children.[6,7]

Medical advances have had an impact on reducing the mortality rate and outcome in burn and inhalation injury. However, prevention remains the most important aspect of lowering the risk of these injuries to children. Important measures in preventing pediatric thermal-related injuries are having working smoke detectors, keeping matches out of reach, lowering hot water temperatures, covering electrical outlets, and using flame-resistant children's clothing.[4,8]

Independently cited as high–mortality risk factors in children are burn injuries exceeding 30% body surface area (Figure 38-1), associated smoke inhalation, and age younger than 4 years.[9] However, with improved treatment of inhalation injury, advancements in early wound repair techniques, effective antibiotics, precise fluid resuscitation and metabolic control, and avoidance of high pulmonary pressure and oxygen concentrations, the pediatric mortality rate and outcomes continue to improve.[3,10] With these advances, the mortality rate has dropped 45% over 20 years, and the likelihood is that a child will survive even after burn exposure of up to 60% of the body surface area.[5]

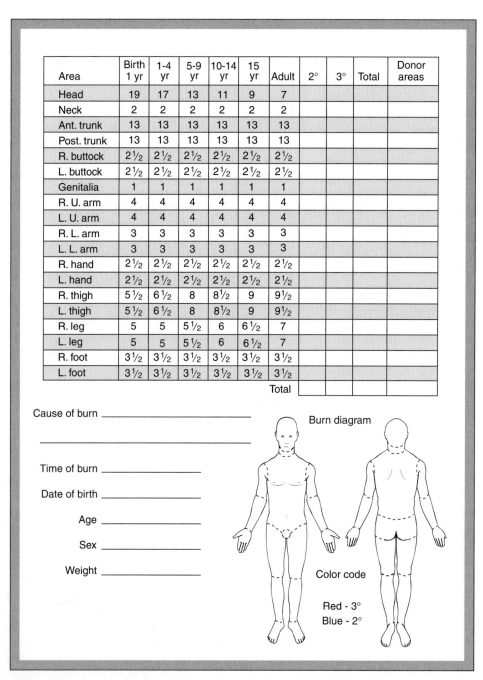

Area	Birth 1 yr	1-4 yr	5-9 yr	10-14 yr	15 yr	Adult	2°	3°	Total	Donor areas
Head	19	17	13	11	9	7				
Neck	2	2	2	2	2	2				
Ant. trunk	13	13	13	13	13	13				
Post. trunk	13	13	13	13	13	13				
R. buttock	2½	2½	2½	2½	2½	2½				
L. buttock	2½	2½	2½	2½	2½	2½				
Genitalia	1	1	1	1	1	1				
R. U. arm	4	4	4	4	4	4				
L. U. arm	4	4	4	4	4	4				
R. L. arm	3	3	3	3	3	3				
L. L. arm	3	3	3	3	3	3				
R. hand	2½	2½	2½	2½	2½	2½				
L. hand	2½	2½	2½	2½	2½	2½				
R. thigh	5½	6½	8	8½	9	9½				
L. thigh	5½	6½	8	8½	9	9½				
R. leg	5	5	5½	6	6½	7				
L. leg	5	5	5½	6	6½	7				
R. foot	3½	3½	3½	3½	3½	3½				
L. foot	3½	3½	3½	3½	3½	3½				
						Total				

Cause of burn _____

_____

Time of burn _____

Date of birth _____

Age _____

Sex _____

Weight _____

Burn diagram

Color code

Red - 3°
Blue - 2°

FIGURE 38-1 Body surface area estimates of burn size based on age. Note the decrease in the surface area of the head and the increase in the areas of the legs from infant to adult. Using this table provides the most accurate percentage for burn size estimates when calculating fluid and nutritional requirements.

Pathophysiology

The skin provides four essential functions that are necessary for survival:

1. protecting the body from infection and injury
2. preventing fluid loss
3. regulating body temperature, and
4. providing sensory input from the environment.[4]

It is composed of two layers: the epidermis and the dermis. The epidermis is the thin outer layer. Below it is the dermis, which is a deeper, thicker layer. The dermis contains hair follicles, sweat glands, sebaceous glands, and sensory fibers for touch, pain, pressure, and temperature. Beneath the dermis lies the subcutaneous tissue, which is composed of connective tissue and fat.

Classification of Burn Injury

The depth of the burn injury classifies the degree of burn and depends on the temperature and duration of contact with the skin. Contact with flame, heat, chemicals, or electrical current results in varying degrees of tissue destruction. Burn depths also vary as a result of body position and skin thickness. Very young children and elderly patients are especially vulnerable to more severe, full-thickness burns because of their particularly thin skin.

First-degree burns are superficial, involving only the epidermis. The skin appears red without blisters and is hypersensitive and painful.

Second-degree burns are partial-thickness by definition and involve the epidermis and part of the dermis. These burns are usually very painful because nerve endings in the mid and superficial dermal layer survive the injury. Blistering is often present. Healing generally occurs quickly and completely because epithelial cells survive in deeper portions of hair follicles and migrate to the surface.

Third-degree burns are classified as full-thickness burns. They involve injury and necrosis beyond the depths of the hair follicles, through the entire thickness of the skin, and into the subcutaneous tissue. The area swells less rapidly than a second-degree burn and is usually blanched in appearance. Sensory nerves are destroyed, causing local anesthesia.

Percent of Body Surface Area Burn

An estimate of burn size and depth assists in determining the severity, prognosis, and disposition of the patient. Because fluid resuscitation requirements, nutritional support, and surgical interventions are all based on the size of the burn, an accurate assessment of the percent of body surface area burned is critical. The size of the burn wound is described in terms of the percent of total body surface area.

The "rule of nines" is the method most frequently used to estimate percent body surface area burned. This estimate is based on various anatomic regions representing 9% of body surface area, or a multiple of nine. However, infants and younger children have body proportions different from those of an adult and a modified "rule of nines" may be used. Figure 38-1 describes the percentages of various anatomic regions as the child ages.[3,9]

Management

First-degree burns heal spontaneously, usually within 2 weeks, and do not require surgical intervention. Excision and grafting of partial- and full-thickness burns, along with topical antimicrobial therapy, have decreased the incidence of burn wound sepsis. Topical agents most commonly used are sulfadiazine (Silvadene), silver nitrate, and mafenide acetate (Sulfamylon).

After burn injury, the area of deepest burn contains cells that are dead without hope of salvage. The dead skin forms an eschar, which is tough and leathery. Because the eschar layer does not expand well, circumferential burns of the limbs often swell and occlude perfusion to peripheral portions of the extremities. In the same manner, circumferential burns of the thorax can restrict ventilation. An escharotomy, which consists of making long incisions into the eschar to allow for wound expansion, relieves the tight, restricting band created by the eschar (Figure 38-2).[3,9] It is important to prevent both early edema and infection that can destroy dermal remnants and convert a burn wound from partial thickness to full thickness.

A crucial component of burn care is initiating accurate fluid resuscitation as soon as possible after the injury. Several formulas for resuscitation are available, with children younger than 10 years of age requiring a modified formula. Delays in resuscitation often lead to increased fluid requirements. Overaggressive fluid resuscitation may result in increased extravascular

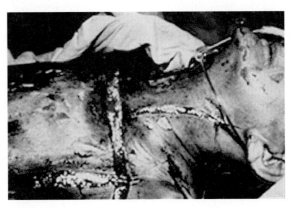

FIGURE 38-2 Escharotomy incisions on the chest and neck.

hydrostatic pressure, pulmonary edema, and soft tissue swelling. Urine output is the usual indicator of adequate resuscitation. Careful hemodynamic monitoring is required, along with intubation for most patients with severe burns. It is important to view the formulas as simply guidelines to fluid resuscitation and not substitutes for diligent monitoring of urine output, electrolytes, and volume status.[11,12]

The metabolic rate can increase as much as two to three times normal after burn injury and is generally related to the size of the burn. This is accompanied by constant hyperthermia. Nutritional support is extremely important and is best accomplished by calculating caloric needs and correcting electrolyte disturbances that are common to burn patients. Pharmacologic support of the hypermetabolic response consists of using anabolic agents to alleviate muscle wasting and preserve lean body mass and antiadrenergic drugs to decrease myocardial oxygen consumption and cardiac work.[11]

INHALATION INJURY

Over the past decade there have been many advances in the critical care of burn patients. Burn shock, which in the 1930s and 1940s accounted for nearly 20% of burn deaths, is now treated with early, vigorous fluid resuscitation and rarely leads to loss of life.[6,12] Invasive sepsis originating from the burn wound was at one time found to be the major cause of mortality in 80% of autopsies.[13] Aggressive wound excision and grafting, along with the use of topical antibiotics, have dramatically decreased the incidence of burn wound sepsis. Inhalation injury has now emerged as the most frequent cause of death in patients with severe burns.[13-17]

Although the mortality from smoke inhalation alone is low (0% to 11%), smoke inhalation injury in combination with cutaneous burns is fatal in 30% to 90% of patients.[18] Inhalation injury impairs the mucociliary transport mechanism in the lung, predisposing the patient to retain secretions, which leads to pneumonia and atelectasis. The combination of inhalation injury and pneumonia has been shown to carry a mortality rate of 60%.[19,20] Along with burn size and the patient's age, inhalation injury is one of the most significant predictors of burn-related mortality.[21]

Pathophysiology

Airway injury after smoke inhalation is complex and can occur at any level of the respiratory system, resulting in impaired ventilation and oxygenation. Box 38-1 lists the physiologic consequences that accompany smoke inhalation.

Box 38-1	Physiologic Consequences of Inhalation Injury

- Hypoxemia
- Bronchospasm
- Airway edema
- Airway obstruction
- Impaired ciliary activity
- Impaired surfactant production
- Increased dead space
- Increased airway resistance
- Increased mucus production
- Increased work of breathing
- Increased oxygen consumption
- Increased intrapulmonary shunting
- Increased ventilation/perfusion mismatch
- Decreased lung and chest wall compliance

Upper Airway Injury

Direct thermal trauma is limited to the upper airway and results in obstruction from edema, hemorrhage, and ulceration of the mucosa. In only a few hours, mild pharyngeal edema can rapidly progress to complete upper airway obstruction with asphyxia.[22,23] The worsening of upper airway edema is most prominent in supraglottic structures. Serial nasopharyngoscopic evaluations demonstrate obliteration of the aryepiglottic folds, arytenoid eminences, and interarytenoid areas created by edematous tissue that prolapses and occludes the airway.[24,25]

Smoke particles vary in size and most often deposit in the upper airway. The type of gas released during combustion depends on the material burned, the temperature, and the amount of oxygen present. Many of the gases, such as ammonia and hydrogen chloride, are chemical irritants and cause intense coughing, bronchospasm, and upper airway edema.[26]

Lung Parenchyma Injury

Direct thermal trauma after inhalation injury is not responsible for the pathophysiologic changes in the parenchyma of the lung, and the carbonaceous material present in smoke is not directly responsible for parenchymal damage, although it can serve as a carrier for other agents.[27] Only steam, with a heat-carrying capacity many times that of dry air, is capable of overwhelming the extremely efficient heat-dissipatory capabilities of the upper airways and transmitting heat to the subglottic airways.[28]

The damage to the lung parenchyma is caused by inhalation of incomplete products of combustion. There is direct cellular injury to the respiratory epithelium and pulmonary macrophages, resulting in an inflammatory response. The inflammatory mediators cause bronchoconstriction, an increase in tracheobronchial blood flow with edema formation, and leukocyte infiltration. Bronchoscopic study of the airways in the first 24 hours after inhalation injury shows gradual evolution of an edematous tracheobronchial mucosa.[29] As large portions of the respiratory epithelium slough, necrotic cellular debris accumulates in the airways. Progressive separation of the epithelium with formation of pseudomembranous casts causes partial or complete airway obstruction that can be fatal.[30]

The pulmonary parenchyma surrounding injured airways shows varying degrees of congestion, interstitial and alveolar edema, occasional hyaline membranes, and dense atelectasis. Systemic effects of inhalation injury are manifested by

1. an increase in airway resistance, ventilation-perfusion mismatch, and oxygen consumption
2. a decrease in lung compliance, oxygenation, and surfactant production.[31,32]

Carbon Monoxide Poisoning

Carbon monoxide (CO) is a colorless, odorless, tasteless gas produced by the incomplete combustion of carbon-containing compounds. Smoke inhalation from all types of fires often results in significant CO exposure. The majority of immediate deaths that occur at the scene of building fires are caused by CO poisoning. Every patient received from a fire scene should be evaluated for CO poisoning.

The affinity of CO for the binding sites on the hemoglobin molecule is 200 to 280 times that of oxygen. The formation of carboxyhemoglobin (COHb) leads to a tremendous reduction in the oxygen-carrying capacity of the blood.[33] This shortage of oxygen is made worse by a concomitant shift of the oxyhemoglobin dissociation curve to the left, reducing the ability of hemoglobin to release oxygen to the tissues.[34-36]

Pulse oximetry measurement does not accurately reflect oxygen saturation in the presence of COHb. The pulse oximeter equates COHb with oxygenated hemoglobin and measures the percentage of saturation of available binding sites, regardless of whether the sites are occupied by CO or oxygen. This causes the pulse oximeter to read falsely elevated oxygen saturation values in the presence of COHb.[37] Direct measurement of COHb using co-oximetry is recommended.

The symptoms of CO poisoning correlate roughly with the percentage of COHb in the blood. Table 38-1 lists the expected symptoms based on CO blood concentrations. The major effects are on organs that are most susceptible to anoxia, such as the brain, heart, and central nervous system.

TABLE 38-1

Symptoms of Carbon Monoxide Poisoning

Carboxyhemoglobin (%)	Symptoms
0-10	None
10-20	Frontal headache, tightness across forehead
20-30	Dyspnea, headache, throbbing temples
30-40	Dizziness, blurred vision, nausea, vomiting, severe, headache
40-50	Tachypnea, tachycardia, confusion, collapse
50-70	Depressed consciousness level, seizures, bradycardia
>70	Respiratory failure, death

Modified from Lacey DJ: Neurologic sequelae of acute carbon monoxide intoxication, *Am J Dis Child* 1981;135:145. Copyright 1981, American Medical Association.

Evaluation of Injury

Clinical Manifestations

The clinical diagnosis of inhalation injury has traditionally rested on various unreliable observations. Smoke inhalation injury is more likely to be present in those with a history of burn injury in an enclosed space, the appearance of facial burns, singed nasal vibrissae and facial hair, erythema of the oropharynx, and the presence of carbonaceous sputum and debris around the nose, mouth, and pharynx.[38] Rhonchi, crackles, wheezes, stridor, dyspnea, cough, and hoarse voice are seldom present on admission, occurring only in persons with the most severe injury and implying an extremely poor prognosis.[39] The admission chest radiograph is often normal and is a very poor indicator of severity of acute lung injury.[40] However, two thirds of patients develop changes of diffuse or focal infiltrates or pulmonary edema within 5 to 10 days of injury.

Bronchoscopy

The current gold standard for the diagnosis of inhalation injury in most burn centers is fiberoptic bronchoscopy.[41] Direct visualization of the upper airway provides information concerning the extent of upper airway injury. The diagnosis of inhalation injury is confirmed in the presence of soot, charring, mucosal erythema and ulceration, hemorrhage, airway edema, and inflammation.[42] The widespread use of bronchoscopy has led to an approximately twofold increase in diagnosis over that based on the traditional clinical signs.

Xenon Scan

The xenon scan is a safe, rapid test used to evaluate parenchymal damage.[43] Requiring minimal patient cooperation, it involves serial chest scintiphotograms after an initial intravenous injection of radioactive xenon gas. It demonstrates areas of decreased alveolar gas washout, which identifies sites of small airway destruction caused by edema or cast formation. Both false-negative and false-positive results are possible, occurring mainly in patients in whom scanning is delayed for 4 or more days or who have preexisting lung disease. The most important limitation is the logistic problem of transporting the unstable patient to the hospital's nuclear medicine department. Although reported in the literature, few burn centers currently use the xenon scan for diagnosis of inhalation injury.

Spirometry

Although not routinely used for the diagnosis of inhalation injury in children, pulmonary function studies are abnormal after inhalation injury. Reductions in the forced expiratory volume in 1 second (FEV_1) and the ratio of FEV_1 to vital capacity (FEV_1/VC) are seen within 24 hours of injury.[44] Over the next several days, vital capacity and peak flow are reduced and pulmonary resistance is increased.[45,46]

Thermal and Dye Dilution

A more recent method of evaluating inhalation injury is the estimation of extravascular lung water by simultaneous thermal and dye dilution measurements. This procedure has been unable to quantify the severity of injury but has proven useful in separating parenchymal injury from upper airway injury.[47]

Management

The management of any patient with an inhalation injury is determined by the degree of hypoxia, airway obstruction and edema, sepsis, and respiratory failure. Current treatment includes oxygen therapy, adequate airway maintenance, aggressive bronchial hygiene therapy, pharmacologic management, and mechanical ventilatory support.

Oxygen Therapy

The goal of oxygen therapy in a patient with inhalation injury is to increase the oxygen content of the blood. All patients should be given 100% oxygen through a nonrebreathing mask immediately after inhalation injury. Oxygenation is monitored by arterial blood gas analysis, and COHb level is analyzed with co-oximetry. The use of hyperbaric oxygen is widely debated.

Airway Maintenance

Acute upper airway obstruction occurs in one fifth to one third of hospitalized burn victims with inhalation injury. Stridor, hoarseness, wheezing, retractions, and tachypnea are all signs of upper airway compromise and mandate prompt intervention. Whenever airway obstruction is suspected, the most experienced clinician should perform endotracheal intubation. It is better to intubate early than to wait and find that the obstruction has progressed to where visualization of the larynx is reduced.

Securing the endotracheal tube can be difficult, owing to burn wounds and the rapid airway swelling that occurs within the first 72 hours after the injury. A nasotracheal tube is often more readily secured than an orotracheal tube. Reintubation after an accidental extubation may be difficult if not impossible if facial and oropharyngeal edema is severe. It is important to secure the tube in a manner that avoids trauma to the skin, especially when the face and neck are burned.[47]

Burns of the neck, especially in children, can cause unyielding eschars that externally compress and obstruct the airway. Escharotomies to the neck may be helpful in reducing the tight eschar and therefore decreasing the pressure exerted on the trachea.

Bronchial Hygiene Therapy

Aggressive bronchial hygiene therapy is an essential component of the respiratory management of patients after inhalation injury. Retained secretions may result in life-threatening airway obstruction. They can also lead to atelectasis and ventilation-perfusion mismatch and, ultimately, contribute to the development of pneumonia, which has been shown to increase mortality after burns and inhalation injury.[48] Early ambulation, therapeutic coughing, chest physiotherapy, airway suctioning, therapeutic bronchoscopy, and pharmacologic agents are used to mobilize and remove retained secretions and fibrin casts.

Early ambulation includes having the patient stand, walk, and sit in a chair. Patients with inhalation injury are routinely gotten out of bed and allowed to sit in a chair to improve lung function. Parents are encouraged to hold and rock their children as a means of therapy and to provide patient comfort.

Tracheobronchial suctioning and lavage are imperative for the removal of secretions and casts in the patient who has an ineffective cough or incapacitated mucociliary apparatus. When secretions or casts become thick and adhere to the airways, bronchial lavage is used as an adjunct to suctioning. Care is taken not to use excessive lavage fluid. Nasotracheal suctioning may be used as a mechanism to stimulate coughing and remove secretions in patients who are not intubated.

Chest physiotherapy, postural drainage, and routine repositioning of the patient every 2 hours have been effective in secretion removal. However, positioning is often limited because of the location of fresh skin grafts and donor sites.

When these techniques fail to remove secretions, the use of fiberoptic bronchoscopy has proven effective. Bronchoscopy allows for visualization of the airway and enables meticulous pulmonary toilet for retained secretions. The presence of inspissated secretions and fibrin casts may require repeated bronchoscopy to maintain airway patency and adequate gas exchange.[42,49]

Pharmacologic Management

Inhalation injury to the lower airways results in a chemical tracheobronchitis that can cause intense bronchospasm and wheezing. This is best managed with β₂-agonists, especially in patients who also have preexisting asthma or reactive airway disease. Aerosolized bronchodilators are effective by providing bronchial smooth muscle relaxation and stimulating mucociliary clearance.

Racemic epinephrine may be used as an aerosolized vasoconstrictor, bronchodilator, and secretion bond breaker. The vasoconstrictive action of racemic epinephrine is useful in reducing mucosal and submucosal edema within the walls of the pulmonary airways. A secondary bronchodilator action serves to reduce potential spasm of the smooth muscle of the terminal bronchioles. Racemic epinephrine has also been used in the treatment of postextubation stridor.

Investigators have suggested that of corticosteroids may be administered to decrease mucosal edema and bronchospasm, maintain surfactant function, and decrease the inflammatory response that occurs after inhalation injury. Prospective studies showed no benefit in morbidity and mortality in patients who received intravenous corticosteroids after inhalation injury. Some researchers have suggested that there might be an increase in infection-related complications in patients who receive corticosteroid therapy.[50,51]

N-Acetylcysteine is a powerful mucolytic agent used in respiratory care. It contains a thiol group, the free sulfhydryl radical of which is a strong reducing agent that ruptures the disulfide bonds that stabilize the mucoprotein network of molecules in mucus. Agents that break down these disulfide bonds produce the most effective mucolysis.[52] N-Acetylcysteine has been proven effective in combination with aerosolized heparin for the treatment of inhalation injury in animal studies.[53] Heparin and N-acetylcysteine combinations have been used as scavengers for the oxygen free radicals produced when alveolar macrophages are activated, either directly by chemicals in smoke or by one or more compounds in the arachidonic cascade.[54] Animal studies have shown an increased ratio of Pa_{O_2} to Fi_{O_2}, decreased peak inspiratory pressures, and a decreased amount of fibrin cast formation with heparin/N-acetylcysteine combinations.[55] Pediatric patients treated with aerosolized heparin/N-acetylcysteine combinations showed a reduction in the incidence of atelectasis, number of ventilator days, incidence of reintubation for progressive respiratory failure, and mortality.[56]

Although pneumonia occurs in as many as 50% of children with inhalation injury, the prophylactic use of antibiotics is not recommended. Instead, antibiotic therapy is directed by sputum Gram's stain and blood cultures, with culture specimens obtained when infection or pneumonia is suspected.

Mechanical Ventilatory Support

Despite conservative efforts to support unassisted ventilation, patients with moderate or severe inhalation injury may develop respiratory failure and require mechanical ventilation.[57] Patients with severe inhalation injury are at a substantial risk for iatrogenic, ventilator-induced lung damage. Airway resistance is increased secondary to edema and obstruction caused by cast formation. The increased resistance requires higher airway pressures to maintain sufficient flow to support minute ventilation. Ideally, the optimal treatment of any disease should reverse the pathophysiologic process without causing further injury. When inhalation injury is severe enough to require conventional mechanical ventilation, such an outcome is rarely achieved.

Conventional Mechanical Ventilation

Conventional mechanical ventilation does not reverse the pathologic process, is not characterized by improved clearance of secretions, and may actually compound the existing injury.[58] Conventional volume-limited ventilation in patients with inhalation injury is usually instituted at a tidal volume of 6 to 8 ml/kg.[47] Numerous factors, such as lung/thorax compliance, system resistance, compressive volume loss, oxygenation, ventilation, and barotrauma must be considered when tidal volumes are selected. Positive end-expiratory pressure (PEEP) is applied to recruit lung volumes, elevate mean airway pressures, and improve oxygenation. The level of PEEP used varies with the disease process. High levels of PEEP are often required with severe smoke inhalation injury.

Over the past 30 years, and especially in the past decade, there has been an increase in new ventilator techniques that present alternatives for the treatment of patients with inhalation injury. Unfortunately, although the number of options available to the clinician has appeared to increase exponentially, well-controlled prospective trials defining the specific role for each mode of ventilation and then comparing them with other modes of ventilation have not been forthcoming, particularly in the pediatric population.

Other ventilator modes have been employed in both animal models and clinical trials of inhalation injury. Pressure-limited ventilation with and without inverse inspiratory:expiratory ratios has been studied in an ovine smoke inhalation model.[59] Although gas exchange was not significantly improved with this mode, adequate ventilation was achieved at lower mean airway pressures, suggesting that ventilator-induced lung injury may be reduced. Excellent results have been reported using pressure-controlled ventilation in a cohort of pediatric burn patients.[60] Their results suggest that the incidences of barotrauma, pneumonia, and deaths were all considerably less than that expected based on historic controls.

High-Frequency Percussive Ventilation

High-frequency ventilation has also been employed after inhalation injury. This mode provides oxygenation at lower inspired oxygen concentrations and adequate ventilation at lower peak and mean airway pressures. In addition, a few reports have indicated increased secretion clearance with some forms of high-frequency ventilation.[61]

The terms *high-frequency flow interruption* and *high-frequency percussive ventilation* (HFPV) are used to describe a technique in which ventilation is accomplished by a positive-phase percussion delivered at the proximal airway. In clinical trials, HFPV was found to permit adequate ventilation and oxygenation without increasing barotrauma in a small cohort of patients for whom conventional ventilatory support after inhalation injury had failed.[62,63] Studies in adult patients with burns and inhalation injury reported optimal ventilation, decreases in pneumonia, and improved survival with HFPV when compared with conventional volume-limited ventilation.[64] A retrospective study of the effects of HFPV and conventional ventilation in pediatric patients with inhalation injury found that those patients treated with HFPV showed a decrease in the incidence of pneumonia, a lower peak inspiratory pressure, and improvement in the ratio of Pa_{O_2} to FI_{O_2}.[65]

Complications

The most common complications of inhalation injury that lead to increased mortality are infection and respiratory failure. Patients with inhalation injury have a high incidence of pneumonia. Burn-wound infection and sepsis place the patient at extremely high risk for multiple organ system failure.

Early Complications

The reported early complications of inhalation injury are usually mechanical or infectious. Immediate recognition of these complications is imperative so that appropriate treatment can begin and thus decrease the severity of the injury.

Mechanical complications are usually manifestations of barotrauma. Barotrauma can result from a variety of injuries caused by mechanical ventilation, especially when high peak inspiratory pressures are maintained. Patients with inhalation injury often develop sloughing of the tracheobronchial mucosa, which results in a ball-valve type obstruction. This type of obstruction acts as a one-way valve. The volume from the mechanical ventilator is allowed to enter the lungs; however, expiration is only allowed to partially occur. If this problem is left untreated, further barotrauma may occur and a pneumothorax may result.

Infectious complications may result in tracheobronchitis or pneumonia. The injured trachea is known to be at risk for infections, with respiratory infections being the most common complication after inhalation injury.[66]

The diagnosis of tracheobronchitis or pneumonia can be difficult to establish, owing to the presence of inhalation injury and bacterial colonization of the airways. The diagnosis of tracheobronchitis rests on the presence of fever, leukocytosis, and productive cough, as well as on organisms and white blood cells on Gram's stain of sputum specimens. Additionally, parenchymal infiltrates must be present on the chest radiograph to make the diagnosis of pneumonia.

Late Complications

Late complications of inhalation injury may be related to mechanical damage or to the consequences of an inflammatory response. Mechanical complications occur most often as a result of iatrogenic injury from endotracheal or tracheostomy tube cuffs. This damage may cause erosion of the tracheal cartilage and result in tracheomalacia. Injuries to the tracheal epithelium may result in fibrosis and stenosis of the trachea, which lead to subglottic stenosis. Cuff erosion into adjacent structures (e.g., innominate artery) may result in exsanguinating hemorrhage. The injuries are difficult to diagnose and often develop slowly. Endotracheal tube instability, high cuff pressures (>20 cm H_2O), and duration of intubation all contribute to airway damage. Meticulous attention to detail regarding tube security and cuff pressures can reduce the incidence of mechanical damage that occurs with artificial airways.

Inflammatory complications, such as bronchiectasis and bronchial stenosis, are thought to occur as a result of neutrophil activation at the site of the airway damaged by inhalation injury. Activated neutrophils produce proteases and oxygen radicals, which may cause severe damage to the already injured bronchial mucosa and extracellular matrix. Although most proteases are produced by neutrophils, other cells—including alveolar macrophages, mast cells, eosinophils, and fibroblasts— all may participate in protease secretion. Normal host defense mechanisms protecting mucosal integrity have been shown to function poorly after inhalation injury.[67] Damage of both smoke-injured and normal tissues by proteases and oxidants may lead to persistent worsening of the inflammatory response, which may prevent healing.

LONG-TERM OUTCOMES

Early reports in the literature indicate that long-term pulmonary parenchyma dysfunction after inhalation injury appears to be uncommon. Patients with inhalation injury alone have significant obstructive defects, whereas those patients with both inhalation and burn injury have a mixed obstructive and restrictive pattern. Although the abnormalities may persist in the early convalescent period, in general most patients have normal lung parenchyma within 5 months of injury.

A study of children with inhalation and burn injury reported pulmonary function changes for up to 8 years after injury. The results indicated that:

1. resting lung function showed some degree of residual pulmonary pathology
2. altered lung mechanics, impaired gas exchange, chest wall scarring, and respiratory muscle weakness may have contributed to the decrease in lung function; and
3. children with severe thermal injury and smoke inhalation may not regain normal lung function.[68]

Children evaluated with cardiopulmonary stress testing after thermal and inhalation injury showed an increased ratio of physiologic dead space to tidal volume during exercise as late as 2 years after the injury.[69] The physiologic insults that occur as a result of thermal injury may limit exercise endurance in children.[70] Data from exercise stress testing showed evidence of a respiratory limitation to exercise. This was confirmed by a decrease in maximal heart rate, decreased maximal oxygen consumption, and increased respiratory rate.

Although thermal and inhalation injuries present a challenge to the health care team, an orderly, systematic approach can simplify management. Successful outcome requires careful attention to treatment priorities, protocols, and meticulous attention to details in all areas of care.

ASSESSMENT QUESTIONS

See Evolve Resources for the answers.

1. What is the function of normal skin?
   I. Protect the body from infection and injury
   II. Prevent fluid loss
   III. Regulate hemodynamics
   IV. Provide mass and form
   V. Provide sensory input
   A. I, II, III
   B. II, III, IV
   C. III, IV
   D. I, II, V
   E. III, IV,V
2. How are second-degree burns defined?
   A. Necrotic epidermal layer
   B. Partial-thickness and involve the epidermis and part of the dermis
   C. Blisters
   D. Also known as eschar
   E. Minor burn injuries and are not very serious
3. How are third-degree burns classified?
   A. Full-thickness burns involving injury and necrosis into the subcutaneous tissue
   B. Swells rapidly and appears black in color
   C. Anesthetized since sensory nerves are destroyed
   D. A and B
   E. A and C
4. What does the rule of nines estimate?
   A. The percent of body surface that is burned in infants and young children
   B. Fluid requirements for burn injury fluid resuscitation
   C. The weight of the patient for total body surface area
   D. Ideal body weight for ventilator management
   E. The Pao2 related to a specific oxygen saturation on the oxyhemoglobin dissociation curve
5. The metabolic rate is generally related to the size of the burn injury and
   A. Increases further with the use of metabolic colloids
   B. Responds best by using diet suppression drugs
   C. Can increase as much as two to three times normal
   D. Is used to estimate wound healing
   E. Is calculated from the amount of sodium and protein
6. Mortality rate from burns injuries increases
   A. As burn surface area and degree increases
   B. With burn size and the presence of inhalation injury
   C. Exponentially with the amount of fluid resuscitation required
   D. A and C
   E. A and B

Continued

ASSESSMENT QUESTIONS—cont'd

7. Inhalation injury to the peripheral airways and parenchymal lung damage are due to
   A. Carbonaceous material present in the inhaled smoke
   B. Direct thermal trauma from smoke inhalation
   C. Incomplete combustion of toxic materials
   D. Direct contact with flames
   E. Heated dry air below the glottic opening
8. Fiberoptic bronchoscopy is the gold standard for diagnosing inhalation injury by
   A. Directly visualizing the extent of upper airway injury
   B. Taking bronchoalveolar lavage and biopsy specimens
   C. Confirming the presence of soot, mucosal erythema, hemorrhage, or edema in the airway
   D. None of the above
   E. A and C
9. The main pharmacologic management of smoke inhalation is the use of
   A. N-Acetylcysteine aerosol to break down the disulfide bonds present in mucus
   B. Albuterol sulfate and DNA-ase to thin the mucosal sol layer
   C. Aerosolized antiinflammatory agents to reduce airway swelling
   D. Aerosolized heparin and N-acetylcysteine combination to act as a scavenger for the oxygen free radicals produced by alveolar macrophagatosis
   E. Albuterol sulfate and aerosolized steroids to reduce airway swelling and inflammation
10. Carbon monoxide inhaled into the lungs and transferred to the blood stream
    A. Combines with hemoglobin and reduces the oxygen-carrying capacity
    B. Has a higher affinity for binding to hemoglobin than oxygen
    C. Shifts the oxyhemoglobin dissociation curve to the left and reduces the ability of hemoglobin to offload oxygen to the tissues
    D. Is responsible for the majority of immediate deaths occurring at the scene of building fires
    E. All of the above

References

1. Faxon NW, Churchill ED: The Coconut Grove disaster in Boston, *JAMA* 1942; 120:1385.
2. Brigham PA, McLoughlin E: Burn incidence and medical care in the United States: estimates, trends, and data sources, *J Burn Care Rehabil* 1996;17:95.
3. Herndon DN, Spies M: Modern burn care, *Semin Pediatr Surg* 2001;10:28.
4. Joffe MD: Burns. In Fleisher GR, Ludwig S, editors: *Textbook of pediatric emergency medicine*, ed 4, Philadelphia: Lippincott Williams & Wilkins; 2000. p 1427.
5. O'Neill JA: Advances in the management of pediatric trauma, *Am J Surg* 2000;180:365.
6. Cope O, Ruinelander FW: The problem of burn shock complicated by pulmonary damage, *Ann Surg* 1943;117:915.
7. Aub JC, Pittman H: The pulmonary complications: a clinical description, *Ann Surg* 1943;117:834.
8. Barillo DJ et al: The fire-safe cigarette: a burn prevention tool, *J Burn Care Rehabil* 2000;21:162.
9. Finkelstein JL et al: Pediatric burns: an overview, *Pediatr Clin North Am* 1992;39:1145.
10. Sheridan RL, Schnitzer JJ: Management of the high-risk pediatric burn patient, *J Pediatr Surg* 2001;36:1308.
11. Ramzy PI, Barret JP, Herndon DN: Thermal injury, *Crit Care Clin* 1999;15:333.
12. Henriques FC Jr: Studies of thermal injury: V. The predictability and significance of thermally induced rate process leading to irreversible epidermal injury, *Arch Pathol* 1947;43:489.
13. Linares HA: A report of 115 consecutive autopsies in burned children: 1966-1980, *Burns* 1982;8:270.
14. Brown JM: Respiratory complications in burned patients, *Physiotherapy* 1977;63:151.
15. Clark WR Jr et al: The pathophysiology of the acute smoke inhalation, *Surg Forum* 1977;177.
16. Foley FD, Moncriff JA, Mason AD Jr: Pathology of the lung in fatally burned patients, *Ann Surg* 1968;167:251.
17. Moylan JA: Inhalation injury: a primary determinant of survival. *J Burn Care Rehabil* 1981; 3:78-84.
18. Haponik EF, Summer WR: Respiratory complications in burned patients: Pathogenesis and spectrum of inhalation injury, *Crit Care* 1987;2:49.
19. Pruitt BA Jr et al: The occurrence and significance of pneumonia and other pulmonary complications in burned patients, *J Trauma* 1970;10:519.
20. Shirani KZ, Pruitt BA Jr, Mason AD Jr: The influence of inhalation injury and pneumonia on burned mortality, *Ann Surg* 1987;205:82.
21. Thompson PB et al: Effects on mortality of inhalation injury, *J Trauma* 1986;26:163.
22. Haponik EF, Lykens MG: Acute upper airway obstruction in burned patients, *Crit Care Rep* 1990;2:28.
23. Waymack JP et al: Acute upper airway obstruction in the post burn period, *Arch Surg* 1985;120:1042.
24. Haponik EF et al: Upper airway function in burn patients, *Am Rev Respir Dis* 1984;129:251.
25. Haponik EF et al: Acute upper airway injury in burn patients; serial changes of flow volume curves and nasopharyngoscopy, *Am Rev Respir Dis* 1987;135:360.
26. Wald PH, Balmes JR: Respiratory effects of short-term, high-intensity toxic inhalations: smoke, gases, and fumes, *J Intensive Care Med* 1987;2:260.
27. Zirka BA et al: What is clinical smoke poisoning? *Ann Surg* 1975;181:151.
28. Moritiz AR, Henriques FC Jr, McLean R: The effects of inhaled heat on the air passages and lungs: an experimental investigation, *Am J Pathol* 1945;21:311.
29. Head JM: Inhalation injury in burns, *Am J Surg* 1980;139:508.

30. Walker HL, McLeoud CG, McManus WL: Experimental inhalation injury in the goat, *J Trauma* 1981;21:962.
31. Demling RH: Initial effect of smoke inhalation injury on oxygen consumption (response to positive pressure ventilation), *Surgery* 1994;115:563.
32. Liu Z-Y et al: Pulmonary surfactant activity after severe steam inhalation in rabbits, *Burns* 1986;12:330.
33. Rodkey F, O'Neal J, Collison H: Relative affinity of hemoglobin S and hemoglobin A for carbon monoxide and oxygen, *Clin Chem* 1974;20:834.
34. Emmans HW: Fire and fire protection, *Sci Am* 1974;231:21.
35. Zirka BA, Ferre JM, Floch HF: The chemical factors contributing to pulmonary damage, *Surgery* 1972;71:704.
36. Parish RA: Smoke inhalation and carbon monoxide poisoning in children, *Pediatr Emerg Care* 1985;2:36.
37. Barker SJ, Tremper KK, Hyatt J: The effect of carbon monoxide inhalation on pulse oximetry and transcutaneous Po2, *Anesthesiology* 1987;66:677.
38. Moylan JA, Chan CK: Inhalation injury an increasing problem, *Surgery* 1978;188:34.
39. Stone HH, Martin JD Jr: Pulmonary injury associated with thermal injury, *Surg Gynecol Obstet* 1969;129:1242.
40. Putman CE et al: Radiological manifestations of acute smoke inhalation, *AJR Am J Roentgenol* 1977;129:865.
41. Wanner A, Cutchauarece A: Early recognition of upper airway obstruction following smoke inhalation, *Am Rev Respir Dis* 1973;108:1421.
42. Moylan JA et al: Fiberoptic bronchoscopy following thermal injury, *Surg Gynecol Obstet* 1975;140:541.
43. Moylan JA et al: Early diagnosis of inhalation injury using xenon scan, *Ann Surg* 1972;176:477.
44. Whitener DR et al: Pulmonary function measurements in patients with thermal injury and smoke inhalation, *Am Rev Respir Dis* 1980;122:731.
45. Petroff PA et al: Pulmonary function studies after smoke inhalation, *Am J Surg* 1976;132:346.
46. Garzon AA et al: Respiratory mechanics in patients with inhalation injury, *J Trauma* 1970;10:57.
47. Mlcak RP, Desai MH, Nichols RJ: Respiratory care. In Herndon DA, editor: *Total burn care*, London: WB Saunders; 1996. pp 193-204.
48. Sirani KZ, Pruitt BA, Mason AD: The influence of inhalation injury and pneumonia on burn mortality, *Ann Surg* 1986;205:82.
49. Pruitt BA Jr et al: Evaluation and management of patients with inhalation injury, *J Trauma* 1990;30:563.
50. Levine BA, Petroff PA, Slade CL: Prospective trials of dexamethasone and aerosolized gentamicin in the treatment of inhalation injury, *J Trauma* 1978;18:118.
51. Nieman GF, Clark WR, Hakim T: Methylprednisolone does not protect the lung from inhalation injury, *Burns* 1991;17:384.
52. Hirsh SR, Zastrow JE, Korg RC: Sputum liquification agents: a comprehensive in vitro study, *J Lab Clin Med* 1969;74:346.
53. Brown M et al: Dimethylsulfoxide with heparin in the treatment of smoke inhalation injury, *J Burn Care Rehab* 1988;9:22.
54. Desai MH et al: Reduction of smoke injury with dimethylsulfoxide and heparin treatments, *Surg Forum* 1985;36:103.
55. Desai MH, Brown M, Mlcak RP: Nebulization treatments of inhalation injury in the sheep model with dimethylsulfoxide/heparin combinations and N-acetylcysteine, *Crit Care Med* 1986;14:321.
56. Desai MH et al: Reduction in mortality in pediatric patients with inhalation injury with aerosolized heparin/N-acetylcysteine therapy, *J Burn Care Rehabil* 1998;19:210.
57. Reynolds EM, Ryan DP, Doody DP: Mortality and respiratory failure in a pediatric burn population, *J Pediatr Surg* 1993;28:1326.
58. Mammel MC, Boros SJ: Airway damage and mechanical ventilation: a review and commentary, *Pediatr Pulmonol* 1987;3:443.
59. Ogura H, Cioffi WG, Okerberg C: *Effects of pressure-controlled, inverse-ratio ventilation on smoke inhalation injury in an animal model.* San Antonio, TX. US Army Institute of Surgical Research, 1991.
60. Sheridan RL et al: Permissive hypercapnia as a ventilatory strategy in burned children, *J Trauma* 1995;39:854.
61. Arnold JH: High-frequency oscillatory ventilation: theory and practice in paediatric patients, *Paediatr Anaesth* 1996;6:437.
62. Cioffi WG et al: Prophylactic use of high-frequency ventilation in patients with inhalation injury, *Ann Surg* 1991;213:575.
63. Rue LW et al: Improved survival of burned patients with inhalation injury, *Arch Surg* 1993;128:772.
64. Cioffi WG et al: High-frequency percussive ventilation in patients with inhalation injury, *J Trauma* 1989;29:350.
65. Cortiella J, Mlcak RP, Herndon D: High-frequency percussive ventilation in pediatric patients with inhalation injury, *J Burn Care Rehabil* 1999;20:232.
66. Demarst GB, Hudson LD, Altman LC: Impaired alveolar macrophage chemotaxis in patients with acute smoke inhalation, *Am Rev Respir Dis* 1979;119:279.
67. Gadek JE et al: Antielastase of the human alveolar structures, *J Clin Invest* 1981;68:889.
68. Mlcak RP et al: Lung function following thermal injury in children: an 8-year follow-up, *Burns* 1998;24:213.
69. Mlcak RP et al: Increased physiological dead space: tidal volume ratio during exercise in burned children, *Burns* 1995;21:337.
70. Desai MH et al: Does inhalation injury limit exercise endurance in children convalescing from thermal injury? *J Burn Care Rehabil* 1993;14:12.

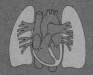

Chapter 39

Head Injury and Cerebral Disorders

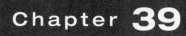

PAUL MATHEWS

LEARNING OBJECTIVES

After reading this chapter the reader will be able to:
- Discuss the three general causes of brain damage
- Define and characterize the concept of "plasticity" applied to brain function
- Cite two blood tests used to diagnose Reye's Syndrome

- List three signs of child abuse
- Classify various types of paralysis
- Describe and provide examples of the Monroe-Kellie doctrine

Damage to the brain or skull is among the most potentially serious and handicapping of all traumatic injuries. Head injuries are a primary cause of trauma deaths in both adults and children. A brain injury occurs in the United States every 15 seconds, and more than 1 million people with head injury are seen in emergency departments (EDs) each year. More than 5.3 million Americans are disabled from traumatic brain injury (TBI).[1] A substantial percentage of these patients are infants and children. The number of people disabled or killed is even higher when nontraumatic organic causes are factored into the epidemiology of brain injury.

Because a child's head is large and heavy in relation to the body, the center of gravity shifts toward the head. And because balance, coordination, gait, and judgment are immature, children are especially vulnerable to falls with head injury[2] (Figure 39-1). Because of these factors, children fall more frequently than adults and thus have a higher percentage of head injuries. The size and weight of the head also tends to rotate the child's body into a head-down position, frequently leading to headfirst impacts.

Inertial injuries, such as what is commonly seen in automobile accidents or shaken baby syndrome (SBS), account for a large number of head and central nervous system (CNS) injuries, especially in infants less than 1 year of age. Because of poorly developed neck muscles, when a baby is shaken, the head moves like a pendulum or church bell, whipping back and forth or side to side, with resulting brain injury as the brain impacts the sides of the skull with each movement. Health care professionals, including respiratory therapists, are required by law to report suspected incidents of SBS to legal authorities.

This chapter covers the general causes of brain injury; the anatomic, biophysical, and physiologic factors that influence the type and severity of injury; and the diagnosis and treatment of brain injury. Preventive actions to reduce brain injury and respiratory care procedures to treat and manage head injuries are also discussed.

CAUSES AND ANATOMIC CONSIDERATIONS

Damage to the brain may be classified in many ways. One useful way to classify brain injury is by *general cause*. Brain injury results from one of three general causes:

1. genetic-developmental
2. toxic-infective
3. traumatic (Box 39-1).

Although the causal agent may be different in each of these classes, the potential worst-case end results are the same: death or disability. Between the worst-case outcome and a no-harm result lays a continuum of possible outcomes.

The outcome and potential disability caused by each injury may vary in effect and seriousness based on many factors. Age is a major factor in some cases, allowing infants and young children to compensate for injuries when adults might sustain a permanent injury. Also, repetitive injuries have a cumulative effect, as evidenced by "punch drunk" boxers or football players with multiple concussions.

The brain has functional specificity (Figure 39-2). That is, certain areas of the brain are responsible for certain functions. However, the brains of infants and children apparently have a large degree of *plasticity* in redistributing function from a damaged area to an undamaged area. In adults the ability of the brain segments to adapt to new functions seems to be rarely, if ever, present. This flexibility of assigned purpose provides protection and enhances rehabilitative potential for infants and children but decreases with age as the maturing brain becomes patterned and locked into its distribution of functional capacity.

Infants and young children also have malleable skulls because of the large fontanels ("soft spots") and the flat bones of the skull, which have not yet fused and

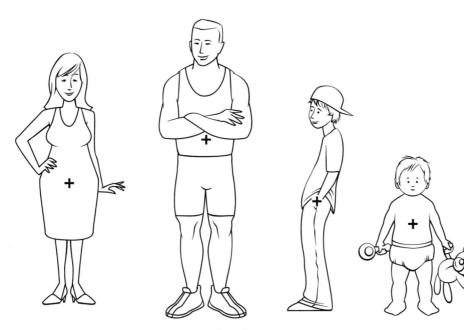

FIGURE 39-1 Centers of gravity by age and gender.

Box 39-1	General Causes of Brain Injury

GENETIC-DEVELOPMENTAL
- Microcephaly
- Down syndrome
- Hydroencephaly
- Cerebral palsy
- Cerebral aneurysm
- Seizures

TOXIC-INFECTIVE
- Meningitis
- Lead poisoning
- Carbon monoxide poisoning
- Septicemia
- Drug overdose

TRAUMATIC
- Subarachnoid hemorrhage
- Anoxia of childbirth
- Penetrating head wounds
- Blunt force injury
- Falls
- Abuse
- Suffocation, strangulation

still may be cartilaginous before ossification (Figure 39-3). These factors allow for elasticity of the cranial vault and lessen or prevent both fractures and pressure-related brain injuries during passage through the birth canal. Skull malleability also protects against damage from other sources, such as trauma or illness causing increased pressures in the cranial vault. This protection occurs by allowing a degree of expansion of the cranial

volume. These normally transitory anatomic features can provide important diagnostic clues as well. (See later discussion in the section on Volume Displacement Injuries and Increased Intracranial Pressure).

When the body is ill or injured, it strives to minimize damage, maintain as much function as possible, and stabilize, maintain, or regain homeostasis. Many signs and symptoms are the result of these survival attempts. These clinical features may provide valuable clues as to which part of the brain is injured.

The normal newborn brain and spinal cord are immature and not completely myelinated until about 18 months of age (Figure 39-4). As interbrain connections (synapses) are completed and the integrative functions of the brain begin to mature, more of the brain becomes active and functional. Knowledge of these processes and conditions are crucial when assessing neurologic status in infants and children with incomplete CNS development and integration. Their reactions and responses will change as the children age and gain maturity.

INITIAL ASSESSMENT AND DIAGNOSIS

Rapid Assessment

On arrival at the injury scene by emergency medical services (EMS) personnel and on arrival in the ED, a rapid assessment of the head-injured patient is performed to
1. establish a baseline to measure progress or deterioration and
2. quickly provide information about resources needed to stabilize and treat the patient.

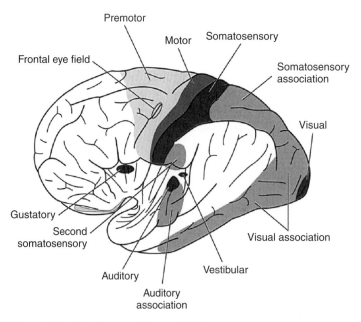

FIGURE 39-2 General functional areas of the cerebral cortex.

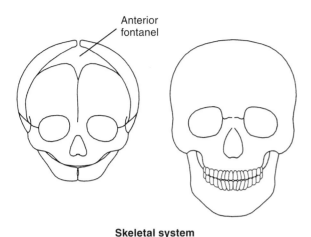

FIGURE 39-3 Comparative bone structure in infant and adolescent skulls.

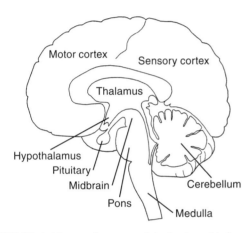

FIGURE 39-4 Most active parts of the brain at birth.

In addition to head trauma assessment the cervical spine should be stabilized and assessed for possible injury.

Rapid assessment protocols vary from region to region but generally include certain accepted variables (Box 39-2). On completion of the rapid assessment and initiation of emergent stabilization procedures and therapies, a more detailed assessment should be performed to arrive at a provisional diagnosis. This diagnostic workup includes physical and cognitive examinations, history (previous and causative event specific), and laboratory/radiologic testing.

Diagnostic Assessment

As in other conditions, the proper diagnosis of the cause, type, and extent of cerebral injury depends on both the subjective and objective data associated with the patient's condition.

Box 39-2	Rapid Trauma Assessment in Head Injury

Airway: clear and patent
Breathing: present with good rate and volume
Circulation: pulses present with adequate perfusion at an acceptable rate
Bleeding: no overt bleeding or abdominal rigidity
Level of consciousness (**AVPU**):
- **A**lert
- Responds to **V**oice
- **P**ain response
- **U**nresponsive

Pupillary response: equally reactive and midline bilaterally

Subjective Data

Subjective data cannot be collected by the assessor's senses (e.g., sight, touch, smell) without input from the patient. The presence, extent, and magnitude of pain and fear status are examples of subjective data that the patient must be asked to reveal. Because infants and young children often cannot effectively verbalize these factors, the assessor must be alert for clues that suggest a problem. For example, an exaggerated response to the examiner's touch may indicate pain.

Parents may be the best sources of information about variations from normal behavior. The exception would be if a high index of suspicion of child neglect or abuse exists. Abuse should be suspected if the patient draws away or cringes when the parent approaches, the patient has multiple bruises of varying ages, and/or suddenly becomes nonverbal or otherwise shows change in behavior when the parent or caregiver approaches. "Accidental falls rarely produce significant head injuries" according to Dr. Karl Johnson. A study of 94 patients ages 4 months to 5 years who had been witnessed falling from heights ranging from 20 cm (8 inches) to more than 3 meters (9.9 feet) found that 89% to 95% had "no significant long-term problems." Severe head injury in patients below 5 years of age blamed on falls or household accidents should raise suspicions about the possibility of abuse.[3] Further, head injury, according to Rubin et al, is the leading cause of death in abused children under 2 years of age.[4]

In these cases the law requires that, among others, licensed health care professionals including RTs notify legally designated authorities.

Objective Data

Objective data relate to the mechanism of injury, the patient's medical history (past and present), and the situation that led to injury event. The child's past medical history indicates the body's preinjury state. The present medical history may reveal exposure to harmful substances or activities.

Additional objective data help the clinician track the patient's physiologic response to injury and treatment. Objective data are measurable and allow discovery and recording of trends in the treatment and recovery process. Such data include laboratory studies, radiographs, computed tomography (CT) scans, magnetic resonance imaging (MRI), electrocardiograms (ECGs), electroencephalograms (EEGs), and lumbar puncture (LP). Objective data also include pulse, blood pressure, temperature and respirations. Recently two other "vital signs" have been added to this list. One, pulse oximetry, is objective (measurable and quantifiable) and the other, pain, is considered subjective. Pain, however, is often measured using "pain scales" (these are discussed on p. 661 under "Neurologic Assessment"). The use of these scales is a method of objectifying this symptom.

Mechanism of Injury

Knowledge of the mechanism of injury (MOI) provides the clinicians with information on the traumatic external event and the potential internal injuries. MOI includes the object causing or the reason for the injury, the amount of force applied, and the vector or direction of that force. For example, "The patient was the front seat passenger in a two-car motor vehicle accident (MVA). The car in which she was riding was hit on the driver's side at 30 mph while entering an intersection at 5 to 10 mph when the light had just turned green. Both she and the driver were wearing seat belts." This explanation of the mechanism of the patient's injuries provides information concerning potential pathophysiologic impact and helps determine the type and extent of possible injuries.

Head injuries can be classified in several ways according to cause. A primary classification is to distinguish between direct and indirect trauma. Direct trauma, such as striking one's head as a result of a fall, is further classified as either a blunt force or a penetrating injury. Indirect trauma occurs when the head is not the primary site of impact. A further distinction should be made to determine, by radiologic assessment, the presence or absence of space-occupying lesions. A space-occupying lesion is an injury that causes a shift in the position of normal tissues to make room for the blood or tissues affected by the injury.

Another, complementary, method is to classify the injury by the *direction* or *vector* of impact. For example, torsion and inertia are terms used to describe the application of force by vector, each with the potential to be either direct or indirect. In the example above, the vector or direction of force was from left to right (i.e., from driver's to passenger's side).

Torsion Injuries

Torsion, or rotational, CNS injuries occur when the head is rotated or twisted around the longitudinal axis of the vertebral column. If severe, such injuries can result in total paralysis and death. The rotation or torsion may occur not only in the lateral plane but also in the anterior-posterior plane. These injuries tend to sever, transect, or partially transect the spinal cord and/or the lower structures of the brainstem, resulting in catastrophic injuries (Figure 39-5). Less severe twisting may result in muscle strains and tears that are painful but are usually limited in terms of length of disability. These may be commonly referred to as "whiplash" injuries.

Because of the potential for damage to the spinal cord and brainstem, trauma patients should by moved only by trained and properly prepared individuals, unless risk of loss of life is imminent. It is critically important to prevent further damage to the cervical spine (see later discussion in the section on spinal injuries). Use of cervical collar (C-collar) or other fixation devices will help to protect the spine until the patient has been "cleared" for spinal injuries or until definitive measures can be instituted.

Effects of spinal cord injury depend on three factors: first, the type of injury, second, the level of the injury, and third, the extent of the injury. The type of injury refers to the mechanism of injury that caused the injury. The level of injury refers to the area of the spinal cord that is injured; extent of injury means how severe the injury is and the effects of injuries in that location on the rest of the body. There are five subdivisions to the spine. These roughly correspond to the normal curves of the spinal column. The sections of the spinal cord are:

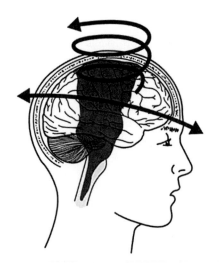

FIGURE 39-5 Torsion mechanism of injury.

- cervical (C1-C7)
- thoracic (T1-T12)
- lumbar (L1-L5)
- sacral (S1-S5)
- coccyx with 3 fused bones.

Each of the numbers represents a vertebral body. The lower the injury, the more function and sensation will be salvaged. ("C3, 4, and 5 keep the diaphragm alive. S2, 3, and 4 urine and feces hit the floor."[5])

Inertial Injuries

Inertial injuries are caused by sudden changes in the velocity of the head. When the head stops moving, the brain continues moving until it strikes the inside of the skull in the original direction of movement—remember Newton's Laws of Motion. In addition to movement-related injuries, assaults can cause significant inertial injuries as the force exerted by the weapon is dissipated on the skull and its contents. The sudden change in acceleration or application of force can also result from automobile accidents, sports, falls, or deliberate assaults.

Any blow to the head or sudden change in direction or speed of travel can result in a rebound injury from inertia. This secondary injury is called a contrecoup injury, referring to the side opposite (contre) the contact (coup) side. If there is a bruise on the right side of the skull, the practitioner should examine for trauma on the left side of the brain, because the brain will continue to move at the speed the head was moving before deceleration. The skull may stop moving but its contents can still be moving in the original direction of the force. The damage may be more severe on the *contrecoup*, or *contralateral*, side (Figure 39-6). The degree of damage is related to the magnitude of the abrupt change in force on the skull. The potential damage from a deceleration from 2 to 1 mph is much less than the damage potential when abruptly slowing from 50 to 5 mph.

Volume Displacement Injuries

Volume displacement injuries are the space-occupying lesions referred to above. They occur when lesions cause an increased volume of tissue or fluids to accumulate in the skull, including tumors, spinal fluid, and blood. Cerebral edema secondary to head injury is a major cause of this increased tissue mass in the skull. In these space-occupying lesions, the space that the lesion occupies reduces the space available for other tissues in the skull (see later discussion about the Munroe-Kellie doctrine).

Data Gathering

Age-specific subjective and objective data are gathered simultaneously during the patient assessment process. Children are often poor historians because of age, emotional/psychiatric problems, or the injury itself. It is often necessary to rely on eyewitness accounts of the events or reports or educated guesses of accompanying adults to determine cause and mechanism of injury. Trends and alteration from the norm are particularly important in this and other noncommunicative populations. Cultural or language differences may markedly affect both data gathering and interpretation. Care should be taken to ensure that patients and their families understand what information is needed and what care methods are to be employed during the diagnosis and treatment process. Time spent gathering data may not seem important to parents awaiting focused treatment for their child but they should be informed that the more knowledge about the child, the child's medical and social history, and the details of the circumstances of the injury the medical staff have, the better and more focused the care for their child.

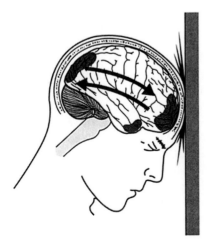

FIGURE 39-6 Posterior to anterior coup-contrecoup mechanism of injury.

STABILIZATION

A complete head-to-toe assessment of the patient is desirable but may have to be postponed or abbreviated until the patient's condition is stabilized. For patients of any age, head injuries are often critical, and assessment should at least include the *ABCs plus C*:

- **A**irway patency
- **B**reathing support
- adequacy of **C**irculation
- stability of the **C**ervical spine.

All children who have injured their upper torso, neck, or head should be assumed to have a cervical spine injury, and precautionary measures should be taken to prevent further spinal cord damage. As discussed above, cervical spine stabilization should be the first order of business in trauma situations.

Airway Patency

Without a patent (open or clear) airway, other interventions are of little value. A patent airway

- maintains physiologic integrity
- allows intervention to reduce cerebral swelling
- protects the brain from hypoxemia.

A patent airway can be initiated by means of a jaw thrust maneuver to open the airway. Maintain the airway with orotracheal intubation, nasotracheal intubation, cricothyrotomy, or tracheostomy. **Do not use the head tilt, sniff position, or chin lift maneuvers until the neck is "cleared," since these procedures change the orientation of the spinal column and increase the risk of additional spinal injury. The jaw thrust technique may be used in these children unless otherwise contraindicated.**

In patients with direct cranial trauma avoid nasotracheal intubation, nasotracheal suctioning, or inserting nasogastric tubes because inadvertent cranial intubation may result through open fractures of the cranial vault, especially in patients who may have basilar skull injuries or paranasal fractures. Extreme care should also be taken not to manipulate the head and neck any more than necessary until radiologic tests definitively rule out cervical spine injuries. Caution is necessary when moving or positioning the patient to prevent further displacement of any spinal fractures and cause additional damage to the spine, spinal cord, and cranial or spinal nerves. Therefore the head, neck, spine, and body should be treated as a single entity and moved in unison and in the same plane.

Breathing Support

Breathing support includes providing supplemental oxygen. The patient may require only a nasal cannula or possibly artificial ventilation with bag-valve-mask resuscitators. Breathing support may progress to intubation with bag-valve-tube ventilation and eventually to mechanical ventilation. Skull and facial fractures or lacerations may preclude mask ventilation.

Provide for all possible adverse airway events by having the appropriate equipment on hand. Give high concentrations of oxygen, and monitor oxygen saturation with a pulse oximeter (Spo_2) and ventilation with a capnometer ($ETco_2$). Correlate Spo_2 and $ETco_2$ with arterial blood gas (ABG) measurements to determine the adequacy of oxygenation and ventilation. Even with adequate ABG values, continue administering high concentrations of oxygen to maximize cerebral oxygenation after consultation with the physician. If the patient is breathing without difficulty and is not likely to vomit and aspirate, a face mask is appropriate. Remember to protect the airway from aspiration of blood, vomit, and other substances.

If respirations deteriorate or the patient's state of consciousness declines, mechanical ventilation should be instituted immediately. Minimize peak inflation pressure (PIP) and mean airway pressure (Paw), and select inspiratory and expiratory times that favor prolonged expiration if possible. Decreasing Paw minimizes outflow tract resistance from the cerebral vasculature, enhancing cerebral perfusion by minimizing effects on intracranial pressure (ICP). Minimize suctioning to prevent coughing and gagging on the tracheal tube or suction catheter, which may increase ICP.

Adequacy of Circulation

Assess pulse rate and pressure at all pulse points and note significant discrepancies. Pulse oximetry is a valuable adjunct for this purpose. Both manual and automatic blood pressure monitors are appropriate for head-injured patients. Blood pressure should be monitored for adequacy and bilateral symmetry. ECG monitoring is mandatory: head injury often results in secondary cardiac and cardiovascular effects. Carefully examine carotid pulses on both the right and left side: force and duration should be equal bilaterally. The practitioner must not take both carotid pulses or obstruct the carotid arteries simultaneously because this may cut off the blood supply to the brain.

Assessing capillary refill is a quick and specific method of checking the adequacy of peripheral circulation. One method of determining capillary refill is to depress the patient's thumb nail with moderate force. This will cause the underlying tissue to blanch (turn white or pale pink) by forcing blood from the tissue. Releasing the pressure allows blood to refill the tissue's capillaries. Normal capillary refill time is less than 2 seconds. Inadequate capillary refill on initial assessment may be caused by regional perfusion problems. To rule out this possibility, repeat the capillary refill test on the opposite hand.

Failure of the patient to maintain blood pressure, heart rate, and rhythm indicates the need for vasopressors, fluid administration, or cardiopulmonary resuscitation (CPR) and consideration of the use of cardiac assist devices such as a pacemaker. It is essential that adequate pulse and perfusion pressures be maintained. A delicate balance may exist between maintaining adequate blood pressures and fluid overload and increasing cerebral vascular and cerebrospinal fluid (CSF) pressure. These procedures are performed only while ensuring that the head and neck orientation is stable and as motion free as possible.

When assessing pulse rate remember to differentiate between electrical activity (ECG) and pulsate beats. ECG measures the electrical activity of the heart, not necessarily the beating of the heart. In this case pulse oximetry, which detects pulsate flow (blood flow caused by the heart's beating action), is a better assessment of perfusion that the ECG.

Cervical Spine Precautions

Due to the lack of muscle tone and lack of muscular control infants are at particular risk for these injuries. However, teenagers are the age cohort with the greatest risk of devastating spinal cord injury. This is due to their propensity for undertaking risky activities and behaviors. As expected teen males have the greatest risk of cervical spine (C-spine) damage, although teen girls appear to be increasingly closing the risk gap.

The neck and cervical spine are easily involved in injury when the head is struck or shaken. Injuries to the cervical spine can result in paralysis and loss of sensation. This paralysis and sensory loss can range from limited to profound and may involve the entire body from the neck down. Severe injuries to the first (C1) and second (C2) cervical vertebrae are overwhelmingly fatal. Complete cord transections result in paralysis and sensory loss below the transected area. Partial transections are problematic, with outcomes varying from almost complete recovery to severe residual limitations. Bruising, edema, and hematoma formation may result in damage that is either permanent or completely or partially reversible as the swelling, bruising, and hematoma resolve.

Cervical spine precautions are taught in all life support and first-aid courses in the United States. Basic techniques for spinal immobilization address support for intubation, transportation, and movement during care and transport. If movement of the patient is necessary, keep the head and neck immobilized in a straight line using a cervical collar, backboard and/or sandbags to ensure that the neck is not rotated, flexed, or abducted. Do not apply traction to the head and neck because of the high probability of further damage if neck injuries are present. Body and head should only be moved in the same plane and as a supported unit.

Use of head and neck protective devices is an important method for reducing postinjury spinal or head trauma. An often-overlooked safety feature in modern automobiles is the head restraint. Given the restraint's proper adjustment and use, head and neck injuries are likely to decrease markedly. The adjustment of head restraints should become part of the starting ritual of seat and mirror adjustment and seat belt donning for both drivers and passengers.

NEUROLOGIC ASSESSMENT

Keep several factors in mind when diagnosing and caring for neurologically injured individuals. Patients with neurologic damage, at least initially, may react in an

exaggerated fashion to outside stimuli. Bright lights, loud sudden sounds, and touching may all evoke hyperreactive responses. Avoid hypothermia because sensitivity to temperature variations is a hallmark of head and spinal injuries. Changes in temperature may result in a cascade of diaphoresis, chills, and shivering. When tactile, auditory, and visual stimuli are limited, the brain is allowed to focus on reintegrating itself and regaining physiologic balance.

Once the ABC plus Cs of trauma life support are under control, the examination and assessment can begin in earnest. Assessment of the patient with probable head injury or brain damage must be thorough, systematic, and repetitive.

The standardized assessment mechanisms are powerful trend and tracking tools for the injured patient. Frequently, altered vital signs and level of consciousness indicate deterioration of cerebral control that demands intervention. Historically, vital signs have included pulse rate, blood pressure, respiratory rate, temperature, and oxygen saturation (Spo_2) using a pulse oximeter. Assessment of the patient's level of pain recently was added to this growing list of vital signs and symptoms.

The six "Ps" are another method to assess nervous system function in the injured patient:
1. Pain
2. Position
3. Paralysis
4. Paresthesia
5. Ptosis
6. Priapism.[6]

Pupils can be considered a seventh *P*. This assessment system is subject to an individual observer's bias and perception. In addition, the following are signs of spinal cord injury in the young child: flaccid extremities, paralysis, numbness or paresthesia, incontinence of urine or stool, and loss of rectal tone.[7]

Pain

Pain may be localized or disseminated over large areas. The pain sensations may range from deep, almost unbearable discomfort to a total lack of sensation.

Assessing pain is a difficult task in the infant and pediatric population for several reasons, including the inability to communicate due to age or injury. For children who are responsive and alert, even as young as 2 or 3 years old, a simple visual analog scale (VAS) can help assess quantity of pain. For older children, adolescents, and adults the use of the VAS or a modified Borg scale can help to quantify and trend pain (Figure 39-7, *A*, and Table 39-1). Another helpful tool is using a trend graph of pain sensations (Figure 39-7, *B*). Construct this by using a line to indicate the limits of a continuum of pain at either end. Label the left end No Pain and the right end

FACES SCALE

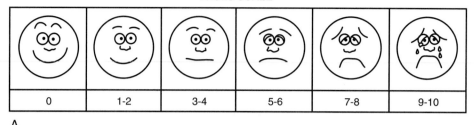

| 0 | 1-2 | 3-4 | 5-6 | 7-8 | 9-10 |

A

NUMERIC PAIN SCALE

No pain   Moderate pain   Worst pain

0   1   2   3   4   5   6   7   8   9   10

B

FIGURE 39-7 **A**, Visual analog pain scale. **B**, Linear pain scale.

Most Pain Ever. Next, instruct patients to mark an "x" at the point on the line that indicates where they feel they are on the line related to how much pain they feel. Then simply measure and record the distance from one end of the line. Each time pain is assessed have the patient perform the same selection. Compare the placement of the "x" from each assessment. It is important to use the same length scale every time to record the patient's response.

Each type of scale allows the patient to indicate a level of pain or discomfort for repeated testing and measurement over time, thus providing the ability to track or trend the data as indicated by the patient. In addition to the three previous examples, a fourth method uses a *color bar* with bright red being the most discomfort and a pale blue the best possible comfort. All four of these methods are highly repeatable and have a high reliability.

TABLE 39-1

Modified Borg Scale

Scale	Severity
0	None
0.5	Extremely slight, just noticeable
1	Very slight
2	Slight
3	Moderate
4	Slightly severe
5	Somewhat severe
6	Moderately severe
7	Severe
8	Very severe
9	Extremely severe, almost maximum
10	Maximum

Modified from Borg G. Perceived exertion as an indicator of somatic stress. *Scand J Rehab Med* 1970;2:92-98. Pub Med www.ncbi.nlm.nih.gov.

Position

The position that reproduces the location of pain, or paresthesia, may indicate the level of injury in the cervical spine. With severe brain injury the posture of the body also indicates the section of the brain that is injured. The position that a person's body assumes after head injury can be diagnostic of the level of brain function, with damage to cortical structures forcing one telltale posture while damage to the cerebellum results in a different, but equally specific, position.

Trunk and limb position at rest, spontaneous movements, and response to painful stimuli must be carefully observed. Spontaneous movement of all limbs generally indicates a mild depression of hemispheric function without structural disturbance. Monoplegia or hemiplegia, except in the postictal state, suggests a structural disturbance of the contralateral or opposite side hemisphere. In other words right monoplegia suggests left hemisphere damage and visa-versa.

An extensor response to a painful stimulus by the trunk and limbs is termed decerebrate posturing, or rigidity. The most severe form is called opisthotonos, in which the neck is hyperextended and the teeth are clenched; the arms are adducted, hyperextended, and hyperpronated; and the legs are extended with the feet plantar flexed. Decerebrate posturing indicates lesions at the level of the cerebrum and is characterized by rigid extension of the limbs, hands turned outward, and head retracted toward the sternum. This rigidity should be considered an ominous sign whether present at rest or in response to painful stimuli. Decerebrate posturing is uncommon in children except after head injury and indicates hemispheric dysfunction with a decrease in or a loss of brainstem integrity.

Decorticate posturing indicates lesions at or above the brainstem and is characterized by rigid extended legs, rigid flexed arms, and fists tightly clenched in the middle of the chest.

Rarely, unilateral or mixed presentation of these symptoms is seen, caused by either unilateral trauma or a well-defined disease process. The characteristics of decerebrate and decorticate posturing allow comparison of the various positions associated with specific brain injuries (Figure 39-8).

Paralysis

The inability to move a limb or limbs can be unilateral or bilateral, affecting either the right side, left side, or both. Paralysis can be defined by its vertical extent. Paraplegia, for example, refers to paralysis of the lower limbs, whereas paralysis of both upper and lower limbs is called quadriplegia or tetraplegia. Paralysis may also be complete or may be incomplete, sometimes termed paresis. The patient with paresis may either have partial voluntary range of motion in one or more of the affected limbs or have involuntary motions. The location and completeness of paralysis are determined by the location of the CNS lesions or the damage to peripheral nerves in the case of single-limb or partial-limb paralysis.

Paresthesia, Ptosis, and Priapism

Paresthesia is a sensation of numbness, tingling, "prickly or needles and pins" sensations, or heightened sensitivity that is often associated with lesions of the peripheral or central nervous system.

Ptosis ("toe sis") is a drooping of a tissue due to paralysis or weakness of a muscle. The term is usually used when referring to the eyelids. Ptosis and a partially contracted pupil is called Horner's syndrome, suggestive of cervical sympathetic nerve trunk injury on the affected side.

Priapism is partial or complete painful erection of the penis that fails to relax. It is not associated with sexual stimulation. This condition may indicate lesions in the supralumbar region. Priapism is considered a medical emergency.

Pupils

An additional *P*, the seventh, is pupils. Abnormal pupil size and reactivity are indicative of drug interference or brain injury location (Figure 39-9). The clinician should be familiar with pupil variation in each type of brain injury.

Metabolic disturbances usually do not affect the pupillary light reflex; its absence in a comatose patient indicates a structural abnormality. The major exception is drug use; fixed, dilated pupils in an alert patient are caused by topical administration of mydriatics. In a comatose patient, hypothalamic damage causes unilateral pupillary constriction. In Horner's syndrome a midbrain lesion or a lateral medullary lesion causes midposition fixed pupils; a pontine lesion (injury located in the pons) causes small but reactive pupils. Tonic lateral deviation of both eyes indicates a seizure originating in the hemisphere opposite the direction of gaze or a destructive lesion in the hemisphere in the direction of gaze.

Glasgow Coma Scale and Other Monitoring

The Glasgow Coma Scale (GCS) is sufficiently accurate for use in adults, older children, and adolescents (Box 39-3). Coma scales for younger children have proven to be unreliable when compared to vital signs and neurologic assessment trending (Box 39-4). The age-specific GCS is a third system that combines the adult and child forms of the GCS (Table 39-2). This scale allows decision making as to coma level regardless of the patient's age.

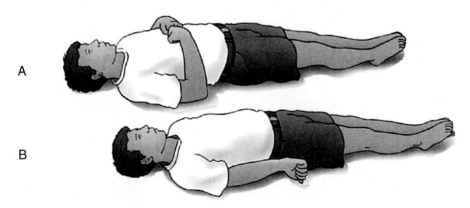

FIGURE 39-8 Neurogenic posturing. **A,** Decorticate posturing. **B,** Decerebrate posturing.

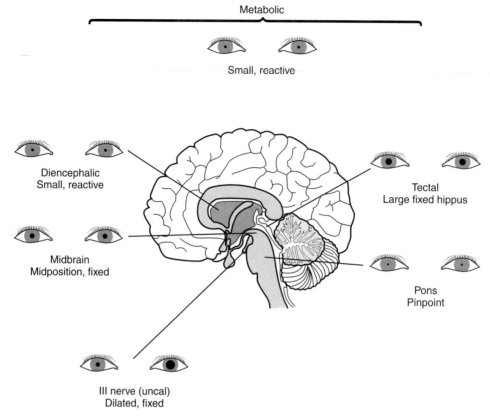

Metabolic

Small, reactive

Diencephalic
Small, reactive

Tectal
Large fixed hippus

Midbrain
Midposition, fixed

Pons
Pinpoint

III nerve (uncal)
Dilated, fixed

FIGURE 39-9 Abnormal pupil response.

Intravenous Access

In addition to vital signs and neurologic monitoring, insertion of an intravenous (IV) line for peripheral access is essential. This access allows the clinician to give the patient fluids, blood, and medications. The encephalic patient is often ventilator dependent. IV medications are administered to sedate the patient, reduce swelling in the brain, reduce cellular damage to the brain, and promote healing. Preexisting IV access also permits blood sampling without causing painful stimuli as well as rapid infusion of resuscitation drugs if needed.

Box 39-3	Glasgow Coma Scale*

I. Best Motor Rosponse
5 = Obeys
4 = Localizes
3 = Withdraws (flexion)
2 = Abnormal flexion
1 = Extensor response
II. Verbal Response
4 = Oriented
3 = Confused conversation
2 = Inappropriate words
1 = Incomprehensible sounds
III. Eye opening
4 = Spontaneous
3 = To speech
2 = To pain
1 = Nil

From Ghajar J, Hariri RJ: Management of pediatric head injury, *Pediatr Clin North Am* 1992;39:1093.
*Score = Score from Column I plus score from Column II, plus score from Column III = GCS (i.e., I + II + III). Maximum score = 13; minimum score = 3.

Box 39-4	Children's Coma Scale*

I. Ocular Response
4 = Pursuit
3 = Extraocular movement intact, reactive pupils
2 = Fixed pupils or extraocular movement impaired
1 = Fixed pupil and extraocular movement paralyzed
II. Verbal Response
3 = Cries
2 = Spontaneous respirations
1 = Apneic
III. Motor response
4 = Flexes and extends
3 = Withdraws from painful stimuli
2 = Hypertonic
1 = Flaccid

*Score = I + II + III. Maximum score = 11; minimum score = 3.

TABLE 39-2

Age-Specific Glasgow Coma Scale*

Points	Infant/Preverbal Child	Verbal Child/Adult
Eye Opening (E)		
4	Spontaneous	Spontaneous
3	To speech	To speech
2	To pain	To pain
1	None	None
Verbal Response (V)		
5	Coos, babbles	Oriented
4	Irritable cries	Confused
3	Cries to pain	Inappropriate words
2	Moans to pain	Incomprehensible sounds
1	None	None
Motor Response (M)		
6	Normal, spontaneous	Obeys commands
5	Withdraws to touch	Localizes pain
4	Withdraws to pain	Withdraws to pain
3	Abnormal flexion	Abnormal flexion
2	Abnormal extension	Abnormal extension
1	None	None

Modified from Laskowsi-Jones L, Salati DS: Responding to pediatric trauma, *Nursing* 2001;31:37.
*Score = E + V + M. Normal, 15 or 16 points; mildly impaired consciousness, 13 or 14 points; moderate impairment, 9 to 12 points; severe impairment, 3 to 8 points.

Respirations

Variation in the respiratory pattern also helps reveal the location of brain injury and the body's attempt to compensate for physiologic change. In some patients the abnormal respiratory patterns are the body's attempt to alter cerebral perfusion pressure and distribution. In other patients these changes in respiration are the direct result of injury to respiratory control centers in the brain and pons. A more complete discussion of these patterns is found in the Respiratory Effects section.

Physical Signs

Some classic "signs" are associated with certain head injuries. These signs indicate fractures of the basilar skull. Traumatic head injury may be highlighted by the presence of Battle's sign or "raccoon eyes." Battle's sign represents ecchymosis or bruised areas behind the ear that indicate basilar skull fractures. The self-explanatory term raccoon eyes represent bruising discolorations around the orbits. Both Battle's sign and raccoon eyes are the body's attempts to show internal injury with as simple a sign as a small bruise.

As a result of a meta-analysis conducted by Bergman and colleagues and published in *Pediatrics*, a joint Subcommittee on Minor Closed Head Injury of the American Association of Family Practice (AAFP) Committee on Quality Improvement suggests that "Among children with minor closed head injury and no loss of consciousness, a through history and appropriate physical and neurologic examination should be performed. Subcommittee consensus was that observation in the clinic, office, emergency department or home and under the care of a competent observer should be used as the primary treatment strategy."[8]

Greenes and Schutzman report the results of a prospective study of infants with head injuries in which 608 infants (ages 11.2 ± 6.8 months) were studied. The authors' findings "suggest" that radiology screening of head-injured infants should be directed at two groups of patients: those with symptoms and signs of brain injury, and those without symptoms or signs of brain injury but with significant scalp hematomas."[9]

TREATMENT PLAN

After assessment and stabilization, a plan is developed for definitive treatment and evaluation. Before and throughout treatment, a comprehensive plan should be in place that includes goals, outcomes, and evaluation criteria. Preferably these plans are developed by an interdisciplinary team of acute care and rehabilitation professionals and will be reviewed with the patient's family as care progresses.

As previously discussed, protection of the airway and cervical spine, protection from further injury, and progress toward recovery goals guides the plan of care for the brain injury patient. The plan encompasses three major goals, as follows:

1. Determine the correct diagnosis.
2. Treat the injuries and sequelae in an appropriate, caring, and resource-sparing manner.
3. Develop and implement a rehabilitation plan that is timely, centers on increasing quality of life, and employs strategies that maximize the patient's control of and autonomy in the rehabilitation process.

Evaluation of any plan of care is based on the desired outcomes. This evaluation should result in improvements and should be adaptable to make both the assessment and the plan dynamic processes. Outcomes goals and evaluation objectives should be dynamic guides which are revised as the clinical situation changes with the patient's response to treatment. The evaluation process should be based on achievable and measurable therapeutic goals and objectives. For example, a goal in the brain-injured patient might be to reduce positional hypertension or hypotension. The associated objective might be to reduce blood pressure swings to 10 mm Hg with position changes.

Clearly, all members of the care team, the patient, and family should be aware of the plan, its goals and objectives, and the progress toward fulfillment of the goals. This requires open and honest communications beginning early in the process and maintained throughout the stabilization and rehabilitation phases.

Other Body Systems

In addition to neurologic care, the incapacitated patient needs care for the eyes, the skin, gastrointestinal tract, urinary tract, and pulmonary and cardiovascular systems. Keep the head of the bed elevated to control cerebral edema. In some cases hyperventilation or hypoventilation assists in controlling edema as well as maintaining body integrity. Nutritionally, caloric demands need to be met. Preventing skin and muscle deterioration helps to prevent further injury. Additionally, head of the bed elevation to 30 to 45 degrees helps prevent aspiration and hospital-acquired pneumonia. All these systems must be functional when the patient's brain recovers.

CEREBRAL DISORDERS

Cerebral disorders are the result of trauma, altered cellular function secondary to drugs, metabolic problems, anoxia, or genetic-developmental disorders. Cerebral disorders range from inconsequential to profoundly debilitating, from not being able to remember a distant relative's phone number to being in a persistent vegetative state (PVS).

The term encephalopathy is used to describe a diffuse disorder of the brain with many causes. The prominent features of encephalopathy are a decreased state of consciousness, abnormal response to external stimulus, and seizures. An encephalopathy is called encephalitis when

inflammatory cells are found in the CSF. These altered states of consciousness and rationality may be constant or transitory; they may be temporary disabilities or permanent life-altering conditions.

Encephalopathy secondary to oxygen deprivation is called anoxic or hypoxic encephalopathy (anoxic brain damage) and is the cause of many serious brain injuries. The primary goal of management of head injury in children is to prevent secondary injury to the brain. Prevention of hypoxia, ischemia, and increased intracranial pressure is essential.[10]

Lethargy and Coma

A progressive decline in consciousness can be caused by diffuse or multifocal disturbances of the cerebral hemispheres or by focal injury to the brainstem. Specific characteristics are used to describe and delineate various states of decreased consciousness (Table 39-3).

The GCS, although originally designed for trauma cases, is now used to provide clinicians with a standardized system to assess a patient with an altered level of consciousness (see Box 39-3). The Children's Coma Scale was developed to assess infants and toddlers who are unable to speak or follow commands (see Box 39-4). Although pupil diameter and light reactivity are not addressed in the coma scales, they are important indicators of cerebral herniation and should be assessed during a neurologic examination.[10] Combining the pediatric and adult GCS scoring method may be helpful in evaluating transitionally aged children or when age is uncertain (see Table 39-2).

The clinical features that localize the anatomic site of disturbed brain function are state of consciousness, pattern of breathing, pupillary size and reactivity, eye movements, and motor responses.[11] Lethargy and *obtundation* are generally caused by mild depression of the cerebral hemispheres. Stupor and coma occur when hemispheric dysfunction is more extensive or when the diencephalon

---

TABLE 39-3

Classifications of Stupor and Coma

Grade	State of Awareness	Responds Appropriately to:		
		Name	Light Pain	Deep Pain
1	Drowsy, lethargic, indifferent; does not lapse into sleep	Yes	Yes	Yes
2	Stuporous; lapses into sleep; may be disoriented	No	Yes	Yes
3	Deep stupor; responds to deep pain	No	No	Yes
4	Does not respond to appropriate stimuli; possible decorticate and decerebrate posturing; retains deep tendon reflexes	No	No	No
5	Nonresponsive, flaccid, no deep tendon reflexes, apneic	No	No	No

or upper brainstem is involved. Abnormalities in the dominant hemisphere have a greater effect on consciousness than those in the nondominant hemisphere.

Respiratory Effects

Hypothalamic and midbrain damage results in rapid, sustained, deep hyperventilation (central neurogenic hyperventilation). Injury to the medulla and the pons affects the respiratory centers and produces several different patterns:

1. apneustic breathing, with a prolonged pause at full inspiration;
2. ataxic breathing, which consists of random, ineffective, haphazard breaths and pauses without a predictable pattern; and
3. primary alveolar hypoventilation (Ondine's curse), a failure to breathe while sleeping, which is the failure of automatic breathing centers when asleep.

Cheyne-Stokes respirations, during which periods of hyperpnea alternate with periods of apnea, result from an extensive, usually bilateral, diencephalic disturbance with an intact brainstem.

The most common cerebral causes of respiratory insufficiency are increased ICP and drugs that depress brain function. Barbiturates are often used to put the brain into an inactive state, inducing a coma to treat encephalopathies and intractable seizures (status epilepticus). Intubation and mechanical ventilation must be initiated before barbiturates are given.

Persistent Vegetative State

The terms *persistent vegetative state* (PVS) and *neocortical death* are used interchangeably to describe patients who, after recovery from coma, return to a state of wakefulness without cognition. PVS is "a form of eyes-open permanent unconsciousness in which the patient has periods of wakefulness and physiological sleep/wake cycles, but at no time is the patient aware of him or herself or the environment."[12] Brainstem functions such as respiration and circulation are intact, and with good nursing care, survival is indefinite. With intensive and aggressive therapy, patients tend to maintain basic vital signs but are usually technology dependent and have an apparent poor quality of life.

PVS occurs in 12% of adults who survive nontraumatic coma but is probably less common in children. The usual causes, in order of frequency, are anoxic and ischemic brain injury, metabolic or encephalitic coma, and head trauma. Recovery is rare when the vegetative state has persisted for 1 month in adults. The prognosis may be better in children, although recovery after 3 months is unlikely.

The American Academy of Neurology has adopted the policy that all medical treatment, including the provision of nutrition and hydration, may be ethically discontinued when

1. a patient's condition has been diagnosed as a PVS
2. it is clear that the patient would not want to be maintained in this state, and
3. the family agrees to discontinue therapy.[13]

Recent adult cases have brought these issues to the forefront of public and professional debate without a clear consensus on the discontinuation of medical support technologies and techniques used to accomplish life sustaining activities.

Reye's Syndrome

Douglas Reye, an Australian pathologist, defined the clinical and pathologic features of Reye's syndrome in 1963. Reye's syndrome involves multiple organ systems and is a combination of fatty infiltrates in the internal organs, especially in the liver, and progressive encephalopathy.[14] Reye's syndrome is not a primary neurologic disorder but, if left untreated, has fatal neurologic consequences. During later stages the neurologic care plan for Reye's syndrome is similar to that for other conditions producing increased ICP.

Reye's syndrome is predominantly a pediatric disease occurring in infancy through adolescence, with males and females affected equally. It usually follows a febrile viral illness such as a respiratory tract infection, gastroenteritis, or chickenpox—conditions usually caused by influenza B or varicella viruses. Epidemiologic studies have associated Reye's syndrome with the use of aspirin or other salicylates used to control aching, temperature and other flulike symptoms during the initial illness.[15]

Stages

Mortality is related to the severity of the disease, which is classified by five stages (Table 39-4). Early diagnosis and treatment may also contribute to a decrease in mortality. Patients who move rapidly from Stage I to Stage III Reye's syndrome have been reported to have a poor prognosis, as have patients with an initial blood ammonia level greater than 300 mg/dl.[16]

Differential Diagnosis

Although it may be difficult to differentiate Reye's syndrome from other types of encephalopathy, it is important to consider this diagnosis when a patient presents with clinical symptoms of encephalopathy, especially when vomiting is present after a viral-type illness. Elevated serum ammonia and elevated liver enzyme levels are hallmarks of Reye's syndrome. Therefore, the syndrome should be highly suspected in children who present with acute encephalopathy after a viral illness and who also have evidence of hepatic dysfunction.

TABLE 39-4

Clinical Stages of Reye's Syndrome

Stage	Consciousness	Motor Response	Seizures	Other Features
I	Lethargy; responds to pain	None	None	Vomiting, rash, hepatic dysfunction, hyperventilation
II	Delirium, combativeness	None	None	Hepatic dysfunction, hyperactive reflexes, hyperventilation
III	Coma, decorticate rigidity, sluggish pupils, doll's eye reflex	None	None	Hepatic dysfunction, hyperventilation
IV	Coma, decerebrate rigidity, sluggish large pupils	No OR	Minimal	Hepatic dysfunction
V	Coma, flaccid, fixed pupils	No reflexes	Present	Respiratory arrest; serum ammonia >300 mg/ml

OR, Oculocephalic reflex.

Symptoms appear within 1 week after the onset of the viral illness and may initially include sudden onset of vomiting, a rash, and confusion with personality changes. As the encephalopathy becomes more acute, seizures may occur; the patient becomes lethargic, and the lethargy frequently progresses to coma. During the first stages, neurologic status may be assessed by behavioral changes; however, coma progresses throughout Stages III to V. Hyperventilation usually occurs when the patient becomes confused or combative, or both, and is reflected in ABG values, but metabolic acidosis may also be present. Staging of Reye's syndrome is accomplished by frequent neurologic examinations and monitoring of laboratory values.[17]

Treatment

Treating Reye's syndrome focuses on individual symptoms and supportive therapy. Patients in an intensive care unit (ICU) have frequent neurologic monitoring, which includes level of consciousness, reflex activity, and reactions to stimuli. Laboratory values should include coagulation studies and blood urea nitrogen levels. Patients in Stages III to V require more intensive monitoring and treatment for the increased ICP, including arterial lines, mechanical ventilation with hyperventilation, hypothermia, osmotic diuretics (e.g., mannitol), and pentobarbital coma.[17] Increased public awareness of the association between salicylates and Reye's Syndrome has lead to a decrease in the number of cases seen in recent years.

INCREASED INTRACRANIAL PRESSURE

Anatomic Considerations

The size of a normal infant's skull is determined by its contents. The normal skull contents consist of three substances: brain tissue, blood, and cerebral spinal fluid (CSF). The growing brain causes the skull to increase in size. Normal circumferential head growth in the term newborn is 2 cm per month for the first 3 months, 1 cm per month for the second 3 months, and 0.5 cm per month for the next 6 months. Excessive head growth resulting from separation of the cranial sutures is an important feature of increased ICP throughout the first year of life. When the separation of cranial sutures is no longer sufficient to decompress increased ICP, the infant becomes lethargic, does not take feedings, and vomits.

After infancy or when the suture lines and fontanels close, the skull can no longer increase in size, and the total pressure within the skull is caused by the size of its contents—the brain tissue (80% to 90% of the intracranial content by volume), CSF (5% to 10%), and blood (5% to 9%). The Monroe-Kellie doctrine or hypothesis may be paraphrased as follows: in a closed system, such as the skull, an increase in the size of one component requires compression of the other components to maintain a constant ICP.[18] If the internal volume of the skull is 500 ml, for example, and the brain, blood, and CSF volume is 450 ml, then 50 ml of expansion volume remains in the skull. According to the Monroe-Kellie doctrine, if the volume of these three components increases by more than 50 ml, compression of the skull contents occurs.[19] Because CSF and blood are fluids and thus almost incompressible at physiologic pressures, the compression will occur in the brain tissue. Compression of the brain tissue inhibits blood flow by reducing cerebral perfusion pressure (CPP) and causes cerebral tissue hypoxia, ischemia, and coma. CPP = mean BP − ICP and averages 85 ± 15 mm Hg.

The patient whose condition has progressed to coma requires testing to determine the presence of increased intracranial pressure (ICP). Normal ICP is 130 mm H_2O (10 mm Hg). Computerized tomography (CT) scans or magnetic resonance imaging (MRI) are used to evaluate the brain for evidence of fluid buildup, displacement of the brain, or displacement of the ventricles of the brain. Alternatively, direct pressure measurements may be obtained by lumbar puncture (LP) or by inserting a needle into the interspinal spaces between L3 and L4 or L4 and L5 and attaching a pressure monitor. Other methods of measuring ICP include using an intracranial pressure monitor (subarachnoid screw) or a cerebral ventricular catheter. Because these direct methods are invasive and potentially dangerous, CT or MRI are the preferred, at least as screening tools.

Increased ICP can be a life-threatening feature of an encephalopathy. CSF and blood acting on the brain and bony structures of the skull generate ICP. In the newborn and infant, measuring the head circumference and palpating the anterior fontanel allow rapid assessment of ICP. Bulging of the fontanels may be a key sign of increased ICP that requires a response by caregivers. Gentle palpation of the fontanels may reveal pulsations of the fontanels that may occur normally at a frequency equal to the pulse rate. It is unusual for these pulsations to be either absent or of bounding force.

Clinical Features
Headache
A common symptom of increased ICP at all ages is headache, primarily caused by traction and displacement of intracranial arteries. When increased ICP is generalized, as from cerebral edema or obstruction of the ventricular system, headache is generalized and is more prominent in the morning on awakening. The pain is constant but varies in intensity. Coughing, sneezing, straining, and other maneuvers that transiently increase ICP exaggerate the headache. The quality of pain is often difficult to describe. Vomiting in the absence of nausea, especially on arising in the morning, is often a concurrent feature. Vomiting itself is, of course, also a source of increased ICP. With knowledge of the MOI, the clinician is able to assess the potential pathophysiologic impact on the patient.

Diplopia and Strabismus
Diplopia is characterized by double vision caused by a disruption of the extraocular muscles or the muscle nerves. Strabismus, caused by paralysis of one or both abducens nerves so that the eye cannot turn outward, is a relatively common feature of generalized increased ICP. Strabismus may be a more prominent feature than headache in children with increased ICP.

Papilledema
Papilledema is passive swelling of the optic disc caused by increased ICP. Examining the eye with an ophthalmoscope allows visualization of the disc. The edema is usually bilateral; unilateral edema suggests a mass lesion behind the affected eye. Early papilledema is asymptomatic, and the patient experiences transitory disturbances of vision only with advanced disease. Preservation of visual acuity differentiates papilledema from primary optic nerve disturbances, such as optic neuritis, in which blindness occurs early in the course of disease.[20]

As edema progresses, the optic disc swells and is raised above the plane of the retina, causing the disc margin to be obscured. Tortuosity (twisted appearance) of the veins also results. If the process continues, the retina surrounding the disc becomes edematous so that the disc appears greatly enlarged and retinal exudate radiates from the fovea. Eventually the exudate clears; however, optic atrophy ensues and blindness may be permanent. Even if increased ICP is relieved during the early stages of disc edema, 4 to 6 weeks are required before the retina appears normal again.

Herniation
Increased ICP may cause portions of the brain to shift from their normal location into other compartments, compressing structures already occupying that space. Such shifts may occur under the falx cerebri, through the tentorial notch, and through the foramen magnum. Brain stem herniation is an emergency condition that, if not rapidly addressed, will almost surely result in major injury and probable death.

Lumbar puncture (LP) is generally contraindicated in patients with increased ICP because of the concern that a change in fluid dynamics will cause brain stem herniation. LP is especially hazardous when pressure between cranial compartments is unequal. This prohibition is relative, and early LP is the rule in infants and children with suspected CNS infections, despite the presence of increased ICP. LP is also used to diagnose and treat increased ICP in pseudotumor cerebri.

Monitoring
Enthusiasm is declining for the continuous monitoring of ICP in children. Despite advances in technology, the effect of pressure monitoring on outcome is questionable. It is not indicated in children with hypoxic-ischemic encephalopathies and has marginal value in children with other types of encephalopathy.[11] Use of LP to obtain CSF pressure readings is a dangerous and risky procedure in infants with disorders such as hydrocephalus— a condition that causes increased production or reduced clearance of cerebral spinal fluid leading to markedly increased ICP as evidenced by a large swollen skull. The symptoms and prognosis of increased ICP depend more on the *cause* than on the level of pressure attained. Systemic arterial blood pressure should be monitored along with ABG values and oxygen saturation.

Treatment

Head Elevation

Elevating the head of the bed 30 to 45 degrees above horizontal decreases ICP by improving jugular venous drainage. The head should also be kept in the midline position so that the vasculature on each side of the neck is not compressed. Systemic blood pressure is not affected, so the overall result is increased CPP.

Hyperventilation

ICP declines within seconds of beginning hyperventilation. The mechanism is vasoconstriction resulting from hypocarbia. The goal is to lower the partial pressure of arterial carbon dioxide ($Paco_2$) from 40 to 25 mm Hg. Further reduction can result in cerebral ischemia and is contraindicated. Vasoconstriction is maintained as long as hyperventilation is continued. When hyperventilation is withdrawn, however, the vessels again dilate and blood flow returns to normal. To prevent a rebound effect, in which blood flow increases above baseline, hyperventilation should be withdrawn gradually. Disponde writes "The limits of cerebral autoregulation may be shifted to significantly lower values (mean arterial pressure [MAP] 20-60 mm Hg) in the neonates and infants. The "margin of safety" is narrower as the infant is less well able to compensate for acute hypo- or hypertension. Low MAP presents the risk of ischemia while hypertension in infants may present risk of intracranial hemorrhage. Response to hyperventilation (low Paco2) in infants may be brisk, with a risk of inducing cerebral ischemia with extremely low Paco2 (<20 mm Hg)."[12]

Hyperventilation is achieved by endotracheal intubation or tracheostomy and mechanical ventilation. Use of hyperventilation should be limited to the first few hours of care to protect against rebound vasoconstriction and increased ICP. Careful monitoring of ICP and $Paco_2$ should always accompany hyperventilation. Colorimetric end tidal carbon dioxide monitoring is not appropriate in these cases as that technique does not provide accurate numerical data for use in either monitoring or trending the hyperventilated patient.

Also, be aware that intubation and tracheostomy, in addition to the risks of damage to the tracheal mucosa and development of tracheoesophageal fistula, carry the risk of ventilatory-associated pneumonia (VAP). A strong correlation exists between nosocomial pneumonia and aspiration of oropharyngeal and gastric emesis. These fluids travel down the exterior of the artificial airway into the open airway past the epiglottis, which is propped open by the tracheal tube. In older children with a cuffed tube, these secretions pool between the larynx and the top of the cuff, poised to flow down the airway into the lungs. The use of continuous positive airway pressure (CPAP) may help prevent this type of pneumonia by increasing the pressure gradient between the airway and the oral cavity, thus restraining the fluid flow.[21]

Osmotic Diuretics

Mannitol and glycerol are the two osmotic diuretics most widely used in the United States. Mannitol is given intravenously as a 20% solution. It does not cross the blood-brain barrier and remains in the plasma, creating an osmotic gradient that draws water from the brain into the capillaries thus reducing cerebral fluid volume and therefore ICP. Onset of action is within 30 minutes, with the peak effect generally lasting 1 to 2 hours after administration. The effect is short term, and infusions must be given 3 to 6 times each day to keep serum osmolality at less than 320 mOsm/L (320 nmol/L). Repeated infusions of mannitol also cause dehydration as well as fluid and electrolyte imbalances. Rebound may occur when mannitol is discontinued.

Glycerol is given intravenously as a 10% solution 3 to 4 times per day. The onset of action is within 30 minutes, with the effect usually lasting 24 hours or longer. As with mannitol, dehydration and electrolyte disturbances may follow repeated administration. Rebound is less prominent than with mannitol.

Corticosteroids

Corticosteroids, such as dexamethasone, are effective in the treatment of vasogenic edema. Onset of action is 12 to 24 hours, and peak action may be delayed even longer. The mechanism is uncertain, but cerebral blood flow (CBF) is not affected. Corticosteroids are most useful for reducing edema surrounding mass (space-occupying) lesions. These agents are not beneficial in cytotoxic edema, as seen after hypoxic-ischemic injuries. The delay in onset of action limits the usefulness of corticosteroids in patients needing emergent or urgent cerebral volume reduction.

Hypothermia

Hypothermia decreases CBF and is frequently used concurrently with pentobarbital coma. Body temperature is generally kept between 27° and 30° C. It is not clear how much improvement is gained by hypothermia in addition to other measures that decrease CBF, such as head elevation, hyperventilation, and pentobarbital coma.

In a recent well-designed study in adults, 392 subjects (16 to 65 years of age), all sustaining closed head trauma, were randomly assigned to a control (normothermic) group or an experimental group (hypothermia within 6 hours of injury to 33° C for 48 hours), with the patients in each group having similar injuries by type and severity and mean age. The outcomes were poor in 57% of each group (resulting in a vegetative state, disability, or death). The death rates were 27% in the normothermic subjects and 28% in the hypothermic group. The hypothermic subjects also had more complications and more hospital days but fewer episodes of increased ICP. The authors concluded that hypothermia was not advantageous in this group of patients.[22, 23, 24]

Although the applicability of this study to neonates and children is not known, it suggests a need to examine practices for safety, efficacy, and cost-benefit considerations. The infant and child's greater body surface–to body mass ratio, heat loss, and labile temperature control must be considered in the head-injured infant and child. Hypothermia applied early in the course of injury may be protective in that the lower body temperature may prevent or slow production of cellular end products usually released after tissue injury.[22] This reduction in metabolic end products may occur secondary to low temperature–induced metabolic rate reduction.

Pentobarbital Coma

Barbiturates such as pentobarbital reduce CBF, decrease edema formation, and lower the brain's metabolic rate. These effects do not occur at anticonvulsant plasma concentrations but require brain concentrations sufficient to produce a burst-suppression pattern on the EEG. Pentobarbital medically induced coma is particularly useful in patients with increased ICP resulting from disorders of mitochondrial function, such as Reye's syndrome. In adults medically induced coma is increasingly being seen as a way of "resting the brain" to aid healing of the fragile brain tissue.

Ventilatory Maneuvers

The increase in intrathoracic pressure that occurs during positive-pressure ventilation may impede cerebral venous return and increase ICP. Therefore the patient should be mechanically ventilated with the lowest peak pressures possible. A minimal level of positive end-expiratory pressure (PEEP) should be used to maintain adequate ventilation at low mean airway pressures. Chest physical therapy and postural drainage positioning may also exaggerate the ICP and should be used with caution. Care should be taken to monitor and maintain inflation of newly recruited alveoli. Suctioning may increase the ICP and should be performed minimally and must be preceded with oxygen-supplemented hyperventilation. It is also important to prevent Valsalva maneuvers and coughing, each of which can cause marked increases in ICP.

STATUS EPILEPTICUS

The condition in which seizures are repetitive and do not stop spontaneously is called status epilepticus. Seizures begin with abnormal neurons that discharge repeatedly. Repetitive seizures increase the body's requirements for adenosine triphosphate (ATP), which in turn increases metabolic needs for oxygen and glucose. Apnea, hypoxemia, and hypoglycemia may result, along with increased oxygen consumption and lactic acidosis. Anoxic injury to the brain and other organs, as well as cardiac arrhythmias and traumatic injuries (e.g., tongue laceration, concussion), may also occur.

Status epilepticus is a medical emergency that requires prompt attention. A controlled airway must be established immediately, and supplemental oxygen and mechanical ventilation should be rapidly available. Venous access must be established and blood withdrawn for measurement of glucose and electrolyte levels. Other tests, such as anticonvulsant drug concentrations and toxicology screens, are performed as indicated. After blood is withdrawn, an IV infusion of saline solution is started for the administration of anticonvulsant drugs. An IV bolus of a 50% glucose solution is also administered to replenish the glucose stores and allow for metabolic needs.

The ideal drug for treating status epilepticus is one that acts rapidly, has a long duration of action, and does not produce sedation. Diazepam and lorazepam are widely used for this purpose, but their duration of action is brief. In addition, children who receive IV benzodiazepines after a prior load of barbiturate often experience respiratory depression.

IV *phenytoin* is a preferable drug because of its long duration of action. A slow rate of administration is necessary to avoid causing cardiac arrhythmias. Phenytoin is usually effective unless status epilepticus is caused by severe acute encephalopathy. If phenytoin fails, the patient should be given a loading dose of phenobarbital. This dose may be repeated, but respiratory depression may ensue. If this fails, medically induced pentobarbital coma is a reasonable next treatment.

The patient should be intubated and mechanically ventilated in the ED and then transferred to the ICU. After an arterial line is placed, the patient's blood pressure, cardiac rhythm, body temperature, and oxygen saturation should be monitored.

To achieve pentobarbital coma in the patient with status epilepticus, boluses of pentobarbital are infused until a burst-suppression pattern appears on the ECG monitor, which is continuously recording. Hypotension occurs with large doses, and vasopressor support may be necessary. The coma can be safely maintained for 3 days; longer coma periods may cause pulmonary edema. The ECG should be checked several times each day for the burst-suppression pattern. The coma can be lifted every 48 to 72 hours to see whether the seizures have stopped. Mechanical ventilation should be continued until the patient regains consciousness and can spontaneously support ventilation and until reflexive airway protection is adequate.

The above discussion of head injury is not exhaustive but should serve to illustrate to the reader that these injuries and conditions are potentially life threatening and life altering. The mastery of skills relate to ventilator and airway control are often among the most crucial in the care and survival of these patients.

CLINICAL SCENARIO

12-year-old male is watching a golf match when a club slips out of a golfer's hand and strikes him on the left temporal region of his head. Answer the following questions about his injury and its treatment.

1. He falls to the ground unconscious, and is not able to be aroused. He is breathing, nonresponsive to verbal stimuli (although he pulls away from pain), he exhibits tachycardia at 128, his pulse full and bounding. His eyes are nonreactive and midline. There is no bleeding at the injury site. The patient's Glasgow Coma Score would be:
    A. 10
    B. 15
    C. 6*
    D. 8
2. Which of the following do you do next?
    A. Stat—this is a standard medical term meaning right away head and spine CT scan, electrolytes, pulse oximetry, and spinal tap.
    B. Immobilize head and spine, cover with jackets, call EMS, and monitor vital signs.*
    C. Move to the clubhouse on golf cart, put ice on impact point, and give aspirin for headache.
    D. Penalize golfer two strokes for loss of club control and failing to call "fore."
    E. Start large bore IV, insert airway, sit him up at 45° angle, and monitor vital signs.
3. On arrival to the hospital the patient was found to have less muscle tone on his left side than on his right. This suggests:
    A. A contrecoup injury to the right side of the brain.*
    B. A left subdural hematoma.
    C. An orbital fracture.
    D. A crush injury to the carotid bulb outflow track.

4. Over the next few hours the patient becomes increasingly arousable although he is confused about time and place. He complains about a right-sided headache that seems to be localized near the right temple. CT scan and MRI are negative for bleeding or fractures. What is the likely Diagnosis?
    A. A Munroe-Kellie class 4 closed head injury.
    B. A severe interosseous skull injury.
    C. Grade III (Severe) concussion.*
    D. Traumatic migraine headache.
5. What is/are the most likely future actions with regard to the patient and his injury?
    A. Observe in hospital for 24 to 48 hours.
    B. Vital signs and neurologic checks Q1 × 4, Q2 × 2, Q4 × 4 until discharge
    C. Reduced activity level and observe at home for 2 days after discharge.
    D. All of the above are standard and appropriate actions.*

ASSESSMENT QUESTIONS

See Evolve Resources for the answers.

1. Which organ or organs could be injured in response to the Monroe-Kellie doctrine?
    A. The brain
    B. The heart
    C. The lungs
    D. All of the above
2. Injuries to which levels of the spine affect the diaphragm?
    A. S1 and S2
    B. C1 and C2
    C. T1 and T2
    D. C3 and T1
3. How many children suffer head injury every minute?
    A. One
    B. Four
    C. Three
    D. Five
4. Contrecoup injuries
    A. Are examples of inertial injuries
    B. Appear on the side the damaging force was applied
    C. Occur on the opposite side from the applied force
    D. A and C

Continued

ASSESSMENT QUESTIONS—cont'd

5. The Glasgow Coma Score (GCS) includes the following variable(s)
   A. Grip strength, Babinski response, eyes closed nose touch
   B. Temperature, Pulse Rate, SpO_2, Systemic BP
   C. Eye opening, verbal response, motor response
   D. Children's Coma Scale + SpO_2
6. Which of the following pain assessment scales is most appropriate for a 3-year-old child?
   A. FACES scale
   B. Borg scale
   C. Numeric pain scale
   D. Color bar scale
7. Which of the following suggests possible child abuse?
   A. Multiple bruises of various ages
   B. Withdrawal from caregiver contact
   C. "Flat" affect (not responsive to people or location)
   D. All of the above are possible signs of abuse
8. Decorticate posturing is characterized by
   A. Toes pointed, hands clenched and at midline
   B. Toes clenched, arms at sides, hands clenched and rotated outwards
   C. Feet rotated inwards, fingers extended and spread, head turned to side of injury
   D. Jaw toward chest, mouth open, tongue protruding to uninjured side
9. Reye's syndrome is associated with which of the following?
   A. Penicillin
   B. Aspirin
   C. Pentamidine
   D. Ibuprophen
10. Ataxic breathing patterns are characterized by
    A. Ineffective breaths with haphazard pauses and no predictable cause
    B. Continual full inspirations and full expiration with slight pauses
    C. Respirations that start with small volumes then rise in volume in a stair step pattern with an abrupt return to small volume breaths
    D. Gasping respirations

References

1. Newsbytes, *Case Manager* 2001;12:6.
2. Laskowski-Jones L, Salati DS: Responding to pediatric trauma, *Nursing* 2001; 31(9):37.
3. Norton PGW. Accidental falls don't often cause severe head injuries, *Pediatric News* June 1, 2003. *http://www.merckmedicus.com/pp/us/newsarticleprint.jsp?newsid=311832* accessed 1/26/2006.
4. Rubin DM et al: Occult head injury in high risk children, *Pediatrics* 2003;111:1382.
5. Carey MG, Lasko M: Acute stages of spinal cord injuries. *Perspectives: recovery strategies from the OR to home* 2005:6:1.
6. Strange GG et al: *Pediatric emergency medicine*, New York: McGraw-Hill, 1998.
7. Hayes JS, Arriloa T: Pediatric spinal injuries, *Pediatric Nursing* 2005;31:464.
8. Bergman DA et al: The Management of minor closed head injury in children, *Pediatrics* 1999:104:1407.
9. Greenes DS, Schutzman SA: Clinical indicators of inter-cranial injury in head-injured infants, *Pediatrics* 1999;104:861.
10. Ghajar J, Hariri RJ: Management of pediatric head injury, *Pediatr Clin North Am* 1992;39:1093.
11. Plum F, Posner JB: *The diagnosis of stupor and coma*, ed 3. Philadelphia. Davis, 1980.
12. Deshpande JK: Anesthesia for neurosurgery in infants and children. Accessed March 17, 2008. *http://www.csaol.cn/img/2007asa/RCL_src/328_Deshpande.pdf.*
13. American Academy of Neurology: Position of the American Academy of Neurology on certain aspects of the care and management of the persistent vegetative state patient, *Neurology* 1989;39:125.
14. LeRoux PD, Jardine DS, Loeser JD: Pediatric intracranial pressure monitoring in hypoxic and nonhypoxic brain injury, *Child Nerv Syst* 1991;7:34.
15. Reye RDK, Morgan G, Baral J: Encephalopathy and fatty degeneration of the viscera: a disease entity in childhood, *Lancet* 1963;2:749.
16. Surgeon General's advisory on the use of salicylate in Reye's syndrome, 1981: Reye's syndrome and salicylate usage, *MMWR* 1982;31:51.
17. Corey L, Rubin RJ, Hattwick MAW: Reye's syndrome: clinical progression and evaluation of therapy, *Pediatrics* 1977;60:708.
18. Crocker JFS, Bagnell PC: Reye's syndrome: a clinical review, *CMA J* 1981;124:375.
19. Morki B: The Monro-Kellie hypothesis: applications in CSF volume depletion, *Neurology* 2001;56:1746.
20. Greitz D et al: Pulsatile brain movement and associated hydrodynamics studied by magnetic resonance phase imaging: the Monro-Kellie doctrine revisited, *Neuroradiology* 1992;34:370.
21. Fenichel GM: *Clinical pediatric neurology*, ed 3. Philadelphia: Saunders; 1977. pp 93-95.
22. Finder JD, Yellon R, Charron M: Successful management of tracheotomized patients with chronic saliva aspiration by use of constant positive airway pressure, *Pediatrics* 2001;107:1343.
23. Clifton GL et al: Lack of effect of hypothermia after acute brain injury, *N Engl J Med* 2001;22:556
24. Narayan RK: Hypothermia for traumatic brain injury: a good idea proven ineffective, *N Engl J Med* 2001 (editorial);344:602.

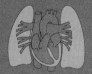

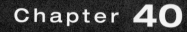

Chapter 40

Thoracic Trauma in Children

BRADLEY M. RODGERS • EUGENE D. McGAHREN

OUTLINE

LEARNING OBJECTIVES

After reading this chapter the reader will be able to:
- Recognize the spectrum of thoracic injuries seen in pediatric practice
- Evaluate methods to avoid thoracic birth trauma
- Appraise the most common forms of thoracic birth trauma and their treatment
- Explain the causes of blunt thoracic trauma in children

- Recognize the spectrum of penetrating thoracic injuries seen in children
- Describe imaging strategies for penetrating thoracic trauma
- Recognize the spectrum of the most common forms of iatrogenic thoracic trauma in infants and children and their treatment

Thoracic trauma encompasses a broad range of injuries in the pediatric population, from those iatrogenic injuries encountered in the newborn infant through acquired traumatic injuries seen in adolescents. The traumatic thoracic injuries encountered in children generally present in a somewhat different fashion from those encountered in adults and usually are better tolerated, within a background of normal pulmonary function. Overall, thoracic trauma accounts for about 5% to 10% of admissions in pediatric trauma centers.[1] This chapter covers the more common forms of thoracic birth trauma,

acquired blunt and penetrating thoracic trauma, and special forms of iatrogenic thoracic trauma, perhaps seen more commonly in children than adults.

BIRTH TRAUMA

The fetus is exposed to considerable compression stresses in passage through the birth canal for vaginal delivery. The flexibility of the fetal thoracic skeleton allows considerable pulmonary compression in this process and occasional pulmonary trauma.[2]

Nerve Injury

Distortion of the axial skeleton during delivery can stretch and damage the nerves involved with the respiratory mechanics of the newborn, particularly the phrenic nerve, which arises from the C4 level in the neck.[3] Flexion and extension of the neck during the delivery process can stretch the origin of the phrenic nerve and cause diaphragmatic paralysis. Depending on the degree of injury, this may be transient or permanent.

The newborn infant, with diminutive extrathoracic musculature, is primarily a diaphragmatic breather. Paralysis of the diaphragm may cause significant respiratory embarrassment. Abdominal pressure is always greater than pleural pressure in the newborn, and the paralyzed diaphragm tends to elevate in the chest, compressing the ipsilateral lung and shifting the mediastinum to compress the contralateral lung. In this setting the infant may have a tidal volume sufficiently restricted to require intubation and mechanical ventilation. In general, one should wait for 3 to 6 weeks to judge if the phrenic nerve will recover from the injury before considering surgical treatment.

The surgical therapy for persistent diaphragm paralysis consists of plication of the diaphragm, performed either through an open thoracotomy or by thoracoscopic techniques.[4] The plication shortens the diaphragm fibers and flattens the diaphragm on that side to allow better expansion of the ipsilateral lung and movement of the mediastinum to a more central position. Even in neonates without severe respiratory compromise, one must be concerned with persistent compression of the pulmonary parenchyma as this can interfere with postnatal pulmonary development.

There is a congenital condition of the newborn in which muscle ingrowth never occurs into the hemidiaphragm and the resultant physiology is identical to that of phrenic nerve palsy. Infants with so-called eventration of the diaphragm will never recover function and consideration should be given to early plication in these patients.

Congenital Chylothorax

It is thought that another pulmonary injury that may occur during the birth process is congenital chylothorax. This condition occurs in approximately one in every 20,000 live births and the infants are noted to have a significant pleural effusion that develops shortly following delivery. It is felt that elevation of the venous pressure by thoracic compression in the birth canal causes an elevation of pressure in the thoracic duct and actually ruptures branches or perhaps congenital malformations of this duct, allowing chyle to leak into the thoracic cavity. Chyle is a fluid rich in protein and lymphocytes and its loss may cause a significant protein deficit for the newborn infant, in addition to presenting significant pulmonary compression.

Infants with congenital chylothorax frequently present with severe respiratory compromise secondary to compression of the ipsilateral lung and shift of the mediastinum. They should be treated with immediate chest tube drainage and they should be placed NPO to minimize the formation of thoracic duct lymph. Their nutrition should be supplied by total parenteral nutrition until the chyle leak ceases.

In approximately 30% of these patients the leak will not stop with these measures and surgical treatment will be required, either by placement of a pleuroperitoneal shunt to drain the fluid into the peritoneal cavity, where it can be absorbed, or by thoracotomy with thoracic duct ligation to cease all lymphatic flow through the chest. Both of these techniques have approximately an 80% success rate in managing infants with congenital chylothorax.[5,6]

Pneumothorax

Pneumothorax occurring in the newborn infant will be discussed in more detail in the section on iatrogenic trauma since in most cases this is caused by overzealous positive pressure ventilation of the newborn.

Transition from fetal life—with a fluid-filled, consolidated lung—to newborn life with an expanded and aerated lung is a complicated process. Compression of the thorax in the birth canal can begin to mobilize fluid from the pulmonary parenchyma, but many infants will require positive pressure assistance to fully expand their lung. This is particularly true in the premature infant in whom pulmonary surfactant levels may be quite low. Positive pressure ventilation of these small infants must be performed at very low peak inspiratory pressures. If high pressures are employed to rapidly expand regions of consolidated lung, the portions of the lung that are aerated will expand more rapidly. Occasionally this expansion is sufficient to rupture the visceral pleura and cause a pneumothorax, with sudden deterioration in pulmonary function. These infants must be treated with prompt placement of a chest tube and reduction of the peak inspiratory pressures.

BLUNT THORACIC TRAUMA

Pulmonary Contusion

Significant blunt thoracic trauma is relatively less common in the pediatric population than in adults. Overall, blunt chest trauma accounts for 80% of the chest injuries that occur in civilian populations.[7] The child's ribs and cartilage are more flexible than the adult's, and the thorax can be quite significantly compressed without fracturing ribs. This compression causes trauma to the underlying pulmonary parenchyma with resultant edema and occasional hemorrhage into the parenchyma. As children get older and approach adolescence the ribs begin to calcify and stiffen and rib fractures are seen more commonly in this population. If the fractured end of a rib penetrates the visceral pleura of the lung beneath it, a pneumothorax is produced. These patients can present to the emergency room in extreme respiratory distress and improvement in ventilation is often seen immediately with placement of a chest tube.

Flail Chest

When several adjacent ribs are fractured in two areas, a flail segment of the chest wall may be produced. This segment of the chest moves in paradoxical fashion with respiratory effort, collapsing with inspiratory effort and expanding with expiration. This paradoxical motion interferes with tidal ventilation of the ipsilateral lung and, in conjunction with pulmonary parenchymal contusion, may cause serious respiratory embarrassment.

Although in the past attempts had been made to wire the rib ends together to stabilize this segment of the thoracic wall, these were difficult operations requiring multiple incisions and often did not provide sufficient stability. Likewise, merely strapping that segment of the chest wall with stiff bandages may prevent the flail segment from expanding with expiration, but will not prevent the collapse and pulmonary compression with inspiration. Children with significant segments of flail chest wall are best treated with intubation and positive pressure ventilation with paralysis.[8] Over a 5- to 7-day interval, the inflammatory healing process stabilizes the ends of the ribs and minimizes the flail and these patients can usually be successfully extubated at that point.

PENETRATING THORACIC TRAUMA

Although the majority of thoracic trauma in children occurs from blunt injury, penetrating thoracic trauma carries a significantly higher mortality for these patients. Isolated penetrating trauma, without significant associated injury, carries approximately 5% mortality in pediatric patients, while the mortality with multiple injuries may be as high as 15% to 20%.[9] The range of injuries encountered with penetrating trauma in children varies considerably, depending upon the offending object and the axis of injury. In general, stab wounds, particularly those with pocket knives having short blades, cause the least severe injuries, while high velocity missiles, such as occur in hunting accidents, cause the most severe tissue damage and internal injury.

Incidence

The incidence of penetrating thoracic trauma varies with age, with older children and adolescents having a significantly higher incidence than infants and younger children. A greater proportion of injuries in the older children are associated with handguns or knives used in criminal activity, although a small percentage are secondary to hunting or industrial accidents. The most common injury sustained with penetrating thoracic trauma is a pneumothorax or hemothorax with accumulation of air or blood within the pleural space.

Resuscitation

Often the extent of intrathoracic injury is difficult to predict from the mechanism of injury, particularly in those cases with gunshot wounds, in which the missile may be deflected by bony structures and take a circuitous route. All of these patients should be stabilized in the emergency room before any diagnostic studies are obtained. An adequate airway must be ensured, with many of these children requiring immediate intubation. The adequacy of ventilation should be monitored with transcutaneous oxygen saturation, and mechanical ventilation may be required for those individuals who are hypoxic (Sao_2 <80%) or tachypneic (respiratory rate > 45 per minute). Two large bore IV catheters should be inserted for fluid resuscitation to maintain adequate tissue perfusion. Several clinical studies in the past decade have suggested more favorable clinical outcomes in individuals resuscitated with limited intravenous volume administration prior to control of the source of bleeding.[10] For most pediatric patients systolic blood pressures of 80 to 100 mm Hg should be sufficient to maintain adequate tissue perfusion during this interval.

Imaging

Although the diagnosis of penetrating thoracic trauma is usually rapidly evident from the history of the mechanism of injury and the physical examination, specific information with regard to intrathoracic organ injuries will require further radiologic and interventional procedures. Patients presenting with severe respiratory distress should be treated immediately by intubation and ipsilateral tube thoracostomy, before any radiologic studies are obtained. Patients with less severe symptoms and those who have been stabilized are initially investigated with an AP chest radiograph. Although this should ideally be obtained with the patient in a semiupright position, in practice it is usually acquired with the patient supine. Small collections of blood and air may be difficult to appreciate in the supine chest radiograph as blood tends to layer posteriorly and air collections accumulate anteriorly. Subtle changes in the density of the radiograph on the ipsilateral side, compared to the contralateral side, may be the only clue to these injuries. Careful attention to the ribs, cardiac shadow, mediastinal space, and diaphragm contours should be observed on this initial radiograph. The position of the endotracheal tube and nasogastric tube, if present, should also be noted. A chest CT scan may be more sensitive for identifying small pneumothoraces and pneumomediastinum. CT arteriogram may define major vascular injuries, although aortography may be necessary to provide more precise anatomic details in some of these injuries.[11,12] The evacuation of more than 300 cc of blood from the pleural space after placement of a chest tube, or continuous bleeding through the chest tube, should prompt evaluation for a major vessel injury. Patients with penetrating injuries suspected of involving the mediastinum should undergo esophagoscopy or contrast esophagography. These patients also should undergo fiberoptic bronchoscopy. Patients with penetrating injury in whom either entrance wounds or exit wounds are below the level of the nipples should be suspected of having diaphragm and intraabdominal injuries. These patients should undergo abdominal CT scan to assess for that possibility.

Pneumothorax/Hemothorax

The injuries associated with penetrating thoracic trauma include pneumothorax, hemothorax, pulmonary parenchymal injuries, major airway injuries, great vessel injuries, esophageal injuries, and diaphragmatic injuries. Pneumothorax is seen as a consequence of virtually all penetrating thoracic trauma as the pleural space is opened to atmospheric pressure, even if the visceral pleura is not violated. The presence of both blood and air in the pleura space is referred to as hemopneumothorax. Air under pressure in the pleural space, as might occur with a ball valve–type injury of the visceral pleura, is termed a tension pneumothorax.[13]

In any instance where intubation is considered in the presence of a traumatic thoracic injury, attention should be paid to the possibility of a tension pneumothorax being present, as positive pressure ventilation may increase the pressure within the chest and further compromise the patient's respiratory and hemodynamic status. Otherwise healthy young individuals can generally tolerate a moderate unilateral pneumothorax, but may be quite symptomatic with a tension pneumothorax because of the mobility of the mediastinum in children. Although some patients with a small unilateral pneumothorax may be treated expectantly, most children with pneumothorax as a consequence of penetrating trauma should be treated with a chest tube. Likewise, all children with a significant hemopneumothorax should receive a chest tube for drainage of the pleural blood. Some of these children will not require intubation and most will not require thoracotomy for control. On the other hand, children who suffer high-velocity penetrating injuries of the chest wall will require intubation and often thoracotomy to control bleeding and pulmonary parenchymal injuries. See Clinical Scenario 1.

CLINICAL SCENARIO 1

J K: This 16-year-old young woman suffered severe blunt chest trauma when a horse from which she had fallen tripped and fell on her chest. She was intubated at the scene because of respiratory distress and was hand ventilated with 100% oxygen while transported.

On arrival her transcutaneous oxygen saturation was 83% on a ventilator (PIP 20 cm H_2O, PEEP 5 cm H_2O R12 and F_{IO_2} 1.00). A chest x-ray demonstrated a large tension pneumothorax on the right side with bilateral pulmonary contusions (Figure 40-1). She had multiple rib fractures and fractures of T1 and T2 transverse processes. Bilateral chest tubes were placed immediately with improvement in saturations, but continuous air leak from the right side.

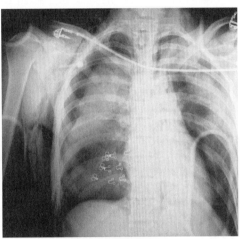

FIGURE 40-1

She was weaned to a F_{IO_2} of 0.23 in the next 12 hours. The patient underwent flexible bronchoscopy through the endotracheal tube, which demonstrated a laceration of the right bronchus intermedius. This was treated nonoperatively, but healed with a stricture, which subsequently required a sleeve resection.

Question:
1. Suspicion of a traumatic pneumothorax is best confirmed by which physical signs?
   A. Hyperexpansion of the ipsilateral chest
   B. Subcutaneous emphysema
   C. Diminished breath sounds on the ipsilateral chest
   D. Elevated jugular venous pressure
2. Treatment of an adolescent with a symptomatic pneumothorax secondary to blunt thoracic trauma is best accomplished immediately by
   A. Insertion of a 12 Fr chest tube in the midclavicular line
   B. Insertion of a 12 Fr chest tube in the posterior axillary line
   C. Carefully monitored observation
   D. Insertion of a 24 Fr chest tube in the midclavicular line
   E. Insertion of a 24 Fr chest tube in the posterior axillary line

Airway Injury

Patients with penetrating thoracic trauma, presenting with a significant pneumothorax in which there is a continuous air leak through the chest tube, should be suspected of having major airway injuries. The majority of these patients will be found to have a pneumomediastinum on plain chest radiographs or chest CT scans. Airway penetration should be confirmed by bronchoscopy. If the patient has been intubated for respiratory distress, this may be performed with a flexible bronchoscope passed through the endotracheal tube. One must be aware that the injury may be proximal to the level of the end of the endotracheal tube; in some cases the flexible bronchoscope may need to be passed through the larynx, beside the endotracheal tube, to examine for this possibility. Patients who are not intubated may undergo either flexible or rigid bronchoscopy. Most major airway lacerations will require open exploration and repair, although smaller injuries may be stented with the endotracheal tube and may heal without significant stricture.[14]

Vascular Injury

Patients with high-velocity penetrating injuries and significant ongoing blood loss should be suspected of having major vessel injuries. Many of these patients may require urgent thoracotomy for control of the bleeding, while some may be stable enough to obtain a CT angiogram or arteriogram to help localize the area of injury.

Some patients with penetrating thoracic trauma may also have sustained significant intra-abdominal injury. In most of the respiratory cycle the apex of the diaphragm is as high as the fourth intercostal space. This is because intra-abdominal pressure always exceeds intrapleural pressure, throughout all phases of ventilation. Penetrating injuries at or below this level, the level of the nipples, must be suspected of having diaphragm penetration and potential intra-abdominal injuries. These patients should be evaluated with a chest-abdomen CT scan. In otherwise stable individuals, thoracoscopy has been reported to be helpful in diagnosing traumatic diaphragm lacerations.[15]

Children with penetrating thoracic injuries who require intubation may present significant ventilatory difficulties because of a massive air leak. To minimize the air leak ventilator strategies in these patients generally attempt to reduce peak inspiratory pressures and mean airway pressures. This can often be accomplished by reducing the tidal volume and using a minimal level of PEEP, with an increase in respiratory rate. Patients with very large air leaks may benefit from the use of high-frequency or oscillating ventilators. Further reduction of mean airway pressure is possible using these ventilators, thereby reducing the volumes of air lost across the chest wall. Most children can be successfully ventilated with these strategies, but on rare occasions emergency surgery and control of the pulmonary leak or pulmonary resection may be necessary.

IATROGENIC THORACIC TRAUMA

Many of the same types of injuries that may be encountered with blunt or penetrating thoracic trauma may be seen as a consequence of iatrogenic trauma. As physicians perform more and more invasive procedures around the chest, the incidence of iatrogenic thoracic trauma has increased.

Pneumomediastinum

Pneumomediastinum, the collection of air in the mediastinal space in the central chest, may be seen as a consequence of sudden Valsalva maneuvers or even asthma. Iatrogenic perforation of the esophagus during esophagoscopy may result in accumulation of mediastinal air and fluid, often rupturing into one of the pleural spaces. Pneumomediastinum may be an isolated clinical finding or it may be associated with a pneumothorax or subcutaneous emphysema. Patients with iatrogenic pneumomediastinum may be asymptomatic, but symptoms of dyspnea, cough or cervical pain are not uncommon. The primary importance of the finding of pneumomediastinum is that it manifests a significant underlying injury and indicates that appropriate investigation must be undertaken. These investigations may include chest CT scans, contrast studies of the esophagus, or panendoscopy.

Pneumothorax

There are a variety of the iatrogenic causes of pneumothorax. These may include overly deep endotracheal suctioning, laceration of the trachea during intubation, penetration of the airway during endoscopy, high-pressure mechanical ventilation (Clinical Scenario 2), central venous catheter placement, or thoracentesis.

A small pneumothorax may be asymptomatic, but larger pneumothoraces usually present with ipsilateral chest pain, dyspnea, tachypnea, and oxygen desaturation. The severity of these symptoms will increase as the magnitude of the pneumothorax increases. Breath sounds from the ipsilateral chest will be diminished or absent and, with tension pneumothorax, the trachea will be shifted to the contralateral side in the suprasternal notch. Chest radiographs will show a collapsed lung and may show shift of the mediastinum.

Treatment of symptomatic pneumothorax requires immediate decompression. In the absence of a hemopneumothorax, this can be accomplished with a small

CLINICAL SCENARIO 2

Baby Boy P: This infant was the product of a 36-week gestation with little prenatal care. He was born with a precipitous vaginal delivery, and had Apgar scores of 3 and 6. He was noted to have meconium-stained amniotic fluid and meconium in the trachea, below the level of the vocal cords. The infant was intubated and surfactant was administered. Progressively higher peak inspiratory pressures and F_{IO_2} were required to adequately ventilate him. He was transferred to the University of Virginia for potential ECMO.

On arrival in the NICU he was noted to be in severe respiratory distress with transcutaneous oxygen saturation of 20%, being hand ventilated, with an F_{IO_2} of 1.00. Immediate radiograph demonstrated a tension left pneumothorax (Figure 40-2), undoubtedly secondary to the high peak inspiratory pressures required for ventilation during transport. Saturations immediately improved with chest tube placement. The patient was placed on the oscillating ventilator with progressively increasing Delta Ps.

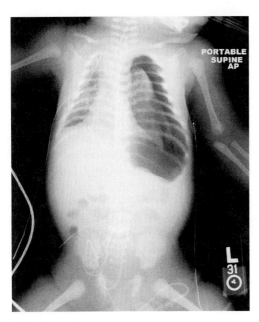

FIGURE 40-2

Eighteen hours later a second episode of acute respiratory deterioration occurred and a radiograph demonstrated massive pneumoperitoneum (Figure 40-3), treated with immediate placement of an intraperitoneal drain, with decompression. The patient was subsequently placed on ECMO for respiratory support. He was decannulated 6 days later and managed on a conventional ventilator until extubated.

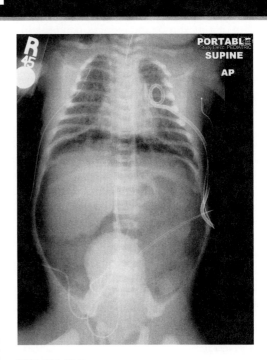

FIGURE 40-3

Question:
1. Extrathoracic causes of acute respiratory decompensation in an infant may include
   A. Obstruction of the endotracheal tube
   B. Massive pneumoperitoneum
   C. Gastric distension
   D. Ventilator malfunction
   E. All of the above

pigtail catheter (8 to 12 Fr), placed in the anterior second intercostal space. This catheter is connected to an underwater seal drainage system and may be connected to suction. Patients with a hemopneumothorax should receive a larger chest tube (16 to 24 Fr) to avoid clotting.

Endotracheal Suctioning

Iatrogenic airway injuries are known to occur as a consequence of overzealous endotracheal suctioning in young infants.[16] The suction catheter should be carefully measured and only passed down to the level of the end of the endotracheal tube in order to avoid direct tracheal or bronchial injury. The most common site of injury is in the medial-basal segment of the right lower lobe. This segmental bronchus is on a straight line beyond the end of the endotracheal tube, and catheters that are passed without attention to the depth will puncture the visceral pleura in this segment. A right pneumothorax is a consequence and an infant will develop sudden respiratory compromise. Since most of these patients are intubated and ventilated, air accumulates in the hemithorax quite rapidly. These patients should be treated with prompt placement of a chest tube and reduction in peak inspiratory pressure.

Esophageal-Pharyngeal Injuries
Nasogastric Tube Placement

Esophageal injuries from catheters usually occur during attempts to pass nasogastric tubes, but occasionally may be seen with vigorous postpartum suctioning to clear the posterior pharynx.[17] These injuries typically manifest with the finding of pneumomediastinum on chest radiograph, although pneumothorax, pleural effusion, or subcutaneous emphysema may also be present. If the tube has been left in place, it may be noted to be in the pleural space on chest radiograph. These injuries will almost uniformly heal spontaneously if the tube is removed and the patient is kept NPO. A chest tube is placed to evacuate a pneumothorax and intravenous antibiotics are administered.

Central Venous Pressure Catheter Placement

Central venous pressure (CVP) catheters have become a mainstay for pediatric patient care, particularly in young infants. Most of these catheters may be considered "temporary," in that they are expected to be used for only a few days and may be easily removed. More "permanent" central venous catheters may be expected to last for weeks or months if needed. These catheters typically are tunneled before entering the vein and have a Dacron cuff that is placed in midtunnel to allow tissue ingrowth and catheter fixation. Access to the venous system for placement of all of these catheters is typically accomplished by percutaneous puncture of one of the subclavian or internal jugular veins. A wire is then threaded through the needle under fluoroscopic control into the right heart and the catheters are passed over this wire to ensure intravascular placement. The vast majority of the iatrogenic injuries of this procedure occur with attempts to percutaneously access the vein and the most common complication is a pneumothorax.[18,19] Hemothorax can be seen from accidental arterial puncture; rarely, cardiac tamponade may be seen if the right atrium or ventricle is punctured by the catheter or the introducing sheath. Precautions that may minimize the frequency of these complications include an appreciation of the inherent risks of the procedure, familiarization with the anatomy of the region, and ensuring that the child is under appropriate sedation or anesthesia and does not move during placement. Fluoroscopic assistance in guiding the advancement of the wire is invaluable. Some operators have found real-time ultrasound to be helpful in accessing the vein. The development of hemody-namic or respiratory changes during the placement of a central catheter should prompt an evaluation for possible pneumothorax, hemothorax, hemopneumothorax, or even pericardial tamponade. Since the majority of these procedures are done with fluoroscopic control, immediate fluoroscopy of the chest can be helpful in making these diagnoses.

Intubation

Intubation injuries, although rare, can create life-threatening conditions, particularly in small infants. The predisposing factors include inappropriate use of a stylet, with the rigid stylet extending beyond the end of the endotracheal tube, or multiple attempts at intubation.[20] The injury usually occurs in the vallecula, posterior and lateral to the laryngeal opening, and the endotracheal tube may be advanced into the pleural space. The symptoms include significant respiratory decompensation as well as shift of the trachea to the contralateral side. Treatment should include immediate chest tube placement and withdrawal of the improperly placed endotracheal tube with control of the airway either through placement of a new endotracheal tube or a tracheostomy.

Endoscopy

Injury to the airway or the esophagus may occur as a consequence of bronchoscopy or esophagoscopy, with both rigid and flexible endoscopes. Injuries may be a consequence of penetration of the trachea or esophagus by the endoscope itself or perforation by injudicious use of biopsy or laser therapy.[21] The risks of injury increase if there is already an anatomic distortion of the trachea or esophagus, such as stricture or displacement. The injury may be suspected at the time of the procedure by the presence of unusual bleeding, or, more commonly, may be discovered afterward on a postprocedure radiograph or by the development of postprocedure symptoms. Risk of injury from endoscopic procedures can be reduced by avoiding passage of the instrument when resistance is met and ensuring that the lumen is visualized before the endoscope is advanced. The postprocedural chest radiograph should always be obtained to assess for the presence of pleural, mediastinal, or subcutaneous air.

Ventilator-Induced Injuries

Injuries from mechanical ventilation are not uncommon in the pediatric population. This is particularly true for infants who develop pulmonary disease from prematurity and those who have been ventilated for long periods of time.[22] Acute presentations of pneumothorax, pneumomediastinum, or subcutaneous emphysema may occur. These complications are usually accompanied by oxygen desaturation and possibly hemodynamic compromise. The mechanism of injury is usually secondary to alveolar overdistention, caused by high peak inspiratory pressures or tidal volume. These abnormalities are complicated by patchy areas of consolidation in these infants, allowing the airway pressure to be transmitted to the small volume of ventilated lung. Since tidal volumes are often calculated from body weight, premature babies are particularly prone to injuries secondary to the lower volume of lung and alveoli. Lung injury can be minimized by judicious use of respiratory settings, particularly keeping tidal volumes at the lowest effective level and peak inspiratory pressures low. Inability to safely ventilate with a standard ventilator may prompt the use of the oscillating ventilator to achieve adequate minute ventilation. These injuries are treated by placement of a chest tube and adjustment of ventilator settings to minimize continued injury. Pneumomediastinum and subcutaneous emphysema, if present, should resolve spontaneously and should not require aggressive treatment.

ASSESSMENT QUESTIONS

See Evolve Resources for the answers.

1. Paralysis o f the hemidiaphragm caused by birth trauma is secondary to
   A. Distortion of the thoracic spine during delivery
   B. Distortion of the cervical spine during delivery
   C. Direct rupture of the diaphragm with increased intrathoracic pressure during delivery
   D. Damage from obstetrical forceps
2. What is the most appropriate treatment for congenital chylothorax?
   A. Institution of a high-fat diet
   B. Intubation and ventilation with a high MAP
   C. Intubation and ventilation with a high PEEP
   D. Place NPO, with total parenteral nutrition
   E. Ligation of the thoracic duct at the base of the left neck
3. Children with penetrating thoracic trauma in the right anterior 7th intercostal space should have the following:
   A. Immediate thoracotomy and control of bleeding from the right lower lobe
   B. Chest CT scan
   C. Chest and abdominal CT scan
   D. Immediate bronchoscopy
   E. Immediate pericardiocentesis
4. Children with posttraumatic pneumothorax may exhibit which of the following symptoms?
   A. Dyspnea
   B. Chest pain
   C. Cough
   D. Hemoptysis
   E. All of the above

ASSESSMENT QUESTIONS—cont'd

5. What is the most common site for perforation of the aerodigestive tract with an endotracheal tube?
   A. Vallecula
   B. Posterior pharynx
   C. Proximal esophagus at the cricopharyngeus
   D. Posterior larynx immediately below the cords
   E. Cricothyroid membrane
6. What is the most common cause for pneumothorax as a consequence of central venous pressure catheter placement?
   A. Puncture of the pleura during passage of the guide wire
   B. Puncture of the pleura during passage of the vein dilator
   C. Puncture of the pleura during venous access
   D. Puncture of the pleura during passage of the peel-away sheath
   E. Puncture of the pleura during passage of the catheter
7. What is the most common site of visceral pleural injury with improper endotracheal suctioning?
   A. Medial basal segment of the left lower lobe
   B. Medial basal segment of the right lower lobe
   C. Medial segment of the right middle lobe
   D. Apical segment of the right upper lobe
   E. Lingula

References

1. Stafford PW, Harmon CM: Thoracic trauma in children, *Curr Opin Pediatr* 1993;5:325.
2. Nakaqawa H et al: Cervical emphysema secondary to pneumomediastinum as a complication of childbirth, *Ear Nose Throat J* 2003;82:948.
3. Schullinger JN: Birth Trauma, *Pediatr Clin NA* 1993;40:1351.
4. Rodgers BM, Hawks P: Bilateral Congenital Eventration of the Diaphragms: Successful Surgical Management, *J Ped Surg* 1986;21:858.
5. Johnstone DW, Ferns RH: Chylothorax. *Chest Surg Clin NA* 1994; 4:617-628.
6. Wolff AB et al: Treatment of refractory chylothorax with externalized pleuroperitoneal shunts in children, *Annals Thor Surg* 1999;68:1053.
7. Collins J: Chest wall trauma, *Jour Thor Imag* 2000;15:112.
8. Tsai FC et al: Blunt trauma with flail chest and penetrating aorta injury, *EurJ Cardiothorac Surg* 1999;16:374.
9. Bliss D, Silen M: Pediatric thoracic trauma, *Critical Care Med* 2002;30:S409.
10. Bickell WH et al: Immediate versus delayed fluid resuscitation for hypotensive patients with torso injuries, *NEJM* 1994;331:1105.
11. LeBlang SD, Dolich MO: Imaging of penetrating thoracic trauma, *Jour Thor Imag* 2000;15:128.
12. Mayberry JC: Imaging in thoracic trauma: the trauma surgeon's perspective, *J Thor Imag* 2000;15:76.

13. Barton ED: Tension pneumothorax, *Curr Opin Pulm Med* 1999;5:269.
14. Self ML et al: Nonoperative management of severe tracheobronchial injuries with positive end-expiratory pressure and low tidal volume ventilation, *J Trauma* 2005;59:1072.
15. Kern JA et al: Thoracoscopy: A potential role in the subacute management of patients with thoraco-abdominal trauma, *Chest* 1993;104:942.
16. Thakur A et al: Bronchial perforation after closed-tube endotracheal suction, *J Pediatr Surg* 2000;35:1353.
17. Sapin E et al: Iatrogenic pharyngo-esophageal perforation in premature infants, Eur J *Pediatr Surg* 2000;10:83.
18. Bagwell CE et al: Potentially lethal complications of central venous catheter placement, *J Pediatr Surg* 2000;35:709.
19. Flores JC et al: Complications of central venous catheterization in critically ill children, *Pediatr Crit Care Med* 2001;2:57.
20. Cordero AMG et al: Possible risk factors associated with moderate or severe airway injuries in children who underwent endotracheal intubation, *Pediatr Crit Care Med* 2004;5:364.
21. Redleaf MI, Fennessy JJ: Pneumomediastinum after rigid bronchoscopy, *Ann Otol Rhinol* Laryngol 1994;104:955.
22. Ricard JD et al: Ventilator-induced lung injury, *Curr Opin in Critical Care* 2000;8:12.

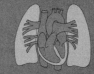

Chapter 41

Drowning in Children

KRISTINA H. DEETER • JOHN K. McGUIRE

OUTLINE

Incidence
Pathophysiology
    Central Nervous System Effects
    Pulmonary Effects
    Cardiovascular Effects
    Other Effects

Treatment
    At the Scene
    Emergency Department
    Inpatient
Outcome
Prevention

LEARNING OBJECTIVES

After reading this chapter the reader will be able to:
- Define drowning and other terms used to describe submersion injury
- Discuss the epidemiology of drowning and which groups of children are at highest risk
- Explain the pathophysiology of drowning and its effects on the various organ systems
- Describe treatment priorities for pediatric drowning victims in the field, at the emergency department, and as inpatients

- Discuss strategies for respiratory management of drowning victims
- Describe various factors that contribute to mortality and morbidity in drowning victims
- Discuss outcomes of drowning and predictors of good neurologic recovery
- Describe strategies for prevention of drowning in children

Drowning is a significant cause of childhood morbidity and mortality around the globe. In some countries, drowning is the first or second leading cause of death among children.[1] *Drowning* is the process of experiencing respiratory impairment from submersion/immersion in a liquid medium. Drowning outcomes are classified as death, morbidity, and no morbidity. Although historically many terms have been used to describe submersion events and subsequent morbidity, an international consensus conference was convened in 2002 in order to develop guidelines for definitions and reporting of data related to drowning.

This definition of drowning was adopted by the World Congress on Drowning and should be widely used.[2] It was also the consensus opinion that drowning without aspiration does not occur. Previously used terminology to describe alternative outcomes such as "dry," "wet," "secondary," and "near-drowning," have been discouraged in future research and publication.[3] Therefore, for the purposes of this discussion, we use the World Congress consensus term of "drowning" to refer to all forms of submersion injury leading to respiratory impairment, including nonfatal events that previously have been described as "near-drowning."

683

A drowning may be classified as "witnessed" when the episode is observed from onset, or "unwitnessed" if the victim is found in the water. *Immersion* is to be covered in water, that is, the face and airway are immersed in order for a drowning to occur. *Submersion* occurs when the entire body is under water.

Injuries may be further classified as cold-water or warm-water drowning. Warm-water drowning occurs at water temperatures of 20° C or higher, and cold-water drowning occurs at water temperatures of less than 20° C. Some references include very cold water drowning, which refers to submersion in water at temperatures of 5° C or less. Additional classification may include the type of water in which the submersion occurred, such as freshwater and saltwater drowning. The distinction between freshwater and saltwater drowning, however, is primarily academic, as initial treatment is not affected by water type.[4-6]

INCIDENCE

Worldwide estimates of drowning incidence indicate that approximately 500,000 such deaths occur yearly. According to the Centers for Disease Control and Prevention (Atlanta, GA), in 2005 there were 3582 fatal unintentional drownings in the United States, averaging 10 deaths per day.[7] More than one in four fatal drowning victims were children 14 years of age and younger. For every child who died of drowning, another four received emergency department (ED) care for nonfatal submersion injuries. During this year, males were four times more likely than females to die of an unintentional drowning episode. Reviewers estimate 8000 hospitalizations and more than 31,000 emergency department visits per year because of childhood immersion.[8] Hospitalization costs have been estimated at $23,000 per death and $7000 per survivor. In an extensive review of a national hospital database, total hospital costs for these patients in 2003 alone were close to $10 million.[9]

Many factors affect the exact nature and circumstances surrounding submersion events. The most extensive review of autopsied drowning cases was published in 2005 and covered a 20-year period in Canada.[10] In this review, the most common site of drowning was open water, followed by residential pools and bathtubs. The largest single group affected was male preschoolers. Factors implicated in drowning deaths included intoxication of victim or supervising adult, recreational boating, epilepsy, cervical spine injury after a high velocity dive, overestimation of swimming abilities, and hypothermia. Inadequate or lapsed supervision of infants and toddlers results in accidental submersion in bathtubs and other small amounts of water. These incidents should always raise suspicion of child abuse and neglect.[11] Drowning in

younger children is witnessed in less than 20% of cases, although more than 80% of victims are in the care of a responsible adult. Adolescent submersions have the highest mortality rate at about 70%, despite being witnessed by adolescent peers about 60% of the time.[12-15]

PATHOPHYSIOLOGY

The drowning process begins when the victim's airway moves below the surface of the liquid, at which time the victim has a period of voluntary apnea, or breath holding. This is usually followed by an involuntary period of laryngospasm secondary to the presence of liquid in the oropharynx or larynx. If immersion continues, the victim becomes hypercarbic, hypoxemic, and acidotic and begins to swallow large amounts of water. As the victim becomes more hypoxic, the laryngospasm relaxes, and the victim actively breathes in liquid. Aspiration of water leads to destruction of surfactant, impaired alveolar capillary gas exchange, intrapulmonary shunting, and pulmonary edema.[16,17] The ongoing hypoxia quickly produces unconsciousness, apnea, and finally cardiac arrest. The duration of this hypoxia and cardiac arrest is the primary determinant of outcome after a submersion injury.[8] Victims often become hypothermic, which leads to extravascular fluid shifts and renal diuresis resulting in increased fluid losses and decreased systemic perfusion. If the victim is not rescued early on in this continuum, multiple organ dysfunction will ensue, and death will result from tissue hypoxia.[16,17]

Central Nervous System Effects

CNS injury remains the major determinant of subsequent survival and long-term morbidity in cases of near drowning.[8,18] Primary CNS injury is initially associated with tissue hypoxia and ischemia. If the period of hypoxia and ischemia is brief or if the person is a very young child who rapidly develops core hypothermia, primary injury may be limited. The patient may actually recover with minimal neurologic sequelae.[19] Submersion injuries that are associated with prolonged hypoxia or ischemia, however, are likely to lead to both significant primary injury and secondary injury from reperfusion, sustained acidosis, cerebral edema, hyperglycemia, release of excitatory neurotransmitters, seizures, hypotension, and impaired cerebral autoregulation.[18]

Autonomic instability (diencephalic/hypothalamic storm) is common after severe traumatic, hypoxic, or ischemic brain injury, often presenting with signs and symptoms of hyperstimulation of the sympathetic nervous system (including tachycardia, hypertension, tachypnea, diaphoresis, agitation, and muscle rigidity).[18] CNS infection is an uncommon but serious complication of near drowning. Infection may result from unusual soil and waterborne bacteria and fungi and is usually insidious in onset, typically occurring more than 30 days after the initial submersion injury.[20]

Pulmonary Effects

Fluid aspiration of as little as 1 to 3 ml/kg can result in significantly impaired gas exchange and a decrease in compliance of 10% to 40%, primarily secondary to altered surfactant function.[5,21,22] Aspiration of either fresh- or saltwater can produce surfactant destruction, damage and blockage of alveolar–capillary gas exchange, and increased intrapulmonary shunt. This contributes to atelectasis, lower functional residual capacity, and pulmonary edema and ultimately leads to profound hypoxia. Hypoxia results in decreased cardiac output, arterial hypotension, and increased pulmonary arterial pressure and pulmonary vascular resistance.[21,23]

Acute respiratory distress syndrome (ARDS) from altered surfactant function and neurogenic pulmonary edema is a common complication among survivors of submersion injury.[8] Increased airway resistance secondary to plugging of the patient's airway with debris, as well as release of inflammatory mediators that result in vasoconstriction, also impair gas exchange. Ventilator-associated lung injury can further compromise noncompliant, edematous lung tissue. Pneumonia is a rare consequence of submersion injury and is more common with submersion in stagnant, warm, and fresh water. As with CNS infections, uncommon pathogens, including *Aeromonas, Burkholderia,* and *Pseudallescheria,* cause a disproportionate percentage of cases of pneumonia.[24]

Cardiovascular Effects

During the drowning event, aspiration of water produces a reflex pulmonary vasoconstriction as detailed previously with pulmonary hypertension and impaired cardiac output. Hypoxia and acidosis may lead to cardiac dysrhythmias and impaired myocardial function both at the time of the injury and later as the clinical course progresses. In a large review of out-of-hospital pediatric cardiac arrest it was noted that in drowning events asystole is the first recorded rhythm in 61% of patients, ventricular tachycardia or fibrillation in 20%, and bradycardia in 16%.[25] Pulmonary hypertension may result from the release of pulmonary inflammatory mediators, increasing right ventricular afterload and thus decreasing both pulmonary perfusion and left ventricular preload. Hypovolemia is primarily secondary to fluid losses from increased capillary permeability and hypothermia during the drowning episode. Profound hypotension may occur during and after the initial resuscitation period, especially when vasodilation occurs as the patient is rewarmed. Although

cardiovascular effects may be severe, if the victim is rescued during the event, they are usually transient, unlike severe CNS injury.

Other Effects

Differences in the fluid and electrolyte changes seen in saltwater submersion and freshwater submersion have been stressed in the past. The theory was that the hypertonicity of saltwater aspirated into the lung may cause an influx of fluid from the vascular space, resulting in intravascular volume depletion and hemoconcentration with hypernatremia.[4,5] Aspirated freshwater may have the opposite effect on fluid balance, producing volume overload, hyponatremia, and hemolysis due to decreased serum osmolality. This has been demonstrated in laboratory models experimentally, but more recent studies have shown that the volumes of fluid actually aspirated during human drowning are inadequate to produce these effects.[6,8,22,26,27] Most patients have fluid aspiration of less than 4 ml/kg.[5] Fluid aspiration of at least 11 ml/kg is required for alterations in blood volume to occur, and aspiration of more than 22 ml/kg is required before significant electrolyte changes develop.[26,27] Ingestion, rather than aspiration, is more likely to cause clinically significant electrolyte imbalances, including hyponatremia from ingestion of large volumes of fresh water (especially in children).[4,12,26,27]

The clinical course after a drowning episode may be complicated by multiorgan system failure resulting from prolonged hypoxia, acidosis, rhabdomyolysis, acute tubular necrosis, or infection or from the treatment modalities. Patients may also be at risk of disseminated intravascular coagulation, hepatic and renal insufficiency, metabolic acidosis, and gastrointestinal injuries and should be appropriately managed.[6,12]

TREATMENT

At the Scene

The most important point in treatment is the quality of resuscitation at the scene of a drowning event. Airway management and rescue breathing should begin before the victim is out of the water, if possible, and cardiopulmonary resuscitation (CPR) should be started as soon as an adequate surface is available. Care should be taken to stabilize the cervical spine if there is any risk of cervical spine injury (i.e., boating or diving accident). If the airway is not patent, standard maneuvers should be used to clear the airway. The Heimlich maneuver, however, should not be used to remove water from the lung.[28] Any efforts to remove water from the lungs, including the Heimlich maneuver, only delay initiation of effective rescue efforts. As soon as trained emergency personnel are available, more advanced techniques should be used, including endotracheal intubation, positive-pressure ventilation, intravenous access, and resuscitation drugs if needed. Hypoxia may be underrecognized, so 100% oxygen should be administered to all victims.

Rapid and appropriate response at the scene may result in the return of spontaneous heart rate and respirations; however, resuscitation is likely to be prolonged if hypoxia has been present for several minutes. Even if spontaneous respiration is restored, the need for continued assisted ventilation should be expected. The presence of hypothermia, hypoxia, and acidosis makes treatment of dysrhythmia more difficult and their recurrence more likely until these factors are corrected. Once a perfusing rhythm has been restored, inotrope and pressor therapy may be needed along with volume resuscitation.[16,22] Cardiac monitoring and management of dysrhythmia should be priorities. Hypothermia is difficult to reverse in the field, but every effort should be made to prevent further cooling during the resuscitation.

Emergency Department

In the emergency department (ED), stability of the airway and adequacy of ventilation should be assessed. The first priority for managing drowning victims is to reverse hypoxemia by restoring adequate oxygenation and ventilation. All victims should be assumed to be hypoxic, acidotic, and hypothermic. Arterial blood gas sampling reveals critical information regarding oxygenation, ventilation, and the severity of acidosis. An arterial line is often invaluable for management of severely affected victims. Electrolytes, blood urea nitrogen, creatinine, and hemoglobin should also be serially monitored.

Indications for intubation include rising arterial carbon dioxide pressure ($Paco_2$; >35 mm Hg), a ratio of arterial oxygen pressure to inspired fraction oxygen (Pao_2:Fio_2) less than 300, arterial oxygen saturation (Sao_2) less than 90%, or tachypnea (compared to normal respiratory rate for age). It is also common for drowning victims to have swallowed a large amount of water and therefore be at high risk of vomiting.[29] Unconscious patients or those with respiratory compromise should be intubated by a rapid sequence induction technique using minimal bag–mask ventilation. Mechanical ventilation with the use of a cuffed endotracheal tube is the most effective method for reversing hypoxemia and preventing further aspiration. Aspiration of liquid, development of pulmonary edema, and decreased lung compliance may make effective ventilation difficult. Positive end-expiratory pressure should be initiated at 5 cm H_2O and increased in 2- to 3-cm H_2O increments to 15 cm H_2O as cardiac output and blood pressure allow.[22]

If ventilation is adequate, treatment of metabolic acidosis with tromethamine (THAM) or sodium bicarbonate is advisable. Cardiac dysrhythmias should continue to be treated but may be refractory in the presence of significant hypothermia. Tissue perfusion and blood pressure should be assessed to determine the adequacy of cardiac output. Intravascular volume expansion is often necessary in the presence of postarrest myocardial dysfunction, and inotrope and vasopressor therapy should be used if indicated, often necessitating placement of a central line.

Some degree of hypothermia (core temperature less than 35° C) is almost always present after a significant submersion, and severe hypothermia is associated with characteristic physical examination findings (Box 41-1). The goals of management are to prevent a further fall in core temperature and establish a safe and steady rewarming rate while maintaining cardiovascular stability. The health care team should attempt to rewarm the patient 1° C to 2° C per hour to a range of 33° C to 36° C.[30] Aggressive rewarming above this range should be avoided as hyperthermia has been shown to worsen underlying cerebral injury in postcardiac arrest patients.[31] When warming is attempted, cardiac dysrhythmia, electrolyte abnormalities, and hypotension due to vasodilation should be anticipated. Increasing core body temperature is the goal, and simple warming of the skin surface alone should be avoided. Warmed intravenous fluid and ventilator gases should be used.

Box 41-1	Key Findings at Various Degrees of Hypothermia
Temperature (° C)*	**Clinical Findings**
37	Normal oral temperature
36	Metabolic rate increased
35	Maximum shivering seen/impaired judgment
33	Severe clouding of consciousness
32	Most shivering ceases and pupils dilate
31	Blood pressure may no longer be obtainable
28-30	Severe slowing of pulse/respiration
	Increased muscle rigidity
	Loss of consciousness
	Ventricular fibrillation
27	Loss of deep tendon, skin, and capillary reflexes
	Patients appear clinically dead
	Complete cardiac standstill

*As documented by low-registering thermometer.
Data from Weinberg AD: Hypothermia, *Ann Emerg Med* 1993;22:370.

Irrigation of the stomach, urinary bladder, and peritoneal cavity with warmed saline is effective and relatively low risk. Irrigation of the pleural space with warmed saline has the advantage of warming the central circulation but may compromise ventilation and oxygenation. Extracorporeal bypass is the most effective means of increasing body temperature for patients presenting with temperature less than 28° C, and in some cases this technique should be considered early in the course of management, although evidence of success in the pediatric population has not been thoroughly studied to date.[32] An algorithm for initial resuscitation is presented in Figure 41-1.

Victims evaluated in the ED who are minimally affected with no history of loss of consciousness, no altered mental status, and no respiratory signs and symptoms may be observed for a period of hours in the ED and discharged home if no complications arise. Patients with any degree of respiratory compromise, history of need for rescue breathing, or loss of consciousness should be admitted to the hospital even if stable in the ED, because both neurologic injury and lung injury may progress over the first hours to days.[19]

Inpatient

For victims requiring admission to the hospital, intensive care unit (ICU) treatment is primarily supportive. Most ICU patients will require invasive monitoring with a central venous catheter, an arterial line, a nasogastric tube (to prevent further aspiration), and a Foley catheter (to monitor urine output). Neurologic injury is the most serious consequence of submersion injury and should be the focus of care. In more severely affected victims, progression of cerebral edema with resultant increased intracranial hypertension (ICP) should be anticipated through the first 3 to 5 days. Seizures and fever may occur and should be aggressively treated as both will exacerbate ICP. Although cerebral edema is a common consequence of prolonged submersion (or submersion followed by prolonged circulatory insufficiency), retrospective reviews and animal studies have not demonstrated any benefit from the use of intracranial pressure monitoring with diffuse axonal injury.[33-35] Therefore, as with any hypoxic brain injury, ICP monitoring and aggressive pressure-directed therapy for drowning victims is not recommended.[34,35]

Basic measures to decrease ICP should be employed (Box 41-2). In patients who have a functional recovery, a slow return of neurologic function occurs over weeks to months as the cerebral edema resolves.

Fever and chest radiograph changes should be expected early in the chemical course of submersion injury. Lung infiltrates, fever, and leukocytosis are common after submersion injury and do not necessarily indicate an infectious pneumonia. It has been widely studied and accepted that early or prophylactic treatment with antibiotics increases the likelihood of later infection with resistant organisms and is therefore discouraged.[5,24] If strong evidence of bacterial pneumonia develops, such as persistent fever, evolving focal infiltrates on chest radiograph, or positive bacterial cultures for likely organisms, then antibiotic therapy should be tailored to treat those organisms most likely in this setting or those found in bacterial culture. Foreign bodies should be suspected if lung changes are focal or if segmental air trapping is present. Bronchoscopy may be indicated in order to evaluate and remove foreign bodies.

Pulmonary edema and ARDS may progress rapidly in the first 24 hours and complicate management, but as with most causes of ARDS, the patient usually responds to careful and aggressive respiratory management. Acute respiratory distress in the context of submersion injury is managed as in any other setting. Adequate positive end-expiratory pressure (PEEP) is the key element of the ventilator strategy, along with minimizing tidal volume and peak inspiratory pressure to reduce the risk of secondary lung injury.[22,24] PEEP should be increased from 5 cm H_2O with the goal of a Pao_2:Fio_2 ratio of 300 or more. The level of PEEP or continuous positive airway pressure needed to maintain oxygenation should be continued for 24 to 48 hours before attempting to decrease it in order to permit adequate surfactant regeneration. To minimize oxygen toxicity, the delivered Fi_{O_2} should also be reduced to 50% or less as tolerated. Newer modes of ventilation, including high-frequency oscillatory ventilation and airway pressure release ventilation, may support ventilation and oxygenation with less risk of ventilator-associated lung injury than is associated with older methods of ventilation. Use of artificial surfactant is usually not indicated in ARDS caused by drowning. Although providing temporary improvement in lung function in many reports, surfactant most likely does not change outcome and is an ongoing focus of investigation.[16] There is also no specific indication for early use of corticosteroids in submersion injury.

Myocardial dysfunction requiring inotropic support may persist for days after a significant hypoxic insult.[2] Recurrent dysrhythmia may also occur but is less likely after the initial hypothermia, acidosis, and hypoxia are corrected. Although it is not especially common in submersion injury, acute renal failure and other organ dysfunction may occur after cardiac arrest from any cause and may require any level of support, including hemodialysis or continuous venovenous hemofiltration and dialysis.

As the patient becomes more stable, early involvement of physical and occupational therapy is appropriate. The need for extensive rehabilitation is common.

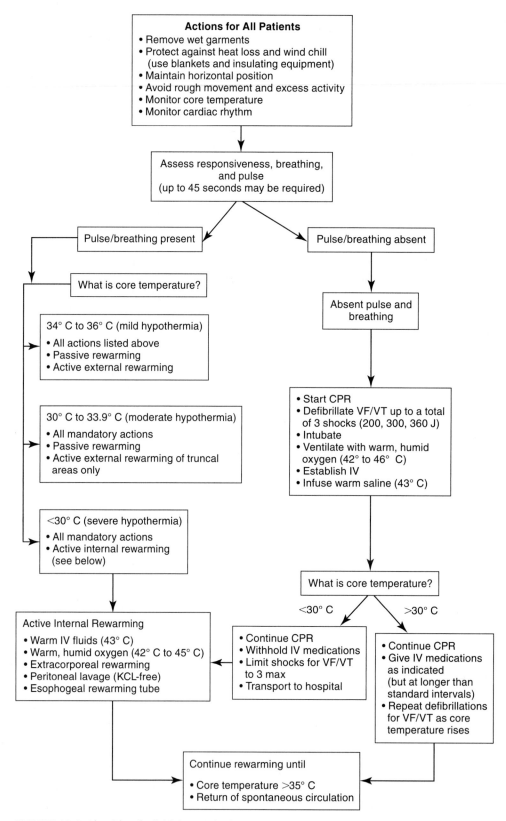

FIGURE 41-1 Algorithm for initial resuscitation.

Box 41-2	Initial Strategies to Control Intracranial Hypertension

1. Elevate the head 15° to 30°.
2. Maintain the head in the midline.
3. Avoid hypercarbia.
4. Ensure adequate blood pressure and oxygenation.
5. Provide adequate sedation and analgesia.
6. Avoid volume overload and hypovolemia.
7. Avoid hyperglycemia.

Data from Weinberg AD: Hypothermia, *Ann Emerg Med* 1993;22:370.

Attention to the emotional and social needs of the parents is also important. Anger and guilt are common because most submersions are preventable accidents. Family dysfunction should be anticipated and appropriate referral made when needed.

OUTCOME

The topic of outcome fits comfortably at the end of most clinical discussions. With submersion injury, however, outcome may have been more appropriately discussed first. As with any condition that includes hypoxic–ischemic brain injury as a primary part of its pathology, submersion injury has a tragically poor prognosis. It is within the context of this poor prognosis that decisions and management plans are made. A frequent question is, "How far should treatment go?" Much of the most recently published literature on submersion injury attempts to answer this difficult question.

Traditionally, all critically ill patients, including submersion victims, are approached with aggressive resuscitation and life support so that each potential survivor has the best chance of eventual recovery. This minimizes the risk of allowing a potential survivor to die because maximal support has been withdrawn. This approach, however, also ensures that many patients whose best possible outcome is persistent vegetative state will also survive. As early resuscitation is associated with improved outcomes, many studies have attempted to determine clinical, laboratory, or other variables to identify which patients would benefit from resuscitative efforts.[36,37] Although no individual characteristics have been found to predict survivability, the Orlowski score is an example of an attempt to identify the likelihood of neurologically intact survival.[37] In using the Orlowski score, one point is given for each item; scores of two or less are associated with a 90% likelihood of complete recovery, and submersion-injury patients with scores of three or more have only a 5% chance of survival. The items in the Orlowski score are as follows:

- Age 3 years or older
- Submersion time of more than 5 minutes
- No resuscitative efforts for more than 10 minutes after rescue
- Comatose on admission to the emergency department
- Arterial pH of less than 7.10

Habib and colleagues[38] predicted outcome in a retrospective case series. Patients arriving in the ED comatose and pulseless had a uniformly poor outcome, whereas those with a pulse and blood pressure in the ED completely recovered. In addition, patients who remained comatose longer than 200 minutes had poor outcomes, and those who were not comatose had normal recovery. A 48-hour period of observation in the pediatric ICU, in addition to the variables seen in the first hours after submersion, may improve our ability to predict outcome. Reliably predicting which patients will experience which outcome early in the clinical course would be helpful in counseling families regarding prognosis and in making decisions about initiating or withdrawing expensive or limited therapeutic resources.

The neuroprotective effects of cold-water drowning are poorly understood. We know that hypothermia profoundly decreases the cerebral metabolic rate. Neuroprotective effects seem to occur only if the hypothermia occurs at the time of submersion and only if rapid cooling occurs in water with a temperature of less than 5° C.[31,34,39] Intact survival of comatose patients after cold-water submersion injuries still is quite uncommon. Anecdotal reports of survival exist for children with moderate hypothermic submersion (core temperature <32° C), but most persons experiencing cold-water submersion do not develop hypothermia rapidly enough to decrease cerebral metabolism before severe, irreversible hypoxia and ischemia occur.[39]

PREVENTION

Submersion events and death from drowning are, in most cases, preventable. A majority of victims are young, previously healthy people. There have been no recent breakthroughs in medical technology or treatment modalities that have improved survival rates for submersion victims. As with all accidental injuries, prevention is the only effective means of reducing morbidity and mortality. This is especially true of submersion injury because outcomes are often poor regardless of therapy.[35] Health care workers can play a major role in educating the public as a whole and individual patients and families. Efforts to prevent deaths from drowning are appropriately focused on improved supervision, proper fencing around pools, and CPR training. Children and adults should be instructed never to swim alone or unsupervised. A recent Cochrane Library review demonstrated that isolation fencing (self-closing latched gate around the pool) is superior to perimeter fencing (enclosing the house and yard together).[40] Pool alarms and covers have not been shown to prevent drowning. Lowering rates of alcohol use around bodies of water and educating parents on the importance of constant supervision of children in the bathtub are also important. Submersion injuries may even occur in toilets and water buckets.[11,13,14] Appropriate measures must be taken to ensure that children are never unsupervised in bathrooms, and water buckets must be emptied when not in use. Training families in CPR may decrease the duration of hypoxia experienced by a submersion victim. Infant swimming or water-adjustment programs do not prevent submersion injuries and are potentially hazardous, providing parents with a false sense of security if they believe their infant can swim.[14]

ASSESSMENT QUESTIONS

See Evolve Resources for answers.

1. The 2002 World Congress on Drowning consensus statement defines drowning as:
   A. Death from asphyxia caused by submersion in water.
   B. The process of experiencing respiratory impairment from submersion in a liquid medium.
   C. A witnessed episode of submersion.
   D. Respiratory injury occurring when the whole body is under water.
2. Males are how many times more likely to die of unintentional drowning than females?
   A. No difference
   B. Two
   C. Four
   D. Ten
3. The primary determinant of neurologic outcome after submersion injury is:
   A. Duration of hypoxia and cardiac arrest
   B. Duration of submersion in water
   C. Temperature of water in which victim was immersed/submerged
   D. Volume of water aspirated into the lungs
4. The major determinant of subsequent survival and long-term morbidity in drowning is:
   A. Initial body temperature
   B. Severity of electrolyte abnormalities
   C. Extent of central nervous system injury
   D. Presence of multiorgan system failure

ASSESSMENT QUESTIONS—cont'd

5. Priorities in initial management of the drowning victim in the field include:
   A. Prompt initiation of airway management, rescue breathing, and CPR
   B. Stabilization of the cervical spine
   C. Administration of 100% oxygen when available
   D. Prevention of progressive hypothermia
   E. All of the above.
6. Patients with hypothermia after submersion should be aggressively rewarmed to 37° C as soon as possible:
   A. True
   B. False
7. Indications that stable patients should be hospitalized after submersion injury include all of the following *except*:
   A. History of loss of consciousness
   B. Persistent respiratory signs and symptoms
   C. History of need for rescue breathing
   D. Emesis at the scene
8. Ventilator management for respiratory disease caused by submersion injury includes which of the following strategies:
   A. Aggressive hyperventilation
   B. Judicious use of PEEP
   C. Maintenance of F_{IO_2} above 50% to increase oxygen delivery to the brain
   D. Rapid reduction in PEEP when gas exchange improves
9. Proven therapies to improve outcome in near drowning include:
   A. Surfactant replacement
   B. Therapeutic hypothermia
   C. Corticosteroid therapy
   D. Prophylactic antibiotic therapy
   E. None of the above
10. The initial arterial blood pH at the time of admission reliably predicts long-term neurologic outcome in drowning victims:
    A. True
    B. False

References

1. Smith G: Global burden of drowning, presented at the World Congress on Drowning, June 26-28, 2002, Amsterdam, The Netherlands.
2. Bierens JJLM, editor: *Handbook on drowning: prevention, rescue, treatment*, Amsterdam: Springer; 2005. Available at http://www.drowning.nl. Retrieved October 2008.
3. Idris AH et al: Recommended guidelines for uniform reporting of data from drowning: the "Utstein style," *Circulation* 2003;108:2565.

4. Modell JH: Serum electrolyte changes in near-drowning victims, *JAMA* 1985;253:253.
5. Harries MG: Drowning in man, *Crit Care Med* 1981;9:407.
6. Modell JH: Drowning, *N Engl J Med* 1993;328:253.
7. National Center for Injury Prevention and Control, Centers for Disease Control and Prevention: Web-based Injury Statistics Query and Reporting System (WISQARS) [online]. Available at www.cdc.gov/ncipc/wisqars. Retrieved October 2008.
8. Orlowski JP: Drowning, near-drowning and ice-water submersions, *Pediatr Clin North Am* 1987;34:75.
9. Cohen RH et al: Unintentional pediatric submersion-injury–related hospitalizations in the United States, 2003, *Inj Prev* 2008;14:131.
10. Somers GR et al: Pediatric drowning: a 20-year review of autopsied cases. I. Demographic features, *Am J Forensic Med* 2005;26:316.
11. Lavelle JM et al: Ten-year review of pediatric bathtub near-drownings: evaluation for child abuse and neglect, *Ann Emerg Med* 1995;25:344.
12. DeNicola LK et al: Submersion injuries in children and adults, *Crit Care Clin* 1997;13:477.
13. Quan L et al: Ten-year study of pediatric drownings and near-drownings in King County, Washington, *Pediatrics* 1989;83:1035.
14. Wintemute GJ: Childhood drowning and near-drowning in the United States, *Am J Dis Child* 1990;144:663.
15. Brenner RA, Committee on Injury, Violence, and Poison Prevention: Prevention of drowning in infants, children, and adolescents, *Pediatrics* 2003;112:440.
16. Bierens JJ et al: Drowning, *Curr Opin Crit Care* 2002;8:578.
17. Levin DL et al: Drowning and near-drowning, *Pediatr Clin North Am* 1993;40:321.
18. Miyamoto O, Auer RN: Hypoxia, hyperoxia, ischemia, and brain necrosis, *Neurology* 2000;54:362.
19. Causey AL et al: Predicting discharge in uncomplicated near-drowning, *Am J Emerg Med* 2000;18:9.
20. Leroy P, Smismans A, Seute T: Invasive pulmonary and central nervous system aspergillosis after near-drowning of a child: case report and review of the literature, *Pediatrics* 2006;118:e509.
21. Giamona ST, Modell JH: Drowning by total immersion, effects on pulmonary surfactant of distilled water, isotonic saline and sea water, *Am J Dis Child* 1967;114:612.
22. Orlowski JP, Szpilman D: Drowning: rescue, resuscitation, and reanimation, *Pediatr Clin North Am* 2001;48:627.
23. Karch SB: Pathology of the lung in near drowning, *Am J Emerg Med* 1980;4:4.
24. Ender PT, Dolan MJ: Pneumonia associated with near-drowning, *Clin Infect Dis* 1997;25:896.
25. Donoghue AJ et al: Out-of-hospital pediatric cardiac arrest: an epidemiologic review and assessment of current knowledge, *Ann Emerg Med* 2005;46:512.
26. Modell JH, May F: Effects of volume aspirated fluid during chlorinated fresh water drowning, *Anesthesiology* 1966;27:662.
27. Modell JH, Davis JH: Electrolyte changes in human drowning victims, *Anesthesiology* 1969;30:414.
28. Rosen P, Stoto M, Harley J: The use of the Heimlich maneuver in near drowning: Institute of Medicine report, *J Emerg Med* 1995;13:397.
29. Manolios N, Mackie I: Drowning and near-drowning on Australian beaches patrolled by life-savers: a 10-year study, 1973-1983, *Med J Aust* 1988;148:165, 170.
30. Nolan JP et al: Therapeutic hypothermia after cardiac arrest: an advisory statement by the Advancement Life support Task Force of the International Liaison Committee on Resuscitation, *Resuscitation* 2003;57:231.
31. Hickey RW et al: Hypothermia and hyperthermia in children after resuscitation from cardiac arrest, *Pediatrics* 2000;106:118.
32. International Liaison Committee on Resuscitation, American Heart Association: Guidelines for cardio-pulmonary resuscitation and emergency cardiovascular care—an international consensus on science, *Resuscitation* 2000;46:3.
33. Sarnaik AP et al: Intracranial pressure and cerebral perfusion pressure in near-drowning, *Crit Care Med* 1985;13:224.
34. Bohn DJ et al: Influence of hypothermia, barbiturate therapy, and intracranial pressure monitoring on morbidity and mortality after near-drowning, *Crit Care Med* 1986;14:529.
35. Spack L et al: Failure of aggressive therapy to alter outcome in pediatric near-drowning, *Pediatr Emerg Med* 1997;13:98.
36. Graf WD et al: Predicting outcome in pediatric submersion victims, *Ann Emerg Med* 1995;26:312.
37. Orlowski JP: Prognostic factors in pediatric cases of drowning and near-drowning, *JACEP* 1979;8:176.
38. Habib DM et al: Near-drowning: morbidity and mortality, *Pediatr Emerg Med* 1996;12:255.
39. Corneli HM: Hot topics in cold medicine: controversies in accidental hypothermia, *Clin Ped Emerg Med* 2001;2:179.
40. Thompson DC, Rivara FP: Pool fencing for preventing drowning in children, *Cochrane Database Syst Rev* 1998;1:CD001047.

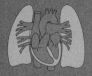

Chapter **42**

Pediatric Poisoning

KATHLEEN D. BONGIOVANNI

LEARNING OBJECTIVES

After reading this chapter the reader will be able to:

- Define intentional poisoning and describe associated risk factors
- Define unintentional poisoning and describe associated risk factors
- Describe common methods of poison diagnosis
- Identify the three main goals of poison exposure management
- Describe the various routes of gastrointestinal decontamination and explain the pros and cons of each

- List the top 10 substances involved in young child poison exposures
- Identify several common poisoning agents that are associated with adverse clinical outcomes
- Describe the causes and risk factors associated with several common poisoning agents
- Describe the clinical manifestations of several common poisoning agents
- Describe and analyze the routes of decontamination and treatment associated with several common poisoning agents

EPIDEMIOLOGY

All substances are poisons; there is none which is not a poison. The right dose differentiates a poison from a remedy.

—*Paracelsus (1493-1541)[1]*

In 2006, the American Association of Poison Control Centers (Alexandria, Va) reported more than 2.4 million cases of poison exposure and 1229 fatalities. Of the 2.4 million poison exposures, 64.3% occurred in the pediatric population (defined as patients under the age of 20 years), and 50.9% occurred in children under the age of 6 years. Exposures in children less than 13 years of age were predominantly male, with females making up the majority of poison exposures among children aged 13 to 19 years. Although the majority of poison exposures occurred in children, most of the fatalities occurred in adults, with children younger than 6 years compromising only 2.4% of the verified fatalities.[2] The lack of correlation between poison exposure and resulting fatality highlights the unique nature of pediatric poisoning, and can be explained by the differences in poison consumption and exposure between children, adolescents, and adults.

There are two general categories of poison exposure: accidental and intentional. Accidental or unintentional poisoning most frequently occurs in children less than 6 years of age (60.6% of unintentional exposures), and represented 83.4% of total poison exposure for all age groups in 2006.[2] Unintentional poison exposure in children less than 19 years of age resulted in only 2.6% of the 1229 total fatalities in 2006, possibly because unintentional poison exposures in children generally involve only a single substance and victims are brought in for medical treatment earlier than intentional poisoning victims.[2-4] Unintentional poison exposures can be broken down into several categories: unintentional misuse, such as oral exploration by a young child; therapeutic error, such as a miscalculation of drug dose; animal bites and stings; environmental exposure, which includes plant poisonings and the presence of heavy metals in the environment; occupational exposures, which are associated with a caregiver's use of industrial cleaning products or pesticides; and food poisoning.

Intentional poisoning represents only 12.8% of total poison exposure, yet results in 71.3% of total poison fatalities, and more frequently involves multiple substances and a delay in seeking medical treatment.[2,4] Intentional exposures occur most frequently in adults (69.5% of intentional exposures took place in adults less than 19 yr old) and adolescents (25.9% of intentional exposures took place in adolescents aged 13 to 19 yr). Intentional poison exposures can be broken down into three categories: suspected suicide, intentional misuse, and intentional abuse. It is important to note that of the 49 intentional exposure fatalities reported in the adolescent age group in 2006, 53.1% were classified as suspected suicide. In some cases of unintentional poisoning in children, it is appropriate to manage symptoms and treatment at home through consultation with a Poison Control Center (1-800-222-1222 in the United States) without admitting the victim to a health care facility.[5,6] However, if a suicide attempt is suspected it is always recommended to take the individual to a hospital for treatment and evaluation.

The addition of child-resistant packaging to containers of hazardous substances became widespread after the Poison Prevention Packaging Act was enacted in 1970. The effort succeeded in reducing the fatality rate due to childhood poisoning from 2.0/100,000 children to 0.5/100,000 children; however, unintentional poison exposures still pose a significant threat to children today.[7] The main route of poison exposure is through ingestion (77.1%), and ingestion accounts for 75.3% of fatal poisonings.[2] Features that make a substance a potential risk for accidental ingestion in the pediatric population are as follows:

- Bright and colorful
- Similar appearance to candy or other familiar safe substances
- Good smell or taste
- Easy access, such as storage under the kitchen counter

There are numerous reasons why unintentional poisoning, especially of children 3 years of age and less, continues to persist. These can include the tendency for parents to rely on packaging that may be child-resistant but not child-proof, as well as parents who base their level of caution and prevention efforts in the home on the child's previous behaviors and skill levels.[8,9]

GENERAL MANAGEMENT

Although there are ways to limit the harm that some poison exposures can cause, for many poisons the only currently available treatment is supportive care. For this reason the primary goal of any treatment regimen is stabilization of the respiratory and cardiovascular systems, ranging from simple monitoring to a full resuscitation. Good venous access is necessary for drug and fluid administration in any patient who has ingested a toxic substance. Formal weight measurement is also important to avoid treatment errors related to dosing. Information regarding the dose and type of poison is an important component for determining proper clinical care. Infants and young children cannot always provide this information; therefore a thorough history from the parents or guardians is extremely valuable.

The use of common toxidromes may aid clinicians in poison exposure diagnosis; however, pediatric poison exposures do not closely mirror those of the adult population, so classical toxidromes may be of limited use.[2,3] Table 42-1 details some of the toxidromes that have been applied successfully in the treatment of pediatric patients. Toxicologic screening may aid in poison diagnosis. Laboratory tests that are frequently obtained include the following[10]:

- Serum glucose and electrolyte levels
- Blood gas analysis
- Anion gap calculations
- Renal and hepatic function tests

These tests are helpful when evaluating the response to various management strategies during the treatment course.

Once hemodynamic and respiratory stabilization has been achieved, the main goals[11] are as follows:

TABLE 42-1

Toxidromes

Possible Toxin	Clinical Manifestations
Anticholinergics	Agitation, hallucinations, dilated pupils, dry skin, flushed color
Opiates	Bradypnea, pinpoint pupils, coma
Organophosphates	Salivation, urination, lacrimation, pulmonary congestion
Tricyclic antidepressants	Coma, convulsions, cardiac arrhythmias
Salicylates	Vomiting, fever, hyperpnea
Barbiturates	Sleepiness, slurred speech
Tranquilizers	Ataxia (without alcohol on breath)

Modified from Mofenson HC, Greensher J: The unknown poison, *Pediatrics* 1974;54:336.

• Limit further drug absorption
• Enhance elimination
• Manage the complications

These maneuvers have variable success; thus the most important therapy is still continued respiratory, cardiovascular, and neurologic support.[12] Initial decontamination consists of removing any remaining agent from the child's skin and mouth. This includes removing all chemical- or toxin-saturated clothing. It is important to appropriately train emergency department staff in the use of personal protective equipment to avoid contaminating health care personnel during the decontamination process. Further toxin absorption can be limited by gastrointestinal decontamination through the removal or dilution of gastric contents and the use of gastric adsorptive agents. Figure 42-1 shows a gastrointestinal decontamination (GID) decision tree that may aid in the process of deciding which, if any, method of decontamination to use on a pediatric patient.

Syrup of Ipecac

The administration of ipecac syrup induces forced vomiting and used to be a standard treatment for poison ingestion; however, syrup of ipecac is no longer an accepted part of routine acute poisoning treatment in the emergency department.[13] Studies have shown that there is little clinical benefit gained from the administration of syrup of ipecac, and emesis may delay other, more effective decontamination procedures.[14-16] It may still play a small role in prehospital management of severe poison exposure when there are no contraindications to the use of ipecac (decreased level of consciousness, convulsions, and ingestion of hydrocarbons or other caustic agents), if it can be administered within 30 minutes of poison ingestion, and there is no alternative therapy or a hospital is more than 60 minutes away.[13] For the most part, syrup of ipecac should not play a role in the treatment of poison exposures, and the American Academy of Pediatrics (Elk Grove Village, Ill) recommends that syrup of ipecac currently in homes be disposed of.[17]

Gastric Lavage

Gastric lavage is the mechanical removal of gastric contents via suction through a nasogastric or orogastric tube. Gastric lavage, like syrup of ipecac, is no longer recommended in the routine treatment of poisoned patients.[13,18] It is associated with procedural risks such as aspiration (especially hydrocarbons), and less common complications include esophageal and gastric perforation. It is limited in the amount of drug recovered, may not remove solid matter such as undissolved pills, shows little evidence of improved outcomes, and may be psychologically harmful.[18]

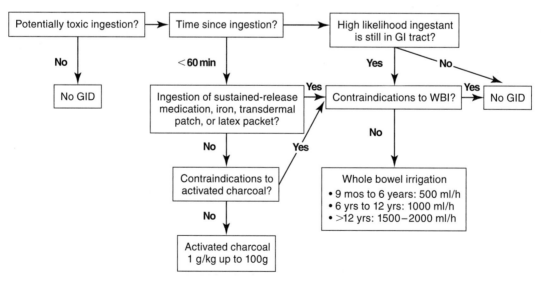

FIGURE 42-1 Gastrointestinal decontamination (GID) decision tree.

Activated Charcoal

Activated charcoal is highly adsorptive and is commonly administered in single or multiple doses, usually in slurry form. Single-dose activated charcoal is the most commonly used gastrointestinal decontamination method used today.[2] In addition to binding the toxin in the stomach, it is useful in absorbing drugs that undergo enterohepatic recirculation, and in these cases multiple-dose activated charcoal treatment may be more appropriate.[19] Charcoal administration is time sensitive and its ability to reduce gastrointestinal absorption is reduced 1 hour postingestion.[14,20] Charcoal is relatively safe, but complications include vomiting, diarrhea, constipation, and aspiration. The main contraindication to its use is the presence of any form of gastrointestinal obstruction. Activated charcoal will not adsorb well to any of the following: alcohols, hydrocarbons, organic solvents, caustic agents, iron, cyanide, heavy metals, and potassium.[3,11]

Cathartic Agents

The only cathartic agent currently used is sorbitol, and it is used only in conjunction with other therapies. Sorbitol is an osmotically active agent that causes diarrhea and may improve the palatability of activated charcoal as well as prevent constipation stemming from activated charcoal administration; however, its use is not routinely recommended. Contraindications include abdominal trauma or obstruction, electrolyte imbalance, and compromised airway reflexes or potential aspiration.[13,21]

Whole-bowel Irrigation

Whole-bowel irrigation with polyethylene glycol electrolyte solution (such as GoLYTELY or Colyte) involves the administration of large amounts of fluid in a short time frame and results in bowel cleansing. There is no conclusive evidence that whole-bowel irrigation improves clinical outcome on poison exposure, and it is not recommended as a routine procedure.[22] It offers no benefit when ingested poisons are rapidly absorbed; however, whole-bowel irrigation may aid in the clearance of sustained-release medications and metals such as iron, lead, and lithium. Bowel irrigation may be effective when activated charcoal is not, as with iron, lead, and lithium; transdermal patches; and latex packets containing drugs.[13]

Other Decontamination Methods

Methods to enhance toxin elimination include alteration of urinary pH, hemodialysis, hemofiltration, hemoperfusion, and the use of specific drug antagonists that either block the drug at its site of action or enhance its elimination from the circulation.[3,11] Forced diuresis is no longer a recommended method for toxin elimination as its clinical benefit has not been supported and it can lead to electrolyte imbalances, pulmonary edema, and increased intracranial pressure. Some toxins are more readily soluble and excreted in alkaline solutions (e.g., salicylates and phenobarbital). In these situations, administering sodium bicarbonate alkalinizes the urine to a pH of 7 to 8.[11] Hemodialysis, hemoperfusion, and peritoneal dialysis remove toxins across either a membrane gradient or an adsorptive surface. Drugs that are more amenable to extracorporeal removal have a small molecular size, low lipid solubility, low levels of protein binding, and a low volume of distribution.[23] The effectiveness of these therapies is highly dependent on the specific characteristics of the ingested substance, and because of potential complications they are appropriate only in situations of serious toxicity.[10]

There are also several antibodies and antidotes available for some toxins. These include the following: atropine, pralidoxime, and benzodiazepines for nerve gas exposure; N-acetylcysteine for acetaminophen overdose; CroFab for snake bites; fomepizole for methanol and ethylene glycol poisoning; and naloxone for opioid overdose.[24,25]

COMMON POISONING AGENTS

The top 10 substances involved in child and adult poison exposures can be seen in Table 42-2. These numbers highlight common poison exposures, not fatalities, and

TABLE 42-2		
Top Ten Substances Involved in Poison Exposure		
Rank	Children ≤ 5 yr	Adults > 19 yr
1	Cosmetics/personal care products	Analgesics
2	Household cleaning substances	Sedatives/hypnotics/antipsychotics
3	Analgesics	Household cleaning substances
4	Foreign objects/toys/miscellaneous	Antidepressants
5	Topical preparations	Bites and envenomations
6	Cold and cough preparations	Cardiovascular drugs
7	Vitamins	Alcohols
8	Pesticides	Pesticides
9	Plants	Food products/food poisoning
10	Antihistamines	Cosmetics/personal care products

Modified from Bronstein AC et al: 2006 annual report of the American Association of Poison Control Centers' National Poison Data System (NPDS), *Clin Toxicol (Phila)* 2007;45:815.

as such it is important to note that the substances represented here may serve as an indicator of availability, rather than toxicity. Many pediatric poison exposures are nontoxic, may result in only minor gastrointestinal upset, and can be managed at home with guidance from a poison control center.[5,6] Other sources of poisoning, such as those listed in the following sections, can be more serious and often require more thorough monitoring and care.

Organophosphates

Organophosphates (such as the nerve gas Sarin) were originally developed for chemical warfare but are now commonly used as insecticides and herbicides. Concerns about the use of these chemicals for purposes of mass destruction or in accidental mass casualty settings make exposure management and treatment highly relevant.[26] Poisoning can occur through skin exposure, inhalation, or ingestion. Organophosphates work by inactivating an important step in neurotransmission: nerve conduction and muscle contraction induced by acetylcholine. Acetylcholine is broken down by the action of acetylcholinesterase, which is found in the neurons, neuromuscular junctions, and red blood cells. Organophosphates irreversibly bind to acetylcholinesterase, and the resultant lack of this enzyme causes an initial increase in the availability of acetylcholine and an overstimulation of neurotransmission. Continued inhibition of acetylcholinesterase activity leads to a depletion of acetylcholine and neurotransmission ceases. Normal hydrolysis of acetylcholine returns only when new acetylcholinesterase is produced.[24,26]

There are three distinct manifestations of organophosphate poisoning: acute cholinergic crisis (occurring within hours of poison exposure), intermediate syndrome (occurring 24 to 96 h after exposure), and organophosphate-induced delayed neurotoxicity (occurring 2-3 wk after exposure[27,28]). Because most deaths are due to respiratory failure, the standard ABCs of resuscitation must be a part of initial treatment.[29] The symptoms of organophosphate exposure vary depending on the dose and route of exposure, and include both muscarinic and nicotinic effects. Mild inhalation effects include miosis, rhinorrhea, and mild dyspnea, whereas more severe exposures can lead to bronchoconstriction, excessive bronchial secretions, seizures, loss of consciousness, muscle fasciculations, flaccid paralysis, central apnea, and death (usually secondary to respiratory failure from bronchoconstriction, bronchorrhea, and central apnea). Liquid and dermal exposure effects are variable in onset (can be delayed up to 18 h) and can include sweating, muscular fasciculations at the site of contact, nausea, vomiting, diarrhea, and weakness, with more severe exposures also leading to seizures, loss of consciousness, muscle fasciculations, flaccid paralysis, central apnea, and death.[24,26,30]

Decontamination depends on the route of entry, and should be initiated concurrently with atropine treatment.[29] Heath care personnel should take care to avoid toxin exposure during decontamination. For topical exposures remove all contaminated clothing and place in an impermeable plastic container, and thoroughly scrub the patient with liberal amounts of soap and water. Gastric lavage and activated charcoal have not been proven to have a beneficial effect, but these are still frequently used.[29] Use caution because vomited organophosphates can be aspirated by the patient and absorbed through the skin of health care personnel.

Atropine inhibits the effects of acetylcholine on muscarinic receptors by competitively antagonizing acetylcholine and should take effect quickly. Atropine administration results in decreased secretions and smooth muscle contraction as well as decreased bronchorrhea and bronchoconstriction and can relieve respiratory depression. In patients with severe twitching and muscle weakness, pralidoxime (2-PAM), a cholinesterase reactivator, should be administered to stimulate the production of new acetylcholinesterase. Table 42-3 has additional dosing information.[24,26] In mass casualty situations involving nerve agents, it may be more effective for emergency medical personnel to use auto-injector kits for antidote delivery. These kits, such as the MARK-1 kit, which consists of two separate injectors containing atropine (2 mg) and 2-PAM (600 mg), have been approved by the U.S. Food and Drug Administration (FDA) for use in adults, but not in children. There is currently no combination autoinjector kit approved for pediatric patients; however, there is a pediatric atropine autoinjector available in three different doses (AtroPen). In chaotic situations, during which IV antidote administration is not available for pediatric patients, it is recommended to use the adult MARK-1 autoinjector.[24,31]

One respiratory medication that affects acetylcholine is theophylline. As such, avoid theophylline-containing preparations during the management of symptoms. In addition, many insecticides are dissolved in a hydrocarbon solution. Treatment for hydrocarbon pneumonitis may be required in addition to organophosphate poison treatment. Other supportive therapy may include treating subsequent pneumonias, treating pulmonary edema, or supporting respiratory efforts with intubation and mechanical ventilation.

Antidepressants

Antidepressants are among the top 10 most common substances involved in human poison exposures (4.0% of all exposures), and in children 5 years of age or younger they represent 1.1% of all poison exposures.[2] Tricyclic antidepressants (TCAs) have historically been

TABLE 42-3

Guideline for Nerve Agent Antidote Administration

Patient (Age)	Antidote		
	Mild-Moderate Symptoms*	Severe Symptoms†	Other Treatments
Infant (0-2 yr)	Atropine: 0.05 mg/kg IM or 0.05 mg/kg IV (minimum, 0.1 mg)	Atropine: 0.1 mg/kg IM or 0.05 mg/kg IV (minimum, 0.1 mg)	• Assist ventilation • Repeat atropine at 5- to 10-min intervals until secretions have decreased and breathing is comfortable and/or airway resistance has returned to near normal
Child (2-10 yr)	2-PAM Cl: 25 mg/kg IV‡ Atropine: 1 mg IM	2-PAM Cl: 25 mg/kg IV‡ Atropine: 2 mg IM	
Adolescent (>10 yr)	2-PAM Cl: 25 mg/kg IV‡ Atropine: 2 mg IM 2-PAM Cl: 25 mg/kg (maximum, 1 g IV, 2 g IM)‡	2-PAM Cl: 25 mg/kg IV‡ Atropine: 4 mg IM or 2 mg IV or 2-PAM Cl: 25 mg/kg IV (maximum, 1 g IV, 2 g IM)‡	
Adult	Atropine: 2-4 mg IM 2-PAM Cl: 1 g IV,‡ 2 g IM	Atropine: 6 mg IM or 2-PAM Cl: 1 g IV,‡ 2 g IM	

Autoinjectors			
	AtroPen >10 yr: 2 mg for 40 kg‡ 5-10 yr: 1 mg for 20 kg‡ 6 mo to 10 yr: 0.5 mg for 10 kg	MARK-1§ Atropine: 2 mg IM 2-PAM Cl: 600 mg IM	For seizures caused by nerve agent poisoning: Diazepam: 0.05-0.3 mg/kg IV/PR (maximum, 10 mg/dose), 5-10 mg/dose IV (adult), repeat every 15-30 min, as needed or Midazolam: 0.15-0.2 mg/kg IV/IM (maximum, 10 mg), repeat as necessary or start continuous intravenous drip or Lorazepam: 0.1 mg/kg (maximum, 4 mg) IV/IM/PR

From White ML, Liebelt EL: Update on antidotes for pediatric poisoning, *Pediatr Emerg Care* 2006;22:740; quiz 747.
2-PAM Cl, pralidoxime chloride; IM, intramuscular; IV, intravenous; PR, rectally.
*Mild-moderate symptoms include nausea, vomiting, salivation, lacrimation, weakness, and dyspnea.
†Severe symptoms include seizures, apnea, unconsciousness, and flaccid paralysis.
‡2-PAM Cl should be administered slowly for 20 minutes. Rapid intravenous administration can cause laryngospasm and rigidity. 2-PAM Cl may be repeated within 30 to 60 minutes, as needed, and then again every 1 hour for 1 or 2 doses, as needed, for persistent weakness and/or high atropine requirements.
§See text.

widely prescribed for the treatment of depression and other neurologic disorders in both adults and children; however, they have become increasingly replaced by selective serotonin reuptake inhibitors (SSRIs) because of their lower toxicity. TCAs are still prescribed for other uses and may therefore be a source of poison exposure. The wide availability of these drugs increases the risk that a young child may be exposed through exploratory behavior, or that an adolescent with suicidal intent could gain access to the drugs.[32,33]

SSRI toxicity is typically mild and includes nausea, vomiting, diarrhea, and central nervous system depression, and can lead to serotonin syndrome.[33,34] Serotonin syndrome is characterized by altered mental status (confusion, agitation), autonomic instability, and neuromuscular dysfunction. SSRI overdose treatment relies mainly on supportive care.[33,35] TCA overdose can lead to seizures, coma, confusion, ataxia, and central respiratory depression. Patients who overdose on TCAs are six times more likely to die than patients who overdose on SSRIs.[36] TCAs cause direct myocardial depression with hypotension and conduction abnormalities, and cardiovascular derangements account for the majority of fatal complications.[37,38] Patients may be asymptomatic for up to 12 hours after ingestion. Conduction is slowed, with increased PR and QRS intervals and an increase in the refractory period, which causes a decrease in the heart rate. The width of the QRS complex is often used as an indicator of the severity of TCA toxicity, with a QRS width greater than 100 milliseconds being an indication for concern and an important marker of mortality.[37,39]

Treatment includes immediate decontamination with charcoal administration (up to 1 h postingestion), and support of the cardiorespiratory system takes precedence over all other treatment. TCAs are well absorbed orally, and 98% of the drug is bound to glycoproteins (highly pH dependent) and concentrates in the tissues.[37] Administration of sodium bicarbonate is the mainstay of TCA poisoning treatment; however, optimal doses have yet to be determined.[25] Sodium bicarbonate bolus administration should generate systemic alkalinization to a range of pH 7.50 to 7.55, which decreases the amount of free drug and may help reduce the cardiac effects.[23,40,41] Sodium bicarbonate should be given to any patient exhibiting QRS prolongation greater than 120 milliseconds, hypotension, or cardiac arrhythmia, even in the absence of acidosis.[39] Antiarrhythmics, particularly classes Ia and Ic, are contraindicated in TCA poisoning; however, class Ib (lidocaine, phenytoin) may prove useful.[42]

Hydrocarbons

Hydrocarbons include substances such as petroleum distillates, gasoline, kerosene, turpentine, lighter fluid, and pine oil. They are present in lamp oil, spot remover, pine cleaner, furniture polish, nail polish, and glue. Many of these products are in the home and are therefore easily available for accidental ingestion. Hydrocarbon exposures are typically due to the exploratory behavior of young children and intentional misuse by adolescents and adults.[43] Ingestions by young children typically involve small amounts of liquid, as most substances containing hydrocarbons have a foul taste. Although severe gastrointestinal irritation results from hydrocarbon ingestion, little systemic absorption occurs.

Death resulting from hydrocarbon ingestion is almost always due to pulmonary complications, rather than CNS involvement. A major complication of hydrocarbon ingestion is toxic exposure directly to the lungs secondary to aspiration or through vaporization of solvents during ingestion or vomiting, as these products frequently produce gasping, gagging, choking, and vomiting.[44] The low surface tension and viscosity of hydrocarbons allows a small amount in the lung to spread over a large area, and can result in hydrocarbon pneumonitis. Because some of these compounds are highly volatile, vapors may also produce inebriation or alterations in mental status.[44,45] Because of complications arising from aspiration of gastric contents in patients with hydrocarbon poisoning, gastric emptying is contraindicated and should not be routinely performed.[45]

Symptoms of hydrocarbon poisoning appear to be the same regardless of the poison ingested, and include respiratory distress with dyspnea, tachypnea, intercostal retractions, fever, and cyanosis. Chest auscultation may reveal wheezing and rales.[46] CNS findings such as somnolence, coma, and seizures are rare and are secondary to the pulmonary injury with hypoxia and acidosis. Gastrointestinal irritation may produce diarrhea, blood-tinged stools, nausea, and vomiting. Symptoms can appear within 30 minutes of the aspiration or 12 to 24 hours later. The chest radiograph is consistent with aspiration pneumonitis with poorly defined patchy infiltrates, and almost all patients with lung involvement show evidence of chemical pneumonitis within 12 hours. Respiratory symptoms are usually progressive over the first 24 to 48 hours and then subside after 2 to 5 days.[44,47] Complications found in patients who survive hydrocarbon ingestion include the formation of pneumatoceles and pulmonary function abnormalities.[45]

Treatment consists of supportive care and prevention of further aspiration.[46] Airway control and mechanical ventilation may be required because of either respiratory distress or failure to protect the airway. Administer oxygen and continuous positive airway pressure for hypoxemia and pulmonary edema. Bronchodilators may be helpful in patients with bronchospasm. Exercise caution with bronchodilator administration because hydrocarbons predispose the myocardium to fibrillation, and catecholamine administration may worsen this effect. Routine use of steroids and antibiotics has no proven efficacy; however, antibiotics can be administered if fever and leukocytosis increase after 2 to 3 days, indicating a secondary bacterial infection. If conventional supportive measures are ineffective, extracorporeal membrane oxygenation has been used with success in pediatric patients for hydrocarbon pneumonitis.[48]

Salicylates

Salicylates (such as aspirin, methyl salicylate, and various topical preparations) persist as a source of poison exposure despite regulations that mandate child-resistant packaging and impose limitations on the number of tablets allowed per bottle of pediatric flavored aspirin. Salicylates have a number of toxic effects, including direct stimulation of the respiratory center, uncoupling of oxidative phosphorylation, inhibition of the Krebs cycle, inhibition of lipid and amino acid metabolism, stimulation of gluconeogenesis, interference with normal glucose homeostatic mechanisms, and interference with hemostatic mechanisms.[49] Both acute (unintentional or intentional ingestion of a single large dose) and chronic (repeated subtherapeutic doses or chronic dermal application) salicylate poisoning can occur.

In acute ingestion, symptoms affecting the gastrointestinal tract can include abdominal pain, vomiting, and occasional hematemesis. Acute systemic toxicity may result in tinnitus, hyperpyrexia, diaphoresis, lethargy, confusion, hyperpnea, tachypnea, coma, and seizures. Complications include dehydration, electrolyte imbalances, acid–base disturbances, hepatitis, cerebral edema, gastrointestinal ulcers, noncardiogenic pulmonary edema, and cerebrospinal fluid hypoglycemia. Chronic exposures can present with similar symptoms; however, they can appear at lower doses, gastrointestinal symptoms may be less evident, and CNS symptoms may be more pronounced.[10,50,51] Unlike adults, children quickly lose their respiratory drive and may present with both metabolic and respiratory acidosis by the time they reach the hospital.[49]

Doses greater than 150 mg/kg are mildly toxic and doses greater than 500 mg/kg are severely toxic.[10] Peak plasma salicylate concentrations correlate roughly with toxicity; however, the salicylate levels may not peak until 12-18 hours after presentation, and therefore salicylate levels need to be measured every 2-4 hours and the patient's clinical features need to be taken into account when assessing toxicity.[10,25] The Done nomogram is available to assess toxicity, but must be used with caution because it does not account for enteric coated products. Patients who succumb usually die from CNS injury secondary to hypoglycemia, hypoperfusion, or intractable seizures.[49]

Controversy exists over the use of gastrointestinal decontamination in cases of salicylate poisoning; however, multiple-dose activated charcoal administered until the plasma salicylate levels peak may be beneficial if administered immediately and contraindications such as vomiting are not present.[50] Treatment of salicylate exposure can include urinary alkalinization with sodium bicarbonate to enhance elimination or hemodialysis to correct fluid and electrolyte disorders.[52] When severe CNS depression and loss of cardiorespiratory function occur, mechanical ventilation is required.

Acetaminophen

Acetaminophen has lower toxicity when compared with salicylates and is widely used in children as an analgesic and antipyretic. Toxic exposures do take place, however, and acetaminophen poisoning can occur as a result of a single acute dose or after repeated subtherapeutic ingestions. Acetaminophen is one of the most commonly used drugs for intentional suicide by adolescents, and in these cases toxic exposure is often due to the ingestion of multiple drugs; therefore it is important not to overlook acetaminophen exposure in multiple drug suicide attempts. Repeated subtherapeutic exposures can also result in toxicity, and in children younger than 6 years this type of exposure is the most common.[53]

Acetaminophen is rapidly absorbed and is metabolized by the liver. One of the metabolites is N-acetyl-p-benzoquinone imine, which can accumulate in the liver and lead to necrosis. Normally, glutathione conjugates N-acetyl-p-benzoquinone imine and it is excreted in the urine; however, in cases of acetaminophen overdose glutathione is used more rapidly than it can be replaced, and hepatocellular necrosis results, which can lead to liver failure.[54] Symptoms of acetaminophen poisoning occur in four distinct stages[55]:

Stage 1: The first 24 hours of exposure, includes nausea, vomiting, and abdominal pain

Stage 2: Occurring between 24 and 72 hours, is typified by transient improvement in gastrointestinal symptoms and onset of increased bilirubin levels, prothrombin time, and liver transaminase levels

Stage 3: Occurring 72 to 96 hours postexposure; patients with severe exposure exhibit fulminant hepatic failure with encephalopathy and coma. Liver transaminases, aspartate aminotransferase, and alanine aminotransferase are highly elevated, and death can occur 3 to 5 days after exposure from multiple organ system failure

Stage 4: Typically the recovery stage for surviving patients

Decontamination with activated charcoal does not have proven clinical efficacy, but can be administered within 1 hour of toxic exposure as long as no contraindications are present. Diagnostic nomograms can be used to evaluate toxin exposure and the need for treatment. Administration of N-acetylcysteine (NAC), a glutathione precursor, has been the long-standing treatment for acetaminophen exposure.[55,56] The dose and time schedule for NAC administration is controversial and in the United States has traditionally consisted of a 72-hour dosing protocol. In 2004 the FDA approved a 20-hour NAC administration protocol (Acetadote). Studies have shown that intravenous administration in pediatric patients results in seizures

TABLE 42-4

Pediatric N-Acetylcysteine (NAC) Dose Guidelines

Body Weight		Loading Dose		Second Dose		Third Dose	
Kilograms	Pounds	Acetadote (ml)	5% Dextrose (ml)	Acetadote (ml)	5% Dextrose (ml)	Acetadote (ml)	5% Dextrose (ml)
30	66	22.5	100	7.5	250	15	500
25	55	18.75	100	6.25	250	12.5	500
20	44	15	60	5	140	10	280
15	33	11.25	45	3.75	105	7.5	210
10	22	7.5	30	2.5	70	5	140

From White ML, Liebelt EL: Update on antidotes for pediatric poisoning, *Pediatr Emerg Care* 2006;22:740; quiz 747.
Loading dose, 150 mg/kg for 60 minutes; second dose, 50 mg/kg for 4 hours; third dose, 100 mg/kg for 16 hours.
Acetadote is hyperosmolar (2600 mOsm/L) and is compatible with 5% dextrose, 0.5 N saline (0.45% sodium chloride injection), and water for injection.

due to free water load. The conventional pediatric dilution scheme is shown in Table 42-4.[24] The doses are the same as in adult treatments (loading dose, 150 mg/kg for 1 h; second dose, 50 mg/kg for 4 h; third dose, 100 mg/kg for 16 h), but the free water is less.

Iron

Iron ingestions have historically been a significant source of pediatric toxin morbidity and mortality; however, deaths due to iron overdose have decreased as a result of changes in tablet packaging (unit-dose packaging was mandated by the FDA in 1997, and later revoked in 2003, but some manufacturers continue to voluntarily package their products this way) and coating (from sugar coatings to film coatings).[57] In 2006 there were 1845 exposures to iron as a single substance in children less than 6 years old, and 21,035 iron-containing multivitamin exposures (43.8% of all multivitamin exposures included iron, and vitamin exposures represent 3.9% of all exposures in children ≤5 years). There were no reported deaths.[2]

Systemic iron toxicity is secondary to free radical formation. Normally, iron binds to transferrin; however, in acute exposures the binding capacity of transferrin is exceeded and free ferrous iron circulates in the blood, binds with peroxides, and forms free radicals. These free radicals affect aerobic cellular respiration in the mitochondria and lead to metabolic acidosis. The gastrointestinal tract, cardiovascular system, liver, and CNS are also directly affected by the unbound iron.[58] Ingestion of elemental iron at less than 20 mg/kg is considered nontoxic, 20 to 60 mg/kg is mildly toxic, greater than 60 mg/kg is severely toxic, and greater than 200 mg/kg is lethal.[59] Symptoms of iron poisoning follow a multistage process, which can be seen in Table 42-5.[60] The chronic sequelae of iron intoxication include hepatic cirrhosis, chronic bowel obstruction, and CNS damage.

Serum levels can predict toxicity, but they must be obtained within 2 to 6 hours of ingestion because iron

is rapidly cleared from the plasma. Treatment includes protection of the airway, fluid resuscitation, and chelation therapy. Gastric lavage has not been shown to improve clinical outcome and activated charcoal will not bind iron well, so these therapies are not usually administered. Whole-bowel irrigation may be effective, and decreases iron absorption and reduces the potential for direct mucosal damage in the gastrointestinal tract. Abdominal radiographs can be used to visualize the location of pills, and surgery to prevent bowel perforation and sepsis could be necessary if tablets are not dislodged.[61,62]

Chelation therapy uses deferoxamine, which binds the ferric form of iron and is then excreted in the urine (sometimes turning urine a "vin rose" color). Deferoxamine is indicated in children who have signs of systemic poisoning, and is usually administered via continuous intravenous infusion at a rate of 15 mg/kg

TABLE 42-5

Stages and Symptoms of Iron Toxicity

Stage	Symptoms	Time From Ingestion
1	Vomiting, diarrhea, gastrointestinal blood loss	0-6 h
2	Transient resolution of gastrointestinal symptoms	12-24 h
3	Recurrence of gastrointestinal symptoms, metabolic acidosis, shock, acute respiratory syndrome	24-48 h
4	Hepatotoxicity to recovery	48+ h
5	Vomiting, gastric outlet obstruction	2-4 h

From Madiwale T, Liebelt E: Iron: not a benign therapeutic drug, *Curr Opin Pediatr* 2006;18:174.

per hour, up to 35 mg/kg per hour. Side effects include hypotension. Chelation therapy is continued until measured iron levels return to normal.[63]

Alcohols

Toxic alcohols include methanol, ethylene glycol, and isopropanol. These alcohols are readily available in the home as components of many cleaning solutions. Ingestions in young children are commonly due to exploratory behavior and similarities between brightly colored cleaning fluids and sweet drinks. These alcohols are responsible for initial CNS depression, and are metabolized by alcohol dehydrogenase and aldehyde dehydrogenase. Metabolites of methanol (formaldehyde and formic acid) and ethylene glycol (glycolic acid, glyoxylic acid, and oxalic acid) are responsible for end-organ toxicity and acidosis, and exposures can be serious. The high concentration (95%) of these alcohols in windshield washer fluid and antifreeze, respectively, means that ingestion of even small quantities can be deadly. Isopropanol metabolizes into acetone, and although isopropanol is involved in the majority of ingestions, serious outcomes are rare.[25]

Symptoms of methanol ingestion may be delayed 8 to 24 hours, and can include CNS depression, high anion gap metabolic acidosis, and visual symptoms including blindness. Ethylene glycol symptoms appear more rapidly, within 4 to 8 hours, and include high anion gap metabolic acidosis, cranial nervous system depression, renal failure, and cardiac failure. The main toxic effects of isopropanol are myocardial depression and shock.[64]

Alcohol is rapidly absorbed from the gastrointestinal tract, so activated charcoal is rarely effective. Treatment is initially supportive, with intubation and mechanical ventilation instituted if the airway or respirations are compromised. Alcohol dehydrogenase is the rate-limiting enzyme in the generation of toxic metabolites, and ethanol competes with methanol and ethylene glycol as a substrate for this enzyme, effectively inhibiting the metabolism of these toxins when at a sufficient concentration (100 to 150 mg/dl).[24] Traditional ethanol therapy has fallen out of favor, however, with the advent of fomepizole, which is indicated when alcohol levels are greater than 20 mg/dl. Fomepizole is an approved treatment for methanol and ethylene glycol poisoning, and acts as a safe and effective competitive inhibitor for alcohol dehydrogenase. An initial dose of 15 mg/kg followed by 10 mg/kg every 12 hours for 4 doses, followed by 15 mg/kg every 12 hours thereafter until alcohol levels drop below 20 mg/dl, is indicated.[65,66]

Carbon Monoxide

Carbon monoxide (CO) is a colorless, tasteless, and odorless gas that has a higher affinity for hemoglobin than does oxygen, leading to the formation of carboxyhemoglobin and a reduction of oxygen in the blood. CO exposure has also been associated with platelet–neutrophil activation and perivascular oxidative stress, which may explain some of the neurologic effects.[67] CO is formed by the incomplete combustion of hydrocarbon-containing fuels such as oil, wood, coal, and natural gas, and sources of CO are commonly found in homes and places of work.[68] CO is a significant threat to children and adults in developing countries because of their increased dependence on biomass combustion for heating and cooking inside the home.[69] CO exposure also occurs when charcoal briquettes are burned for heating or cooking purposes without ventilation, as is sometimes done in the United States during power outages. Intentional CO exposure can occur through the inhalation of motor vehicle exhaust.[70]

Symptoms of acute CO exposure tend to be nonspecific and can include headache, nausea, drowsiness, dizziness, fatigue, and chest pain, as well as delayed neurologic sequelae.[71] These symptoms are often overlooked, especially by elderly patients who misclassify them as flu symptoms.[68] The traditional method for detecting CO exposure relied on blood carboxyhemoglobin concentration; however, these measurements depend greatly on the time interval between exposure, sampling, and analysis. Measurements of expired air can be helpful but rely on trained personnel and are difficult to perform accurately in the field. A new method of noninvasive pulse co-oximetry has been validated and is potentially useful for rapid testing in the hospital and emergency rescue setting, or as a routine screening method.[72]

Decontamination involves removal from the source of poison. Treatment for CO exposure includes the administration of 100% humidified normobaric oxygen (which reduces the half-life of CO from 5 or 6 h to between 30 and 90 min) or hyperbaric oxygen therapy (which further reduces the half-life to 20 min). Levels of carboxyhemoglobin do not correlate with clinical severity, and therefore all patients with suspected CO exposure should be administered normobaric oxygen, and those patients with severe poisoning should receive hyperbaric oxygen therapy.[73] Prevention of CO poisoning in the home can be accomplished with a CO detector; however. these devices were designed on the basis of adult data and the higher respiration rate of children as well as the presence of fetal hemoglobin might put them at higher risk.[71]

Cyanide

Cyanide poisoning is increasingly being recognized as an important source of pediatric toxin exposure because of its widespread availability, potency, and potential for fatal outcomes. Cyanide poisoning can be both acute and chronic, and cyanide and its precursors are present in some plants, household products, and in fire smoke. Cyanide also poses a threat as a potential chemical weapon, as it can be easily obtained and disseminated.

Cyanide binds to ferric iron in the mitochondria, which inhibits oxidative phosphorylation and leads to the exhaustion of available ATP. The inhibition of aerobic metabolism causes a shift to anaerobic metabolism, which generates high amounts of lactic acid and can lead to high anion gap metabolic acidosis.[74] The prevention of normal cellular oxygen use, even in the presence of high blood oxygen levels, leads to cellular hypoxia and damage to the brain and heart. Specific symptoms of cyanide poisoning can be seen in Table 42-6.

Poisoning can occur through the ingestion of plants containing cyanogenic compounds, which can be metabolized to form hydrogen cyanide. Almonds, sorghum, cassava, lima beans, and the stone pits of fruits are some examples of food containing cyanogenic glycosides.[75] Historically, cyanide has been an underappreciated factor in smoke inhalation–related deaths. Carbon monoxide is traditionally considered to be the greatest inhalation risk in household fires; however, high levels of cyanide have consistently been found in the blood of people exposed to smoke.[76] The combustion of textiles and plastics releases cyanogenic compounds and subsequent inhalation and serious poison exposure can occur. Cyanide poisoning can also be due to accidental ingestion of household products such as acetonitrile-containing fingernail polish remover, or from ingestion of nitroprusside.[75]

Decontamination involves removal from the source of poison, and mouth-to-mouth resuscitation is contraindicated if inhalation of smoke containing cyanide is suspected.[77] Treatment includes intensive supportive care and 100% supplemental oxygen. Antidotes are available for cyanide poisoning, but it is important to note that the rapid toxicity of cyanide often necessitates empiric dosing before blood cyanide concentrations can be evaluated.[78]

At present two different antidote kits are available: a three-drug kit (containing amyl nitrite, sodium nitrite, and sodium thiosulfate), and hydroxocobalamin. The three-drug kit has been approved for use since the 1950s, and although it has proven efficacy it also presents considerable side effects, especially in pediatric patients.[75] Amyl nitrate, packaged in a crushable glass ampoule that is inhaled for 30 seconds, serves as a stabilizing agent while an intravenous line is being placed and sodium nitrite and sodium thiosulfate administration can begin. The goal of sodium nitrite is to generate methemoglobin, which functions as a preferential binding site for cyanide and restores aerobic metabolism. The formation of methemoglobin can have toxic side effects, however, especially in children, as they are more susceptible to nitrite-induced methemoglobinemia and hemolysis due to the presence of fetal hemoglobin.[75] Methemoglobinemia reduces the amount of hemoglobin available for oxygen transport, and in cases of concordant carbon monoxide poisoning this can have an additive effect to already reduced oxygen-carrying capacity. Sodium thiosulfate acts as a sulfur donor and facilitates the excretion of cyanide in the urine by forming thiocyanate; however, this process has a slow onset of action.[74]

The hydroxocobalamin kit was approved by the FDA in 2006, and functions in a different manner than the three-drug antidote kit. Hydroxocobalamin is a vitamin B_{12} precursor that binds cyanide to form cyanocobalamin, which is then excreted. For children the initial dose is 70 mg/kg by intravenous line, followed by 35 mg/kg if needed. Side effects are rare and include reddening of the skin and urine.[74,79] In addition, hydroxocobalamin can interfere with CO-oximetry measurements of carboxyhemoglobin, which may be clinically relevant for the care of patients with carbon monoxide poisoning.[80]

TABLE 42-6

Signs and Symptoms of Cyanide Poisoning

System	Sign or Symptom
Dermatologic	Cherry-red color of skin
Neurologic	Headache, agitation, disorientation, confusion, weakness, malaise, dizziness, lethargy, seizures, coma, cerebral death
Cardiovascular	Hypotension, tachycardia or bradycardia, ST-T wave changes, dysrhythmias, atrioventricular block, cardiovascular collapse
Respiratory and metabolic	Tachypnea or apnea, venous hyperoxemia, red venous blood, increased mixed venous oxygen content and decreased oxygen consumption resulting in narrow arteriovenous oxygen differential
Gastrointestinal	Nausea, vomiting, abdominal pain
Other	Bitter, almond-like breath odor in some patients

From Geller RJ et al: Pediatric cyanide poisoning: causes, manifestations, management, and unmet needs, *Pediatrics* 2006;118:2146. Data from Ruangkanchanasetr S et al: Cyanide poisoning: two case reports and treatment review, *J Med Assoc Thai* 1999;82(suppl 1):S162; Mégarbane B et al: Antidotal treatment of cyanide poisoning, *J Chin Med Assoc* 2003;66:193; and Dart RC, Bogdan GM: Acute cyanide poisoning: causes, consequences, recognition and management, *Frontline First Responder* 2004;2:19.

NOTE ON COUGH AND COLD PREPARATIONS

There has been an increase in debate over the efficacy and safety of common over-the-counter cough and cold medicines for children. Cough and cold medications are often combinations of several drugs, usually decongestants, antihistamines, antitussives, and expectorants.[81] Cough and cold preparations rank sixth among the top 10 substances most frequently involved in pediatric poison exposures (5.7% of all exposures in children ≤5 years old), and were responsible for 43 deaths in 2006 (all age groups).[2] There is controversy regarding the therapeutic benefit of these medications in young children; however, studies have shown that cough and cold medications do alleviate discomfort in adolescents and adults. Numerous literature reviews have come to the conclusion that there is no clear efficacy derived from the use of cough and cold medications in children, and that the potential for harmful overdose outweighs the possibility of clinical benefit.[82-85] At present the FDA advises that cough and cold preparations are contraindicated in children less than 2 years old, and a review of their safety in children aged 2 through 11 years is ongoing.[86]

ASSESSMENT QUESTIONS

See Evolve Resources for answers.

1. Which of these does *not* describe a common risk factor for unintentional poison exposure?
   A. Age less than 6 years
   B. Age between 13 and 19 years
   C. Presence of candy-like medication in the home
   D. Lack of child-proof containers for hazardous chemicals
2. Categories of intentional poisoning include:
   A. Suspected suicide
   B. Intentional misuse
   C. Intentional abuse
   D. All of the above
3. Which of the following is *not* an important feature of poison diagnosis?
   A. Blood gas analysis
   B. Questioning only the child and not the parents
   C. Anion gap calculations
   D. Toxicologic screening
4. Match each gastrointestinal decontamination method with its description:

A. Syrup of ipecac	I. Leads to bowel cleansing, useful in sustained release poison exposure
B. Gastric lavage	II. Adsorbs numerous poisons, time-sensitive application

ASSESSMENT QUESTIONS—cont'd

C. Activated charcoal	III. Causes emesis, not routinely recommended
D. Whole-bowel irrigation	IV. Mechanical removal of stomach contents, not routinely recommended

5. Which of the following are in the top 10 poison exposures for children not more than 5 years of age?
   A. Cold and cough preparations
   B. Pesticides
   C. Vitamins
   D. Cosmetic/personal care products
   E. All of the above
6. Which statement is true regarding organophosphates?
   A. Examples include petroleum distillates, gasoline, kerosene, turpentine, lighter fluid, and pine oil.
   B. Organophosphates were originally developed for chemical warfare.
   C. Organophosphates irreversibly bind to transferrin.
   D. Symptoms are often overlooked, especially by elderly patients who misclassify them as flu symptoms.
7. Which of the following is a sign of severe TCA poison exposure?
   A. Pinpoint pupils
   B. "Vin rose"-colored urine
   C. QRS interval greater than 100 milliseconds
   D. Hepatitis
8. What method of decontamination is recommended for salicylate poisoning if performed immediately and no contraindications are present?
   A. Whole-bowel irrigation
   B. Nothing
   C. Single dose of activated charcoal
   D. Multiple doses of activated charcoal
9. What is the correct order of the following five stages of iron poisoning?
   I. Hepatotoxicity to recovery
   II. Transient resolution of GI symptoms
   III. Vomiting, diarrhea, GI blood loss
   IV. Vomiting, gastric outlet obstruction
   V. Recurrence of GI symptoms, metabolic acidosis, shock, acute respiratory syndrome
   A. III, IV, II, V, I
   B. IV, II, V, III, I
   C. III, II, V, I, IV
   D. IV, I, V, II, III
10. Cyanide exposure can occur as a result of which of the following?
    A. Smoke inhalation from a house fire
    B. Eating improperly prepared cassava
    C. Aspirin overdose
    D. Both A and B
    E. A, B, and C

References

1. Langman LJ, Kapur BM: Toxicology: then and now, *Clin Biochem* 2006;39:498.
2. Bronstein AC et al: 2006 annual report of the American Association of Poison Control Centers' National Poison Data System (NPDS), *Clin Toxicol (Phila)* 2007;45:815.
3. Criddle LM: An overview of pediatric poisonings, *AACN Adv Crit Care* 2007;18:109.
4. Fazen LE III et al: Acute poisoning in a children's hospital: a 2-year experience, *Pediatrics* 1986;77:144.
5. Zaloshnja E et al: The impact of poison control centers on poisoning-related visits to EDs: United States, 2003, *Am J Emerg Med* 2008;26:310.
6. Muller AA: Common nontoxic pediatric ingestions, *J Emerg Nurs* 2005;31:494.
7. Walton WW: An evaluation of the Poison Prevention Packaging Act, *Pediatrics* 1982;69:363.
8. Gibbs L et al: Understanding parental motivators and barriers to uptake of child poison safety strategies: a qualitative study, *Inj Prev* 2005;11:373.
9. Ozanne-Smith J et al: Childhood poisoning: access and prevention, *J Paediatr Child Health* 2001;37:262.
10. Greene SL, Dargan PI, Jones AL: Acute poisoning: understanding 90% of cases in a nutshell, *Postgrad Med J* 2005;81:204.
11. Mokhlesi B et al: Adult toxicology in critical care. I. General approach to the intoxicated patient, *Chest* 2003;123:577.
12. Fine JS, Goldfrank LR: Update in medical toxicology, *Pediatr Clin North Am* 1992;39:1031.
13. Greene S, Harris C, Singer J: Gastrointestinal decontamination of the poisoned patient, *Pediatr Emerg Care* 2008;24:176; quiz 187.
14. Liebelt EL, Deangelis CD: Evolving trends and treatment advances in pediatric poisoning, *JAMA* 1999;282:1113.
15. Bond GR: Home use of syrup of ipecac is associated with a reduction in pediatric emergency department visits, *Ann Emerg Med* 1995;25:338.
16. Krenzelok EP, McGuigan M, Lheur P; American Academy of Clinical Toxicology; European Association of Poisons Centres and Clinical Toxicologists: Position statement: ipecac syrup, *J Toxicol Clin Toxicol* 1997;35:699.
17. American Academy of Pediatrics Committee on Injury, Violence, and Poison Prevention: Poison treatment in the home, *Pediatrics* 2003;112:1182.
18. Vale JA; American Academy of Clinical Toxicology; European Association of Poisons Centres and Clinical Toxicologists: Position statement: gastric lavage, *J Toxicol Clin Toxicol* 1997;35:711.
19. Burns MM: Activated charcoal as the sole intervention for treatment after childhood poisoning, *Curr Opin Pediatr* 2000;12:166.
20. Chyka PA, Seger D; American Academy of Clinical Toxicology; European Association of Poisons Centres and Clinical Toxicologists: Position statement: single-dose activated charcoal, *J Toxicol Clin Toxicol* 1997;35:721.
21. Barceloux D, McGuigan M, Hartigan-Go K; American Academy of Clinical Toxicology; European Association of Poisons Centres and Clinical Toxicologists: Position statement: cathartics, *J Toxicol Clin Toxicol* 1997;35:743.
22. Tenenbein M; American Academy of Clinical Toxicology; European Association of Poisons Centres and Clinical Toxicologists: Position statement: whole bowel irrigation, *J Toxicol Clin Toxicol* 1997;35:753.
23. Steinhart CM, Pearson-Shaver AL: Poisoning, *Crit Care Clin* 1988;4:845.
24. White ML, Liebelt EL: Update on antidotes for pediatric poisoning, *Pediatr Emerg Care* 2006;22:740; quiz 747.
25. Michael JB, Sztajnkrycer MD: Deadly pediatric poisons: nine common agents that kill at low doses, *Emerg Med Clin North Am* 2004;22:1019.
26. Lynch EL, Thomas TL: Pediatric considerations in chemical exposures: are we prepared? *Pediatr Emerg Care* 2004;20:198.
27. Yang CC, Deng JF: Intermediate syndrome following organophosphate insecticide poisoning, *J Chin Med Assoc* 2007;70:467.
28. Senanayake N, Karalliedde L: Neurotoxic effects of organophosphorus insecticides: an intermediate syndrome, *N Engl J Med* 1987;316:761.
29. Eddleston M et al: Early management after self-poisoning with an organophosphorus or carbamate pesticide: a treatment protocol for junior doctors, *Crit Care* 2004;8:R391.
30. Aardema H et al: Organophosphorus pesticide poisoning: cases and developments, *Neth J Med* 2008;66:149.
31. Foltin G et al: Pediatric nerve agent poisoning: Medical and operational considerations for emergency medical services in a large American city, *Pediatr Emerg Care* 2006;22:239.
32. Rosenbaum TG, Kou M: Are one or two dangerous? Tricyclic antidepressant exposure in toddlers, *J Emerg Med* 2005;28:169.
33. Nelson LS et al: Selective serotonin reuptake inhibitor poisoning: an evidence-based consensus guideline for out-of-hospital management, *Clin Toxicol (Phila)* 2007;45:315.
34. Whyte IM, Dawson AH, Buckley NA: Relative toxicity of venlafaxine and selective serotonin reuptake inhibitors in overdose compared to tricyclic antidepressants, *Q J Med* 2003;96:369.
35. Bijl D: The serotonin syndrome, *Neth J Med* 2004;62:309.
36. McKenzie MS, McFarland BH: Trends in antidepressant overdoses, *Pharmacoepidemiol Drug Saf* 2007;16:513.
37. Henry JA: Epidemiology and relative toxicity of antidepressant drugs in overdose, *Drug Saf* 1997;16:374.
38. Woolf AD et al; American Association of Poison Control Centers: Tricyclic antidepressant poisoning: an evidence-based consensus guideline for out-of-hospital management, *Clin Toxicol (Phila)* 2007;45:203.
39. Shannon MW: Duration of QRS disturbances after severe tricyclic antidepressant intoxication, *J Toxicol Clin Toxicol* 1992;30:377.
40. Braden NJ, Jackson JE, Walson PD: Tricyclic antidepressant overdose, *Pediatr Clin North Am* 1986;33:287.
41. Liebelt EL: Targeted management strategies for cardiovascular toxicity from tricyclic antidepressant overdose: the pivotal role for alkalinization and sodium loading, *Pediatr Emerg Care* 1998;14:293.
42. Bradberry SM et al: Management of the cardiovascular complications of tricyclic antidepressant poisoning: role of sodium bicarbonate, *Toxicol Rev* 2005;24:195.

43. Wyse DG: Deliberate inhalation of volatile hydrocarbons: a review, *Can Med Assoc J* 1973;108:71.

44. Eade NR, Taussig LM, Marks MI: Hydrocarbon pneumonitis, *Pediatrics* 1974;54:351.

45. Klein BL, Simon JE: Hydrocarbon poisonings, *Pediatr Clin North Am* 1986;33:411.

46. Karlson KH Jr: Hydrocarbon poisoning in children, *South Med J* 1982;75:839.

47. Foley JC et al: Kerosene poisoning in young children, *Radiology* 1954;62:817.

48. Chyka PA: Benefits of extracorporeal membrane oxygenation for hydrocarbon pneumonitis, *J Toxicol Clin Toxicol* 1996;34:357.

49. Snodgrass WR: Salicylate toxicity, *Pediatr Clin North Am* 1986;33:381.

50. Chyka PA et al; American Association of Poison Control Centers, Healthcare Systems Bureau, Health Resources and Services Administration, Department of Health and Human Services: Salicylate poisoning: an evidence-based consensus guideline for out-of-hospital management, *Clin Toxicol (Phila)* 2007;45:95.

51. Brenner BE, Simon RR: Management of salicylate intoxication, *Drugs* 1982;24:335.

52. Davis JE: Are one or two dangerous? Methyl salicylate exposure in toddlers, *J Emerg Med* 2007;32:63.

53. Dart RC et al; American Association of Poison Control Centers: Acetaminophen poisoning: an evidence-based consensus guideline for out-of-hospital management, *Clin Toxicol (Phila)* 2006;44:1.

54. American Academy of Pediatrics Committee on Drugs: Acetaminophen toxicity in children, *Pediatrics* 2001;108:1020.

55. Zed PJ, Krenzelok EP: Therapy update: treatment of acetaminophen overdose, *Am J Health Syst Pharm* 1999;56:1081.

56. Krenzelok EP, Leikin JB: Approach to the poisoned patient, *Dis Mon* 1996;42:509.

57. Manoguerra AS et al: Iron ingestion: an evidence-based consensus guideline for out-of-hospital management, *Clin Toxicol (Phila)* 2005;43:553.

58. Aldridge MD: Acute iron poisoning: what every pediatric intensive care unit nurse should know, *Dimens Crit Care Nurs* 2007;26:43; quiz 49.

59. Banner W Jr, Tong TG: Iron poisoning, *Pediatr Clin North Am* 1986;33:393.

60. Madiwale T, Liebelt E: Iron: not a benign therapeutic drug, *Curr Opin Pediatr* 2006;18:174.

61. Singhi SC, Baranwal AK, Jayashree M: Acute iron poisoning: clinical picture, intensive care needs and outcome, *Indian Pediatrics* 2003;40:1177.

62. Goldstein LH, Berkovitch M: Ingestion of slow-release iron treated with gastric lavage: never say late, *Clin Toxicol (Phila)* 2006;44:343.

63. Baranwal AK, Singhi SC: Acute iron poisoning: management guidelines, *Indian Pediatrics* 2003;40:534.

64. Velez LI et al: Ethylene glycol ingestion treated only with fomepizole, *J Med Toxicol* 2007;3:125.

65. Velez LI, Gracia R, Neerman MF: Ethylene glycol poisoning: current diagnostic and management issues, *J Emerg Nurs* 2007;33:342.

66. Burns MJ et al: Treatment of methanol poisoning with intravenous 4-methylpyrazole, *Ann Emerg Med* 1997;30:829.

67. Thom SR et al: Intravascular neutrophil activation due to carbon monoxide poisoning, *Am J Respir Crit Care Med* 2006;174:1239.

68. Centers for Disease Control and Prevention (CDC): Unintentional non-fire-related carbon monoxide exposures: United States, 2001-2003. *MMWR Morb Mortal Wkly Rep* 2005;54:36.

69. Rumchev K et al: Indoor air pollution from biomass combustion and respiratory symptoms of women and children in a Zimbabwean village, *Indoor Air* 2007;17:468.

70. Mendoza JA, Hampson NB: Epidemiology of severe carbon monoxide poisoning in children, *Undersea Hyperb Med* 2006;33:439.

71. Baum CR: What's new in pediatric carbon monoxide poisoning? *Clin Pediatr Emerg Med* 2008;9:43.

72. Coulange M et al: Reliability of new pulse CO-oximeter in victims of carbon monoxide poisoning, *Undersea Hyperb Med* 2008;35:107.

73. Prockop LD, Chichkova RI: Carbon monoxide intoxication: an updated review, *J Neurol Sci* 2007;262:122.

74. Shepherd G, Velez LI: Role of hydroxocobalamin in acute cyanide poisoning, *Ann Pharmacother* 2008;42:661.

75. Geller RJ et al: Pediatric cyanide poisoning: causes, manifestations, management, and unmet needs, *Pediatrics* 2006;118:2146.

76. Silverman SH et al: Cyanide toxicity in burned patients, *J Trauma* 1988;28:171.

77. Cummings TF: The treatment of cyanide poisoning, *Occup Med (Lond)* 2004;54:82.

78. Riordan M, Rylance G, Berry K: Poisoning in children. 5. Rare and dangerous poisons, *Arch Dis Child* 2002;87:407.

79. Hall AH, Dart R, Bogdan G: Sodium thiosulfate or hydroxocobalamin for the empiric treatment of cyanide poisoning? *Ann Emerg Med* 2007;49:806.

80. Lee J et al: Potential interference by hydroxocobalamin on co-oximetry hemoglobin measurements during cyanide and smoke inhalation treatments, *Ann Emerg Med* 2007;49:802.

81. Kelly LF: Pediatric cough and cold preparations, *Pediatr Rev* 2004;25:115.

82. Wingert WE et al: Possible role of pseudoephedrine and other over-the-counter cold medications in the deaths of very young children, *J Forensic Sci* 2007;52:487.

83. Gunn VL et al: Toxicity of over-the-counter cough and cold medications, *Pediatrics* 2001;108:E52.

84. Schaefer MK et al: Adverse events from cough and cold medications in children, *Pediatrics* 2008;121:783.

85. Carr BC: Efficacy, abuse, and toxicity of over-the-counter cough and cold medicines in the pediatric population, *Curr Opin Pediatr* 2006;18:184.

86. U.S. Food and Drug Administration: Public Health Advisory: nonprescription cough and cold medicine use in children [Internet]. Available from: http://www.fda.gov/cder/drug/advisory/cough_cold_2008.htm. Retrieved September 2008.

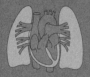

Chapter 43

Disorders of the Pleura

PAUL C. STILLWELL

OUTLINE

Pleural Effusions
Pneumothorax

Thoracostomy Drainage
Surgery in the Pleural Space

LEARNING OBJECTIVES

After reading this chapter the reader will be able to:

- Describe the normal function of the pleural space in healthy children
- List the causes of pneumothorax in neonates and children

- Recognize the causes of pleural effusions and empyema in children of all ages
- Discuss the principles of managing abnormal air or fluid in the pleural space in children

The pleura surround the outer surface of the lungs and the mediastinum as well as the inner surface of the chest wall and the diaphragm. This sliding surface provides minimal resistance between the lung and chest wall during respiratory movements. The pleural "space" is generally only a *potential* space with a normal fluid volume of 1 to 5 ml. The pleural membranes, however, are permeable to both liquid and gas; an estimated 5 to 10 L of fluid per day crosses from the parietal pleura to the visceral pleura in a normal adult.[1]

The pleura lining the chest wall, mediastinum, and diaphragm is called the *parietal pleura*. Its blood supply is from the systemic circulation, and its venous drainage is through the azygos, hemiazygos, and internal mammary veins. The *visceral pleura* covers the surface of the lungs, with its blood supply from the pulmonary arteries or bronchial arteries and its venous drainage through the pulmonary veins. In the healthy subject a *positive* (+) 9 cm H_2O of hydrostatic pressure drives fluid from the parietal pleura capillary bed into the pleural space, and a negative (–) 10 cm H_2O of hydrostatic pressure favors absorption of fluid into the visceral pleura capillaries.[1,2]

Several factors determine the amount of fluid in the pleural space. The *intracapillary* hydrostatic pressures tend to drive fluid out of the capillaries, whereas the *pericapillary* hydrostatic pressures tend to counterbalance this force. The *plasma* colloid osmotic pressures exert a force to retain fluid within the capillaries, whereas the *pericapillary* colloid osmotic pressure tends to favor fluid movement out of the capillaries. Changes in the balance of these forces determine how much fluid is retained within the pleural space. Increased capillary permeability (e.g., acute respiratory distress syndrome), decreased intravascular colloid osmotic pressure (e.g., low serum albumin), and increased pulmonary venous pressure (e.g., heart failure) are common contributors to accumulation of fluid in the pleural space. Obstructed lymphatic drainage is another factor that favors accumulation of fluid in the pleural space.[1,2] *Chylothorax* is an uncommon cause of pleural effusion in children, except when they have undergone thoracic surgery with interruption of the thoracic duct.[3]

In healthy individuals the chest radiograph seldom demonstrates any pleural fluid. An estimated 4% of normal adults may have minor radiographic evidence of pleural fluid if the films are taken in the decubitus or Trendelenburg's position. A pleural effusion has typical radiographic features (Figures 43-1 and 43-2). Ultrasound examination or computed tomography (CT) of the chest may be more sensitive in identifying small accumulations of pleural fluid.[2] The CT scan may also provide more information about the underlying lung parenchyma than is available from the plain chest radiograph, especially when large amounts of fluid are present. However, ultrasound and CT usually are not required to identify a clinically significant effusion. Ultrasound may be used to facilitate finding the optimal location to perform a thoracentesis.

PLEURAL EFFUSIONS

Pleural effusions may be suspected clinically when there is an area of decreased-intensity breath sounds on chest auscultation with an associated dullness to percussion over the corresponding area.[4,5] Comparison with the contralateral lung can help distinguish the normal boundaries of the thoracic cavity unless the effusion is bilateral. The patient may experience few symptoms from a small pleural effusion but usually has symptoms of respiratory distress with larger accumulations. Chest pain, chest wall tenderness, dyspnea, and pain with coughing or deep breathing are often associated with pleural effusions. In addition to decreased intensity of breath sounds with dullness to percussion, crackles may be appreciated immediately superior to the effusion, where the lung may be involved with underlying pneumonia, or the normal lung may be partially compressed by the effusion. The location of these abnormal examination findings may change when the position of the patient is changed if the fluid is flowing freely within the pleural space. The respiratory care practitioner may be the first to detect the findings of a pleural effusion during auscultation.

When an effusion is found on a chest radiograph, the initial diagnostic procedure to determine its cause is often a *thoracentesis*.[2,4-6] This procedure consists of placing a needle into the pleural space and withdrawing the pleural fluid for both diagnostic and therapeutic purposes. On occasion an underlying disease such as overt

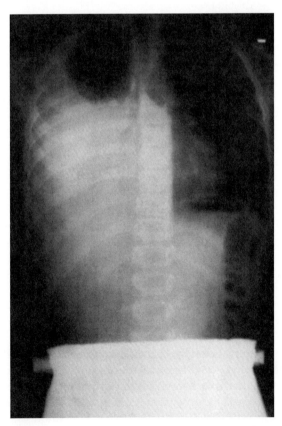

FIGURE 43-1 Upright chest radiograph of child with a large pleural effusion on the right. The majority of the hemithorax is white with a rounded superior margin (meniscus sign). The diaphragm is obscured, and there are air bronchograms in the right lower lung zone. This parapneumonic effusion was caused by *Haemophilus influenzae* pneumonia.

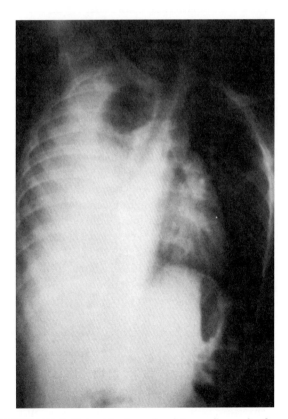

FIGURE 43-2 Right-side-down decubitus radiograph of the child in Figure 43-1. The fluid is more prominent on the lateral chest wall margin, indicating free movement of the fluid in the pleural space.

TABLE 43-1

Distinguishing Transudate From Exudate

Measurement	Transudate	Exudate
Protein (g/dl)	<3	>3
Effusion/serum protein ratio	<0.5	>0.5 protein
LDH (units/L)	<250	>250
Effusion/serum LDH ratio	<0.6	>0.6

LDH, lactate dehydrogenase.

Box 43-2	Causes of Transudative Pleural Effusions

- Congestive heart failure
- Nephrotic syndrome
- Cirrhosis or liver failure
- Acute glomerulonephritis
- Hypoproteinemia
- Myxedema
- Sarcoidosis
- Peritoneal dialysis

Box 43-1	Common Pleural Fluid Analyses

- Total protein
- Lactate dehydrogenase
- Cell counts and differential cell count
- pH
- Cytology
- Studies for infection
  - Gram's stain, bacterial culture
  - Acid-fast stain and culture
  - Fungal stains and culture
- Glucose
- Amylase

Box 43-3	Causes of Exudative Pleural Effusions

- Parapneumonic effusion or empyema
- Pulmonary embolism
- Neoplasm
- Collagen vascular disease
- Trauma
- Drug hypersensitivity
- Lung transplant rejection
- Chylothorax
- Gastrointestinal diseases
- Lymphatic disease
- Postcardiac injury syndrome

heart failure or nephrotic syndrome will leave little doubt as to the cause and nature of the pleural effusion, thereby decreasing the need for thoracentesis.[4-6] After thoracentesis has been performed, the fluid is generally categorized as either a transudate or an exudate on the basis of specific criteria (Table 43-1 and Box 43-1). Disease processes associated with transudates and exudates in children are listed in Boxes 43-2 and 43-3.[2,7]

If a pleural effusion is detected on the chest radiograph, consideration should be given to thoracentesis in all cases. This procedure is usually performed by a physician, with the patient under conscious sedation or general anesthesia. In pediatrics, thoracentesis is not usually done without the assistance of nurses or respiratory care practitioners, or both, to provide stabilization, comfort, and reassurance to the patient. They also handle the drained pleural fluid and monitor the child's cardiovascular status during the procedure. The procedure is performed under sterile conditions, so care must be taken that the physician and assistants do not inadvertently contaminate the field or the specimens. The patient is positioned so that the fluid will be in a dependent position; thus the favored position is either sitting and leaning forward or the lateral decubitus position (effusion side down). The area of dullness should be carefully

percussed in an effort to insert the needle into the spot most likely to provide a return of fluid.[6]

Ultrasound can be helpful to direct the needle into the area most likely to yield fluid. Care must be taken to pass the needle over the rib to prevent injury to the neurovascular bundle, which generally traverses the inferior margin of the ribs. While the needle is being advanced, gentle suction is applied to the attached syringe so that fluid rapidly flows into the syringe when the effusion is entered. Care must be taken to keep the system closed so that no air is sucked back into the pleural space on inspiration. Fluid is withdrawn as long as it drains easily.[6]

Complications of thoracentesis include pneumothorax, hemorrhage, and infection. A *pneumothorax* may be created by nicking the lung with the needle or by not maintaining a closed system and allowing air to enter the chest cavity. *Hemorrhage* may result from nicking a vessel during needle insertion.[6] If sterile technique is not followed, *infection* can be introduced into the pleural space, or the sample sent for microbiology evaluation will be contaminated, or both. Other complications include an allergic reaction to the sedating medicines or hypoventilation resulting from oversedation. It is important for the respiratory care practitioner to be familiar with these complications because he or she may be monitoring the patient's cardiovascular status during the procedure and will be able to auscultate the chest during the procedure without breaking the sterile field. Any deterioration in the patient's clinical status during the procedure should be immediately called to the attention of the physician performing the procedure so that it can be determined whether it is safe to continue.

Several laboratory tests are performed on the pleural fluid to identify the cause of effusion.[2,7] Perhaps the most common type of pleural effusion in pediatrics is a *parapneumonic effusion*,[8,9] which indicates that the pleural fluid is the result of an underlying pneumonia. Although typically a bacterial pneumonia, parapneumonic effusion can also result from a viral, fungal, or parasitic infection, or from tuberculosis (Box 43-4).[9] If the pneumonia extends to infect the pleural space as well, the effusion is then termed an *empyema*.[2] This entity is diagnosed by the presence of frank pus in the pleural space, by a positive culture of the pleural fluid, by a positive Gram's stain of the pleural fluid, or by a white blood cell count greater than 15,000/mm[3]. *Steptococcus pneumoniae* is the most common organism causing pneumonia and empyema in children.[10]

Box 43-4	Causative Organisms in Pleural Effusions

AEROBIC BACTERIA
- (both methicillin sensitive and methicillin resistant)
- *Haemophilus influenzae*
- *Streptococcus pneumoniae*
- *Streptococcus pyogenes*
- Group A, β-hemolytic streptococci

ANAEROBIC BACTERIA
- *Bacteroides* species
- *Peptostreptococcus* species
- *Peptococcus* species
- *Fusobacterium* species

TUBERCULOSIS
- *Mycobacterium tuberculosis*

VIRUSES/MYCOPLASMA
- Adenoviruses
- Parainfluenza viruses
- *Mycoplasma pneumoniae*

FUNGI/FUNGAL ORGANISMS
- *Coccidioides immitis*
- Actinomyces species
- Nocardia species

PARASITES
- *Paragonimus* species
- *Cysticercus* species
- *Entamoeba histolytica*
- *Echinococcus multilocularis*

In adult patients the presence of an empyema suggests that a chest tube should be placed to prevent subsequent fibrous entrapment of the lung.[2] In children it is less clear how often entrapment occurs after empyema. It is becoming less common for physicians to perform repeated thoracenteses or to wait for the antibiotic therapy alone to resolve both the pneumonia and the empyema (see the section Surgery in the Pleural Space).[11-13] In addition to chest tube drainage, prolonged antibiotic therapy is often administered (e.g., 4 to 6 wk).[11] The availability of long-term indwelling intravenous catheters allows transition of intravenous therapy from hospital to home. The duration of combined intravenous and oral antibiotics necessary for successful resolution is not well defined. Eventual healing with normal lung function and a normal chest radiograph is the usual outcome for children, although the chest radiograph may not return to normal for several months.[14,15] Because of the wide variation in success with different management strategies, the decision regarding drainage, fibrinolytic therapy, or surgery in the child with empyema should be individualized.[11-13]

Although less common, other causes of pleural effusion besides infection should be considered; malignancy, acute chest syndrome from sickle cell disease, and postsurgical effusions can also create exudative effusions.[8]

Additional studies besides total protein and lactate dehydrogenase levels may help identify the cause of the effusion. Cell counts and special stains may be helpful. Malignant cells are found in 60% to 90% of effusions caused by malignancy.[2] The respiratory care practitioner may be asked to determine the pleural fluid pH, using a blood gas machine. The specimen must be collected anaerobically in a heparinized syringe and kept on ice until it is analyzed. A pH less than 7.0 or less than 0.15 pH unit below the arterial pH in a patient with parapneumonic effusion may indicate that the patient is at risk for prolonged effusion and subsequent lung entrapment. This has not been extensively studied in children.[7,16]

PNEUMOTHORAX

Air in the pleural space is called a *pneumothorax*.[17] It is termed a *tension pneumothorax* if the pleural air increases with each breath, subsequently pushing the heart and mediastinal structures into the opposite hemithorax. This is generally a life-threatening situation unless the tension is relieved. The patient with a tension pneumothorax will subsequently go into shock from decreased venous return to the heart and from compromised cardiac output caused by the shift of the mediastinum.[4,5] Sometimes the pleural air is not under tension and causes only minimal or moderate respiratory distress.

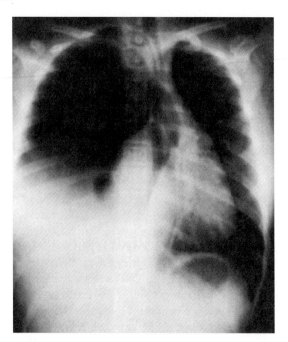

FIGURE 43-3   Chest radiograph showing a right hydropneumothorax (combination of pleural fluid and free air in the pleural space). There are no lung markings in the right chest cavity, and the mediastinal structures are shifted to the left. Fluid fills the lower portion of the right side of the chest cavity. The collapsed right lung is seen as a density to the right of the heart border overlying the spine.

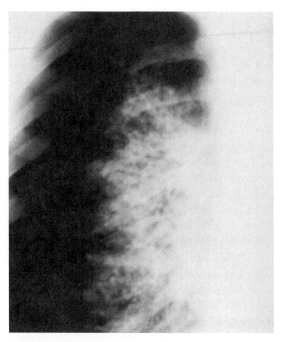

FIGURE 43-4   Portion of chest radiograph from a young man with cystic fibrosis who has a right-sided pneumothorax. The lung stays partially expanded because it has poor compliance (i.e., it is too stiff to collapse completely). A chest tube has not yet been inserted. The outline of the visceral pleura and lung is clearly seen, and there is a lack of lung markings near the chest wall.

A small percentage of patients with a pneumothorax are asymptomatic or have only mild and vague symptoms; however, it is much more common for chest pain and shortness of breath to accompany the pneumothorax. On examination, breath sounds will have decreased intensity on the affected side, and the percussion note will be hyperresonant. With a mediastinal shift the location of the heart's point of maximal impulse may change, and the patient is usually cyanotic with severe respiratory distress. Air under the skin is called *subcutaneous emphysema*, which usually indicates a pneumothorax or pneumomediastinum.

A pneumothorax has a characteristic radiographic appearance (Figure 43-3). Lung markings are lost toward the peripheral chest wall, with evidence of a collapse of the underlying lung. In diseases in which the lung is stiff from underlying disease, such as respiratory distress syndrome of the newborn or cystic fibrosis, the lung may stay partly expanded (Figure 43-4). Pneumothorax and pneumoperitoneum may also result from diaphragmatic hernia and barotrauma (Figures 43-5 and 43-6). The common causes of pneumothorax in neonates and children are listed in Boxes 43-5 and 43-6.[4-6,17] Other conditions associated with pneumothorax are listed in Box 43-7.

Treatment of the pneumothorax depends on whether it is under tension.[6,17,18] The tension pneumothorax is an emergency and should be relieved as soon as possible. The pleural space is drained with a large-bore needle while awaiting more definitive therapy (see the next section). Some small pneumothoraces in patients with chronic lung disease (e.g., cystic fibrosis) might only be observed if there is no clinical deterioration. If the patient is stable, noninvasive therapy with 100% oxygen may be given a brief trial before a more definitive therapy is considered. In rare cases it may be appropriate to withdraw the air by thoracentesis, similar to removing pleural fluid but without resorting to thoracostomy tube drainage.[6,17,18]

THORACOSTOMY DRAINAGE

Tube thoracostomy drainage, or chest tube drainage, is the placement of a tube in the pleural space to drain air or fluid, or both, out of the pleural space. Chest tubes are routinely placed after many thoracic surgeries to ensure appropriate drainage of air, fluid, or blood.[6,18] A chest tube is usually placed for an empyema in adults and chest tubes are often used to drain empyemas in children.[6,11-13] The decision to place a chest tube for drainage of a pleural effusion is based on the patient's

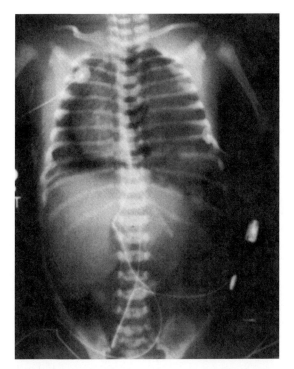

FIGURE 43-5 "Whole baby" radiograph of infant with left diaphragmatic hernia and left pneumothorax. Endotracheal and nasogastric tubes are in place. A chest tube is in the right pleural space. Umbilical artery and vein catheters are in place. The abdominal contents are in the left side of the chest with free air evident at the apex. The heart and mediastinum are shifted to the right. There is free air in the abdominal cavity.

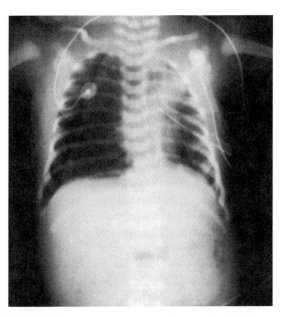

FIGURE 43-6 The same infant as in Figure 43-5 after surgical correction of the diaphragmatic hernia. The density in the left upper lung field is the hypoplastic left lung. There is now a chest tube in the left pleural space as well. There is a persistent pneumothorax on the right despite the chest tube.

Box 43-5	Causes of Pneumothorax in Neonates

- Respiratory distress syndrome
- Meconium aspiration
- Barotrauma
- Spontaneous onset
- First breath
- Congenital anomaly
  - Cystic adenomatoid malformation
  - Pulmonary hypoplasia
  - Congenital lobar emphysema
- Iatrogenic

Box 43-6	Causes of Pneumothorax in Children

- Chronic obstructive lung disease
  - Cystic fibrosis
  - Bronchopulmonary dysplasia
  - Asthma
- Trauma
- Surgery
- Foreign body or ball-valve effect
- Tumor
- Infection
- Pneumatocele
- Barotrauma
- Spontaneous onset
- Congenital anomaly
  - Bronchogenic cyst
- Iatrogenic

Box 43-7	Conditions Associated With Air Leakage in Pneumothorax

- Interstitial emphysema
- Pneumomediastinum
- Pneumopericardium
- Pneumoperitoneum
- Subcutaneous emphysema

clinical status and whether the physician thinks that the respiratory system is compromised by the presence of the pleural fluid. Tension pneumothoraces almost always require chest tube drainage.

The insertion of chest tubes outside of the operating room is generally done in an intensive care unit or in a specialized treatment area because of the seriousness of the underlying illness and the risk of complication. The duties of the respiratory care practitioner during a thoracostomy are similar to those during a thoracentesis, that is, to monitor the patient's cardiopulmonary status during insertion of the chest tube. The complications of chest tube insertion are similar to those of thoracentesis and may occur more frequently in small premature infants.[6,18,19] Some patients require more than one chest tube per side, especially if the pleural fluid is very viscous or loculated or if a pneumothorax persists.[18,20]

The procedure is carried out under conscious sedation or general anesthesia. A small incision is made in the skin with a scalpel. Blunt dissection is used to tunnel into the subcutaneous space over one or two ribs to help secure the position of the tube as well as to provide a seal at skin level. The pleural space is then entered just above a rib either by blunt dissection with forceps or with a trocar placed inside the chest tube. When the tube is placed in an appropriate position, there is frequently a gush of air or fluid out of the tube, which is then temporarily clamped to prevent entrance of air into the pleural space with the next inspiration. The tube is then advanced into the desired position and sutured into place at skin level. The end of the tube is connected to commercially available devices that provide both a water seal and a collection chamber (Figure 43-7). There is a port for wall suction so that continuous negative pressure can be provided to the pleural space to help evacuate its contents. The level of water in the suction control chamber determines the amount of negative pressure applied to the pleural space. Bubbling in the water seal chamber indicates ongoing air leaks, which are usually from the pleural space.[18,19]

While caring for the patient, the practitioner must not disrupt the chest tube and its attachments. A change in the patient's clinical status during evaluation by the respiratory care practitioner may indicate either a new problem with the lung or a malfunction of the chest tube system, which demands immediate evaluation. The practitioner should also anticipate patient discomfort at the site of the chest tube while manipulating the patient or surrounding equipment during chest physical therapy or ventilator tubing changes.

The *bronchopleural fistula* presents a difficult management problem. When the integrity of the lung is not reestablished after an air leak or injury, a large portion of the volume of inspired gases may pass directly through the air leak, thus bypassing the gas-exchanging units of the lung. This can cause hypoventilation in the affected lung and a very large air leak through the chest tube. The bronchopleural fistula may be so severe that

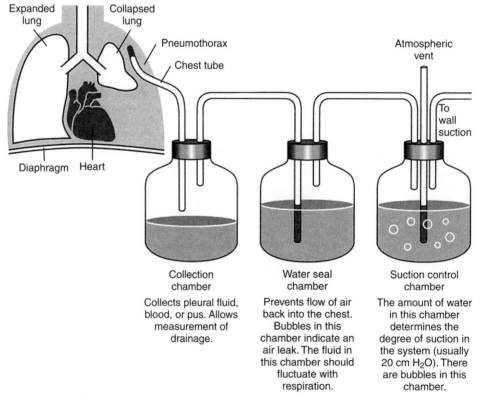

Collection chamber	Water seal chamber	Suction control chamber
Collects pleural fluid, blood, or pus. Allows measurement of drainage.	Prevents flow of air back into the chest. Bubbles in this chamber indicate an air leak. The fluid in this chamber should fluctuate with respiration.	The amount of water in this chamber determines the degree of suction in the system (usually 20 cm H_2O). There are bubbles in this chamber.

FIGURE 43-7 Example of the three-bottle system for thoracostomy drainage. Most current systems include all three components in a single plastic container. Not all systems include the three components, and occasionally two components are combined (collection chamber and water seal chamber).

hypoventilation occurs despite increasing mechanical ventilatory support and the presence of several chest tubes.[21] Spontaneous healing of a bronchopleural fistula may take several days or even weeks. Surgical intervention may be required to oversew the air leak. In the interim, every attempt is made to reexpand the affected lung and minimize the interference with ventilation. In extreme cases, independent lung ventilation may be required or special valves inserted between the chest tube and wall suction to occlude the chest tube drainage intermittently during the inspiratory cycle of the mechanical ventilator.[20] Special glues and patches have been used to seal the bronchopleural fistula.[22,23]

SURGERY IN THE PLEURAL SPACE

The indications for pleural space surgery in pediatric patients with empyema are less well established than in adults.[11,24] A basic infectious disease tenet is that *pus in a closed space should be drained.* This tenet is partly the basis for recommending closed-tube thoracostomy drainage for an empyema. Failure to drain the empyema adequately risks the development of a trapped lung, which subsequently may require pleural decortication.[11] In children treatment with appropriate antibiotic therapy usually avoids the need for subsequent decortication.[14,15] The child with an empyema who has had a slow clinical response to broad-spectrum intravenous antibiotics may benefit from a surgical procedure to evacuate the purulent material and consider a pleural decortication.[24] The use of fibrinolytics is an alternative option for children with slowly improving empyema despite chest tube drainage.[11-13]

No clear consensus exists on the most appropriate management of the difficult problem of surgery in the pleural space, so each patient should receive the benefit of an individualized therapeutic plan with flexibility to change depending on therapeutic success.

If a chest tube placed to drain an empyema stops functioning, often the empyema fluid is loculated and the chest tube is in the wrong place.[6,18,20] Repositioning the chest tube or adding another may allow better drainage. Injecting fibrinolytics (streptokinase, urokinase, or alteplase) into the pleural cavity may facilitate drainage by liquefying the organizing empyema and dissolving the fibrin septations that are causing loculation of fluid.[12]

Thoracoscopy is the direct visualization of the pleural space through either rigid or flexible surgical equipment.[25] This technique has had increasing utilization for a wide variety of pediatric pulmonary problems since the initial use nearly 30 years ago.[24,25] The video-assisted thorascopic surgery (VATS) technology is now commonly utilized for the following:[26]

- Biopsy in patients with diffuse lung disease
- Evaluation and biopsy of mediastinal masses
- Diagnosis and management of pleural disease
- Treatment of spontaneous pneumothorax
- Intrathoracic resections

The major advantage of this approach is the avoidance of a thoracotomy, resulting in less postoperative pain and a shorter recovery period.

In larger children, some surgical interventions are possible through the thoracoscope.[24,25] The major advantage of this approach is the avoidance of a thoracotomy, resulting in less postoperative pain and a shorter recovery period. Because the surgeon inserts a video camera into the pleural space to allow visualization of the surgical field, the procedure is called video-assisted thoracoscopic surgery (VATS).

The current size limitations of the equipment may limit the usefulness of thoracoscopy in premature infants and neonates, and some have recommended that it not be used in children less than 6 months of age or in those who weigh less than 8 kg.[26] General anesthesia is required, and unilateral lung ventilation must be used. This may be accomplished by using a double-lumen endotracheal tube in larger patients (adolescents) or by performing mainstem intubation or bronchial blocking with a balloon catheter in the smaller child.[24,25] However, many children younger than 4 years of age cannot tolerate unilateral ventilation and become hypoxic because of their relatively limited functional residual capacity. Pneumothorax, infection, and bleeding are the most often reported complications, although complications often depend on the patient's preoperative condition.[25]

Surgical intervention is seldom needed for persistent pneumothorax or bronchopleural fistula in children. Borrowing from the experience with malignant pleural effusions, *chemical pleurodesis* has been attempted in children who have persistent pneumothorax or recurrent pneumothorax due to cystic fibrosis.[27] This procedure uses agents such as tetracycline or talc to produce a pleural abrasion that results in the adhesion of pleural surfaces. There has been no clear consensus as to whether surgical intervention or chemical pleurodesis is the most appropriate approach to this problem.[28] An individualized patient management plan should be offered, with flexibility to consider alternative options if the initial plan is unsuccessful. The use of chemical or surgical pleurodesis may complicate or prohibit subsequent lung transplantation.

The respiratory therapist should be aware of the wide variety of pleural space diseases that might compromise the patient's respiratory function. Familiarity with these diseases will help the practitioner understand the reason for the patient's deterioration or improvement and will contribute to the health care team's management of these problems.

ASSESSMENT QUESTIONS

See Evolve Resources for answers.

1. Which of the following statements regarding the pleural space in a normal child is *true*?
   A. There is usually no fluid in the pleural space.
   B. There is normally a small amount of free air in the pleural space that can be seen only on a decubitus chest radiograph.
   C. There is a small amount of fluid in the pleural space that represents a balance of the fluid flux between the parietal and visceral pleura.
   D. The parietal pleura is thick and leathery to prevent penetration by sharp objects.
2. What is the most common cause of pneumothorax in the small premature infant with respiratory distress syndrome (hyaline membrane disease)?
   A. Neonatal pneumonia
   B. Barotrauma from mechanical ventilation and poorly compliant lungs
   C. Complication from subclavian intravenous line placement
   D. Meconium aspiration
3. The lung disease that is most commonly associated with spontaneous pneumothorax in adolescents is:
   A. Langerhans cell histiocytosis X (eosinophilic granuloma)
   B. Pulmonary alveolar proteinosis
   C. Congenital tracheo-esophageal fistula
   D. Cystic fibrosis
4. Which of the following pleural fluid measurements indicates the fluid is an exudate rather than a transudate?
   A. Total protein = 5.0 g/dL
   B. Lactate dehydrogenase (LDH) = 120 IU/L
   C. White blood cell count (WBC) = 860 cells/mm³
   D. pH 7.30
5. When assessing the function of a chest tube draining air from the pleural space of a pediatric patient, which of the following suggests an ongoing intrapleural air leak?
   A. Bubbling in the water seal chamber
   B. Fluid in the collection chamber
   C. Fluctuating fluid in the chest tube
   D. Bubbling in the suction control chamber
6. Which of the following organisms most commonly causes empyema in toddlers and school age children?
   A. *Mycobacterium tuberculosis*
   B. Adenovirus
   C. *Streptococcus pneumoniae*
   D. *Aspergillus fumigatus*

ASSESSMENT QUESTIONS—cont'd

7. Which of the following pleural fluid characteristics determines that the fluid represents and empyema?
   A. Appearance of gross pus
   B. WBC ≥ 15,000 cells/mm³
   C. Positive Gram's stain of the pleural fluid
   D. All of the above
8. Which of the following statements about video-assisted thoracoscopic surgery (VATS) in the management of empyema is *true*?
   A. VATS will likely hasten the resolution of empyema compared with chest tube drainage alone.
   B. VATS requires the same skill level and equipment as standard chest tube insertion.
   C. VATS has been shown to be superior to the instillation of fibrinolytic agents (e.g., urokinase, streptokinase, alteplase) in the management of pediatric empyema.
   D. VATS should be performed early in the evaluation and management of pleural effusion regardless of whether or not the fluid is a transudate, an exudate, or an empyema.
9. What are the current limitations to VATS in pediatric patients?
   A. Size of equipment
   B. Necessity for general anesthesia
   C. Requirement of unilateral lung ventilation with a double-lumen endotracheal tube (ETT).
   D. All of the above
10. What are three congenital anomalies that may cause a pneumothorax in a neonate?
    A. Cystic adenomatoid malformation, pulmonary hypoplasia, lobar emphysema
    B. Surfactant-deficient respiratory distress syndrome, first-breath malfunction, meconium aspiration syndrome
    C. Ventilator-induced trauma, ETT suctioning, spontaneous onset
    D. None of the above

References

1. Black LF: The pleural space and pleural fluid, *Mayo Clin Proc* 1972;47:493.
2. Sahn SA: State of the art: the pleura, *Am Rev Respir Dis* 1988;138:184.
3. Büttiker V, Fanconi S, Burger R: Chylothorax in children: guidelines for diagnosis and management, *Chest* 1999;116:682.
4. Panitch HB, Papastomelos C, Schidlow DV: Abnormalities of the pleural space. In Taussig LM, Landau LI, editors: *Pediatric respiratory medicine*, St. Louis: Mosby; 1999. pp 1178-1196.
5. Montgomery M: Air and liquid in the pleural space. In Chernick V, Boat TF, Kendig EL, editors: *Kendig's*

disorders of the respiratory tract in children, Philadelphia: WB Saunders; 1998. pp 389-411.

6. Tucker WY: Thoracentesis and tube thoracotomy. In Hilman B, editor: *Pediatric respiratory disease: diagnosis and treatment*, Philadelphia: WB Saunders; 1993. pp 839-844.

7. Heffner JE: Evaluating diagnostic tests in the pleural space: differentiating transudates from exudates as a model, *Clin Chest Med* 1998;19:277.

8. Hardie W et al: Pneumococcal pleural empyemas in children, *Clin Infect Dis* 1996;22:1057.

9. Freij BJ et al: Parapneumonic effusions and empyema in hospitalized children: a retrospective review of 227 cases, *Pediatr Infect Dis J* 1984;3:578.

10. Buckingham SC, King MD, Miller ML: Incidence and etiologies of complicated parapneumonic effusions in children, 1996-2001, *Pediatr Infect Dis J* 2003;22:499.

11. Balfour-Lynn IM et al: BTS guidelines for the management of pleural infection in children, *Thorax* 2005;60(suppl 1):i1.

12. Barnes NP, Hull J, Thompson AH: Medical management of parapneumonic pleural disease, *Pediatr Pulmonol* 2005;39:127.

13. Hilliard TN, Henderson AJ, Langton Hewer SC: Management of parapneumonic effusion and empyema, *Arch Dis Child* 2003;88:915.

14. McLaughlin FJ et al: Empyema in children: clinical course and long-term follow up, *Pediatrics* 1984;73:587.

15. Redding GJ et al: Lung function in children following empyema, *Am J Dis Child* 1990;144:337.

16. Givan DC, Eigen H: Common pleural effusions in children, *Clin Chest Med* 1998;10:363.

17. Sahn SA, Heffner JE: Spontaneous pneumothorax, *N Engl J Med* 2000;342:868.

18. Miller KS, Sahn SA: Chest tubes: indications, technique, management, and complications, *Chest* 1987;91:258.

19. Moessinger AC, Driscoll JM, Wigger HJ: High incidence of lung perforation by chest tube in neonatal pneumothorax, *Pediatrics* 1978;92:635.

20. Cohen S, Stack M: How to work with chest tubes, *Am J Nurs* 1980;80:685.

21. Baumann MH, Sahn SA: Medical management and therapy of bronchopulmonary fistulas in mechanically ventilated patients, *Chest* 1990;97:721.

22. Dumire R et al: Autologous "blood patch" pleurodesis for persistent pulmonary air leak, *Chest* 1992;101:64.

23. Berger JT, Gilhooly J: Fibrin glue treatment of persistent pneumothorax in a premature infant, *J Pediatr* 1993;122:958.

24. Milanez de Campos JR et al: Thoracoscopy in children and adolescents, *Chest* 1997;111:494.

25. Avansino JR et al: Primary operative versus nonoperative therapy for pediatric empyema: a meta-analysis, *Pediatrics* 2005;115:1652.

26. Rothenberg SS: Thoracoscopic pulmonary surgery, *Semin Pediatr Surg* 2007; 16(4):231.

27. Rodgers BM: Pediatric thoracoscopy: where have we come and what have we learned? *Ann Thorac Surg* 1993;56:704.

28. McLaughlin FJ et al: Pneumothorax in cystic fibrosis: management and outcome, *Pediatrics* 1982;100:863.

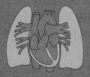
Neurologic and Neuromuscular Disorders

MARY E. HARTMAN • PETER H. MICHELSON • MICHAEL P. CZERVINSKE

LEARNING OBJECTIVES

After reading this chapter the reader will be able to:
- Discuss the components of the central and peripheral nervous systems that control normal respiration
- Explain how the nervous system interacts with the muscles of respiration during normal and pathologic breathing
- Identify which muscle groups are enervated by the brainstem and how bulbar weakness interferes with protecting the airway and clearing secretions
- Identify the most common central nervous system conditions that affect respiratory pattern and neuromuscular impairment
- Identify the most common peripheral nervous system conditions that cause neuromuscular and respiratory impairment

- Describe the important features of the respiratory physical examination for children with neuromuscular weakness
- Describe the tests available to quantify respiratory compromise for children with neuromuscular weakness
- Describe the respiratory aids available to support respiration for children with neuromuscular weakness
- Explain the indications and proper use of respiratory aids for children with neuromuscular weakness
- Identify the multisystem and nonrespiratory complications related to neuromuscular disease

Although there are many congenital and acquired neuromuscular conditions that present in childhood, the uniting feature of all these disorders is their effect on the respiratory system. The primary cause of morbidity and mortality for children with neuromuscular disease is respiratory compromise.[1] As such, health care providers should have a comprehensive understanding of the physiology of normal breathing, its derangements in neuromuscular disorders, the evaluation of patients with weakness, and specific aspects of their care.

NEUROMUSCULAR CONTROL OF RESPIRATION

Advances over the previous century provided detailed understanding of the control of respiration and the various components involved in breathing, but there remain significant gaps in our comprehension of the overall system.[2,3] The presence of a "neuromuscular respiratory system" was first recognized by the second-century anatomist and physician Galen.[4] Central and reflex control of breathing has been subsequently described by investigators including Hering, Breuer, and Head, with significant contributions in the early twentieth century by Haldane and Priestley on the role of carbon dioxide in chemical respiratory control.[5] This chapter focuses on the present state of understanding of the neuromuscular control of respiration.

Central Nervous System

The respiratory system brings oxygen into the body to fuel energy production and removes carbon dioxide, a metabolic waste product. Central nervous system control occurs in the cerebral cortex, which supports voluntary breathing actions, and incorporates input from the brainstem, which is involved with automatic breathing actions.[3,6] Central nervous system (CNS) signals are transmitted to the anterior horn cells of the spinal cord and then to the motor neurons that supply the respiratory muscles. Separate pathways in the spinal cord support both voluntary (corticospinal) and involuntary (reticulospinal) ventilation and transmit signals through descending pathways to motor neurons in the cervicothoracic portion of the spinal cord. These motor neurons transmit signals through peripheral nerves and across the neuromuscular junction to the muscles of respiration.[7] Dysfunction in any part of this control system, from brainstem to respiratory muscles, can result in respiratory failure.

Peripheral Nervous System

Each lower motor neuron arises from the cell body in the spinal cord (anterior horn cell) to supply the respiratory muscles. The efferent nerves extend to the diaphragm and intercostal muscles, and to the accessory muscles of the neck. The diaphragm is supplied by the phrenic nerve, the intercostal muscles by the intercostal nerves, the accessory muscles of the neck from the cervical plexus, and the abdominal muscles from the lumbar nerve roots.[3,8]

The nerves divide into branches when reaching the muscle fiber and apply themselves to the muscle membrane at the motor endplates. At these junctions, the chemical transmitter acetylcholine is released to depolarize the muscle membrane and causes intracellular calcium release, which in turn serves to initiate contraction of the muscle fiber.[9]

Respiratory Muscles

The muscles of respiration are divided into three groups: the inspiratory muscles, expiratory muscles, and accessory muscles. Although not formally classified as accessory muscles of respiration, the muscles of the upper airway are also important in maintaining airway patency and may lose function with certain neuromuscular disorders.

The main inspiratory muscle is the diaphragm, which contributes almost three quarters of the inspiratory capacity. Cervical nerves 3 to 5 contribute to form the phrenic nerve, which drives the diaphragm. Additional inspiratory force is provided by the external intercostal muscles, which contract to expand the rib cage during inspiration. The innervation of the intercostals muscles is via the intercostal nerves, which come off the thoracic spinal nerve roots.

The expiratory muscles include the internal intercostals, which help to reduce the thoracic volume, as well as the accessory abdominal muscles. These include the internal and external obliques and the transversus abdominus, which contract to displace the diaphragm into the thoracic cavity, and the rectus abdominus, which also contributes to increasing pleural pressure during exhalation.

The accessory muscles of respiration include the sternocleidomastoid, scalenes, trapezii, latissimus dorsi, and platysma and pectoralis groups. These groups are active predominantly with increased respiratory work, such as exercise, or loss of functional residual capacity, which occurs with infection or neuromuscular weakness. By contributing to rib cage expansion, these muscles support inspiration during active ventilation, although function during quiet breathing also exists.[3,6]

Respiratory Control System

Respiratory control is divided into both voluntary and metabolic control systems. Voluntary control originates in the cerebral cortex and is mediated by tracts in the dorsolateral spinal cord; voluntary control regulates ventilation affected by sleep, pain or anxiety. Metabolic control, mediated by the ventrolateral pathways, incorporates inputs from central chemoreceptors within the medulla. Peripheral receptors in the carotid and aortic bodies respond to fluctuations in arterial oxygen pressure (Pao_2), arterial carbon dioxide pressure ($Paco_2$), and pH. These various receptors operate via feedback loops that help to contribute to respiratory drive and regulate the ventilatory pattern in most normal physiologic states.[3]

In addition, mechanical receptors in the lung and airways provide feedback to the respiratory centers as well as stimulate spinal reflexes that further regulate the breathing pattern. Examples of mechanical receptor control include the Hering-Breuer reflex, which prevents overinflation, coughing, bronchoconstriction, and the recruitment of accessory muscles during respiratory distress. Related mechanical receptors in the upper airway also induce coughing, glottic closure, vagal stimulation, and singultus (hiccups).

Bulbar Muscles

The bulbar muscles are not related to ventilation, but are important in protecting the airway and secretion clearance. The bulbar muscles are enervated by the motor neurons emanating from the brainstem. This muscle group controls the epiglottis and other glottic structures, tongue, mouth, larynx, and throat. Bulbar muscle weakness impairs swallowing, coughing, speech, and other throat and pharyngeal activities. Bulbar muscle weakness also leads to severe fixed and variable extrathoracic upper airway obstruction on forced inspiratory and expiratory respiratory efforts. Examples of forced respiratory efforts include coughing, sneezing, respiratory distress, and pulmonary function testing.

NEUROMUSCULAR DISEASES THAT AFFECT THE RESPIRATORY SYSTEM

Neuromuscular disease is a broad term that encompasses many diseases that affect muscle function either directly, via muscle pathology, or indirectly, via nerve pathology. The diseases themselves are associated with a diverse range of muscle impairment from increased muscle tone with rigidity and spasticity to muscle weakness and flaccidity. This chapter covers primarily those affecting infants and children with muscle weakness or paralysis, because these conditions affect the respiratory system by impairing ventilation and airway clearance.

Central Nervous System

Conditions in the CNS that affect respiration include either those that impact the brainstem respiratory centers, or the pathways connecting these centers to the motor neurons in the spinal cord.[3]

Disorders of the Brain

One of the best examples of a CNS disorder that affects breathing is congenital central hypoventilation syndrome (CCHS). Also known as "Ondine's curse," this represents a condition of hypoventilation associated with sleep. The name refers to the mythical character Ondine, who after professing his love "with every waking breath" was cursed by the water nymph he betrayed, to stop breathing on falling asleep.[10] Although almost all cases of CCHS are congenital, affecting approximately 1 in 200,000 live births, it can also be acquired through spinal cord or other central nervous system injury.[10] CCHS, manifested by nocturnal hypoventilation and respiratory arrest, is diagnosed by polysomnography and treated with lifetime nocturnal mechanical ventilation or phrenic nerve pacing.[10,11]

Other cranial conditions affecting respiration in infants and children include congenital disorders such as hydrocephalus and anencephaly, along with genetic neurodegenerative disorders such as Tay-Sachs disease and Friedreich's ataxia.[3,12,13] Acquired CNS disorders include neoplasms, infarction, hemorrhage, and anoxic injury.[3] All of these conditions are associated with multiple organ system symptomatology, resulting from diffuse neurologic injury and loss of autonomic control. Respiratory symptoms of these conditions include changes in respiratory drive or pattern, respiratory and upper airway muscle weakness with loss of airway clearance ability, and chronic aspiration.

Disorders Affecting the Spinal Cord

Trauma. Almost 11,000 Americans sustain a spinal cord injury every year, costing an approximated 9.7 billion dollars in health care expenditure.[14] The spinal cord nerve roots that control diaphragm function exit the spine at the level of the cervical vertebrae.[8,15] Spinal cord injury above cervical vertebra 3 will require tracheostomy and mechanical ventilation or phrenic nerve pacing.[16] Spinal cord injuries between vertebrae 3 and 5 will have variable amounts of respiratory impairment, and those below the fifth vertebra almost always allow independent breathing.[3] However, the abdominal and intercostal rib muscles involved in cough function exit the spinal cord lower in the thoracic spine.[15] Therefore, lower spine injuries may permit spontaneous respiration but have significant impact on airway clearance mechanisms.[3]

Chiari Malformations. Chiari malformations are congenital malformations characterized by a small or misshapen skull, causing the cerebellum to protrude through the bottom of the skull into the spinal canal. Under these circumstances, the brainstem, spinal cord, cranial nerves, or the cerebellum may be stretched or compressed. In addition, the flow of cerebrospinal fluid around the brain and spinal cord can be obstructed, causing hydrocephalus or a cyst to form within the spinal cord, known as *syringomyelia*.[17] Estimates indicate that between 0.5% and 1% of live births in the United States may be affected by a Chiari malformation.[17] Symptoms of Chiari malformations are variable and related to the affected areas. Many patients with Chiari malformations report no symptoms, but those that do complain of headaches, dizziness, vision changes, muscle weakness, or balance problems.[18] Younger children may present with difficulty swallowing, choking, irregular breathing patterns, or apnea.[17] Chiari malformations can be easily diagnosed by magnetic resonance imaging scan and are treated by surgical decompression.

Other Conditions. Other, less common causes of spinal cord impairment include spinal tumors, infections, and birth injury. Spinal tumors either originate locally in the CNS or are metastatic. Meningiomas are primary CNS tumors that develop from the meninges, the membrane that surrounds the brain and spinal cord. They are rare in children, with pediatric cases accounting for only 1.5% of all cases.[19] Metastatic spinal tumors are also rare in children, but may be seen with invasive lymphomas and have been reported in other childhood cancers.[20] Central nervous system infections, such as epidural abscesses, can have both local inflammatory and mass effect on the spinal cord, causing neuromuscular symptoms to develop. Finally, spinal cord injury may be a rare complication of the birthing process. In this situation, traction applied to the infant's head while assisting delivery may result in nervous system trauma. These injuries include cervical spinal cord hematomas as well as direct nerve and nerve root stretch injury.

Peripheral Nervous System
Disorders of the Motor Nerves

Acute paralytic poliomyelitis was once the most common neuronopathy in the United States.[21] However, massive immunization campaigns have been effectively instituted and all but eliminated community-acquired poliovirus infections in the United States. As a result, the *spinal muscular atrophies* are now the most common cause of degenerative nerve cell disease in children.

Spinal Muscular Atrophy. The spinal muscular atrophies (SMAs) include a number of different disorders that clinically manifest as muscle weakness due to progressive destruction of the motor neurons of the spinal cord and brainstem.[22,23] The SMAs are hereditary disorders transmitted by autosomal recessive inheritance, with three recognized forms categorized by severity and age of onset.[22,23] All types are caused by defects at the same site on chromosome 5, and the overlap in

clinical features is considerable.[24-26] SMA type I, also called Werdnig-Hoffmann disease, is the acute infantile form, which usually presents within the first 6 months of life.[27] In these children, limb weakness develops rapidly, whereas the facial muscles are slower to fail and the extraocular muscles are essentially spared. The result is a child who appears alert and responsive but cannot move. The respiratory effects of SMA type I include weakness of the bulbar, abdominal, and intercostal muscles, which makes feeding difficult and leads to aspiration and a weak, ineffective cough. A weak cough results in recurrent pneumonias and poor airway clearance. Even relatively minor viral infections result in severe airway and ventilator compromise. Without intervention, most infants will die of respiratory insufficiency and infection before reaching 1 year of age.[26]

SMA type II, the *chronic childhood form*, has a later onset and often more insidious course.[27] Some affected children may be able to sit unsupported, but usually proximal muscle weakness prevents these children from standing or walking independently, and leads to scoliosis; these children eventually become wheelchair dependent.[28] The course of SMA type II is unpredictable; long intervals without progression of weakness are expected and survival into adulthood is common.[29] SMA type III (Kugelberg-Welander disease) is the mildest form; affected patients are able to stand and walk independently, and have much slower progression of muscle weakness compared with the other two forms.[27]

Poliomyelitis. Poliomyelitis is an infection caused by the polio virus, and was one of the most dreaded childhood diseases of the 20th century in the United States.[21] The vast majority of infected individuals are asymptomatic or experience only mild, nonspecific viral symptoms. However, in a small proportion of patients, the virus enters the central nervous system, where it infects and destroys motor neurons in the spinal cord, leading to muscle wasting and weakness.[30] Most commonly, this causes a self-limited case of nonparalytic viral meningitis, but in a small proportion of patients the infection causes permanent wasting and paralysis. Depending on the site of paralysis, paralytic polio is classified as *spinal*, affecting the nerves of the trunk and extremities; *bulbar*, affecting the nerves that control breathing, speaking, and swallowing; or *bulbospinal*, representing a combination of these two forms.[30] Bulbospinal polio is particularly problematic because it affects the nerves in the cervical spine region that control diaphragm function. Destruction of these nerves makes independent respiration, swallowing, and effective coughing impossible. Lifelong ventilator support and airway clearance is essential for the survival of these patients.[30]

Guillain-Barré Syndrome. Guillain-Barré syndrome (GBS), or acute inflammatory demyelinating polyradiculoneuropathy, is an acute, autoimmune process that affects the peripheral nervous system. Guillain-Barré syndrome is not hereditary, affects persons of all ages, and has an approximate population incidence that ranges from 1 to 3 per 100,000 population.[31,32] Although its cause is not completely understood, GBS is probably triggered by an acute infectious process, which leads to antibody-mediated destruction of the myelin sheaths that coat peripheral nerves.[33] This demyelination leads to nerve conduction block, which causes weakness, and often sensory and autonomic changes as well.[34] Guillain-Barré syndrome usually presents as an ascending weakness or paralysis that starts in the legs and spreads to the upper limbs and the face. The weakness is frequently preceded by sensory symptoms such as "pins and needles" and muscle tenderness, followed by a complete loss of deep tendon reflexes.[33] Patients often experience rapid progression of symptoms; more than three quarters of patients reach a nadir in strength within 3 weeks of symptom onset.[33] Autonomic dysfunction, characterized by dysrhythmias, blood pressure lability, and gastrointestinal dysfunction, may also be present.[35] Respiratory paralysis occurs in roughly 14% to 18% of children with GBS, and approximately 20% of all patients with GBS require intensive care during the acute phase of illness.[32,33] Treatment is mainly supportive, although corticosteroids, plasmapheresis, and intravenous immunoglobulin have all been used with variable success.[32,36] Although plasmapheresis is considered the treatment of choice in adults, certain technical factors may limit its usefulness in children. Careful monitoring of patients' respiratory status, accompanied by intubation and mechanical ventilation when required, constitutes the mainstay of acute supportive care. If the child is well ventilated during the critical time of profound paralysis, complete recovery can be expected.[31] Most children fully recover within 6 months, and fewer than 10% have symptom recurrence.[31,34]

Disorders of the Neuromuscular Junction

Infantile Botulism. Human botulism results from eating food contaminated with the organism *Clostridium botulinum* or the toxin it produces.[37] The clinical spectrum of infantile botulism ranges from asymptomatic carrier states, mild hypotonia, and failure to thrive to severe with progressive, life-threatening paralysis and/or sudden death.[38] Most infants experience a prodromal syndrome of constipation and poor feeding, followed by progressive bulbar and skeletal muscle weakness and loss of tendon reflexes. Typical features on examination include diffuse hypotonia, ptosis, dysphagia, and a weak cry. Respiratory history and examination are often notable for respiratory insufficiency and apnea. Diagnosis is confirmed by the isolation of *C. botulinum* organisms from the stool. In general, botulism is a self-limited disease lasting 2 to 6 weeks, and even with the use of immunoglobulin therapy the infant requires meticulous supportive respiratory care. In severe cases, this support is life-saving. Recovery is often complete, but relapse can occur in as many as 5% of affected infants.[39]

Myasthenia Gravis. Myasthenia gravis is an autoimmune disorder characterized by fluctuating muscle weakness and easy fatigability.[40] The pathophysiology of the disorder occurs at the neuromuscular junction, where circulating antibodies block synaptic receptors, inhibiting the effect of neurotransmitter chemicals, most notably acetylcholine; this prevents muscle contraction.[40] The current prevalence of myasthenia gravis in the United States is estimated to be about 20 per 100,000 population, although frequent misdiagnosis means that the true prevalence is likely higher.[41] Juvenile myasthenia describes the immune-mediated form of myasthenia gravis that occurs in late infancy through adult life.[42] Two forms are recognized[43]:

- *Ocular myasthenia*: In which the eye muscles are primarily or exclusively affected
- *Generalized myasthenia*: In which moderate to severe weakness occurs in bulbar, limb, trunk, and even respiratory muscles

The initial features of both the ocular and generalized forms are usually ptosis, diplopia, or both.[41] Prepubertal onset is associated with a slight male bias and ocular symptoms only, whereas postpubertal onset is associated with a strong female bias and generalized myasthenia.[44] Patients with myasthenia gravis often have little chronic respiratory compromise, and are symptomatic only during periods of myasthenia crisis, when symptoms, particularly bulbar symptoms, suddenly escalate. During a crisis patients may have sudden paralysis of the respiratory muscles, temporarily requiring assisted ventilation. Treatment also includes using cholinesterase inhibitors to help transmission of acetylcholine, and immune suppressants such as corticosteroids and cyclosporine. Exchange transfusions and intravenous immunoglobulin therapy rapidly restore function, but are temporary measures.[41]

Congenital myasthenia and *familial infantile myasthenia* are terms used to describe clinical syndromes that are caused by several different genetic defects and are generally rare. Respiratory insufficiency and feeding difficulty may be present at birth or develop during infancy. Usually, ptosis and generalized weakness are present at birth. Many affected newborns require mechanical ventilation, but over a course of weeks most infants become stronger and no longer need ventilator support.[45]

A *transitory myasthenic syndrome* is observed in 10% to 15% of offspring of myasthenic mothers. The syndrome is believed to be caused by the transfer of antibody from the myasthenic mother to her normal fetus. Symptoms are generally observed within hours of birth. The severity of newborn symptoms correlates with the newborn's antibody concentration and not the severity of weakness in the mother, which is generally exacerbated during pregnancy.[46] Difficulty feeding and generalized hypotonia are the major clinical features; they are eager to feed, but suckling quickly causes fatigue. Respiratory insufficiency is uncommon and weakness becomes progressively worse in the first few days of life and then improves. Recovery is complete, and transitory neonatal myasthenia does not develop into myasthenia later in life.

Other Conditions Affecting the Neuromuscular Junction. In the medical setting, there are a number of other causes of incomplete or failed transmission at the neuromuscular junction related to drug exposure. These medications include antibiotics, corticosteroids, antirheumatics, lidocaine, lithium, and anesthetic agents.[3]

Myopathies

Myopathies are diseases of the skeletal musculature causing muscle weakness and degeneration. Myopathies are caused by inherited genetic defects and by inflammatory, endocrinologic, and metabolic disorders.

Duchenne and Becker Muscular Dystrophy

The muscular dystrophies are a group of genetic disorders with multisystem symptoms involving the cardiac, respiratory, gastrointestinal, endocrine, and nervous systems.[47] Although there are more than 100 diseases that have similarities to muscular dystrophy, the two most common muscular dystrophies that present in childhood are Duchenne and Becker muscular dystrophy.[47] Duchenne muscular dystrophy (DMD) is the most common childhood form of muscular dystrophy, occurring in roughly 1 in 3500 live male births.[47,48] The male preponderance is related to its inheritance pattern: DMD is an X-linked genetic disorder, resulting in female carriers and affected males. DMD presents in early childhood with proximal muscle weakness, which is manifest as difficulty in running, climbing stairs, and standing.[47] The muscle weakness is progressive and eventually leads to profound skeletal and respiratory muscle weakness in all cases. By adolescence, all patients with DMD are wheelchair bound and require assistance with ventilation.[47] Becker muscular dystrophy is also an X-linked inherited muscular dystrophy, with a distribution of muscle wasting and weakness similar to that of DMD.[47] However, Becker muscular dystrophy typically has a milder course with symptom onset in the second decade or later.

There is no cure for any of the muscular dystrophies, and current therapy is supportive. Treatment goals are to maintain function, prevent contractures, and provide psychological support for the child and family. Traditional estimates suggest that up to 90% of patients with DMD die of respiratory failure before reaching 20 years of age.[49] Muscular dystrophy affects the heart as well, and the second leading cause of death in DMD is cardiomyopathy and cardiac failure, or arrhythmia.[48] However, aggressive intervention with noninvasive ventilation, airway clearance techniques, and surgical correction of spine deformation to improve lung volumes at the onset of respiratory symptoms has been demonstrated to significantly reduce morbidity and prolong life for patients with muscular dystrophy.[49]

Myotonic Dystrophies

Myotonic dystrophy is a highly variable inherited disease characterized by chronic, slowly progressive muscle wasting and weakness, cataracts, heart conduction defects, and endocrine disorders.[50] The muscles most commonly affected are the voluntary muscles in the face, neck, and lower arms and legs, and in more severe cases the intercostal muscles and the diaphragm.[50] Myotonic dystrophy most commonly presents in adolescence or adulthood, but a severe congenital form exists and is associated with mental retardation, orthopedic problems, and other developmental delays.[50] Affected infants are extremely hypotonic and may have difficulty feeding. They often require ventilatory support, at least temporarily, because of muscle weakness and decreased central ventilatory drive.[50] Similar to the muscular dystrophies, the overwhelming majority of affected children die in infancy. However, supported ventilation, corrective surgery, and tube feeding have all extended the life span of patients and dramatically improved quality of life for these children and their families.[50]

Glycogen Storage Diseases

The glycogen storage diseases are a family of 12 inherited errors of metabolism that result in enzyme defects in glycogen synthesis or breakdown. In general, clinical classifications can be made on the basis of whether affected organs include the liver only, or additionally the muscles, blood cells, connective tissue, heart, brain, and/or kidneys. In terms of respiratory involvement, glycogen storage disease type II (also called Pompe disease or acid maltase deficiency) has the most severe symptoms. Pompe disease is a rare, autosomal recessive disorder occurring in roughly 1 in 40,000 to 100,000 live births.[51,52] It is caused by a deficiency in the enzyme α-1,4-glucosidase, which causes glycogen accumulation in cellular lysosomes and leads to progressive weakness in all muscles.[52] Like all of the congenital disorders, the severity of symptoms of Pompe disease are related to age at onset. Infantile onset is the most severe form, and is characterized by the development of marked hypotonia, hepatomegaly, and severe cardiomegaly within several months of birth. Mental development is usually normal, although most children die of respiratory or cardiac complications before 2 years of age.[53] Late-onset Pompe disease occurs in patients with minimal—as opposed to absent—levels of the acid maltase enzyme.[51,52] Symptoms in these affected individuals present in adolescence or adulthood, tend to progress somewhat more slowly, and include primarily weakness of muscles in the trunk, lower limbs, and the diaphragm. A small number of adult patients live relatively normal lives without major limitations.[52]

Electrolyte Abnormalities

Other, less common causes of muscle weakness in the outpatient setting include electrolyte abnormalities—most commonly caused by insufficient dietary intake. Potassium is essential for many body functions, including muscle and nerve activity. Maintenance of the electrochemical gradient of potassium between the intracellular and extracellular space is essential for normal nerve function. Mild hypokalemia is often asymptomatic; however, moderate hypokalemia may cause diffuse muscular weakness, myalgias, and arrhythmias.[54] Severe hypokalemia has been associated with respiratory depression from severe impairment of skeletal muscle function.[55] Similarly, hypomagnesemia can cause weakness and muscle cramps, and may contribute to impairments in respiratory muscle function.[54] Hypomagnesemia, which can be seen in the presence of hypokalemia, hypocalcemia, and/or hypophosphatemia, should prompt the evaluation of other electrolyte disturbances that can further exacerbate these clinical symptoms.[56]

RESPIRATORY EVALUATION OF CHILDREN WITH NEUROMUSCULAR DISEASE

Pulmonary Function Testing

Neuromuscular weakness affecting the respiratory system initially develops as impaired cough and airway clearance, with gradual progression to nocturnal and eventually daytime hypoventilation. Monitoring the respiratory status of a patient with neuromuscular weakness depends on the underlying disease, its rate of progression, and extent of involvement. Because most conditions involve weakness of the inspiratory and expiratory muscles, pulmonary function testing including muscle strength assessment is the main mode of testing, with polysomnography and noninvasive measures of hypoventilation as the disease progresses in severity.

The use of pulmonary function tests in diagnosing and monitoring the progression of the neuromuscular disease has been well established in adults, but pediatric testing remains a challenge. Although newer techniques in respiratory muscle strength testing are being introduced, the majority of school-age children and adolescents are best monitored by standard spirometry with maximal inspiratory and expiratory pressure monitoring (Figure 44-1).[57,58] Additional testing includes assessment of cough flows, as it is the main determinant of respiratory compromise. However, because peak cough flows have been well correlated with forced vital capacity (FVC) and forced expiratory volume at 1 second, these tests remain the mainstay of pulmonary function testing in this population.[8,59]

Standard spirometry is performed according to the standards of the American Thoracic Society (New York, NY). Measurements include FVC, forced expiratory volume at 1 second, and forced inspiratory volume displayed primarily as a flow–volume loop. Including forced inspiratory volume allows for separate evaluation of extrathoracic and upper airway obstruction in children with bulbar weakness. Measuring maximal expiratory pressure and maximal inspiratory pressure and, in some instances, static mouth pressures allows monitoring of diaphragm and other cough-related strength.[60] For patients with Duchenne muscular dystrophy, a decline in FVC has been demonstrated to be a useful predictor of worsening respiratory muscle weakness and death, so that

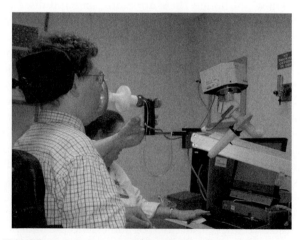

FIGURE 44-1 Spirometry. The majority of school-age children and adolescents are best monitored by standard spirometry with maximal inspiratory and expiratory pressure monitoring. In this image a mask has been substituted for a mouthpiece because of bulbar weakness and inability to use or create a seal around a standard mouthpiece.

interventions such as pulmonary clinical monitoring, secretion clearance, and ventilatory assistance devices can be recommended to be initiated at specific rates of decline.[61] An FVC less than 20% of predicted, or 1 L, is associated with significant carbon dioxide retention and a limited survival rate past 3 years.[48] Last, static lung volume measurements in this population usually reveal restriction, which may be the result of multiple factors including diminished chest wall compliance, reduced inspiratory muscle strength and kyphoscoliosis if present.

Measuring carbon dioxide tension and oxygen analysis are useful adjuncts when determining whether an assisted ventilation device may be required. Noninvasive capnography and pulse oximetry are easily applied in the clinic, but arterial gas analysis should be performed if these are not available. In addition, noninvasive monitoring of cardiac output, using capnometry and a modified Fick equation, may be done to determine the cardiac function of patients with cardiac involvement, but should not replace echocardiography for definitive analysis. Daytime monitoring should be performed every 3 months, or more frequently with diminished mucus mobilization, decline in lung function, and reduced peak cough flows.[48,62] With further progression of carbon dioxide retention and muscle weakness, and advancing concerns regarding nighttime hypoventilation, home overnight oximetry or polysomnography may be useful in determining the early need for assisted respiratory support.

Measurement of cough effectiveness and lung volume, combined with monitoring for hypoventilation, may provide an assessment of trends that could facilitate the timeliness of initiating airway clearance and ventilatory support. With patient and caregiver education, these studies may help patients sustain more normal daily activities and direct the care needed to minimize the complications associated with respiratory muscle weakness.

Sleep Studies

Polysomnography needs to be performed and sleep-disordered breathing monitored in all patients with neuromuscular weakness. Nighttime sleep–disordered breathing often precedes diurnal respiratory failure in affected patients. Polysomnography is the most complete diagnostic test available to assess for the nature and severity of the sleep disturbance.[63] Sleep assessment allows for anticipatory evaluation and more timely recognition and management with assisted ventilation. Full polysomnography should include sleep stage recording, arousal documentation, and monitoring of oxygen saturation, hypoventilation, and hypercapnia.[64] Together, this testing allows for monitoring of sleep complaints and treatable conditions in an otherwise progressive disease process.

General Considerations

The onset of pulmonary symptoms of children with neuromuscular disease largely depends on the underlying disease.[59] For example, a boy with Becker muscular dystrophy is likely to have few respiratory symptoms until late adolescence or adulthood, whereas an infant with SMA type I will almost certainly develop symptoms in the first few months of life. In either case, however, a predictable sequence of events will occur, leading each child to experience progressive respiratory insufficiency and eventually respiratory failure.[65] Initially, respiratory muscle weakness is manifested as a weak cough and impaired airway clearance, which leads to recurrent atelectasis and chest infections.[59] As respiratory muscle weakness progresses, patients experience nocturnal hypoventilation and symptoms related to hypercapnia. These symptoms include nightmares, frequent wakening, early morning headaches, and daytime sleepiness.[47] At this point, most patients maintain relatively normal daytime respiration and are eucapnic while awake. However, further deterioration in respiratory muscle strength eventually leads to daytime respiratory insufficiency and daytime hypercapnia.[59] Complete respiratory failure follows shortly thereafter; the trajectory of this decline, however, is unique to each patient and disease, and is usually hastened by serious illness or concomitant conditions such as scoliosis. With the institution of cough assist devices or mechanical ventilatory support, this trajectory may be effectively slowed.

Many of the interventions used to support airway clearance and ventilation in adults have also been used to assist children; however, limitations in size and the inability of young children to cooperate with or comprehend respiratory therapies can present unique challenges. While respiratory insufficiency or some form of cardiopulmonary disease is the most common cause of death among children with almost any congenital or acquired neuromuscular disorders, innovations in pediatric ventilatory assistance have considerably extended survival and improved quality of life for affected children.[48,66]

Airway Clearance Mechanisms

Airway clearance is achieved in a healthy individual via two mechanisms: mucociliary transport and cough clearance. The mucociliary escalator lining the bronchial tree moves a thin layer of mucus upward toward the proximal airway, where the mucus and entrapped particles are sensed and expelled via cough clearance. Normal coughing is a highly controlled reflex with defined phases. The initial phase is inspiration, when a maximal inspiration is performed in order to get air behind the mucus or debris that needs to be cleared. The next phase is the compressive phase, during which the glottis is closed and the abdominal muscles contract. This allows intrathoracic pressure to rise and narrows the central airways, making the velocity of the airflow higher. The last phase of coughing is expulsion, during which the glottis is opened and air is released at a high velocity, carrying with it collected mucus and debris.

Children with neuromuscular weakness may have trouble with each phase of coughing; inspiratory muscle weakness reduces vital capacity and maximal inhaled volume, bulbar muscle weakness can lead to impaired glottic closure, and expiratory muscle weakness reduces the maximal intrathoracic pressure and expulsive force.[59,67] The significance of this cannot be overstated: in patients with neuromuscular disease, most episodes of acute respiratory failure result from the inability to eliminate airway secretions and mucus during otherwise benign chest infections.[68] A peak cough flow less than 160 L/minute is associated with impaired secretion clearance, but early intervention at 250 to 270 L/minute is recommended for beginning cough assistance.[48]

Facilitating Clearance of Mucus

Mucus mobilization can be facilitated both by use of medications that reduce mucus viscosity, and by assisted maneuvers to clear secretions from the airways. These maneuvers include manual physiotherapy, mechanical or vibratory chest percussion, and postural drainage. The goal of these therapies is to transport secretions in the peripheral airways centrally to larger airways, where assisted coughing can more easily expel them from the respiratory tract. Commercially available mucolytics commonly used for this purpose include Pulmozyme and *N*-acetylcysteine (NAC). Pulmozyme (dornase alfa) is an aerosolized enzyme that hydrolyzes the DNA in sputum, reducing sputum viscoelasticity. Similarly, NAC cleaves the disulfide bonds in mucoproteins, reducing their chain lengths and thinning lung mucus. These medications can be used as daily maintenance therapy or on an as-needed basis during infections. If necessary, NAC can be used up to six times a day to facilitate mucus clearance.

Chest percussion is the manual clapping performed by a caregiver to the patient's thorax, alternating from the ventral, lateral, and dorsal aspects of the chest for periods usually lasting 10 to 20 minutes at a time.[68] Chest vibration is similar in application, but instead of manual clapping the thorax is vibrated via a hand-held device or a circumferential chest vest. A third option is intrapulmonary percussive ventilation (IPV), in which

high-frequency percussive ventilation is delivered through an IPV device used either alone or in conjunction with aerosol therapy.[69] Percussion and vibration maneuvers are often repeated several times every day, depending on the quantity of mucus, its viscosity, and its adhesiveness to the airway and the patient's health status.[68] In particular, more frequent use of percussion and/or vibration is an important component of therapy during respiratory tract infections, when mucus production can frequently overwhelm a weak child's clearance mechanisms.[70]

Assisted Coughing

For effective coughing, sufficient strength is needed in bulbar, inspiratory, and expiratory muscles. For patients with generalized weakness, manually assisted coughing (MAC) can permit successful long-term use of noninvasive ventilatory support.[68] For effective MAC, the patient inspires maximally, augmented by either breath stacking or assisted insufflation, and an abdominal thrust or thoracic squeeze, timed to glottic opening, is applied by an assistant or caregiver.[68] For those using abdominal thrusts, a one-handed technique with counterpressure applied to the thorax with the other hand can further increase cough strength. If upper limb weakness is not involved, a patient can employ either maximal insufflation or abdominal thrust in isolation and augment cough peak flow.[67] There are some limitations to assisted cough, however; MAC requires a cooperative patient willing and able to provide adequate physical effort, and a committed caregiver, able to assist multiple times a day.[68]

Mechanical in-exsufflators are cough assist devices that attach to the patient via an oronasal interface. These work by helping to deliver deep insufflations until the lungs are fully expanded, followed by an immediate negative pressure exsufflation that helps to facilitate mucus mobilization (Figure 44-2).[68] When mechanical cough assist devices are used for secretion clearance, multiple cycles are given in one sitting, until no further secretions are induced.[68] Some patients with severe bulbar weakness may not tolerate mechanical assistance and require manual cough assistance.

Glossopharyngeal Breathing

Glossopharyngeal breathing (GPB), sometimes called "frog breathing," can be used to provide brief periods of normal alveolar ventilation for a patient with neuromuscular weakness who spends periods off a ventilator, or during times of unexpected ventilator failure.[68] The technique of GPB is to augment insufflation by "gulping" air in a series of breaths, closing the glottis between "gulps" to entrap air in the lungs.[68] Using this method, one glossopharyngeal "breath" often consists of six to

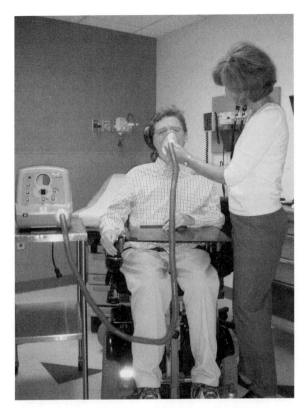

FIGURE 44-2 Mechanical cough assist. Mechanical cough assist devices attach to the patient via an oronasal interface and deliver deep insufflations until the lungs are fully expanded, followed by an immediate negative pressure exsufflation until the lungs are fully deflated.

nine gulps of air. Although severe bulbar muscle weakness can limit the effectiveness of GPB, previous reports of its use in patients with almost no independent breathing and no vital capacity have been published.[68] Bach[71] and Bach and Alba[72] reported that after a period of training to develop proficiency, even patients with ventilator dependence and no autonomous breathing capability have successfully used GPB to facilitate independent breathing for periods ranging from minutes to all day.

Mechanical Ventilatory Support
Noninvasive Ventilation

In the early 1980s, noninvasive ventilation was pioneered first by Rideau and colleagues in France and subsequently by Bach and colleagues in the United States.[73] Since that time, several large studies have shown that noninvasive ventilation is not only effective and well tolerated, but is a preferred method of respiratory support for patients with progressive neuromuscular disease.[68,73] Indeed, work has demonstrated that chronic noninvasive ventilation can extend the average life expectancy for patients with DMD by an average of

6 years, and even restore normal life expectancy for older patients with static weakness, such as long-term polio survivors.[73] Noninvasive ventilation appears to succeed because it allows fatigued respiratory muscles to rest, improves pulmonary mechanics, and restores normal ventilatory sensitivity to carbon dioxide levels.[73]

The goals of assisted ventilation in children are to maintain pulmonary compliance, and normal lung and thoracic growth, and to maintain normal alveolar ventilation. Lung and thorax growth is particularly important when the onset of weakness is in infancy, as is the case with patients with SMA type I. In these cases, the lungs and chest wall do not grow normally because of the inability to take deep breaths. As children age and hypoventilation develops, assessment of pulmonary function determines when assisted ventilation support is indicated, usually with progression from nocturnal-only ventilation to around-the-clock assistance as muscle weakness progresses.

Nocturnal Ventilation

Generally accepted indications for initiating nocturnal ventilation include rapid progression of weakness, hypercapnia or end-tidal carbon dioxide levels exceeding 45 to 50 mm Hg during or at the end of sleep, arterial desaturation below 95% during sleep, and symptoms of respiratory insufficiency.[68,74] The level of nocturnal support is adjusted until there is satisfactory resolution of symptoms and saturations consistently remain greater than 95%.[75] Because of the thoracic deformities that are frequently present, tidal volume or pressure calculation may be inaccurate. In these cases auscultating the basilar lung regions provides a baseline for initial pressure or volume settings.

Initial means of respiratory support include a variety of noninvasive methods. In children, choice of assist device or ventilator mode and patient interface is likely to be dictated by patient age and size. Although the mouthpiece intermittent positive pressure ventilation (IPPV) with lipseal to minimize leak may be preferred in certain instances, these are available only in adolescent and adult sizes.[68] Therefore, nasal ventilation is the most practical means of noninvasive ventilatory support for small children. Younger children and infants can often be easily fitted with nasal interfaces such as adapted continuous positive airway pressure circuits or nasal pillows, nasal masks, or full face masks, although custom headgear might be necessary (Figure 44-3). With any of these designs, the clinician must ensure that a proper fit not only minimizes leaks, but avoids pressure on the bridge of the nose, and prevents future face deformity.[68] Nocturnal ventilation is often best instituted via IPPV with a portable volume ventilator.[68,75] Ventilator settings should be adjusted to mimic age- and weight-based norms for tidal

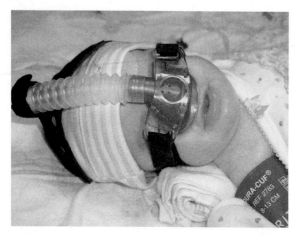

FIGURE 44-3 Infant nasal bilevel positive airway pressure. Nasal ventilation is the most practical means of noninvasive ventilatory support for small children. Although fittings for custom headgear may be necessary, younger children and infants can often be easily fitted with nasal interfaces such as adapted continuous positive airway pressure circuits or nasal pillows, nasal masks, or full face masks.

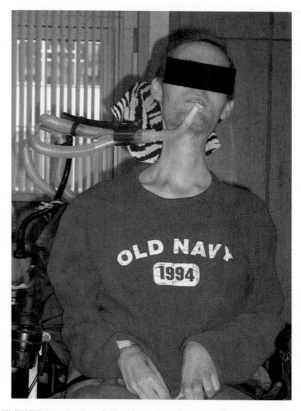

FIGURE 44-4 Mouthpiece ventilation. Mouthpiece intermittent positive pressure ventilation is a safe and effective means of chronic ventilation, even in patients with respiratory failure and no reserve. This mode of support is often preferred by adolescents and adults because it both provides adequate respiratory support and permits normal social interaction.

volume and respiratory rate. In older children, bilevel respiratory assist devices may be used, but because pressure levels are set, they do not accommodate progressive changes in muscle weakness. However, new volume-targeted pressure devices offer a suitable, more compact alternative that can automatically accommodate increasing muscle weakness.

Often, nocturnal ventilatory assistance improves both nocturnal and diurnal ventilation, and the overnight rest allows the respiratory muscles to improve daytime stamina.[68] In fact, most patients use diurnal IPPV for the first time during chest infections, weaning off and returning to isolated nocturnal use, for periods lasting up to several years.[75,76]

Diurnal Ventilation

Daytime use of ventilatory assistance becomes necessary when patients develop end-diurnal hypoventilation.[76] Again, the goal of ventilatory assistance is normalization of arterial blood gas and elimination of respiratory symptoms.[68,76] Ample evidence exists that children, adolescents, and adults who are able to cooperate overwhelmingly prefer noninvasive ventilation.[76,77]

Mouthpiece IPPV has now been studied in several cohorts of end-stage patients, and has been demonstrated to be a safe and effective means of chronic ventilation, even in patients with respiratory failure and no reserve (Figure 44-4).[68,76] It is extremely well tolerated by patients, even in sleep,[68] is a user-friendly system during eating and social activities, and is also relatively inexpensive.[76]

Tracheostomy

Tracheostomy has long been a part of traditional management for patients with progressive neuromuscular weakness.[68,78] Often, tracheostomy tubes are placed during times of respiratory crisis, during or after bouts of respiratory failure triggered by chest infections.[79] Newer therapeutic approaches to patients with neuromuscular weakness discourage tracheostomy, not only because it is often unnecessary, but also because noninvasive support is overwhelmingly preferred by patients. Tracheostomy tubes present numerous disadvantages by impeding normal swallowing and phonation and limiting social interactions; in addition, more advanced in-home health care assistance and intensive follow-up is required. Hygiene issues are also a concern when considering a tracheostomy tube. Tube and stoma care can be uncomfortable, skin breakdown at the stoma site leads to cutaneous infections, and tracheostomy tubes risk sudden plugging with mucus, which can be life-threatening.[68]

Although adolescents and adults prefer noninvasive ventilatory aids for all the reasons given previously, it is important to mention that tracheostomy has also been favorably viewed by many patients. For example, in a 2000 survey in which patients with DMD and amyotrophic lateral sclerosis were surveyed on their quality of life, more than two thirds were satisfied with their lives and 84% believed they had made the right choice.[80] In general, we recommend that as patients demonstrate a need for ventilatory assistance, noninvasive ventilation be pursued first. Tracheostomy is probably best reserved for those patients with severe bulbar weakness and chronic aspiration, if arterial blood gas tensions can no longer be controlled, if there are patient–interface difficulties, or if there is failure to thrive.[70] It is also important to remember that a subpopulation of patients—those with spinal cord injury and Guillain-Barré in particular—may benefit from temporary tracheostomies to facilitate hospital discharge and entry into a rehabilitation program. The long-term goal in these cases is to improve respiratory muscle strength, permitting successful decannulation.

Although more and more centers are developing expertise with chronic noninvasive ventilation, a survey of Jerry Lewis Muscular Dystrophy Association clinics from 1997 showed that few used any form of cough assist and only 20% used mouthpiece positive pressure ventilation.[81] The reasons for this are explained by a combination of family and practitioner unfamiliarity with noninvasive methods, and poor availability or uncertainty about how to use home cough assist devices. This underscores the importance of connecting patients and their families early in the course of the disease with an accredited center caring for a high volume of patients with neuromuscular disease.

Nonrespiratory Care

General medical concerns will cross all stages of growth and development for children with neuromuscular weakness, and attention must be paid to nutritional and cardiac status, extent of scoliosis and restrictive respiratory disease, the contribution of weakness to other organ system functioning, the need for communication assistance, and mental health care. Some of these concerns, such as cardiomyopathy and dysrhythmias, relate to the multisystem effects of the neuromuscular conditions. Others, such as surgical correction of contractures and scoliosis, can be an important strategy in maintaining mobility and preserving lung function.[47]

End-of-life care issues are inevitable in the course of progressive neuromuscular disease. In the discussion of these events it is important to provide the facts and answer every question fully and in terms the parents or patient can understand, without frightening technical language. This communication is one of the most difficult tasks in providing care to these patients. It requires

tact, skill, empathy, and complete support of any decisions made by the parents or patient. The three primary goals include deciding on end-stage pain and dyspnea control, providing spiritual and psychiatric support, and respecting choices concerning tests and treatments.[48]

TRANSITION TO ADULTHOOD

Improved technology and advances in respiratory care have significantly increased the life expectancy of children with neuromuscular weakness.[82] Transition to adulthood requires increasing reliance on ventilator assistance, nursing support, and assistive technologies to help achieve independent living.[59] Another issue that persists across all childhood chronic illnesses is the need for age-appropriate caregivers, so that older adolescents and adults can begin to receive care in an adult health care environment.[83]

Children with neuromuscular weakness require more life-sustaining equipment and assistance in achieving independence. More personal assistance, either from family or skilled nursing, is required in providing basic care needs.[68] Increased support has been associated not only with extended life expectancy but improved quality of life as well.[61,84] Unfortunately, the timing of instituting these assistive technologies and skilled nursing care remains dependent on the individual patient and clinical scenario.[64]

Successful transition requires attention to the challenges associated with providing ventilatory assistance to the young adult with neuromuscular weakness. Additional issues during the transition process include facilitating coordination of care amongst multiple subspecialists, establishing a cadre of skilled caregivers, and arranging support for maintaining activities of daily living. If successful, the transition is likely to result in continued maintenance of a high quality of life despite the physical limitations associated with the underlying condition.[84]

ASSESSMENT QUESTIONS

See Evolve Resources for answers.

1. Which of the following are muscles of inspiration?
    I. The diaphragm
    II. The internal intercostals
    III. The external intercostals
    IV. The external oblique muscles
    V. The rectus abdominus

Continued

A. I and II
B. I and III
C. I, III, and V
D. II and IV
E. II, IV, and V

2. Which condition(s) of the central nervous system affect(s) respiration?
   A. Tay-Sachs disease
   B. Congenital hydrocephalus
   C. Congenital central hypoventilation syndrome
   D. A, B, and C
   E. B and C

3. Which condition is the most common myopathy affecting respiratory muscle function in childhood?
   A. Spinal muscular atrophy
   B. Myasthenia gravis
   C. Muscular dystrophy
   D. Guillain-Barré
   E. Scoliosis

4. Guillain-Barré is an acute, autoimmune process that affects the peripheral nervous system and causes
   A. Inevitable respiratory failure, tracheostomy, and mechanical ventilation
   B. Hereditary weakness that progresses from the legs to the arms
   C. Mild hydrocephalus and confusion along with chest wall weakness
   D. Demyelination of the peripheral nerve sheaths, leading to conduction abnormalities
   E. Pain, starting in the arms and chest and leading to arm and chest weakness

5. Which of the following is an autoimmune disorder of infancy and childhood, which occurs when antibodies block synaptic receptors at the neuromuscular junction?
   A. Myotonic dystrophy
   B. Pediatric botulism toxicity
   C. Infantile spinal muscular atrophy
   D. Juvenile myasthenia gravis
   E. Infantile transitional myasthenia gravis

6. A neuromuscular disease evaluation of the respiratory system of a child with neuromuscular weakness might include which of the following?
   I. Spirometry with a flow–volume loop
   II. Polysomnography
   III. Electroencephalogram
   IV. Mixed venous blood gases
   V. Maximal inspiratory and expiratory pressures
   A. I and V
   B. I, II, and V
   C. III and V
   D. II, III, and V
   E. II, III, and IV

7. There are several phases of a normal cough to create sufficient cough flow for effective pulmonary clearance. The patient with neuromuscular weakness
   A. Is unable to produce peak cough flows
   B. May have difficulty with any of the phases of an effective cough
   C. Is able to produce high expiratory flows, but does not generate enough volume for an effective cough
   D. Has impaired glottic closure and diaphragmatic force for an effective cough
   E. Does not have true impairment of cough flows, because it is relative to the reduced vital capacity

8. Glossopharyngeal breathing
   A. Is known as "frog breathing," which inflates the lungs by gulping air
   B. Has limited effectiveness in patients with bulbar weakness
   C. May provide normal alveolar ventilation in the case of a malfunctioning mechanical ventilator
   D. A and B only
   E. All of the above

9. Select the two indications for initiating nocturnal ventilatory assistance for a pediatric patient with neuromuscular weakness:
   I. Supine negative inspiratory force of 60 to 90 cm H_2O
   II. Hypercapnia during sleep with end-tidal carbon dioxide levels in excess of 50 mm Hg
   III. Documented evidence of right-sided heart failure with peaked P waves on ECG
   IV. Arterial oxygen tension less than 88 mm Hg during 20% of the sleep study
   V. Oxygen desaturation to less than 95% during sleep and symptoms of respiratory insufficiency
   A. I and III
   B. I and V
   C. II and IV
   D. II and V
   E. III and IV

10. Placing a tracheostomy tube to facilitate mechanical ventilation for progressive neuromuscular weakness
    A. Is reserved only for patients with severe bulbar weakness, chronic aspiration, and inability to maintain acceptable blood gas values
    B. May be temporary in children with spinal cord injury or Guillain-Barré
    C. May be temporary to provide rest of the respiratory muscles and aggressive pulmonary hygiene
    D. A and B
    E. B and C

References

1. Shahrizaila N, Kinnear W, Wills A: Respiratory involvement in inherited primary muscle conditions, *J Neurol Neurosurg Psychiatry* 2006;77:1108.
2. Widdicombe J: Reflexes from the lungs and airways: historical perspectives, *J Appl Physiol* 2006;101:628.
3. Benditt JO: The neuromuscular respiratory system: physiology, pathophysiology, and a respiratory care approach to patients, *Respir Care* 2006;51:829; discussion 837.
4. Derenne JP et al: History of diaphragm physiology: the achievements of Galen, *Eur Respir J* 1995,8:154.
5. Remmers JE: A century of control of breathing, *Am J Respir Crit Care Med* 2005;172:6.
6. Phillipson E, Duffin J: *Hypoventilation and hyperventilation syndromes*, ed 4, Philadelphia: Elsevier Saunders; 2005.
7. Sivak ED, Shefner JM, Sexton J: Neuromuscular disease and hypoventilation, *Curr Opin Pulm Med* 1999;5:355.
8. Robinson D, Esau S: Assessment of ventilatory function in patient with neuromuscular disease, *Clin Chest Med* 1994;18:751.
9. Polkey MI, Moxham J: Clinical aspects of respiratory muscle dysfunction in the critically ill, *Chest* 2001;119:926.
10. Gaultier C et al: Genetics and early disturbances of breathing control, *Pediatr Res* 2004;55:729.
11. Chen ML et al: Diaphragm pacers as a treatment for congenital central hypoventilation syndrome, *Expert Rev Med Devices* 2005;2:577.
12. Williams H: A unifying hypothesis for hydrocephalus, Chiari malformation, syringomyelia, anencephaly and spina bifida, *Cerebrospinal Fluid Res* 2008;5:7.
13. Gravel RA, Triggs-Raine BL, Mahuran DJ: Biochemistry and genetics of Tay-Sachs disease, *Can J Neurol Sci* 1991;18(3 suppl):419.
14. National Center for Injury Prevention and Control, Centers for Disease Control and Prevention: *Spinal cord injury (SCI): fact sheet*, Bethesda, Md: Centers for Disease Control and Prevention; 2008. Available at http://www.cdc.gov/ncipc/factsheets/scifacts.htm. Retrieved October 2008.
15. Netter F: *Atlas of human anatomy*, ed 4, Philadelphia: WB Saunders; 2006.
16. Hirschfeld S, Exner G, Luukaala T, Baer GA: Mechanical ventilation or phrenic nerve stimulation for treatment of spinal cord injury–induced respiratory insufficiency, *Spinal Cord* 2008;46(11):738-742.
17. Fenoy AJ, Menezes AH, Fenoy KA: Craniocervical junction fusions in patients with hindbrain herniation and syringohydromyelia, *J Neurosurg Spine* 2008;9:1.
18. Halawa A, Krishnaswamy G: Tussive headache with weakness and atrophy of the right hand, *Rev Neurol Dis* 2007;4:224.
19. Kumar V, Abbas AK, Fauto N: *Robbins and Cotran pathologic basis of disease*, ed 7, Philadelphia: WB Saunders; 2004.
20. Laningham FH et al: Childhood central nervous system leukaemia: historical perspectives, current therapy, and acute neurological sequelae, *Neuroradiology* 2007;49:873.
21. De Jesus NH: Epidemics to eradication: the modern history of poliomyelitis, *Virol J* 2007;4:70.
22. Bach JR et al: Spinal muscular atrophy type 1: management and outcomes, *Pediatr Pulmonol* 2002;34:16.
23. Ioos C et al: Respiratory capacity course in patients with infantile spinal muscular atrophy, *Chest* 2004;126:831.
24. Munsat TL et al: Phenotypic heterogeneity of spinal muscular atrophy mapping to chromosome 5q11.2-13.3 (SMA 5q), *Neurology* 1990;40:1831.
25. Russman BS et al: Spinal muscular atrophy: new thoughts on the pathogenesis and classification schema, *J Child Neurol* 1992;7:347.
26. Kaindl AM et al: Spinal muscular atrophy with respiratory distress type 1 (SMARD1), *J Child Neurol* 2008;23:199.
27. Chng SY et al: Pulmonary function and scoliosis in children with spinal muscular atrophy types II and III, *J Paediatr Child Health* 2003;39:673.
28. Lunn MR, Wang CH: Spinal muscular atrophy, *Lancet* 2008;371:2120.
29. Gozal D: Pulmonary manifestations of neuromuscular disease with special reference to Duchenne muscular dystrophy and spinal muscular atrophy, *Pediatr Pulmonol* 2000;29:141.
30. Kasper DL, Braunwald E, Fauci AS: *Harrison's principles of internal medicine*, ed 16, New York: McGraw-Hill; 2004.
31. Hauck LJ et al: Incidence of Guillain-Barré syndrome in Alberta, Canada: an administrative data study, *J Neurol Neurosurg Psychiatry* 2008;79:318.
32. Ehroni E et al: Guillain-Barré syndrome in Greece: seasonality and other clinico-epidemiological features, *Eur J Neurol* 2004;11:383.
33. Kleyweg RP et al: The natural history of the Guillain-Barré syndrome in 18 children and 50 adults, *J Neurol Neurosurg Psychiatry* 1989;52:853.
34. Sarnat H: *Guillain-Barré syndrome*, Philadelphia: Elsevier Saunders; 2007.
35. Finkelstein JS, Melek BH: Guillain-Barré syndrome as a cause of reversible cardiomyopathy, *Tex Heart Inst J* 2006;33:57.
36. Winer JB: Treatment of Guillain-Barré syndrome, *QJM* 2002;95:717.
37. Tseng-Ong L, Mitchell WG: Infant botulism: 20 years' experience at a single institution, *J Child Neurol* 2007;22:1333.
38. Sobel J: Botulism, *Clin Infect Dis* 2005;41:1167.
39. Glauser TA, Maguire HC, Sladky JT: Relapse of infant botulism, *Ann Neurol* 1990;28:187.
40. Conti-Fine BM, Milani M, Kaminski HJ: Myasthenia gravis: past, present, and future, *J Clin Invest* 2006;116:2843.
41. Vern JC, Massey JM: Myasthenia gravis, *Orphanet J Rare Dis* 2007;2:44.
42. Kothari MJ: Myasthenia gravis, *J Am Osteopath Assoc* 2004;104:377.
43. Thanvi BR, Lo TC: Update on myasthenia gravis, *Postgrad Med J* 2004;80:690.
44. Batocchi A et al: Early-onset myasthenia gravis: clinical characteristics and response to therapy, *Eur J Pediatr* 1990;150:66.
45. Misulis KE, Fenichel GM: Genetic forms of myasthenia gravis, *Pediatr Neurol* 1989;5:205.
46. Djelmis J et al: Myasthenia gravis in pregnancy: report on 69 cases, *Eur J Obstet Gynecol Reprod Biol* 2002;104:21.

47. Emery AE: The muscular dystrophies, *Lancet* 2002; 359:687.

48. Birnkrant DJ et al: American College of Chest Physicians consensus statement on the respiratory and related management of patients with Duchenne muscular dystrophy undergoing anesthesia or sedation, *Chest* 2007;132:1977.

49. Bach JR, Ishikawa Y, Kim H: Prevention of pulmonary morbidity for patients with Duchenne muscular dystrophy, *Chest* 1997;112:1024.

50. Cardamone M, Darras DT, Ryan MM: Inherited myopathies and muscular dystrophies, *Semin Neurol* 2008;28:250.

51. Kishanni PS, Chen Y-T: *Glycogen storage diseases*, ed 15, Philadelphia: WB Saunders; 1996.

52. Katzin LW, Amato AA: Pompe disease: a review of the current diagnosis and treatment recommendations in the era of enzyme replacement therapy, *J Clin Neuromuscul Dis* 2008;9:421.

53. Pellegrini N et al: Respiratory insufficiency and limb muscle weakness in adults with Pompe's disease, *Eur Respir J* 2005;26:1024.

54. Marino PL: *The ICU book*, ed 2, Philadelphia: Lippincott Williams & Wilkins; 1998.

55. McCarty M, Jagoda A, Fairweather P: Hyperkalemic ascending paralysis [report], *Ann Emerg Med* 1998;32:104.

56. Pathare N et al: Deficit in human muscle strength with cast immobilization: contribution of inorganic phosphate, *Eur J Appl Physiol* 2006;98:71.

57. Nicot F et al: Respiratory muscle testing: a valuable tool for children with neuromuscular disorders, *Am J Respir Crit Care Med* 2006;174:67.

58. Koessler W et al: Two years' experience with inspiratory muscle training in patients with neuromuscular disorders, *Chest* 2001;120:765.

59. Panitch HB: Respiratory issues in the management of children with neuromuscular disease, *Respir Care* 2006;51:885; discussion 894.

60. Steier J et al: The values of multiple tests of respiratory muscle strength, *Thorax* 2007;62:975.

61. Finder JD et al: Respiratory care of the patient with Duchenne muscular dystrophy: ATS consensus statement, *Am J Respir Crit Care Med* 2004;170:456.

62. Gauld LM, Boynton A: Relationship between peak cough flow and spirometry in Duchenne muscular dystrophy, *Pediatr Pulmonol* 2005;39:457.

63. Dhand UK, Dhand R: Sleep disorders in neuromuscular diseases, *Curr Opin Pulm Med* 2006;12:402.

64. Toussaint M, Chatwin M, Soudon P: Mechanical ventilation in Duchenne patients with chronic respiratory insufficiency: clinical implications of 20 years published experience, *Chron Respir Dis* 2007;4:167.

65. Birnkrant DJ: The assessment and management of the respiratory complications of pediatric neuromuscular diseases, *Clin Pediatr* 2002;41:301.

66. Simonds AK: Respiratory complications of the muscular dystrophies, *Semin Respir Crit Care Med* 2002;23:231.

67. Panitch HB: Airway clearance in children with neuromuscular weakness, *Curr Opin Pediatr* 2006;18:277.

68. Bach JR: *Management of patients with neuromuscular disease*, Philadelphia: Hanley & Belfus; 2004.

69. Toussaint M et al: Effect of intrapulmonary percussive ventilation on mucus clearance in Duchenne muscular dystrophy patients: a preliminary report, *Respir Care* 2003;48:940.

70. Simonds AK: Recent advances in respiratory care for neuromuscular disease, *Chest* 2006;130:1879.

71. Bach JR: New approaches in the rehabilitation of the traumatic high level quadriplegic, *Am J Phys Med Rehabil* 1991;70:13.

72. Bach JR, Alba AS: Noninvasive options for ventilatory support of the traumatic high level quadriplegic patient, *Chest* 1990;98:613.

73. Rideau Y et al: Prolongation of life in Duchenne's muscular dystrophy, *Acta Neurol* 1983;5:118; and Bach JR, Alba AS, Saporito LR: Intermittent positive pressure ventilation via the mouth as an alternative to tracheostomy for 257 ventilator users, *Chest* 1993;103:174. As cited in Simonds AK et al: Impact of nasal ventilation on survival in hypercapnic Duchenne muscular dystrophy, *Thorax* 1998;53:949.

74. Laub M, Berg S, Midgren B: Symptoms, clinical and physiological findings motivating home mechanical ventilation in patients with neuromuscular diseases, *J Rehabil Med* 2006;38:250.

75. Tzeng AC, Bach JR: Prevention of pulmonary morbidity for patients with neuromuscular disease, *Chest* 2000;118:1390.

76. Toussaint M et al: Diurnal ventilation via mouthpiece: survival in end-stage Duchenne patients, *Eur Respir J* 2006;28:549.

77. Bach JR, Alba AS, Saporito LR: Intermittent positive pressure ventilation via the mouth as an alternative to tracheostomy for 257 ventilator users, *Chest* 1993;103:174.

78. Bach JR: Medical considerations of long-term survival of Werdnig-Hoffman disease, *Am J Phys Med Rehabil* 2007;86:349.

79. Bach J et al: Neuromuscular ventilatory insufficiency: effect of home mechanical ventilator use v. oxygen therapy on pneumonia and hospitalization rates, *Am J Phys Med Rehabil* 1998;77:8.

80. Narayanaswami P et al: Long-term tracheostomy ventilation in neuromuscular diseases: patient acceptance and quality of life, *Neurorehabil Neural Repair* 2000;14:135.

81. Bach JR, Chaudhry SS; Muscular Dystrophy Association: Standards of care in MDA clinics, *Am J Phys Med Rehabil* 2000;79:193.

82. Scal P et al: Trends in transition from pediatric to adult health care services for young adults with chronic conditions, *J Adolesc Health* 1999;24:259.

83. Denboba D et al: Achieving family and provider partnerships with children with special health care needs, *Pediatrics* 2006;118:1607.

84. Kohler M et al: Quality of life, physical disability, and respiratory impairment in Duchenne muscular dystrophy, *Am J Respir Crit Care Med* 2005;172:1032.

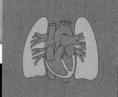

Chapter **45**

Transport of Infants and Children

GARRY SITLER

LEARNING OBJECTIVES

After reading this chapter the reader will be able to:
- Discuss and recognize the importance of team composition, roles, and education
- Review and compare the caveats of each mode of transport
- Explain the role of communication during a medical transport

- List the specific equipment needed for pediatric transport
- Demonstrate how to provide a patient assessment in a nontraditional environment
- Review safety and accreditation requirements for pediatric transport agencies

Since the late 1980s the care of the critically ill pediatric patient has seen rapid development in technology and improvement in patient outcomes. Today many infants and children, who previously would have died, are surviving. The cost of such care has necessitated regionalization of intensive care centers to larger tertiary care centers. This regionalization has led to the need for safe and effective patient transport systems. For neonatal transport, antenatal transport of the mother and high-risk fetus to a tertiary center is preferable. However, antenatal referral is not always possible and the critically ill neonate must often be transported after birth. In most states the operation of a neonatal/ pediatric transport team will fall under the auspices of the state health department as an emergency medical services (EMS) provider. Each state will have its own specific rules and regulations for staffing, training, equipment, and safety. There are few things more challenging to clinicians than transporting critically ill infants and children from a local hospital to a tertiary care medical center. Respiratory therapists must change their focus to monitoring the status of patients and performing procedures while operating in a changing and often hostile environment, such as a moving ambulance or aircraft.

The transport of neonatal and pediatric patients requires a multidisciplinary approach that may involve

- Respiratory therapists
- Nurses
- Pilots/drivers
- Physicians
- Emergency medical personnel

The ages, sizes, and diagnoses of transported neonatal and pediatric patients encompass virtually the entire scope of the critically ill population, from the 500-g infant to the 100-kg adolescent.

The skilled, rapid transport of neonatal and pediatric patients suffering from serious illness or trauma to facilities specializing in the care of these patients has resulted in significantly improved outcomes.[1,2] The skilled transport of critically ill patients is an intervention of the highest value and an activity in which respiratory therapist should be proud and enthusiastic to participate.

TEAM COMPOSITION

Staffing

Critical care transport requires experienced personnel with advanced clinical skills, additional training, and education. If the team is to function autonomously, they must work together with others involved in the transport process. Personnel are the single most valuable assets of any transport system. Because the stabilization and critical care skills required for the critically ill pediatric patient are specialized, the composition of the team is important. Team composition varies among different health care institutions across the country. More important than the exact credentialing of the transport personnel is the training and skills of the team. A qualified transport team should consist of individuals who have pediatric/neonatal critical care experience and training in the special needs of children during transport, and who have participated in the transport of these patients with the frequency to maintain their expertise.[3] Most transport teams are composed of one or more of the following health care team members:

- A registered nurse
- A respiratory therapist
- An emergency medical technician
- A neonatal nurse practitioner, and/or
- A staff physician, resident, or fellow

Data show that most pediatric transport teams in the United States are led by a nurse and accompanied by a respiratory therapist.[4] The use of a specialized pediatric transport team (registered nurse and respiratory therapist) has been shown to result in lower morbidity then the traditional EMS helicopter staffed with a flight/trauma nurse and a paramedic.[5] An respiratory therapist is at an advantage because of the large number of transported pediatric patients who require respiratory support. The background and training of nurses and respiratory therapist are so different that such a team creates a broader scope of knowledge and experience when both are used. This combination works successfully in the majority of the routine transports.

All pediatric transport teams should have a mechanism to identify critical patient transports that require the addition of a physician to the transport team. Most pediatric transport teams in the United States report that a physician accompanies their team on 10% to 15% of all transports.[4] All team members should be cross-trained so that each member of the team can function at the other's skill level. The medical director of the pediatric transport program should be a critical care intensivist or a neonatologist (or both) with an interest in transport medicine.

Though most exclusive neonatal/pediatric transport teams are affiliated with children's hospitals, the administrative home of the transport team varies with each institution. *Unit-based* transport teams are staffed and scheduled within the intensive care units (ICUs) or, in the case of respiratory therapist, with in the respiratory care department. The transport staff are generally given a patient care assignment and then "pulled" from that assignment when a transport call is received. From an administrative standpoint this is the most cost-effective use of personnel resources.

Dedicated transport teams are scheduled and staffed separately from the ICU personnel. These staff members generally "float" throughout the hospital without a patient assignment when they are not on transport. They are there to assist other hospital personnel but can leave immediately when a transport call is received. A large volume of transports is necessary to justify a dedicated transport team. Most transport programs have found that once volumes exceed 1000-1200 transports per year, it is fiscally advantageous to allocate the resources for a dedicated transport team. Personnel accustomed to managing transport coordination are the best suited for accomplishing the relatively complex logistics of transporting critically ill patients. The objective of adequate staffing is to ensure that each member of the transport team has the opportunity to participate in enough transports per month (15 to 20 per month) to maintain a high level of competency while at the same time making sure not to overwork the staff and create "burnout."

Training

The qualities of the team members are as important as the team composition. The selection process should include interviews not only with the nursing and respiratory leadership, but with the medical director of the transport team under whose license the person will operate. Ideal candidates should have exemplary clinical skills, leadership and decision-making abilities, flexibility, compassion, and assertiveness, all while working in a high-stress transport service.

See Box 45-1 for a list of minimal requirements for transport team members.

Inadequate training of pediatric caregivers has been correlated with increased morbidity.[5] Several different professional organizations have developed training/educational requirements for pediatric transport teams. The Air & Surface Transport Nurses Association (ASTNA, Greenwood Village, Colo), American Association for Respiratory Care (AARC, Irving, Tx), Commission on Accreditation of Medical Transport Systems (CAMTS, Anderson, SC), and American Academy of Pediatrics (AAP, Elk Grove Village, Ill) are commonly recognized. In general, they recommend that transport nurses and respiratory therapists have at least 2 years of pediatric critical care experience. Annual recurrent training should include didactic material and hands-on training in procedures that are used during transport (Box 45-2).

Box 45-2	Annual Recurrent Training Topics*

- Advanced airway management
- Central line/umbilical artery line insertion
- Thermoregulation
- Identification and treatment of pneumothorax
- Stabilization of critically ill pediatric patients
- Acid–base balance
- High-altitude physiology (for air transport)
- Transport equipment operation
- Ambulance safety procedures
- Aircraft evacuation drills
- Community relations

*Not exclusive.

Box 45-1	Minimal Requirements for Transport Team Members

TRANSPORT NURSE
- Licensed by the state
- Two years of experience as an registered nurse, including 12 months of neonatal intensive care unit/pediatric intensive care unit (NICU/PICU) experience
- Current Basic Cardiac Life Support (BCLS) certification
- Current Neonatal Resuscitation Program (NRP) certification
- Current Pediatric Advanced Life Support (PALS) certification
- Has participated in a pediatric transport course and has demonstrated a working knowledge of transport equipment and transport supplies
- Has observed two or three transports

TRANSPORT RESPIRATORY THERAPIST
- Registered by the National Board for Respiratory Care (NBRC)
- Licensed by the state
- Two years of NICU/PICU experience
- Current BCLS certification
- Current NRP certification
- Current PALS certification
- Has participated in a pediatric transport course and has demonstrated a working knowledge of transport equipment and transport supplies
- Has observed two or three transports

MODES OF TRANSPORTATION

The single largest expense of a transport program is in the operation and maintenance of its transport vehicles. The selection of specific vehicles is an important decision that must include many different factors. The vehicles must be safe and have the operational characteristics appropriate for the program requirements. All vehicles used to transport patients must comply with local, state, and federal guidelines for both air and ground ambulances. The vehicles must have 110-V AC electrical power available for the medical equipment used during transport. There should be sufficient medical gas (medical air and oxygen) capacity for all transport operations plus reserve capacity for use in the event of mechanical breakdown. The vehicles must also have provisions for suction equipment. The medical equipment used in transport, as well as the stretcher/incubator, must be safely secured within the vehicle during transport. The vehicle must have interior room, which will allow the transport team to treat and assess the patient, and on occasion, perform procedures safely during transport.[6] All transport vehicles must have two-way communication capability, using radios or cellular phone. Each mode of transport—ground, rotor wing (helicopter), and fixed wing (airplane)—has advantages and disadvantages. The vehicle chosen should be appropriate for the patient population and geographic area served.

Ground Transport

Ground transport should be considered when distances are 30 miles or less one way for critical patients and, for stable patients, less than 80 miles one way. The ground transport vehicle should be an ambulance equipped with the special equipment needed for intensive care transport. The ambulance should have a hydraulic or electrical lift for loading the heavy transport incubators used in neonatal transport (Figure 45-1). The incubator should be secured with four-point restraint straps. The

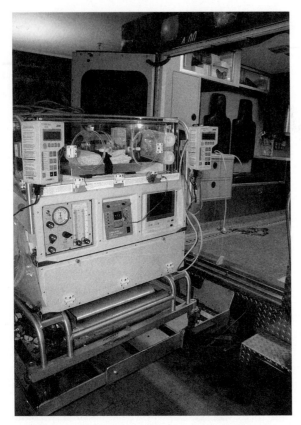

FIGURE 45-1 Ambulance with a hydraulic lift loading a neonatal transport incubator.

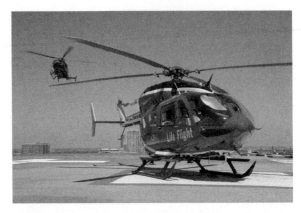

FIGURE 45-2 A midsized twin-engine helicopter that has the capacity to transport a neonatal transport team with a transport incubator.

ambulance interior should be large enough to secure two transport incubators for transport of twins and room to seat the transport team members required for the care of two patients.

Advantages and disadvantages of ground transportation are listed in Box 45-3.

Air Transport
Rotor Wing

Helicopters are effective for rapid transport of critical patients within a 30- to 150-mile radius.[7] The size of the helicopter and the corresponding size of the cabin within the helicopter must be adequate to handle the equipment and transport team members. The transport team must be able to access and treat the patient during flight should an emergency arise. A neonatal transport team with a transport incubator will require a midsized twin-engine aircraft in order to have enough room for proper patient care (Figure 45-2). These larger aircraft are expensive to operate and the aircraft may not be able to land at all of the hospitals serviced by the program, because of their size.

Advantages and disadvantages of helicopters are listed in Box 45-4.

Fixed-wing Aircraft

Airplanes are effective for long-distance patient transport. Because airplanes fly from airport to airport, the increased coordination of ground ambulances for two airports, the time required to load and unload at both airports, and the additional ground transport time must be balanced against the time required to drive from

---

Box 45-3   Advantages and Disadvantages of Ground Transportation

ADVANTAGES
- Lowest operating cost
- Ability to go directly from hospital to hospital
- Ability to carry a large number of staff and equipment
- Ability to transport in poor weather

DISADVANTAGES
- Slower response time over greater distances
- Can be slowed or stopped by traffic congestion

Box 45-4   Advantages and Disadvantages of Rotor Wing Transportation

ADVANTAGES
- Rapid response time within a 30- to 150-mile radius
- Ability to fly directly from hospital to hospital

DISADVANTAGES
- High operating and capital expense to operate
- Small operating radius without refueling
- Small cabin area allows limited medical procedures (no cabin pressurization)
- Limited payload for personnel and equipment
- Inability to fly in inclement weather

hospital to hospital. Under normal circumstances the time needed to drive 120 miles is greater than the fixed-wing aircraft transport time for the same distance. All airplanes used for critical patient transport should have the ability to control the cabin altitude (pressurization), which makes the transport of critically ill patients with marginal arterial oxygenation possible (Figure 45-3).

Advantages and disadvantages of airplanes are listed in Box 45-5.

EQUIPMENT

The equipment, both communication and medical, carried on board an ambulance, helicopter, or airplane will need to meet various standards. In general, the equipment should be as lightweight as possible, both

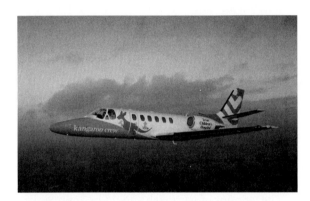

FIGURE 45-3 A twin-engine turboprop aircraft that has the ability to transport two patients and five medical crewmembers within a pressurized cabin.

Box 45-5	Advantages and Disadvantages of Airplanes

ADVANTAGES
- Rapid response time for distances greater than 120 miles
- Ability to fly long distances
- Larger cabin area to allow for more medical procedures
- Ability to control cabin altitude (pressurization)
- Larger payload for personnel and equipment
- Ability to fly in inclement weather

DISADVANTAGES
- Moderate operating and capital expense to operate
- Requires an airport to land, and thus an ambulance at both ends of the flight

electrical and battery operated, and should not interfere electromagnetically with aircraft navigation or communication equipment.[8] It should be as ruggedly constructed as possible.[9] All equipment should be well secured for the duration of transport.

Communications

The transport team should always have the ability to communicate with the online medical control physician who is supervising the transport. This communication has traditionally been accomplished via radio for both ground and air transport. However, the use of cellular phones in ground ambulances has steadily increased, especially with more cellular companies offering a "walkie talkie"-type option. Both helicopters and airplanes are equipped with VHF radios for communicating with air traffic control. EMS helicopters are generally equipped with another type of radio, called a *UHF/AM transceiver*. This additional radio allows communication with ground support agencies (fire, police, etc.) and their dispatch centers. The transport teams on the helicopter can contact their online medical control via this UHF radio. Because of the short-range limitations of UHF radios, fixed-wing air ambulances should be equipped with a satellite-type cell phone for air-to-hospital communication. This will allow communication from just about any location around the world.

Medical
Monitoring Equipment
Electrocardiogram monitoring, pulse oximetry monitoring (Sao_2), and blood pressure monitoring are standard practice during the transport of critically ill patients. Most modern transport monitors incorporate the following:
- ECG (electrocardiograph)
- Sao_2 (pulse oximeter)
- Noninvasive blood pressure monitoring (blood pressure cuff)
- Invasive blood pressure monitoring (pressure transducers)
- Patient temperature monitoring (skin or rectal probes)

End-tidal carbon dioxide ($ETco_2$) monitoring is a valuable option on most transport monitors; monitoring end-tidal carbon dioxide provides the transport team with a visual method to ensure effective ventilation in the intubated patient during transport. Alarm limits should be set for each transport. Visual alarm indicators are usually more helpful than audible alarms in a noisy transport environment. Monitors with interchangeable battery packs allow for quicker turnaround times as an alternative to waiting for batteries to recharge.

Ventilator

Use of a transport ventilator will allow the transport team to provide the same level of care given or already established in an ICU. Transport ventilators are now available with most of the intensive care parameters (i.e., positive end-expiratory pressure, synchronized intermittent mandatory ventilation, adjustable fraction of inspired oxygen, and pressure support) in small, portable, lightweight cases. Ventilators with external battery packs allow for quicker turnaround times compared with waiting for an internal battery to recharge. The decision to use a volume- limited or a pressure-limited ventilator should be based on the patient's size and ventilatory requirements. A manual resuscitation bag should always be carried on transport in the event of ventilator malfunction. Transport team members should be reminded that studies have shown there are tendencies to hyperventilate the patient while using a manual resuscitator.[10]

Transport Incubator

The ability to transport an infant with a body weight of 5 kg or less in a neutrothermal environment requires the use of a transport incubator. There are several commercially available transport incubators at present. They are modular units that allow customers to select among different models of heart monitors, ventilators, infusion pumps, and oxygen/air sources. When considering the purchase of a transport incubator, the first concern should be the type of vehicle in which the incubator will be transported. For example, the primary factor if planning to use the incubator in an aircraft (especially a helicopter) would be the weight and size of the incubator. Other factors to consider include the following: battery power, which should be able to power the incubator for 2 to 3 hours; easy access to the infant without excessive heat loss; ability to visually monitor the infant at all times; and adequate lighting of the patient in dark areas.

Infusion Pumps

The syringe pump–type infusion pump is popular with transport teams because it requires no special tubing or cassette. A standard syringe (anywhere between 1 and 60 cc) is loaded onto the pump. The pump applies constant pressure to the plunger of the syringe and can be programmed for infusion rates from 0.1 to 999 ml/hour. These pumps are lightweight and battery powered, capable of running for 3 to 4 hours between charges.

Point of Care Testing

Pediatric transport teams are gradually moving to the use of a commercially available portable blood gas analyzer. Studies have shown that point of care testing reduces stabilization times and can have the potential to improve the quality of care during transport.[11] Most analyzers have a small, battery-powered, handheld unit and a variable set of testing cartridges. Transport teams are able to do blood analysis either during transport or at small outlying hospitals, which do not have the ability to analyze small blood samples. The following parameters can be determined with three or four drops of blood: pH, carbon dioxide pressure (Pco_2), oxygen pressure (Po_2), sodium (Na), potassium (K), ionized calcium (iCa), glucose (Glu), hematocrit (Hct), and hemoglobin (Hb).

Medications

The type and quantity of medications carried by the transport team should meet the requirements for care of the various patients transported. If the team operates under medical protocols, each medication carried should have its own protocol for use. Proper attention should be given to the storage of medication. Medications should be stored to prevent extreme temperatures of heat or cold. A process must be developed to handle drugs requiring refrigeration.

Medical Gas Supply

Pediatric transport teams who transport low birth weight infants will need to have both medical oxygen and medical air available while on transport. This will allow for the use of a blender to titrate the inspired oxygen of low birth weight infants. It is critical that the amounts of gas needed be calculated on the basis of projected use. The amount of gas taken should be approximately double that required. This allows for emergency usage in the event of mechanical breakdown of a vehicle. In ground ambulances, where weight is less of a consideration, the gases are usually provided by size H cylinders. In aircraft, where weight is a significant consideration, the use of aluminum and Kevlar cylinders has become the standard because of their low weight. Most fixed-wing aircraft have electrical air compressors to provide medical air, and liquid oxygen systems for medical oxygen, thus providing gases over a long duration.

Supplies

The type and quantity of disposable supplies carried by the transport team should be sufficient for the proper care of the various patients transported.

PATIENT ASSESSMENT AND STABILIZATION

Assessment of the patient begins with the first phone call from the referring hospital. The basic information required to initiate a transport should include the following[12]:

- Name
- Weight
- General description of the patient's condition
- Any relevant past medical history
- Current vital signs including oxygen saturation
- Any major clinical problems currently presenting

The referring hospital should be given any recommendations for changes in medical management and the estimated time of arrival of the transport team. The referring hospital should also be given phone numbers and instructions to call back with any questions or significant changes in the patient condition prior to the transport team's arrival.

On arrival, assessment of the patient by the transport team should be thorough yet rapid. Stabilization at the referring hospital has become a much-discussed topic. The question of "Stay and Play" or "Scoop and Run" is debated in transport conferences across the country. The goal of the transport team should be to transport the patient in the most stable condition possible. Proper stabilization should be designed to minimize the number of adverse incidents (hypoxic events, hypotensive events, etc.) that occur during the transport. At the same time, the team should avoid the temptation to perform time-consuming therapeutic testing procedures while on transport.

ADVANCED TRANSPORT

High-altitude Physiology

A complete understanding of flight physiology is essential in order to provide optimal patient care in the air-medical environment.[13] Normal physiological responses to changing altitude are further complicated when transporting an already compromised patient.

Boyle's law states that at constant temperature, volume is inversely proportional to pressure. As the aircraft and patient rise in altitude, the volume of contained gases will expand. This expansion has the following clinical implications for patient care: increased respiratory rate and depth, changes in intravenous flow rates, nausea and vomiting, increased need to urinate, increased pain, endotracheal tube cuff expansion (prevented by filling the cuff with normal saline), and increased sinus pressure in the case of head colds or blocked sinuses.

Dalton's law of partial pressure states that the pressure of a gas mixture equals the sum of the partial pressures of gases making up the mixture. As the aircraft climbs to altitude the barometric pressure within the aircraft will drop, the fraction of inspired oxygen will remain the same (21%), but the delivery of oxygen to the patient will be reduced because of decreased partial pressure.

Cabin pressurization will allow the transport team to compensate for the decreased barometric pressure at flight altitude. Each aircraft manufacturer designs a maximal pressurization limit for their aircraft. This limit is based on the maximal pressure differential between cabin pressure and actual barometric pressure at flight altitude, which is expressed as a ratio of flight altitude to cabin pressure, each expressed as pounds per square inch (psi). Cabin pressurization creates an artificial atmospheric pressure inside the aircraft, known as *cabin altitude*. The cabin altitude can be adjusted from sea level to a maximal differential (usually 5000 to 6000 ft) depending on patient requirements and aircraft operations. An aircraft flown with a sea-level cabin altitude will not experience any of the effects of high altitude, but this could have a negative effect on the operation of the aircraft. Because of the pressure differential the aircraft might need to be flown at a lower flight altitude to allow for the sea-level cabin pressurization. This lower flight altitude might increase the fuel burn (possibly requiring a fuel stop), slow the aircraft and thus increase transport time, and expose the aircraft to more severe weather concerns.

Most large twin-engine airplanes have pressurization systems. There are no helicopters with pressurization systems. It is imperative that the transport team be aware of an aircraft's abilities before employing the vehicle in patient care.

Nitric Oxide

At many community hospitals, nitric oxide may be administered to some very low birth weight premature infants to lower the risk of lung and brain damage. In addition, there is the use of nitric oxide for the treatment of some cardiac diseases and pulmonary hypertension in the pediatric population. Therefore, it is likely that the number of requests to transport a patient already receiving nitric oxide will continue to increase. Furthermore, the beneficial effects of nitric oxide in the stabilization and transport of critically ill neonatal and pediatric patients may require transport teams to initiate the use of nitric oxide before transport.[14] The transport RT must be able to integrate the nitric oxide delivery device with the patient's ventilator and monitor the various gas levels.

As with all transport equipment, the nitric oxide delivery device should be as lightweight as possible, should be both electrically and battery operated, should not interfere electromagnetically with aircraft navigation or communication equipment, and be ruggedly constructed. The nitric oxide delivery device and the cylinder should be well secured for the duration of transport. A considerable amount of study has been focused on the exposure of the transport team to exhaled nitric oxide, and on the scenario of a catastrophic release of gas from a nitric oxide cylinder within the small working area of an ambulance or aircraft. The results have shown that the high air exchange rates within ambulances and aircraft, and the low doses of nitric oxide used, make environmental nitric oxide toxicity unlikely.

SAFETY OF TRANSPORT

Every transport program (air or ground) must provide a safe work environment. There should be a structured safety program in place to protect both the patient and the transport team members.[15] This program should include the following:

- A safety officer
- An incident reporting process
- Strict safety policies that are enforced
- Annual safety training
- Regularly scheduled transport safety committee meetings
- Regular safety assessments

Recommendations and actions from the transport safety committee must be linked to the transport program's performance improvement program. Safe performance in the transport environment starts with properly trained and educated personnel.[16] Didactic education should include the following:

- Disease physiology and how it relates to transport
- Safety
- Communications
- Stress management
- Survival training
- Legal aspects of transport

Whenever possible, opportunities to practice classroom instruction in the back of an aircraft/ambulance during actual operations are invaluable.

Every transport program should have an "Accident/Incident Action Plan." The plan should include the process for notification of the following in the event of an accident involving the transport team:

- Transport team management
- Hospital administration
- Physicians
- Risk management
- Public affairs
- The media
- The transport team families

ACCREDITATION

The transport program must be in compliance with local, state, and federal regulations related to the transport of neonatal/pediatric patients. Regulations that involve the following all have an effect on the transport

of patients, documentation requirements, team composition, equipment and supplies, and transfer/transport consent forms.

- Certificates of need
- City/county/state/federal licensure
- Emergency medical services state health departments
- Consolidated Omnibus Budget Reconciliation Act (COBRA)
- Emergency Medical Treatment and Active Labor Act (EMTALA)
- Centers for Medicare and Medicaid Services (CMS)
- Federal aviation regulations (FARs)
- The Federal Aviation Administration (FAA)

The program director needs to be knowledgeable about all these regulations and requirements. The transport staff must also be aware of and understand the regulations that influence the day-to-day operations of the program.

The Commission on Accreditation of Medical Transport Systems (CAMTS) is a peer review organization that offers a program of voluntary evaluation of compliance with a set of accreditation standards. The core elements of the standards include aircraft/ambulance configuration, communications, legal requirements, maintenance, management, pilots and drivers, medical direction, scope of care, safety program, scheduling, and training and education of personnel. By participating in the voluntary accreditation process, transport teams can verify their adherence to quality standards to themselves, their peers, medical professionals, insurance companies, and the general public. At present several different states are considering adopting the CAMTS standards as the minimal standards required of transport teams for state licensing.

ASSESSMENT QUESTIONS

See Evolve Resources for answers.

1. Rapid transport of a neonate or a pediatric patient with a serious illness or trauma to a specialty facility can result in which of the following?
   A. Improved outcomes
   B. No difference
   C. Worse outcomes
   D. Unknown
2. Which of the following is the single most important asset in transport?
   A. Aircraft
   B. Life-saving equipment
   C. Ambulance
   D. Personnel

Continued

ASSESSMENT QUESTIONS—cont'd

3. How many transports are typically required to justify a dedicated team?
   A. 300 to 500
   B. 500 to 700
   C. 700 to 900
   D. 1000 to 1200
4. What is the single largest expense of a transport team?
   A. Personnel
   B. Transport vehicles
   C. Transport ventilators
   D. Cardiopulmonary monitors
5. What types of alarms are preferred in transport?
   A. Audible
   B. Visual
   C. Both audible and visual
   D. None
6. Why should mechanical ventilators be used during transport?
   A. Many of them offer the same level of support as ICU ventilation.
   B. They help prevent hyperventilation associated with manual ventilation.
   C. Monitoring of pressure, tidal volume, and minute ventilation can be achieved with appropriate alarm functions.
   D. All of the above
7. Many transport teams are offering point of care testing with a portable blood gas analyzer for what reasons?
   A. It reduces stabilization times and improves quality of care.
   B. Many blood gas analyzers are small and battery powered.
   C. It compensates for clinical assessment skills.
   D. A and B
8. The simple goal of the transport team is to:
   A. Transfer the patient in the most stable condition possible
   B. Transfer the patient within the "golden hour"
   C. Scoop and run
   D. None of the above
9. According to Boyle's law, what will the endotracheal tube cuff pressure do when the aircraft climbs in altitude?
   A. Remain the same
   B. Increase in pressure
   C. Decrease in pressure
   D. The pilot balloon pressure will increase, but the ETT cuff pressure will remain constant
10. Every transport program should have a(n)
    A. Rescue plan
    B. Back-up plan
    C. Accident/Incident Action Plan
    D. Media coverage plan

References

1. Reynolds M et al: The nuts and bolts of organizing and initiating a pediatric transport team, *Crit Care Clin* 1992;8:465.
2. Pon S et al: The organization of a pediatric critical care transport program, *Pediatr Clin North Am* 1993;40:241.
3. Kronick JB et al: Pediatric and neonatal critical care transport: a comparison of therapeutic interventions, *Pediatr Emerg Care* 1996;12:23.
4. Sitler CG, Graf JM: Pediatric transport team composition: a dynamic paradigm (unpublished manuscript, 2004).
5. Orr R et al: Pediatric specialty care teams are associated with reduced morbidity during pediatric interfacility transport (unpublished manuscript, 1999).
6. Scott S et al: A multidisciplinary approach to neonatal ambulance design, *Neonatal Network* 1994;13:13.
7. Brink LW et al: Air transport, *Pediatr Clin North Am* 1993;40:439.
8. Nish WA et al: Effect of electromagnetic interference by neonatal transport equipment on aircraft operation, *Aviat Space Environ Med* 1989;60:599.
9. Macnab A et al: Vibration and noise in pediatric emergency transport vehicles: a potential cause of morbidity? *Aviat Space Environ Med* 1995;66:212.
10. Dockery WK et al: A comparison of manual and mechanical ventilation during pediatric transport, *Crit Care Med* 1999;27:694.
11. Macnab AJ et al: Cost:benefit of point of care blood gas analysis vs. laboratory measurement during stabilization prior to transport, *Prehosp Disaster Med* 2003;18:24.
12. Reimer-Brady J: Legal issues related to stabilization and transport of the critically ill neonate, *J Perinat Neonatal Nurs* 1996;10:59.
13. Raszynski A: Aviation physiology and international transport of infants and children, *International Pediatrics* 1999;14:99.
14. Dhillon JS et al: A portable nitric oxide scavenging system designed for use on neonatal transport, *Crit Care Med* 1996;24:1068.
15. O'Brien DJ et al: The effectiveness of lights and siren use during ambulance transport by paramedics, *Prehosp Emerg Care* 1999;3:127.
16. King BR et al: Pediatric critical care transport—the safety of the journey: a five-year review of vehicular collisions involving pediatric and neonatal transport teams, *Prehosp Emerg Care* 2002;6:449.

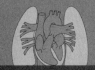

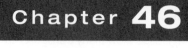

Chapter **46**

Home Care

SHERRY L. BARNHART

LEARNING OBJECTIVES:

- Discuss the critical components of a discharge plan for the child who is respiratory technology-dependent.
- Recognize barriers that may delay the hospital discharge of a child who is respiratory technology-dependent.
- Compare the three types of oxygen systems available for use in the home.
- Describe the procedure used to attach the apnea-bradycardia monitor and the scenarios in which a monitor is indicated.

- List the essential components of a trach-to-go bag.
- Recognize the need for decannulation and changing the tracheostomy tube.
- Discuss how caregivers are best prepared in caring for a ventilator-dependent child at home.
- Discuss the considerations needed in selecting the home ventilator and the home medical equipment provider.

dvances in pharmaceuticals and medical devices have now made it possible for parents and health care professionals to care for infant and pediatric patients who are technology-dependent. Today an unprecedented amount of that medical care is being provided in the child's home. The reasons are many for this shift toward care at home. Medical equipment is now more portable and better able to accommodate home care needs. There is also the ever-increasing pressure to reduce health care costs and shorten hospital stays by expediting the transition from hospital to home. Perhaps most importantly is the growing belief that prolonged hospitalizations have a negative impact on the development of infants and children, and therefore the home is the optimal setting for the medically stable, technology-dependent patient.[1]

In 1981, the move toward caring for technology-dependent children at home caught national attention when, during a press conference, President Ronald Reagan cited the case of 3-year-old Katie Beckett. Katie had been hospitalized since she was admitted at 3 months old with viral encephalitis. Regulations at that time mandated that she remain in the hospital in order for Medicaid to cover her medical bills. Two days after that press conference, the Secretary of Health and Human Services waived the rules that were preventing Katie from being discharged to her home, where she could be treated far less expensively. Only a few months after that, a waiver program was established that enables a child living at home to receive Medicaid-funded long-term care services. That program remains in place today and is often referred to as the *Katie Beckett waiver*.[2]

DISCHARGE PLANNING: THE DECISION TO GO HOME

Discharge planning should begin on admission to the hospital and continue through the hospital stay and transfer to an alternative site of care. Alternative sites include the child's home, foster care, long-term care facilities, and hospice care. The goals of discharge planning include the following:

- Reducing the length of stay in the hospital
- Ensuring successful transition to an alternative site of care
- Reducing unplanned readmissions and postdischarge medical costs
- Coordinating community services to support the child at home

Central to the discharge planning process is a multidisciplinary team of health care professionals that works together to establish an appropriate discharge plan (Box 46-1). Extensive collaboration between the team and the parents is necessary to ensure that discharge planning is achieved properly.[3]

Before making the decision to provide home care for a child dependent on technology, a discharge plan is developed.[4] Critical components of this plan include the following:

- Assessment of the patient and family needs
- Identification and education of in-home caregivers
- Assessment of available financial resources
- Evaluation of the home environment

Box 46-1	Multidisciplinary Discharge Planning Team

- Patient and family/caregivers
- Physician
- Staff nurse
- Pulmonary nurse specialist
- Social worker
- Respiratory care discharge planner
- Nurse discharge planner
- Respiratory therapist
- Physical therapist
- Occupational therapist
- Speech pathologist
- Child development/education specialist
- Nutritionist
- Pharmacist
- Chaplain
- Case manager (funding source)
- Home medical equipment provider
- Home health agency representative
- Alternative site representative (if needed)

- Availability of medical equipment and health care resources
- Identification of home care personnel and community resources
- Open communication and a strong relationship between the parent/caregivers and the discharge planning team
- Recognition of barriers that will delay the discharge home

Patient and Family Assessment

The entire discharge planning team should meet and assess the needs of both the child and family. Before discharge home, the child must be medically stable and receiving optimal ventilatory, nutritional, and developmental support.[5] Assessment includes evaluation of the family's ability, availability, and commitment to care for their child as well as a psychosocial assessment for parenting risk factors that could potentially result in adverse outcomes.[6] Language barriers and physical or cognitive limitations that will impact the family's ability to understand and participate in the discharge process are best dealt with immediately.

The family's involvement is critical to the health and well-being of the child.[7] Parents or caregivers must be informed of the implications of home care and the physical, emotional, social, and financial aspects it entails. Frank discussions about confidentiality and privacy issues, the impact on other family members, and the time demands of home care should also occur.[8] Caregivers must be willing and capable of making such a courageous commitment. This includes providing constant direct care in a home environment that is safe and suitable for the medical equipment as well as being able to successfully complete the necessary training. Including them early in the decision-making and care provided for the child at the hospital has been shown to have a positive effect on their confidence and readiness to assume full responsibility for their child's care at home.[6]

A discharge contract or agreement that describes mutual responsibilities and obligations has been found to be an invaluable tool. The agreement includes specific expectations that the parents must meet in order to demonstrate their ability to provide safe care for their child after discharge. The contract may also describe consequences for noncompliance with any aspect of the discharge plans. Caregivers must demonstrate willingness to work together with the hospital team, home medical equipment (HME) provider, and home health staff. Despite a family's best intentions, however, there are situations in which sending the child home may not be appropriate and may actually put the child's life at risk.

Identification and Education of In-home Caregivers

In most situations at least two people, usually the parents, are identified as the primary caregivers. These caregivers must have the ability and commitment to learn and actively participate in the child's care at home. The educational component of the discharge plan includes training not only the primary caregivers but also any other individuals who identify themselves as a support person for the child (e.g., grandparents, teachers) and even the child to the greatest extent possible. Training ideally begins at least 1 month before discharge and does not end when the child goes home. It is an ongoing process to reinforce all the skills that the caregivers have been taught. Caregivers must understand the child's medical condition, emergency plans, and the function of all medical equipment, including maintenance and troubleshooting procedures.

All education, whether knowledge or skill based, must be consistent and at the level of understanding of each participant.[9] Keep in mind that the level of care that parents of technology-dependent children are expected to provide is far beyond that normally expected of parents. Mastery of the skills requires both material knowledge and practical experience. Training should be provided by an experienced professional who can also recognize unvoiced needs of the primary caregivers. Use of a training manual that includes a detailed checklist is a useful tool to organize the required skills and help avoid missing any essential steps. It also assists in providing consistent education while serving as a resource for the

> **Box 46-2** **Essentials of a Home Care Training Manual**
>
> - Basics of anatomy and physiology
> - Disease pathophysiology (specific to child's condition)
> - Assessment of clinical status
> - List of equipment and supplies
> - Special care procedures (tracheostomy care, suctioning, manual ventilation, respiratory treatment)
> - Medication administration (dosage, frequency, storage, recognition of adverse effects)
> - HME operation, maintenance, and troubleshooting
> - Infection control
> - Emergency phone numbers
> - Scope of services offered by HME provider
>
> HME, Home medical equipment.

caregivers (Box 46-2). Because most individuals obtain more information by actually performing procedures, it is imperative that the caregivers be given the opportunity to perform hands-on care with the child in a controlled hospital environment. With the hospital staff assuming a supportive role, the caregivers should provide as much hands-on care of the child as possible. Participating in mock scenarios also provides opportunities to problem solve and practice skills and emergency techniques.[10]

Caregivers, especially those with children who require a tracheostomy or ventilator, are required to participate in an in-hospital trial or rooming-in period in which they are responsible for the total care of their child. The goal of this period is to build confidence in their ability to care for their child while also offering an opportunity for backup assistance and coaching. While rooming-in, the caregivers are responsible for all routine care (i.e., feeding, bathing, dressing), respiratory care (i.e., treatments, ventilator checks, suctioning), medication delivery, equipment cleaning and troubleshooting, and arranging for relief periods with cocaregivers. Before discharge, they must have demonstrated knowledge and competency as well as be independent in successfully handling all aspects of their child's care.[11-13]

Financial Resources

In today's managed care arena, high cost and inadequate funding of care are usually the major obstacles to providing quality care at home. Funding necessary to provide long-term care to the technology-dependent child varies, depending on the complexity of care required, the level of parental capability, and responsibilities the parents may have (e.g., other children, work outside the home). Although home care costs are usually less expensive than cost for care in the hospital, parents often find that their insurance does not cover 100% of the cost at home as it did in the hospital. These nonreimbursable costs may be for home equipment and supplies, transportation to and from the hospital and clinics, and even changes made to the home so it will accommodate the child and equipment. Inadequate reimbursement creates a financial hardship for families and may be cause for HME providers and nursing agencies to refrain from providing services to the child. Limited payment for home care equipment and personnel has in many cases limited the scope and practice of mechanical ventilation in the home and delayed discharge for months. This has led professional societies to work together to create expert guidelines for mechanical ventilation outside the intensive care unit.[14]

Because professional care can be costly, it is essential to establish a solid financial plan to fund this care long before discharge. It should be determined early whether the insurance policy has a limit on medical equipment and home care resources. The funding source must cover the cost of equipment, supplies, and professional services, such as skilled nursing and physical, occupational, and speech therapies. In most cases, insurance will fund these needs as long as the patient meets the criteria of medical stability, and the physician certifies a plan of care and completes a certificate of medical necessity. There should be continued communication with the child's insurers. A case manager is usually assigned by the payer to monitor care and ensure it is cost-effective. Notifying the case manager early in the discharge process is essential in order to maximize the available dollars. In many cases, the home medical equipment provider is the expert on reimbursement for home medical supplies.[15,16]

Evaluation of Home Environment

Depending on the home equipment needed, an on-site evaluation of the patient's home may be required before discharge to address any concerns or problems in the home environment. The evaluation includes assessment of the physical space, electrical capabilities, heating/cooling system, in-house water supply, availability of 24-hour telephone access, and the geographic location of the home (Box 46-3). It is best to address these issues early in the discharge planning process so that adequate time is available to make any necessary changes.

It is essential that the house be fully accessible for the child and the home care staff. There must be enough room for the child and equipment to be easily moved in and out of the home. Children who are ventilator dependent ideally need a bedroom of their own so that family members are not disturbed by the care needed during sleep or the nursing staff. The bedroom must

---

Box 46-3   Checklist for Home Assessment

- Adequate electrical power and wiring
- Appropriate heating/cooling system
- Working smoke detectors
- Adequate lighting
- Adequate space in bedroom for equipment
- Counter space to clean equipment
- Storage space for equipment
- Adequate physical space for nurse/caregiver to work
- Door sizes to accommodate child and equipment entry
- Steps or wheelchair ramps to access home
- Telephone service
- 9-1-1 service

---

be large enough to accommodate the medical equipment as well as a comfortable chair for the nurse to use. An area for supplies and equipment storage should be designated and counter space made available for cleaning small equipment and reusable items. The room must be climate controlled with proper ventilation and free of drafts. The amount of medical equipment in the room can cause a small room to heat up quickly and some mechanical ventilators will shut down if the temperature exceeds a certain level.

The electrical circuitry of the home must be evaluated to determine whether there are a sufficient number of grounded electrical outlets to provide safe operation of the equipment. Because multiple pieces of equipment may be running simultaneously, the household circuitry must support the total amperage of the equipment to be supplied. If not, another circuit breaker must be installed.

The geographic location of the patient must be considered to plan for transportation systems and emergency care. The family must have a telephone in working condition and live in an area that has 24-hour access to emergency medical services.

Home Medical Equipment

Home medical equipment includes any product or device that is used in the home environment by a child who is ill or has disabilities. The equipment required depends on the child's medical condition. Examples of home medical equipment are air compressors, oxygen concentrators, mechanical ventilators, continuous positive airway pressure systems, wheelchairs, infusion pumps, blood glucose meters, and apnea monitors. The company that supplies this equipment is referred to as the HME provider. Additional equipment may be needed for availability at each site that the child attends (e.g., daycare, school). Equipment that will be used at home should be used in the hospital first so that caregivers can become familiar and proficient with its use. Any differences in its use at home should be addressed before discharge.[8]

When selecting an HME provider, the following must be considered. Does the provider supply all of the equipment needed? Many providers are no longer supplying apnea monitors. It may also prove difficult to find one that provides tracheostomy and ventilator supplies. Does the provider have a contract with the child's health care insurer, or is it considered out-of-network? Caregivers are required to pay much less for the equipment and supplies when an in-network provider is selected. Does it employ respiratory therapists who are trained to provide the patient/caregiver education, psychosocial support, and physical assessment needed for children who require specialized respiratory equipment and supplies? Does it provide service to the area in which the child lives? It is essential that the selected HME provider have a pediatric staff that is available for consultation and emergency coverage 24 hours a day, 7 days a week.

Home Care Personnel and Community Resources

Home care involves cooperation and collaboration between the hospital and the home nursing and community services. The visiting nurse or home care agency that will be supporting the child at home is contacted before discharge and given therapy and medication regimens, a follow-up appointment schedule, and instructions on general care of the child. These instructions include recognizing signs that would indicate the child is becoming ill and how to seek medical help. Acknowledgment of the parents as experts in the care of the child is an essential point during the education of the nursing and HME providers. Some caregivers may even choose to assist in teaching the home care staff about the needs of their child. Home care nurses must be educated on use of the medical equipment that will be in the home. This training is most often made available by the HME provider. If the child is of school age, the teachers and school nurse also need to understand any special needs and limitations the child may have. Respite services and emergency staffing in case the caregiver is ill should also be included in the discharge plan.[8]

Before discharge a primary care provider is identified and an initial appointment scheduled. It is imperative that the designated primary care provider be one who is agreeable to caring for a technology-dependent child. Not every physician is willing to assume responsibility for a medically fragile child who is moving into the home environment. Unfortunately, failure to obtain a primary care provider can delay discharge home. Appointments for follow-up care with each physician specialist (e.g., surgery; pulmonary; otolaryngology)

Box 46-4	Health Care and Community Resources Telephone List

The resource telephone list should include phone numbers for the following:

- Primary care physician
- Pulmonologist
- Other physician specialists
- Emergency room: local hospital and children's hospital
- Pharmacy
- Home medical equipment provider
- Home health agency: nursing
- Therapies: occupational, physical, speech
- School and daycare
- Insurance contact
- Utility companies

---

should also be arranged before discharge, with every effort made to schedule the appointments together on the same day. This not only decreases the burden on the family but has also proven to improve compliance. Each family is given a telephone list that includes the office and emergency phone numbers of the child's physicians and community resources (Box 46-4).

Public awareness is a vital part of the technology-dependent child's acceptance back into the community. The local utility company must be informed that for medical reasons the child is dependent on electricity. This information is provided through a letter signed by the physician. Having the letter on file allows the company to make it a high priority to restore electricity to the home in the event of a power outage and may even qualify the family for a discounted rate. A similar letter stating that the child needs a functioning communication system is sent to the telephone company. The water and sewage company as well as the local emergency medical service providers are also contacted and provided with information concerning the child's medical condition. Some emergency medical service or volunteer departments have little or no experience in caring for a child with a tracheostomy or who is ventilator dependent. In that case special training should be arranged and a plan developed for the child's needs before discharge. Such community awareness allows for a smooth transition from the hospital to the home and even to the school environment.

Communication With Discharge Planning Team

When parents are overwhelmed by the uncertainty of their child's condition and future, they often develop unrealistic expectations of outcomes, time frames, and discharge dates. Open communication and a strong relationship with the discharge planning team are keys to providing a successful discharge home and preventing readmission to the hospital. The purpose of the initial meeting is often simply to determine whether or not home care is suitable and manageable for the child. Patient care conferences in which the family and the discharge planning team candidly discuss the needs of the child and what they will face at home should continue at strategic points during the discharge process. These conferences provide an opportunity for the family to meet the home health providers, including nurses and respiratory therapists, and to voice any questions or concerns they may have. The meetings should focus on establishing the needs of the family and the child as well as providing a detailed plan for discharge and discussing any problems that may affect success. It is during these meetings that the home care therapist clarifies the time frame in which training and equipment setup must be completed. Because the child and family's needs often change over time, this also provides an opportunity to review the family's needs, how they are managing, and progress toward the home care goals.[8]

Barriers That Delay Discharge

Many technology-dependent children remain hospitalized for extended periods of time even though they are considered medically stable. Unfortunately, it is often a nonmedical reason that delays the discharge. These barriers may include the inability to obtain a safe home environment or alternative care site, lack of financial resources, or uncooperativeness within the family. Diverse sociocultural backgrounds, including problems stemming from language, can impact communication and the learning needs of the caregivers. Delays in obtaining medical equipment or a provider for the equipment will in turn delay beginning the education for the caregivers. Other barriers to discharge include the inability to provide home nursing or community resources as well as failing to identify all pertinent problems or needs.[4,17-19]

OXYGEN THERAPY AT HOME

Unlike adults, in whom measurement of the arterial partial pressure of oxygen is considered critical, the need for home oxygen therapy for infants and children is established on the basis of oxygen saturation as measured by pulse oximetry.[1,20] Although there are those children who will require oxygen for many years, the majority who are discharged home with oxygen need it for a limited period, eventually requiring it only at night and then weaning off completely.

The three types of oxygen system available for the home environment are liquid oxygen, oxygen concentrators, and compressed oxygen cylinders. Selection of the particular system is commonly the responsibility of the HME provider. Regardless of the type of oxygen system provided, it is essential that the HME provider be advised of the specific flow rate the child requires. This will determine which flowmeter to use with the system. Although there are flowmeters available that provide "microflows" with readings as low as 0.025 L/minute, some clinicians do not advocate using them. When weaning from oxygen begins, the majority of infants are often decreased to 0.1 L/minute and do not require lower flows before going to room air. There is also some concern that a caregiver could become confused by the decimal points and inadvertently administer the incorrect flow.[20]

Before discharge home, the child's caregivers must receive the oxygen equipment and successfully complete training in its use. If the child attends daycare or school, then arrangements should also be made to instruct responsible staff and teachers in use of the equipment. Safety issues are stressed, including the need for a nonsmoking environment in the home and for keeping the patient 4 to 6 ft away from any heat source including fireplaces, heaters, cooking stoves, and even candles on a birthday cake.[21]

Liquid Oxygen System

The liquid oxygen system consists of a base unit reservoir and a small, portable canister used for patient transport (Figure 46-1). The canister weighs 8 to 10 lb and is carried with a shoulder strap or rolling cart. When the canister becomes empty it is refilled from the base unit.

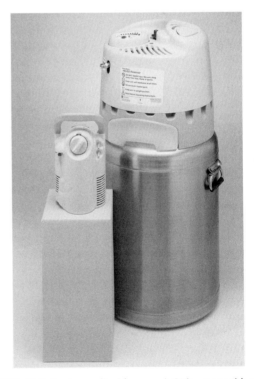

FIGURE 46-1 Stationary liquid oxygen (LOX) system with a portable system capable of being refilled by the patient or family.

The base unit has a flowmeter that can deliver oxygen at low to high flow rates. Most systems have interchangeable flowmeters that range from 0.08 to 15 L/minute.

Advantages to this system are that no electricity is required and little noise is produced. Also, some caregivers prefer to use the canister for transport rather than an oxygen cylinder. A disadvantage to using this system is that the base unit requires regular refilling by the HME provider. Frequency depends on both the oxygen flow rate and the size of the reservoir and can be as often as once a week to every other month. Another disadvantage to the liquid oxygen system is that it vents continually to prevent pressure from building within the reservoir, resulting in a loss of oxygen regardless of whether the flow is on or off. Caregivers must therefore be reminded that liquid oxygen will evaporate and portable units should be checked for contents and filled just before use.

Oxygen Concentrators

First produced in the 1960s, the oxygen concentrator is an electric device capable of separating oxygen from nitrogen in room air, collecting the oxygen, and then dispensing it through a flowmeter (Figure 46-2).[22] Most concentrators provide greater than 90% oxygen. On some concentrators the flowmeters can be changed to provide low flow rates (Figure 46-3) whereas others have dual flowmeters to accommodate the varied needs of the patient (Figure 46-4). The HME provider needs to evaluate each concentrator's specifications before use

with pediatric patients to ensure it can be used with low flows. When using concentrators, oxygen cylinders are provided for the patient to use for transport and for backup in the case of an electrical power outage.

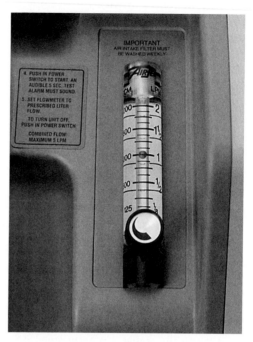

FIGURE 46-3 Close-up view of the low-range flowmeter on an oxygen concentrator.

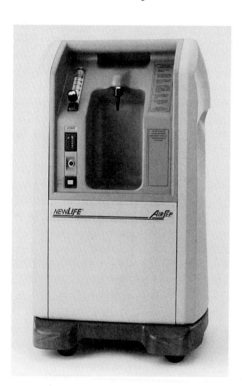

FIGURE 46-2 Oxygen concentrator.

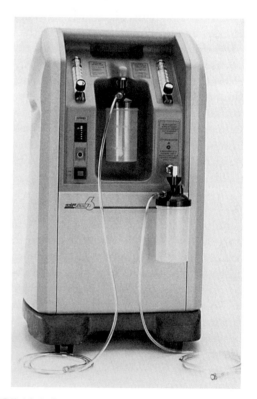

FIGURE 46-4 Oxygen concentrator with dual flowmeters set at different flow rates.

As long as there is an electrical source, an oxygen concentrator provides an unlimited supply of oxygen and does not need to be refilled. It can be easily moved from room to room and requires minimal maintenance. However, the concentrator's motor may produce additional heat and noise. Caregivers may also complain that use has resulted in an increase in their monthly electrical bill.

Oxygen Cylinders

A compressed gas cylinder is usually made of seamless aluminum or fiberglass so that it can be as lightweight as possible. Oxygen cylinders are considered a cost-effective method of providing oxygen because they do not require electricity and can be stored for a long period without leakage. The major disadvantages of cylinders are the storage space required and the potential safety hazards due to the gas being contained under high pressure. Although the cylinders are smaller, they may still seem a bit more bulky than the liquid oxygen canister.

Portable cylinders are available in a variety of sizes and are identified by letter designations At one time the E cylinder was the smallest available in portable cylinders, making liquid oxygen the number one choice for pediatric patients. Today, however, compressed gas cylinders are gaining in popularity thanks to the availability of smaller cylinders with custom carrying cases and regulators with flowmeters that allow for very low flow rates.

APNEA–BRADYCARDIA MONITORS

An apnea–bradycardia monitor, more commonly referred to as an *apnea monitor*, is a portable machine that noninvasively monitors an infant's respiratory rate and heart rate. When there is apnea beyond a preset time limit (usually 20 s), or when the infant's heart rate falls below or exceeds preset limits, an alarm will sound to notify the caregivers. Rather than being purchased by the caregiver, an apnea monitor is usually rented from an HME provider. More recently introduced to the market are apnea–bradycardia monitors that also incorporate a pulse oximeter.

For effective monitoring, monitors should be equipped with an event recorder that is able to capture and store cardiopulmonary events. The events are provided in a printout, commonly known as a *download*. Downloading is the process by which the information stored in the monitor is retrieved. The HME provider usually downloads this information over the phone. The download contains a printout of waveforms, a log of the events including the frequency of alarms and how low the heart rate dropped, and the frequency of monitor use. The information obtained can be used to distinguish the type of apnea, decide the type of medical treatment needed, and determine compliance and when to discontinue the monitor. When the infant lives a far distance from the HME provider, a second monitor may be placed in the home. To have consistent, consecutive data when downloading the memory, it is recommended that only one monitor be used and the other kept solely for backup in case of monitor malfunction.

Monitor Placement

An apnea monitor may be considered medically necessary for infants who:

- Have apnea of prematurity, which is defined as documented episodes of periodic breathing that result in prolonged apnea (20 s or greater) or bradycardia (heart rate less than 80 beats/min). Because the neurologic breathing control mechanisms may not have matured by the time a newborn is ready for discharge home, an apnea monitor may be required to monitor the infant at home during unattended sleep. The monitor is indicated until the infant is 43 weeks of gestational age or is event free for at least 2 weeks.
- Are receiving caffeine or theophylline for treatment of apnea or bradycardia. The monitor is considered medically necessary until the infant is event free for 2 weeks after the medication is discontinued.
- Have experienced an apparent life-threatening event, which is defined as an episode characterized by a combination of apnea, color change, choking, gagging, or muscle tone change that required mouth-to-mouth resuscitation or vigorous stimulation. The monitor is used until the infant is event free for 2 to 3 months.
- Have pertussis with positive cultures. The monitor is used for 1 month after the diagnosis.
- Are diagnosed with gastroesophageal reflux disease accompanied by apnea, bradycardia, or oxygen desaturation. The monitor is indicated until the infant is event free for 6 weeks.
- Have neurologic or metabolic disorders affecting respiratory control.
- Have chronic lung disease and are requiring noninvasive or invasive ventilatory support.
- Have two siblings who died of sudden infant death syndrome (SIDS). These infants may be monitored until they have remained event free and are 1 month older than the age at which their siblings died. Because there is no proof that apneic episodes are related to SIDS, the American Academy of Pediatrics (Elk Grove Village, Ill) released a policy statement in 2003 that does not recommend apnea monitoring in infants with only one SIDS sibling.[23]

Although an apnea–bradycardia monitor may be a helpful adjunct to monitoring the infant requiring mechanical ventilation, use of this monitor is redundant and caution should be advised when interpreting alarm conditions. The reverse is also true: As long as heart rate is maintained and minimal chest excursion occurs, the alarm on the monitor will not be activated. However, this does not necessarily indicate that the ventilator is functioning properly. An infant with a tracheostomy is frequently prone to mucous plugging or decannulation. During these potentially life-threatening events, the apnea alarm will not be activated as long as the infant can struggle against an occlusion in the tracheostomy tube or breathe through an open stoma after accidental decannulation. Likewise, the bradycardia alarm usually becomes activated late during this type of event. When monitoring an infant with a tracheostomy, the clinician and parents must be aware of the potential hazards and the limitations of the monitor.

Caregiver Education

The HME provider usually trains the parents in the use and care of the monitor. Parents are instructed to use the monitor whenever the infant is sleeping (naps and at night), riding in the car, and anytime the infant is not being held or closely watched. To monitor the infant, electrodes are either stuck on the infant's chest or held in place with a soft belt and the heart rate and respiratory pattern are measured by means of a method known as *impedance pneumography* (Box 46-5). The monitor should be placed on a table near the infant, not on

the floor, and at least 1 ft away from electrical devices such as televisions, air conditioners, telephones, electric water bed heaters, nursery monitor intercoms, oscillating fans, and humidifiers. Interference from these devices, although uncommon, may affect the monitor's performance. If items (e.g., diapers, toys) are near the monitor, they should be placed so that they do not block the displays or muffle the alarms. Caregivers should be advised not to allow the infant to sleep with adults, children, or pets while being monitored because their movement may prevent the monitor from working properly. Parents should check daily that the monitor's alarms sound by disconnecting the leads from the infant. They should also perform a daily inspection of the electrodes, lead wires, and power cords. A logbook should be provided for parents to record the date and time of all events, unique observations about the monitor, and any intervention required (i.e., stimulation, resuscitation). The Velcro belt can be washed by hand in soapy water, rinsed well, and hung to air dry. Moving the patches just slightly can help minimize skin irritation. The belt should be tight enough to fit only one finger between the belt and the infant's chest. If the belt is too loose, signals for breathing and heart rate will not be picked up and may result in frequent loose lead or false alarms. If the belt is too tight, it may interfere with the infant's breathing. Powder, oil, and lotion can disrupt the monitor's conduction and result in false alarms. Unless traveling outside the home, the apnea monitor should be plugged into an electrical outlet so that the batteries can remain fully charged.

Education for parents also includes infant cardiopulmonary resuscitation (CPR) and recognizing the signs of apnea. Parents should be instructed to respond to alarms by turning on the light if the room is dark and immediately checking the infant for signs of breathing. If the infant is breathing and skin color is good, parents should check the electrode placement, lead wires, and the cable. If the infant is pale, cyanotic, or is not breathing, stimulation is immediately required. It is essential that parents be taught not to shake their infant as a form of stimulation because vigorous shaking may result in severe head and neck injury and even death. If the infant does not respond, then CPR is indicated immediately. Any time CPR is performed, the infant should be seen immediately by a physician.

Most monitors have built-in algorithms that differentiate precordial movement from chest wall movement, but false alarm conditions are frequent. The most common reason for a false alarm is shallow breathing. An infant may be having abdominal breathing and the chest wall is not moving enough to be recognized as a breath. Lead wires that connect the electrodes to the

Box 46-5	Lead Placement for Apnea Monitors

1. Wash and dry infant's chest. Do *not* use lotions, oil, or powders.
2. Connect electrodes to lead wires, making sure metal tips of lead wires are pushed all the way in.
3. Place foam belt on a flat surface, then place infant's back on the belt. Line the belt up with infant's nipples.
4. Position electrodes on belt (smooth side up) with each electrode under an armpit lined up with infant's nipples. White lead is on infant's right side, *not* the caregiver's right (hint "White is Right") and black is on the infant's left side, *not* the caregiver's left.
5. Wrap belt around infant's chest and fasten with Velcro tab. Check belt to make sure it is tight, so caregiver can fit only one finger between belt and infant's chest wall. Belt may be shortened by cutting it.
6. Connect lead wires to patient cable. White lead goes to cable for right arm (marked RA). Black lead goes to cable for left arm (marked LA).
7. Turn monitor to "ON."

monitor can become loose during vigorous infant activity, often resulting in false alarms. There is an increased chance of obtaining false alarms when the infant is playing, burping, being fed, and moving. Other causes of false alarms are crying, the Valsalva maneuver, incorrect lead or belt placement, poor skin contact, broken lead wires, and a low battery. Although there is no way for a parent to distinguish between a real and a false alarm when it initially sounds, especially if the infant is breathing by the time the parent arrives, information obtained from a download will include the amount of time the infant did not breathe and what the heart rate was at that time. The download can allow for differentiation between real apneas and loose lead wires, because there is an abrupt drop in the heart rate with a loose lead wire instead of the gradual drop that occurs with a true apneic event.

Changes in heart rate may be the source of annoying intermittent alarms for which a cause is difficult to find. Usually this is from an apneic episode that may not be long enough to alert the parents of apnea but that causes the heart rate to decelerate and briefly activate the bradycardia alarm. A rare cardiac arrhythmia may also cause a similar situation. Proper settings to minimize false alarms are important because parents become conditioned to most alarms being false. They must be constantly reminded of this phenomenon and encouraged not to delay in responding to the monitor when it alerts them.

PULSE OXIMETERS

The pulse oximeter is used for continuous monitoring as well as "spot checks." Its use in the home is indicated for infants and children who require continuous oxygen therapy and whose oxygen need varies from day to day or with activities, including feeding, sleeping, and playing. By monitoring the oxygen saturation, the caregiver has the ability to increase or decrease the oxygen flow rate to maintain a specific oxygen saturation range.[1] Use of a pulse oximeter may also be indicated during the process of weaning from oxygen therapy and to monitor infants and children who have a tracheostomy and/or are using mechanical ventilation at home. Potential inaccuracies associated with oximeter readings may result from poor perfusion and excessive movement of the child.[24]

For infants with hypoplastic left heart syndrome, daily pulse oximetry spot checks along with daily weighing is often part of the home surveillance program following stage 1 of the Norwood procedure. On discharge from the hospital, parents are given a notebook to record their infant's daily weights and oxygen saturations. They are also provided with guidelines about when to notify

the health care provider with concerns, including contacting their physician if the oxygen saturation is less than 70%, if the infant's weight drops more than 30 g in 24 hours, or if the infant fails to gain at least 20 g during a 3-day period. The daily home surveillance of both oxygen saturation and weight in infants who are at increased risk of death before they return for stage 2 of the Norwood procedure has resulted in improved interstage survival.[25]

THE CHILD WITH A TRACHEOSTOMY

Although children receive a tracheostomy for a variety of medical conditions, there are three primary indications for placement: to provide a stable airway for children with upper airway obstruction, to provide an interface for long-term invasive mechanical ventilation, and to allow for more effective pulmonary toilet in children with excessive secretions or aspiration. Placement of a tracheostomy in a child may be a life-saving maneuver but it has a significant impact on the family as well as on socialization and health of the child. Parents are concerned that they will never hear their baby cry or their child speak. Because of the small diameter of the infant and pediatric tracheostomy tube, there remains the potential hazard of airway obstruction and the child requires constant observation. To minimize this risk, adequate humidification, effective suctioning, CPR, tracheostomy care with regular tube changes, and decannulation are essential components of home care management. Because there is little research to guide the care of a child at home with a tracheostomy, in the absence of scientific data many recommendations are based on consensus, the care performed in the hospital, and local clinical practice. Unfortunately, many times procedures are determined by insurance coverage policies when payment limits the type and amount of supplies that will be reimbursed.[26]

At least two family members, usually the parents, must be identified as primary caregivers and education should begin as early as possible. Caregivers must understand basic airway anatomy, recognize the signs of respiratory distress, and demonstrate how to respond to an emergency. They must also be able to demonstrate proper use of the home medical equipment (Box 46-6), suctioning technique, how to clean and change out the tracheostomy tube, and proper placement and care of the speaking valve. The HME provider will educate the caregivers on the respiratory and tracheostomy equipment. The hospital staff will provide the remaining education. Caregivers are encouraged to frequently visit the hospital and to participate in as much of their child's bedside care as possible. The child with a tracheostomy must have emergency supplies readily available at all times. An emergency bag, or trach-to-go bag, should accompany the child at all times (Box 46-7). The contents of this bag should not be used at the bedside but instead used only when the child is away from the home. Caregivers must attend a CPR class that includes training with an emphasis on emergency management of the airway and tracheostomy tube. They must be able to recognize respiratory distress, such as accidental decannulation and a plugged tube, and respond to emergency situations quickly, including changing the tube.[27]

Airway Suctioning

Simplicity is an essential component of successful home medical management, especially with suctioning. Home suctioning differs from the aseptic, *sterile technique* used in the hospital, where a sterile glove and a sterile catheter are used for each suctioning procedure. Two methods are used at home: one is referred to as the *modified clean technique*, defined as using a sterile catheter with clean, nonsterile, disposable gloves. The other is the *clean technique*, and is defined as the use of a clean but nonsterile catheter with clean, nonsterile gloves or freshly washed, clean hands.[28] When performing suctioning by the clean technique, the hands are washed thoroughly before beginning the procedure. The suction catheter begins as a sterile catheter but instead of being discarded, it is washed, disinfected, and reused (Box 46-8). There is some variation among caregivers regarding how long a catheter is used before it is cleaned. Some clean the catheter after every suctioning procedure whereas others change the catheter ever 8 to 24 hours. Should the catheter be contaminated (i.e., dropped on the floor), it should be cleaned at that point.[28] If other individuals in the home are ill, the modified clean technique, using a sterile catheter and clean glove, should be used temporarily. Some professional clinicians may choose to use sterile technique in the home while the child is ill.

In addition to learning the suctioning techniques, caregivers must be able to recognize the need for

---

Box 46-6	Home Medical Equipment and Supplies Needed for a Child with a Tracheostomy

- Self-inflating manual resuscitation bag
- Oxygen supplies
  - Stationary and portable oxygen supply systems
  - Oxygen tubing and bleed-in adapters
- Heated humidifier with a tracheostomy collar (to use at night)
- Air compressor or high-pressure concentrator to power humidifier
- Heat and moisture exchangers (to use during day)
- Suction supplies
  - Portable and stationary suction machines
  - Suction collection canister and connecting tubing
  - Suction catheter kits
  - Single-dose normal saline units
  - Sterile water
  - Gloves
- Tracheostomy supplies
  - Tracheostomy tubes: current size
  - Tracheostomy tubes: next smaller size
  - Tracheostomy ties: Velcro or twill tape
  - Cotton tip applicators or gauze
  - Tracheostomy cleaning kits
  - Water-soluble lubricant
- Disinfectant solution
- Monitoring systems
  - Pulse oximeter (optional)
  - Apnea monitor (optional)

Box 46-7	Contents of a "Trach-to-Go" Bag

- DeLee suction trap to use if suction machine fails
- Suction catheters and gloves
- Small bottle of sterile water for cleaning suction catheter
- Single-dose normal saline units for irrigation
- Lubricant for tracheostomy tube insertion
- Two tracheostomy tubes (current size, one size smaller)
- Extra obturator
- Tracheostomy ties (Velcro or twill tape)
- Blunt-nosed scissors for cutting tracheostomy ties
- Self-inflating resuscitation bag with mask
- Heat and moisture exchangers
- Stethoscope

Box 46-8	Cleaning Suction Catheters in the Home

1. Using a 20-cc syringe, flush the catheter clean with either sterile/boiled water or 3% hydrogen peroxide.
2. Soak in one (not all) of the following to disinfect:
   A. 1:50 dilution of bleach for 3 minutes (1 teaspoon of bleach to 1 cup of water)
   B. 70% isopropyl alcohol for 5 minutes
   C. 3% hydrogen peroxide for 30 minutes
   D. Commercial disinfectant, such as Control III, for 15 to 20 minutes
3. Rinse the inside and outside of catheter with sterile/boiled water.
4. Place on a clean paper towel to air dry and then store in a clean, sealed plastic bag.

suctioning. Suctioning is based on clinical assessment and should be performed on an as-needed basis rather than scheduled. Typically caregivers are taught to suction when the child wakes up in the morning or after a nap because secretions accumulate in the airway during sleep. They should suction after chest physiotherapy and respiratory treatments when indicated and when secretions can be heard in the tube. Suctioning should be performed if the child seems restless or uncomfortable or exhibits signs and symptoms of respiratory distress. If the child has an effective cough, suctioning is performed infrequently. If the child exhibits copious amounts of secretions or is ill, more frequent suctioning may be required, as often as every 2 to 4 hours.

Caregivers should be taught to note the amount, color, and consistency of the secretions and to report significant changes to their physician. To prevent injury to the tracheal mucosa, the suction catheter is inserted in the tracheostomy to only ¼ to ½ inch beyond the tip of the tube.[29] A suction catheter should be premeasured and marked, and then set aside for caregivers to use as a measuring guide. Routine use of normal saline for lavage is *not* recommended.[28] Caregivers must demonstrate proficiency at suctioning when the child is in the hospital, before the rooming-in period.

All children with a tracheostomy should have a stationary and portable suction machine (Figure 46-5). In addition to an internal battery that can be charged from AC power, the portable suction unit must have a cigarette lighter adapter to charge off of the car battery. The caregiver is advised to take the trach-to-go bag with the patient whenever leaving the house. A DeLee suction trap should be kept in the bag for use in case the suction unit fails. Suction catheters, oral suction tubes, and suction canisters are supplied by the HME provider. A manual self-inflating resuscitation bag with an

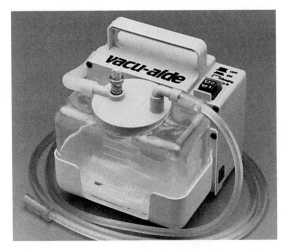

FIGURE 46-5 Battery-powered portable suction machine.

Box 46-9	Emergency Tracheostomy Supplies Kept at the Bedside

- Extra tube, same size currently using
- Extra tube, one size smaller
- Obturator
- Tracheostomy tube ties
- Scissors
- Manual resuscitator bag and appropriate-size mask
- Standby oxygen, if ordered

appropriate-size mask, oxygen, and extra suction canisters should be kept in the home and readily available in case of an emergency (Box 46-9).

Decannulation and Tube Changes

The purpose of changing the tracheostomy tube in the home is to minimize infection and the formation of granulation tissue.[30] As a general rule for children, the tube is changed once a week or as needed should it become obstructed. All caregivers must be taught to change the tube routinely and during an emergency if the child suddenly experiences signs and symptoms of respiratory distress (Box 46-10).[31] Before the rooming-in period and before a child can be discharged home, both primary caregivers are required to demonstrate that they can correctly and independently change the tracheostomy tube. Caregivers are strongly encouraged to be available to change the tracheostomy tube as often as possible while the child is in the hospital.

If at all possible tube changes should be performed in the early morning before the child eats (Box 46-11). It is best for two caregivers to be present when changing the tracheostomy tube: one to remove the tube and the other to insert the clean one. All equipment, including the emergency supplies, should be gathered and readily available at the bedside. To change the tube, a blanket or towel roll is placed under the child's shoulders to extend the neck. While one caregiver holds the tube in place, loosens the ties, and then removes the tube, the other caregiver inserts the clean tube. The clean

Box 46-10	Indications for Changing a Tracheostomy Tube

- Scheduled change is due
- Suction catheter does not pass freely (plugging)
- Respiratory distress is unresolved by suctioning or other interventions
- Oxygen desaturation is unresolved by suctioning or other interventions
- Accidental decannulation

Box 46-11	Steps in Performing Tracheostomy Change

1. Wash hands.
2. Gather equipment.
3. Suction patient, then wash hands again.
4. Arrange workspace with adequate lighting.
5. Place obturator in the extra identical tracheostomy tube; thread ties or collar through one side of tube.
6. Lightly coat tip of tube with water-soluble lubricant.
7. Place child on back with a rolled towel under the shoulders.
8. Cut and remove old ties and pull tube out with a curved, downward motion.
9. Gently insert tube into the stoma, using a downward and forward motion that follows the curve of the tube.
10. Remove the obturator immediately after inserting the tube.
11. Secure the ties.
12. Suction as needed.
13. Assess the child's respiratory status.

tracheostomy ties are attached, the child's work of breathing is assessed, and assurance is made that the airway is intact.

Two tracheostomy tubes should always be available at the bedside and in the trach-to-go bag. One tube should be the size the child is currently using and the other tube should be one size smaller. The smaller tube is available in case a situation exists in which the current size cannot be reinserted. If resistance is met when attempting to replace the current tube, then the smaller tube is placed until further medical assistance can be obtained. A child's stoma can close quickly, so placement of a smaller tube will preserve the opening. Cuffless tubes are preferred in children; however, a cuffed tube may be required if the child is being mechanically ventilated.

Humidification Systems

Several types of humidification systems can be used in the home care environment. Humidification during mechanical ventilation is necessary to prevent destruction of airway epithelium, hypothermia, atelectasis, and thickening of secretions. The humidification system chosen should provide a minimum of 30 mg of H_2O/L of delivered gas at 30° C and meet specifications of the American National Standards Institute (Washington, DC). These are especially important in the pediatric population requiring continuous mechanical ventilatory support that uses high peak inspiratory flow rates.[32]

A portable, 50-psig air compressor or a 20-psig high-flow/high-pressure oxygen concentrator with a heated humidifier and tracheostomy collar is an excellent humidification system. The humidifier should be stabilized near the child's bed, either attached to the bed or to a table or pole located nearby. Many HME providers will assist families with obtaining a table or microwave cart that can be placed beside the bed to hold the ventilator and humidifier. They will also instruct the parents in preparing sterile water and normal saline at home (Box 46-12). The tracheostomy collar is often bulky and limits the child's mobility. Therefore it is suggested that unless the child is being mechanically ventilated, the collar and heated humidity should be used during sleep at night and that a *heat and moisture exchanger* be used during transport and daytime hours. The first attempt at using the heat and moisture exchanger should take place in a controlled setting several days before the child is discharged home. The caregivers should be taught to observe for signs and symptoms of respiratory distress associated with the lack of humidification. The heat and moisture exchanger should never be used with another humidification system. The added moisture will wet the exchanger and increase the child's work of breathing through the exchanger. The caregiver should understand that airway obstruction may occur if secretions are trapped in the heat and moisture exchanger. If the child requires oxygen, the addition of a T-ring

Box 46-12	Preparing Sterile Distilled Water and Normal Saline at Home

1. Buy distilled water from a local store.
2. Obtain clean glass jars with lids. Baby food jars work well for saline.
3. Boil the distilled water for 15 minutes.
4. For normal saline, add 1 tablespoon of noniodized salt to 1 quart of distilled water (or ¼ teaspoon of salt to 1 cup of distilled water) and boil for 15 minutes.
5. Sterilize the jars by completely immersing them in water and boiling for 15 minutes.
6. Sterilization must be done on a stove. Do not use a dishwasher or a microwave.
7. Pour the water out of the pan and allow the jars and lids to cool in the pan.
8. Remove the jars and lids from the pan without touching the inside of the jars or lids.
9. Place the jars and lids upright on a clean towel.
10. Pour the boiled distilled water into the jars and place the lids on tightly.
11. Do not pour any used solution back into the jar.
12. After 3 days, discard any leftover solution and resterilize the jar and lid.

adapter around the tracheostomy tube can reduce the amount of oxygen flow necessary to maintain the child's oxygen saturation levels. The T-ring adapter can be used with the heat and moisture exchanger and with the tracheostomy collar

Communication and Speaking Valves

Children begin to communicate from the moment they are born. Communication is an innate component of every human who interacts with the environment and is part of the bonding process for parents and caregivers. Research also shows that speech and language development is interdependent on and interactive with motor and cognitive development. The child with a tracheostomy is limited in its ability to vocalize and speech therapy becomes an essential part of the home care plan. The goal of speech therapy is to improve deficits in speech and language development. Therapy assists in developing oral motor skills, maximizing language, and encouraging nonvocal behavior. Many forms of communication are used with the pediatric tracheostomy patient, including computers, sign language, and speaking valves. The benefits of combining all forms of effective communication are critical to the child's development.

A tracheostomy tube not only causes the child's vocal cords to remain in the open position, resulting in a diminished ability to vocalize and cough, but it also impacts a child's swallowing function. These factors can lead to a higher susceptibility to aspiration, subsequent pneumonia, and atelectasis, which can in turn result in longer placement of the tracheostomy tube and need for mechanical ventilation.[33] Use of a speaking valve provides a form of communication, enhances the ability to cough effectively, and also filters and protects the airway from particles.[34] The effective cough reduces the need for suctioning and the potential for infection and airway trauma.[31] Restoration of airflow through the upper airway also restores sensation to the oropharynx as well as the sense of smell and taste. In turn this improves appetite, overall nutritional intake, and swallowing efficiency.[35]

The Passy-Muir tracheostomy swallowing and speaking valve (PMV) allows a child to speak without occluding the tracheostomy stoma. The valve was developed in the 1980s by David Muir, a patient with muscular dystrophy who had a tracheostomy. Opening only during inspiration, the PMV allows air to enter the airway. On expiration the valve closes, which results in air being forced out of the airway through the vocal cords, nose, and mouth (Figure 46-6). The patient can resume speaking, which enhances social interaction and decreases frustration by making it easier

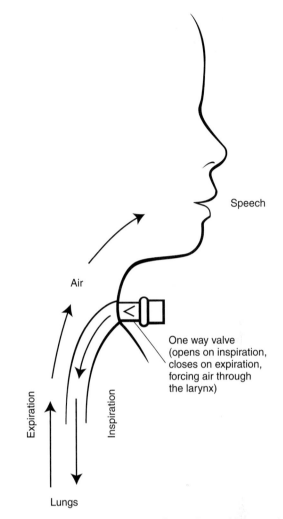

FIGURE 46-6 Tracheostomy speaking valve enables speech by redirecting exhaled air around the tracheostomy tube and through the larynx and upper airway.

to vocalize spontaneously. Ideally the speaking valve should be placed within a few days of receiving the tracheostomy so that the child will consider it part of the tracheostomy tube. Successful transitioning techniques used when placing the valve include play therapy and distractions such as coloring books, whistles, and toys. Techniques for training children to exhale through the valve include blowing whistles, bubbles, and feathers. If the tracheostomy tube does not allow the child to exhale through the valve, then the tube should be downsized. A speaking valve is contraindicated in patients who have severe tracheal stenosis or excessive secretions, require continuously inflated cuffed tubes, or are unconscious or heavily sedated.

Activities of Daily Living

Pediatric patients with a tracheostomy should be treated as normal children. A child who is overprotected will feel different from other children and may become demanding. This child is "special" only in the way he or she breathes; helping others to understand this is important.[36] The child with a tracheostomy can take part in most play activities suitable for that age. With an infant or small child, all small toy parts or objects should be removed from the play area because the child might put these into the tube. During outdoor play the caregivers must protect the child's tracheostomy from extreme temperatures and dirt in the air. Extremely cold or hot air may be irritating to the child's lungs. An artificial mask, a disposable mask, or a scarf tied around the neck works well to protect the child's tracheostomy tube. The child should not go swimming unless closely supervised. The pediatric patient may still go to the beach, when it is not windy, as long as the child wears a heat and moisture exchanger to keep sand out of the tube.

When bathing a child with a tracheostomy, the child may be placed in a tub but care must be taken not to allow water into the tube. To wash a child's hair, hold the child on his back over a sink or tub. Wash and rinse the hair with a cup of water and washcloth, or spray the hair carefully. The child can play in the water, but never submerge the child in the water or leave the child alone in the tub. An older child can take a shower as long as the tracheostomy is protected.

There is no need to buy special clothing for the child with a tracheostomy. However, parents are instructed to buy clothes that do *not* cover the tracheostomy. Items to avoid include turtlenecks, necklaces, scarves, or any type of material with fibers that could be released into the tracheostomy opening. The home environment should be kept as free of lint, dust, and animal hair as possible. It is imperative that no one smokes, uses powders, or sprays aerosols around or on the child. Particles and fumes can enter the lungs through the tube and cause breathing problems.

Some children require suctioning at night, so an intercom system is helpful to notify the parent easily. If the child has limited strength, proper positioning and monitoring with an apnea monitor or a pulse oximeter should be done.

Because every caregiver or parent needs a break, qualified providers, or respite care, must be available to care for the child in the absence of the primary caregiver. This is a major reason why more than one caregiver should be trained to care for the child. Also, the primary caregiver may become ill and be unable to care for the child for an extended time.

Transporting the child may require extra precautions and planning (Box 46-13). It is recommended that another individual besides the driver be in the vehicle

Box 46-13	Equipment Needed for Travel

- Trach-to-go bag
- Portable suction machine
- Extra suction canister and tubing
- Prescriptions (medicine, oxygen, and respiratory equipment)
- Pulse oximeter, extra probes
- Oxygen
- List of phone numbers (physician, HME provider, pharmacy)

with the child. Standard car seat restraints may not work for the child with a tracheostomy. A survey on the methods of transporting technology-dependent children found that the children were restrained appropriately; however, in 66% of the cases the heavy medical equipment was not secured.[37]

MECHANICAL VENTILATION IN THE HOME

As neonatal and pediatric respiratory care continues to evolve, we have seen an increase in the number of children with chronic respiratory failure who are medically stable. Many of these children require some level of ventilatory assistance, ranging from noninvasive night-time ventilation to 24-hour ventilatory support. The clinical conditions resulting in respiratory failure and chronic ventilatory support are varied and include chronic lung disease, acquired or congenital neuromuscular impairment, airway abnormalities, and ventilatory control disorders. And even though the number of ventilator-assisted children is relatively small compared with other groups, the cost of care is substantial when specialized equipment and education are required and especially when hospital stays are prolonged. There is no argument that the hospital is an unsuitable environment for the ventilator-assisted child who is medically stable. The benefits of having the child at home are many, including an enhanced quality of life. Yet the discharge process for a ventilator-assisted child can be long and complicated. In few other situations does it require a more coordinated multidisciplinary team approach.

Family Preparation

The decision to provide care at home must be family centered, not staff generated. Successful home management of the ventilator-assisted child depends largely on the parents' willingness and capacity to meet the needs of their child.[32] Care at home is time-consuming, labor-intensive, and expensive. Parents should be told that care at home will require more than normal parenting skills. It will impact every aspect of each family member's lifestyle and quality of life. Siblings often feel neglected and marriages are challenged. An even heavier burden is imposed on single-parent families. But time and again families agree that overcoming the challenges and finally arriving home is justified and worthwhile.

Before the discharge process begins for a ventilator-assisted child, the following criteria must be met:

- At least two adult caregivers must be willing to commit to participate in the necessary training and the child's ongoing care.
- Parents must be in agreement on taking the child home.
- Caregivers must be physically and mentally capable of providing home care for the child.

Once a family makes the decision to commit to caring for their ventilator-assisted child at home, a formal discharge process begins. The first step is often a meeting with all, or select, members of the discharge planning team. Parents should be informed that the discharge process may take several weeks or even months, depending on the individual child's needs. Identification of the two primary caregivers is essential at this point. Because transition to home for a ventilator-assisted child involves such an extensive commitment from the caregivers, they may be asked to sign contracts agreeing to the education/training, hospital rooming-in period, and the steps involved in discharge home. The caregivers should be given an overview of the discharge process with projected dates and timelines for certain steps in the process.

Moving the child from the intensive care unit to an area where the caregivers can be more involved in their child's care is an enormous step in beginning the discharge process. Even though formal teaching by the HME provider may not have begun, the caregivers can learn a great deal about the care of their child from the respiratory therapists, nurses, physical therapists, speech therapists, and occupational therapists who care daily for the child. Once teaching begins, the caregivers have more time to begin practicing their skills in their child's room. Quite often the most successful transitions home are with those families who have spent the most time at their child's bedside, taking an active part in the daily care.

Parents with ventilator-assisted children have commented on how they initially feel shocked and crushed by the uncertainty of their child's illness and their family's future. It may be helpful for the caregivers to be in contact with other parents who have a similar experience. The parents' ability and commitment to be involved in their child's care may vary during the course of the hospitalization, especially when the hospital stay extends into months. Parents struggle with their own adjustment and coping abilities and other aspects of their life. Research has shown that families of ventilator-assisted children face profound burdens in household management, social relations, and financial issues.[38] Because many caregivers must work outside the home, it is common for employment issues to become complicated during the discharge process. This is especially true when caregivers live and work quite some distance from the hospital, yet they are being asked to be with their child to receive training and to become more familiar with the bedside care.

Selection of the Ventilator and HME Provider

There is no standard approach for selecting a ventilator for the pediatric patient. The ventilator and the settings chosen must be tailored to meet the needs of each child. The overall goal is to choose a ventilator capable of maintaining clinical stability with arterial blood gas levels as close to physiologic values as possible. Ideally, ventilators chosen for home care should be user-friendly, compact, and portable and operate on a variety of power sources.[4,39] The device should incorporate a reliable alarm system, and should be trouble free for extended periods. Home care ventilators should have hidden controls or a locked panel to prevent pediatric patients or siblings from inadvertently altering the settings.

Always consider the child's needs when selecting a suitable ventilator. Factors to be considered include, but are not limited to, home versus public school, distance to the health care provider, and how well it will meet the growing needs of the child. If the ventilator selected for home mechanical ventilation is not available in the hospital, the HME provider may be asked to supply the appropriate machine for a trial period before discharge.

Another factor to be considered when selecting a home ventilator concerns the compatibility of the circuit and the positive end-expiratory pressure (PEEP) valve. PEEP is often accomplished by using an external PEEP valve, which can be heavy and may also have exhalation ports that can be easily blocked. The combination of the PEEP valve and circuit must have minimal exhaled resistance. The PEEP valve must also be able to function at any angle; this precludes gravity and water columns for home use.

A major advantage of a portable ventilator is the ability to use a variety of power sources including house current, an internal battery for short periods, and an external battery for extended periods. Some portable ventilators can operate from a car battery by connecting to the cigarette lighter. A 12-V battery should be available for use during trips away from home and as an extended backup during an electric power failure. A 12-V 74-A/hour, deep-cycle battery can power a ventilator for about 20 hours without recharging. A 12-V 34-A/hour, gel-cell battery can power a ventilator for about 10 hours before recharging is required. It is important to note how heavy the battery is and whether the combined weight of the battery and ventilator still allows portability. In rural areas where power outages frequently occur, or where it may take extensive time for electricity to be restored, it is often advisable to purchase a backup electricity generator. Another alternative is to have portable backup batteries or power packs.

The HME provider should be selected as soon as it is determined that the child will go home. Caregivers should be given the option of selecting the provider; however, there may be few choices, because many may not provide ventilators for children. To obtain one that is an in-network provider with the child's insurance carrier or one that will accept Medicaid reimbursement may narrow the field even more. It is essential, though, that the chosen HME provider have home care personnel who are familiar with the care of infants and children with tracheostomies and who are also familiar with pediatric mechanical ventilation. If the provider agrees to accept the patient, then the home assessment can be scheduled and a list of needed supplies provided. The supply list should be given to the provider as soon as possible so that equipment can be ordered (Box 46-14).

A second ventilator, or backup ventilator, should be provided in the home for the child who[40]

- Cannot maintain spontaneous ventilation for four or more consecutive hours

- Lives in an area where a replacement ventilator cannot be provided within 2 hours
- Requires mechanical ventilation during mobility

An emergency backup ventilator must be available in the event of a ventilator malfunction. Without a backup ventilator in the home, the home care company must assume the responsibility for providing immediate service. It is also best to have extra ventilator circuits and a spare temperature probe in the home. Although it is not practical to duplicate all equipment, it may be reasonable to have a second suction machine and oxygen source to use at the school or at daycare.

User and clinician manuals should be available from the manufacturer, along with training materials such as videotapes. The user information manual and audiovisual material should be left in the home for parents to use as a reference. All educational materials should be well organized and easy to understand. Various factors must be considered to achieve the goals of pediatric ventilatory support in the home environment (Box 46-15).

Common Delays to Discharge Home

In spite of the most valorous attempts at organization, communication, and planning within the discharge process, obstacles to discharge will still occur. The major barriers for chronically ventilated children include failure to obtain qualified nursing staff, delays in approval for home care funding, an unsuitable home environment, complex family issues, and arrangements for out-of-home placement.[41,42]

Recruitment of qualified nursing is a problem no matter where the child's home may be. Some areas are better staffed than others, but there always tends to be a shortage of nurses who can care for the ventilator-assisted child. In some cases, the discharge date is set, the caregivers have completed all training and assessments, and the parents have roomed-in; and then, for various reasons, nursing staff is no longer available and the child cannot go home. When nursing shortage is an issue, some families have resorted to advertising for

---

Box 46-14	**Home Medical Equipment and Supplies for Ventilator-assisted Children**

- Mechanical ventilator
  - Primary ventilator
  - Backup ventilator
  - 12-V battery and connecting cable
  - Ventilator circuits
- Humidification supplies
  - Humidifier and heater
  - Heat and moisture exchangers
- Tracheostomy supplies
- Suctioning supplies
- Self-inflating manual resuscitation bag
- Monitoring systems
  - Pulse oximeter (optional)
  - Apnea monitor (optional)

Box 46-15	**Goals of Pediatric Home Mechanical Ventilation**

- Enhance quality of life
- Extend life
- Provide an environment that promotes individual growth
- Improve psychological function
- Improve physical function
- Reduce morbidity
- Be cost beneficial

their nurses. Although it is not an option for most families, some have just opted to go home without nursing care.

Funding delays are often the greatest hurdle to getting the child home. Without reimbursement, home equipment cannot be obtained. The greatest difficulty arises when there is little or no reimbursement for the ventilator. Community resources, such as nursing, speech therapy, physical therapy, and occupational therapy, are also unattainable without funding. Without reimbursement, discharge is delayed indefinitely.

The sooner it is known that housing is unsuitable, the more likely solutions can be made. That is why it is so important that the HME provider obtain the home assessment as soon as it is determined that the child intends to be sent home. Many times the problems are simply that electrical outlets are not in compliance, or a ramp needs to be built to accommodate the wheelchair. There are situations in which the home is in an area that nursing or the HME provider refuses to travel to, because it is too far away or it is unsafe. Other situations include not having electricity or air conditioning, not enough space for the child's equipment, or even extreme situations in which the caregivers have been evicted. The social worker is an invaluable member of the discharge planning team when these issues arise.

Family issues are all too often the most difficult barriers to overcome. The longer the hospital stay, the more likely that family dynamics will change. Strained finances, guilt, fatigue, worry, and emotional distress are all issues faced by most families of ventilator-assisted children. However, issues such as divorce, which often results in loss of one of the primary caregivers, and drug abuse and mental illness are the types of issues that tend to result in the longest delays.

Although it is not a commonly faced obstacle, making arrangements to discharge the ventilator-assisted child to an alternative site often leads to extensive delays. It may take weeks if not months to find a medical foster home for the child, which in turn requires home assessment and education of the foster parents. Locating an institution that accepts ventilator-assisted children may be difficult if the child resides in a state that does not have such a facility. It is often difficult for parents to agree to send their child to a facility that is hours away, much less in another state. It may be even more difficult to find a facility that has an opening available for the child.

Home at Last

Before a ventilator-dependent child can be discharged home, the following criteria must be met. Ventilator settings must be stable for at least 1 week. The oxygen concentration must be less than 40%, and blood gas analysis must be stable and within normal limits.[32] The home environment must be acceptable and the home equipment available either at the hospital or at the child's home. It is also essential that there be adequate home care available. This includes two primary caregivers who have successfully completed all of the training and the rooming-in period, as well as adequate home nursing staff. On the day of discharge, transportation home or to the alternative site of care is usually provided by an ambulance. It is recommended that the respiratory therapist from the HME provider meet the child when they arrive home and assist the family with "settling in" at home.

Children requiring mechanical ventilation have not only complex medical problems but home medical equipment that requires frequent evaluation (Box 46-16). Although equipment malfunction may be minimal, there can be no delay in troubleshooting when problems arise. For this reason it is imperative that these children be provided with appropriate medical expertise. This includes 24-hour availability of the HME provider's staff as well as nurses and respiratory therapists from a pulmonary center.

Ventilator-assisted children should be evaluated by a pulmonologist every 3 to 6 months. During the visits the child's ventilatory status and oxygenation requirements are evaluated to determine optimal ventilator settings and the potential for weaning. Because children often have large leaks associated with uncuffed

Box 46-16	Problems Associated with Home Mechanical Ventilation

- Disconnected ventilator circuit
- Leaks in ventilator circuit
- Obstructions in ventilator circuit
- Water in ventilator circuit
- Water in exhalation valve
- Water in external PEEP valve
- Dirty filter
- Leak around tracheostomy tube
- Ventilator autocycling
- Power surge
- Increased suctioning requirement
- Increased oxygen requirement
- Change in child's pulmonary status
- Change in child's nutritional status
- Change in child's activity level
- Development of infection
- Extensive time required to adjustment to home/ environment

PEEP, Positive end-expiratory pressure.

tubes, the child's tracheostomy is assessed for correct size and placement. In fact, studies have shown that 9 of 11 children with uncuffed tubes are inadequately ventilated, resulting in chronic hypercapnia and fatigue.[43-48] Problems with equipment are addressed and continuing education of the caregivers is provided if necessary.

A SUCCESSFUL TRANSITION HOME

Caring for technology-dependent children in the home often presents challenges for their families, their community, and the health care system. Every caregiver of a technology-dependent child is at risk of physical burnout, financial and emotional stress, depression, and social isolation, especially when support and resources are insufficient or inaccessible.[49,50] Many of these challenges can be resolved by interdisciplinary discharge planning, the use of discharge protocols, case management approaches, respite care, psychological counseling, and adequate financial provisions for sustaining home care.[51] A successful transition home often depends on when the discharge process begins. Waiting to the last minute often ends in failure. The advances in care and equipment that make a child's survival possible in the first place are many times the greatest challenges in the transition home. The family's central role in the discharge planning process must be recognized and supported because in the end, successful transitions may have less to do with the child's medical condition than with the family's commitment to the child and their ability to adapt, work as a team, and persevere.

ASSESSMENT QUESTIONS

See Evolve Resources for answers.

1. A 12-year-old male with Duchenne's muscular dystrophy is admitted to the hospital for a planned tracheostomy and preparation for home mechanical ventilation. Discharge planning should begin for this child and his family
   A. Immediately after placement of the tracheostomy
   B. On admission to the hospital
   C. After transition to the home mechanical ventilator
   D. Once the child is medically stable

ASSESSMENT QUESTIONS—cont'd

2. The parents of an infant who is ventilator dependent have missed several educational sessions that are required before discharge home. They have also been sporadic in visiting their child and practicing bedside skills. What action should the discharge planning team take *next*?
   A. Submit a report to the local child neglect hotline.
   B. Ask the infant's physician to counsel with the parents.
   C. Provide the parents with a discharge contract/agreement.
   D. Suggest that the parents attend a parenting class together.
3. Which of the following is usually the major obstacle to providing quality care in the home of a technology-dependent child?
   A. High cost and inadequate funding of home care services
   B. HME providers that do not employ respiratory therapists
   C. Inability to provide home nursing
   D. Lack of two committed in-home caregivers
4. The need for home oxygen therapy for infants is most often established by
   A. Arterial blood gas analysis
   B. Oxygen saturation measured by pulse oximetry
   C. Sleep scoring from polysomnography studies
   D. Capillary blood gas analysis
5. An infant requires oxygen with a nasal cannula at 0.5 L/minute. The mother states that because of financial difficulties they have moved to a one-bedroom house. Which of the following oxygen systems would be most appropriate to provide in this home?
   A. Liquid oxygen with a base unit reservoir
   B. An oxygen concentrator
   C. A compressed gas H cylinder of oxygen
   D. Multiple compressed gas E cylinders of oxygen
6. An infant will be discharged home with an apnea–bradycardia monitor. Which of the following instructions should the parents be given?
   A. "Your baby only needs the monitor during naps and when sleeping at night."
   B. "The belt is tight enough if you can fit two fingers between it and your baby's chest."
   C. "When the monitor alarms, immediately check for correct electrode placement."
   D. "Do not place lotion on your baby's chest."
7. During use of a home apnea–bradycardia monitor, which of the following is the most common cause of a false alarm?
   A. The baby is crying.
   B. The lead wires are loose.
   C. The baby is breathing shallowly.
   D. The baby is burping.

Continued

ASSESSMENT QUESTIONS—cont'd

8. How often should a cuffless tracheostomy tube in a child be changed when at home?
   A. Once a day
   B. Once a week
   C. Once each month
   D. Only when it becomes obstructed

9. After placing a speaking valve on a child with a 4.5 cuffless pediatric tracheostomy tube, the child exhibits signs of difficulty in exhaling. Which of the following changes should be made?
   A. Change to a 4.5 cuffed tracheostomy tube.
   B. Replace the tracheostomy tube with a fenestrated tube.
   C. Change to a 4.0 cuffed tracheostomy tube.
   D. Downsize to a 4.0 cuffless tracheostomy tube.

10. In which of the following situations should a second (backup) ventilator be placed in a child's home?
   A. The child requires the ventilator only at night while sleeping.
   B. The child's home is within a 1-hour drive of the HME provider.
   C. The child is sprinting from the ventilator for 2 hours twice each day.
   D. The home nursing agency can provide nurses only at night.

References

1. American Thoracic Society: Statement on the care of the child with chronic lung disease of infancy and childhood, *Am J Respir Crit Care Med* 2003;168:356.
2. Social Security Administration: Supplemental security income for the aged, blind, and disabled; deeming of income and resources [20 CFR Part 416], *Fed Regist* 1982;47:24274.
3. Gracey K et al: The changing face of bronchopulmonary dysplasia. 2. Discharging an infant home on oxygen, *Adv Neonatal Care* 2003;3:88.
4. American Association for Respiratory Care: Clinical practice guidelines: discharge planning for the respiratory care patient, *Respir Care* 1995;40:1308.
5. DeWitt PK et al: Obstacles to discharge of ventilator-assisted children from the hospital to home, *Chest* 1993;103:1560.
6. American Academy of Pediatrics: Statement on hospital discharge of the high-risk neonate—proposed guidelines, *Pediatrics* 1998;102:411.
7. Gilmartin MR: Transition from the intensive care unit to home: patient selection and discharge planning, *Respir Care* 1994;39:456.
8. American Academy of Pediatrics, Committee on Children with Disabilities: Guidelines for home care of infants, children, and adolescents with chronic disease, *Pediatrics* 1995;96:161.
9. Czervinske MP: Ensuring quality care for infant tracheostomy patients: part 1, *AARC Times* 1999;23:31.
10. Fiske E: Effective strategies to prepare infants and families for home tracheostomy care, *Adv Neonatal Care* 2004;4:42.
11. American Association for Respiratory Care: Clinical practice guidelines: providing patient and caregiver training, *Respir Care* 1996;41:658.
12. Glenn KA, Make BJ: *Learning objective for positive pressure ventilation in the home*, Denver, Colo: National Center for Home Mechanical Ventilation and National Jewish Center for Immunology and Respiratory Medicine; 1993.
13. American Medical Association Home Care Advisory Panel: *Physicians and home care: guidelines for the medical management of the home care patient*, Chicago: American Medical Association; 1992.
14. American Academy of Pediatrics, Committee on Children with Disabilities: Managed care and children with special health care needs: a subject review, *Pediatrics* 1998;102:657.
15. Hill L, Thompson M: Case management of technology-dependent children: a family-centered approach, *J Home Care Pract* 1994;6:37.
16. McCarthy M: A home discharge program for ventilator-assisted children, *Pediatr Nurs* 1986;1986:331.
17. American Academy of Pediatrics, Medical Home Initiatives for Children with Special Needs Project Advisory Committee: The medical home, *Pediatrics* 2002;110:184.
18. American Academy of Pediatrics, Committee on Child Health Financing: Guiding principles for managed care arrangements for the health care of newborns, infants, children, adolescents, and young adults, *Pediatrics* 2000;105:132.
19. American Academy of Pediatrics, Committee on Children with Disabilities: Managed care and children with special health care needs: a subject review, *Pediatrics* 1998;102:657.
20. Balfour-Lynn IM, Primhak RA, Shaw BNJ: Home oxygen for children: who, how, and when? *Thorax* 2005;60:76.
21. Laubscher B: Home oxygen therapy: beware of birthday cakes, *Arch Dis Child* 2003;88:1125.
22. Harris ND, Stamp JM: Current developments in oxygen concentrator technology, *J Med Eng Technol* 1987;11:103.
23. American Academy of Pediatrics, Committee on Fetus and Newborn: Policy statement 2003: apnea, sudden infant death syndrome, and home monitoring, *Pediatrics* 2003;111:914.
24. American Association for Respiratory Care: Clinical practice guidelines: pulse oximetry, *Respir Care* 1991;36:1406.
25. Ghanayem NS et al: Home surveillance program prevents interstage mortality after the Norwood procedure, *J Thorac Cardiovasc Surg* 2003;126:1367.
26. Lewarski J: Long-term care of the patient with a tracheostomy, *Respir Care* 2005;5:534.
27. Fiske E: Effective strategies to prepare infants and families for home tracheostomy care, *Adv Neonatal Care* 2004;4:42.
28. American Thoracic Society: Care of the child with a chronic tracheostomy, *Am J Respir Crit Care Med* 2001;161:297.
29. Hodge D: Endotracheal suctioning and the infant: a nursing care protocol to decrease complications, *Neonatal Network* 1991;9:7.

30. Fitton CM: Nursing management of the child with a tracheotomy, *Pediatr Clin North Am* 1994;4:513.

31. Miyasaka K et al: Interactive communication in high-technology home care: video phones for pediatric ventilatory care, *Pediatrics* 1997;99:1e.

32. American Association for Respiratory Care, Mechanical Ventilation Guidelines Committee: Clinical practice guidelines: humidification during mechanical ventilation, *Respir Care* 1992;37:887.

33. Torres LY, Sirbegovic DJ: Problems caused by tracheostomy tube placement, *Neonatal Intensive Care* 2004;16:52.

34. Miyasaka K et al: Interactive communication in high-technology home care: video phones for pediatric ventilatory care, *Pediatrics* 1997;99:1e.

35. Dettelbach MA et al: Effect of the Passy-Muir valve on aspiration in patients with tracheostomy, *Head Neck* 1995;17:297.

36. Keen SE et al: Effect of in-home nursing care on distress and coping resources in caregivers of ventilator-assisted children at home, *Am Rev Respir Dis* 1991; 143:A257.

37. Jansen MT et al: Caregiver's safety restraint practices for technology-dependent children during motor vehicle transportation, *Am Rev Respir Dis* 1993;147:A410.

38. Tsara V et al: Burden and coping strategies in families of patients under noninvasive home mechanical ventilation, *Respiration* 2006;73:61.

39. University of Illinois: *Conference proceedings: strategies for success in home for medically fragile children*, Springfield, Ill: University of Illinois, Division of Services for Crippled Children; 1989.

40. American Association for Respiratory Care: Clinical practice guidelines: long-term invasive mechanical ventilation in the home, *Respir Care* 2007;52:1056.

41. DeWitt PK et al: Obstacles to discharge of ventilator-assisted children from hospital to home, *Chest* 1993; 103:1560.

42. Edwards EA, O'Toole M, Wallis C: Sending children home on tracheostomy dependent ventilation: pitfalls and outcomes, *Arch Dis Child* 2004;89:251.

43. Kacmarek RM et al: Imposed work of breathing during synchronized intermittent mandatory ventilation (SIMV) provided by five home care ventilators, *Respir Care* 1990;35:405.

44. Robert P et al: Work of breathing imposed during spontaneous breathing in the SIMV mode of home care ventilators [abstract], *Respir Care* 1992;37:1358.

45. Gilgoff IS, Peng RC, Keens TG: Hypoventilation and apnea in children during mechanically assisted ventilation, *Chest* 1992;101:1500.

46. Chatburn RL, Volsko TA, El-Khatib M: The effect of airway leak on tidal volume during pressure- or flow-controlled ventilation of the neonate: a model study, *Respir Care* 1996;41:728.

47. Bach JR, Alba AS: Tracheostomy ventilation: a study of efficacy with deflated cuffs and cuffless tubes, *Chest* 1998;978:679.

48. Keens TG et al: Frequency, causes, and outcomes of home ventilatory failure, *Am Rev Respir Dis* 1993;147:A408.

49. Leonard BJ, Brust JD, Nelson RP: Parental distress: caring for medically fragile children at home, *J Pediatr Nurs* 1993;8:22.

50. Thyen U, Kuhlthau K, Perrin JM: Employment, child care, and mental health of mothers caring for children assisted by technology, *Pediatrics* 1999;103:1235.

51. Capen CL, Dedlow ER: Discharging ventilator-dependent children: a continuing challenge, *J Pediatr Nurs* 1998;13:175.

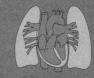

Credits

Chapter 1

Figure 1-1   From Moore KL, Persaud TVN: *The developing human,* ed 5. Philadelphia, 1993, WB Saunders.

Figure 1-2   Langston C, Kida K, Reed M, et al. Human lung growth in late gestation and in the neonate. *Am Rev Respir Dis* 1984 Apr; 129(4):607-13.

Figure 1-3   Langston C, Kida K, Reed M, et al. Human lung growth in late gestation and in the neonate. *Am Rev Respir Dis* 1984 Apr; 129(4):607-13.

Figure 1-4   Langston C, Kida K, Reed M, et al. Human lung growth in late gestation and in the neonate. *Am Rev Respir Dis* 1984 Apr; 129(4):607-13.

Figure 1-5   Langston C, Kida K, Reed M, et al. Human lung growth in late gestation and in the neonate. *Am Rev Respir Dis* 1984 Apr; 129(4):607-13.

Chapter 2

Figure 2-1   From Blechschmidt E, editor: *The stages of human development before birth.* Philadelphia, 1961, WB Saunders.

Figure 2-2   From Moore KL, editor: *The developing human: clinically oriented embryology,* ed 3. Philadelphia, 1982, WB Saunders.

Figure 2-3   Modified from Moore KL, editor: *The developing human: clinically oriented embryology,* ed 3. Philadelphia, 1982, WB Saunders.

Figure 2-4   Modified from Moore KL, editor: *The developing human: clinically oriented embryology,* ed 3. Philadelphia, 1982, WB Saunders.

Figure 2-5   From Moore KL, Persaud TVN: *The developing human: clinically oriented embryology,* ed 8. Philadelphia, 2008, WB Saunders.

Figure 2-6   Modified from Moore KL, editor: *The developing human: clinically oriented embryology,* ed 3. Philadelphia, 1982, WB Saunders.

Chapter 3

Figure 3-1   Courtesy Frank Fox, RDMS.

Chapter 4

Figure 4-1   From American Academy of Pediatrics and AHA: *Neonatal resuscitation textbook,* ed 5. Chicago, American Heart Association, 2006.

Figure 4-2   Courtesy Neotech Products, Valencia, Calif.

Figure 4-3   From American Academy of Pediatrics and AHA: *Neonatal resuscitation textbook,* ed 5. Chicago, 2006, American Heart Association.

Figure 4-4   From Bahar PM, Todd NW: Resuscitation of the newborn with airway compromise. *Clin Perinatol,* Sept., 1999; 26[3]:727.

Figure 4-5   From Bahar PM, Todd NW: Resuscitation of the newborn with airway compromise. *Clin Perinatol,* Sept, 1999; 26[3]:727.

Chapter 5

Figure 5-1   From Ballard JL: New Ballard score, expanded to include extremely premature infants. *J Pediatr* 1991; 119:417-423.

Figure 5-2   Adapted from Lubchenco L.: *The high risk infant.* Philadelphia, 1976, WB Saunders.

Figure 5-4   From Wilkins RL, Stoller JK, Kacmarek RM: Egan's fundamentals of respiratory care, ed 9, 2009, Mosby. Modified from Silverman WA, Anderson DH: A controlled clinical trial of effects of water mist on obstructive respiratory signs, death rate and necropsy findings among premature infants. *Pediatrics* 17:1-6, 1956.

Chapter 10

Figure 10-8   From *Understanding hemodynamic measurements made with the Swan-Ganz catheter.* Irvine, Calif, Baxter Edwards Laboratories, 1989.

Figure 10-9   From Oski FA: Fetal hemoglobin, the neonatal red cell, and 2,3-diphosphoglycerate. *Pediatr Clin North Am* 1972; 19:907-917.

Chapter 11

Figure 11-1   From *Pulse oximetry,* note 7. Image used by permission from Nellcor Puritan Bennett, LCC, Boulder, CO, part of Covidien.

Figure 11-2   From *Clinical reference card,* no 1. Hayward, Calif, Nellcor, 1988.

Figure 11-5   From Stock MC: Non-invasive carbon dioxide monitoring. *Crit Care Clin* 1988; 4:511.

Figure 11-6   From *Advanced concepts in capnography.* Image used by permission from Nellcor Puritan Bennett, LCC, Boulder, CO, part of Covidien.

Figure 11-7   From Stock MC: Non-invasive carbon dioxide monitoring. *Crit Care Clin* 1988; 4:511.

Figure 11-8   From Stock MC: Non-invasive carbon dioxide monitoring. *Crit Care Clin* 1988; 4:511.

Figure 11-9   From Stock MC: Non-invasive carbon dioxide monitoring. *Crit Care Clin* 1988; 4:511.

Figure 11-10   From Curley MA, Thompson JE: End tidal CO_2 monitoring in critically ill infants and children. *Pediatr Nurs* 1990; 16:397.

Figure 11-11   From Stock MC: Non-invasive carbon dioxide monitoring. *Crit Care Clin* 1988; 4:511.

Unn. Figure 11-1   Modified from *Advanced concepts in capnography.* Image used by permission from Nellcor Puritan Bennett, LCC, Boulder, CO, part of Covidien.

Chapter 12

Figure 12-2   Courtesy Neotech Products, Inc., Valencia, CA.

Figure 12-9   Courtesy Timeter Instrument, St. Louis.

Figure 12-11   Courtesy Nova Health Systems, Blackwood, NJ.

Chapter 13

Figure 13-1   Adapted from Wildhaber JH, Janssens HM, Pierart F, et al. High percentage lung delivery in children from detergent-treated spacers. *Pediatr Pulmonol* 2000; 29: 389-393.

Figure 13-2   Redrawn from Dolovich MB. Assessing nebulizer performance. *Respir Care* 2002; 47(11):1290-1301.

Figure 13-3   Redrawn from Fok TF, Monkman S, Dolovich M, et al. Efficient of aerosol medication delivery from a metered dose inhaler versus jet nebulizer in infants with bronchopulmonary dysplasia. *Pediatr Pulmonol* 1996; 21(5): 301-309.

Figure 13-6   Courtesy ICN Pharmaceuticals, Costa Mesa, Calif.

Figure 13-7   From Fink J, Cohen N: Humidity and aerosols. In Eubanks DH, Bone RC, editors: *Principles and applications of cardiorespiratory care equipment*. St. Louis. 1994, Mosby.

Figure 13-8   Modified from Rau JL Jr: *Respiratory care pharmacology*, ed 5. St. Louis, 1998, Mosby.

Figure 13-9   From Fink J, Cohen N: Humidity and aerosols. In Eubanks DH, Bone RC, editors: *Principles and applications of cardiorespiratory care equipment*. St. Louis, 1994, Mosby.

Figure 13-10   Modified from Dhand R, Fink J: Dry powder inhalers. *Respir Care* 1999; 44:940-951.

Figure 13-11   From Smith KJ, Chan H-K, Brown KF: Influence of flow rate on particle size distributions from pressurized and breath actuated inhalers. *J Aerosol Med* 1998; 11:231-245.

Figure 13-12   From Pederson S: Delivery options for the inhaled therapy in children over the age of 6 years. *J Aerosol Med* 1997; 10:41-44.

Figure 13-13   From Qureshi F, Pestian J, Davis P, et al: Effect of nebulized ipratropium on the hospitalization rates of children with asthma. *N Engl J Med* 1998; 339: 1030-1035. Copyright 1998 Massachusetts Medical Society. All rights reserved.

Figure 13-14   Redrawn from Fink J, Cohen N: Humidity and aerosols. In Eubanks DH, Bone RC, editors: *Principles and applications of cardiorespiratory care equipment*. St. Louis, 1994, Mosby.

Figure 13-15   Redrawn from Clinical Trial, Fok TF, Lam K, Ng PC, So HK, Cheung KL, and Wong W: Delivery of salbutamol to nonventilated preterm infants by metered-dose inhaler, jet nebulizer, and ultrasonic nebulizer. *Eur Respir J* Jul 1998; 12(1):159-164.

Chapter 14

Figure 14-1   From Waring WW: Diagnostic and therapeutic procedures. In Chernick V, editor: *Kendig's disorders of the respiratory tract in children*, ed 5. Philadelphia, 1990, WB Saunders.

Figure 14-2   From Waring WW: Diagnostic and therapeutic procedures. In Chernick V, editor: *Kendig's disorders of the respiratory tract in children*, ed 5. Philadelphia, 1990, WB Saunders.

Chapter 15

Figure 15-5   From Cairo JM, Pilbeam SP. *Mosby's respiratory care equipment*, ed 8, St. Louis, 2010, Mosby.

Figure 15-9   Courtesy Neotech Products, Inc., Valencia, Calif.

Figure 15-10   From Handler SD: Craniofacial surgery: otolaryngological concerns. *Int Anesthesiol Clin North Am* 1988; 26:62. (www.lww.com)

Figure 15-11   From Handler SD: Craniofacial surgery: otolaryngological concerns. *Int Anesthesiol Clin North Am* 1988; 26:62. (www.lww.com)

Figure 15-12   From Handler SD: Craniofacial surgery: otolaryngological concerns. *Int Anesthesiol Clin North Am* 1988; 26:63. (www.lww.com)

Figure 15-14   From Gray RF, Todd NW, Jacobs IN: Tracheostomy decannulation in children: approaches and techniques. *Laryngoscope* 1998; 108:10. www.lww.com

Figure 15-19   From Gray RF, Todd WN, Jacobs IN: Tracheostomy decannulation in children: approaches and techniques. *Laryngoscope* 1998; 108:10. http://lww.com

Figure 15-20   From Myer CM, O'Connor DM, Cotton RT: Proposed grading system for subglottic stenosis based upon endotracheal tube sizes. *Ann Otol Rhinol Laryngol* 1994; 103:319. www.lww.com

Figure 15-21   Redrawn from Cotton RT, Myer CM, editors: *Practical pediatric otolaryngology*, Philadelphia, Lippincott-Raven, 1999, p.528. www.lww.com

Figure 15-22   Redrawn from Walner DL, Cotton RT: Acquired anomalies of the larynx and trachea in Cotton RT, Myer CM, editors: *Practical pediatric otolaryngology*, Philadelphia, Lippincott-Raven, 1999 p.528. www.lww.com

Figure 15-23   Redrawn from Walner DL, Cotton RT: Acquired anomalies of the larynx and trachea. In Cotton RT, Myer CM, editors: *Practical pediatric otolaryngology*, Philadelphia, Lippincott-Raven, 1999 p.532. www.lww.com

Chapter 16

Figure 16-1   From Hills BA: *Biology of surfactant*. Cambridge, UK. Cambridge University Press, 1988.

Figure 16-3   From Murray JF: *The normal lung*, ed 2. Philadelphia. WB Saunders, 1986. Courtesy Dr. Mary C. Williams.

Figure 16-4   Redrawn from Batenburg JJ: Biosynthesis, secretion, and recycling of surfactant components. In Robertson B, Taesch HW, Editors: *Surfactant therapy for lung disease*. New York. Courtesy Marcel Dekker, Inc., 1985.

Figure 16-6   From Jobe AH, Ikegami M: Surfactant and acute lung injury. *Proc Assoc Am Phys* 1998; 110:489-495.

Figure 16-7   Photos courtesy Drs. Kaufman and Robin LeGallo (Departments of Neonatology and Pathology, respectively, University of Virginia).

Figure 16-8   From Willson DF, Zaritsky A, Bauman LA, et al: Instillation of calf's lung surfactant extract (Infasurf) is beneficial in pediatric acute hypoxemic respiratory failure. *Crit Care Med* 1999; 27:188-195.

Chapter 17
Figure 17-1   From Chatburn RL: Classification of mechanical ventilations. *Respir Care* 1992; 37:1009-1025.
Figure 17-2   From Wilkins RL, Stoller JK, Kacmarek RM. Egan's fundamentals of respiratory care, ed 9, St. Louis, 2009, Mosby. Redrawn from Chatburn RL: Classification of mechanical ventilations. *Respir Care* 1992; 37:1009-1025.
Figure 17-3   From Wilkins RL, Stoller JK, Kacmarek RM. Egan's fundamentals of respiratory care, ed 9, St. Louis, 2009, Mosby. Redrawn from Chatburn RL: Classification of mechanical ventilations. *Respir Care* 1992; 37:1009-1025.
Figure 17-4   Courtesy Dräger, Telford, Penn.
Figure 17-5   Courtesy Sechrist Industries, Anaheim, Calif.
Figure 17-6   From Cairo JM, Pilbeam SP. Mosby's respiratory care equipment, ed 8, St. Louis, 2010, Mosby. Courtesy Cardinal Health, Yorba Linda, Calif.
Figure 17-7   Courtesy Dräger, Telford, Penn.
Figure 17-8   From Cairo JM, Pilbeam SP. *Mosby's respiratory care equipment,* ed 8, St. Louis, 2010, Mosby. Image used by permission from Nellcor Puritan Bennett, LCC, Boulder, CO, part of Covidien.
Figure 17-9   From Cairo JM, Pilbeam SP. *Mosby's respiratory care equipment,* ed 8, St. Louis, 2010, Mosby. Courtesy Siemens Medical Solutions, Inc., Danvers, Mass.
Figure 17-10   Courtesy Hamilton Medical, AG, Bonaduz, Switzerland.
Figure 17-11   Courtesy GE Healthcare, Waukesha, Wisconsin.
Figure 17-12   Image used by permission from Nellcor Puritan Bennett, LCC, Boulder, CO, part of Covidien.
Figure 17-14   From Cairo JM, Pilbeam SP. *Mosby's respiratory care equipment,* ed 8, St. Louis, 2010, Mosby. Courtesy Pulmonetic Systems, Colton, Calif.
Figure 17-15   From Cairo JM, Pilbeam SP. *Mosby's respiratory care equipment,* ed 8, St. Louis, 2010, Mosby. Courtesy Newport Medical Instruments, Newport Beach, Calif.

Chapter 18
Figure 18-3   Robertson NJ, McCarthy LS, Hamilton PA, et al. Nasal deformities resulting from flow driver continuous positive airway pressure. *Arch Dis Child Fetal Neonatal Ed* 1996; 75(3):209-212.
Figure 18-6   Courtesy VIASYS Healthcare, Yorba Linda, Calif.
Figure 18-7   Courtesy SensorMedics, Inc., Yorba Linda, Calif.
Figure 18-8   **A,** Courtesy VIASYS Healthcare, Yorba Linda, Calif
Figure 18-9   Courtesy VIASYS Healthcare, Yorba Linda, Calif.
Figure 18-10   Courtesy VIASYS Healthcare, Yorba Linda, Calif.
Figure 18-11   Courtesy VIASYS Healthcare, Yorba Linda, Calif.

Chapter 19
Figure 19-15   Modified from *Advanced Concepts in Capnography.* Image used by permission from Nellcor Puritan Bennett, LCC, Boulder, CO, part of Covidien.
Figure 19-20   From Wolf GK and Arnold JH: Noninvasive assessment of lung volume: respiratory inductance plethysmography and electrical impedance tomography. *Crit Care Med* 2005; 33(3):p.145.

Chapter 20
Figure 20-3   Modified from McCulloch PR, Forkert PG, Froese AB: Lung volume maintenance prevents lung injury during high-frequency oscillatory ventilation in surfactant deficient rabbits. *Am Rev Respir Dis* 1988;137:1185.
Figure 20-4   Courtesy Bunnell, Salt Lake City, Utah.
Figure 20-5   Courtesy Bunnell, Salt Lake City, Utah.
Figure 20-6   Courtesy SensorMedics, Yorba Linda, Calif.

Chapter 22
Figure 22-1   From Aranda A, Pearl RG: The biology of nitric oxide. *Respir Care* 1999; 44:157.
Figure 22-2   Redrawn from Hess D et al: Use of inhaled nitric oxide in patients with acute respiratory distress syndrome. *Respir Care* 1996; 41:428.
Figure 22-3   A, Courtesy Bedfont Scientific, Rochester, Kent, UK; B, Courtesy Pulmonox, Tofield, Alberta, Canada.
Figure 22-4   Courtesy Datex-Ohmeda, Helsinki, Finland.
Figure 22-5   Courtesy Pulmonox, Tofield, Alberta, Canada.

Chapter 23
Figure 23-2   From Short BL: Physiology of extracorporeal membrane oxygenation. In Polin RA, Fox WW, editors: *Fetal and neonatal physiology.* Philadelphia. WB Saunders, 1992.
Figure 23-3   Courtesy Medtronic Perfusion Systems, Plymouth, Minn.
Figure 23-4   Redrawn from Short BL: Physiology of extracorporeal membrane oxygenation. In Polin RA, Fox WW, editors: *Fetal and neonatal physiology.* Philadelphia. WB Saunders, 1992.

Chapter 25
Figure 25-2   Data from United Network for Organ Sharing, www.UNOS.org, November 2005.
Figure 25-3   Redrawn from Waltz DA, et al. Registry of the International Society for Heart and Lung Transplantation: ninth official pediatric lung and heart-lung transplantation report–2006. *J Heart Lung Transplant* 2006; 25:904-911.
Figure 25-4   The U.S. Organ Procurement and Transplantation Network and the Scientific Registry of Transplant Recipients website. www.optn.org
Figure 25-7   From Moodie DS, Stillwell PC: Thoracic organ transplantation in children: the state of heart, heart-lung, and lung transplantation. *Clin Pediatr* 1993; 32:322-328.

Chapter 27
Figure 27-1   Redrawn from Wiswell TE, Bent RC: Meconium staining and the meconium aspiration syndrome. Pediatr Clin North Am 1993; 40:957; modified from Bacsik RD: Meconium aspiration system. *Pediatr Clin North Am* 1977; 24:467.

Chapter 28
Figure 28-10   From Kumar V, Abbas A, Nelson F. Robbins and Cotran: *Pathologic basis if disease,* ed 7, Saunders, 2005, Philadelphia.

Chapter 29

Figure 29-1   From Bland JD, Coalson JJ. *Chronic lung disease in early infancy.* London, 2007, Taylor & Francis.

Figure 29-2   From Bland JD, Coalson JJ. *Chronic lung disease in early infancy.* London, 2007, Taylor & Francis.

Figure 29-3   From Bland JD, Coalson JJ. *Chronic lung disease in early infancy.* London, 2007, Taylor & Francis.

Figure 29-4   Redrawn from Björklund LJ, Ingimarsson J, Curstedt T, et al. Manual ventilation with a few large breaths at birth compromises the therapeutic effect of subsequent surfactant replacement in immature lambs. *Pediatr Res* 1997 Sep; 42(3):348-55.

Figure 29-7   Courtesy Dr. J. Bertsch, Kansas University Medical School, Department of Radiology.

Chapter 30

Figure 30-1   From Mullin CE, Mayer DC: *Congenital heart disease: a diagrammatic atlas.* New York. This material used by permission of Wiley-Liss, Inc., a subsidiary of John Wiley & Sons, Inc. 1988.

Figure 30-3   Redrawn from Guntheroth WG, et al. Physiology of circulation: fetus, neonate and child. In Kelly VC, editor: *Practice of pediatrics.* Harper-Row, Philadelphia. 1983.

Figure 30-4   From *Congenital heart abnormalities.* Clinical Education Aid No. 7. Columbus, Ohio. Ross Products Division, Abbott Laboratories, 1970.

Figure 30-5   From Mullin CE, Mayer DC: *Congenital heart disease: a diagrammatic atlas.* New York. This material used by permission of Wiley-Liss, Inc., a subsidiary of John Wiley & Sons, Inc 1988.

Figure 30-6   From *Congenital heart abnormalities.* Clinical Education Aid No. 7. Columbus, Ohio. Ross Products Division, Abbott Laboratories, 1970.

Figure 30-7   From Mullin CE, Mayer DC: *Congenital heart disease: a diagrammatic atlas.* New York. This material used by permission of Wiley-Liss, Inc., a subsidiary of John Wiley & Sons, Inc.1988.

Figure 30-8   From *Congenital heart abnormalities.* Clinical Education Aid No. 7. Columbus, Ohio. Ross Products Division, Abbott Laboratories, 1970.

Figure 30-9   Modified from Mullin CE, Mayer DC: *Congenital heart disease: a diagrammatic atlas.* New York. This material used by permission of Wiley-Liss, Inc., a subsidiary of John Wiley & Sons, Inc.1988.

Figure 30-10   From Mullin CE, Mayer DC: *Congenital heart disease: a diagrammatic atlas.* New York. This material used by permission of Wiley-Liss, Inc., a subsidiary of John Wiley & Sons, Inc 1988.

Figure 30-11   From: Park MK, Troxler RG. *Pediatric cardiology for practitioners.* Mosby. St. Louis. 2002:386.

Figure 30-12   Redrawn from Castaneda AR, Jonas RA, Mayer JE, Hanley FL. *Cardiac surgery of the neonate and infant.* W.B. Saunders. New York 1994:377.

Figure 30-14   Redrawn from Sano S, Ishino K, Kawada M, et al. Right ventricle-pulmonary artery shunt in first-stage palliation of hypoplastic left heart syndrome. *J Thorac Cardiovasc Surg.* 2003 Aug;126(2):504-9.

Figure 30-16   From Mullin CE, Mayer DC: *Congenital heart disease: a diagrammatic atlas.* New York. This material

used by permission of Wiley-Liss, Inc., a subsidiary of John Wiley & Sons, Inc 1988.

Figure 30-17   From Mullin CE, Mayer DC: *Congenital heart disease: a diagrammatic atlas.* New York. This material used by permission of Wiley-Liss, Inc., a subsidiary of John Wiley & Sons, Inc. 1988.

Figure 30-18   From Mullin CE, Mayer DC: *Congenital heart disease: a diagrammatic atlas.* New York. This material used by permission of Wiley-Liss, Inc., a subsidiary of John Wiley & Sons, Inc.1988.

Figure 30-19   From Mullin CE, Mayer DC: *Congenital heart disease: a diagrammatic atlas. New York.* This material used by permission of Wiley-Liss, Inc., a subsidiary of John Wiley & Sons, Inc. 1988.

Figure 30-20   From Mullin CE, Mayer DC: *Congenital heart disease: a diagrammatic atlas.* New York. This material used by permission of Wiley-Liss, Inc., a subsidiary of John Wiley & Sons, Inc. 1988.

Figure 30-21   From Mullin CE, Mayer DC: *Congenital heart disease: a diagrammatic atlas.* New York. This material used by permission of Wiley-Liss, Inc., a subsidiary of John Wiley & Sons, Inc. 1988.

Figure 30-22   From Mullin CE, Mayer DC: *Congenital heart disease: a diagrammatic atlas.* New York. This material used by permission of Wiley-Liss, Inc., a subsidiary of John Wiley & Sons, Inc.1988.

Figure 30-23   From Mullin CE, Mayer DC: *Congenital heart disease: a diagrammatic atlas.* New York. This material used by permission of Wiley-Liss, Inc., a subsidiary of John Wiley & Sons, Inc.1988.

Figure 30-24   From Mullin CE, Mayer DC: *Congenital heart disease: a diagrammatic atlas.* New York. This material used by permission of Wiley-Liss, Inc., a subsidiary of John Wiley & Sons, Inc. 1988.

Figure 30-25   From Mullin CE, Mayer DC: *Congenital heart disease: a diagrammatic atlas.* New York. This material used by permission of Wiley-Liss, Inc., a subsidiary of John Wiley & Sons, Inc. 1988.

Chapter 31

Figure 31-6   From Kelly DH, Pathak A, Meny RG: Sudden severe bradycardia in infancy. *Pediatr Pulmonol* 1991; 10:203, John Wiley & Sons, Inc. From Wiley-Liss, Inc., a subsidiary of John Wiley & Sons, Inc.

Chapter 32

Figure 32-11   Modified from Denny FW, Clyde WA: Acute lower respiratory tract infections in nonhospitalized children. *J Pediatr* 1986; 108:635.

Chapter 33

Figure 33-1   Courtesy Respironics HealthScan Asthma & Allergy Products, Cedar Grove, NJ.

Chapter 38

Figure 38-1   From Hess DR, MacIntyre NR, Mishoe SC, et al: *Respiratory care: principles and practice.* Philadelphia. WB Saunders, 2002.

Chapter 39

Figure 39-2   From Nolte J: *The human brain: an introduction to its functional anatomy.* St Louis, Mosby, 2002; modified from von Economo C: *The cytoarchitectonics of the human cerebral cortex.* Oxford. Oxford University Press, 1929.

Figure 39-3   From MacGregor J: *Introduction to the anatomy and physiology of children,* London. Routledge, 2000.

Figure 39-4   From MacGregor J: *Introduction to the anatomy and physiology of children.* London. Routledge, 2000.

Figure 39-5   From McQuillan KA, Flynn M, Ianuzzi M: *Trauma nursing: from resuscitation through rehabilitation,* ed 3, Philadelphia. WB Saunders, 2002.

Figure 39-6   From McQuillan KA, Flynn M, Ianuzzi M: *Trauma nursing: from resuscitation through rehabilitation,* ed 3, Philadelphia. WB Saunders, 2002.

Figure 39-7   From Hockenberry MJ, Wilson D: Wong's essentials of pediatric nursing, ed 8, St. Louis, 2009, Mosby. Used with permission. Copyright Mosby.

Figure 39-8   From Hess DR, MacIntyre NR, Mishoe SC, et al: *Respiratory care: principles and practice.* Philadelphia. WB Saunders, 2002.

Chapter 41

Figure 41-1   Data from Weinberg AD: Hypothermia. *Ann Emerg* Med, February 1993;22 (Pt 2):370-377.

Chapter 42

Figure 42-1   Redrawn from Greene S, Harris C, Singer J. Gastrointestinal decontamination of the poisoned patient. *Pediatr Emerg Care* 2008 Mar;24(3):176,86; quiz 187-9.

Chapter 44

Figure 44-3   Reprint permission from Dr. Howard Panitch, Children's Hospital of Philadelphia.

Figure 44-4   Courtesy Dr. Howard Panitch.

Chapter 45

Figure 45-1   Courtesy Texas Children's Hospital, Houston, Texas.

Figure 45-2   Courtesy Memorial Hermann Hospital, Houston, Texas.

Figure 45-3   With permission Paul Bowen Photography.

Chapter 46

Figure 46-1   Image used by permission from Nellcor Puritan Bennett, LCC, Boulder, CO, part of Covidien. With permission Paul Bowen Photography.

Figure 46-2   Courtesy AirSep, Buffalo, NY.

Figure 46-3   Courtesy AirSep, Buffalo, NY.

Figure 46-4   Courtesy AirSep, Buffalo, NY.

Figure 46-5   Courtesy Sunrise Medical, Longmont, Colo.

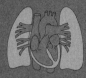
Note: f indicates figures; t, tables, b, boxes.